Textbook of
DIAGNOSTIC
MEDICINE

Textbook of
DIAGNOSTIC MEDICINE

Textbook of
DIAGNOSTIC MEDICINE

Edited and with contributions by

A. H. Samiy, M.D.

Professor of Clinical Medicine
Cornell University Medical College
Director of Division of Medicine
The New York Hospital, Westchester Division
Attending Physician
The New York Hospital-Cornell Medical Center
New York, NY

and Consulting Editors

R. Gordon Douglas, Jr., M.D.

E. Hugh Luckey Distinguished Professor of Medicine
Chairman, Department of Medicine
Cornell University Medical College
Physician-in-Chief
The New York Hospital-Cornell Medical Center
New York, NY

Jeremiah A. Barondess, M.D.

Professor of Clinical Medicine
Associate Chairman
Department of Medicine
Cornell University Medical College
Attending Physician
The New York Hospital-Cornell Medical Center
New York, NY

Lea & Febiger   Philadelphia   1987

Lea & Febiger
600 Washington Square
Philadelphia, PA   19106-4198
U.S.A.
(215) 922-1330

Library of Congress Cataloging-in-Publication Data

Main entry under title:

Textbook of diagnostic medicine.

  Includes bibliographies and index.
  1. Diagnosis, I. Samiy, A. H. II. Douglas, R.
Gordon (Robert Gordon), 1934- . III. Barondess,
Jeremiah A., 1924- . [DNLM: 1. Diagnosis.
WB 141 T355]
RC71.T49 1987   616.07′5   85-23966
ISBN 0-8121-1006-4

PRINTED IN THE UNITED STATES OF AMERICA

Print number: 5 4 3 2 1

This book is dedicated
to the memory of my parents
and
the four outstanding clinicians from whom
I learned the art of clinical diagnosis:
David P. Barr, M.D., Walter Bauer, M.D.,
Harold G. Wolff, M.D., and Aaron Feder, M.D.

PREFACE

The Textbook of Diagnostic Medicine is the first comprehensive textbook of medicine fully devoted to a problem-oriented approach to clinical medicine. It has been conceptualized for the specific purpose of filling a gap in clinical diagnosis by providing physicians with an expert guide in the evaluation of the patient's problem, with particular emphasis on the evaluation of symptoms and signs.

Past decades have witnessed a remarkable technical revolution in diagnostic medicine with the proliferation of diagnostic devices such as ultrasound, computed tomography, positron-emission tomography and nuclear magnetic imaging, and other newer techniques in laboratory tests.

These imaging and laboratory procedures have increased the physician's diagnostic capability to an unimaginable and unprecedented standard of reliability and accuracy. Paradoxically, with these advances the practice of clinical diagnosis may have declined to a new level of neglect. Over-reliance on diagnostic tests may have contributed to reduced attention to and diminished skill in history-taking and physical examination, despite their continued value in the practice of medicine.[1] For example, a significant number of errors in physical examination was detected in two thirds of all patients examined by interns and residents.[2]

Inappropriate ordering of laboratory and other diagnostic tests has also contributed to a substantial increase in national health expenditure. False positive results from unnecessary tests may readily lead to additional costly and sometimes harmful diagnostic or therapeutic interventions. Laboratory or diagnostic tests may be ordered witout sufficient attention to their proper sequences or patterns.[3] Above all, the physician-patient relationship may be depersonalized by excessive reliance on ancillary diagnostic procedures.

Most patients come to physicians because of a subjective complaint. In this context the initial and most important task of the physician is to investigate the underlying cause of the complaint before instituting treatment. In dealing with clinical diagnosis the physician has access to many excellent textbooks of medicine, which are basically disease-oriented. It may be presumed that the physician has made a working diagnosis prior to using these resources, to which he is referring for additional information on the specific disease process. Thus, these books are helpful chiefly after a tentative diagnosis has been made or is at least being entertained. Even in the final stages of diagnostic evaluation, however, textbooks of medicine may be of limited help because in actuality disease processes frequently do not conform to their typical and classic descriptions. In the clinical situation the physician must deal with a constellation of signs, symptoms, and test results when attempting to develop a working diagnosis.

A textbook has not been available as a reference source for medical students during the period of clinical clerkship in Medicine, Pediatrics, Surgery, and Psychiatry.

Accordingly, the purposes and aims of the Textbook of Diagnostic Medicine are:

1. To provide a reference for practicing physicians in order to facilitate diagnostic evaluation of the patient's complaints.
2. To serve as a textbook of medicine for medical students during the clinical clerkship.
3. To rekindle an interest in clinical diagnosis.

The approach of the Textbook of Diagnostic Medicine reflects the way clinicians proceed with diagnostic problem-solving. In developing the organization of the book, a master list of patients' complaints or problems, consisting of signs, symptoms, and abnormal laboratory tests, was prepared from many sources. Contributors were selected on the basis of their expertise in subspecialty areas. Each contributor was asked to identify major signs and symptoms of disease in the particular specialty. The list was compared to the master list to make certain that no significant clinical finding was left out. In certain areas, such as infectious disease, immunology, allergy, metabolic disorders, and others in which disturbed function could not be expressed in terms of specific signs and symptoms, contributors were asked to include important pathophysiologic entities, abnormal laboratory findings, or major syndromes of particular or current clinical significance.

The Textbook of Diagnostic Medicine covers more

than 500 patient complaints, including symptoms, signs, abnormal laboratory results, and syndromes. Most topics are discussed in terms of:

1. Definition
2. Pathophysiologic considerations
3. Clinical presentation
4. Differential diagnosis
5. Diagnostic evaluation and workup of the patient's complaint.

In this era of biomedical technology, in the current climate of cost-control efforts and marked specialization, the need for expertise in clinical diagnosis is of increasing importance. Generalists and specialists must continue to play a pivotal role in diagnostic decision-making by employing the bedside techniques of clinical data–gathering as the primary basis for organizing diagnostic thought and for appropriately utilizing the various laboratory and imaging procedures that are available. For this crucial task, it is hoped that the Textbook of Diagnostic Medicine will be of value as a reference source book in clinical diagnosis.

Finally, I am indebted to all contributors for their devoted participation in this book, for giving their valuable time, and for sharing with us their widely recognized expertise.

This book could not have been completed without the professional support of Lea & Febiger's editorial and production staff. My special thanks to Mr. R. Kenneth Bussy, Executive Editor, Mr. Samuel A. Rondinelli, Assistant Production Manager, and Ms. Amy Norwitz, Copy Editor. Last but not least my thanks to Patricia Weeks for her careful and efficient secretarial assistance.

New York, NY   A.H. Samiy, M.D.

REFERENCES

1. Kern, D.C., Parrini, T.A., and Korst, D.R.: The lasting value of clinical skills. JAMA *254*:70, 1985.
2. Wray, N.P. and Friedland, J.A.: Detection and correction of house staff error in physical diagnosis. JAMA *249*:1035, 1983.
3. Wong, E.T., McCarron, M.M., and Shaw, S.T.: Ordering of laboratory tests in a teaching hospital. JAMA *249*:3078, 1983.

CONTRIBUTORS

Charles F. Abboud, M.D., B.Ch.
Associate Professor of Medicine
Mayo Medical School
Consultant, Division of Endocrinology and
    Internal Medicine
Mayo Clinic
Rochester, MN

Gerard Addonizio, M.D.
Assistant Professor of Psychiatry
Cornell University Medical College
Assistant Attending Psychiatrist
The New York Hospital-Cornell Medical Center,
    Westchester Division
White Plains, NY

Wilhelmina V.S.I. Akman, M.D.
Assistant Professor of Medicine in Psychiatry
Cornell University Medical College
Assistant Attending Physician
The New York Hospital-Cornell Medical Center,
    Westchester Division
White Plains, NY

George Alexopoulos, M.D.
Associate Professor of Psychiatry
Cornell University Medical College
Associate Attending Physician
The New York Hospital-Cornell Medical Center,
    Westchester Division
White Plains, NY

Jeffrey S. Berns, M.D.
Associate Research Scientist
Department of Physiology
Yale University School of Medicine
Fellow in Nephrology
Yale-New Haven Hospital
New Haven, CT

John J. Caronna, M.D.
Professor and Vice-Chairman
Department of Neurology
Cornell University Medical College
Attending Neurologist
The New York Hospital-Cornell Medical Center
New York, NY

D. Jackson Coleman, M.D.
John McLean Professor of Ophthalmology
Cornell University Medical College
Ophthalmologist-in-Chief
The New York Hospital-Cornell Medical Center
New York, NY

Burke A. Cunha, M.D.
Associate Professor of Medicine
State University of New York at Stony Brook
Chief, Division of Infectious Diseases
Vice-Chairman, Department of Medicine
Winthrop University Hospital
Mineola, NY

Jerry M. Earll, M.D.
Professor of Medicine
Georgetown University School of Medicine
Chief, Division of Internal Medicine
Georgetown University Medical Center
Washington, DC

Richard J. Francis, M.D.
Formerly Associate Professor of Clinical Psychiatry
Cornell University Medical College
Associate Attending Psychiatrist
The New York Hospital-Cornell Medical Center,
    Westchester Division
White Plains, NY

Stephen K. Gerard, M.D., Ph.D.
Chief Resident in Laboratory Medicine
    (Nuclear Medicine)
Department of Laboratory Medicine
University of California, San Francisco
San Francisco General Hospital Medical Center
San Francisco, CA

Lewis Goldfrank, M.D.
Associate Professor of Clinical Medicine
New York University School of Medicine
Director, Emergency Medical Services
Bellevue Hospital Center and
    New York University Medical Center
New York, NY

Eugene L. Gottfried, M.D.
Clinical Professor and Vice Chairman
Department of Laboratory Medicine
University of California, San Francisco
Director, Clinical Laboratories
San Francisco General Hospital Medical Center
San Francisco, CA

Murk-Hein Heinemann, M.D.
Assistant Professor of Ophthalmology
Cornell University Medical College
Assistant Attending Ophthalmologist
The New York Hospital-Cornell Medical Center
New York, NY

Hira Chand Jain, M.D.
Instructor of Psychiatry
Cornell University Medical College
Clinical Instructor of Psychiatry
The New York Hospital-Cornell Medical Center,
    Westchester Division
White Plains, NY

Graham H. Jeffries, M.D.
Professor and Chairman
Department of Medicine
The Pennsylvania State University College
    of Medicine
Hershey, PA

Marie-Louise Johnson, M.D., Ph.D.
Clinical Professor of Dermatology
Yale University School of Medicine
New Haven, CT
Director of Medical Education
Benedictine Hospital
Kingston, NY

Harvey L. Katzeff, M.D.
Assistant Professor of Medicine
Cornell University Medical College
New York, NY
Director, Diabetes Education and Treatment Center
Department of Endocrinology
Assistant Attending Physician in Medicine
North Shore University Hospital
Manhasset, NY

Homayoun Kazemi, M.D.
Professor of Medicine
Harvard Medical School
Chief, Pulmonary Unit
Massachusetts General Hospital
Boston, MA

Alan S. Kliger, M.D.
Associate Professor of Clinical Medicine
Yale-University School of Medicine
Medical Director, Dialysis Services
Yale-New Haven Hospital
New Haven, CT

Arnold Meisler, M.D.
Associate Professor of Medicine
University of Pittsburgh School of Medicine
Member, Pittsburgh Cancer Institute
Chief of Hematology/Oncology
V.A. Medical Center
Pittsburgh, PA

Barnett S. Meyers, M.D.
Assistant Professor of Psychiatry
Cornell University Medical College
Assistant Attending Psychiatrist
The New York Hospital-Cornell Medical Center,
    Westchester Division
White Plains, NY

Raj Mittal, M.D.
Formerly Assistant Professor of Medicine
University of Pittsburgh School of Medicine
Staff Physician
V.A. Medical Center
Pittsburgh, PA

Valerie Ng, M.D., Ph.D.
Chief Resident in Laboratory Medicine
Department of Laboratory Medicine
University of California, San Francisco
San Francisco General Hospital Medical Center
San Francisco, CA

William P. Owen, M.D.
Formerly Assistant Professor of Psychiatry
Cornell University Medical College
Assistant Attending Psychiatrist
The New York Hospital-Cornell Medical Center,
    Westchester Division
White Plains, NY
Director, Eating Disorder Program
Stonylodge Hospital
Briarcliff Manor, NY

Stephen A. Paget, M.D.
Associate Professor of Clinical Medicine
Cornell University Medical College
Associate Attending Physician
Department of Medicine
The New York Hospital and Hospital for
    Special Surgery
New York, NY

Thomas G. Pickering, M.D., D. Phil.
Professor of Medicine
Cornell University Medical College
Attending Physician
The New York Hospital-Cornell Medical Center
New York, NY

Charles P. Pollak, M.D.
Assistant Professor of Neurology in Psychiatry
    and Neurology
Cornell University Medical College
Head, Sleep-Wake Disorders Center
Acting Director
Institute of Chronobiology
The New York Hospital-Cornell Medical Center,
    Westchester Division
White Plains, NY

A. H. Samiy, M.D.
Professor of Clinical Medicine
Cornell University Medical College
Director of Division of Medicine
The New York Hospital-Cornell Medical Center,
    Westchester Division
Attending Physician
The New York Hospital-Cornell Medical Center
New York, NY

Robert W. Selfe, Jr., M.D.
Professor and Chairman
Department of Otorhinolaryngology
Cornell University Medical College
Otorhinolaryngologist-in-Chief
The New York Hospital-Cornell Medical Center
New York, NY

Charles A. Shamoian, M.D., Ph.D.
Professor of Clinical Psychiatry
Department of Psychiatry
Cornell University Medical College
Director of Geriatric Services
The New York Hospital-Cornell Medical Center,
    Westchester Division
White Plains, NY

Gillian M. Shepherd, M.D.
Assistant Professor of Medicine
Cornell University Medical College
Assistant Attending Physician
The New York Hospital-Cornell Medical Center
New York, NY

B. Taylor Thompson, M.D.
Instructor of Medicine
Harvard Medical School
Assistant in Medicine
Massachusetts General Hospital
Boston, MA

Robert E. Whalen, M.D.
Professor of Medicine
Duke University School of Medicine
Director, Cardiovascular Disease Service
Duke University Medical Center
Durham, NC

Robert C. Young, M.D.
Assistant Professor of Psychiatry
Cornell University Medical College
Assistant Attending Psychiarist
The New York Hospital-Cornell Medical Center,
    Westchester Division
White Plains, NY

CONTENTS

Chapter 4. Hematologic and Oncologic Problems   Arnold Meisler, M.D.
Raj Mittal, M.D.

Clinical Problems

Chapter 5. Infectious Diseases   Burke A. Cunha, M.D.

Clinical Problems

Chapter 10. Water, Electrolyte, and Acid-Base Problems

Charles F. Abboud, M.D., B.Ch.
Alan S. Kliger, M.D.

Clinical Problems

Chapter 11. Endocrine and Metabolic Problems

Charles F. Abboud, M.D., B.Ch.

Clinical Problems

Chapter 12. Gastrointestinal and Liver Problems   Graham H. Jeffries, M.D.

Clinical Problems

CHAPTER 1

PRINCIPLES OF CLINICAL DIAGNOSIS

A.H. Samiy, M.D. and Wilhelmina V.S.I. Akman, M.D.

INTRODUCTION TO CLINICAL DIAGNOSIS

System, or as I shall term it, the virtue of method, is the harness without which only the horses of genius can travel.

William Osler

Patients usually consult physicians seeking alleviation of symptoms or treatment of problems. Before any treatment is instituted, however, the physician must determine the nature of the complaint. Diagnosis, or the clinical evaluation of the problem, is usually the initial and always an important element in patient management. By its nature, clinical diagnosis is one of the most challenging and intellectually demanding tasks in the practice of medicine. The course and the outcome of the illness are often influenced by the physician's ability to reach an early and correct diagnosis.

Recent advances in biomedical technology have had a tremendous impact on the diagnostic aspect of medical practice. In the past decade, a technologic revolution has occurred in the areas of diagnostic laboratory and diagnostic imaging with the introduction of diagnostic equipment such as ultrasonography, computed tomography, positron-emission tomography, and, most recently, magnetic resonance imaging. Remarkably accurate diagnoses can now be made with delineation of the location, size, physiologic function, and even the pathologic structure of lesions.[1,2] These technologic advances, however, may have had some undesirable effects on the practice of medicine. Overreliance on diagnostic tests and procedures may have weakened the once enviable personal nature of the patient-physician relationship. Skills in history-taking and physical examination, still of great importance for the diagnosis and treatment of patients, may have suffered significantly. Inappropriate, unnecessary, or redundant use of diagnostic tests, occasionally the result of practicing defensive medicine, may have resulted in additional health hazards and financial costs to the patient and in a substantial increase in national health expenditure.[3]

While a return to the ''horse and buggy'' era of medical practice is not being advocated, a balanced approach to the use of diagnostic tests should be maintained. The physician should still play the leading role in the process of clinical diagnosis, only employing diagnostic tools with appropriate clinical justification. Diagnostic studies should complement our clinical assessments, by achieving a higher standard of diagnosis and treatment and not by becoming a substitute for our clinical skills and expertise.

One of the complexities in the practice of medicine is that patients usually do not consult the physician with a known diagnosis, but present with common, complex, or atypical symptoms. To make matters more complicated, symptoms of disease are subjective and are often influenced by the patient's sex, age, socioeconomic status, and cultural and ethnic background. Symptoms may also be forgotten, suppressed, or exaggerated by patients and modified by the disease itself and by its treatment.

The process of formulating a diagnosis is not unlike putting together a complicated jigsaw puzzle. In fact, it is like trying to do a jigsaw puzzle with only a few pieces in the box, with no knowledge of its ultimate dimensions or configuration, and with no picture on the cover of the box to guide us. Signs and symptoms of the patient and the results of diagnostic tests constitute the pieces required for constructing the puzzle. But the pieces are not conveniently available in the box, and must be collected by the physician by carefully taking a history and performing a complete physical examination, and by ordering appropriate laboratory tests. Therefore, a successful diagnostic workup is initiated by collecting relevant clinical data. Since we are not given the ultimate design of the puzzle, the process of putting pieces together requires the ability to project the configuration of the puzzle, based on our knowledge of disease pathophysiology and with continued reference to the available clinical clues. The clinical puzzle, unlike the ordinary static and two-dimensional jigsaw puzzle, has a dynamic nature. One must go through a series of reconstructions of the design before the final shape of the puzzle, or a diagnosis, is realized. The final configuration of the puzzle needs to be continuously redesigned as newer clinical clues become available by further clinical observation and additional diagnostic studies.

In brief, there are five major requirements for the successful practice of diagnostic medicine.[4-8]
1. Ability to collect clinical data.
2. Competence and skill in peforming an appropriate physical examination.
3. Familiarity with diagnostic tests—their interpretation, indications, proper ordering sequence, contraindications, hazards, and costs.
4. Medical knowledge base, including pathophysiology and clinical manifestation of disease.
5. Cognitive ability to analyze and integrate clinical data in order to develop problem lists, to formulate a differential diagnosis, and to establish a working diagnosis.

DIAGNOSTIC STRATEGIES

Two alternative strategies are employed by experienced clinicians in approaching diagnostic formulation: pattern recognition and pathophysiologic analysis.

Pattern Recognition. As with our exemplary jigsaw puzzle, pieces of clinical data, consisting of signs, symptoms, clinical clues, and laboratory data, are put into recognizable configurations, such as syndromes or specific disease entities. This strategy requires a strong knowledge base derived from past clinical encounters and reading of textbooks and recent literature. This active process begins with the initial patient contact and continues during interviewing and history-taking and the physical examination, during which clinical clues suggest new diagnostic possibilities.

Pattern recognition is a dynamic process that generates and discards diagnostic possibilities at all stages of clinical evaluation of the patient. For instance, evaluation of a patient complaining of cough, irritation of the eyes, and skin eruption may by pattern recognition bring to mind the diagnostic possibilities of sarcoidosis, Sjogren's syndrome, and systemic sclerosis. As more information is obtained from the history and the physical examination, certain diagnostic possibilities will come into focus and others may become more remote. If our hypothetical patient is a black woman in whom physical examination reveals enlarged lymph nodes, the possibility of sarcoidosis will be most likely. The physician must consider other possibilities if the chest x-ray does not reveal hilar adenopathy. In pattern recognition, the ability to identify clusters of signs and symptoms with recognizable disease entities determines the success in reaching a correct diagnosis. In the interpretation of diagnostic data, demographic evidence such as age, sex, race, geographic location, etc., should be taken into account.

Pathophysiologic Analysis. Symptoms and abnormal signs are manifestations of disturbed functions of organs or systems. By analyzing signs and symptoms and abnormal laboratory findings, specific pathophysiologic entities can be recognized. This strategy is often helpful in problem-oriented differential diagnosis. The purpose of pathophysiologic analysis is to generate diagnostic possibilities if pattern recognition is unsuccessful.

Regardless of what diagnostic strategies are employed, appropriate diagnostic studies are selected and pursued until the nature, severity, and cause of the disease have been established. It is essential that laboratory studies are ordered with the necessary attention to their indications, proper sequence, contraindications, hazards, and costs.

CLINICAL DATA BASE

Patient History. The history is still the most valuable source of diagnostic information. A patient's history probably serves as a basis for 70 to 80% of correct diagnoses, particularly in the ambulatory setting.[6]

History-taking is a skill that requires considerable experience for full development. The first and most important step in history-taking is to establish a sympathetic and understanding relationship with the patient. The physician must attempt to make patients comfortable and relaxed. In successful history-taking a patient's confidence and trust in the physician are essential. Thus, any indication of indifference or haste by the physician will establish an atmosphere of mistrust and lack of confidence.

Patients should be given sufficient time to discuss their problems and complaints, but physicians should also provide direction to the interview whenever feasible or necessary. Additional information should be obtained by direct questioning of the patient for further clarification of the symptoms. Although patients should be encouraged to describe symptoms in their own words, the terminology employed by patients may have different interpretations and therefore be misleading to the physician. To illustrate the point, the case of a woman who was referred to Duke University Medical Center with a chief complaint of "falling out spells" can be cited. When extensive neurologic and diagnostic studies did not reveal any abnormality, further careful history-taking revealed that the patient was complaining about a prolapse of the uterus.[9] Or when a patient refers with a complaint of "dizziness," careful history-taking may identify the symptom more clearly as weakness, fatigue, syncope, lightheadedness, lack of coordination, or vertigo. During the period of history-taking the physician should be alert to observe nonverbal clues in the patient's general appearance, demeanor, tone of voice, movements, and affect.

In case of a medical emergency, however, treatment must obviously assume the first priority. History-taking should be brief and limited to the immediate problem, so that treatment of life threatening medical emergency is not delayed. A more complete history must be taken after the patient's condition becomes stable.

Symptoms are clinical manifestations of the disorder of organs or systems as experienced by patients. It is important to realize that symptoms of disease are not experienced similarly or expressed with the same intensity by all patients. In fact, patients vary widely in their response to the same disease process, based on age, sex, social and cultural background, and constitutional or genetic makeup. In addition, demographic factors influence the prevalence and the incidences of the disease.

In general, symptoms are either localized (specific) or nonlocalized (nonspecific). Localized symptoms such as diarrhea, cough, and chest pain usually indicate a disorder of a specific organ or system. In contrast, nonspecific symptoms, such as fatigue, weakness, anorexia, or weight loss, do not by themselves suggest diseases of a specific organ or system. Nonspecific symptoms may result from a generalized or multisystem disease or from the accumulated effects of several disturbed functions. Specific symptoms, however, such as diarrhea or cough, point to the diseases of specific organs, such as the gastrointestinal tract or the respiratory tract, respectively.

In most illnesses, nonspecific symptoms will not be decisive in the diagnosis, whereas specific symptoms may be helpful in narrowing the diagnostic possibilities. The concomitant presence of specific symptoms may render nonspecific symptoms diagnostically more meaningful. Fatigue and anorexia alone suggest a wide spectrum of diagnostic possibilities, but the concomitant presence of the symptoms or signs of fever and cough will reduce the number of diagnostic possibilities to infectious diseases of the pulmonary system. Certain nonspecific symptoms may at times represent specific signs and symptoms of a group of disease entities. For instance, fever, which is a nonspecific symptom and is seen in a wide range of diseases, is often a manifestation of an infectious disease process.

Physical Examination. The importance of the physical examination in clinical diagnosis is generally recognized. As opposed to revealing symptoms, which are subjective and often difficult to quantify, physical examination reveals information that is comparatively more objective, measurable, and reproducible. A positive finding on physical examination may occasionally become the single clue to a diagnosis. For example, finding an enlarged lymph node in the supraclavicular area in an elderly patient affected by weight loss and anorexia may serve as a very valuable clue to the possible diagnosis of carcinoma of the stomach or pancreas.

A careful examiner not only must have searching

eyes, hearing ears, and sensitive fingers, but above all must possess an agile and inquisitive mind to direct him or her toward important physical clues in diagnostic evaluation of the patient's problem. The physician is more likely to search for a Roth's spot, to hear a faint diastolic murmur, or to palpate an enlarged spleen when he or she is actively considering the possibility of subacute infective endocarditis. Expertise in physical examination is thus not merely dependent on technical skill, but requires a prepared and knowledgeable mind.

Nevertheless, physical examination should ordinarily be complete and should be performed systematically to cover all parts of the body, although in acutely ill patients the physician should initially perform a limited physical examination so as not to delay the treatment of an emergency medical problem. Obviously, patients should subsequently have a thorough physical examination. The physician may need to reexamine the patient, not only to confirm his initial findings, but to look for changes in physical signs during the course and with the progression of the disease. After completing the initial physical examination, the physician may be guided by the history to pursue closer examination of specific relevant organs.

Laboratory Diagnostic Tests. Diagnostic tests are essential not only to the diagnostic process, but in determining the cause of disease, its severity, and its prognosis. Laboratory tests may also be used to monitor therapy.

After a careful history and a thorough physical examination, a diagnostic plan should be developed to exclude or confirm various diagnostic possibilities. The need for each diagnostic test should be evaluated in terms of its sensitivity, specificity, predictive values, cost, and safety, and patient's comfort. Before a diagnostic test is ordered the physician should seriously contemplate these points:

1. What test should be ordered?
2. How does the test clarify the patient's problem?
3. In what sequence should these tests be ordered?
4. What is the relative sensitivity and specificity of the test and what are its predictive values?
5. What underlying pathophysiologic mechanism of disease will be explained by the test?
6. What are the costs, benefits, and hazards of the diagnostic test?

It should be remembered that a sensitive test, when negative, is helpful in excluding the presence of a disease, whereas a specific test, when positive, will confirm its presence.[3] Occasionally physicians are not familiar with or neglect the proper sequence of test ordering. Not only does faulty test ordering increase the cost of a patient's care and drain limited resources, but tests ordered improperly may not provide the necessary diagnostic information or may generate redundant or even misleading diagnostic data.

DATA PROCESSING AND FORMULATION

Although data processing and formulation of a patient's problems are being considered separately from data collection, in real-life situations the clinician analyzes and integrates the clinical data as it is being generated from the first contact with the patient. Clinical data collection and data processing and formulation, which are the most critical parts of the diagnostic workup, are highly interdependent. Data processing and formulation may reveal an information gap requiring the collection of additional clinical data, by history or re-examination of the patient. Similarly, the history may provide an additional guide in the search for subtle or easily missed physical signs. With the introduction of newer clinical data, the diagnostic formulation may have to be revised.

The patient must be continually observed and reexamined. If subsequent findings do not correlate with the initial impression, the diagnostic possibilities should be reassessed. The adage "when you hear hoofbeats, think of horses, not zebras" still holds. However, when further careful examination reveals demarcated black and white stripes, perhaps you should consider zebras.[11]

As history-taking proceeds and as physical examination is performed, the physician begins to formulate an initial impression about the diagnosis. At this point the history and the physical examination should unravel essential clues to diagnosis. With additional information from the diagnostic tests, working diagnoses may begin to emerge.

Basic knowledge of pathophysiology and clinical manifestations of disease is crucial to diagnosis, and data processing and diagnostic formulation are the final links in the chain of clinical problem-solving. It requires the knowledge base and the proper reasoning process with which to apply that knowledge to solving the patient's problem.[12]

The relationship between clinical problem-solving and medical knowledge has been the subject of recent studies. In one such study, the similarity between clinical problem-solving and the game of chess has been noted. A chess master does not recognize the randomly arranged chess board any better than the less experienced player, but he has a greater knowledge of various patterns of the chess pieces.[13,14] The process of becoming a chess master, it is estimated, requires learning by experience approximately 50,000 different configurations. Similarly, physicians must learn thousands of diagnostic "configurations" of clinical data to achieve the status of a master diagnostician. An investigation involving the study of subspecialists in internal medicine revealed that problem-solving skills were considerably reduced when physicians were dealing with problems outside of their subspecialty.[15]

Diagnostic formulation of the patient's problems reflects the physician's analysis of clinical data, obtained from history, physical examination, laboratory diagnostic tests, and other clinical observations. Various diagnostic possibilities will begin to emerge, as clinical data are integrated with the physician's basic knowledge of pathophysiology and manifestations of disease. The final working diagnosis should be consistent with the clinical data, the knowledge of disease process, and the course of the illness.

If in the evaluation of a patient's problems a specific diagnosis is initially apparent, physicians may initiate diagnostic evaluation by considering the differential diagnosis of each relevant clinical data, including symptoms, physical signs, and abnormal laboratory results. For instance, a problem list may consist of abdominal pain, fever, and hepatomegaly. The pathophysiologic consideration and differential diagnosis of each abnormality should be considered and integrated to suggest a disease entity or a clinical syndrome.

As already indicated, symptoms are either localized (specific) or nonlocalized (nonspecific). Localized clues are usually more helpful in formulating a diagnosis. In case of the aforementioned patient with abdominal pain, fever, and hepatomegaly, fever is a nonlocalized or nonspecific symptom and is not initially a helpful diagnostic clue. But the presence of abdominal pain, as a localized or specific symptom, will guide the physician to a specific anatomic site or organ. The finding on physical examination of an enlarged liver may provide an additional specific clue for explaining fever and abdominal pain.

If the symptoms are referable to the same system, it is likely that they are related. If the symptoms occur in different systems or organs, however, the physician should consider several possibilities:

1. A single disease involving several systems or a multisystem disease, such as diabetes mellitus, affecting kidneys, peripheral nerves, and the retina.
2. The existence of more than one disease process.
3. A single disease with effects on distant or un-

related organs, such as cancer of the lung with paraneoplastic syndrome or with metastasis to the liver and the brain.

In analyzing clinical data, attention should be paid to the presence of positive and negative clues. Clues may be so specific that their presence confirms the diagnosis or so sensitive that their absence effectively eliminates certain diagnoses.[3,8]

Astute clinicians may be able to integrate an apparently unrelated cluster of symptoms, signs, and laboratory abnormalities into well-recognized syndromes as the initial step in clinical diagnosis. It should be emphasized, however, that diagnosis based on syndrome identification may not necessarily be the final diagnosis. The syndromic approach, however, narrows the gap between analysis of clinical data and formulation of problems and final diagnosis. For instance, presence of obesity, acne, abdominal stria, hypertension, and glucose intolerance may suggest Cushing's syndrome, but these findings do not by themselves indicate various diagnostic possibilities such as ACTH-producing pituitary or adrenal tumor or hyperplasia, or an ectopic ACTH-secreting tumor. When clinical findings do not fit into a recognizable syndrome, the diagnostic problem is usually more difficult and may require additional clinical data or diagnostic studies.

Certain diagnostic problems are straightforward and can be resolved by a careful history, a complete physical examination, and the use of appropriate diagnostic tests. In this process the physician proceeds from collection of clinical data to their analysis and interpretation, and, finally, to establishing a diagnosis.

In more complicated problems, most of the information does not appear to fit into an easily recognizable disease entity or syndrome. When confronted with this situation, the physician should develop a list of major clinical findings and consider the differential diagnosis of each problem. Additional clinical data and clues, diagnostic tests, and observation of the course of the illness may be required before a working diagnosis can be made. The correct diagnosis may be reached by successive reappraisal of the working diagnosis.

In dealing with diagnostic problems, it should be kept in mind that common problems do occur commonly, and even uncommon manifestations of a common problem are encountered more frequently than a common presentation of an uncommon disease.

Although it is a great source of satisfaction (and essential to treatment) for a physician to make a diagnosis of an uncommon disease, it is critically important not to miss the clinical manifestations of a common and treatable disease.

Demographic information, particularly as related to the patient's age, sex, race, and family history, knowledge of the prevalence and the geographic distribution of the disease process are commonly employed by experienced physicians to exclude or to confirm certain apparent diagnostic possibilities.

Having briefly reviewed the principles of clinical diagnosis, we will now proceed with a more detailed discussion of the various elements of clinical data base, including the medical history, physical examination, and the initial laboratory tests.

COLLECTION OF CLINICAL DATA

As noted earlier, the clinical data base includes the patient history, the physical examination, and initial laboratory tests.

PATIENT HISTORY

The patient's medical history is the most important part of the clinical data base.[8] Obtaining it also requires the greatest skill. The examiner needs to perfect his ability to inquire, listen, and observe, and he must be able to modify his use of these three components to accommodate individual patients.[16] When the history is taken correctly, the essential data obtained direct the subsequent physical examination and laboratory testing, making an accurate diagnosis more likely. The interview is the physician's first opportunity for establishing a good rapport with the patient.[16] Gaining the patient's trust, confidence, and respect (i.e., a positive transference) promotes honesty about historic facts, discourages the withholding of information that may be embarrassing, and serves as a basis for encouraging the patient to endure the future discomforts and inconveniences of diagnostic testing and treatment.[17] The systematic method of history-taking includes the following:[16–19]

1. Biographic data
2. Chief complaint
3. History of present illness
4. Past medical history
5. Family history
6. Review of organ systems
7. Social and personal history

Traditionally the various components of the medical history have been recorded sequentially, however, the physician may deviate from the stereotyped method in order to follow the patient's general direction of thought and conversation. It is the ability to be flexible and accommodating without sacrificing thoroughness that largely contributes to good rapport with the patient. The ultimate objective is, of course, to compile a comprehensive medical history as the initial step in the diagnostic process.

Biographic Data. Biographic data includes the patient's name, age, sex, race, occupation, place of birth, and permanent home address. This information allows the physician to understand the patient's background and other demographic facts that may provide some clues to the correct diagnosis. For example, a jaundiced bartender, by virtue of his occupation, is more likely to suffer from alcohol-related liver disease than from viral hepatitis. A young Vietnamese refugee with chronic weight loss, low-grade fever, and cough probably has active tuberculosis, while bronchogenic carcinoma underlies similar symptoms in a long-standing heavy smoker. Some diseases are relatively specific to certain age groups. Benign febrile convulsions are not seen in adults, whereas atherosclerotic coronary artery disease is rarely seen in children.

There are times when a patient cannot give his own history, such as in cases of coma or confusion. Language barriers may also interfere with the accurate communication of facts. Thus, it is sometimes necessary to depend on information provided by a relative, a friend, or an observer. In addition, valuable information can be obtained from old hospital records and from a previous physician. Compiling a complete history requires utilization of all resources and helps steer the physician down the pathway most likely to yield a correct diagnosis.

Chief Complaint. The chief complaint, or the primary reason for seeking medical attention, should be recorded in the patient's own words. It consists of the symptom or symptoms that cause discomfort. The physician must not only listen to the patient, but must also observe him closely while he or she relates the problem. For example, a tightly clenched fist held over the chest while a patient describes chest pain (Levine's sign) is characteristic of true angina pectoris. Emotional flatness while describing sudden paralysis of an extremity may suggest a hysterical personality.

History of Present Illness. The history of the present illness is a chronologic elaboration of the patient's complaints. Each symptom should be characterized according to date and time of onset; mode of onset; location; quantity; quality; duration; frequency of recurrence; precipitating factors; aggravating factors; alleviating factors; and associated symptoms.

A painstaking effort in history-taking on the part of the examiner will usually be rewarded, but it is not an easy task; it requires a broad cognitive awareness of disease manifestations, an ability to constantly scrutinize and delete nonessential information, and the skill to integrate the relevant points into a limited number of diagnostic possibilities. For example, chest discomfort can be a manifestation of dysfunction in a variety of organ systems and may even represent different pathophysiologic entities in the same organ. Ischemic cardiac chest pain typically has the quality of "heaviness" or "tightness" of varying severity. Its typical location is in the center of the chest, often with radiation to the jaw and/or the left upper extremity. Physical activity and emotional upsets are common precipitating factors. The pain may be aggravated by cold weather and associated with shortness of breath and palpitations. Relief occurs within minutes after resting and/or with sublingual nitroglycerin. On the other hand, chest pain, arising from mitral valve prolapse, may be "pinching" or "knifelike" in quality. Radiation to the jaw or left upper extremity is usually absent, there are no distinct precipitating factors, duration is often prolonged, and relief is not obtained with rest and nitroglycerin. The demographic setting is also different: ischemic pain occurs in older adults with coronary artery disease risk factors, whereas pain of mitral valve prolapse occurs in young adult women.

Chest pain of pericardial origin is precipitated or alleviated by changes in position, whereas pain of a pleural nature classically is worsened by inspiration. Diseases of the esophagus may also present with chest discomfort. Esophageal spasm may have the same intensity and distribution as pain of myocardial ischemia, and may even be relieved with nitroglycerin, whereas the pain of reflux esophagitis may occur when the patient is supine. Chest pain may also be the presenting symptom of many other diseases, including spinal disc disease, rib fracture, herpes zoster, and intra-abdominal disorders such as cholecystitis and pancreatitis. The above examples underscore the extensive fund of medical information that the physician must have in order to succeed in history-taking.

Past Medical History. The past medical history includes all prior medical illnesses, surgical procedures, and injuries. A review of the prenatal, parturient, and postnatal history is also of value when congenital and inherited disease are involved.

Many important clues may surface here. For example, a 50-year-old woman complaining of lethargy, weight gain, and constipation may have hypothyroidism secondary to radioiodine treatment of an overactive thyroid gland performed a decade before. Constipation and bloating, intermittent abdominal pain in a 62-year-old man may well relate to intestinal adhesions from a prior appendectomy. A knee injury in childhood may become one of the precipitating causes of osteoarthritis in old age, and maternal use of steroids can explain a cleft palate in her newborn baby.

One disease is sometimes simultaneously associated with the presence of others. Pseudogout occurs more often in patients with hyperparathyroidism. Peripheral vascular disease with intermittent claudication of a lower extremity or a frank gangrene is not uncommon in patients with diabetes mellitus. Hypertension frequently occurs in patients with renal disease.

Not to be forgotten is a detailed account of allergic reactions, especially noting associated symptoms and signs related to the use of certain medications, for example, antibiotics. Careful documentation of allergies will help avoid potentially fatal hypersensitivity reactions.

Finally, immunization history allows for exclusion of many diseases.

Family History. Certain diseases are genetically transmitted. Offspring of diabetic patients are more likely than others to develop diabetes mellitus. A history of myocardial infarction at a young age in a parent is a strong risk factor for early coronary artery disease in the offspring. Sometimes there is a clear-cut pattern of inheritance, such as in Huntington's chorea, which is transmitted as an autosomal dominant trait, or in hemophilia, which is transmitted as a sex-linked recessive trait.

It is therefore important to document the health status of all close family members. This group should include, at a minimum, parents, siblings, and children. Specific illnesses, age of occurrence, and cause of death should all be noted where applicable. Construction of a family tree can be a helpful adjunct in this regard.

Review of Organ Systems. The review of systems is a comprehensive listing of symptoms related to each organ system of the body. Detailed inquiry about all possible symptoms is made with the intent of eliciting complaints that have been suppressed, forgotten, or considered unimportant. Complete questionnaire formats are found in most of the standard textbooks of physical diagnosis, and all questions should be asked of all patients. This is particularly true of elderly patients. For example, a 76-year-old housewife who took two aspirins every morning ''to keep her strength'' and two aspirins at bedtime ''to go to sleep'' was brought to the office by her son because she seemed weak and showed little interest in doing anything, including looking after her general hygiene. The review of systems revealed that her stools were black. She turned out to be suffering from severe iron deficiency anemia secondary to gastrointestinal bleeding.

Not to be overlooked is an inquiry into weight changes. A 50-year-old man complaining of cough with a long-standing history of smoking and a 20-lb weight loss over the past 15 months is likely to have bronchogenic carcinoma. Weight loss in an 18-year-old girl who is brought by her mother because of postprandial vomiting is probably self-induced and secondary to bulimia and anorexia nervosa.

The systems review may put the complaints of the present illness into proper perspective. It may also change the focus of interest from originally established trivial or nonspecific problems to a specific organ system. Generally, the systems review helps to identify multisystem disease and often allows for the discovery of additional diagnostic problems.

Social and Personal History. The social and personal history characterizes the patient's environment and his reaction to it. It includes the patient's level of education, financial situation, employment history, marital status, habits, recreational activities, and interpersonal relationships, as well as information concerning diet, weight changes, sleeping patterns, exercise, sexual preference, alcohol intake, and drug abuse. This knowledge is crucial to the understanding of the patient as an individual and often provides strong support for the suspected diagnosis. For example, a history of intravenous drug use in a patient presenting with chills and fever suggests a diagnosis of bacteremia with endocarditis. A diffuse pulmonary infiltrate on a chest x-ray is likely to be pneumocystis pneumonia in a male homosexual, tuberculosis in a homeless chronic alcoholic, and bird fanciers' lung in a person who breeds parakeets as a hobby.

A man with abdominal pain who has suffered a recent series of personal misfortunes may well have a peptic ulcer, and a patient who has changed jobs frequently, has not managed his finances well, and has recently been estranged from his wife may be in the early stage of an emotional breakdown, or may be suffering from an organic brain syndrome secondary to alcohol abuse, neurosyphilis, or Alzheimer's disease.

PHYSICAL EXAMINATION

There are many books that describe the detailed techniques of physical examination at which each physician should be adept.[16-21] Of equal importance is the development of expertise in correlating the physical findings with the medical history so that a synthesis of one or more likely diagnostic hypotheses can be made.

The basic principles of physical examination include inspection, palpation, percussion, and auscultation. Although emphasis is often placed on being systematic, orderly, and observant, the physician must not overlook the importance of being considerate and sensitive to the patient's needs. For example, when a male physician examines a female patient, it is appropriate not only to have a female nurse in the room, but also to use a combination of gown and bedsheet to limit bodily exposure at any one time. Comments about positive findings should not be made during the examination, even if the findings are normal. Imagine the agony a patient must feel when the physician's eyes light up as he tells his nurse, "Mrs. Jones has a functional heart murmur and her breath sounds are bronchovesicular!"

Errors in physical examination may not necessarily arise from deficits in medical knowledge, but from a lack of organization during the procedure. Inadequate facilities and equipment may also play a role. Poor lighting would make jaundice difficult to see. A weak battery precludes a comprehensive examination of the fundus, and unless the size of the blood pressure cuff is appropriate to the arm circumference of the patient, readings will be inaccurate.

An uncomfortable and uncooperative patient can interfere with the smoothness and success of the physical examination. He can tense his abdomen, precluding palpation of an enlarged liver or spleen. He can refuse to hold his breath long enough for the physician to hear the carotid bruit. He can prevent the muscular relaxation needed for testing the deep tendon reflexes. In short, the patient can work against himself unless a good rapport has been established during the history-taking interview and the physician has created an atmosphere that encourages full patient cooperation.

There are occasions when an abbreviated form of history and physical examination, with emphasis on only the organ system indicated by the history of the present illness, is more appropriate. This method is often used in treating acute, brief, and minor ailments like sore throat, hay fever, or earache in a clinic setting. Although this method effectively saves time, quality of care is certainly compromised. Similarly, medical emergencies are initially dealt with in this manner, but only to expedite the delivery of urgent treatment. Once the patient is stabilized, a complete history and physical examination should be performed if at all possible.

Systematic Approach to Physical Examination

The routine physical examination is a complete assessment of the functioning of the entire body. Although it is best performed in a ritualistic fashion, progressing in a predetermined order from one organ system or one region to another, often emphasis is placed on specific aspects, depending on the history.

The traditional starting point is the recording of vital signs. Pulse rate and rhythm, blood pressure, temperature, respiratory rate, height, and weight should all be documented. Sometimes, definitive clues to an underlying illness become apparent after these simple measurements are done. A slow or irregular heart rate in an elderly person may suggest that a cardiac arrhythmia underlies the chief complaint of dizziness, or an elevated blood pressure may explain the patient's headaches. Even if the vital signs are normal, they serve as a baseline for reference on subsequent visits.

The initial blood pressure reading should be measured on the right arm. In younger patients, if the blood pressure is high, recording the pressure in the left upper extremity and a lower extremity is important in the diagnosis of coarctation of the aorta. Geriatric patients are more likely to have atherosclerotic involvement of the subclavian arteries. This can preclude hypertensive readings in the affected extremity. Taking blood pressure measurements in both arms is therefore of value in this age group. In some instances, comparison of systolic blood pressure in the supine and standing positions may reveal orthostatic hypotension and can confirm the suspicion of dehydration or an adverse reaction to antihypertensive drugs. A systolic pressure drop in excess of 30 mm Hg from the supine to upright position, especially if accompanied by a rise in pulse rate, is significant.

General inspection is the next area of focus, although it in fact begins with the first patient contact and is elaborated upon during the entire history and physical examination. It is pertinent to note all aspects of appearance and behavior. These may include the degree of patient discomfort, the severity of respiratory distress, a general assessment of physique, abnormal posturing, body movements, speech, breath and body odors, general hygiene, appropriateness of dress, cooperativeness, and so on. These observations form an integral part of the diagnostic synthesis. For example, a pulse rate of 45 can be physiologic in a 20-year-old athletic muscular male but may point to a diagnosis of sick sinus syndrome or heart block in an 80-year-old female with syncope. Similarly, the presence of alcohol on the patient's breath can be the most important finding of the entire physical examination.

Abnormalities involving the ears may also be related to a variety of illnesses. Congenital malformations of the external ear frequently accompany anomalies of the urinary tract, especially those involving the collecting system.[22] Gouty tophi, deposited in the helix or antihelix, are a valuable clue in the diagnosis of hyperuricemia. Certain common symptoms, such as headache and tinnitus, may be related to swelling and inflammation of the tympanic membrane caused by otitis media. Hearing loss may be caused by problems in the external auditory canal (such as an impacted foreign body or impacted cerumen) or in the middle ear (sclerosis of the oscillating bones), as well as in the inner ear and auditory nerve.

Nasal discharge is one of the commonest symptoms suffered by patients. Usually it is related to a viral upper respiratory tract infection, but one must not forget that unilateral whitish nasal mucus, particularly when occurring in children, may be caused by a foreign body, and an intermittent or persistent unilateral discharge occurs when there is cerebrospinal fluid leakage through the cribriform plate or adjacent sinuses. If the latter is not treated, serious sequelae such as meningitis or brain abscess may ensue.

Bloody nasal discharge is most commonly caused by nose picking which damages the rich network of veins in the anterior nares (Kiesselbach's plexus). Hypertension or a bleeding diathesis are other causes. The saddle nose deformity suggests the diagnosis of congenital syphilis, and flaring of the alae nasi is an important clinical clue of respiratory distress in pneumonia.

The head, eyes, ears, nose, mouth, and throat are generally grouped together for purposes of examination because of their close anatomic location. The head is first inspected for skull configuration, palpated for abnormalities such as exostosis or depressions secondary to a fracture, and auscultated for vascular bruits.

The eyes may reveal important clues to a variety of neurologic and medical conditions. An orderly approach begins with inspection and palpation of the orbit and adnexa, always comparing one eye to the other. Pupil size and equality, as well as response to light and accommodation, are noted. Eyelids are inspected for evidence of ptosis, edema, and hematoma. The sclera and conjunctiva are assessed for jaundice and increased vascularity.

Corneal deposits of cholesterol are responsible for arcus senilis, which when present in a young or middle-aged adult may suggest the diagnosis of hypercholesterolemia.[22] Band keratopathy, resulting from the presence of calcium phosphates and carbonates under the corneal epithelium, is seen in both primary hyperparathyroidism and hypercalcemia secondary to sarcoidosis and vitamin D intoxication. Green or golden deposits of copper (Kayser Fleischer rings) in Descemet's membrane occur in Wilson's disease. Hurler's disease causes gross cloudiness of the cornea secondary to polysaccharide deposits, and crystals of chloroquine are sometimes deposited in the cornea when patients with discoid lupus are treated with the drug.

The blink reflex and visual acuity are also evaluated,

and extraocular eye muscle movements are carefully assessed. The latter is an integral part of the eye examination, allowing for clues pertaining to neurologic disease, muscle disease, and even endocrine (Graves') disease. Finally, a funduscopic exam may reveal the first evidence of diabetes or hypertension.

The presence of collagen vascular diseases, metabolic and endocrine disorders, infections, hematologic disorders, reactions to medications, malnutrition, vitamin deficiency, and even poisoning may all be suspected after examining the oral cavity. For example, leukemia can cause oral mucosal ulcerations and gingival bleeding. Malnutrition and pernicious anemia are associated with a beefy red tongue. Lead and bismuth poisoning are associated with a dark line along the gingival margin. Dilantin therapy is associated with gingival hyperplasia. Macular brown areas on the buccal mucosa are characteristic of Addison's disease, and Koplik's spots are pathognomonic of measles. Pigmentation of the lips and oral muscosa is seen in association with intestinal polyposis (Peutz-Jeghers syndrome).

The neck is inspected for abnormal swelling or masses as well as for jugular venous pulse and pressure. Palpation of masses, lymph nodes, the thyroid, the carotid arteries, and the trachea is also an important part of the examination of this region, which is a prime anatomic landmark. Palpation of the carotid pulse not only is useful in the diagnosis of aortic stenosis, aortic regurgitation, or asymmetrical septal hypertrophy, but also is essential in monitoring the progress of cardiopulmonary resuscitation. Cervical lymph nodes may contain important histologic clues to the diagnosis of neoplastic disease, tuberculosis, and sarcoidosis. Tracheal deviation may suggest a pneumothorax or a large lung mass, and a tracheal tug is sometimes felt with a thoracic aortic aneurysm. A vascular bruit over the thyroid is sometimes heard in hyperthyroidism, and a carotid bruit may be the first sign of atherosclerotic carotid artery narrowing.

The most common cause of a mass in the anterior cervical triangle of the neck is thyroid enlargement. Swelling in the posterior cervical triangle may be caused by carotid artery aneurysms, cystic hygromas, branchial cleft cysts, and enlarged lymph nodes. Aneurysms, of course, are pulsatile. Cystic hygromas are more commonly seen in children and transilluminate brightly. Branchial cleft cysts, usually appearing in adults, are firm, cystic, palpable masses located beneath the sternocleidomastoid.

The four basic components of the physical examination—inspection, palpation, percussion, and auscultation—can be used to full advantage in the examination of the chest and lungs. Pectus carinatum or excavatum may be congenital or acquired, and pectus excavatum may be a clue to the presence of mitral valve prolapse. A large anteroposterior diameter of the chest is seen with emphysema. Symmetry of chest expansion is evaluated by inspection and palpation. The presence of tactile fremitus may lead one to suspect pneumonia, pleural effusion, atelectasis, and even tumors. Chest percussion helps define any of the abnormalities detected with inspection and palpation. When these examinations are combined with careful auscultation for rales, rhonchi, wheezes, pleural friction rubs, vocal resonance, and egophony, a fairly accurate assessment of underlying pathologic processes can usually be made.

Some symptoms that relate to pulmonary dysfunction, such as dyspnea, are quite nonspecific. Anemia, muscle disease, any debilitating illness, acidosis, pulmonic valvular stenosis, and simple deconditioning can all have dyspnea as a presenting symptom. Careful examination of the lung is therefore necessary to exclude or confirm the diagnosis of pulmonary disease. For example, obstructive airway disease such as asthma is characterized by diffuse wheezes and prolonged expiration. Left sided congestive heart failure causes rales, and if pulmonary edema is present the patient often coughs up blood-tinged frothy sputum. Rales along with the findings of consolidation are found in pneumonia. Decreased breath sounds and dullness to percussion are demonstrated in pleural effusion.

Perhaps the most challenging part of the physical examination is examination of the heart. The location and nature of the apical impulse of the heart and the presence of ventricular lifts, cardiac thrills, and even abnormal heart sounds can be discovered by careful palpation. The loud first heart sound of mitral stenosis can often be palpated, and it is not uncommon to feel gallop sounds through the chest wall even when they cannot be heard with the stethoscope because of their low frequency.

Percussion is the least utilized component of the physical examination of the heart. Its main purpose is to delineate the left cardiac border, but inherent inaccuracy has all but led to its abandonment.

Although cardiac auscultation is one of the most difficult parts of the physical examination to master, it is the most exciting and probably the most rewarding in terms of reaching a correct diagnosis. An organized approach and careful technique are required. Each area should be listened to with the diaphragm and the bell of the stethoscope so that both high-pitched and low-frequency sounds and murmurs are detected. Timing is essential in interpreting what is heard, and it is a good practice to keep a finger on the carotid pulse during auscultation. Lack of facility in cardiovascular physiology will preclude an adequate examination.

One of the commonly forgotten aspects of the cardiac exam is auscultation while the patient is doing different maneuvers. For example, the click and murmur of mitral valve prolapse may not be heard in the supine position, whereas it becomes readily audible when the patient stands up. A widely split second heart sound that appears to be fixed in the supine position, suggesting an atrial septal defect, may become narrowly and physiologically split in the sitting position. An S_3 may be heard only in the left lateral decubitus position. Valsalva's maneuver may bring on the typical murmur of asymmetrical septal hypertrophy, and the murmur of aortic insufficiency may not be appreciated until the patient squats.

The traditional order of the components of the physical examination is altered in the examination of the abdomen because palpation and percussion may result in decreased or absent bowel sounds. Thus, inspection is the first step, followed by auscultation, palpation, and percussion. Many organs and structures are contained within the abdomen, and many diagnostic tests are available to evaluate the multiplicity of symptoms that may arise. Therefore, appropriate diagnostic testing depends on a very careful examination. Pain in the epigastrium suggests peptic ulcer, leading the physician to select a gastroscopy and upper gastrointestinal series as the first diagnostic tests. A palpable painful gallbladder is compatible with acute cholecystitis. An enlarged and painless gallbladder, on the other hand, should focus attention on the possibility of carcinoma of the pancreas.

Too often, the rectal examination is omitted. Nevertheless, it is an essential part of the physical examination on all middle-aged and elderly patients, both male and female. It would be regrettable to miss a rectal or prostatic carcinoma, or to miss the diagnosis of anemia resulting from blood loss, if examination for occult blood in the stool was not performed.

Like the rectal exam, examination of the genitalia is frequently overlooked during the general physical examination, deferred to a urologist or gynecologist that the patient (especially the male) may never see. Encouragement in performing this part of the examination in male patients should come from the fact that more than 7.5% of all males have intrascrotal masses.[22] The commonest of these is the hydrocoele, which occurs most often in children. It is characterized by its cystic nature and is readily transilluminated. Malignant testicular tumors, on the other hand, appear as painless, asymmetrical firm enlargements without the property of transillumination. Careful examination is warranted in young and old alike because testicular carcinoma has incidence peaks in childhood, young adult life, and old age.

When the pelvic examination is being done in a female it is generally prudent to have the patient empty her bladder before the exam is attempted and to have a female assistant present. A pap smear should be a routine part of the procedure.

Examination of the extremities, skin, nails, muscles, and joints may show abnormalities as manifestations of local or systemic illness. Generally, gross inequality and asymmetry are associated with congenital disorders, neurologic diseases, or traumatic injuries. The lower extremities are more likely to accumulate edema because of their dependent position. Bilateral leg edema is seen with congestive heart failure, nephrotic syndrome, cirrhosis of the liver, and venous insufficiency. Unilateral leg edema is often caused by venous thrombosis, whereas unilateral upper extremity edema is usually the result of localized lymphatic or venous obstruction. Because venous thrombosis is rare in the veins serving the upper limbs, another cause, such as neoplasm, must be considered.

Examination of the nails and nail beds may suggest such diagnoses as psoriasis, iron deficiency anemia, arsenic poisoning, and the hyperdynamic states accompanying aortic insufficiency, hyperthyroidism, and severe anemia of any cause (Quincke's pulse).

Typical skin lesions are seen with acute rheumatic fever. Urticaria and erythema nodosum may be the first indication of primary tuberculosis, sarcoidosis, and even regional enteritis. Firm thickened skin overlying fingers that have a leathery appearance is characteristic of scleroderma, whereas thin shiny skin with hair loss over the legs suggests arterial vascular insufficiency.

Bacterial endocarditis may be associated with splinter hemorrhages, Osler's nodes, and Janeway lesions. Joint deformities with ulnar deviation of the metacarpophalangeal joints are seen in rheumatoid arthritis, Heberden's nodes are found in osteoarthritis, and tophi are not uncommonly deposited behind the elbow. Congenital varus and valgus deformities of the lower extremities may account for the patient's complaint of lower back pain. Arthralgia and digital clubbing are associated with hypertrophic osteoarthropathy, which commonly occurs when lung and pleural neoplasms, pulmonary abscess and empyema, cyanotic cardiac malformations, biliary cirrhosis, regional enteritis, or ulcerative colitis are present. The idiopathic and familial causes occur less frequently.[22]

Just as the carotid pulses are examined when the neck is being evaluated, pulses in the limbs should be evaluated at this time. The brachial, radial, femoral, popliteal, dorsalis pedis, and posterior tibialis pulses should all be palpated bilaterally and their presence and strength documented. One should listen for bruits over both femoral arteries.

Although the detail with which the neurologic examination is done will depend on the nature of the complaint, an evaluation of gait, cerebellar function, muscle strength, deep tendon and plantar reflexes, posterior column function, sensation, and cranial nerves can all be done in a short time.

A mental status evaluation is also an integral part of the examination, although it will actually be gleaned in bits and pieces as the physician goes through the history and physical examination. Evaluating mental status should include observing the patient's behavior, appearance, manner and attitude, expression, speech, and motor activity, as well as assessing his intellectual function with particular emphasis on his memory, orientation, and concentration, his insights and judgments, and his ideational content. It is not sufficient simply to document that the patient is oriented and has no obvious disorders of thought processes. One must also try to learn about the patient's anxieties, moods, and affects because they have so much to do with the causation or the expression of illness.

Mental stress is considered by some as an important risk factor to the development of coronary artery disease and peptic ulcer. Anxiety may underlie abdominal discomfort produced by swallowing air or by the irritable bowel syndrome. A chronic alcoholic who has lost his insight and judgment may deny his problem and refuse help. A patient presenting with fatigue, exhaustion, and headache may not have an organic disorder, but such symptoms may rather be a manifestation of underlying affective disorders, like anxiety, depression, etc.

LABORATORY DIAGNOSIS

The fundamental reason for ordering a test following the history and physical examination is to arrive at the most likely diagnosis so that a prudent therapeutic decision can be made.[8,23] In addition to determining the diagnosis, tests are done to prognosticate the severity and extent of disease, to monitor treatment and clinical status, to screen for other disease processes, and to direct the decision-making regarding management.

As an example, a 50-year-old man with a 25-pack/year history of cigarette smoking complained of chronic cough, hemoptysis, and weight loss. On physical examination, localized wheezes at the posterior left mid lung field were found. The suspicion of bronchogenic carcinoma would be supported by the presence of a left hilar mass lesion on the chest x-ray.

Additional tests are still needed to define the nature of the mass; a bronchoscopy with positive tissue biopsy would confirm the diagnosis. The patient's prognosis as well as the appropriate treatment now depends on the extent of the disease, i.e., whether the cancer has metastasized. Staging of carcinoma can be accomplished by a CT scan of the chest,[24,25] by mediastinoscopy with mediastinal node biopsy, and by evaluation of organs where metastasis is most likely (for example, the liver).[26] Evidence of metastasis alters the decision to operate by placing the patient in a nonresectable category and mandates other modes of palliative therapy. Experience also dictates that certain routine tests like a complete blood count (CBC), SMA-6, SMA-12, ECG, and urinalysis be used to screen for other disease processes that may be independent of or a result of the carcinoma. Failure to recognize the presence of diabetes mellitus, even if it is mild, may result in complications if the patient goes to surgery. The detection of hyperuricemia would allow for appropriate management before initiation of chemotherapy, which in itself can cause hyperuricemia and acute gout. Hyponatremia caused by inappropriate secretion of antidiuretic hormones can cause symptoms of lethargy, unresponsiveness, and even seizures. With the use of chemotherapy or radiation, periodic CBC, platelet counts, and liver function tests are indicated to monitor toxic side effects that may necessitate temporary suspension of treatment or a change in therapeutic approach. Follow-up chest x-rays would be a way of measuring the response to therapy.

Few tests are without morbidity. Even the drawing of blood has the risks of hematoma formation, infection, and phlebitis. All tests have a cost, and most are quite expensive. Many are painful, time consuming, and embarrassing to the patient. Therefore, all laboratory investigations should be ordered for appropriate reasons, and it is important to resist the temptation in our present litigious society to practice defensive medicine by ordering a multiplicity of unnecessary studies for fear of a lawsuit.[23] It is equally important not to limit testing because of pressures by insurance companies and government agencies to control cost. Limited testing usually devalues the quality of medical care given to the less financially fortunate members of our society.

From the above it can be concluded that the effective practitioner must be expert in understanding the meaning of the various laboratory tests that he employs and in utilizing the findings to establish a diagnosis. Physiologic disorders and anatomic abnormalities are often revealed by laboratory tests. Nevertheless, most tests are not perfect in that they do not establish definitively the normality of a parameter.

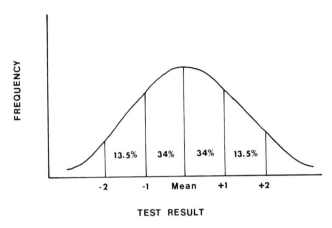

Fig. 1–1. The normal frequency distribution. Standard deviations are abscissa. Frequency of distributions within the corresponding standard deviation segments are indicated by percentages.

Sensitivity and Specificity. Laboratory values have an inherent variation, termed the normal range or reference range.[23,27] A frequency distribution of values obtained from a healthy reference or control population typically assumes a bell shaped curve known as a normal or Gaussian curve (Fig. 1–1). The mean is a central location around which most results fall. As values get farther from the mean there is a symmetrical decrease in their frequency, and a standard deviation can be calculated to express variations from the mean. Values falling within two standard deviations of the mean constitute the reference range and are considered normal. The reference range includes approximately 95% of the population sample. It is apparent that the reference range is rather arbitrary; it depends on the study population and the testing method and hence is liable to substantial error.

Predictive Value. The clinical implications of a particular laboratory test arise from knowledge not only of the reference range, but also of the test's ability to separate patients into diseased groups (i.e., the test's

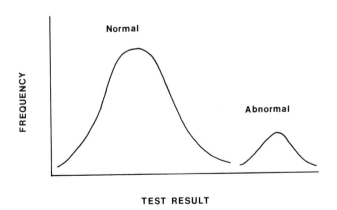

Fig. 1–2. Frequency distribution of an ideal test.

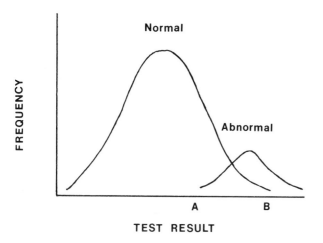

Fig. 1–3. Frequency distribution of a typical laboratory test.

Table 1–1. Influence of Disease Prevalence

	N = 100 Prevalence = 60% Sensitivity = 90% Specificity = 90%	N = 100 Prevalence = 10% Sensitivity = 90% Specificity = 90%
True Positives*	54	9
False Negative*	6	1
True Negatives**	36	81
False Positives**	4	9

$$*\text{Sensitivity} = \frac{TP}{(TP + FN)}$$

$(TP + FN) = \text{Prevalence}$

$TP = \text{Sensitivity} \times \text{Prevalence}$

$FN = \text{Prevalence} - TP$

$$**\text{Specificity} = \frac{TN}{(TN + FP)}$$

$(TN + FP) = (N - \text{Prevalence})$

$TN = \text{Specificity} \times (N - \text{Prevalence})$

$FP = (N - \text{Prevalence}) - TN$

sensitivity) and nondiseased groups (i.e., the test's specificity). Sensitivity is the ratio of the true positive tests to the sum of the true positive and false negative tests (sensitivity = TP/TP + FN). It refers to the proportion of patients who have the disease that the test has correctly identified. Specificity, which is calculated by the ratio of negative tests to the sum of true negative and false positive tests (specificity = TN/TN + FP) defines patients without the disease who are correctly identified by the test.

The ideal test has a sensitivity of 1 (100%) and a specificity of 1 (100%). It separates all normal from all affected patients. In the perfect test, normal and abnormal results are completely separated, and there are no false positives or false negatives (Fig. 1–2). Usually, however, normal and abnormal values overlap, reducing both sensitivity and specificity (Fig. 1–3). For example, if the upper limit of the reference range were at point A, all true positive patients would be identified at the expense of many false positives, and there would be no false negatives. Sensitivity would be 100%, but specificity would be low because of the large number of false positives. On the other hand, if the upper limit of normal were at point B, there would be a large number of false negatives, but all true negative patients would be correctly identified. A calculated specificity of 100% would occur because of no false positives, but sensitivity would be low. By way of compromise between these two extremes, the reference range is generally defined as two standard deviations above and below the mean. This has the effect of decreasing both specificity and sensitivity, but it makes the test more clinically useful by limiting the number of false negatives and false positives.

False positive and false negative tests are also determined by disease prevalence (Bayes' theorem). If, for example, the prevalence of an abnormality in a

population of 100 was 60%, and the sensitivity and specificity were both 90%, the number of true positives would be 54 (60 × 90%), 6 people would be incorrectly identified as not having the disease (false negative), 36 people (40 × 90%) would be correctly labeled as negative, and 4 would be placed in the false positive group (Table 1–1). Compare this when the disease prevalence is only 10%, using the same test with similar sensitivity and specificity. The number of true positives (10 × 90%) would be 9, with 1 false negative, and the number of true negatives would be 81 (90 × 90%), with 9 false positives. What, then, is the meaning of a positive test when there is an equal number of true positive and false positive results?

Thus there are difficulties in interpreting laboratory tests. Normal values are not completely separated from abnormal values because reference ranges are imperfect, with overlapping normal and abnormal results. Sensitivities and specificities of less than 100% create difficulties in determining the significance of both positive and negative tests.

The interpretation of laboratory tests is to some extent an ''art'' in the science of medicine, creating so many differences of opinions among physicians and increasingly bringing physicians in conflict with those whose interests are mainly in lowering medical expenditures. The physician's understanding of the sensitivity and specificity of the tests that he orders is crucial. With this knowledge, a physician can plan a rational series of laboratory investigations for each patient. Cautious interpretation in the context of the clinical situation is prudent. It is often useful to categorize the results as ''definitely positive,'' ''definitely negative, '' or ''equivocal.'' The first two categories will confirm disease or rule it out, respectively. An equivocal result should be repeated. If the finding persists, more definitive testing and clinical correlation must be used in order to ascertain the presence of disease. To illustrate, in the search for bone disease, skeletal x-rays are far less sensitive than a total body bone scan, which detects cancer in its earliest stages. But bone scans are also positive for bone disease secondary to old trauma or degenerative joint disease. Bone scans are therefore less specific than skeletal x-rays, requiring careful interpretation in the clinical context.

A very popular noninvasive method to determine the presence of coronary artery disease in patients with chest pain is the treadmill exercise test.[28] The interpretation of the results is fraught with difficulties, however. To begin with, there is considerable debate concerning the criteria for a positive test. Although most cardiologists consider 1 mm of ST depression significant, others argue that at least 2 mm of ST depression is necessary to indicate coronary artery disease. Even if we assume that the former criterion is correct, the sensitivity of the test is still only in the range of 55 to 75%. The specificity of exercise tests is quite variable. In a group of middle-aged men with typical angina-like chest pain who are on no medication, specificity may be as high as 80 to 90%. But many false positive tests occur in patients who have resting ST-T wave abnormalities in their electrocardiograms, are on a variety of drugs, or have mitral valve prolapse, all of which markedly decreases specificity. The use of thallium scanning in conjunction with electrocardiogram does increase sensitivity to levels of 80 to 90%, but it virtually doubles the cost.

Breast cancer can be diagnosed with a sensitivity of 80% and specificity of 90% by mammography.[29] The sensitivity and specificity of fine needle aspiration of a breast mass followed by cytologic examination are 90% and 98%, respectively. A sensitivity of 98% can be achieved if the fine needle aspiration is repeated in those cases in which the first cytology is doubtful but malignancy is clinically suspected. These tests are highly superior to thermography (sensitivity and specificity of 70%), ultrasonography (sensitivity and specificity of 38% and 90%, respectively), and breast self-examination (sensitivity and specificity of 38% and 0%, respectively). On the negative side for mammography is the cost and radiation, while needle aspirations have the potential risks of hematoma, infection, tumor spread, and even pneumothorax. Are these tests worth the increased cost and risk? The answer is probably "yes" when one considers how common breast cancer is in women, and how important it is to correctly diagnose and remove a malignant cancer before it spreads.

Be Aware and Beware of New Diagnostic Tests and Procedures

Diagnostic Imaging. Technology in medicine has experienced a boom within the last decade. Imaging techniques have perhaps undergone the greatest advances. Whereas x-rays and radionuclide scans used to be our modality to visualize parts of the body, we now have ultrasonography, computed tomography, magnetic resonance, and positron-emission tomography. The practicing physician is thus faced with the task of evaluating new tests, many of which are very expensive and can be done only in specialized centers by specially trained technicians and physicians. Familiarity with the sensitivity and specificity for various groups of patients as well as the cost and risk to the patient must all be considered. In fact, because of the numerous recent advances in diagnostic testing, the American College of Physicians has recently rated many of the more commonly used tests and procedures for their applicability to the practice of medicine in the 1980s.[30] Several of the newer diagnostic methods will be described here.

Ultrasonography. Ultrasonography is a noninvasive procedure utilizing reflection of high-frequency sound waves from organs of the body to derive images. It is safe and inexpensive. The technique is highly specific in the diagnosis of subphrenic abscess, gallstones, and dilated intrahepatic ducts caused by obstruction.[31] It can detect retroperitoneal nodes and masses, measure size and configuration of the liver, spleen, and kidney, and even determine the nature of a mass (cystic or solid). Ultrasonography can be safely used during pregnancy to detect fetal abnormalities, fetal gender, fetal size and position, and ectopic pregnancy. Differentiation of cystic and solid breast masses is accurate 70 to 80% of the time.

Two-dimensional and M-mode ultrasonography are excellent in the diagnosis of a variety of cardiac diseases, particularly mitral and aortic stenosis, mitral valve prolapse, atrial myxoma, ventricular aneurysm, pericardial effusion, and congenital heart abnormalities.[32] They are also useful in the detection of valvular vegetations in endocarditis and mural thrombus. However, the value of the tests depends on several factors. Poor-quality echocardiography studies may occur because the technology to compensate for obesity or emphysema has not been perfected. Technical skill in performing the studies varies, and of course the accuracy of the result will depend on the expertise of the interpreter.

CT Scan. Computed tomography, since its introduction in 1972, has become a major method of visualizing almost all parts of the body.[26] It has eliminated the need for pneumoencephalography and is very often used in place of invasive procedures such as angiography, lymphangiography, and myelography. It is accurate in the diagnosis of brain disorders such as tumors, hemorrhages, vascular occlusion, and vascular anomalies. It is quite specific in differentiating mediastinal disorders, including aneurysms, nodes, metastases, primary tumors (thymoma and teratoma), and substernal thyroid glands. The CT scan can determine the stage of bronchogenic carcinoma by demonstrating the presence or absence of pleural, mediastinal, thoracic wall, and lung metastases. Herniated intervertebral discs and spinal stenosis can be visualized.

In the abdomen, the CT scan is used to identify subphrenic abscess, liver, spleen, and kidney size, tumors, congenital anomalies, and retroperitoneal tumors, nodes, and hemorrhages. In trauma cases in which multiple-organ injury is suspected, the CT scan will detect lacerations to the liver, as well as fractures of the spleen (and subcapsular hematoma), kidney, vertebrae, and pelvis.

To enhance tissue attenuation, iodinated radiographic contrast material can be injected intravenously before the CT scan is performed. Accuracy is high and the test is safe except for an occasional allergic reaction to the dye. This is a test par excellence. Although it is costly and exposes the patient to radiation similar to that of a barium enema, it hastens the diagnosis and often saves the patient from a surgical procedure. Also of note is that ultrasonography and CT scanning have enhanced the value of needle biopsy. Inaccessible or dangerous areas have been safely aspirated and biopsy performed under the guidance of these techniques.

Digital Subtraction Angiography. Digital subtraction angiography is the visualization of the arterial system using an intravenous injection of a contrast material. Through a computer, the digitized preinjection image is stored and subtracted from the postinjection image, allowing the dye in the arteries to be seen. It can be used instead of a potentially dangerous arteriogram in the diagnosis of carotid artery stenosis, and it also has been used in pulmonary arterial thrombosis and embolism and in the detection of renal vascular disease.

Advances in radionuclide imaging have also recently been made. Multiple gated acquisition (MuGa) scans measure the ejection fraction of the ventricle as a determinant of cardiac function. The technique is used to detect wall motion abnormalities and even mitral regurgitation. Technetium scans can detect the presence of acute myocardial infarctions. Postexercise thallium heart scans have enhanced the sensitivity of the treadmill exercise test in diagnosing coronary ar-

tery obstruction and myocardial ischemia. Total body bone scans are used to detect osteomyelitis or bone metastasis. Technetium-labeled compounds such as diisopropyl imidodiacetic acid (DISIDA) provide a sensitive method for detecting acute cholecystitis. Thrombophlebitis can be demonstrated by radioiodinated fibrinogen. Tagging the red blood cells may give some information on their survival and sequestration and may help locate the site of gastrointestinal bleeding; tagged white blood cells may locate occult abscesses.

Magnetic Resonance Imaging. The two newest radiologic modalities are nuclear magnetic resonance imaging (MRI) and positron-emission tomography (PET). Magnetic resonance imaging gives structural and biochemical information about tissue. It involves the computer imaging of released energy signals from body sites previously subjected to giant magnetic fields and subsequently stimulated by short bursts of radiofrequency waves. The application of this totally noninvasive but extremely expensive procedure has been highly successful in detecting cerebral edema, in delineating the spinal cord, in differentiating the white matter from the gray matter, and in detecting carcinomas early.

Positron-Emission Tomography. Positron-emission tomography is a technique that scans the in vivo distribution of substrate labeled with short-half-life positron-emitting radionuclides. Thus are characterized, for example, cerebral blood flow, oxygen utilization, glucose metabolism, and protein synthesis. It is highly sensitive and specific for the diagnosis of stroke, multiple sclerosis, and epilepsy.

In conclusion, the principles of clinical diagnosis are based on: (1) accurate clinical data collection, by history and physical examination and the appropriate use of laboratory and other diagnostic tests, and (2) analysis and integration of these data into meaningful diagnostic possibilities. Both are supported by knowledge of pathophysiology and clinical manifestations of the disease.

Diagnosis of the disease can be simple and straightforward or it can demand all of our clinical skills, cognitive abilities, depth of knowledge, and experience. Clinical diagnosis, in the present complex inpatient setting and in busy outpatient practice, can be a challenging and rewarding task. It should not, however, be idle intellectual exercise or an end in itself. On the contrary, clinical diagnosis should be an ongoing part of the patient management and should include the detection of disease at its early stages, the identification of its nature and severity, and the monitoring of its course and response to treatment.

REFERENCES

1. Palmer, P.E.S., and Cockshott, W.P.: The appropriate use of diagnostic imaging: Avoidance of the red goggle syndrome. JAMA *252*:2753, 1984.

2. Jacobson, H.G.: Machines and People: Who and what are important? JAMA *252*:1181, 1984.

3. Griner, P.F., and Glaser, R.J.: Misuse of laboratory tests and diagnostic procedures. N Engl J Med *307*:1336, 1982.

4. Weinstein, M.C., and Fineberg, H.V.: Clinical Decision Analysis. Philadelphia, W.B. Saunders Company, 1980.

5. Fineberg, H.V.: Medical decision making and the future of medical practice. Med Desic Making. *1*:4, 1981.

6. Blacklow, R.S.: MacBryde's Signs and Symptoms. 6th Ed. Philadelphia, J.B. Lippincott & Company, 1983.

7. Hurst, J.W.: Osler as visiting professor: House pupils plus six skills. Ann Intern Med *101*:546, 1984.

8. Cutler, P.: Problem Solving in Clinical Medicine. 2nd Ed. Baltimore, Williams & Wilkins, 1985.

9. Rothstein, M.S.: Listening to the patient. Ann Intern Med *101*:406, 1984.

10. Wong, E.T., and Lincoln, T.L.: Ready! Fire! Aim!: An inquiry into laboratory test ordering. JAMA *250*:2510, 1983.

11. Rabiner, C.J.: An unusual case of depression. Hospital Psychiatry *16*:11, 1985.

12. Kassirer, J.P., Kuipers, B.J., and Gorry, G.A.: Toward a theory of clinical expertise. Am J Med *73*:251, 1982.

13. Chase, W.G., and Simon, H.A.: The mind's eye in chess. *In* Visual Information Processing. Edited by W.G. Chase. New York, Academic Press, 1973.

14. DeGroot, A.D.: Thought & Choice in Chess. Mouton, The Hague, 1965.

15. Kassirer, J.P., and Gorry, G.A.: Clinical problem solving: A behavioral analysis. Ann Intern Med *89*:245, 1978.

16. Judge, R.D., Zuidema, G.D., and Fitzgerald, F.T.: Clinical Diagnosis. 4th Ed. Boston, Little, Brown & Company, 1982.

17. Prior, J.A., Silberstein, J.S., and Stang, J.M.: Physical diagnosis: The History and Examination of the Patient. 6th Ed. St. Louis, The C.V. Mosby Co., 1981.

18. Delp, M.H., and Manning, R.T.: Major's Physical Diagnosis: An Introduction to the Clinical Process. 9th Ed. Philadelphia, W.B. Saunders Co., 1981.

19. Burnside, J.W.: Physical Diagnosis. 16th Ed. Baltimore, Williams and Wilkins, 1981.

20. Bates, B.: A Guide to Physical Examination. 3rd Ed. Philadelphia, J.B. Lippincott Co., 1983.

21. DeGown, E.L., and DeGown, R.: The Bedside Diagnostic Exam. 4th Ed. New York, Macmillan, 1981.

22. Petersdorf, R.G., Adams, R.D., Braunwald, E., Isselbacher, K.J., Martin, J.B., and Wilson, J.D.: Harrison's Principles of Internal Medicine. 10th Ed. New York, McGraw-Hill, 1983.

23. Statland, B.E.: Clinical Decision Levels for Laboratory Tests. 3rd Ed. New Jersey, Medec Books, 1983.

24. Pugatch, R.D., Falling, L.J., Robins, A.H., and Snider, G.L.: Differentiation of pleural and pulmonary lesions using computed tomography. J Comput Assist Tomogr *2*:606, 1978.

25. Baron, R.L., Levit, R.G., Sagel, S.S., and Stanley, R.J.: Computed tomography in the evaluation of mediastinal widening. Radiology *138*:107, 1981.

26. Wittenburg, J.: Computed tomography of the body. (two parts). N Engl J Med *309*:1224, 1983.

27. Sox, H.P.: Probability theory in the use of diagnostic tests. Ann Intern Med *104*:60, 1986.

28. Goldschlager, N.: Use of the treadmill test in the diagnosis of coronary artery disease in patients with chest pain. Ann Intern Med *97*:383, 1982.

29. Mushlin, A.I.: Diagnostic tests in breast cancer. Clinical strategies based on diagnostic probabilities. Ann Intern Med *103*:79, 1985.

30. Clinical Efficacy Assessment Project. Statement summaries, 1978–present. Recommendation American College of Physicians. October, 1985.

31. Baron, R.L., Stanley, J.K.T., et al.: A prospective comparison of the evaluation of biliary obstruction using computed tomography and ultrasonography. Radiology *145*:91, 1982.

32. Feigenbaum, H.: Echocardiography. 4th Ed. Philadelphia, Lea & Febiger, 1986.

CHAPTER 2

SELECTION AND INTERPRETATION OF LABORATORY TESTS AND DIAGNOSTIC PROCEDURES

Eugene L. Gottfried, M.D. and Stephen K. Gerard, M.D., Ph.D.

INTRODUCTION

Laboratory tests and diagnostic procedures play a major role in modern medical practice, both in the diagnosis and management of disease and in the overall cost of health care. Many physicians—and their patients—regard a battery of tests as a normal part of even the most routine checkup. This was not always the case. Until the 1950s, most laboratory tests were done individually or in small batches by relatively slow and labor-intensive manual methods. Routine testing was often limited to procedures such as a urinalysis and a hematocrit that could be done in the physician's own office. Patients hospitalized with acute illnesses were likely to have chest x-rays and a number of biochemical analyses from a relatively restricted list. "Stat" testing—especially outside of regular working hours—was often limited to procedures that an intern was willing and able to perform personally.

Over the past three decades, the development of high-capacity automated analyzers and the growth of commercial medical laboratories has been accompanied by a steady rise in the number of laboratory tests performed. Although the yearly increase of 10 to 15% went almost unnoticed for a long time, the cumulative effect on the total volume of laboratory tests has been enormous. In one teaching hospital, for example, the clinical laboratory's test volume multiplied fifteenfold over the course of two decades (Fig. 2–1). This trend toward increased testing has affected both patients in hospitals and those attending outpatient clinics and doctors' private offices. Studies have demonstrated increased numbers of tests and procedures in all categories of patients, whether calculated from the standpoint of tests per patient visit, or tests per case or category of disease.[1,2]

The rising number of laboratory tests and procedures has contributed to the dramatic increase in the overall cost of health care in the United States, which climbed from $13 billion (4.4% of the gross national product [GNP]) in 1950 to $355 billion (10.8% of the GNP) in 1983[3,4] (Fig. 2–2). Laboratory tests and procedures alone account for about 1% of the gross national product.

With increasing public awareness of this alarming increase in the cost of health care, there has been mounting pressure to reverse the trend by cost containment schemes such as prospective payment plans, restrictions on the indications for hospitalization and the length of stay, and increasing scrutiny of patients'

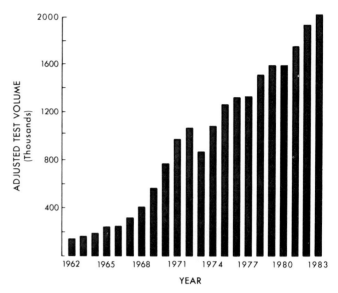

Fig. 2–1. Test volume of the Clinical Laboratories of the San Francisco General Hospital Medical Center, 1962–1983. The figures have been adjusted to account for changes in the method of counting test panels.

records by regulatory agencies. Physicians must now be prepared to justify anything that contributes to the cost of medical care, including laboratory tests and diagnostic procedures.

Until recently, few medical schools provided students with any formal instruction in the principles and practice of laboratory testing. Instead, students would imitate the ordering patterns of the interns and residents encountered during the clinical clerkships, thus perpetuating these patterns. Traditionally, the quality of the diagnostic workup has been judged on completeness, with as much emphasis on the number of tests ordered as on the appropriateness of the individual tests.

The growing economic pressures on health care, disturbing as they may be for both the patient and the physician, provide an additional incentive to review the current customs in ordering laboratory tests and procedures and to evaluate more critically the information these tests provide.

WHY LABORATORY TESTS ARE ORDERED

Laboratory tests are ordered for a variety of reasons, some of which are listed in Table 2–1.[5,6] Tests are usually ordered as part of the initial workup, accom-

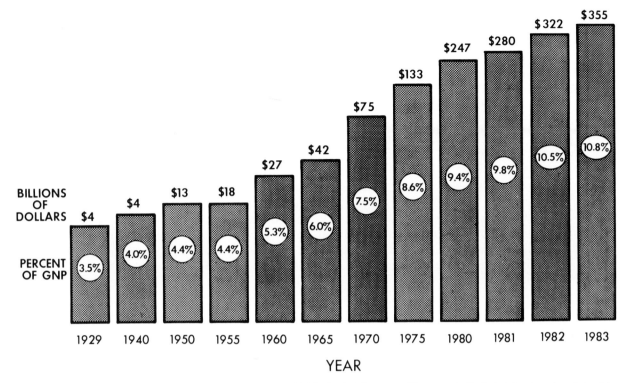

Fig. 2–2. Health care costs as a percentage of the GNP, 1929–1983. Total dollar expenditures are indicated at the top of each bar.[3,4]

Table 2–1. Why Laboratory Tests Are Ordered

Diagnosis
   Screening for potential disease
   Confirming suspected disease
   Excluding possible disease
Management
   Monitoring treatment
   Following the course of disease
   Determining prognosis
Research
Curiosity
Profit
Placebo effect
Fear of criticism ("Defensive medicine")

panying the medical history and physical examination. Some tests are ordered for screening, i.e., to detect an otherwise unsuspected, asymptomatic disorder. Others are done for the purpose of confirming or ruling out a specific disease.

Just how helpful are these tests? In academic training centers, there is a common perception that the diagnosis usually depends on the results of the laboratory tests and procedures. On the other hand, Hampton et al. found just the opposite when they evaluated the relative contributions of the medical history, physical examination, and laboratory tests to the diagnosis and management of 80 outpatients.[7] In 66 of these patients, the diagnosis was immediately apparent from the re-

ferral letter or the medical history alone. In another 7 patients, the correct diagnosis was made after the physical examination had been performed. Laboratory tests were of some help in establishing the diagnosis in 7 patients (9% of the group), but in only one case did the diagnosis depend solely on the laboratory tests. In another report, laboratory studies were instrumental in making the diagnosis in only 1% of the cases studied.[8]

Although laboratory tests are often used to screen for asymptomatic disease, the underlying concepts of screening are often misunderstood. The primary purpose of screening is to identify the disease in question as early as possible and then alter its natural course.[9] The disease should be common enough and serious enough to justify the effort, and there should be some recognizable benefit from treating the patient before the onset of symptoms.[10] As we will demonstrate later in this chapter, some tests are more suitable for screening than others.

Perhaps the widest application of laboratory testing, particularly in the hospital setting, is for monitoring treatment and following the patient's progress.[11] Changing results in a liver function test or blood count may indicate the rate and degree of clinical improvement. Drug levels may provide a useful guide to dosage, particularly for powerful chemotherapeutic agents with a narrow margin between therapeutic and toxic levels. Testing for patient management is appropriate and beneficial, but only to the extent that the tests are selected carefully and not repeated more often than necessary to detect a change that will alter the treatment plan.

Many laboratory procedures (especially in teaching hospitals) are ordered in connection with a research project. The results of these tests may play an important role in medical progress, provided that the research is carefully planned and organized. On the other hand, a poorly developed (or nonexistent) research protocol leads only to the frivolous waste of limited resources. Tests ordered without any visible purpose are sometimes called "educational" by the medical student or resident who is unable to provide a rational justification. This wasteful practice rarely produces any results with real educational or research value, and the costs must be borne by the patient or the laboratory rather than by the intended beneficiary.

A few doctors order laboratory tests as a kind of placebo therapy, to impress patients or colleagues with the thoroughness of the workup, or to increase income. Here, the test results are far less important than the length of the order sheet or the size of the bill.[12]

Another factor in the decision to order laboratory tests is fear, which leads to the attitude commonly called "defensive medicine." The inexperienced intern fears criticism from his older and wiser chief resident or professor if he neglects to order a possibly helpful test. The attending physician, in turn, fears that he may be vulnerable on the same grounds in a malpractice suit. Nevertheless, there is no evidence that using a shotgun approach in a vain attempt to "cover the field" can provide medicolegal protection.[13] As we shall see later in this chapter, too many tests may be just as hazardous as too few, and there may be even more medicolegal vulnerability if the physician neglects to respond to an abnormal test result.[14]

THE FALLACY OF COMPLETENESS

Traditional teaching in medicine holds that the physician should know as much as possible about the patient in order to render the most effective care. It is easy to misinterpret this principle as a signal to order as many laboratory tests as possible in an effort to document the normal findings and rule out even remote diagnostic possibilities. Instead of clarifying the clinical picture, the sheer mass of trivial data may distract

the doctor's attention from the few really important test results. Unnecessary tests may also yield unexpected results that confuse or mislead the physician and delay appropriate treatment.

The potential hazards of unnecessary radiation in the course of diagnostic x-ray studies are well known, as are the risks of invasive procedures. Less well known is the very real possibility of nosocomial anemia, which may result from the repeated collection of blood for laboratory tests. In one study, the volume of blood drawn for laboratory tests in an acute care ward averaged over 400 ml per patient per week.[15] Indeed, patients have occasionally been found to have had the equivalent of three pints of blood withdrawn over a 3-week period of acute-care hospitalization. This practice may account for some of the "unexplained" anemia often observed in hospitalized patients.

THE FALLACY OF THE ABNORMAL TEST

In deciding whether to order a particular laboratory test, one can easily be trapped by the following error in logic:
1. In Disease A, Test B is abnormal.
2. Disease A is suspected.
3. Therefore, Test B should be ordered.

The unstated assumption here is that if Test B is abnormal, then Disease A must be present. Such a conclusion is not warranted. In other words, "If A, then B" is not equivalent to "If B, then A." In order to assess the real value of Test B, more information is needed about the clinical circumstances, the likelihood or prevalence of the disease in question, and the sensitivity and specificity of the test. One quantitative measure of the usefulness of a test is the *predictive value,* which will be discussed later in this chapter.

THE FALLACY OF STATISTICAL SIGNIFICANCE

From time to time, the results of a new test or procedure are reported to show a statistically signifi-

Table 2–2. Proposed Test for "Condition F"

Subjects	N	95% Range	Mean	SD*	SE**
Healthy men	993	184–370	265	50	1.6
Condition F	295	208–406	287	55	3.2

*Standard deviation
**Standard error of the mean

cant difference between a group of healthy people and a group of individuals with a particular disease. On the basis of this statistical significance, the procedure is then recommended as a diagnostic test. The pitfall of this approach can be illustrated by the following example.

EXAMPLE: Table 2–2 summarizes the results of a new test in healthy men and in a group of patients with a hypothetical disorder, "Condition F." The statistical significance of the difference between the mean test values of these two groups is very high ($P < 0.0001$). One might suppose, therefore, that this test would be useful in the diagnosis of "Condition F." Unfortunately, there is so much overlap between the two distributions that the test is of no value in assigning an individual to one of the two groups (Fig. 2–3).

The data for the example cited above were derived from a study of platelet counts in healthy men and women.[16] Thus, despite a statistically significant difference, the platelet count is a poor way to determine the sex of a patient.

EXAMPLE: Merx et al. studied plasma fibrinogen levels before and after intracoronary streptokinase infusion for the treatment of acute myocardial infarction.[17] The average fibrinogen level after treatment was significantly lower in the group of patients who suffered serious hemorrhage than in those who did not ($P < 0.025$). A fibrinogen concentration of 100 mg/dl was selected as the decision level. Nevertheless, 84% of the patients with a fibrinogen concentration below 100 mg/dl did not have serious bleeding; therefore, this test would be a poor predictor of hemorrhage after thrombolytic therapy with streptokinase.

Hartz has proposed a new nonparametric formula, the *overlap index* (O_1), to measure the degree of over-

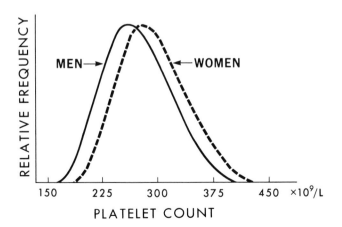

Fig. 2–3. Relative frequency distributions for the blood platelet count in healthy men and healthy women ("Condition F").[16] Compare with Fig. 2–9.

lap between test results in normal and abnormal populations and thereby judge the clinical utility of the test.[18] This approach will probably be more useful for comparing tests than for interpreting a given result.

MEASURES OF TEST PERFORMANCE

ACCURACY AND PRECISION

Accuracy describes the degree of conformity between a test result and the true value (determined by an independent reference method). *Precision*, on the other hand, reflects the ability to achieve the same result time after time. Accuracy and precision are usually expressed quantitatively in terms of inaccuracy (error) and imprecision (standard deviation, coefficient of variation).

High precision is necessary, but not sufficient, to assure accuracy. For example, automated chemical analyzers are capable of determining the serum uric acid level with very high precision, compared with older manual methods. Even so, a poorly adjusted analyzer can give precise—but wrong—results. Not only must the procedure be based on a precise, reliable method, but in addition, the instruments must be calibrated regularly with reference standards of known value.

In the real world, hard choices must often be made between precision, turnaround time, and cost. In general, automated test methods on modern electronic instruments are much more precise than manual procedures that depend on humans to pipette, count, measure, and interpret observations. Some of these instruments, like the automated hematology analyzers, can provide a very rapid turnaround time for "stat" requests. Others, like the Technicon SMAC chemistry system, require so much time for the daily setup, maintenance, and calibration that individual stat tests are impractical.

Sometimes the laboratory (in consultation with the physicians who use it) must balance the need for precise, accurate results against the equally valid need to produce fast results.

EXAMPLE: The total protein concentration of cerebrospinal fluid (CSF) can be determined with good accuracy and precision by the Coomassie Brilliant Blue dye-binding method, but the procedure is relatively time consuming and may not be available in some laboratories as a stat procedure.[19,20] A rough estimate of the CSF protein concentration can be obtained very quickly with a urine dipstick (Stein, Khayam-Bashi, and Gottfried, unpublished). For the physician engaged in the emergency workup of a patient with signs of an acute neurologic disorder, the quick estimate may actually be more useful than a delayed report of the exact value.

Modern electronic hematology analyzers can perform a red blood cell (RBC) count at least seven times more precise than the old manual method, which required the technologist to count individual cells in a hemacytometer.[21] Consequently, manual RBC counts are rarely performed today. On the other hand, the leukocyte differential count is still performed in the majority of laboratories by the time-honored method of examining a stained blood smear under a microscope and counting 100 consecutive leukocytes.

The precision of this 100-cell manual differential count is far worse than most users realize.[22]

EXAMPLE: Consider an imaginary laboratory in which the working conditions are ideal, the instruments always work perfectly, the specimens are collected properly and delivered immediately in optimal condition, and there is never a human error. A physician orders a manual differential count, and the following results are reported:

Total WBC	7800 per μl
Segmented neutrophils	60%
Band neutrophils	4%
Lymphocytes	29%
Monocytes	5%
Eosinophils	2%

A repeat count the following day shows the following results:

Total WBC	8100 per μl
Segmented neutrophils	65%
Band neutrophils	9%
Lymphocytes	22%
Monocytes	3%
Eosinophils	1%

How should these results be interpreted? First, a comparison of the two total leukocyte counts shows a change of less than 4%, well within the expected limits for consecutive counts on separate blood samples. The proportion of segmented neutrophils has increased by 5% and the band count has more than doubled. If the clinical examination is compatible with early infection, the physician may conclude that the differential count has verified his suspicion. Such is not the case.

Table 2–3 lists the range of values that can be expected on repeated 100-cell differential counts under ideal conditions 95% of the time. The table demonstrates that a true value of 5% may be "correctly" reported as low as 1% or as high as 9%. Real laboratories will not do as well.[23] Besides the inherent variability of the method, there is a considerable degree of biologic variability in the leukocyte count. Indeed, in some individuals the absolute neutrophil count may vary by several thousand over the course of a single day.[23] Thus, the 100-cell manual differential count is

Table 2–3. Variability of the 100-Cell Differential Count

True Value (%)	95% Confidence Interval* (%)
2	0– 5
5	1– 9
10	4– 16
20	12– 28
30	21– 39
40	30– 50
50	40– 60
60	50– 70
70	61– 79
80	72– 88
90	84– 96
95	91– 99
98	95–100

*95% confidence interval = p ± 2 SD

$$SD = \sqrt{\frac{p \times q}{N}}$$

where p = true frequency (percent)
q = 100 − p
N = number of cells counted[62]

often an unreliable indicator of a change in the band count or a change in the patient's clinical condition.

Use of the manual differential count as a routine screening test for case finding, in either inpatient or outpatient settings, has been criticized as an inefficient and time-consuming procedure that is no longer appropriate for routine medical practice.[24,25]

As automated equipment for performing differential counts becomes more widely available, the manual differential count will probably fall into disuse, although qualitative examination of the stained smear will continue to be important. Automated differential analyzers, with their ability to examine thousands of cells in a few seconds, have very high precision. Nevertheless, current instruments have distinct limitations, in particular an inability to identify certain cell types, including bands.

SENSITIVITY, SPECIFICITY, AND EFFICIENCY

Sensitivity is the probability of an abnormal test result in a patient who has the disease under investigation. A sensitivity of 95% indicates that 5% of patients with that disease will have false negative test results. The higher the sensitivity, the more likely it is that the disease will be detected and the less likely that someone with a negative test result has the disease.

Specificity is the probability of a normal test result in a person who does not have the disease in question. If the specificity is 98%, 2% of normal subjects will have a false positive test result. The higher the specificity, the smaller the likelihood of a false positive

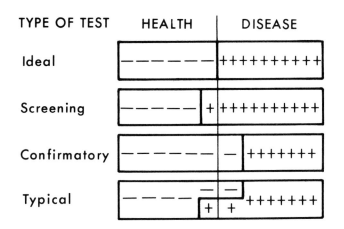

TYPE OF TEST	HEALTH	DISEASE
Ideal	– – – – –	+ + + + + + + + +
Screening	– – – – – +	+ + + + + + + + +
Confirmatory	– – – – – –	+ + + + + +
Typical	– – – – –	+ + + + + +

Fig. 2–4. Expected results in health and disease for ideal and typical laboratory procedures, and for tests with high sensitivity (screening tests) or high specificity (confirmatory tests). "–" indicates a negative test result; "+" indicates a positive result. (Reproduced with permission from Gottfried, E.L. and Wagar, E.A.: Laboratory testing: A practical guide, in Cotsonas, N.J., Jr., et al. (eds.): Disease-a-Month. Copyright 1983 by Year Book Medical Publishers, Inc., Chicago.)

result. In order to know how helpful a test will be in actual clinical use, we need to know not just the specificity in healthy individuals, but also the specificity in the population being tested, e.g., hospitalized patients with similar symptoms who do not have the disease in question.

EXAMPLE: Electrophoretic analysis of cerebrospinal fluid for the detection of oligoclonal bands is a very sensitive test for multiple sclerosis. Positive results have been obtained in up to 95% of patients with definite clinical evidence of the disease, so the sensitivity of the method is considered to be 95%.[26] (The actual sensitivity is probably lower, because the test may be negative in patients who have multiple sclerosis but for whom there is not enough evidence to permit a definite diagnosis.)[27] Oligoclonal bands are rarely seen in healthy individuals, but up to 40% of patients with other inflammatory neurologic disorders may have a positive test.[26,28] Thus, as used for the diagnostic evaluation of patients with possible multiple sclerosis, the oligoclonal band test has a specificity of only 60%.

Efficiency is the proportion of correct test results, that is, true positive plus true negative results. The term is misleading because it seems to imply that a test with high efficiency is a good clinical test. This is not necessarily so, as we will demonstrate later in this chapter.

An ideal laboratory test or diagnostic procedure would always give normal results for healthy people and abnormal results for those with the disease, i.e., both sensitivity and specificity would be 100%. Unfortunately, real tests and procedures fall short of this ideal. Occasionally, there is a choice between one test with high sensitivity and somewhat lower specificity and another with higher specificity at the expense of

reduced sensitivity. The selection should then be made according to the intended application (Fig. 2–4).

A *screening test* is best suited for evaluating a group of subjects in whom the disease is fairly prevalent or an individual in whom the disease is a reasonable possibility but is not the most likely diagnosis. In general, screening tests should have the highest possible sensitivity in order to detect most cases of the disease in the screening program. Some false positives are expected, but a negative test result effectively rules out the disease. Because of the false positives, however, abnormal results usually need to be confirmed by a test with higher specificity.

EXAMPLE: The antinuclear antibody (ANA) test is a sensitive test for systemic lupus erythematosus (SLE), but abnormal results may also be encountered in patients with other collagen-vascular disorders and even in some healthy subjects.[29,30] A positive ANA test is therefore not diagnostic for active SLE, but a negative result effectively excludes this disease.

Confirmatory tests verify a diagnosis already suspected. A good confirmatory test has very few false positive results, i.e., the test must have high specificity. Such a test may lack the high sensitivity of a screening test, so a negative result does not rule out the disease in question.

EXAMPLE: Acute myocardial infarction produces characteristic changes on the electrocardiogram. Some of these abnormalities are highly specific and their presence confirms the diagnosis of acute myocardial infarction. In many patients, however, these diagnostic changes are not observed, so the electrocardiogram alone cannot be used to exclude recent myocardial infarction.[31]

Most of the laboratory tests used in current medical practice are limited in both sensitivity and specificity, and both false positive and false negative results are encountered with some frequency.

WHAT IS "NORMAL"?

It may seem obvious that one cannot determine whether a result is abnormal unless the range of normal values is available for comparison. There are, however, many definitions of "normal."[32–34] As the term is applied to clinical medicine, it may mean anything from "no disorder identified" to "optimal health," or it may be used in a statistical context to describe a Gaussian frequency distribution of test values (Fig. 2–5). These definitions cannot be readily interchanged, and the choice may have an important effect on the interpretation of the test result.

EXAMPLE: A serum cholesterol level of 270 mg/dl in a 50-year-old man is normal in the sense that the value falls within a published "normal range" for men of that age. The normal range in this case was derived from test results on a group of

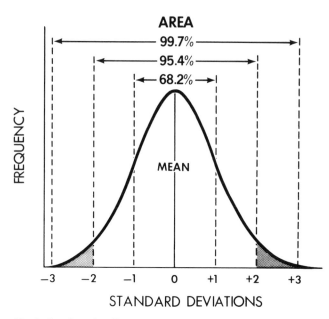

Fig. 2–5. Gaussian ("normal") frequency distribution. (Reproduced with permission from Gottfried, E.L. and Wagar, E.A.: Laboratory testing: A practical guide, in Cotsonas, N.J., Jr., et al. (eds.): Disease-a-Month. Copyright 1983 by Year Book Medical Publishers, Inc., Chicago.)

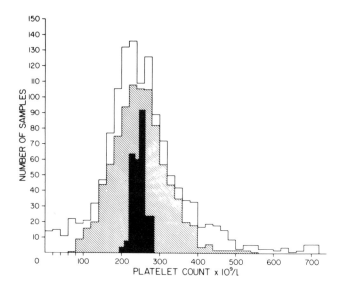

Fig. 2–6. Frequency distribution of platelet counts in a single healthy individual (solid black bars), a group of healthy blood donors (hatched bars), and a group of hospitalized patients (open bars). (From Ross, D.W., Ayscue, L., and Culley, M.: Automated platelet counts: Accuracy, range, and precision. Am J Clin Pathol 74:151, 1980. Reproduced by permission.)

presumably healthy volunteers. Nevertheless, total serum cholesterol concentrations above 240 mg/dl are associated with increased mortality from cardiovascular disease and thus exceed the range associated with optimal health.[35,36]

DEFINING THE REFERENCE RANGE

The range of normal values for a laboratory test is usually taken from a predefined proportion (e.g., 95%) of the results obtained from a group of healthy subjects. By the very nature of this process, it is inevitable that some healthy people will have results that fall outside the accepted limits. Moreover, there is no assurance that patients with normal results are free of disease. The term "reference range" is now preferred instead of "normal limits" in order to avoid unwarranted inferences.

For a given laboratory procedure, the reference range may vary considerably, depending on such factors as the subjects' states of health, ages, sex, nutritional status, ethnic origins, etc. Ross et al. showed that one person's platelet count varies relatively little when the count is repeated (Fig. 2–6).[37] In comparison, platelet counts performed on a group of healthy blood donors cover a much broader range of values, and the range among the patients in a general hospital population is wider still. Matching the reference range to the patient's own set of normal values remains a troublesome aspect of laboratory medicine.

Because of all the variables encountered in setting

up reference ranges, various laboratories may adopt different limits for the same procedure, and published tables of normal values may show apparent discrepancies. For example, Table 2–4 gives the reference ranges for hemoglobin in adult men as reported in three separate studies. The values reported by Wintrobe are the oldest and most widely used, but the range is higher than those derived from larger groups of subjects with modern automated test methods.[16,39] The diagnosis of mild anemia may well depend on the reference range with which the patient's hemoglobin level is compared.

If the results of a laboratory test follow a Gaussian frequency distribution, about 95% of the results will fall in the interval between 2 standard deviations (SD) below the mean value and 2 SD above the mean (Fig. 2–5). Many of the reference ranges commonly used for clinical laboratory tests have been derived in this fashion, by calculating the mean and standard deviation of a group of tests performed on healthy people. It follows that 2.5% of equally healthy individuals will have results below the lower limit and 2.5% will have

Table 2–4.   Reference Limits for Hemoglobin in Adult Men

Reference	N	Mean	95% Limits (g/dl)
Wintrobe[38]	86	16.0	14.0–18.0
Godwin and Jencks[39]*	2089	14.9	12.6–17.1
Gottfried and Nigro[16]	993	15.4	13.5–17.3

*Data derived from the authors' tables for 20- to 69-year-old men.

results exceeding the upper limit. Alternatively, instead of this "two-tailed" approach, the reference range can be treated as a "one-tailed" curve, and only results exceeding some limit (e.g., the 95th percentile) are considered abnormal. An example of this application is the prothrombin time.

Depending on the specific reason for ordering the test, it may be desirable to use broader or narrower limits than those provided by the customary 95% reference range. This choice will, of course, determine the proportion of healthy individuals whose test results fall outside the accepted limits. Changing the reference range is one way to improve the specificity of the test at the expense of decreased sensitivity, or vice versa, without changing the method itself.

Contrary to popular belief, most laboratory tests follow not the Gaussian model of frequency distribution, but a skewed distribution like that shown in Figure 2–7 for the total leukocyte count.[16]

When the test values do not follow a Gaussian distribution, the reference range cannot be determined accurately by calculation of the mean and standard deviation. It is then necessary either to manipulate the raw data mathematically (e.g., logarithmic or square-root transformation) to approximate a Gaussian distribution, or (better) to use a nonparametric method to

find the central 95% (or some other fraction) of the distribution. The method selected can make a real difference in the reference range. For example, the upper 2.5% limit for serum ALT levels in healthy men may range from 49 to 63 I.U./L depending on the method selected.[40] The effect of the method on the reference range for the total leukocyte count is shown in Figure 2–8.

For most laboratory tests, there is a certain amount of overlap between the ranges of values encountered in patients with the disease in question and those who do not have the disease. In Figure 2–9, Curve 1 represents the frequency distribution of test results in a group of healthy subjects, and Curve 2 represents the range of results in patients with the disease. Depending on where we set the upper limit, we can make the test either highly sensitive or highly specific without changing the method, but not both at once. For example, if we set the upper limit at X, all patients with the disease will be detected by this test, and the sensitivity will be 100%. At the same time, healthy subjects with values between X and Y (Interval B) will have false positive results, so the test will not be highly specific. On the other hand, if we set the upper limit at Y, specificity will rise to 100%, but sensitivity will suffer, and the test will not detect any patients whose

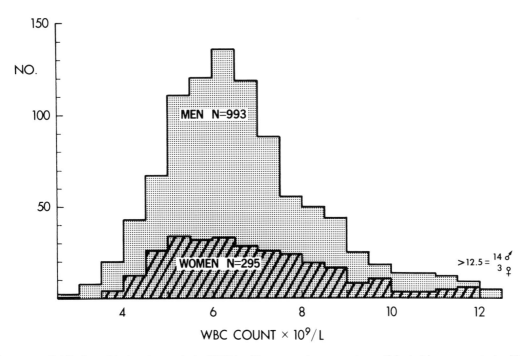

Fig. 2–7. Frequency distribution of leukocyte counts in 1288 healthy men and women who participated in a corporate health survey in New York City in 1981.[16] Stippled bars indicate the total leukocyte counts in 993 men; hatched bars, 295 women. (Reproduced with permission from Gottfried, E.L. and Wagar, E.A.: Laboratory testing: A practical guide, in Cotsonas, N.J., Jr., et al. (eds.): Disease-a-Month. Copyright 1983 by Year Book Medical Publishers, Inc., Chicago.)

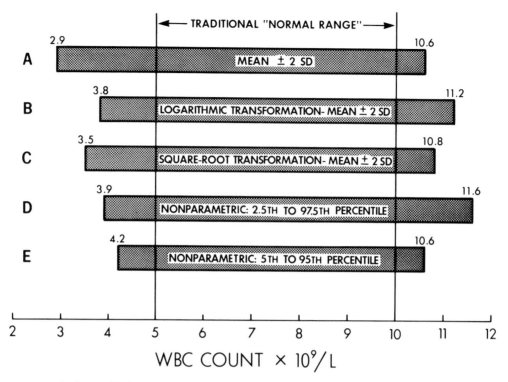

Fig. 2–8.   Reference range for the total leukocyte count in 1288 healthy subjects.[16] *A,* assuming a Gaussian frequency distribution of the raw data; *B,* after logarithmic transformation; *C,* after square-root transformation; *D,* nonparametric central 95% range; *E,* nonparametric central 90% range. The vertical lines delineate the traditional "normal range" of 5-10 × 10⁹/L.

results fall in Interval B. In practice, the upper limit is usually set somewhere between X and Y, a compromise between maximum sensitivity and maximum specificity.

EXAMPLE: Serum uric acid is often included in the multiple-test panels provided by continuous-flow chemical analyzers, such as the Technicon SMA 12/60 and SMAC series. The application of this test in screening for asymptomatic gout is based in large measure on the work of Seegmiller et al.[41] The authors measured serum uric acid in 940 normal subjects and in 60 patients with gout. They recommended a cutoff value of 7.0 mg/dl, based on the uric acid concentrations found in their healthy subjects (mean + 2 SD). With 7.0 mg/dl as the reference limit, 5% of normal individuals had values above this point, whereas 9% of the patients with gout had values within the normal range. The test sensitivity is therefore 91% and the specificity is 95%.

A diagnostic decision could be made with greater confidence if multiple decision levels instead of fixed reference limits were available for each test. Thus, in Figure 2–9, results below X rule out the disease and those above Y are diagnostic. Results in Interval B cannot reliably distinguish healthy subjects from those with the disease and so would be disregarded. In the example of serum uric acid cited above, the lower level (X) is 6.0 mg/dl, and the upper level (Y) is 9.5 mg/dl.[41]

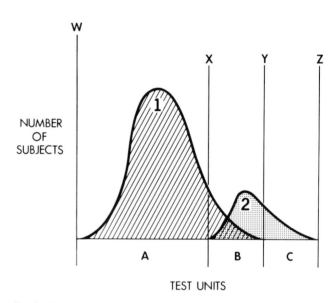

Fig. 2–9.   Frequency distributions for a hypothetical test in health (curve 1, hatched area) and disease (curve 2, stippled area). All values less than X (interval A) exclude disease under investigation, whereas values greater than Y (interval C) are diagnostic for the disease. Values between X and Y (interval B) are inconclusive. (Reproduced with permission from Gottfried, E.L. and Wagar, E.A.: Laboratory testing: A practical guide, in Cotsonas, N.J., Jr., et al. (eds.): Disease-a-Month. Copyright 1983 by Year Book Medical Publishers, Inc., Chicago.)

Table 2–5. Predictive Value Matrix

	Test Results		
Disease	Positive	Negative	Totals
Present	True +	False −	Total with disease
Absent	False +	True −	Total without disease
All patients	Total +	Total −	Total tests

MORE TESTS MEAN MORE ABNORMAL RESULTS

For the typical clinical test, the reference range includes 95% of healthy subjects. The probability of a true negative result is, therefore, $P = 0.95$. When a series of N unrelated tests is performed on a healthy individual, the probability that all the results will be negative is $P = 0.95^N$, and the probability of at least one false positive result is $P = 1 - 0.95^N$.

In a large screening panel, the effects can be considerable. For example, in the Technicon SMAC biochemical panel, $N = 20$ and (assuming that there is no interaction between the tests) $P = 1 - 0.95^{20} = 0.64$. Thus, about two thirds of healthy people will have at least one abnormal result. If the test group consists mostly of acutely or chronically ill patients, a much larger proportion of abnormal results will be seen, even though the tests are not directly related to the disease under consideration.

BAYES' THEOREM AND THE PREDICTIVE VALUE MODEL

PREDICTIVE VALUE

Probably the most powerful mathematical tool now available for judging the usefulness of a clinical test is the *predictive value*.[42,43] If the sensitivity, specificity, and prevalence (or the pretest probability) of the disease are known, one may easily calculate the effect of the test result on the probability of a correct diagnosis. The calculation is based on Bayes' theorem, a formula developed by the 18th century mathematician, the Reverend Thomas Bayes.[44] The predictive value of a positive test (PV +) is the probability that the disease is present when the test result is positive (abnormal). Similarly, the predictive value of a negative test (PV −) is the probability that the disease is absent when the test result is negative (normal).

Predictive value can be readily calculated by first listing the data in the format shown in Table 2–5.

Then,

Sensitivity = True +/Total with disease
Specificity = True −/Total without disease
Prevalence = Total with disease/Total tests

And predictive value is calculated as follows:

PV + = True +/Total +
PV − = True −/Total −

$$\text{Efficiency} = \frac{(\text{True }+) + (\text{True }-)}{\text{Total tests}}$$

The predictive value model can be easily applied to tests in the published literature, if enough information is provided. Newer procedures, especially biochemical tests, are more likely than the older, traditional tests to undergo extensive evaluation, and good estimates of sensitivity and specificity are more readily available.

EXAMPLE: Serologic tests for syphilis are widely used in connection with screening programs. One popular version, the rapid plasma reagin (RPR) card test, has a sensitivity for seropositive syphilis of 96.8% and a specificity of 98.8%.[45] Given a prevalence of about 35 cases of syphilis per 100,000 in the general population,[46,47] we can calculate the predictive value of the RPR card test as follows:

	RPR CARD TEST		
	Positive	Negative	Totals
Syphilis	33.9	1.1	35
No syphilis	1,199.6	98,765.4	99,965
All patients	1,233.5	98,766.5	100,000

PV + = 33.9/1233.5 = 2.7%
PV − = 98765.4/98766.5 = 99.999%
$$\text{Efficiency} = \frac{33.9 + 98765.4}{100000} = 98.8\%$$

A negative RPR card test accurately rules out seropositive syphilis and so serves as an excellent example of a screening test as defined earlier. Most of the positive test results, however, are false positives. A confirmatory follow-up test must be done in order to establish the diagnosis of syphilis.

EXAMPLE: The use of serum uric acid as a screening test for asymptomatic gout was cited earlier. The effectiveness of this approach can be measured by applying the predictive value model.

Using the values for sensitivity (91%) and specificity (95%) from the data provided by Seegmiller et al.,[41] and assuming a prevalence of 0.0025,[46] we can calculate the predictive value as in the previous example:

	URIC ACID (mg/dl)		
	> 7.0	< 7.0	Totals
Gout	227.5	22.5	250
No gout	4,987.5	94,762.5	99,750
All patients	5,215	94,785	100,000

PV + = 227.5/5215 = 4.4%
PV − = 94762.5/94785 = 99.98%
$$\text{Efficiency} = \frac{227.5 + 94,762.5}{100,000} = 94.99\%$$

These results demonstrate that a normal serum uric acid level on a routine screening test effectively excludes asymptomatic gout. On the other hand, a high value (> 7.0 mg/dl) usually does *not* mean that the patient has gout, because over 95% of the high values are false positives.

The low positive predictive value makes this test a poor one in screening for asymptomatic gout. Yet the efficiency is high, and one might argue that the test serves a useful purpose by ruling out the disease in patients with a normal result. But consider an alternative "test," the negative guess. Because the prevalence is so low, we can simply guess that a given asymptomatic individual does not have gout. Then, with the data given above, our guess will be correct 99,750 times out of 100,000. We will miss every case of asymptomatic gout, but the efficiency of the guess is 99.75% (better than that of the actual analysis). Moreover, the predictive value of a normal uric acid level is only 0.23% higher than that of the guess.

We demonstrated earlier that the specificity of the serum uric acid level as a test for gout can be increased by raising the reference limit to 8.0 mg/dl. Let us now examine the effect of this maneuver on the predictive value. The new reference limit of 8.0 mg/dl reduces the test sensitivity to 84% and increases the specificity to 99%. Using the same value of 0.0025 for prevalence, we obtain the following results:

	URIC ACID (mg/dl)		
	> 8.0	< 8.0	Totals
Gout	210	40	250
No gout	997.5	98,752.5	99,750
Totals	1,207.5	98,792.5	100,000

PV + = 210/1207.5 = 17.4%
PV − = 98752.5/98792.5 = 99.96%

Raising the reference limit for serum uric acid from 7.0 mg/dl to 8.0 mg/dl increase the predictive value of a positive test from 4.4% to 17.4%, a fourfold improvement, with virtually no change in the negative predictive value. The trade-off is a decrease in sensitivity from 91% to 84%, leading to negative results in 40 cases of asymptomatic gout for each 100,000 subjects screened.

The predictive value model can be applied just as readily to diagnostic procedures as to laboratory tests.

EXAMPLE: Freitas et al.[48] evaluated the utility of cholescintigraphy in the diagnosis of acute cholecystitis in 211 patients with acute right upper quadrant pain or epigastric pain. From the data provided, we can construct the following table:

	CHOLESCINTIGRAPHY		
	Positive	Negative	Totals
Cholecystitis	60	1	61
No cholecystitis	5	145	150
All patients	65	146	211

Sensitivity = 60/61 = 98.4%
Specificity = 145/150 = 96.7%
PV + = 60/65 = 92.3%
PV − = 145/146 = 99.3%

These calculations demonstrate that cholescintigraphy is a reliable method for either confirming or ruling out the diagnosis of acute cholecystitis.

EXAMPLE: Ultrasonography is a noninvasive diagnostic procedure that appears to be especially useful in the detection of cystic lesions. Clayman et al. examined the effectiveness of this technique by comparing ultrasound interpretations with histologic findings in 260 successive patients with renal masses that had been discovered by intravenous urography.[49] The results were as follows:

	CYST ON ULTRASOUND		
	Present	Absent	Totals
Renal cyst	168	0	168
No cyst	2	90	92
All patients	170	90	260

Sensitivity = 168/168 = 100%
Specificity = 90/92 = 97.8%
PV + = 168/170 = 98.8%
PV − = 90/90 = 100%

The results indicate that ultrasonography is a very sensitive and reliable way to identify a benign renal cyst, thus providing a means to avoid the additional expense and hazards of an invasive diagnostic procedure. Conversely, the absence of a cyst on the ultrasonogram justifies further studies to rule out a malignancy.

In order to calculate the predictive value of a test or procedure, we need to know not only the sensitivity and specificity of the method, but also the probability of finding the disorder in the group of patients being tested. For population screening, this value is the same as the prevalence of the disease. For the diagnostic evaluation of a specific patient, however, we use the *pretest probability* (also known as prior probability) of the disease in question. This is the likelihood that the patient actually has the disease, based on all the information already available from the history, physical examination, and other tests and procedures. The physician's subjective estimate, based on experience and clinical judgment, is usually the most reliable indicator available, and it should be used without hesitation.

Pretest probability has a profound effect on both the predictive value and the real clinical usefulness of the test. Figure 2–10 shows the effect of the pretest probability on the post-test probability of disease (sometimes called the posterior probability) for both positive and negative test results. The test result is most likely to influence the diagnosis when the pretest probability is moderately high (in the example shown, between 15% and 85%). If the likelihood of the disease is very high before the test is performed, a positive result will not make much difference, whereas a negative result will have too low a predictive value to influence the diagnostic decision. Conversely, when the pretest probability is very low (as in screening for a rare disease), most positive results will be false positives.

EXAMPLE: The measurement of urinary metanephrines is an exquisitely sensitive test for pheochromocytoma. According to Gitlow et al., the level is increased in 100% of patients with

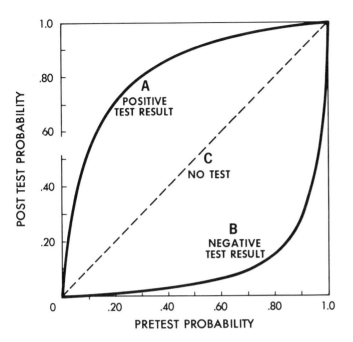

Fig. 2–10. Effects of pretest probability (prior probability) of disease on post-test probability (posterior probability) for a hypothetical test with a sensitivity of 0.95 and specificity of 0.90. Curve A indicates the probability of disease when the test is positive; Curve B, when the test is negative. For a positive test result, post-test probability equals the predictive value; for a negative result, 1 − predictive value. These curves should be compared with the line of identity, C, which would be observed if the test result were unrelated to the probability of disease, i.e., both sensitivity and specificity were 0.50.

pheochromocytoma and in 2% of other hypertensive patients.[50] The prevalence of pheochromocytoma among patients with hypertension is 0.0004,[51] so the predictive value calculations are as follows:

| | URINARY METANEPHRINES | | |
	Increased	Normal	Totals
Pheochromocytoma	40	0	40
No pheochromocytoma	1,999	97,961	99,960
All patients	2,039	97,961	100,000

PV + = 40/2039 = 2%
PV − = 97961/97961 = 100%

These calculations demonstrate that a negative test for urinary metanephrines rules out pheochromocytoma. On the other hand, 98% of the positive results will be false positives, and further diagnostic studies will be required to exclude the disease in those patients. Since 99,960 out of 100,000 patients will not have pheochromocytoma, we can guess "no pheochromocytoma" with a predictive value of 99.96%—almost as good as that of the normal urinary metanephrine test.

EXAMPLE: In a previous example of the predictive value model, we showed that the RPR card test, despite its high sensitivity and specificity, has a positive predictive value of only 2.7% when used as a screening test for syphilis. If, instead of testing the general population, we were to test only patients

attending a venereal disease clinic where the prevalence of seropositive syphilis is 20%, the results would be as follows:

| | RPR CARD TEST | | |
	Positive	Negative	Totals
Syphilis	19,360	640	20,000
No syphilis	960	79,040	80,000
All patients	20,320	79,680	100,000

PV + = 19360/20320 = 95.3%
PV − = 79040/79680 = 99.2%

Used in a population with a high prevalence of syphilis, the RPR card test shows a thirty-five fold improvement in positive predictive value, and in this setting a positive test result is virtually diagnostic.

LIKELIHOOD RATIO

Another estimate of the probability of disease, based on Bayes' theorem, is the *likelihood ratio,* L(x).[52,53] The likelihood ratio indicates the relative odds in favor of the disease at any given test value, x. If the sensitivity and specificity of the test at value x are known, L(x) can be calculated as follows:

$$L(x) = \frac{Sensitivity}{1 - Specificity}$$

EXAMPLE: For serum uric acid, the likelihood ratio at 7 mg/dl (sensitivity = 91%, specificity = 95%) is:

L (7 mg/dl) = 0.91/(1 − 0.95) = 18.2

At 8 mg/dl (sensitivity = 84%, specificity = 99%), the likelihood ratio is:

L (8 mg/dl) = 0.84/(1 − 0.99) = 84

Thus, gout is over four times as likely at the higher serum uric acid level as at the lower level.

For a test that yields numeric results, physicians recognize intuitively that an extreme value is generally more important than a mere borderline abnormality.[54] The predictive value model is limited by its dependence on a fixed reference limit that permits only a "yes/no" decision. The resulting estimate is the average probability of disease for all test results beyond the selected limit. With enough data, one could calculate the likelihood ratio for any value of x (Fig. 2–11). Then, the predictive value at x is equal to L(x) times the pretest probability or prevalence. This approach has potential for providing a more useful prediction for the individual patient than an estimate based on a fixed limit. The calculations require more data than are currently available for most applications in clinical

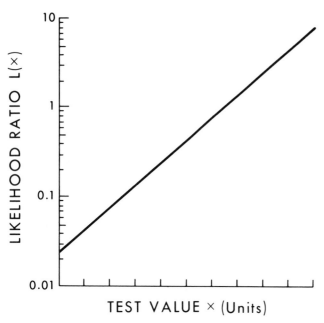

Fig. 2–11. Likelihood ratio, L(x), an expression of the relative probability of disease, based on Bayes' theorem, that varies continuously with the value (x) of the test result.[52,53]

medicine; the concept offers exciting possibilities for the computer-assisted diagnostic systems of the future.

STRATEGIES IN DIAGNOSTIC TESTING

SINGLE TESTS

Screening tests should have as high a sensitivity as possible, in order to avoid missing patients with the disease under investigation. If the prevalence of the disease is low, there will inevitably be many false positive results, as we demonstrated in the example of urinary metanephrines for pheochromocytoma. In order to minimize the number of false positives, the test group should be selected with care *before* testing, so as to include only the subjects most likely to have the disease. For any disease with very low prevalence in the group selected for testing, the predictive value of a positive test will also be very low, and the predictive value of a negative test will be not much better than that of a negative guess.

Confirmatory tests should have high specificity in order to limit the number of false positives. A confirmatory test is most useful when there is already a

reasonably high clinical suspicion of the disease, i.e., pretest probability is greater than 15%. On the other hand, when there is already a strong clinical suspicion of the disease (pretest probability 60 to 75%), the next test may not add enough new information to be of real use. If the test result is positive, it may improve the physician's confidence in the diagnosis but will probably not alter the management of the case. On the other hand, a negative result could be confusing enough to delay necessary treatment, even though the predictive value of the negative result is relatively low.

MULTIPLE TESTS

In practice, combinations of tests are often used to reach a diagnostic decision. Apart from the irrational "shotgun" approach, several strategies may be employed to achieve the desired results most effectively.

Simultaneous Testing

It is common to order several tests at once and then to interpret the results as a group. This approach is often used for the initial workup, but the interpretation of various combinations of test results deserves more attention than is usually given. For example, consider the following pairs of hypothetical tests:

	TEST PAIR			
	1	2	3	4
FIRST TEST	+	+	−	−
SECOND TEST	+	−	+	−

In pair 1, both tests are positive, and we conclude that the disease is present. Similarly, in pair 4, both test results are negative, and the disease can be ruled out. The decision is not as clear-cut in pairs 2 and 3, however, since the test results are divergent. We have the following choices:

(1) If either test is positive, the results will be considered positive.

(2) If either test is negative, the results will be considered negative.

(3) If the test results disagree, then they are uninterpretable and will be disregarded.

Once we are committed to one of these choices, we can then treat the test combination as a unit and calculate the sensitivity, specificity, and predictive value of the combination just as if it were a single test.

EXAMPLE: Two hypothetical tests, A and B, give the following results:

TEST RESULTS (A/B)

DISEASE	+/+	+/−	−/+	−/−	TO-TALS
Present	765	135	85	15	1,000
Absent	90	1,710	360	6,840	9,000
All patients	855	1,845	445	6,855	10,000

Then, for Test A alone:

Sensitivity = (765 + 135)/1000 = 90%

Specificity = (360 + 6840)/9000 = 80%

Prevalence = 1000/10000 = 10%

PV + = (765 + 135)/(855 + 1845) = 33.3%

PV − = (360 + 6840)/(445 + 6855) = 98.6%

For Test B alone:

Sensitivity = (765 + 85)/1000 = 85%

Specificity = (1710 + 6840)/9000 = 95%

PV + = (765 + 85)/(855 + 445) = 65.4%

PV − = (1710 + 6840)/(1845 + 6855) = 98.3%

If *both* Tests A and B must be positive for the results to be considered positive:

Sensitivity = 765/1000 = 76.5%

Specificity = (1710 + 360 + 6840)/9000 = 99%

PV + = 765/855 = 89.5%

PV − = (1710 + 360 + 6840)/(1845 + 445 + 6855) = 97.4%

If the test is considered positive when *either* Test A or Test B is positive:

Sensitivity = (765 + 135 + 85)/1000 = 98.5%

Specificity = 6840/9000 = 76%

PV + = (765 + 135 + 85)/(855 + 1845 + 445) = 31.3%

PV − = 6840/6855 = 99.8%

The effect of requiring both tests to be positive for a positive result is to make a positive result less likely. Sensitivity is reduced and specificity is improved compared to either test alone. On the other hand, simply requiring either of the two tests to be positive creates the opposite effect, i.e., sensitivity is increased at the expense of specificity. An alternative approach is to separate the results into positive (both tests positive), negative (both tests negative), and unclassified (divergent results). In this example, 23% of the patients would remain unclassified, but for the other 77%, the predictive value of either a positive or a negative result would be very high (0.895 and 0.998, respectively).

A real-life example of this concept is provided in the interpretation of two new spot tests recently added to urine dipsticks, the leukocyte esterase test and the nitrite test. These tests are designed to detect leukocytes and nitrate-reducing bacteria in the urine, respectively. In one study, the two spot tests were compared with microscopic examination of the urine sediment, using the urine culture as the reference standard (E.L. Gottfried and C. Hogan, unpublished observations). The following results were obtained with a selected group of 97 specimens (of which 30 yielded positive cultures):

Test	Sensitivity	Specificity	PV +	PV −
Microscopy	80%	63%	49%	88%
LE only	70%	81%	62%	86%
LE or Nitrite	80%	72%	56%	89%

The leukocyte esterase test alone was not as sensitive as microscopy, although the specificity and the positive predictive value were better. Adding the nitrite test (i.e., a positive finding with either test was interpreted as a positive result) resulted in improved sensitivity, equal to that of microscopy, with better specificity and predictive values (both positive and negative) than those of microscopy. For this reason, the combination of two tests was selected as the screening method of choice and reported as the "LN test" with a positive or negative result.

Although the test groups in these examples include only two tests, any number of tests can be combined and treated in the same fashion.

EXAMPLE: England and Fraser proposed a discriminant function (DF′) for the differential diagnosis of beta-thalassemia trait and iron deficiency anemia. The function is derived from the mean corpuscular volume (MCV), red blood cell count (RBC), and hemoglobin concentration (Hb), as follows:[55]

$$DF' = MCV - RBC - (5 \times Hb) - 3.4$$

In appropriately selected patients, a positive value for the DF′ suggests iron deficiency; a negative value, thalassemia trait. For example:

The following results were obtained for a 28-year-old woman with a history of heavy menstrual bleeding: Hb = 10.0 g/dl; RBC = 4.0×10^{12}/L; MCV = 75 fl.*

$$DF' = 75 - 4.0 - (5 \times 10.0) - 3.4 = 17.6$$

The value is greater than zero, and the presumptive diagnosis is iron deficiency.

A 35-year-old healthy man of Greek ancestry had a routine blood count with these results: Hb = 13.5 g/dl; RBC = 6.0×10^{12}/L; MCV = 68 fl.

$$DF' = 68 - 6.0 - (5 \times 13.5) - 3.4 = -8.9$$

The value is less than zero, and the presumptive diagnosis is thalassemia trait.

Sequential Testing

For the most useful results at the lowest total cost, laboratory tests should be conducted in an orderly sequence. A follow-up test is most likely to yield useful information when the likelihood of the disease is around 50%, as explained earlier (Fig. 2–10).

One common pattern of sequential testing is shown in Figure 2–12. Tests are performed one at a time (or, more likely, one combination at a time). At each stage, the disease is either confirmed or ruled out in the majority of those tested, and there are fewer patients remaining without a diagnosis. Only patients who remain unclassified need additional tests.

EXAMPLE: Beck et al. have offered a method for the diagnostic workup of iron deficiency anemia in four stages: (1) serum ferritin plus MCV (determined from the routine blood count), (2) serum iron and iron-binding capacity, (3) erythrocyte sedimentation rate, and (4) bone marrow examination.[56] Among the 416 patients studied, the diagnosis was established in 95% without the need for the last stage. The test sequence

---

*fl = femtoliter (former term: cubic micron)

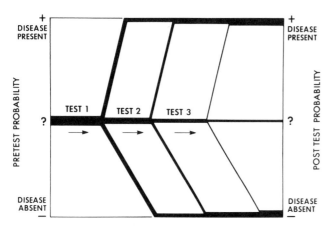

Fig. 2–12. One approach to sequential testing. After each test (or group of tests), a diagnostic decision can be made for the majority of the patients tested, viz., disease is present or absent. Only patients still unclassified require the next level of testing. (Reproduced with permission from Gottfried, E.L. and Wagar, E.A.: Laboratory testing: A practical guide, in Cotsonas, N.J., Jr., et al. (eds.): Disease-a-Month. Copyright 1983 by Year Book Medical Publishers, Inc., Chicago.)

was designed to detect a reduced serum iron level first and then to rule out other conditions such as chronic disease. (Some physicians will prefer other test combinations or a different sequence of testing, but this approach can provide efficient and economical results.)

Another pattern of sequential testing is diagrammed in Figure 2–13. In this method, a sensitive screening test is performed initially. The disease is excluded in most of the patients by the negative test result. Only

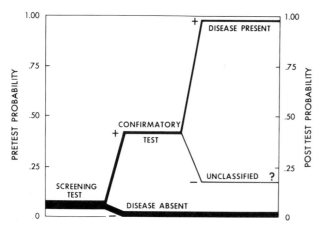

Fig. 2–13. Another approach to sequential testing. A sensitive screening test is used to rule out the disease in most of the patients tested. Those with a positive screening test require a follow-up confirmatory test in order to establish the diagnosis. (Reproduced with permission from Gottfried, E.L. and Wagar, E.A.: Laboratory testing: A practical guide, in Cotsonas, N.J., Jr., et al. (eds.): Disease-a-Month. Copyright 1983 by Year Book Medical Publishers, Inc., Chicago.)

Table 2–6.   Criteria for Evaluating a Laboratory Test

Technical factors
   Accuracy
   Precision
   Lack of interference by drugs or disease
Clinical factors
   Sensitivity
   Specificity
   Predictive value
   Unique information provided
Cost factors
   Simplicity of the method
   Costs of required equipment and reagents
   Cost/benefit ratio

a small proportion of those originally tested will have a positive result. This smaller group will need another, more specific, confirmatory test in order to establish the diagnosis. Patients who have a positive screening test result but a negative confirmatory test are considered either normal or unclassified depending on the particular disease and the clinical circumstances.

The best known application of this test strategy is screening for syphilis. Initial screening is done with a simple, sensitive, but somewhat nonspecific anticardiolipin procedure such as the RPR card test. Positive results must be confirmed by one of the specific antitreponemal tests, such as the immunofluorescence (FTA-ABS) or microhemagglutination (MHA-TP) procedures. Another example is shown below.

EXAMPLE: Urine dipstick tests for leukocyte esterase and nitrite, described in an earlier example, can be used to screen specimens for bacteriuria before the specimens are submitted for urine culture.[57,58] Bartlett et al. evaluated this approach in a study of 2,782 urine specimens that had been submitted for routine urine culture.[58] The culture was positive ($\geq 10^5$ bacteria per ml) in 13.4% of the specimens. The predictive value of a positive LN test was 29%, and that of a negative test was 97%. As a screening method to rule out bacteriuria, the LN test would be quick and reliable when the results are negative. Only positive specimens would require urine culture, and the number of cultures could be decreased by 55 to 65%.

MISCELLANEOUS OBSERVATIONS

GENERAL CRITERIA FOR A GOOD TEST

Some of the characteristics of a good laboratory test are listed in Table 2–6. From the laboratory's viewpoint, the test must be capable of providing accurate and reproducible results, with a minimum of interference by such conditions as jaundice or high serum drug levels.

From the physician's point of view, the test should provide new information about the patient. It should be noted that an additional test that indicates the same disorder or the same metabolic imbalance as a prior test, but in different terms or different units, does not necessarily add new information. When a number of different tests are available to identify the same disorder, one should choose the one best suited to the clinical circumstances instead of striving for "completeness" by ordering all of them.

EXAMPLE: In acute hepatic parenchymal disease, a number of serum enzyme levels may be increased, including alanine aminotransferase (ALT or SGPT), aspartate aminotransferase (AST or SGOT), as well as gamma-glutamyl transpeptidase (GGT), lactic dehydrogenase (LDH), and others. The relative sensitivities and specificities of these enzymes for liver disease vary, and several different tests may be needed initially in order to establish the diagnosis. Follow-up monitoring, on the other hand, can generally be accomplished with just one enzyme type (e.g., AST or ALT), despite the current widespread custom of repeating entire test panels ("LFTs") at frequent intervals.

The test should be appropriate for its intended use. For screening, the sensitivity must be very high, whereas for confirmation of disease, high specificity is most important. With any test, predictive value is usually a more important measure of clinical usefulness than either sensitivity or specificity alone. As we pointed out earlier, however, the predictive value of a given test depends largely on the way the test is used. Even more important is to consider how the results will affect patient care.

EXAMPLE: Earlier in this chapter, serum uric acid was cited as an example of a screening test. The test is often included in routine biochemical test panels, presumably for the purpose of detecting asymptomatic gout. We showed that a normal value for serum uric acid effectively rules out gout but is not much more effective than a simple negative guess, since the prevalence of the disorder is low. Calculation of predictive values demonstrated that most positive results will be false positives. But the most important reason of all for not doing the test is that asymptomatic hyperuricemia requires no therapy.[46]

Economic factors cannot be disregarded in the evaluation of a laboratory test or procedure, particularly when a new procedure is being considered for general use, or when there is a choice between two or more methods. One obvious factor is the cost of performing the procedure. The cost is based in part on the price of the equipment, reagents, and supplies. For laboratory tests, personnel time is usually the most costly single factor. In the long run, the real costs of any procedure must be measured in relation to the benefits derived from it.

EXAMPLE: The introduction of computed tomography (CT) into the practice of medicine has been accompanied by continuing—and often heated—controversy over the high costs and alleged benefits.[1,59] After its introduction, CT scanning immediately impressed physicians with its promise of demonstrating anatomic lesions in an entirely new way, and with images of high quality. The procedure was quickly adopted as a diagnostic method in neurology, and then in other areas of medical practice, before any formal cost/benefit studies had been done.[1] Similar problems have accompanied the introduction into clinical medicine of magnetic resonance and other promising but expensive techniques.

Although a complete cost analysis of these procedures is beyond the scope of this discussion, we can readily determine the effectiveness of computed tomography in a specific application, e.g., the diagnosis of intracranial tumors, by using the predictive value model. The following data are taken from the report of a multicenter study of 2204 patients with clinical suspicion of intracranial tumor, on whom computed tomography was performed with or without contrast enhancement.[60]

| | CT SCAN | | |
	Positive	Negative	Totals
Tumor	1017	54	1071
No tumor	13	1120	1133
All patients	1030	1174	2204

Sensitivity = 1017/1071 = 95%
Specificity = 1120/1133 = 98.9%
PV + = 1017/1030 = 98.7%
PV − = 1120/1174 = 95.4%

These results demonstrate that, in appropriately selected patients, this technique is extraordinarily effective in establishing the diagnosis of intracranial tumor. Moreover, all 13 of the false positive scans proved to be non-neoplastic intracranial abnormalities, so the positive predictive value of CT scanning for an intracranial lesion (not necessarily neoplastic) was an impressive 100%.

STAT TESTS

Most clinical laboratories perform a range of procedures according to a predefined schedule, batching samples in order to save personnel time and reduce the cost of materials (especially standards and control samples). Routine test requests are assigned to the next available run, and reports are distributed periodically. In contrast, stat test orders are accorded priority, in order to make the results available as soon as possible. Each request is usually handled individually at every step, including processing the order, preparing and analyzing the sample, and reporting the results to the physician. As a result, the cost of the analysis (including standards and control specimens run at the same time) can be several times higher than that of an equivalent routine specimen.

EXAMPLE: Serum theophylline levels can be determined in a centrifugal analyzer that has a batch capacity of 20 patient specimens in addition to controls and standards. Each run requires the same number of standards (five) and controls (two), and the same amount of personnel time, regardless of the number of patient samples in the batch. The estimated direct cost to the laboratory for each test performed by this method (for reagents and personnel time only, based on 1984 prices) ranges from $3.50 for a full batch of 20 tests to $32.00 for a single stat test—a 900% difference.

Besides the added cost of materials and labor, there is a hidden cost in stat tests: the limited resources of the laboratory are diverted to perform the stat test, and another patient's results may be further delayed, or another useful laboratory service must be omitted. A stat test request is appropriate only when the result will affect a treatment decision and the patient may be harmed by the wait for routine results. Unfortunately, stat tests are often ordered for reasons other than the one described. In one hospital, for example, over 60% of all orders for automated blood counts and differential counts were stat requests. Many of these orders seemed to be motivated by the doctor's anxiety or impatience rather than on plans for an immediate patient-care decision based on the test results.

TESTS UNDER DEVELOPMENT

There is a tendency, especially in teaching hospitals, to greet each proposed new test or procedure with enthusiasm, even while the technique is still being developed. The new procedure is likely to be tried out in the most complex and puzzling clinical cases. However, until the procedure has been thoroughly evaluated, results obtained for an individual patient will not be reliable enough to use for diagnostic or therapeutic decisions. Indeed, the results will not even be useful for researchers responsible for developing the procedure, unless the patient's diagnosis has already been established from independent criteria. This limitation is expressed in Gottfried's First Law:[61]

You cannot evaluate a test and a patient at the same time.

UNCLASSIFIABLE DISEASE STATES

The goal of the diagnostic workup is to make a firm medical diagnosis for each patient. Although this goal is accomplished much of the time, every physician eventually encounters a patient with atypical signs and symptoms and equivocal laboratory results. Often, this leads to mounting frustration and a rapidly expanding diagnostic order sheet. The results are predictable, according to Gottfried's Second Law[61]:

A test will fail when you need it most.

This rule is not merely a restatement of Murphy's

Law (which is still operable, because anything can and will go wrong in clinical laboratories as elsewhere), but an acknowledgment that unclassifiable clinical states do exist. The disorder may take the form of an ill-defined preclinical condition falling somewhere between normalcy and the full-blown textbook picture of disease, persistently eluding diagnosis. It may be a transient state that will either progress until the diagnosis becomes clear or disappear as the patient recovers. Sometimes, this state is prolonged. When the standard clinical procedures and common laboratory tests have been exhausted, the physician is tempted to try more exotic procedures. Typically, those tests will be more expensive, harder to perform, and less reliable than the more common variety, and the results will be even more difficult to interpret. At some point in the workup, the physician will be forced to choose between the risks of a deferred diagnosis and the costs of still more tests of diminishing value.

FUTURE DEVELOPMENTS

In the next few years, new procedures, instruments, and analytical methods will lead to continuing improvement in diagnostic sensitivity and specificity. The availability of increasingly versatile computers will undoubtedly change the way we examine and interpret test results. Graphic presentation of laboratory reports will make it much easier to evaluate abnormalities and trends. Computer-assisted analysis will enhance our ability to interpret complex interactions among the components of test panels.

Nevertheless, the principles described here will remain valid, and the physician will still need a systematic approach to diagnosis and a clear understanding of the strengths and weaknesses of individual tests and procedures.

For many of the common clinical tests, we still do not have enough reliable data to permit an accurate assessment of sensitivity, specificity, and predictive value, but such information is becoming increasingly available. More work is also needed to develop reference ranges specific for sex, age, ethnic group, and perhaps other characteristics of individual patients.

GUIDELINES FOR LABORATORY TESTING

DIAGNOSTIC TESTS

1. When *screening* for a given disease, test only those patients most likely to have that disease,

and select a test with the highest available sensitivity and negative predictive value.

2. To *confirm* a suspected disease, use a test with the highest available specificity and positive predictive value.

3. Avoid routine screening tests and baseline studies in the absence of a specific indication.

4. Order stat tests only when a patient-care decision depends on the results *and* when the added turn-around time of a routine test report may endanger the patient.

FOLLOW-UP TESTS

1. Order follow-up tests only when the results will influence the treatment.

2. Before repeating the tests, wait long enough to permit a change in the results.

REFERENCES

1. Altman, S.H., and Blendon, R.J. (eds.): Medical Technology: The Culprit Behind Health Care Costs? Washington, D.C., Government Printing Office, DHEW Publication No. PHS 79-3216, 1979.

2. Tydeman, J., Morrison, J.I., Cassidy, P.A., and Hardwick, D.F.: Analyzing the factors contributing to rising laboratory costs. Arch Pathol Lab Med 107:7, 1983.

3. Gibson, R.M., Waldo, D.R., and Levit, K.R.: National health expenditures, 1982. Health Care Financing Rev 5(1):1, 1983.

4. Gibson, R.M., Levit, K.R., Lazenby, H., and Waldo, D.R.: National health expenditures, 1983. Health Care Financing Rev 6(2):1, 1984.

5. Krieg, A.F., and Israel, M.: Why physicians order too many tests. Med Lab Observer 9:46, 1977.

6. Wertman, B.G., Sostrin, S.V., Pavlova, Z, and Lundberg, G.D.: Why do physicians order laboratory tests? A study of laboratory test request and use patterns. JAMA 243:2080, 1980.

7. Hampton, J.R., et al.: Relative contributions of history-taking, physical examination, and laboratory investigation to diagnosis and management of medical outpatients. Br Med J 2:486, 1975.

8. Sandler, G.: Costs of unnecessary tests. Br Med J 2:21, 1979.

9. Griner, P.F., and Glaser, R.J.: Misuse of laboratory tests and diagnostic procedures. N Engl J Med 307:1336, 1982.

10. Griner, P.F., Mayewski, R.J., Mushlin, A.I., and Greenland, P.: Selection and interpretation of diagnostic tests and procedures. Principles and applications. Ann Intern Med 94:553, 1981.

11. Griner, P.F., and Liptzin, B.: Use of the laboratory in a teaching hospital. Implications for patient care, education, and hospital costs. Ann Intern Med 75:157, 1971.

12. Sox, H.C., Jr., Margulies, I., and Sox, C.H.: Psychologically mediated effects of diagnostic tests. Ann Intern Med 95:680, 1981.

13. Danzon, P.M., Manning, W.G., Jr., and Marquis, M.S.: Factors affecting laboratory test use and prices. Health Care Financing Rev 5(4):23, 1984.

14. Altschuler, C.H.: Use of a laboratory database to monitor medical care. *In* Clinical Decisions and Laboratory Use. Edited by D.P. Connelly, E.S. Benson, M.D. Burke, and D. Fenderson. Minneapolis, University of Minnesota Press, 1982.

15. Eyster, E., and Bernini, J.: Nosocomial anemia. JAMA 223:73, 1973.

16. Gottfried, E.L., and Nigro, F.A.: SMAC panel and blood count reference values based on executive health survey. Clin Chem 28:1556, 1982.

17. Merx, W., et al.: Evaluation of the effectiveness of intracoronary streptokinase infusion in acute myocardial infarction. Postprocedure management and hospital course in 204 patients. Am Heart J 102:1181, 1981.

18. Hartz, A.J.: Overlap index. An alternative to sensitivity and specificity in comparing the utility of a laboratory test. Arch Pathol Lab Med 108:65, 1984.

19. Hische, E.A.H., Van der Helm, H.J., Van Meegen, M. Th., and Blanken, H.I.G.: Protein estimation in cerebrospinal fluid with Coomassie Brilliant Blue. Clin Chem 28:1237, 1982.

20. Bozimowski, D., Artiss, J.D., and Zak, B.: Spectrophotometric comparison of several reactions used for cerebrospinal fluid protein determinations. Microchem J 28:285, 1983.

21. Miale, J.B.: Laboratory Medicine: Hematology. 6th Ed. St. Louis, C.V. Mosby Co., 1982.

22. Brecher, G., Anderson, R.E., and McMullen, P.D.: When to do diffs: How often should differential counts be repeated? Blood Cells 6:431, 1980.

23. Dutcher, T.F.: Automated leukocyte differentials: A review and prospectus. Lab Med 14:483, 1983.

24. Connelly, D.P., McClain, M.P., Crowson, T.W., and Benson, E.S.: The use of the differential leukocyte count for inpatient casefinding. Hum Pathol 13:294, 1982.

25. Rich, E.C., Crowson, T.W., and Connelly, D.P.: Effectiveness of differential leukocyte count in case finding in the ambulatory care setting. JAMA 249:633, 1983.

26. Markowitz, H., and Kokmen, E.: Neurologic diseases and the cerebrospinal fluid immunoglobulin profile. Mayo Clinic Proc 58:273, 1983.

27. Bloomer, L.C., and Bray, P.F.: Relative value of three laboratory methods in the diagnosis of multiple sclerosis. Clin Chem 27:2011, 1981.

28. Link, H., and Kostulas, V.: Utility of isoelectric focusing of cerebrospinal fluid and serum on agarose evaluated for neurological patients. Clin Chem 29:810, 1983.

29. Bartholomew, B.A.: Antinuclear antibody tests as a clinically selected screening procedure. Am J Clin Pathol 61:495, 1974.

30. Richardson, B., and Epstein, W.V.: Utility of the fluorescent antinuclear antibody test in a single patient. Ann Intern Med 95:333, 1981.

31. Lott, J.A., and Stang, J.M.: Serum enzymes and isoenzymes in the diagnosis and differential diagnosis of myocardial ischemia and necrosis. Clin Chem 26:1241, 1980.

32. Murphy, E.A.: A scientific viewpoint on normalcy. Perspect Biol Med 9:333, 1966.

33. Rozanski, A., et al.: Alternative referent standards for cardiac normality. Implications for diagnostic testing. Ann Intern Med 101:164, 1984.

34. Werner, M., and Marsh, W.L.: Normal values: Theoretical and practical aspects. CRC Critical Rev in Clin Lab Sci 6(2):81, 1975.

35. Wright, I.: Correct levels of serum cholesterol. JAMA 236:261, 1976.

36. Pooling Project Research Group: Relationship of blood pressure, serum cholesterol, smoking habit, relative weight, and ECG abnormalities to incidence of major coronary events: Final report of the pooling project. J Chronic Dis 31:201, 1978.

37. Ross, D.W., Ayscue, L., and Gulley, M.: Automated platelet counts: Accuracy, range, and precision. Am J Clin Pathol 74:151, 1980.

38. Wintrobe, M.M.: Blood of normal men and women: Erythrocyte counts, hemoglobin, and volume of packed red cells of 229 individuals. Bull Johns Hopkins Hosp 53:118, 1933.

39. Godwin, I.D., and Jencks, J.A.: Normal hematologic values obtained with a Coulter counter, Model S. South Med J 71:47, 1978.

40. Brown, G.W.: What makes a reference range? Diagnostic Med 7:61, 1984.

41. Seegmiller, J.E., Laster, L., and R.R. Howell: Medical progress: Biochemistry of uric acid and its relation to gout. N Engl J Med 268:712, 1963.
42. Vecchio, T.J.: Predictive value of a single diagnostic test in unselected populations. N Engl J Med 274:1171, 1966.
43. Galen, R.S., and Gambino, S.R.: Beyond Normality: The Predictive Value and Efficiency of Medical Diagnoses. New York, John Wiley & Sons, 1975.
44. Bayes, T.: An essay toward solving a problem in the doctrine of chance. Phylos Trans Royal Soc London 53:370, 1763. (Cited by Galen and Gambino.[43])
45. Hambie, E.A., et al.: Comparison of a new rapid plasma reagin card test with the standard rapid plasma reagin 18-mm circle card test and the Venereal Disease Research Laboratory slide test for serodiagnosis of syphilis. J Clin Microbiol 17:249, 1983.
46. Wyngaarden, J.B., and Smith, L.H., Jr. (eds.): Cecil Textbook of Medicine. 16th Ed. Philadelphia, W.B. Saunders Co., 1982.
47. Morbidity and Mortality Weekly Report 33:726, 1985.
48. Freitas, J.E., et al.: Influence of scan and pathologic criteria on the specificity of cholescintigraphy. Concise communication. J Nuclear Med 24:876, 1983.
49. Clayman, R.V. et al.: Pursuit of the renal mass: Is ultrasound enough? Am J Med 77:281, 1984.
50. Gitlow, S.E., Mendlowitz, M., and Bertani, C.M.: The biochemical techniques for detecting and establishing the presence of a pheochromocytoma. Am J Cardiol 26:270, 1970.
51. Tucker, R.M., and Labarthe, D.R.: Frequence of surgical treatment for hypertension in adults at the Mayo Clinic from 1973 through 1975. Mayo Clinic Proc 52:549, 1977.
52. Van der Helm, H.J., and Hische, E.A.H.: Application of Bayes's theorem to results of quantitative clinical chemical determinations. Clin Chem 25:985, 1979.
53. Albert, A.: On the use and computation of likelihood ratios in clinical chemistry. Clin Chem 28:1113, 1982.
54. Durbridge, T.C.: Clinical responsiveness to laboratory results. Am J Clin Pathol 82:725, 1984.
55. England, J.M., and Fraser, P.M.: Differentiation of iron deficiency from thalassaemia trait by routine blood-count. Lancet 1:449, 1973.
56. Beck, J.R., et al.: The ''iron screen'': Modification of standard laboratory practice with data analysis. Human Pathol 12:118, 1981.
57. Loo, S.Y.T., et al.: Urine screening strategy employing dipstick analysis and selective culture: An evaluation. Am J Clin Pathol 81:634, 1984.
58. Bartlett, R.C., O'Neill, D., and McLaughlin, J.C.: Detection of bacteriuria by leukocyte esterase, nitrite, and the automicrobic system. Am J Clin Pathol 82:683, 1984.
59. Evens, R.G.: Computed tomography—a controversy revisited. N Engl J Med 310:1183, 1984.
60. Baker, H.L., Houser, W., and Campbell, J.K.: National Cancer Institute study: Evaluation of computed tomography in the diagnosis of intracranial neoplasms. Radiology 136:91, 1980.
61. Gottfried, E.L., and Wagar, E.A.: Laboratory testing: A practical guide. Disease-a-Month 29(11):1, 1983.
62. Snedecor, G.W., and Cochran, W.G.: Statistical Methods. 6th Ed. Ames, Iowa, Iowa State University Press, 1967.

CHAPTER 3

ALLERGY AND IMMUNOLOGIC PROBLEMS

Gillian M. Shepherd, M.D.

ANAPHYLAXIS

DEFINITION

Anaphylaxis is a reaction characterized by the acute onset of some or all of the following symptoms: flushing, lightheadedness, hypotension, shock, cardiac arrhythmias, urticaria, angioedema, throat tightness, dyspnea, nausea, vomiting, abdominal cramps, and diarrhea.[1,2] It occurs as a result of an immunologically mediated reaction to a specific antigen. Generally it happens within 2 hours of exposure to the antigen in a sensitive patient. Usually, the more severe the reaction, the sooner it occurs. Immunologically mediated reactions occurring after 2 hours are rarely life threatening.

PATHOPHYSIOLOGIC CONSIDERATIONS

The immune mechanism responsible for this reaction is shown in Figure 3–1. The antibody involved is IgE, which is attached by specific receptors to the surface of tissue mast cells and circulating basophils. Antigen must bind to and bridge at least two IgE molecules. This binding triggers the release from the cell of a wide variety of pharmacologically active mediators, for example, histamine and leukotrienes. Histamine causes vasodilatation and bronchoconstriction. Leukotrienes are sulfido-peptide products of the lipoxygenase enzyme pathway in the cell. One of them, leukotriene B (LTB), is a very potent chemotactic factor. LTC, LTD, and LTE (formerly referred to collectively as slow reacting substance of anaphylaxis) are potent bronchoconstrictive agents.

The other mediators released from the mast cells or basophils also generally cause vasodilation and bronchoconstriction. An exception is eosinophilic chemotactic factor of anaphylaxis (ECF-A). This factor recruits eosinophils to the area of the allergic reaction. Once there, eosinophils also release a variety of factors. Some of these, however, function to inactivate mediators from mast cells and basophils; for example, histaminase inactivates histamine and phospholipase D inactivates acetyl glyceryl ether phosphorylcholine (AGEPC, or platelet activating factor). Thus, eosinophils, which are always associated with allergic reactions, appear to act in part to dampen these reactions. Another substance released from eosinophils, however, is major basic protein, which has been shown in vitro to cause damage to human tissue at concentrations encountered in vivo in some disease states, for example, in the sputum of patients with asthma.[3] Hence, it may contribute to the pathogenesis of these disorders.

If the vasodilation resulting from this reaction is local, the patient may experience only urticaria or angioedema. The latter tends to involve the eyelids, lips, tongue, larynx, penis, palms, and soles. If the vasodilatation is widespread, various manifestations of hypotension will result, ranging from mild flushing and lightheadedness to severe shock. Cardiac arrhythmias can develop as a result of hypotension and also as a direct effect of the mediators. Gastrointestinal symptoms of nausea, vomiting, cramps, and diarrhea can be part of the reaction, especially if the allergen has been ingested. Rarely, they can occur as the sole manifestation of a reaction.

There are many substances that have been associated with anaphylactic reactions (Table 3–1). The most

Major Mediators Released	Primary Effects
1. Histamine	Vasodilation and bronchoconstriction
2. Leukotrienes	Bronchoconstriction
3. Prostaglandin D_2 (mast cell only)	Bronchoconstriction
4. AGEPC (acetyl glyceryl ether phosphorylcholine)	Recruits platelets
5. Neutrophil chemotactic factor	Recruits neutrophils
6. Bradykinin factor of anaphylaxis	Activates kinin system
7. Heparin	Anticoagulation
8. Eosinophilic chemotactic factor of anaphylaxis	Recruits eosinophils

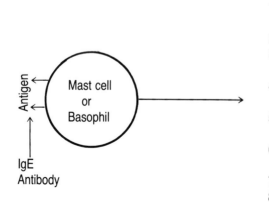

Fig. 3–1. Pathogenesis of anaphylaxis.

Table 3–1. Cause of Anaphylactic Reactions (probably mediated by IgE antibody)*

Idiopathic
Drugs
  Antibiotics
    <u>Penicillin</u> and derivatives
    <u>Cephalosporins</u>
    Sulfas
  Anesthetic agents
    Local anesthetics
  Hormones
    ACTH
    Insulin
  Chemotherapeutic agents
    Cis-platinum
  Other
    Antilymphocyte serum
    Psyllium
Vaccines
  Tetanus toxoid
  Human diploid cell rabies vaccine
  Vaccines grown on eggs
Enzymes
  <u>Chymopapain</u>
  Asparaginase
<u>Hymenoptera stings</u>
  Wasp
  Honeybee
  Vespids
    Yellow Jacket
    Yellow Hornet
    White Faced Hornet
  Fire Ants
Pollen extracts used in diagnosis and treatment
Foods
  <u>Peanut</u>
  Other legumes (e.g., chick-peas, soybeans, peas)
  Shrimp, lobster, crayfish
  Mussel, clams, scallops
  Sunflower seeds
  Camomile tea
  Eggs
  Milk
  Corn
  Citrus fruits
  Banana
  Others
Other
  Human seminal fluid
  Endogenous progesterone

*Common causes underlined. Others are generally rare causes.

Table 3–2. Cause of Anaphylactoid Reactions (non-IgE mediated reactions and/or mechanism currently unknown)*

<u>Idiopathic</u>
<u>Radio contrast media</u>
<u>Blood and blood products</u>
Drugs
  <u>Aspirin</u>
  Nonsteroidal anti-inflammatory agents
    Zomepirac sodium
    Naproxen
    Indomethacin
    Ibuprofen
    Fenoprofen
    Tolmetin
    Sulindac
  Narcotic analgesics
    Morphine
    Meperidine
    Codeine
  Muscle relaxants
    Suxamethonium
    Pancuronium
    Gallamine
  Antibiotics
    Vancomycin
    Streptomycin
    Bacitracin ointment
    Tetracycline
  Chemotherapeutic agents
    Aminopyrine
    Diethylcarbamizine
    Cyclophosphamide
    Nitrogen mustard
    Bleomycin
Exercise
Food-dependent, exercise-induced anaphylaxis
Food
  Strawberries
  Wine
Preservatives/additives
  Sulfites
  Paraben
Other
  DEET (diethyl-meta-toluamide) insecticide
  Rupture of echinococcal cyst
  Cuprophane—membrane dialyzers
  Colloid plasma substitutes
    Dextrans
    Modified fluid gelatins
    Hydroxyethyl starch
  Mannitol
  Ethylene oxide

*Common causes underlined. Others are generally rare causes.

common cause of death from anaphylaxis is penicillin, accounting for 75% (approximately 500) of such deaths per year. Insect stings are the second most common cause, accounting for about 15% of the deaths. The remainder of the large list is therefore responsible for a very small percentage of fatal reactions. In many cases the cause is not found, these reactions are termed ''idiopathic'' anaphylactic reactions.

Additionally, there is a group of substances that cause anaphylact*oid*, as opposed to anaphylact*ic*, reactions (Table 3–2). These substances, through a variety of means, induce a reaction that is physiologically identical to that seen with anaphylaxis. The difference is that no specific IgE antibody appears to be involved. Because these reactions are not specifically mediated by the immune system, there are a variety of differences between these reactions and ''true'' allergic re-

Table 3–3. Evaluation of Anaphylaxis

ECG
CBC
Biochemistry profile
Blood cultures
C4, C2
Indirect laryngoscopy
Lateral neck radiographs
Chest radiograph
Abdominal radiographs
Specific IgE levels by skin testing or RAST

actions. For example, they can occur on first exposure to the substance; generally one cannot desensitize against them or treat them with immunotherapy, although in some cases the reactions can be blocked with pretreatment of steroids and antihistamines. The most frequent cause of death from anaphylactoid reaction is from radio contrast media, accounting, like penicillin, for approximately 500 deaths per year. Aspirin is the second leading cause.

The more common causes of anaphylactic and anaphylactoid reactions are discussed in the section on specific causes of allergic reactions.

DIFFERENTIAL DIAGNOSIS AND DIAGNOSTIC EVALUATION

A patient with an anaphylactic reaction normally presents as an emergency. A brief physical exam should determine the diagnosis rapidly in most patients. Further evaluation should include an ECG to evaluate a primary cardiac problem or the presence of an arrhythmia (Table 3–3). Screening blood tests will usually be normal in anaphylaxis, except for an elevated partial thromboplastin time (PTT) caused by heparin release from mast cells, but they are helpful in ruling out an electrolyte or other abnormality that might cause a comparable clinical picture. If septic shock is considered, a complete blood count (CBC), differential, and blood cultures should be obtained. Total levels of eosinophils and IgE antibody are generally not helpful.

Indirect laryngoscopy and lateral neck radiographs aid in the diagnosis of foreign body aspiration or laryngeal edema. Abdominal radiographs help in the differential diagnosis of abdominal symptoms. Chest radiograph is usually normal in an anaphylactic reaction but is helpful in ruling out cardiac disease, infection, or the presence of a foreign body.

Serum and urine histamine levels may be elevated during the initial moments of the reaction. Histamine assays, however, are usually not routinely available. After the reaction, such testing is not helpful because histamine has a half-life of less than 1 minute. If he-

reditary angioedema (HAE) is suspected, C2 and C4 levels should be drawn initially as a screen. C4 is usually constantly decreased and C2 is decreased during an attack. If either C4 or C2 is found to be low, a C1 inhibitor level can be obtained. This is low in 85% of cases and functionally deficient in 15% of cases of HAE. If the C4 level is normal, HAE is highly unlikely.

Once the diagnosis of an anaphylactic reaction has been made and the patient treated, the physician must attempt to determine the specific cause. The history remains the most important diagnostic tool. One must keep in mind that exposure to the incriminating antigen most likely occurred within 2 hours preceding the reaction. A suspected antigen can sometimes be verified by finding IgE antibody specific for it through skin testing or radioallergosorbent testing (RAST). These tests are readily available for inhalant allergens, foods, insect venoms, penicillin, and insulin. For other substances they either are not available or are available only as a research tool. The amount of IgE may be low immediately following a reaction, as it may have been utilized in large part during that reaction. Therefore it may be best to evaluate the patient several weeks after the anaphylactic reaction.

Double blind, placebo controlled challenge testing, though the definitive diagnostic test, is dangerous and rarely necessary. If it is considered, it should be done by a specialist in a monitored setting.

The differential diagnosis of anaphylaxis is outlined in Table 3–4. There are three key points to this differential. First, an anaphylactic reaction usually develops in a healthy person, producing signs and symptoms within 2 hours. Second, there is often a history of an inciting event. Third, signs and symptoms usually appear in unique combinations that facilitate diagnosis. The difficulty comes mainly when a single sign or symptom occurs.

Hypotension resulting from an anaphylactic reaction is of rapid onset; therefore, the differential usually involves other causes of shock of rapid onset, such as myocardial infarction or blood loss. The fact that the patient was well immediately preceding the reaction is a helpful differentiating point, often enabling the physician to eliminate other kinds of shock, such as septic shock. Patients with anaphylaxis are normally afebrile. It is very rare for a patient to present solely with an arrhythmia.

Laryngeal edema is usually accompanied by facial edema and bronchospasm but may occur alone. The presence of stridor and inspiratory wheezing over the larynx are useful signs in diagnosis. The relatively sudden onset makes suspect foreign body aspiration, especially if no history is available, and makes infec-

Table 3–4. Differential Diagnosis of Anaphylaxis

Signs and Symptoms of Anaphylaxis	Differential Diagnosis
Acute onset of any of the following: Hypotension	Cardiogenic shock, e.g., myocardial infarction, massive bleeding, septic shock including toxic shock syndrome
Cardiac arrhythmias	Intrinsic cardiac pathology Shock Electrolyte imbalance Iatrogenic, medications, etc.
Laryngeal edema	Foreign body aspiration Laryngitis, tracheitis
Bronchospasm	Foreign body aspiration Asthma flare due to factors other than allergy
Urticaria and angioedema	Nonallergic causes of urticaria Hereditary angioedema
Nausea, vomiting, abdominal cramps, and diarrhea	Acute abdominal pathology, e.g., mechanical, obstructive, infective, toxic Hereditary angioedema Familial Mediterranean fever

tions a less likely cause. If no history is available, lack of fever may be a clue.

Bronchospasm can occur as a sole manifestation of an anaphylactic reaction. As with laryngeal edema, if the onset of shortness of breath is sudden, foreign body aspiration should be considered. Generally, foreign body aspiration results in inspiratory wheezing, loudest over the bronchi. If inspiratory and expiratory wheezing or only expiratory wheezing is heard and the expiratory phase is prolonged, all nonallergic causes of asthma, such as exercise, stress, or exposure to an irritant odor, must be considered.

Unlike the other signs and symptoms of anaphylaxis, urticaria (swelling in the dermis) and angioedema (swelling in the deeper tissues) frequently occur alone. Most commonly, urticaria occurs with angioedema, although each can occur separately. By definition, if either occurs within 2 hours of exposure to an antigen, the reaction is termed anaphylactic, albeit not life threatening. The characteristic appearance of urticaria and angioedema makes the diagnosis obvious in most cases. The history holds the clue to distinguishing urticaria caused by IgE mediated mechanisms from other kinds of urticaria, e.g., physical (see urticaria section for detailed discussion).

Hereditary angioedema can occasionally be confused with an anaphylactic reaction. This angioedema can also develop rapidly and can be associated with gastrointestinal symptoms. Important points in the history differentiating hereditary angioedema are lack of associated urticaria, lack of pruritus, frequent positive family history of angioedema, and frequent history of trauma preceding the angioedema.

Abdominal symptoms are rarely the sole manifes-

tation of an anaphylactic reaction. When they occur it is usually after the antigen has been ingested. The cramps can be quite severe, simulating labor cramps. Many causes of an acute abdomen must be considered in the differential diagnosis. The rapid onset of symptoms, again, is a helpful differentiating feature.

SPECIFIC CAUSES OF ALLERGIC REACTIONS

PENICILLIN ALLERGY

Penicillin and its β-lactam derivatives with the exception of the cephalosporins (Table 3–5) are responsible for more than 50% of all drug allergies. Approximately 2% of patients who receive a course of penicillin have an immunologically mediated reaction to it. The incidence of anaphylaxis per course given is approximately 1 in 2500 cases. It has been grossly estimated that there are about 500 deaths per year in the U.S. caused by anaphylaxis from penicillin.[4,5]

This drug causes more allergic reactions than other drugs for several reasons. First, it is given frequently. Second, its metabolic products are highly reactive. Alone, these metabolic products are too small to act as antigens. They are immunogenic because they form stable covalent bonds with endogenous macromolecules and thus act as haptens bound to larger carrier molecules.

Penicillin is metabolized in the body primarily to penicilloyl, the major determinant. The remaining products include penicillin, penicilloate, penilloate, and penicilloyl-n-propylamine. These minor determinants are noteworthy because patients at risk of anaphylactic reactions appear to have IgE antibody specific for these determinants.[6]

Table 3–5. Penicillin Derivatives

Natural derivatives
  Penicillin G
  Benzathine penicillin
  Procaine penicillin
  Phenoxyethyl penicillin
  Phenoxymethyl penicillin
Penicillinase-resistant derivatives
  Cloxacillin
  Dicloxacillin
  Methicillin
  Nafcillin
  Oxacillin
Penicillins active against gram-negative bacteria
  Amoxicillin
  Ampicillin
  Carbenicillin
  Ticarcillin
Newer drugs
  Azlocillin
  Bacampicillin
  Amdinocillin
  Mezlocillin
  Piperacillin

Penicillin can cause a wide variety of immunologically mediated reactions besides anaphylaxis. Some of the more important ones are shown in Table 3–6.

DIAGNOSTIC EVALUATION. The history and physical examination are the mainstays of the evaluation of a drug reaction. Laboratory tests are less helpful. Eosinophilia generally argues for an allergic cause of the reaction, but its absence does not preclude it.

Performing skin tests as part of the initial evaluation to determine if the reaction was due to penicillin may be helpful but because skin tests for IgE antibody specific for penicillin are not commercially available for all the determinants of penicillin, sensitivity to some of the minor determinants may be missed. If skin test-

ing is negative immediately after the reaction, the results are not diagnostic. If positive, it is suggestive but not definitive. Another limitation here is lack of knowledge of the skin test reactivity before the reaction occurred. Blood tests are available to determine IgM and IgG antibodies specific for penicillin, but they are available only for the major determinant, and almost 100% of patients exposed to penicillin in the past have IgM specific for penicillin and 20% have IgG antibody. An additional problem is that there are no reliable tests currently available to determine sensitivity to other drugs except insulin, chymopapain, and ACTH, so establishing if a rash is caused by penicillin or a sulfa drug, for example, can best be determined by noting the timing of the reaction and the propensity of the suspected drugs for causing such a reaction.

A major clinical problem is encountered when the patient needs a penicillin drug but has a history of a possible allergic reaction to penicillin. An approach to this problem is outlined in Table 3–7. The physician should first evaluate the history to determine if the reaction appeared to be immunologically mediated and caused by penicillin. The physician should ascertain the time since the last reaction; studies have shown that 60 to 70% of patients lose their sensitivity to penicillin over the course of 5 to 10 years after their reaction, though the remainder may maintain their sensitivity forever.[4]

The most definitive test to determine if a patient is still allergic to penicillin (Table 3–8) is skin testing. This involves placing 0.01 to 0.02 ml of the reagents intradermally. If there is enough IgE antibody specific for penicillin bound to skin mast cells, a wheal of greater than 5 mm with surrounding erythema will develop in 15 minutes. Studies show that if a wheal develops to testing concentrations, the patient may

Table 3–6. Immunologically Mediated Reactions Associated With Penicillin

Time after Penicillin Administration When Reaction is First Seen	Manifestation	Mechanism	Predominant Specificity of Antibody
Within 2 hours	Anaphylaxis	IgE mediated	Minor determinants
Anytime	Urticaria/angioedema	IgE mediated	Major determinant
After 2 to 3 days	Recurrent urticaria and arthralgias	?	?
After 2 to 3 days	Immune complex disease: rash, fever, arthralgias, myalgias, neuralgias, lymphadenopathy, vasculitis	IgG and IgM Immune complexes	Major determinant
After 1 day	Maculopapular rashes	immune complexes? Delayed hypersensitivity?	Major determinant
After 2 to 3 days	Hemolytic anemia	IgG and IgM bound to penicillin on surface of RBC	Major determinant
After 2 to 3 days	Interstitial nephritis	Immune complexes? Delayed hypersensitivity?	Major determinant
After 2 to 3 days	Fever	Release of pyrogens from sensitized cells?	?

Table 3–7. Approach to the Patient with a History of an Allergic Reaction to Penicillin

1. Evaluate the history to determine
   a. If the reaction was probably due to penicillin
   b. If the reaction was probably immunologically mediated; for example, a maculopapular rash developing in a patient with infectious mononucleosis who is receiving ampicillin is not a true allergy
   c. The severity of the reaction
2. Evaluate the time since the last reaction. Approximately 70% of patients will lose their sensitivity over 5 to 10 years, but some patients maintain it forever.
3. Skin testing:*†
   a. Reagents:
      (1) Benzylpenicilloyl-polylysine = major determinant (Pre-Pen)
      (2) Penicillin G = most important minor determinant (diluted to 5000 units/ml freshly made)
      (3) Histamine as a positive control
   b. Technique: Inject 0.01 to 0.02 ml intradermally (the smallest amount to raise a discernible bleb on the skin) using a 27-gauge needle.
   c. Evaluation: The development of a wheal greater than 5 mm in diameter with an associated flare in 15 to 20 minutes is considered positive.
   d. The test is uninterpretable if:
      (1) The histamine control is negative
      (2) The original injection bleb is greater than 5 mm
      (3) There is no associated flare
      (4) The patient has taken hydroxyzine, prochlorperazine, or diphenhydramine in the preceding 72 hours or other antihistamines in the preceding 24 hours.

*These reagents miss approximately 5% of patients sensitive to the other minor determinants.
†Skin testing shouldn't be done unless penicillin is going to be given within 48 hours, since theoretically the small amount of penicillin G given (50 to 100 units) may be enough to sensitize the patient to develop increased amounts of IgE antibody, a process which takes several days. Commercially available penicilloyl (Pre-Pen) won't do this because it's linked to polylysine, hence preventing sensitization. Also, because sensitivity changes with time, a patient found to be skin test-negative at the time of testing might develop an undetected allergy after an unknown contact with penicillin, for example, in food, and have a reaction if penicillin is administered therapeutically some time after skin testing.

Table 3–8. Treatment Based on Results of Penicillin Skin Testing

History of Past Allergic Reaction to Penicillin	Skin Test Result	Treatment
No	Negative	Full therapeutic dose of drug
Yes	Negative	Test dose* before proceeding with full therapeutic dose
No	Positive	Use alternative antibiotic or desensitize patient
Yes	Positive	Use alternative antibiotic or desensitize patient

*Give a small dose (e.g., 1000 to 5000 units or 3 to 5 mg of penicillin or derivative) by desired route and observe for 1 hour. If no reaction, proceed with therapeutic dose.

have sufficient total body IgE to cause a systemic reaction if given penicillin.

Skin testing is able to predict those patients at risk of developing only an immediate (IgE mediated) reaction if given penicillin. There is currently no way to predict who is at risk of developing a later (greater than 24 to 48 hours) reaction, as IgE production may be stimulated when the drug is given and several days may be required to develop a sufficient quantity to cause a reaction, and there appears to be no correlation between the presence of IgG and IgM antibody specific for penicillin and susceptibility to a later reaction to penicillin.

Despite these limitations, skin testing is useful in helping identify patients at risk of developing an anaphylactic reaction if given penicillin.[7] Currently only penicilloyl, the major determinant, is commercially available for skin testing (benzylpenicilloyll-polylysine. Penicillin G (diluted to 5000 units per ml and made fresh daily) is the most important minor determinant, and used in combination with penicilloyl for skin testing will detect approximately 95% of patients allergic to penicillin.[8] Therefore, approximately 5% of patients sensitive to the other minor determinants will be missed with this combination. A mix of all the significant minor determinants has been found to be very effective in clinical trials and hopefully will be commercially available in a few years. An approach to present treatment based on skin test reactivity is outlined in Table 3–8. As these reagents may miss some sensitive patients, history-positive, skin test-negative patients should receive a test dose before proceeding with full therapeutic dose.

The majority of deaths caused by anaphylaxis from penicillin occur in patients who had no prior history of allergy to the drug. Additionally, a recent multicenter prospective clinical trial using most of the minor determinants found that 4% of patients who had no past history of a reaction to penicillin were skin test positive. Other data suggests that 60 to 70% of this group would be at risk of an immediate reaction if given penicillin. This raises the question of whether all patients should be skin tested before receiving penicillin. The answer awaits further investigation.

Differential Diagnosis. The diagnosis of an allergic reaction to penicillin is usually clear if the onset correlates with the administration of the drug. Difficulty arises when many drugs are given concurrently or when the underlying illness can cause the same reaction. When many drugs are given one has to look at the timing of the reaction's onset very carefully. A maculopapular rash, for example, is more likely to have been caused by the drug started 1 week ago rather than that begun 3 weeks ago. If drugs are started simultaneously one has to consider each one's propensity for causing that reaction. Penicillin and sulfa drugs are much more likely to cause rashes than, for example, the macrolide antibiotics. If the patient was recently exposed to a drug that is being administered again, all immunologic reactions can be accelerated. For example, although maculopapular rashes usually occur after 1 week of treatment, in a patient who received penicillin 1 month ago (without incident) and is receiving it again, the rash may appear on day 2 of treatment.

Penicillin is responsible for approximately 75% of the deaths caused by anaphylaxis per year in the U.S. (approximately 500 patients).[4] The onset of symptoms within 1 hour, rarely 2, after exposure to penicillin facilitates the diagnosis.

Urticaria and angioedema can occur any time after penicillin administration. Usually angioedema is seen in conjunction with urticaria but occasionally is the sole manifestation of a reaction. Most frequently it involves the lips, eyelids, tongue, larynx, penis, palms, and soles.

The syndrome of recurrent urticaria and arthralgias is rare. It usually occurs from 2 to 15 weeks after withdrawal of penicillin and may be caused in extremely sensitive individuals by exposure to penicillin hidden, for example, in food.

Manifestations of immune complex disease are generally seen about 7 to 10 days after starting the drug and may include fever, arthralgias, myalgias, lymphadenopathy, glomerulonephritis, inflammation of serosal surfaces, and rashes. The latter are usually maculopapular or urticarial. Occasionally the palpable purpura associated with vasculitis is present.

Maculopapular rashes are the most common manifestation of penicillin allergy. They are frequently difficult to distinguish from viral exanthems, especially in children. One feature distinguishing allergic rashes is their association with pruritus, which is rarely present with viral exanthems. Also, viral rashes tend to remain macular, whereas penicillin rashes may progress to papular and even exfoliative rashes if the drug is continued. "Fixed" drug eruptions, characterized by a rash developing in the same localized area with each exposure to the drug, can also occur.

The incidence of maculopapular rashes is 2% per course of penicillin administered. This incidence reaches 5 to 10% in patients given ampicillin or amoxicillin. Although still not proven, increasing data suggests that these rashes when occurring in patients treated with ampicillin or amoxicillin may not be immunologically mediated, and that therefore the drug possibly can be continued and the patient may not have to be designated allergic to penicillin. The incidence of maculopapular rashes occurring in patients treated with ampicillin or amoxicillin increases dramatically in patients with concurrent cytomegalovirus infections, with chronic lymphocytic leukemia, and perhaps with elevated uric acid or on allopurinol treatment. It reaches almost 100% if the patient has concurrent infectious mononucleosis. This latter group of patients should not be labeled penicillin allergic. It is very important, however, to differentiate maculopapular rashes from urticaria, which is mediated by IgE antibody and whose presence indicates that the patient should be considered allergic to penicillin.

A positive direct Coombs' test is seen in about 3% of patients receiving high-dose penicillin (10 to 20 million units per day) but is rarely associated with clinically significant hemolytic anemia.

Interstitial nephritis, while commonly associated with methacillin, also can be seen with high doses of other penicillins. Usually it occurs from several days to weeks after starting therapy. It is commonly associated with preceding or concurrent fever, morbilliform rash, arthralgias, and eosinophilia. The urinalysis usually shows hematuria and mild to moderate proteinuria.

CEPHALOSPORIN ALLERGY

Cephalosporins can cause most of the same immunologically mediated reactions associated with penicillin (Table 3–6).[10] The differential diagnosis and evaluation are also the same, except that there are no skin tests currently available for cephalosporins.

Because cephalosporins are structurally similar to penicillin there is cross-reactivity between them, though the nature and extent of this reactivity is still not well defined. Both groups of drugs have a β-lactam ring in the center of their respective structures. It appears that this ring is the primary site of metabolism with the resultant formation of metabolic products, e.g., the major and minor determinants as in the case of penicillin. Hence, one would expect some degree of cross-reactivity. Patients receiving penicillin who have never had a cephalosporin can be shown to have IgE, IgM, and IgG antibodies specific for cephalosporins. Likewise, patients who are receiving cephalosporins can be shown to have an increase in antibody titers specific for penicillin.[11–13]

There are limited clinical studies on this cross-reactivity. One study suggested that patients with a history of a past allergic reaction to penicillin who were given a cephalosporin had four times the incidence of reactions to the cephalosporin (8%) than patients with no prior history of an allergic reaction to penicillin (2%).[12] Other explanations may account for this difference, however, and further studies are clearly needed. Sufficient data does not exist to determine if third generation cephalosporins will differ from the older drugs with regard to cross-reactivity.

At present, the physician has to rely primarily on judgment when evaluating a patient with a history of penicillin allergy who needs a cephalosporin drug. As discussed with penicillin, one has to evaluate the severity of the past history and the time since the last reaction occurred.

Skin testing with at least the major determinant of penicillin will provide additional information. If the test is positive, the chance of reaction to a cephalosporin is greater than normal. If the history shows a vague sense of pruritus 30 years ago and the skin test is negative, one can probably give the drug with limited concern. In all cases it is prudent to give a small test dose first. If the patient had an anaphylactic reaction to penicillin 6 months ago, regardless of the skin test results, the patient should probably be desensitized to the cephalosporin.

In the case of a patient with a history of an allergic reaction to cephalosporins and a current need for a penicillin drug, penicillin skin testing can be performed, as discussed in the penicillin section.

SULFA DRUGS ALLERGY

The sulfa drugs can cause all the hypersensitivity reactions noted for penicillin. Additionally, they can cause renal dysfunction and, rarely, idiosyncratic blood dyscrasias and hepatocellular dysfunction. As with penicillin, the most common hypersensitivity reaction is the development of a maculopapular rash usually occurring after several days of treatment. In patients with the Acquired Immune Deficiency Syndrome (AIDS) receiving sulfonamides, the incidence of this rash is increased substantially.[14]

The evaluation of a patient with a suspected allergic reaction to a sulfa drug is the same as for penicillin, with the exception that there is no skin testing reagent available. Therefore, if sulfa allergy is reasonably suspected, sulfa should not, ideally, be given again.

There is a varying degree of cross-reactivity among sulfa derivatives, so if a patient has a history of sensitivity to one drug, other derivatives (Table 3–9) should be used with caution.

VANCOMYCIN ALLERGY

A variety of reactions including erythema, urticaria, maculopapular rashes, pruritus, fever, hypotension, and, very rarely, cardiac arrest have been associated with vancomycin. The urticaria, maculopapular rashes, and fever are rare and may be immunologically mediated reactions, although this has not been demonstrated.

Table 3–9. Common Sulfa Derivatives

Antibiotics
  Sulfamethoxazole (Bactrim, Septra)
  Sulfisoxazole (Azo Gantrisin)
  Sulfadoxine (Fansidar)
  Sulfasalazine (Azulfidine)
  Sulfinpyrazone (Anturane)
Oral hypoglycemics
  Chlorpropamide (Diabinese)
  Tolbutamide (Orinase)
  Acetohexamide (Dymelor)
  Tolazamide (Tolinase)
Diuretics
  Thiazides (Hydrodiuril, Esidrix)
  Metolazone (Zaroxolyn)
  Furosemide (Lasix)
Antihypertensives
  Diazoxide (Hyperstat)
Carbonic anhydrase inhibitor
  Acetazolamide (Diamox)

More common is the development of diffuse erythema; sometimes a maculopapular rash, especially on the face and neck; hypotension; and, rarely, cardiac arrest coincident with the infusion of the antibiotic. This reaction is sometimes termed the "red-neck syndrome."[15] It seems clearly related to a rapid rate of infusion of the drug.[15a] It is currently recommended that vancomycin be infused over at least 1 hour, although one case of the above reaction has been reported even with this slow rate of administration.[15b]

The mechanism is unknown but may involve histamine release. Because patients with red-neck syndrome frequently tolerate vancomycin again if infused slowly, it is unlikely that the reaction is immunologically mediated. The reaction of flushing and hypotension has also been reported when vancomycin has been administered coincident with anesthetic agents before surgery.

ALLERGY TO LOCAL ANESTHETICS

Local anesthetics are frequently suspected as the cause of allergic reactions, especially those anesthetics associated with dental procedures. True immune mediated reactions to these agents, however, are rare. The development of an immune reaction such as urticaria, angioedema in a site distant from the administration of the anesthetic, bronchoconstriction, or hypotension coincident with administration of the agent makes allergy to that local anesthetic likely. Other, more common reactions such as local swelling, lightheadedness, palpitations, syncope, or dyspnea with normal vital signs and a clear chest on physical exam are rarely caused by an immune mediated reaction. They may result from the dental or other procedure itself, from anxiety with hyperventilation, from a vasovagal reaction, from a toxic reaction, or from the epinephrine that is usually mixed with the local anesthetic to keep it at the site for a longer time.

The history of the nature of the reaction and the timing of its onset associated with administration of the agent is the most important part of the evaluation to determine the likelihood of allergy to the local anesthetic. Laboratory tests are generally not helpful in the diagnosis.

Although skin testing using local anesthetics is available, its efficacy is not completely established because the exact nature of the antigen responsible for the reaction is not known. Nevertheless, many studies suggest that incremental skin tests (starting with a 1:100 dilution by prick test and concluding with 0.02 ml by intradermal injection) followed by incremental challenge doses of the local anesthetic (culminating in 1.0 ml full strength subcutaneously) are a safe and valuable approach.[16] Although there may be an incidence of false positive results as high as a 15%, the incidence of false negative results is extremely low. Local anesthetics used for skin testing should not include epinephrine because the resultant vasoconstriction may either produce a false positive result or blunt a true positive skin test. Because most anesthetics contain epinephrine and because its use diminishes the amount of anesthetic needed, a local anesthetic with epinephrine should probably be used for challenge.

Rarely the reaction may be caused by preservatives (usually parabens) that are present in multidose vials and that should be tested for separately.

Local anesthetics can be classified chemically into those that are benzoic acid esters and those that have other structures (Table 3–10). Anesthetics in the former group (including procaine) appear to cross-react substantially with each other. There may be less cross-reactivity among those benzoic acid esters lacking a p-aminobenzoyl group. Anesthetics in the other group (including lidocaine and mepivacaine) do not appear to cross-react with the benzoic acid esters or react significantly with each other.

Therefore, if a patient is suspected of having had a reaction to a local anesthetic, an anesthetic in another group should be chosen, and skin testing followed by incremental challenge should be undertaken. Using this approach the majority of patients with a history of adverse reactions have been able to tolerate administration of another reagent. This approach is preferable to withholding further local anesthetic administration.

INSULIN ALLERGY

Human insulin differs from pork insulin by one amino acid and from beef insulin by three amino acids. This difference is sufficient to stimulate certain patients

Table 3–10.   Classification of Local Anesthetics

Group I: Benzoic acid esters
  p-Aminobenzoic acid esters
    Benzocaine
    Butacaine (Butyn)
    Butethamine (Monocaine)
    Chlorprocaine (Nesacaine)
    Procaine (Novocain)
    Tetracaine (Pontocaine)*
  Benzoic acid esters lacking p-aminobenzoyl group
    Amydricaine (Alypin)
    Cyclomethycaine (Surfacaine)
    Isobucaine (Kincaine)
    Piperocaine (Metycaine)
    Proparacaine (Ophthaine)
Group II: Others
    Bupivacaine (Marcaine)
    Dibucaine (Nupercaine)
    Dyclonine (Dyclone)
    Diperodon (Diothane)
    Lidocaine (Xylocaine)
    Mepivacaine (Carbocaine)
    Oxethazaine (Oxaine)
    Phenacaine (Holocaine)
    Pramoxine (Tronothane)
    Prilocaine (Citonest)

*Contains substituted p-aminobenzoyl group and exhibits variable cross-reactivity with other benzoic acid esters in the reported studies. (From Schatz, M.: Skin testing and incremental challenge in the evaluation of adverse reactions to local anesthetics. J Allergy Clin Immunol 74:606, 1984, with permission.)

to develop an immune reaction to the administered insulin.[17,18,18a] The manifestations of these reactions are noted on Table 3–11. Reactions occurring within 1 hour are probably mediated by IgE antibody.

The problem should be suspected by the history and confirmed by skin testing productive of an immediate wheal and flare reaction, a reliable indication of IgE mediated insulin allergy. The later reactions more likely involve IgG and IgM antibodies and T cells. IgG antibodies against insulin can be detected serologically. However, because almost all patients on insulin for 2 months or more, regardless of symptoms,

Table 3–11.   Immune Reactions Noted with Insulin Administration

Anaphylaxis
Reactions occurring within 1 hour at the injection site
  Warmth
  Erythema
  Swelling
  Pruritus
  Urticaria
Reactions occurring after several hours at the injection site
  Same as above
Reactions occurring 1 to 2 days later locally or systemically
  Swelling
  Pruritus
  Urticaria

have detectable IgG specific for the hormone, detection of this IgG antibody is not very helpful in diagnosing insulin allergy.[19]

Delayed hypersensitivity testing (placing 0.1 ml of the antigen intradermally and evaluating induration and erythema at 48 hours) likewise is not helpful in diagnosing insulin allergy. A history of reactions occurring consistently several hours after insulin administration is still the most useful diagnostic tool for diagnosing nonimmediate reactions.

Human insulin manufactured by recombinant DNA technology should theoretically not provoke an immune response. Nevertheless, several reports to date document its immunogenicity,[19a] including the development of IgE antibody specific for human insulin associated with clinical symptoms ranging from immediate systemic to local reactions. In fact, one prospective study showed that 6% of diabetics treated with human insulin developed IgE antibodies specific for insulin, versus 17% treated with pork insulin and 19% treated with beef insulin.[20]

Patients treated intermittently or irregularly with insulin may be more prone to develop allergic reactions. If such a reaction is documented, a variety of therapeutic maneuvers can be attempted, including desensitization and changing the source of the insulin.[17]

CHYMOPAPAIN ALLERGY

Chymopapain is a 27,000 M.W. protease derived from papaya. It is used therapeutically for chemonucleolysis of herniated intervertebral discs. Approximately 1% of patients undergoing this procedure have an anaphylactic reaction to the chymopapain.[21,22] The mortality rate has been reported as 0.01%.[23]

The reaction appears to be mediated by IgE antibody,[24] as discussed in the section on anaphylaxis, and studies suggest that skin testing with chymopapain may help predict those patients at risk.[25]

The current protocol for use of chymopapain recommends pretreatment of the patients with antihistamines (both H_1 and H_2 antagonists) in an attempt to modify or prevent an allergic reaction. The extent of efficacy of this treatment is not yet clear.

The likelihood of a reaction might be predicted by taking the patient's history. Prior to undergoing chemonucleolysis, patients should be questioned regarding past possible adverse reactions to other sources of papain (Table 3–12), since it has been shown that papain and chymopapain cross-react.[25a,25b]

PROTAMINE ALLERGY

Protamine sulfate, commonly given to reverse heparin anticoagulation, has been associated with the development of severe hypotension and urticaria/angioedema.[26–28] Bronchospasm has not been reported.

Table 3–12. Sources of Papain Exposure

Chymopapain
Papaya
Meat tenderizers
Beer (used as a clarifying agent)
Contact lens cleaning solutions

Although the hypotension may be related to a rapid infusion rate, the observation that the reaction occurs more frequently in patients commonly exposed to protamine in NPH insulin or salmon suggests an immune mediated reaction.[26–29] NPH insulin contains 0.5 mg protamine per 100 units. Although diabetic patients usually have no history of reaction to the insulin, they may react to protamine when, to reverse the effects of heparin, it is administered in doses about 1000 times greater than they normally receive. In the case of salmon, protamine is present in the sperm and mature testes. Several patients have been described who are allergic to salmon and who have subsequently reacted to protamine.[26,29]

ALLERGY TO ADDITIVES

Before incriminating a particular substance as the source of an allergic reaction, one must entertain the possibility that an additive in the substance caused the reaction. A wide range of additives present in food and drugs can cause a variety of reactions in susceptible patients (Table 3–13).[30] Of the various dye products, FD and C #5 (tartrazine) has in rare cases been implicated in causing asthma in a subset of aspirin-sensitive patients. Penicillin and tetracycline are occasionally found in beef, milk, and other food products and can cause an IgE mediated reaction in susceptible patients. In one case, for example, penicillin was the cause of anaphylaxis after ingestion of a soft drink.[31]

Table 3–13. Selected Factors in Food and Drugs That Can Cause Adverse Reactions

Additives
  Dyes—FD & C #5 (tartrazine)
  Drugs in Foods—Penicillin, Tetracycline, Bacitracin
  Monosodium Glutamate (MSG)
Preservatives
  Parabens
  Sulfites
  Nitrates
Contaminants
  Mold
Toxins in Foods
  Mushrooms
  Fish/Shellfish
Other
  Ingestion of lactose by lactase-deficient patients
  Ingestion of drugs and foods that will cause hemolytic anemia in glucose-6-phosphate dehydrogenase–deficient patients

Monosodium glutamate produces the Chinese restaurant syndrome (see the section on food allergies).

The preservatives parabens and, especially, sulfites can cause significant reactions and are discussed separately below. Occasionally, a reaction to a contaminant like mold or to a toxin, as discussed in the food allergy section, can mimic a true allergic reaction.

Ingestion of lactose in foods by a lactase-deficient patient will lead to a variety of gastrointestinal symptoms, including pain, bloating, and diarrhea, that can be confused with a food allergy. Coincidence with ingestion of milk products and lack of urticaria are helpful differentiating points. Exposure to a wide variety of oxidant drugs and other substances can result in hemolysis in a glucose-6-phosphate dehydrogenase–deficient patient.

PARABEN ALLERGY. Parabens, usually in the form of methylparaben and propylparaben, are widely used as preservatives in medications, foods, and cosmetics. Contact results in dermatitis, thought to be caused by a delayed hypersensitivity reaction. No reactions to orally administered parabens are known, and reactions to parenteral administration, while documented, are extremely rare in view of the ubiquitous presence of the preservatives in parenteral medications, especially multidose preparations.[32]

Sensitivity to parabens should be suspected in any case of dermatitis resulting from contact with a medication or cosmetic. Patch testing with parabens esters can establish the diagnosis.

SULFITE SENSITIVITY. Sulfites are effective antioxidants and hence are present in a wide variety of foods, beverages, and medications (Table 3–14). They are also used as sanitizing agents for fermentation equipment. Sulfur dioxide is a common air pollutant. The various forms have been demonstrated to cause anaphylaxis and bronchospasm and, rarely, have been associated with urticaria and angioedema alone (Table 3–15).[33,34] Although all asthmatics will react to an inhalation challenge of 1 to 5 ppm of SO_2,[35] only a small group, approximately 5%, seems to react routinely to lesser concentrations.[34] Reactions can occur after oral or inhalation exposure.

The mechanism of this reaction is still unclear. It does not appear to involve IgE antibody in most cases. Preliminary data suggest that some patients may be quantitatively deficient in the enzyme sulfite oxidase,[34] which is responsible for the oxidation of HSO_3 to SO_4 (sulfate). HSO_3 can escape as SO_2 gas. It is postulated that sensitive asthmatics may not be able to handle a sulfite load and the resultant development of HSO_3 or SO_2 may cause their symptoms.[34]

A history suggesting a correlation of symptoms with sulfite exposure is currently the best means of diag-

Table 3–14. Possible Sources of Sulfite Exposure*

Foods
  Dried fruit (except dark raisins and prunes)
  Lemon and lime juice (not frozen)
  Salad bar items that discolor with air exposure, e.g., lettuce, avocado
  Shrimp
  Potato products
  Vinegar
  Sauerkraut
  Molasses
  Pickled food
  Corn and beet sweeteners
  Gravies, sauces
  Maraschino cherries
  Some frozen vegetables
Beverages
  Beer
  Wine with corks
  Grape juice
  Some fruit drinks
  Cider
Air Pollution
Medications
  (Certain preparations)
  Epinephrine
  Multidose bronchodilator solutions (not individual dose inhalers)
  Parenteral corticosteroids
  Parenteral antibiotics
  Parenteral antiarrhythmics
  Parenteral pressor agents
  Local anesthetics
  Radio contrast media
  Peritoneal dialysis solutions
  Antiemetics
  Psychotropic drugs

*Those with a high concentration are underlined.

nosis. Challenge testing can be done but is not yet standardized. Public concern about sulfite sensitivity has already led to restrictions on the use of sulfites. Additionally, dipsticks that detect the presence of sulfites are commercially available so that sensitive patients can know what substances to avoid.

FOOD ALLERGY

The incidence of "true" allergic (IgE mediated) reactions to food substances is probably overestimated.[36] When it occurs, it is suggested by anaphylaxis, urticaria, angioedema, and/or bronchospasm; isolated respiratory symptoms are rare. Gastrointestinal symptoms are more difficult to evaluate. Most

Table 3–15. Commonly Encountered Sulfites

Sodium metabisulfite
Potassium metabisulfite
Sodium bisulfite
Potassium bisulfite
Sodium sulfite
Sulfur dioxide

reactions occur within 2 hours after ingesting a particular food. The longer the time interval after the ingestion of the suspected food, the less likely the problem is to be allergy. Occult food allergy responsible for constant symptoms is very rare.

As with most allergic disease, the most important factor in determining a diagnosis is the patient's history. Consistency of symptoms on rechallenge is helpful in making the diagnosis, as is knowledge of which foods frequently cause problems. Because food antigens are generally proteins, some of which will be denatured with cooking, a history of reaction to a raw food, rather than to a cooked one, is useful.

Peanut is one of the strongest food antigens and in adults is a frequent cause of anaphylaxis. Shellfish, milk, egg, wheat, and nuts are other, less common causes. Foods are grouped in biological families, and reactivity to several foods in the group can be found. For instance, patients allergic to peanuts, which are in the legume family, may also experience symptoms with other foods in this group, such as soybeans, other beans, peas, and chick-peas. Reactivity to multiple groups is unusual, so a true allergy to peanuts, walnuts, and almonds (three distinct food groups) would be very uncommon. Certain foods (e.g., wine) have a high histamine content and therefore can cause allergic symptoms without involving IgE antibody. Other foods (e.g., strawberries) may nonspecifically induce histamine release when ingested. Bananas contain high concentrations of other vasoactive amines.

The suspicion that the reaction may be due to something other than the food substance itself should be kept in mind (Table 3–13). Reactions to a variety of seemingly unrelated substances may be due to a common preservative or additive. If reactions occur only after eating the substance in a restaurant, sulfite preservative sensitivity should be suspected. Nitrite, another common preservative found in cured meats, usually produces a headache. Rarely, milk and meat products may be contaminated with penicillin, tetracycline, or bacitracin. Aspirin-sensitive asthmatics will rarely develop bronchospasm when exposed to FD & C #5 yellow dye (tartrazine), which is widely used commercially in yellow colored foods, beverages, and medications. If the reaction occurs only after consuming Chinese food, it is most probably caused by sensitivity to the monosodium glutamate (MSG) frequently used in its preparation. The symptoms of "Chinese restaurant syndrome" are burning and tingling, especially of the trunk and arms, often associated with severe headaches. These symptoms are very unusual for an IgE mediated reaction. The onset of symptoms often within 10 to 20 minutes in IgE me-

diated reactions and MSG sensitivity can sometimes confuse the diagnosis.

Reactions to fish frequently perceived as being due to allergy may be due to scombroid or ciguatera poisoning. With scombroid poisoning, mackerel, bonita, tuna, and other related fish, if left in a warm temperature for too long, may develop a toxin, saurine, from the breakdown of histidine in their skin by Proteus morgani. Ingestion of the toxins causes urticaria, nausea, vomiting, and abdominal pain, along with headache, dry mouth, dysphagia, and a sense of palpitations. The reaction is generally self-limited.

Ciguatera poisoning can occur from a wide variety of fish. The toxin, which is thought to originate from certain types of algae, collects in the fish tissue. Human ingestion of this results in nausea, vomiting, and a variety of neurologic symptoms that, in severe cases, can lead to respiratory paralysis. Characteristically there is a reversal of temperature sensation. The onset occurs generally within several hours after consuming the fish. Unlike with an allergic reaction, symptoms last for several weeks (if the patient survives the initial reaction).

Lactase deficiency, which is occasionally confused with allergy, is the most common diagnosis in adults presenting with gastrointestinal symptoms of distension, pain, flatulence, and diarrhea after ingestion of milk or milk products. Generally, patients' symptoms of lactase deficiency are directly related to the amount of milk ingested. Most commonly the diagnosis is made by taking the history and by diet manipulation. Diagnostic tests include changes in blood glucose or exhaled hydrogen after a lactose load or, rarely, an intestinal biopsy.

As is the case with most allergic diseases, the history is of primary importance in the evaluation of the patient with possible food allergies. Evaluated levels of serum IgE or eosinophils support the diagnosis of allergy if other considerations, such as parasitic diseases, are eliminated. There is no blood test that specifically documents food allergy. The only completely reliable way to implicate a specific food is by double blind, placebo controlled challenges with the suspected food placed in opaque capsules.

Skin testing may be helpful using an aqueous preparation of the food. The testing suffers from lack of standardization and lack of knowledge of the exact nature of the antigen in most cases. Also, there are many false positive results. False negative reactions, however, confirmed by blind oral challenge, appear to be very rare.

Radioallergosorbent testing (RAST), which involves looking for specific IgE in the blood as opposed to that bound to the surface of the mast cell, is as specific as but generally less sensitive than skin testing. It likewise suffers from lack of standardization of the antigens used, it is expensive, and it requires time for the results to be known in most cases. It is most effective in cases in which patients have significant dermatographism, have a skin problem such as diffuse atopic dermatitis, lack a suitable skin testing site, or have extreme anaphylactic sensitivity to the suspected antigen.

Stimulation of basophils with the antigen in vitro and assaying histamine release is another means of evaluating IgE mediated sensitivity to food. It is available only in research laboratories and also suffers from lack of knowledge about and standardization of the antigens.

Occasionally, food diaries are suggested as a means of evaluating an allergic reaction to food. The patient notes all reactions along with all foods consumed at the time. The physician can then review it looking for possible causes of the reaction. Food diaries rarely supplement a detailed history taken by the physician.

An elimination diet may help in the diagnosis. The suspected food is eliminated from the diet and is reintroduced when symptoms have subsided to see if they recur. In extreme cases the patient can be given an elemental diet such as Vivonex until the symptoms subside, followed by the gradual introduction of suspected foods one by one. This approach is tedious and can lead to malnutrition in children, and it is flawed by a placebo effect that may reach 30%. Hence, the only accurate way to evaluate cause and effect is by the double blind, placebo controlled trial, which, however, requires considerable effort on the part of the physician. In the routine office setting, the elimination from the diet of the suspected food, followed by rechallenge, will probably be of most help, despite its limitations.

HYMENOPTERA ALLERGY

Insect stings are the second most frequent cause (after penicillin) of anaphylactic reactions in the U.S.[37,38] The insects responsible for the allergic reaction belong to the order Hymenoptera (Fig. 3–2) and include the wasp, honeybee, and vespids (Yellow Jacket, Yellow Hornet, and White Faced Hornet). In the southern part of the country, fire ants are also a problem. Although the actual number of deaths caused by anaphylaxis is low (estimated at about 25 to 40 per year), morbidity is high. Many patients who believe they are allergic make drastic changes in their lifestyles to avoid being stung. For those patients who have significant sensitivity to these stinging insects, effective treatment in the form of venom immunotherapy is now available for all the insects except fire ants.

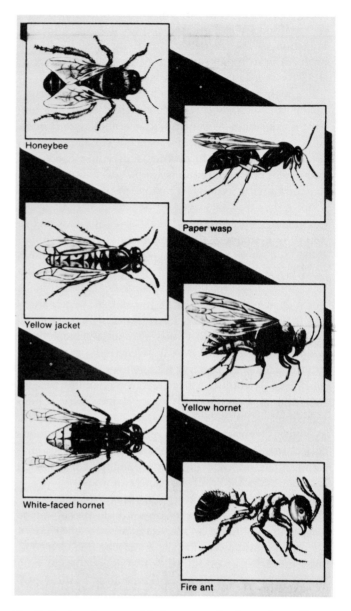

Fig. 3–2. Insects responsible for severe allergic reactions. (From Shepherd, G.: Update on Insect Allergy. Drug Therapy *13*:147, 1983, with permission.)

It is usually difficult to determine which insect was responsible for the reaction without skin testing. Only honeybees leave their stinger in place after a sting. Knowledge of the prevalent insects in one's area and the circumstances of the sting are helpful; for example, stings from stepping on an insect in the grass are usually from yellow jackets, whereas stings from encountering a nest under the eave of a house are more likely to be from wasps or hornets.

The major problem encountered in evaluating a reaction to an insect sting is determining whether it is a true allergic reaction or just an inflammatory reaction to the many proteolytic enzymes and other substances in the venom, and, if it is a true allergic reaction, determining the patient's chances of being at risk of a significant allergic reaction if stung in the future.

If a patient has a small area of erythema, induration, and tenderness at the site of the sting, the reaction is not allergic (Table 3–16). However, if any systemic reaction develops, e.g., urticaria in a site not contiguous with the sting, the reaction is probably IgE antibody mediated. The difficulty in diagnosing arises with patients who have extensive local reactions to a sting, such as a swollen, tender limb after a sting on a finger or toe. If this large local reaction is due to an allergic reaction, the risk of a future systemic reaction to an insect sting is probably quite low, even if the patient has positive venom skin tests.[39]

If there is a history of a systemic reaction, the patient should undergo venom skin testing by a specialist. If that demonstrates the presence of IgE antibody specific for the venom(s), the patient should be treated with venom immunotherapy or should be advised to carry an epinephrine syringe at all times.

ALLERGY TO RADIO CONTRAST MEDIA

Anaphylactoid reactions ranging from mild urticaria to shock are reported to occur in 1 to 2% of procedures in which radiographic contrast media (RCM) is employed. Although the reaction is not thought to be mediated by IgE antibody, the resultant signs and symptoms are indistinguishable from true anaphylaxis. The exact mechanism whereby RCM causes these re-

actions is unknown. If a patient has a history of a reaction in the past, the chance of having a repeat reaction on re-exposure to the RCM is approximately 17 to 35%, with one study suggesting as high as 60%.[40]

At the present time there appears to be no way to identify patients at risk of a reaction upon first exposure to RCM. As the reaction does not appear to be mediated by IgE antibody, a history of atopy is not a predictive factor. Likewise, since the reaction does not appear to be related to iodine or iodide, a history of adverse reactions to shellfish (also probably unrelated to iodine) is irrelevant.

Although there is clearly a greater risk of a reaction if a patient experienced one in the past, there is currently no way to identify that group of patients who will experience the repeat reaction. Studies have shown that patients with a history of a dye reaction, when pretreated with the regimen outlined in Table 3–17, will be at 97% less risk of a repeat reaction.[41]

Hence, the best approach at present is to pretreat with corticosteroids, antihistamines, and ephedrine all patients about to undergo a radiographic contrast dye study who have a history of a prior adverse reaction. There is not sufficient data yet to comment on differential risk between arterial or venous studies or between types of media used. There is no substantial data about patient pretreatment in situations requiring emergent dye studies.

ASPIRIN ALLERGY

Aspirin is a common cause of drug allergy. Sensitive patients will occasionally experience an anaphylactoid

Table 3–16. Management Approaches to Various Types of Insect Sting Reactions

Type of Past Reaction	Risk of Systemic Reaction to Subsequent Stings	Should Skin Testing be Performed?	Results of Skin Testing	Recommended Treatment
Never stung	Minimal	No		None
Minor local reaction (immediate pain, swelling, and itching at sting site; subsides generally in 1 day)	Minimal	No		None
Extensive local reaction (swelling contiguous to sting site; peaking 48 to 72 hr after the sting and resolves within a week)	Approximately 5%	No		Epinephrine syringe (ANA-Kit, Epi-Pen)*
Systemic reaction (adult) (urticaria, angioedema, or anaphylaxis)	Approximately 60%	Yes	+	Venom immunotherapy
			−	Epinephrine syringe
Systemic reaction (child) (urticaria and mild angioedema only)	Low	?	+	Venom immunotherapy or epinephrine syringe
			−	Epinephrine syringe
Systemic reaction (child) (anaphylaxis)	Moderate	Yes	+	Venom immunotherapy
			−	Epinephrine syringe

*ANA-Kit—Hollister-Steir, Spokane, Washington
Epi-Pen—Center Laboratories, Port Washington, NY
(Modified from Shepherd, G.: Update on Insect Allergy. Drug Therapy 13:147, 1983.)

Table 3–17. Pretreatment of Patients with a History of a Reaction to Radiographic Contrast Dye Who Need a Repeat Study

13 hours before the procedure—50 mg prednisone or equivalent
7 hours before the procedure—50 mg prednisone or equivalent
1 hour before the procedure —50 mg prednisone or equivalent
50 mg diphenhydramine (Benadryl) po or IM
25 mg ephedrine po*

*As long as the patient has no contraindication to taking ephedrine, such as significant arrythmias, hypertension, or angina.
(From Greenberger, P.A., Patterson, R., and Radin, R.C.: Two pretreatment regimens for high risk patients receiving radiocontrast media. J Allergy Clin Immunol 74:540, 1984, with permission.)

reaction, the exact mechanism of which is unknown. Most commonly they will experience bronchospasm without associated urticaria, angioedema, or hypotension.[42–44] It has been proposed that the origin of bronchospasm involves aspirin's modification of prostaglandin production. Possible mechanisms of bronchoconstriction include an increased production of prostaglandin $F_{2\alpha}$ or prostaglandin D_2 (bronchoconstriction) relative to prostaglandin E (bronchodilation) and/or an enhanced production of leukotrienes LTC, D, and E, which are potent bronchoconstrictors. Aspirin acts to block the cycloxygenase pathway and hence may shift metabolism to the lipoxygenase pathway, resulting in production of the leukotrienes (Fig. 3–3). Various studies have estimated that from 4 to 40% of patients with asthma will develop bronchoconstriction upon exposure to aspirin, although the 4% figure is more likely.[42–44]

Sensitivity to aspirin has also been associated with rhinosinusitis (sinusitis documented by radiographs, enlarged pale nasal turbinates sometimes with polypoid changes, and nasal polyps). The classic "aspirin triad" consists of sensitivity to aspirin, asthma, and rhinosinusitis; it is now recognized, however, that while the triad exists in some patients, others may have only one or two manifestations of it. Patients may present with rhinosinusitis several years before developing aspirin sensitivity or asthma.

The classic patient with the triad is 20 to 40 years old, either male or female. Presenting symptoms are usual nasal congestion, occasional anosmia, chest tightness, shortness of breath, and wheezing. Physical examination reveals enlarged pale nasal turbinates, polyps, and wheezing. These patients tend to have a high percentage of eosinophils in their nasal secretions. Sinus disease should be evaluated by radiographs or computed tomography, since the physical examination is not reliable. These will demonstrate anything from diffuse periosteal thickening to clouding of the sinuses with air fluid levels. If the diagnosis of aspirin sensitivity is in doubt, oral aspirin challenge followed by symptom and spirometry assessment can be considered. This procedure obviously has inherent risks but in experienced hands has proven to be useful.

Aspirin has also been cited as both a cause of and a factor exacerbating acute and chronic urticaria and angioedema. As with anaphylaxis, the exact mechanism of this reaction is unknown. Sensitive patients tend to develop either urticaria or rhinosinusitis and bronchospasm upon aspirin exposure, but rarely both.

Sodium salicylate rarely seems to cause any of the reactions seen with aspirin. There also appears to be no significant reactivity with acetaminophen. Rarely, asthmatic patients sensitive to aspirin may react in the

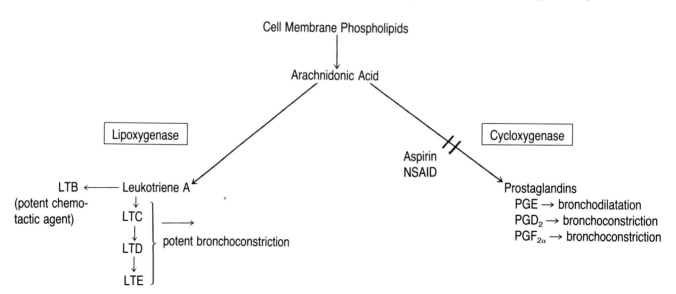

Fig. 3–3. Effect of aspirin and nonsteroidal anti-inflammatory drugs on arachnidonic acid.

Table 3–18.   Nonsteroidal Anti-Inflammatory Agents

Benoxaprofen
Diflunisal (Dolobid)
Fenoprofen (Nalfon)
Ibuprofen (Motrin; Rufen; Advil; Nuprin)
Indomethacin (Indocin)
Meclofenamate sodium (Meclomen)
Mefenamic acid (Ponstel)
Naproxen (Naprosyn)
Naproxen sodium (Anaprox)
Phenylbutazone (Butazolidin)
Piroxicam (Feldene)
Sulindac (Clinoril)
Tolmetin (Tolectin)
Zomepirac (Zomax)

same manner to FD & C yellow dye #5 (tartrazine), which is present in a wide number of commercially prepared foods, beverages, and medications.

ALLERGY TO NONSTEROIDAL ANTI-INFLAMMATORY DRUGS (NSAID)

An increasing number of the NSAIDs have been reported, like aspirin, to cause anaphylactoid, urticarial, and bronchospastic reactions.[45] Although generally chemically unrelated to aspirin, both groups block cycloxygenase synthesis and hence could be expected to have similar effects.[46] These drugs are listed on Table 3–18. Zomepirac sodium is currently off the market since it was associated with a number of deaths from anaphylactoid reactions. Tolmetin is chemically similar to Zomepirac. Benoxaprofen, an inhibitor of the lipoxygenase pathway, is an exception because it does not appear to cause these reactions; it too was taken off the market, however, after it was associated with hepatotoxicity. The extent of cross-reactivity between aspirin and the NSAIDs is not known. It appears to be high, at least for indomethacin. In all cases it is probably of sufficient magnitude to warn aspirin-sensitive patients not to use NSAIDs. The physician may elect to very cautiously challenge a patient with an NSAID in a monitored setting if alternative drugs cannot be used therapeutically.

EXERCISE-INDUCED ANAPHYLAXIS

It is clear that exercise, most frequently jogging, can cause anaphylaxis in certain susceptible individuals. Studies of this problem have been hampered by the fact that the anaphylactic reactions do not happen consistently under common circumstances. Neither can they be reproduced every time by having subjects exercise on a treadmill in an occlusive suit. When the reaction occurs under laboratory observation, it appears to result from mast cell degranulation.[47] At present, susceptible patients are advised to modify their exercise regimens substantially. Although asthma re-

sulting from exercise can be effectively blocked by albuterol or cromolyn sodium inhalation, an anaphylactic reaction cannot be blocked at the present time.

There is a very interesting rare subgroup of these patients that has food-dependent, exercise-induced anaphylaxis. Some of these patients will have anaphylactic reactions if they eat anything within 2 hours of exercise. Others will have it only if they consume a specific food. One recent series documented patients sensitive to celery, a food generally not considered to be a significant antigen. If these patients ate celery and exercised within 2 hours, they experienced anaphylactic reactions. They could tolerate either independently. The mechanism of this reaction is unknown.[48]

IDIOPATHIC ANAPHYLAXIS

There are certain patients who have recurrent episodes of anaphylaxis for which no cause can be found despite exhaustive studies.[49,50] At present this is termed idiopathic anaphylaxis. Since the cause is eventually found in some patients (e.g., endogenous progesterone[51]), it is not clear if other patients have an as yet unrecognized disorder of regulation resulting in "spontaneous" episodes of anaphylaxis or if they are reacting against an unidentified antigen.

The most important factor in diagnosing these patients is the taking of an exhaustive history, looking for any possible association. If this is unrevealing, further evaluation (e.g., skin tests, venom testing, elimination diets, etc.) should be undertaken, as one is dealing with a potentially life threatening disorder. Even so, the results rarely yield a clue to the cause.

URTICARIA AND ANGIOEDEMA (UAE)

DEFINITION

Urticaria is characterized by pruritic raised wheals surrounded by a flare located in the superficial dermis. Individual lesions usually last for a few hours. Angioedema is generally caused by the same mechanism; however, the swelling is in the deeper dermis and subcutaneous tissue, and because there are fewer sensory nerve endings there it is less associated with pruritis. Urticaria can occur anywhere, but angioedema usually affects the eyelids, lips, tongue, larynx, penis, palms, and soles. Erythema multiforme is a form of urticaria and angioedema in which ''iris'' or target lesions develop. Erythema multiforme can also involve mucous membranes and occasionally results in bullae formation (Stevens-Johnson syndrome), if severe.

PATHOPHYSIOLOGIC CONSIDERATIONS

Urticaria is an extremely common disorder, estimated to have affected 10 to 20% of the population at some time. Of patients presenting to a referral practice, 40% had urticaria alone, 11% had angioedema alone, and 49% had both.[52] The lesions of urticaria and angioedema most commonly result from the release of histamine and other mediators from mast cells and basophils.[53] (See the section on anaphylaxis for detailed discussion of the mechanism.) Antigen binding to IgE antibody on the surface of a mast cell or basophil, thus triggering the cell to release vasoactive mediators including histamine, is probably the most common mechanism responsible for acute urticaria. Other factors, including complement and eosinophil major basic protein, can nonspecifically trigger a mast cell or basophil to release its mediators.[54] The pathogenesis of physical urticaria is unknown but is thought to eventually involve histamine release. In the case of hereditary angioedema, the swelling results from an inherited defect of the complement pathway.

Most episodes of UAE are acute and self-limited. The cause, when found, is usually related to food, medication, insect stings, infection, or animal exposure.

In most nonidiopathic cases, urticaria results from ingestion of the antigen or its parenteral introduction by infection or sting. When, on rare occasions, it is associated with inhalation, it is usually accompanied by respiratory tract symptoms. It can also occur as a result of cat scratches or contact with Portuguese man-of-war, nettles, insects (e.g., moth), skin, or hair. It generally does not occur as a result of contact with soaps or lotions.

Chronic UAE (defined as lasting for longer than 6 weeks) presents more of a clinical problem. The majority of cases are idiopathic, with the cause being found in less than 20%. Nevertheless, every patient with chronic UAE should be thoroughly evaluated to determine if there is an identifiable cause.

DIFFERENTIAL DIAGNOSIS AND DIAGNOSTIC EVALUATION

An approach to evaluating the patient with UAE is outlined in Table 3–19. As with all allergic diseases the history is the most important factor in evaluation. Causal associations should be sought carefully. In

Table 3–19. Evaluation of Urticaria and Angioedema

Initial
  History and physical exam
  CBC with differential, biochemistry profile, ESR, ANA, IgE level, protein electrophoresis, chest x-ray.
Other selective tests based on history and physical exam
  Drug or food elimination and challenge trials
  HgBsAg and Ab
  Stool for ova and parasites; serology for parasites
  Immune complex determination (Raji and C1q assay)
  CH_{50}, C4, C1q, C1 esterase inhibitor (quantitative and functional assays)
  Cryoglobulins, cryofibrinogens, cold agglutinins
  Immunoelectrophoresis
  Double-stranded DNA
  T_4
  Skin test or RAST
  Tests for physical urticarias; e.g., ice cube test, metacholine test, red cell protoporphyrin levels
  Biopsy of lesion with immunofluorescence

chronic urticaria (of more than 6 weeks duration) a cause will be found in less than 20% of the cases. If the physical examination is unrevealing and an initial screening evaluation is normal (Table 3–19), the yield in pursuing further evaluation is very low. A total serum IgE level is useful in the initial screening, as an elevation suggests either a specific allergen causing the UAE or a parasitic disease. If there is any suspicion of an underlying disease or specific cause, pertinent tests should be performed as outlined in the section on differential diagnosis. For example, if immune complex mediated disease is considered, a biopsy, a urinalysis, and CH_{50}, C4, cryoglobulins, and immune complex determination assays should be considered. Stool examinations for ova and parasites have traditionally been included in the initial screening of a patient with UAE, although in temperate climates for a patient without suggestive history or symptoms the yield is extremely low. Usually only helminthic infections are associated with UAE as they migrate through tissues. Serology is usually more sensitive than stool examination for these parasites. The patient normally has associated eosinophilia and elevated IgE. Intestinal parasites like Giardia rarely cause UAE.

Authors differ on the need for and timing of a skin biopsy in UAE. Chronic ''idiopathic'' urticaria results in edema and vascular dilatation with a predominantly mononuclear cell infiltrate. Biopsies of urticaria associated with vasculitis show polymorphonuclear cells in and around the vessel wall, with necrosis of the wall and fibrinoid changes. Immunofluorescence is also positive in some cases. If the history and physical and laboratory evaluations are not suggestive of vasculitis, the yield on biopsy is very low. If vasculitis is suspected, a confirmatory biopsy should be done. In

Table 3–20. Differential Diagnosis of Chronic Urticaria and Angioedema

Idiopathic (80 to 90%)
Drugs
Food
Infection
  Viral (Hepatitis B, Epstein-Barr)
  Parasitic (Helminths)
Immune complexes
  Vasculitis
  Hypocomplementemia vasculitic syndrome
  Connective tissue diseases
Neoplasm: Lymphoma?
Hormones: Hyperthyroidism
Physical factors
  Mechanical
    Dermatographism
    Pressure (delayed)
    Vibratory
  Temperature
    Cold
      Idiopathic
      Associated with cryoglobulins and cryofibrinogenemia
      Cold-dependent dermatographism
      Systemic cold induced
      Familial cold urticaria
      Cholinergic
  Light
    Solar
    Associated with abnormal protoporphyrin metabolism
Other
  Aquagenic
  Urticaria pigmentosum
  Urticaria, deafness, and amyloidosis syndrome
  Episodic angioedema associated with eosinophilia
Psychogenic
Hereditary angioedema

chronic idiopathic urticaria, a biopsy should probably be considered if the patient is unresponsive to routine treatment short of corticosteroids. The discovery of vasculitis provides greater rationale for corticosteroid treatment.

As noted on Table 3–20, drugs are one cause of chronic urticaria. A wide variety of drugs has been associated with chronic UAE and should be suspected. If possible, the drugs should be discontinued to see if the urticaria resolves. Some authors have remarked that ingestion of aspirin, if not causal, may exacerbate urticaria and hence should be temporarily discontinued.[53]

Food is frequently suspected by the patient as a cause of chronic UAE. In practice it rarely is. (See the discussion in the section on food allergy.) If a cause and effect relationship is not obvious from the history, keeping a food diary may be helpful. Occasionally it is useful in diagnosing sensitivity to preservatives such as sulfites. If sensitivity to a constantly ingested substance like milk or soybean is suspected, tests to de-

termine the presence of specific IgE antibody or an elimination diet as discussed in the food allergy section can very occasionally be useful.

Urticaria is clearly associated with certain infections such as the prodrome of hepatitis B (in which it is thought to be due to circulating immune complexes), infectious mononucleosis, and helminthic infections. It does not appear to be associated with purely gastrointestinal parasites. It is less clear if urticaria is associated with other viral infections. The causal relationship of hepatitis B and chronic urticaria is unclear. In one study, 2.4% of patients with chronic urticaria were found to have circulating HgBsAg, while 15.3% had HgBsAb; both figures are greater than the percentage of the general population with circulating HgBsAg and HgBsAb.[55]

In the past, UAE was thought to be associated with a wide variety of other infections. In some series, patients with chronic UAE have been shown to have a high incidence of focal infections, although treatment of these infections has usually not altered the urticaria.[53] Association with candida infections appears to be coincidental in most cases.

Rarely, urticaria is a manifestation of immune complex mediated disease. Here the mechanism of urticaria is presumed to be the activation of the complement pathway by the immune complexes, leading to the generation of C3a and especially the potent C5a, which induce mast cells to degranulate and release histamine. UAE can occasionally be associated with the connective tissue diseases. Acute urticaria from a transfusion reaction is also probably due to circulating immune complexes. Biopsies on a series of patients with chronic UAE have revealed underlying vasculitis in a range from 2 to 52% of patients, with most authors supporting the lower number.[56] On the other hand, if one looks at a series of patients with hypersensitivity vasculitis, approximately 12% will have urticaria, but most of these patients have associated palpable purpura.[57] Very rarely, therefore, is urticaria the presenting sign of vasculitis.[57]

Zeiss et al. have described a rare disorder termed hypocomplementemic urticarial vasculitis.[58] Patients have hypersensitivity vasculitis, urticaria with occasionally severe laryngeal edema, arthralgias, arthritis, and low complement values. Typically, Clq is very low, and Clr and Cls are normal. C4, C2, and C3 are generally also low. Recently a 7S protein that may be IgG and that precipitates with Clq has been found associated with the disease.[58]

A variety of neoplasms, particularly lymphomas, have been causally associated with UAE, although the common appearance of both necessitates consideration of a coincidental association. Some neoplasms have recently been associated with an acquired deficiency of Cl esterase inhibitor, resulting in angioedema.[53] Like patients with hypocomplementemic vasculitis syndrome but unlike those with hereditary angioedema, these patients usually also have decreased Clq levels.[59]

Hyper- and, rarely, hypothyroidism have been associated with urticaria. Frequently, UAE in women is exacerbated the week before and during their menses. Whether hormonal factors cause or just exacerbate urticaria is unclear. There is at least one well documented case of anaphylactic reactions from endogenous progesterone.[60]

Physical factors will also induce UAE in susceptible patients. About 2 to 5% of the population has dermatographism. Stroking the skin, particularly of the back, in these patients will induce a wheal and flare formation. Although this may be due to mechanical disruption of the mast cells, it can in some cases be transferred by IgE.

Pressure-induced urticaria is unique, since the UAE occurs 4 to 6 hours after the inciting stimulus. The swelling can be painful and is often accompanied by systemic symptoms of fever, chills, and arthralgias. A leukocytosis can also occur.

Vibratory angioedema can occur after a strong vibratory stimulus such as a jack hammer. It can be hereditary (inherited as autosomal dominant) or sporadic.[54]

Temperature change, both cold and hot, can induce UAE. Cold can induce a variety of symptoms.[61] Idiopathic cold UAE occurs in exposed skin. These patients have a positive ice cube test, in which a wheal and flare develop on the skin after 10 minutes of exposure to an ice cube. Cold urticaria can also be seen in patients with cryoglobulins and, rarely, cryofibrinogens. If these are present, the patient should be investigated more closely for the presence of malignancy or connective tissue disease. Cold-dependent dermatographism has also been described, in which skin stroked at room temperature shows no reaction but will develop a wheal and flare if the patient subsequently enters a cold environment.

Systemic cold urticaria is the development of systemic urticaria after exposure to cold. Unlike in idiopathic cold urticaria, there is usually no urticaria on the particular areas of skin exposed to the cold, and the ice cube test is negative. Cold-induced "cholinergic" urticaria is urticaria resembling the small punctate hives of true cholinergic urticaria, induced by exercise in the cold. Exposure to cold temperature or exercise alone does not result in this type of urticaria.

A very rare syndrome of familial cold urticaria has been described in which cold exposure leads to burning papular eruptions associated with systemic symptoms and a negative ice cube test.

Cholinergic urticaria occurs after a hot shower, exercise, anxiety, or anything that raises core body temperature. The resultant punctate lesions are small compared to those of cold and other types of urticaria. The lesions can be reproduced in a sensitive patient by the injection of 0.01 mg of methacholine in 0.05 ml saline intradermally.[54] Satellite wheals will surround the area of injection in a positive reaction. There is a high rate of false negative reactions. If a patient exercises in an occlusive suit to bring on cholinergic urticaria, airway obstruction will also be noted.[62] Cholinergic urticaria presenting during exercise needs to be differentiated from exercise-induced anaphylaxis. In cholinergic urticaria, the wheals are smaller.

Light can also induce UAE in the sensitive patient. Different groups of patients react to different wavelengths of light. In certain groups of patients the reaction appears to be IgE antibody mediated, although the exact mechanism is unknown. Erythropoietic protoporphyria, a genetic abnormality in protoporphyrin IX metabolism, results in the solar sensitivity. This can be diagnosed by abnormal protoporphyrin levels in red cells or feces.

Aquagenic urticaria is very rare. When water comes in contact with skin at room temperature, tiny hives develop at the area of contact. The lesions can usually be duplicated in the sensitive patient by placing a wet towel on the arm at 27° for 30 minutes.

Urticaria pigmentosum is a benign disorder in which pigmented lesions on the skin that are full of mast cells urticate when stroked (Darier's sign).

A hereditary disorder has been described consisting of chronic urticaria, deafness, and amyloidosis.

The syndrome of episodic angioedema, urticaria, fever, and leukocytosis with prominent eosinophilia is discussed in the section on eosinophilia.[63]

Finally, psychogenic factors clearly play a role in urticaria. Whether they are directly causal or just exacerbate the reaction is unclear. All physicians have seen urticaria flare with stress or resolve when psychosocial factors were resolved. The mechanism may be stimulation of the mast cells by the cholinergic nervous system.

Hereditary angioedema (HAE) is an autosomal dominant disorder that results in angioedema without urticaria or pruritis. A few cases have been described without a family history or obvious neoplasm, suggesting possible genetic mutations. Although there is usually an early onset of symptoms, some patients will present in adulthood. Unlike other forms of angioedema, HAE results from a deficiency of the inhibitor of C1 esterase (Fig. 3–4). When the complement path-

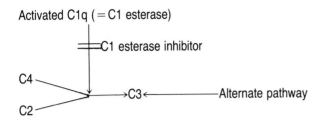

Fig. 3–4. Deficiency of C1 esterase inhibitor in hereditary angio-edema.

Table 3–21. Differential Diagnosis of Conjunctivitis

Allergic conjunctivitis
Atopic keratoconjunctivitis
Vernal conjunctivitis
Contact lens-associated conjunctivitis
Contact dermatoconjunctivitis
Bacterial or viral conjunctivitis
Herpes simplex keratoconjunctivitis
Seborrheic blepharitis
Kertatoconjunctivitis sicca

way is stimulated, the decreased inhibitor level allows the reaction to progress without sufficient regulation. It is now believed that bradykinin, generated during the reaction, may be the substance that causes the swelling.[64] Episodes are frequently precipitated by trauma. During an episode, C1 esterase inhibitor is low, along with C4 and C2, its substrates. In about 15% of the cases, C1 esterase inhibitor is quantitatively normal but functionally abnormal and needs to be measured by a functional assay. Between attacks, only C1 esterase inhibitor and C4 are low.

The angioedema that results from this reaction occurs in the usual locations but also involves the upper respiratory tract, including the larynx and the GI tract.

The diagnosis is usually obvious from the clinical presentation and family history. A CH_{50} should be abnormal, but it is usually helpful to check a C4 level as well. If these are normal, HAE is very unlikely. If the C4 is decreased, the C1 esterase inhibitor level should be checked. If the C1 esterase inhibitor level is normal, a functional assay of the inhibitor should be obtained. During the acute attack C2 will also be decreased. The Clq level is normal in HAE, whereas it may be decreased in certain tumors and in hypocomplementemic vasculitic syndrome.

CONJUNCTIVITIS

DEFINITION

Conjunctivitis is a common clinical problem.[65,65a] Patients usually present with a combination of erythema, irritation, burning, tearing, and, frequently, pruritus. These symptoms involve the conjunctiva covering the lid (palpebral conjunctiva) and the sclera up to the cornea. In conjunctivitis, both surfaces are usually equally affected—if the globe is redder than the lids the condition suggests iritis rather than conjunc-

tivitis. Conjunctivitis involves the dilation of small, snakelike conjunctival vessels that radiate towards the cornea in a halo fashion. Dilated vessels even larger and at right angles to the cornea suggest episcleritis. Dilated vessels that radiate out from the cornea, rather than towards it, are seen with uveitis. Because pure conjunctivitis does not involve the cornea, photophobia and blurred vision are not associated symptoms. Some disorders discussed below, however, can involve both the conjunctiva and the cornea.

PATHOPHYSIOLOGIC CONSIDERATIONS DIFFERENTIAL DIAGNOSIS

The pathophysiology is varied depending on the cause (Table 3–21). Allergic conjunctivitis is the result of an antigen binding to IgE on the surface of a mast cell in the conjunctiva and inducing it to degranulate, releasing a variety of mediators, notably histamine. This action results in pruritus, as well as vasodilation of the palpebral and scleral conjunctiva. If severe, as in the case of cat allergy, for example, the conjunctiva can become edematous (chemosis) and can look like clear jelly covering the sclera. One factor that helps distinguish allergic conjunctivitis from other causes is its frequent association with allergic rhinitis and its frequent seasonal occurrence.

Atopic keratoconjunctivitis, a severe disease, occurs in patients with atopic dermatitis (eczema). The exact pathogenesis is unknown. Although in mild forms it can be confused with allergic conjunctivitis, it is associated with atopic dermatitis rather than rhinitis and there is no associated exposure history. The pruritus tends to be very pronounced in this disorder. In addition to the conjunctiva involvement, the lids are often swollen and lichenified. Tearing is prominent and eventually the cornea can be involved with vascularization. In mild forms it can be confused with allergic conjunctivitis. Both can be associated with atopic dermatitis, though atopic keratoconjunctivitis more frequently and without the rhinitis that accompanies allergic conjunctivitis. However, with atopic keratoconjunctivitis there is no associated exposure history, as there is with allergic conjunctivitis.

Vernal conjunctivitis occurs mainly in children younger than age 14. Three out of four affected patients are male. The pathogenesis is unclear, although the disorder appears to be associated with atopy and is most common in warm climates and seasons. Vernal conjunctivitis can be either palpebral or limbal; both forms are associated with intense pruritus and, usually, photophobia. In the palpebral form, giant papillae develop on the superior palpebral conjunctiva, resulting in a cobblestone appearance on examination. A thick ropy discharge can be pulled from the eye in long strings. In the limbal form, gelatinous masses occur at the scleral-cornea junction. White dots (Trantas' dots) composed of eosinophils are diagnostic. This form occurs more frequently in the nonwhite population. In either form, a scraping of the conjunctiva showing more than two eosinophils per high power field is diagnostic.

Contact lens–associated conjunctivitis can look very similar to vernal conjunctivitis, with giant papillary hypertrophy and thick mucus, but pruritus is much less prominent. It can occur with hard or soft lenses and is thought to be an immune reaction to an allergen imbedded in the lens or to the thimerosal or other preservatives in the disinfecting solution.

Conjunctivitis can also be seen as a manifestation of contact dermatitis. As such it occurs most commonly from topical eye medications, especially antibiotics. Erythema, burning, mild pruritus, and follicular hypertrophy can result. With contactants encountered outside the eye—for example, poison ivy, nail polish, or cosmetics—the eyelid will be erythematous and indurated and will show an eczematous reaction, which can then extend to the conjunctiva.

Viral conjunctivitis is very common. Presenting symptoms are usually erythema, burning, and tearing. Significant pruritus is less common. Follicular hyperplasia, which needs to be differentiated from vernal conjunctivitis by slit lamp examination, can result.

Herpes simplex keratoconjunctivitis presents like viral conjunctivitis but is usually more severe and can involve the cornea, with photophobia, blurred vision, and the presence of dendritic ulcers.

Bacterial conjunctivitis, especially with Staphylococcus aureus, also causes erythema and burning, but there is usually a purulent mucus discharge that will glue the eyes closed, experienced especially upon awakening. Pruritus is not usually associated.

Seborrheic blepharitis is usually associated with seborrheic dermatitis elsewhere. The margins of the eye are scaly and swollen. If they become secondarily infected with S. aureus, the conjunctiva may be involved. There is usually no pruritus.

Keratoconjunctivitis sicca in its early stages can be difficult to differentiate from other types of conjunctivitis. Symptoms are erythema, irritation, mucus discharge, photophobia, and a sense of dry eyes. Corneal epithelial damage can be seen on slit lamp examination, and the decreased lacrimation can be evaluated by Schirmer's test (decreased tear formation leads to decreased wetting of the test strip). Frequently the eye symptoms are accompanied by a dry mouth and arthritis associated with Sjögren's syndrome.

DIAGNOSTIC EVALUATION

As with all allergic diseases, the history is very important in evaluating conjunctivitis. Questions should be asked regarding duration (acute or chronic), appearance (perennial or seasonal), associated diseases (atopic dermatitis, seborrhea), and symptoms (rhinitis, dry mouth). Besides taking the history, noting the symptoms and signs outlined on Table 3–22 is helpful in making the diagnosis. Pruritus is a major distinguishing feature, along with the nature of the discharge and involvement of the cornea. In many cases, especially if the cornea is involved, the patient should be referred to an ophthalmologist for slit lamp examination to confirm the diagnosis. If the diagnosis appears to be allergic conjunctivitis, skin testing (as discussed in the section on anaphylaxis) can determine which antigen is responsible. If a contactant is suspected, patch testing with the suspected antigen can be performed.

RHINITIS

DEFINITION

Rhinitis is a general term referring to symptoms of nasal congestion and rhinorrhea.[66] These may be associated with pruritus and sneezing. The rhinitis may occur alone or in association with conjunctival, sinus, middle ear, or pulmonary disease.

PATHOPHYSIOLOGIC CONSIDERATIONS

Symptoms result from inflammation of the nasal mucosa, vasodilation, edema, and increased mucus secretion. These symptoms can be caused by an allergic reaction resulting in the release of vasoactive mediators, by an infection resulting in inflammation, or by a variety of nonspecific mechanisms including,

Table 3–22.   Signs and Symptoms Associated with Conjunctivitis

Sign/Symptom	Disease Association
Pruritus	
Mild	Contact lens–associated conjunctivitis
Moderate	Allergic rhinitis
Severe	Contact dermatoconjunctivitis
	Atopic keratoconjunctivitis
	Vernal conjunctivitis
Burning	Vernal conjunctivitis
	Herpes simplex conjunctivitis
Scratchy sensation	Keratoconjunctivitis sicca
	Acute viral conjunctivitis
Erythema	Allergic rhinitis
	Atopic keratoconjunctivitis
	Contact dermatographism
	Keratoconjunctivitis sicca
	Chronic Staphylococcus aureus infection
Edema (chemosis)	Allergic rhinitis
Lid swelling	Allergic rhinitis
	Atopic keratoconjunctivitis
	Contact dermatoconjunctivitis
Scales along lid margin	Seborrheic blepharitis
	Chronic Staphylococcus aureus infection
Discharge	
Watery	Allergic rhinitis
	Herpes simplex conjunctivitis
Purulent	Acute viral conjunctivitis
	Contact dermatoconjunctivitis
	Bacterial conjunctivitis
	Contact lens-associated conjunctivitis
	Keratoconjunctivitis sicca
Thick ropy strands	Vernal conjunctivitis
Cobblestone appearance of upper palpebral conjunctiva	Vernal conjunctivitis
Photophobia	Atopic keratoconjunctivitis with corneal involvement
	Vernal conjunctivitis with corneal involvement
	Herpes simplex conjunctivitis/uveitis
	Uveitis
Blurred vision	Herpes simplex conjunctivitis/uveitis
Unilateral symptoms	Allergic rhinitis due to contact with allergen
	Contact dermatoconjunctivitis

possibly, enhanced reactivity to stress of the autonomic nervous system, environmental changes, or inhaled irritants.

DIAGNOSTIC EVALUATION

As discussed in the section on conjunctivitis, the history is very important. Questions should be asked regarding duration (acute or chronic), appearance (perennial or seasonal), associated problems (e.g., sinus, pulmonary, hypothyroid, lack of menses), and use of medication or "recreational" drugs (e.g., cocaine). The physical exam may reveal the presence of enlarged turbinates, polyps, masses, or signs of disease elsewhere. Examination of the nasal mucus may reveal the predominant presence of eosinophils (indicating allergic or nonallergic rhinitis with eosinophilia) or polymorphonuclear cells (indicating chronic rhinitis). If the diagnosis appears to be allergic rhinitis, skin testing (as discussed in the section on anaphylaxis) can determine which antigen is responsible.

The examination of the nose is important in determining the presence of nasal polyps but is less so in differentiating allergic from infectious and chronic causes of the rhinitis. The turbinates, especially the easily visible inferior turbinates, are enlarged in most cases of rhinitis. Classically, it has been taught that pale bluish turbinates were caused by allergy, and erythematous "boggy" turbinates, by infection. Although this guideline is still useful, many overlapping cases

Table 3–23. Differential Diagnosis of Rhinitis

Acute
  Allergy
  Viral infection
Chronic
  Seasonal
  Perennial
    Allergic
    Nasal mastocytosis
    Nonallergic rhinitis with eosinophilia
    Nonallergic rhinitis
      Idiopathic
      Exaggerated physiologic response to
        Stress
        Exercise
        Temperature changes
        Humidity
        Strong odors
        Inhaled particulate matter
      Anatomic
        Nasal polyps
        Deviated nasal septum
        Enlarged tonsils and adenoids
        Cerebrospinal fluid leak
      Endocrine
        Pregnancy
        Hypothyroidism
        Ovarian hormonal changes
      Medications
        Cocaine
        Beta blockers
        Reserpine derivatives
        Hydralazine
        Abuse of nasal decongestants (rhinitis medicamentosum)
      Granulomatous disease
        Sarcoidosis
        Wegener's granulomatosis
        Midline granuloma
      Other
        Kartagener's syndrome
        Cystic fibrosis

will occur. The physical examination, especially trans-illumination, is not reliable in diagnosing the presence of sinus disease; radiographs or a CT scan should be obtained if this disorder is considered. Examination of the ears may reveal associated otitis media.

Acute self-limited episodes of rhinitis usually present no problem in diagnosis if, along with a physical examination, a careful history is taken regarding the circumstances surrounding the episode and the factors effecting its relief. Acute episodes are most frequently due to allergy or viral infections (Table 3–23). Acute allergic rhinitis is likely to be associated with conjunctival edema and pruritus of the nose and, occasionally, of the eyes, soft palate, and external ear canals. The nasal discharge is usually clear. A viral infection, on the other hand, is frequently associated with a sore throat, inflamed pharynx, and enlarged, tender anterior cervical lymph nodes. The nasal discharge is often cloudy or frankly purulent. Both disorders can be associated with sneezing. A useful test to distinguish between the two is a nasal smear showing the predominance of eosinophils or neutrophils. Eosinophils suggest allergy and neutrophils indicate inflammation and possibly infection.

The cause of chronic rhinitis is often more difficult to discern. It is helpful to determine if the problem is seasonal, in which case the cause is usually allergic, or perennial, in which case it may or may not be allergic. If perennial, a history of associated problems of sneezing, pruritus, and conjunctivitis, a history of association with any particular exposure, and a personal history of atopy suggest an allergic cause of the rhinitis. The diagnosis should be further established by intradermal skin testing looking for positive reactions to perennial allergens such as animals, molds, or dust mites. Allergy skin testing is discussed in detail in the section on anaphylaxis. A nasal smear showing a predominance of eosinophils over neutrophils is also helpful in determining the diagnosis.

A rare disorder, nasal mastocytosis, has been described. Patients present with all the symptoms of perennial allergic rhinitis but generally do not have skin test reactivity that correlates with their symptoms. The diagnosis is made by nasal biopsy, which shows increase in mastocytes.

If there is no history suggestive of atopy, and if eosinophils constitute more than 25% on the nasal smear, the diagnosis is most likely nonallergic rhinitis with eosinophilia (NARES).[66a] Whether this is a separate diagnostic entity is still unclear. The importance of diagnosing it lies primarily in predicting its better therapeutic response to corticosteroids, as compared with the response of chronic nonallergic rhinitis. Occasionally NARES may be associated with the presence of nasal polyps, with sinusitis, with asthma, and with aspirin sensitivity.

The remainder of cases of rhinitis are defined as perennial nonallergic rhinitis. Many cases are idiopathic, but a large number of factors need to be considered in the differential diagnosis (Table 3–23).

Patients will frequently complain of increased nasal congestion during times of stress or increased emotional lability, for example, while crying. Nasal congestion and profuse, watery rhinorrhea are also seen with exercise and with changes in temperature and humidity. Exposure to strong odors, such as perfumes, oil based paints, or insecticide sprays, may result in the same symptoms. Inhalation of particulate matter such as cigarette smoke or dust may also cause rhinitis. The common mechanism in this group of patients is thought to be enhanced adrenergic sensitivity, with parasympathetic activity dominating. In the case of inhalation of smoke or dust, this is probably more likely than true allergy (i.e., an IgE antibody mediated reaction) to be the mechanism.

Mechanical factors such as a deviated nasal septum or significant polyposis can lead to rhinitis symptoms. The syndrome of aspirin sensitivity, rhinosinusitis, and asthma is discussed in detail in the section on aspirin.

If the rhinorrhea is unilateral, a break in the cribriform plate with a leak of cerebrospinal fluid (CSF) should always be considered in the diagnosis and can be tested by analyzing the nasal mucus for glucose using the dipstick method. If glucose is present, CSF has leaked, since nasal mucus normally contains none. Rarely, lacrimal fluid will confuse this differentiation, as it also has glucose.

A variety of hormonal states are associated with rhinitis, including rhinitis of pregnancy and hypothyroidism.

Medications should always be suspected as possible causes. Cocaine abuse can frequently lead to rhinitis. Beta blockers can also cause rhinitis, as can reserpine and hydralazine.

Frequent use/abuse of topical vasoconstrictor nose sprays can lead to a rebound congestion phenomenon and rhinitis medicamentosa.

Rarely, rhinitis will be the presenting symptoms of granulomatosus diseases including sarcoidosis and, especially, Wegener's granulomatosis and midline granuloma. Biopsy should be performed on any suspicious mass or polyp that continues to enlarge.

Rhinitis is seen in conjunction with Kartagener's syndrome (situs inversus, bronchiectasis, and rhinosinusitis). It is also seen with cystic fibrosis, although very rarely as a sole symptom; most patients have associated pulmonary symptoms. Diagnosis of cystic fibrosis is made by obtaining an abnormal sodium chloride sweat test.

SHORTNESS OF BREATH WITH WHEEZING (ASTHMA)

DEFINITION AND PATHOPHYSIOLOGIC CONSIDERATIONS

The basic defect in asthma is hyper-reactivity of the bronchi to a variety of factors that elicit no reaction in normal airways.[67] This results in smooth muscle contraction and bronchoconstriction, which, by definition, reverses either spontaneously or as a result of

treatment. If the bronchi remain constricted they tend to become inflamed and produce quantities of mucus. This effect adds to the morbidity of the reaction and, if severe, can lead to mucus plugging of the airway, air trapping, and ventilation perfusion mismatch. As a result of these changes, patients experience a sense of weight or tightness in the chest, shortness of breath with particular difficulty in expiring air, a wheezing sound especially on expiration, and, often, a prominent cough. This reaction can be acute or chronic. The physical examination may reveal tachypnea with a prolonged expiratory phase, use of accessory muscles in respiration, hyperinflation of the chest, decreased expiratory breath sounds, and wheezing on auscultation. Further evaluation usually reveals sputum and serum eosinophilia, chest hyperinflation on radiography, and evidence of an obstructive defect on pulmonary function testing.

The reason for the underlying bronchial hyper-reactivity is not completely clear. Genetic predisposition is clearly a factor, although twin studies showing low concordance suggest that environmental factors are also important. Current data support a possible imbalance in the adrenergic (bronchodilation) and cholinergic or parasympathetic (bronchoconstriction) nervous systems. The cholinergic system may predominate by increased innervation or activity of nerves in the pulmonary and other smooth muscle tissue, resulting in increased bronchial tone. It has also been suggested that asthmatic patients may have a partial blockade of the beta adrenergic (sympathetic) system, resulting in decreased bronchodilation. Though this effect probably exists, it may be a matter of degree, as experimentally induced beta blockade in normal subjects does not result in bronchoconstriction.[68,69] In atopic subjects, allergen-induced release of pharmacologically active mediators in the airways results in bronchoconstriction and inflammation.

The factors that can trigger an asthma attack are numerous and diverse (Table 3–24). Allergens are one of the most prominent factors. It was thought not long ago that all asthma was due to allergies. Although clearly this is not the case, allergy nevertheless plays a significant role in about 35 to 55% of cases of asthma.[67] In general, asthma in juveniles has a significant allergic component, whereas new onset asthma in adults over age 35 rarely involves significant allergies.

As discussed in the section on anaphylaxis, antigen binds with IgE antibody located on the surface of a mast cell or basophil and thus induces the cell to release a variety of pharmacologically active factors. Histamine and, especially, the leukotrienes can induce bronchoconstriction. This mechanism is discussed in detail

Table 3–24. Factors Affecting Asthma

Allergens including allergic bronchopulmonary aspergillosis
Viral infections
Drugs
   Allergy
   Aspirin/tartrazine/nonsteroidal anti-inflammatory drug intolerance
   Sulfite sensitivity
   Pharmacologic effects (e.g., beta adrenergic antagonists)
Exercise
Cholinergic stimulation
Occupational exposure
Nonspecific irritants (e.g., strong odors, cigarette smoke)
Changes in temperature and humidity
Sinusitis
Gastroesophageal reflux
Psychosocial factors

Table 3–25. Diagnostic Features of Allergic Bronchopulmonary Aspergillosis (ABPA)

Asthma
Positive sputum culture for Aspergillus fumigatus (nondiagnostic and may not be present)
Expectoration of brown mucus plugs
Pulmonary infiltrates (can be fleeting or permanent, usually in the upper lobes)
Proximal (central) bronchiectasis
Eosinophilia (usually > 1000/ng/ml) (can be normal in patient on corticosteroids or in remission)
Elevated IgE level (usually > 1000/ng/ml) (increased in 75% of patients)
Skin test reactivity to Aspergillus fumigatus
   Immediate (20 minutes; occurs in 100% of cases of ABPA, 4% of normal patients, 25% of asthmatic patients without ABPA, 25% of patients with aspergilloma, and 39% of patients with cystic fibrosis)
   Late (3 to 6 hours; occurs in 33% of patients)
Ratio of serum IgE and IgG reactivity to Aspergillus fumigatus (as measured by RIA or ELISA and compared with asthmatic patients sensitive to molds[75])
IgG antibody in serum specific for Aspergillus fumigatus
   ("precipitating antibody" as determined by double gel diffusion; occurs in 100% of patients with ABPA, 3 to 6% of normal patients, 25% of asthmatic patients without ABPA, 100% of patients with aspergilloma, and 31% of patients with cystic fibrosis)

(Adapted from Halwig, J.M., Greenberger, P.A., and Patterson, R.: Allergic Bronchopulmonary Aspergillosis. Immunol Allergy Practice 6:292, 1984.)

in the section on anaphylaxis. Generally only allergens smaller than 10 μ induce asthma, possibly because they can reach the smaller airways. Allergic asthma is frequently seasonal, caused by tree and grass pollen in the spring and ragweed, other weeds, and mold in the fall (depending on location). In these cases it is generally associated with rhinitis. It can also be due to exposure to animals, other environmental allergens such as dust mites (which may result in perennial symptoms), or a wide variety of less common substances.

In most cases the bronchoconstriction resulting from antigen exposure occurs within the first 30 minutes. In some patients pulmonary function returns to baseline, and then, 4 to 12 hours after the initial antigen exposure, bronchospasm develops again—the late phase reaction. There are certain notable differences between the two reactions.[70] Like the immediate phase, the late phase reaction appears to be mediated by IgE antibody and factors released from mast cells, although the factors and/or exact mechanisms probably differ. The nature of the infiltrates also differs, since the immediate phase is associated with a predominantly eosinophilic cell infiltrate, and the 4- to 6-hour or late phase reaction is associated with a mixed cell infiltrate of lymphocytes, neutrophils, and eosinophils. Corticosteroids inhibit the late phase but not the immediate phase reaction. It is currently theorized that the late phase reaction may be due to release of mediators from mast cells, which then recruit neutrophils and eosinophils to the area. These cells may then cause the reaction in an as yet unknown manner.[71] The importance of this reaction in asthma is gaining increasing recognition, especially as a cause of persistent increased airway reactivity and symptoms beyond the time of antigen exposure.[71] This late phase response has also been noted in exercise-induced asthma.[72]

Allergic bronchopulmonary aspergillosis (ABPA) is a result of hypersensitivity to the fungus Aspergillus

fumigatus.[73,74] The pathogenesis is due to IgE and IgG antibodies specific for the fungus reacting with it in the lung. Most frequently, the clinical presentation is an asthmatic patient with fever, cough occasionally productive of brown plugs of mucus, pulmonary infiltrates, proximal bronchiectasis, eosinophilia, and evidence of immune reactivity to aspergillus. Many signs and symptoms are associated with ABPA (Table 3–25), though none of them are specific for ABPA. Because all patients have immediate skin test reactivity, skin testing should be used as a screening test. If it is negative, ABPA is unlikely. If it is positive, further evaluation should be done, as the reaction is very nonspecific. Since there is no one sign, symptom, or test that is diagnostic, the presence of a number of abnormal findings need to be documented before the diagnosis of ABPA can be made (Table 3–25).

Viral respiratory infections are also a major trigger of asthma attacks. The exact mechanism of this reaction is not known, but interestingly, IgE antibody specific for respiratory syncytial virus has been noted in the airways of patients with this infection and may play some role in the pathogenesis.[76] Bacterial infections have rarely been noted to cause flares of asthma.[76]

A wide variety of drugs induce or otherwise affect asthma. Aspirin and sulfite sensitivity are discussed in those respective sections. Beta adrenergic antagonist drugs (including timolol maleate eye drops) can induce bronchospasm in susceptible patients. Exercise will clearly induce asthma in certain patients, as has been discussed.

A number of occupational exposures are also associated with asthma.[67] For example, cotton workers can develop byssinosis. This is thought to be due to the nonspecific release of histamine by cotton dust. Workers in the detergent industry used to develop asthma from exposure to the Bacillus subtilis enzyme. Meat wrappers exposed to the plastic used to wrap meat in supermarkets have also been noted to develop asthma. Workers exposed to Western red cedar can develop asthma from plicatic acid. Two chemicals widely used in the production of plastics and other synthetics and shown to cause asthma are trimellitic anhydride (TMA) and toluene diisocyanate (TDI). The former is responsible for a variety of syndromes including rhinitis, asthma, and a flulike illness.

Nonspecific irritants such as cigarette smoke and strong odors like paint or perfume clearly cause flares of asthma in susceptible patients. The mechanism appears to be non-IgE mediated. Air pollution may be a nonspecific irritant, or the reaction may be due to SO_2 sensitivity in some cases (see Additive section). Changes in both temperature and humidity affect many patients with asthma. Most patients are worse on cold, dry days.

There is some data to suggest that sinusitis and gastrointestinal reflux can also adversely affect asthma.[77]

Lastly, it is clear that the emotional state of the patient plays a large role in asthma. Attacks can be precipitated not only by stress or crying, but also by laughter. The mechanism is probably vagal stimulation resulting in bronchial smooth muscle contraction.[67] Hyperventilation may also be a factor.

DIFFERENTIAL DIAGNOSIS AND DIAGNOSTIC EVALUATION

In evaluating the patient with asthma, the history is important, as noted especially to document precipitating factors. Usually dyspnea and wheezing are present, although their absence does not rule out asthma. It is clear in some patients that chronic cough can be the sole presenting symptom. In a series of patients with chronic cough, 25% were diagnosed as having asthma and another 18% as having postnasal drip and asthma.[78] In these cases, the diagnosis is made by abnormal and reversible pulmonary function tests or bronchial challenge testing.

Rarely, the presence of a foreign body or tumor in the chest can lead to dyspnea and possibly wheezing. If the history and physical exam do not distinguish these disorders from asthma, a chest radiograph should be obtained, which should show the former if it is not radiolucent but should be clear in the case of asthma.

The physical examination reveals neck muscle retraction in severe cases and a decreased inspiratory:expiratory ratio, decreased expiratory breath sounds, and wheezing. It has been repeatedly demonstrated, however, that physicians have difficulty determining the severity of asthma from the physical exam. The most reliable test for diagnosis is pulmonary function testing. McFadden noted that when a group of patients with asthma were asymptomatic but still had signs of asthma, their pulmonary function tests were at 40 to 50% of the predicted normal, and that when there were no physical signs of asthma, the tests were still at 60 to 70% of the predicted normal.[79] Many parameters of air flow can be measured from the maximal mid-expiratory flow rate (MMEFR) to the peak flow rate. The latter, although a grosser measurement of flow in large airways, is nevertheless very useful, especially when asthma is severe. In all except very severe cases, one expects to see some reversibility (frequently defined for study purposes as a 20% improvement in the forced expiratory volume in one second [FEV1]) with bronchodilators. If nonreversible obstruction is present, other causes of chronic obstruction should be considered. Asthma, however, should not be totally ruled out. A trial of medications for asthma is often warranted.

If asthma is suspected but pulmonary function testing is normal, bronchial challenge testing should be done. The reagents most commonly used are histamine and methacholine. All asthmatic subjects will have a bronchoconstrictive response to low concentrations of these agents as compared to normal subjects. Short-term reactivity to methacholine can result from several factors causing temporary airway irritability, such as aspiration of a foreign body, a severe upper respiratory infection, chronic bronchitis, and occasionally sarcoidosis or cystic fibrosis. Patients who experience a late phase reaction to an allergen also tend to have heightened methacholine reactivity for at least a week after the challenge.

A chest radiograph is very useful if the diagnosis of asthma is in doubt or if pneumonia, atelectasis, or a foreign body or tumor is suspected as causing a flare of asthma. If the diagnosis is not in doubt and there are no signs upon examination to suggest a further lung disorder, a radiograph is probably unnecessary; it is usually normal or shows only hyperinflation with severe asthma.

Eosinophils are elevated in the sputum and blood of patients with asthma, regardless of the cause. They can also be seen in chronic bronchitis and allergic angiitis with granulomatosis. Because they are not prominent in congestive heart failure or factitious asthma, eosinophils may help differentiate asthma from these disorders. Large numbers of eosinophils in the sputum can turn it yellow (hence yellow sputum is not necessarily a sign of infection).

Serum IgE levels are also not very useful. If significantly elevated they suggest an allergic component to the asthma, a determination that is in any case nearly always obvious from the history. Patients with significant allergies contributing to their asthma can, however, have normal total IgE levels. Very elevated IgE levels can be useful in diagnosing allergic bronchopulmonary aspergillosis.

The differential diagnosis of asthma includes infectious processes. Infiltrates will usually be seen on chest radiographs in these cases, and patients may have fever and leukocytosis, neither of which is seen in asthma. Other types of chronic obstructive pulmonary disease need to be considered. Chronic bronchitis with inflamed airways and mucosal edema can be difficult to distinguish from pure asthma, as both can be associated with similar symptoms, although shortness of breath is less common with chronic bronchitis. Wheezing can be present in both and is not a reliable differentiating feature. In chronic bronchitis the sputum generally contains polymorphonuclear cells rather than eosinophils. Pulmonary function testing may show some obstruction, which usually does not significantly reverse with bronchodilators. Additionally there is no air trapping. Bronchiectasis is diagnosed by history and also by chest radiographs and computed tomography. This will be normal in the case of asthma.

Allergic angiitis and granulomatosis (Churg-Strauss syndrome) can on rare occasions be confused with asthma because wheezing can be present in both. In the former, the disorder is due to vasculitis. Usually there is systemic involvement, possibly preceded by lung symptoms for 2 years. Features distinguishing Churg-Strauss syndrome from asthma include pulmonary infiltrates, eosinophilia, and an elevated erythrocyte sedimentation rate.

Factitious asthma should also occasionally be considered in the differential diagnosis.[80,81] In this disorder, wheezing is usually loudest over the neck, and there is no increase in alveolar-arterial oxygen tension or hyperinflation on chest radiograph. Pulmonary function testing is normal and frequently there is a history of psychiatric disorders.

Congestive heart failure is also confused with asthma, especially in the patient who wakes short of breath in the middle of the night. A thorough examination of cardiac function, examination of the chest for rales at the time of symptoms, and evaluation of therapeutic response to medications is helpful in differentiating the two disorders.

SHORTNESS OF BREATH WITH COUGH, FEVER, AND MALAISE (HYPERSENSITIVITY PNEUMONITIS)

DEFINITION

Shortness of breath with cough, fever, and malaise caused by hypersensitivity pneumonitis (HP), also known as extrinsic allergic alveolitis, can present as an acute, subacute, or chronic pulmonary disease.[82-85] It is caused by immune reactivity to large amounts of inhaled organic dusts. Initially only the terminal bronchioles and alveoli are involved. Duration of symptoms is usually associated with the length and amount of exposure.

In the acute form, previously healthy patients experience a relatively sudden onset (about 4 to 6 hours after exposure) of dyspnea without wheezing, cough, fever, malaise, and weakness. If the exposure is limited, the signs and symptoms spontaneously subside rapidly without treatment. If exposure is recurrent or mild, onset of these signs and symptoms is generally more insidious. If the exposure is mild and frequent, the patient may only have pulmonary symptoms. If it is more severe, systemic signs and symptoms of fever, anorexia, weight loss, and malaise may be prominent along with the pulmonary symptoms. If the entity remains undiagnosed and exposure remains constant or recurrent for a long time (generally years), fibrosis and resultant pulmonary insufficiency can result.

PATHOPHYSIOLOGIC CONSIDERATIONS

The disorder is a result of an immune reaction to an inhaled organic dust. The list of implicated antigens (Table 3–26) is long, but most are rare with the exception of the Thermophilic actinomycetes, which can be found in many places, from moldy hay (Farmer's lung) to forced air systems. The exact nature of the immune reaction is not clear but probably involves both IgG antibody, possibly forming local immune complex reactions at the level of the terminal bronchioles and alveoli, and a cell mediated immune response. IgG antibody specific for the antigen can be demonstrated not only in the serum of patients but also

Table 3-26. Agents of Hypersensitivity Pneumonitis

Agent	Exposure	Disease
Thermophilic actinomycetes		
Micropolyspora faeni	Moldy compost	Farmer's lung
Thermoactinomyces sacchari	Moldy sugar cane	Bagassosis
Thermoactinomyces vulgaris	Moldy compost	Mushroom worker's lung
Thermoactinomyces viridis		
Thermoactinomyces candidus	Contaminated forced air systems	Ventilation pneumonitis
Fungi		
Alternaria species	Moldy wood chips	Wood worker's lung
Pullularia pullulans	Moldy redwood dust	Sequoiosis
Aspergillus clavatus	Moldy malt	Malt worker's lung
Penicillium frequentans	Moldy work dust	Suberosis
Penicillium caseii	Cheese mold	Cheese worker's lung
Penicillium roqueforti		
Phoma species	Moldy shower curtain	Shower curtain lung
Mucor stolonifer	Paprika dust	Paprika splitter's lung
Cryptostroma corticale	Moldy maple bark	Maple bark stripper's disease
Animal proteins		
Avian proteins	Avian droppings	Bird breeder's lung
Bovine and porcine	Heterologous proteins	Pituitary snuff user's lung
Rodent urinary proteins	Rodent urine	Laboratory animal worker's lung
Arthropods		
Sitophilus grainarius	Infested wheat	Wheat weevil lung
Chemicals		
Phthalic anhydride	Epoxy resin	Epoxy resin worker's lung
Toluene diisocyanate	Paint catalyst	Porcelain refinisher's lung
Trimellitic anhydride	Trimellitic anhydride	Plastic worker's lung
Other agents		
Ameba, various fungi	Contaminated systems	Ventilation pneumonitis
Bacillus subtilis	Detergent enzymes	Enzyme worker's lung
Hair dust	Animal proteins	Furrier's lung
Coffee dust	?	Coffee worker's lung
Thatched roof dust	?	New Guinea lung

(From Fink, J.: Hypersensitivity pneumonitis. J Allergy Clin Immunol 74:1, 1984, with permission.)

in the serum of 50% of exposed but asymptomatic individuals, although generally at a lower titer.[82] The onset of the reaction 3 to 8 hours after exposure is suggestive of a local immune complex (Arthus) mediated reaction. Biopsies of lesions, however, while occasionally showing depositions of immunoglobulin or complement, do not show an expected vasculitis. There is also no evidence of complement activation. Instead, one usually sees a mononuclear infiltration suggesting a T-cell mediated reaction. Although lymphocytes are reactive in vitro, patients fail to demonstrate delayed sensitivity (T-cell mediated) reactions on skin testing.

Most likely the pathogenesis may involve a number of aspects of the immune system culminating in inflammation at the level of the terminal bronchiole and alveoli.

There is usually no bronchial constriction and hence no associated wheezing. If the exposure is constant, the inflammatory reaction eventually results in fibrosis.

DIFFERENTIAL DIAGNOSIS AND DIAGNOSTIC EVALUATION

The first and paramount step in the evaluation of a patient with suspected HP is to determine, by taking the patient's history, if there are any suspected exposures. Questions should be asked about the presence of air conditioners or forced air heating systems (Thermophilic actinomycetes) and about any unusual occupational exposure, such as to moldy compost (Thermophilic actinomycetes), malt (Aspergillus clavatus), cheese (Penicillium), or plastics (Trimellitic anhydride), or about exposure from hobbies, especially to birds such as pigeons or parakeets in the home (avian proteins) or work with epoxy resins.

The physical examination is usually not too revealing. Cyanosis and tachypnea may be noted. Acutely basilar end-inspiratory rales are present. Wheezing is not usually a feature.

Diagnostic findings are noted on Table 3-27. A

Table 3–27. Diagnostic Findings in Hypersensitivity Pneumonitis

Leukocytosis to 25,000
Eosinophilia to 10%
Polyclonal gammopathy except IgE
Detectable rheumatoid factor
Serum IgG specific for the antigen (also found in 50% of exposed asymptomatic individuals)
Skin test positivity (relevant antigens generally not available)
   Immediate (10 to 20 minutes)
   Late (3 to 8 hours)
   No delayed reaction (2 to 3 days)
In vitro tests demonstrative of lymphocyte reactivity to the antigen
Chest radiograph
   Acute—Normal or reticulonodular pattern in bases or patchy infiltrates
   Subacute and chronic—varied from infiltrates to diffuse fibrosis
Hypoxemia
Pulmonary function tests
   Obstructive pattern with acute episodes
   Restrictive with chronic disease
Bronchoalveolar lavage: Lymphocytosis to 65% (predominantly T cells[87]) and elevated protein
Lung biopsy: Predominant mononuclear cell infiltrate with granulomas and fibrosis seen in chronic disease

(Adapted from Fink, J.: Hypersensitivity pneumonitis. J Allergy Clin Immunol 74:1, 1984.)

leukocytosis, often with eosinophilia, is often seen, as is polyclonal gammopathy with a positive rheumatoid factor. If HP is suspected, one should analyze the serum for the presence of IgG antibody specific for the implicated antigen. This is usually done as a precipitation reaction in a gel; hence the name ''serum precipitans'' for the IgG. A number of laboratories offer HP ''screening panels'' that test for antibody against some of the Thermophilic actinomycetes and other organic dusts. This testing is limited by the fact that serum IgG specific for the antigen can be found in approximately 50% of exposed asymptomatic individuals. It is also limited by the lack of well-characterized antigens. A screening test using a crude preparation of the suspected antigen in a double gel diffusion is commonly performed.[85] In vitro research techniques such as lymphocyte blast transformation can offer evidence of cellular immune reactivity against an antigen, but again it is unclear if this in vitro reactivity can be correlated with the disease process.

As discussed, the chest radiograph in the acute case can be normal, show fine reticulonodular markings, or show patchy infiltrates most commonly in a basilar distribution. In the subacute and chronic forms, a variety of changes can be noted, from infiltrates to diffuse fibrosis with occasionally a honeycombing pattern.

In the acute episode, pulmonary function testing can show an obstructive defect, despite the lack of clinical signs of bronchoconstriction. Challenge studies show that both an early and late (4- to 6-hour) response can

occur (as discussed on the section on asthma). In the subacute and chronic forms a restrictive defect predominates that, if severe, can be associated with diminished diffusing capacity.

Bronchoscopy and lung biopsy will occasionally be necessary, not so much to establish a diagnosis of HP as to rule out other diagnostic possibilities. This is especially the case in patients with chronic disease or when there is no evidence of specific immune reactivity. The biopsy may reveal a mononuclear cell infiltrate around the terminal bronchioles, interstitium, and alveoli in early cases. Nonspecific granulomata and fibrosis can be seen in chronic cases. Bronchoalveolar lavage may be helpful, as the lavage has been shown to contain an increase in both lymphocytes and protein in patients with HP.[82,86] The predominant phenotypic marker on the lymphocytes is T8 (associated with suppressor activity).[87] Again, increases are also seen in exposed asymptomatic individuals.[87]

The only confirmatory test is an inhalation challenge with the implicated substance with a resultant reproduction of the symptom pattern. Because of the obvious drawback, inducing a significant illness again in a patient, all other reasonable attempts at diagnosis should be exhausted before inhalation challenge is considered.

The differential diagnosis is extensive. The rapid onset of pulmonary embolus may distinguish it from hypersensitivity pneumonitis. A ventilation perfusion scan will show a perfusion defect in the case of pulmonary embolus. Infection is a major consideration. Both infection and hypersensitivity pneumonitis can be associated with a leukocytosis, but HP can also have an eosinophilia to 10%. Usually, as discussed below, the chest radiograph will show nothing or a diffuse reticulonodular pattern, especially at the bases, as opposed to the more localized infiltrate commonly seen with infection, although patchy infiltrates can be seen in HP. Cultures are negative. HP is less frequently associated with fever and constitutional symptoms. If eosinophilia is present, Löffler's syndrome or other causes of pulmonary infiltrates with eosinophilia need to be considered. Subacute and chronic forms may imply chronic infection, causes of chronic eosinophilic pneumonias, drug reactions, sarcoidosis, immune complex mediated diseases (e.g., allergic angiitis with granulomatosis), malignancy, and the remainder of the large differential of interstitial pulmonary diseases.

SYSTEMIC PRURITUS

DEFINITION

Pruritus refers to the sensation of local or systemic itchiness. For purposes of this discussion, pruritus will be considered as a diffuse constant sensation of itchiness in the skin. While this is frequently due to a dermatologic or allergic disorder, it can also be a harbinger of a large number of serious systemic diseases.[88-91] It is incumbent upon the physician to consider these entities when a patient presents with pruritus.

PATHOPHYSIOLOGIC CONSIDERATIONS

The sensation of pruritus is caused by stimulation of cutaneous nerves in the dermis. The exact mechanism of stimulation is not clear; histamine and a variety of other mediators probably have a direct effect on the nerve endings. A variety of factors, including psychogenic factors, temperature, state of hydration, and vasodilatation influence the perception of pruritus.

DIFFERENTIAL DIAGNOSIS AND DIAGNOSTIC EVALUATION

The evaluation of a patient with pruritus should include a careful history of possible allergic exposures, including drugs or any causal association, and a very careful review of systems in search of clues to an underlying disorder. A thorough physical exam should be performed with the same concerns. If neither of these is revealing, screening blood evaluation should be done, including complete blood counts with a differential, screening chemistries including thyroid evaluation, a sedimentation rate, immunoelectrophoresis, chest radiograph, and urinalysis. Other testing, such as for pregnancy, should be done if warranted by the history and exam. Allergic disease is suggested by eosinophilia and elevated IgE antibody levels. If no diagnosis has been made from the above, a skin biopsy can sometimes help, especially to diagnose a dermatologic disorder.

Because of the location of the nerve endings, almost any dermatologic disorder can be associated with pruritus. Some of those particularly associated with pruritus but perhaps less obvious on physical exam are noted on Table 3-28.

Allergic diseases are commonly associated with pruritus. Occasionally an IgE mediated reaction will present only with diffuse pruritus. Pruritus almost always accompanies urticaria but characteristically is not associated with pure angioedema. Itching is always present with atopic dermatitis and frequently with contact dermatitis, but it is rare for these disorders not to have associated skin findings. Drug reactions can become manifest solely with pruritus and should always be considered in the differential diagnosis.

If a patient presents solely with pruritus and there

Table 3-28. Dermatologic Diseases Associated With Severe Pruritus

Atopic dermatitis
Bullous pemphigoid
Contact dermatitis
Dermatitis herpetiformis
Dermatophytosis
Fiberglass dermatitis
Lichen planus
Miliaria
Mastocytosis
Pediculosis
Pityriasis rosea
Scabies
Urticaria
Xerosis

(Adapted from Gilchrest, B.: Pruritus: Pathogenesis, therapy, and significance in systemic disease states. Arch Intern Med *142*:101, 1982.)

is no evidence of a dermatologic or allergic disorder, the possibility of an underlying systemic disease must be considered. A specific cause is found in 10 to 50% of patients in this group, depending on differences in study designs.

Those disorders most frequently associated with

Table 3-29. Systemic Disorders Associated with Pruritus

Systemic Disorders	Frequency of Association with Pruritus, Where Known
Renal	
Chronic renal failure	80 to 90%
Hepatic	
Primary biliary cirrhosis	100%
Cholestasis of pregnancy	<3%
Extrahepatic biliary obstruction	50% (approximately)
Hepatitis	Less common
Drug ingestion	Less common
Hematopoietic	
Polycythemia vera	30 to 50%
Hodgkin's disease	305
Other lymphomas and leukemias	Not known
Multiple myeloma	Rare
Mastocytosis	
Iron deficiency anemia	Rare
Endocrine	
Hyperthyroidism	4 to 11% if severe
Carcinoid syndrome	Rare
Diabetes mellitus	Rare
Miscellaneous	
Malignant neoplasms	
Neurologic syndromes	
Opiate ingestion	
Drug ingestion	
Psychosis	
Parasitic infestations	
Advanced age	

(Adapted from Gilchrest, B.: Pruritus: Pathogenesis, therapy, and significance in systemic disease states. Arch Intern Med *142*:101, 1982.)

pruritus are listed in Table 3–29. Chronic renal failure is probably the most common cause of pruritus in this group, affecting 80 to 90% of patients on maintenance hemodialysis.[88]

Cholestasis with the resultant elevation of bile salts is another very common cause; hence hepatic disorders are associated with pruritus (Table 3–29). In biliary cirrhosis where cholestasis is severe, pruritus is the presenting complaint in approximately 50% of cases.[88] In some cases cholestasis may be the mechanism underlying the pruritus associated with pregnancy.

Hematologic malignancies as listed are also associated with pruritus. It is common in Hodgkin's disease and polycythemia vera, affecting about 30% of patients, especially after a hot bath in the latter case.[88] It is less common with the other disorders and rare in iron deficiency anemia.

Severe hyperthyroidism is associated with pruritus. Patients with diabetes mellitus rarely experience pruritus, except in vaginal infections with candida. A variety of carcinomas have been associated with pruritus, although the incidence of each is unknown. Pruritus restricted to the nostrils is most frequently due to allergic disease but rarely may be the presenting sign of an advanced brain tumor. Pruritus can be the presenting symptom of herpes zoster. Opiates can cause nonspecific release of mast cell mediators, including histamine, resulting in pruritus, as discussed in the section on anaphylaxis. Helminthic infections, which include a tissue migration phase, can rarely be associated with pruritus.

Often there is no evidence of a dermatologic, allergic, or systemic disease associated with the pruritus. Pruritus is very common in elderly patients, whether secondary to xerosis, psychological factors, or an unidentified disorder. Dry skin may be a cause in some cases and, along with substances such as alcohol that cause vasodilation, undoubtedly aggravates other causes. Psychologic factors clearly affect the perception of pruritus. Their role in causing the symptom is less clear.

DISEASES ASSOCIATED WITH EOSINOPHILIA AND ELEVATED TOTAL SERUM IgE ANTIBODY

As noted on Table 3–30 there are a number of disorders, notably allergic and parasitic diseases, associated with a significant increase of both eosinophils

Table 3–30. Diseases Associated with Elevations of Both IgE and Eosinophils

Allergic diseases
Allergic rhinitis
Asthma
Atopic dermatitis
Allergic bronchopulmonary aspergillosis
Infections: Parasitic (Helminths)
Immune deficiency diseases
IgA deficiency
Graft vs host disease
Wiskott-Aldrich syndrome
Other: Hodgkin's disease
Hypereosinophilic syndrome

and serum IgE. These entities are discussed separately in these two sections.

EOSINOPHILIA

Definition

Eosinophilia is generally defined as accumulation of eosinophils greater than 5% of the circulating white blood cells or 350 eosinophils/mm^3 in the blood. Elevations can also be seen in nasal secretions, saliva, effusions, and in certain circumstances in the tissues. Because a large number of diseases are associated with eosinophilia, its diagnostic significance is limited. Worldwide, parasitic diseases are the most frequent cause. In a hospitalized population in the U.S., drug reaction was found to be the most frequent cause.[92]

Pathophysiologic Considerations

The exact nature of the role of the eosinophil is still unclear.[93–95] Eosinophilia is clearly associated with helminth infections, and it is likely that the eosinophil plays a role in killing these parasites. Several eosinophil proteins including major basic protein (pH 11.0) are toxic to schistosomules in vitro. The role of this cell in parasitic infections in vivo is less documented but the available data suggests that it also acts to kill helminths.

Eosinophils are also associated with allergic diseases. One function of the cell in this situation may be to modify mast-cell mediated reactions. Eosinophil chemotactic factor released from mast cells acts to recruit eosinophils to the area. Eosinophils, in turn, release pharmacologically active substances, some of which inactivate substances released from the mast cell; for example, histaminidase inactivates histamine, phospholipase A inactivates acetyl glyceryl ether phosphorylcholine (AGEPC, i.e., platelet activating factor), and major basic protein inactivates heparin. While this neutralization appears beneficial, major basic protein is toxic to tissues at concentrations found in some disease states, for example in the sputum of patients with asthma, and hence may contribute to the pathogenesis of these disorders.[96]

Differential Diagnosis and Diagnostic Evaluation

The evaluation of eosinophilia is facilitated by considering the history and the presenting symptoms and signs. When the cause is still obscure, a chest x-ray and a complete physical examination with CBC, biochemistry profile, sedimentation rate, quantitative immunoglobulins, and immunoelectrophoresis should be done. If the eosinophil count is very high, a vitamin B_{12} level should be obtained to differentiate between hypereosinophilic syndrome and eosinophilic leukemia. Obtaining an IgE level is very helpful because an elevated level narrows the differential, especially toward allergy and parasites. Since drug reaction is a frequent cause of eosinophilia in the U.S., suspected drugs should be discontinued if possible to see if the eosinophilia resolves. If a cause is still not found, parasitic disease should be suspected and should be looked for with appropriate gastrointestinal and serologic tests. Finally, the diagnosis may require a biopsy of the lung, gastrointestinal tract, bone marrow, skin and muscle, or heart.

The differential diagnosis of eosinophilia is extensive (Table 3–31) (see Chapter 4). The majority of cases, however, are due to allergic or parasitic disease. Additionally, eosinophil counts exceeding 3000/ng/ml are usually seen only with allergic bronchopulmonary aspergillosis, tropical pulmonary eosinophilia, helminth infections, hypereosinophilic syndrome, and the rare disorder eosinophilic leukemia. The remainder of the disorders in the differential are usually associated with smaller elevations.

Since the eosinophil appears to help regulate IgE mediated reactions, it is not surprising that eosinophilia usually accompanies allergic reactions such as allergic rhinitis and asthma. Elevated blood levels of eosinophils are also seen in asthma without an obvious allergic origin. In the case of rashes or hepatitis of unknown cause, the presence of eosinophilia implies an allergic cause frequently secondary to medications.

With parasitic infections, eosinophilia usually occurs only when helminths migrate through tissue. Purely intestinal parasites such as Giardia or Enterobius (pinworm) are rarely associated with eosinophilia. Helminth infections with flukes and roundworms are associated with the highest counts. Tropical pulmonary eosinophilia, which is attributed to filaria and visceral larva migrans (which can be due to several helminths), can be associated with up to 10,000 eosinophils/ng/ml

in blood. Frequently the counts rise immediately after treatment.

Eosinophilia is also seen with scarlet fever, usually during the desquamation phase. Less frequently it is seen with tuberculosis if the disease is extensive. It has also been associated with coccidioidomycosis and aspergillosis.

A number of pulmonary disorders are associated with eosinophilia.[97,98] As discussed, elevated counts are seen with asthma regardless of whether allergies are associated. Counts up to 5000/ngm/ml may be seen with allergic bronchopulmonary aspergillosis, vasculitis involving the lung (allergic angiitis and granulomatosis), and chronic pulmonary infiltrates with eosinophilia. Unlike Löffler's syndrome (simple pulmonary eosinophilia), which is self-limited and rarely persists longer than 1 month, chronic pulmonary infiltrates with eosinophilia is a serious illness of unknown origin, usually occurring in women of child-bearing age and characterized by fever, night sweats, weight loss, cough, pulmonary infiltrates, elevated erythrocyte sedimentation rate (ESR), and blood and sputum eosinophilia. It is generally responsive to steroids but can last months to years and can be associated with the development of mild asthma.

Eosinophilic granuloma is also of unknown cause. It typically affects young adult white males and may involve only the lung or may be disseminated. When it involves the lung, mild systemic symptoms, cough, and shortness of breath are present. Chest radiographs show interstitial infiltrates and occasionally a honeycomb appearance. It used to be thought that sarcoidosis was associated with significant eosinophilia but recent studies suggest this probably is not the case.[92]

If severe eosinophilia (usually greater than 2000/ng/ml for 12 months) persists, endomyocarditis can develop. Eosinophils are found on myocardial biopsy. It is speculated that products of the eosinophil gradually damage the heart, resulting in failure.

Eosinophilia is fairly common in myeloproliferative diseases, especially chronic myelogenous leukemia. The elevation is less marked in plasma cell dyscrasias and cyclic neutropenia. Eosinophilic leukemia, defined as eosinophilia with predominance of immature cells, decreased leukocyte alkaline phosphatase, or blast crisis, is a very rare disorder.

Hypereosinophilic syndrome (HES) appears to be a distinct disorder.[99] The eosinophils are mature by light microscopy. Unlike in benign or secondary elevations of eosinophils, the vitamin B_{12} level is generally increased in HES. The syndrome predominantly affects 20- to 40-year-old males. It is generally defined as a level of 1500 eosinophils/ng/ml for greater than 6 months without any obvious cause for the eosinophilia

Table 3–31.   Differential Diagnosis of Eosinophilia

Atopy	Eosinophilic granuloma
Allergic rhinitis	Vasculitis (allergic angiitis and granulomatosis)
Asthma	Tropical pulmonary eosinophilia
Atopic dermatitis (eczema)	Heiner's syndrome
Contact dermatitis	Sarcoidosis?
Drug reactions	Cardiac diseases
Infections	Löffler's endomyocarditis
Parasitic	Hematologic diseases
Helminths	Myeloproliferative diseases
Trematodes (flukes)	Multiple myeloma, heavy chain disease, Waldenström's macro-
Schistosoma	globulinemia
Paragonimus	Cyclic neutropenia
Clonorchis sinensis	Eosinophilic leukemia
Fasciola hepatica	Hypereosinophilic syndrome
Cestodes: (tapeworms)	Solid tumors
Diphyllobothrium latum	Hodgkin's disease
Taenia saginata	Angioimmunoblastic lymphadenopathy with dysproteinemia
Taenia solium	Acinar cell cancer
Hymenolepis nana	Ovarian cancer
Echinococcus	Gastrointestinal diseases
Nematodes (roundworms)	Eosinophilic gastroenteritis
Strongyloides	Chronic active hepatitis
Hookworm	Ulcerative colitis
Ascaris	Immunologic/rhematologic diseases
Trichuris	Immunodeficiency diseases
Trichinella	Wiskott-Aldrich syndrome
Filaria (Loa Loa, Onchocerca volvulus, Wuchereria	Selective IgA deficiency
bancrofti)	Thymic dysplasia syndrome
Angiostrongylus	Graft vs host disease
Toxocariasis	Vasculitis
Gynathostomiasis	Hypersensitivity vasculitis
Bacterial	Allergic angiitis with granulomatosus
Scarlet fever	Polyarteritis nodosa
Tuberculosis	Connective tissue diseases
Fungal	Eosinophilic fasciitis
Coccidioidomycosis	Sjögren's syndrome
Aspergillosis	Skin diseases
Mite: Scabies	Exfoliative reactions
Pulmonary Diseases	Dermatitis herpetiformis
Asthma	Other
Allergic bronchopulmonary aspergillosis	Postradiation treatment
Hypersensitivity pneumonitis	Episodic angioedema associated with eosinophilia
Löffler's (acute eosinophilic pneumonia)	
Chronic pulmonary infiltrates with eosinophilia	

and with evidence of organ involvement, especially the heart and often the liver, spleen, and lungs. A variety of CNS lesions can also occur. About 40% of patients have an associated elevation of IgE. Interestingly this latter group of patients appears more steroid responsive than others.

Hodgkin's disease can be associated with a mild eosinophilia, especially if pruritus is present. About one third of patients with angioimmunoblastic lymphadenopathy with dysproteinemia have an elevation. Pancreatic acinar cell cancer is associated with polyarthritis and panniculitis, as well as elevated eosinophils. Except for ovarian and occasionally thyroid cancer, most other carcinomas and sarcomas are associated with eosinophilia less than 5% of the time.

Irritation of the gastrointestinal tract by inflammation associated with an ulcer or granulomatous disease or by a protozoan infestation may result in tissue but rarely blood eosinophilia. Gastrointestinal symptoms in association with blood eosinophilia should suggest eosinophilic gastroenteritis. Eosinophilia is also associated with Heiner's syndrome of gastrointestinal and respiratory tract symptoms with pulmonary hemosiderosis, iron deficiency anemia, and antibodies to cows' milk.

Immunodeficiency diseases (especially Wiskott-Aldrich syndrome), selective IgA deficiency, and thymic dysplasia syndrome are frequently associated with eosinophilia; they may be related to dysfunction of the immune regulatory network.

Although they do not appear to be involved in the pathogenesis, eosinophils are frequently associated with vasculitis, especially hypersensitivity vasculitis. They are seen much less frequently in connective tissue diseases. In general they are associated much more with IgE than with immune complex mediated diseases.

A number of skin diseases, notably exfoliative reactions and dermatitis herpetiformis, are associated with eosinophilia. Atopic skin disorders, especially atopic dermatitis, can be connected with very high eosinophil levels. Other diseases, such as toxic epidermal necrolysis or scabies infection, have tissue but not blood elevations.

Eosinophilia is associated with radiation treatment, frequently increasing as treatment is increased. The mechanism by which radiation induces eosinophilia is unknown but may involve several possibilities, including the direct triggering of mast cells to release mediators and the changing of tissue antigens, resulting in immune reactivity.

Finally, there is a rare entity, episodic angioedema with eosinophilia.[100] The few patients well described in the literature have episodic severe angioedema with urticaria lasting up to 10 days and associated with weight gain averaging 14% of normal, fever, and marked leukocytosis (up to 108,000/µl) with 40 to 88% eosinophils. Despite recurrence of these attacks, patients do not appear to develop cardiac disease from the eosinophilia and, also unlike with HES, the prognosis appears to be good.

ELEVATED TOTAL SERUM IgE ANTIBODY

Definition

IgE antibody constitutes only 0.001% of the total circulating immunoglobulin. Low levels appear to have no clinical significance. Although an elevation of IgE is defined as more than 200 IU/ml or 240 to 480 ng/ml (1 IU is 2.4 ng of IgE) depending on various factors, the elevation generally has significance only if it is marked. Significant elevations are seen primarily with allergic, parasitic, and immunodeficiency disorders.[101]

Pathophysiologic Considerations and Differential Diagnosis

IgE is produced by plasma cells that are located mainly in lymph tissue and the upper respiratory and gastrointestinal tracts. The antibody enters the blood and secretions and then binds to the surface of mast cells and basophils. Because the production is regulated by class-specific T helper and suppressor cells elevated IgE levels can result from diseases that affect T-cell function.[102,103]

IgE clearly has an adverse role in atopic disease. It may protect against parasitic diseases, although the exact mechanism of this effect is still unclear.[103] Whether it has a further beneficial role in humans is, at present, unknown.

Total serum levels are measured by either radioimmunoassays (RIA) or enzyme-linked immunosorbent assays (ELISA). IgE specific for an individual antigen is measured in vitro by the above techniques, or by skin testing, as discussed in the section on anaphylaxis.

A variety of factors influence IgE levels. A tendency towards an elevated level is inherited recessively. For example, Filipinos born in the U.S. have higher levels than Canadians. There may also be some association with HLA markers. Another factor is the amount of antigen a patient is exposed to, with lower amounts favoring the development of IgE over IgG. Route of exposure to the antigen is also important. If the antigen has to cross a mucosal barrier, atopic patients, as opposed to nonatopic patients, will tend to make IgE antibody against it. However, there seems to be no difference in IgE production between atopic and normal individuals if the antigen is introduced parenterally. Time of year is another factor, as IgE levels increase after the season in the case of inhalant pollen allergies.

Diseases associated with elevations in serum total IgE antibody are listed on Table 3–32. Of these, only hyper IgE syndrome, atopic dermatitis, allergic bronchopulmonary aspergillosis, Wiskott-Aldrich syndrome, and, occasionally, parasitic disease are associated with levels greater than 10,000 IU/ml. Those associated with levels up to 1000 IU/ml include atopic asthma, parasitic disease, other immunodeficiency states, and bullous pemphigoid. Other skin diseases including "neurodermatitis," severe contact dermatitis, psoriasis with arthropathy, and pityriasis rubra can be associated with levels up to 500 IU/ml. Levels below 500 IU/ml, while elevated, have minimal clinical significance in terms of differential diagnosis, as there is a substantial overlap with asymptomatic normal individuals.

While levels are generally increased in atopic disease, the extent depends greatly on the specific entity. Because the increase is minimal in allergic rhinitis, in most cases obtaining a level to determine an allergic origin of the rhinitis is not helpful. They are also generally not increased in chronic urticaria. Levels are increased in 60% of patients with asthma flared by specific allergies and in about 5% of patients with asthma but no demonstrable allergies. Therefore,

Table 3–32. Diseases Associated with Elevated Total Serum IgE Level

Allergic diseases
  Allergic rhinitis
  Asthma
  Atopic dermatitis
  Allergic bronchopulmonary aspergillosis
Infections
  Parasitic (Helminths)
    Trematodes (flukes)
      Schistosoma
      Paragonimus
      Clonorchis sinensis
      Fasciola hepatica
    Cestodes (tapeworms): Echinoccocus
    Nematodes (roundworms)
      Intestinal: Strongyloides, Hookworm, Ascaris, Trichuris
      Tissue: Trichinella, Filaria (Loa Loa, Onchocerca volvulus, Wuchereria bancrofti)
  Fungal: Systemic candidiasis
  Viral: Respiratory syncytial virus
  Bacterial: Leprosy
Immune Deficiency States
  IgA deficiency
  Graft vs host disease
  Wiskott-Aldrich syndrome
  Nezelof's syndrome
Hyper IgE syndrome
Dermatology
  Bullous pemphigoid
  Neurodermatitis
  Contact dermatitis (severe)
  Pityriasis rubra
  Psoriasis with arthropathy
Hematology: IgE myeloma
Oncology
  Hodgkin's disease (nodular sclerosis type)
  Wegener's granulomatosis
Pulmonary
  Cystic fibrosis
  Allergic angiitis with granulomatosis
Other
  Liver disease
  Nephrotic syndrome
  Smoking
  Acute Guillain-Barré syndrome
  Burns
  Mucocutaneous lymph node syndrome

though an elevated IgE level can be helpful in diagnosing allergies associated with asthma, a low value does not rule out an allergic cause.

The level of IgE is increased in 80% of patients with atopic dermatitis, the level roughly correlating with the severity of the disease. The role of IgE in the pathogenesis of atopic dermatitis is unclear. The elevation may reflect only disordered immune regulation. Specific skin tests and RAST will frequently be positive, but because there is a high incidence of false positive results and limited clinical correlation, performing these tests is usually not worthwhile.

Allergic bronchopulmonary aspergillosis (ABPA), a disorder caused by hypersensitivity to the fungus Aspergillus fumigatus, is associated with very high levels of IgE antibody with 90% of patients having levels greater than 2000 IU/ml. This increase is in contrast to hypersensitivity pneumonitis, in which there is no change in IgE levels. ABPA, discussed in detail in the section on asthma, generally occurs in asthmatic patients and is characterized by fleeting pulmonary infiltrates, wheezing and cough productive occasionally of brown plugs, proximal bronchiectasis, hypereosinophilia, elevated IgE, and evidence of IgE and IgG antibody reactivity against aspergillus. Only a small part of the elevated IgE is specific for aspergillus.

Like eosinophils, IgE is elevated in parasitic infections with helminth but not in protozoal infections. Levels seem to correlate with the degree of tissue invasion. With treatment they tend to fall, sometimes after an initial elevation if there is massive parasite death.

Elevated levels have been observed in systemic candidiasis. In this disorder a high percentage of the IgE is specific for candida. A small increase has been noted in upper respiratory infection, especially with respiratory syncytial virus. In this case, IgE specific for the virus can be found in the nasal secretions, leading to interesting speculation on the role of IgE in upper respiratory viral illness.[104] In addition to viral infections, lepromatous and tuberculoid leprosy have been associated with an increase in serum IgE. Both IgE and eosinophils are increased in certain immunodeficiency states. These include IgA deficiency, graft vs host disease, the Wiskott-Aldrich syndrome, and Neselof's syndrome (a modified DiGeorge's syndrome).

Levels greater than 10,000 IU/ml can be seen in hyper IgE syndrome (Job's syndrome).[105] These patients have recurrent severe infections of the skin and respiratory tract, most due to Staphylococcus aureus. Pneumonias may result in pneumatoceles unlike in chronic granulomatous disease. Although most cases described have involved children, many with coarse facial features, it can be seen in adults. Blood tissue and sputum eosinophilia is also prominent. The IgE is polyclonal. These patients have no consistent defect of polymorphonuclear function except for chemotaxis, but they seem to have problems with cell mediated immunity. Current theories suggest that hyper IgE may be a result of an impairment of the immune regulatory system.[106]

A variety of skin disorders other than bullous pemphigoid can cause mild elevations of IgE (Table 3–32).

IgE myeloma is extremely rare. Hodgkin's disease of the nodular sclerosis type has been associated with elevated levels. IgE is increased in about 30% of cases of cystic fibrosis.

A variety of other miscellaneous disorders may result in a mild elevation of IgE. Active smoking may increase it but rarely to over 100 IU/ml. It is seen in approximately 30% of cases of Guillain-Barré syndrome. In burn cases there is a mild increase for 3 weeks, followed by a decline. Mucocutaneous lymph node syndrome (Kawasaki disease) is also associated with a slight increase early in the disease.

Diagnostic Evaluation

If an IgE level is 1000 IU/ml or greater, various disorders should be suspected, as discussed. Hyper IgE syndrome, Wiskott-Aldrich syndrome, bullous pemphigoid, and atopic dermatitis should be obvious from the history and physical examination. If the patient has asthma, allergic bronchopulmonary aspergillosis should be suspected and evaluated, as discussed. If no cause is obvious from the history and physical examination, parasitic diseases should be suspected and thoroughly evaluated. This evaluation can be difficult, requiring appropriate serologic studies as well as frequent stool examinations, especially when helminths are migrating through tissues.

If the level is less than 1000 IU/ml, one should suspect allergic parasitic, or immunodeficiency states, especially IgA deficiency, which may be asymptomatic.

Minimal elevations up to approximately 500 IU/ml, though associated with a wide variety of disorders, are rarely of diagnostic significance because they are rarely the only presenting sign. While such elevations are of help in suggesting an allergic cause of asthma or urticaria, normal values do not rule out allergy in these disorders.

UNUSUAL PREDISPOSITION TO INFECTION SECONDARY TO HUMORAL OR CELL MEDIATED IMMUNODEFICIENCY

DEFINITION

As knowledge about the immune system and its regulation increases, so does knowledge about aberrations of the system. Because the immune network is a vital part of the body's defense system, it is not surprising that immunodeficiency states, whether in-herited or acquired, present most commonly as unusual predispositions to infection, as autoimmune disorders, or as an increased incidence of malignancy.[107-112] This section will focus on the clinical presentation of unusual predisposition to infections. Disorders of regulation resulting in autoimmune diseases or malignancy are discussed elsewhere.

PATHOPHYSIOLOGIC CONSIDERATIONS AND DIFFERENTIAL DIAGNOSIS

Deficiencies associated with each of the four components of the immune system—antibody, cellular immunity, complement, and phagocytosis—result in an increased predisposition to infection, the nature of the clinical presentation and organisms involved differing with each component. Varied presentations and associated disorders should be considered in each case (Table 3–33). It is necessary to recognize, however, that these disorders can be the result of a single or of multiple defects at different points in the immune network. For example, antibody deficiency should be suspected in a patient presenting with recurrent infections with pyogenic encapsulated bacteria. The antibody deficiency, however, may be inherited or acquired, be quantitative or functional, be diffuse or limited to one class of antibody, or occur at one of multiple stages of production in the plasma cell or be the result of disordered immune regulation, e.g., increased suppression, which again could occur at multiple points in the network—just to name a few possible mechanisms. It is beyond the scope of this text to discuss this in detail, but the reader is referred to several recent reviews.[107-112] The purpose of this section is to guide the physician to consider general categories of immunodeficiency when evaluating a patient with an unusual predisposition to infection and, within those categories, to attempt to define the defect more closely by evaluating the patient as outlined below.

In general, immunodeficient patients develop disease with a smaller inoculum of the infectious agent than normal patients and have more severe and prolonged courses. They also tend to develop opportunistic infections (those that rarely cause disease in exposed normal individuals).

Immunoglobulin (antibody) binds to antigens on the surface of organisms and as such "tags" them for removal by the phagocytic system or for cellular- or complement-dependent lysis. Deficiencies of immunoglobulin result primarily in an increased incidence of severe infections with pyogenic encapsulated bacteria.

The cellular immune system (including T cells, macrophages, and Langerhans cells) functions to regulate

Table 3–33. Infections and Associated Immune Disorders

Clinical Presentation	Associated Disorders that May Predispose to Infection
Recurrent infection with bacteria	
Staphylococcus aureus	Hyper IgE syndrome
	Immunoglobulin deficiency
	Chronic granulomatous disease (CGD)
Streptococcus pneumonia	Immunoglobulin deficiency
Streptococcus pyogenes	Phagocyte defect
Escherichia coli	C3b deficiency
Hemophilus influenzae	Sickle cell disease
Klebsiella-Enterobacteriaceae-Serratia	Splenectomy
Pseudomonas aeruginosa	Chronic granulomatous disease, cystic fibrosis
Neisseria meningitidis	Immunoglobulin deficiency
	Deficiency of complement components
	C5, C6, C7, and C8
	Splenectomy
Nocardia	Cell mediated immune defect or CGD
Listeria monocytogenes	Cell mediated immune defect or CGD
Mycobacterium	Cell mediated immune defect or CGD
Salmonella	Cell mediated immune defect plus sickle cell anemia if osteomyelitis present.
Recurrent or severe infection with viruses	
Herpes group (simplex, zoster varicella, Epstein-Barr, cytomegalovirus)	Cell mediated immune defect
Vaccinia	Cell mediated immune defect
Rubella	Cell mediated immune defect
Enteroviruses (polio, coxsackie, ECHO)	Immunoglobulin deficiency
Infections with fungi	
Candida	
Systemic	Cell mediated immune defect, phagocytic defect
Chronic mucocutaneous	Cell mediated immune defect
Cryptococcus neoformans	Cell mediated immune defect
Coccidioides immitis	Cell mediated immune defect
Histoplasma capsulatum	Cell mediated immune defect
Aspergillus fumigatus	Phagocytic defect
Mucor	Phagocytic defect
Infections with parasites	
Pneumocystis carinii	Immunoglobulin and cell mediated immune defect
Toxoplasma gondii	Cell mediated immune defect
Strongyloides stercoralis	Immunoglobulin deficiency
Giardia lamblia	Immunoglobulin deficiency (especially IgA)
Babesia microti	Splenectomy
Infection with opportunistic organisms (e.g., pneumocystis)	Cell mediated immune defect
Infection with catalase positive organisms (S. aureus, most aerobic gram-negative enteric bacteria, candida, and aspergillus)	Chronic granulomatous disease
	Severe glucose-6-phosphate dehydrogenase deficiency
Recurrent skin infection with S. aureus	Phagocytic dysfunction, especially chronic granulomatous disease
	Hyper IgE syndrome
Ulcerative stomatitis	Chronic granulomatous disease
	Cyclic neutropenia
Chronic upper respiratory infections including sinusitis, bronchitis, and bronchiectasis	Diffuse immunoglobulin deficiency
	Specific IgA deficiency
	Cystic fibrosis
	Immobile cilia syndrome
	Chronic granulomatous disease
Chronic bronchitis/bronchiectasis	
Chronic diarrhea/malabsorption	Diffuse immunoglobulin deficiency
	Specific IgA deficiency

antibody production; to mediate delayed hypersensitivity responses, graft vs host reactions, and allograft reactions; and to cause direct cytotoxicity. This system is in large part responsible for the host defense against fungi, facultative intracellular bacteria, protozoa, and viruses; hence, deficiencies in this system result in infections with these organisms.

Complement is discussed in a later section. Deficiencies of the early components tend to be associated with autoimmune disorders. Deficiencies of the late components (C5, C6, C7, and C8) are associated with an increased incidence of Neisseria infections.

The phagocytic system, also discussed in a subsequent section, is comprised of neutrophils, eosinophils, macrophages, and dendritic reticulum cells. It functions mainly to phagocytize and kill invading microbes. As with immunoglobulin deficiencies, deficiencies of this system are associated primarily with chronic bacterial infections.

Because several disorders (for example, common variable immunodeficiency, ataxia-telangiectasia, and Wiskott-Aldrich syndrome) are associated with a variety of defects in the immune system, both humoral and cellular, the clinical presentation may be mixed, reflecting the varied deficiencies. Occasionally a patient may present only with diarrhea, malabsorption or arthritis as a manifestation of immunoglobulin deficiency. Other patients may present with isolated hypogammaglobulinemia without associated infections (discussed below) or with isolated anergy (nonreactivity of delayed hypersensitivity skin tests, discussed in the following section).

Once a particular part of the immune system is suspected of being deficient based on the clinical presentation (Table 3–33), a search should be made for a source of the defect, such as a known syndrome or iatrogenic causes. Some of these syndromes are listed in Table 3–34 and are briefly discussed below. These can be inherited or acquired. The inherited immunodeficiencies almost always present in childhood and, if untreated, are often lethal. It is therefore very rare for an internist to be the first to diagnose one of these disorders. Increasingly, however, internists see patients with a history of a pediatric immunodeficiency disease who were treated (e.g., severe combined immunodeficiency disease treated with bone marrow transplant) and are no longer immunodeficient.

A pure humoral or B-cell deficiency can be the result of a variety of defects, including a stem cell defect in antigen processing or a defect of T-cell regulation.[108] X-linked (Bruton's) agammaglobulinemia affects boys after the age of 6 months. Patients commonly present with severe infections with pyogenic encapsulated organisms. They may live to adulthood if vigorously

Table 3–34. Diseases Associated with Deficiency of Humoral or Cellular Immunity

Humoral immunity
  Primary deficiencies
    Brutons agammaglobulinemia
    Selective class or subclass deficiency. IgA, IgG, IgM
    Immunodeficiency with IgM
    Immunodeficiency with thymoma
  Secondary deficiencies
    Suppressed by malignancy (e.g., multiple myeloma)
    Drugs (e.g., diphenylhydantoin)
    Viral infections
    Nutritional deficit
    Autoimmune disease
    Increased loss by nephrotic syndrome
    Severe burns
    Diarrhea
    Increased catabolism (e.g., cryoglobulinemia)
Cellular immunity
  Primary deficiencies
    Immunodeficiency associated with pregnancy
    Chronic mucocutaneous candidiasis
    Acquired immune deficiency syndrome
    DiGeorge's syndrome
    Nezelof's syndrome
  Secondary deficiencies
    Affected by drugs (e.g., corticosteroids)
      Malignancies (e.g., Hodgkin's disease)
      Viral infections
      Nutritional deficit
      Autoimmune disease
Combined deficiencies
  Common variable immunodeficiency
  Ataxia-telangiectasia
  Wiskott-Aldrich syndrome

treated with gamma globulin; many, however, have severe sinopulmonary disease, and up to 6% develop lymphoreticular neoplasms.[107]

The most common inherited immunodeficiency is absent or decreased IgA (<10 mg/dl). It is reported to be present in 1 out of 886 individuals, although other studies have found it to be more common.[107,108]

Secretory IgA is a dimer found in respiratory and gastrointestinal secretions. It functions partly to block absorption of antigens from these systems as well as to help neutralize viruses. Patients may be completely asymptomatic or have recurrent problems with respiratory and gastrointestinal infections, the latter especially with Giardia lamblia. Diarrhea, malabsorption, nodular lymphoid hyperplasia, autoimmune diseases, atopy, and IgG2 and IgG3 deficiency have been reported associated with IgA deficiency.[113,114]

Selective deficiencies have been described of all the IgG subclasses. IgG4 deficiency appears to be associated with severe recurrent sinopulmonary infections.[115] The other IgG deficiencies are associated with a wide variety of entities, including ataxia-telangiectasia and systemic lupus erythematosus.[116] IgG2 and

IgG3 deficiency may be associated with IgA deficiency.[114]

Immunodeficiency with elevated IgM is another disease that presents in early childhood. Patients develop infections with pyogenic organisms but also have an increased incidence of Pneumocystis carinii pneumonia and verruca vulgaris. The physical exam may reveal lymphoid tissue reactivity. The laboratory evaluation shows low IgG and IgA with a polyclonal elevation of IgM (as opposed to monoclonal with Waldenström's macroglobulinemia). Evidence of autoimmunity and cyclic neutropenia may be observed. It has been shown that B cells from these patients are unable to switch from making IgM to making IgG or IgA. This may be due to an intrinsic defect in the B cell or to a defect in the stimulation signal from a T cell.[117] If treated vigorously with gamma globulin replacement regularly, patients can survive to adulthood, although there is an increased incidence of malignancy.

Immunodeficiency with thymoma occurs in adults and is associated with absent B cells and sometimes pure red cell aplasia or pancytopenia.

There are many causes of secondary deficiencies of immunoglobulin, including the lymphoproliferative malignancies, especially multiple myeloma and chronic lymphocytic leukemia, radiation therapy, and drugs (especially chemotherapeutic agents). Viral infections may depress humoral and cellular immunity. Autoantibodies to various components necessary for antibody production can result in hypogammaglobulinemia. Increased loss can occur from any state in which there is substantial loss of protein (Table 3–34).

In contrast, the immunodeficient state associated with pregnancy appears to be primarily a cellular rather than a humoral defect. An associated decrease in the number of T helper cells has been reported.[118]

Patients with chronic mucocutaneous candidiasis present in a variety of ways, from early to late onset and from juvenile to familial. Characteristically they all have chronic candida infections of the skin and mucous membranes.[111] Associated endocrinopathies and autoimmune diseases may be seen. There appear to be a variety of immune defects. Most patients have a specific lack of immune reactivity to candida.[108]

Acquired Immune Deficiency Syndrome (AIDS) is associated primarily with a cellular immune deficiency caused by a selective infection of and subsequent reduction of the helper/inducer T-cell population by the human immunodeficiency virus HIV-I.[119] Because this is such a central cell in the immune network, many other immune aberrations have also been documented. Most patients eventually develop opportunistic infections that are usually handled by the cell mediated immune system. Additionally there is an increased incidence of aggressive Kaposi's sarcoma. This is most common in patients who are exposed to the virus by inoculation into the blood, e.g., homosexuals by the nature of their sexual practices, intravenous drug users, and infants born to infected mothers.

DiGeorge's syndrome, or thymic hypoplasia, is a cellular immune deficiency that usually presents at birth with hypocalcemia and severe infections, as well as multiple congenital defects. A milder form, "partial DiGeorge's syndrome," is associated with partial hypoplasia.[107] Nezelof's syndrome is a variant of this syndrome.

Cellular immunity can also be suppressed secondarily by a number of factors (Table 3–34). Hodgkin's disease and other malignancies are associated with anergy. Viral infections, severe malnutrition, and autoantibodies can also suppress the system.

A number of disorders are associated with deficiencies of both humoral and cell mediated immunity. Common variable immunodeficiency (adult onset hypogammaglobulinemia) presents mainly with the typical respiratory and gastrointestinal symptoms associated with hypogammaglobulinemia. A variety of T-cell defects can also be present. Several different causes have been reported, ranging from defective production of immunoglobulin to decreased T helper-cell function or increased suppression of the system.[120,121] It seems likely that this is a heterogenous group of diseases with a common presentation.

Patients with ataxia-telangiectasia present in childhood with a combination of symptoms, including ataxia, telangiectasias, and severe chronic respiratory tract infections. It is associated with both B- and T-cell abnormalities. There is a high incidence of malignancies, and patients rarely survive well into adulthood. The Wiskott-Aldrich syndrome is inherited as X-linked recessive and manifests as eczema, thrombocytopenia, and increased susceptibility to infections. Survival to adulthood is rare.

DIAGNOSTIC EVALUATION

The evaluation of a patient with a suspected humoral or cellular immunodeficiency should include a careful history to document frequency, type and location of infections, age at onset, and a family history of comparable problems. Inquiries should be made about associated diarrhea, arthritis, or any symptoms suggestive of an underlying disease process. Medications such as corticosteroids taken by patients should be evaluated for their possible secondary immunodeficiency effects.

The physical examination should focus on the sources and nature of the infectious process. The skin

Table 3–35. General Evaluation of Humoral or Cellular Immunodeficiency

Humoral
1. Quantitate individual immunoglobulins and subclasses, if indicated, by immunodiffusion or nephalometry
2. Perform immunoelectrophoresis to check for presence of a monoclonal protein
3. Quantitate number of B cells by monoclonal antibody specific for surface markers (or by older method of surface immunofluorescence).
4. Measure function by:
   —measuring isohemagglutinin (IgM) titers for anti-A in patients with B blood type, or anti-B in patients with A blood type, or for anti-A and anti-B in patients with O blood type
   —measuring Salmonella anti-H antibody response. If negative, consider immunizing with typhoid and checking 1 month later.
   —performing Schick test.[122] If there is no reaction, a patient has antibodies against diphtheria. If the reaction is positive, consider immunizing with diphtheria and checking 1 month later
   —measuring antitetanus antibodies. Patients can also be immunized and re-evaluated in 1 month.
5. Perform histologic examination of bone marrow or lymph node.
6. Make in vitro measurement of function by assaying lymphocyte response to B-cell mitogens or antigens.

Cellular
1. Quantitate total number of lymphocytes
2. Quantitate total number of T cells by monoclonal antibody specific for cell surface markers (or by older method of agglutination with sheep red blood cells).
3. Quantitate phenotypic subsets of T cells by monoclonal antibody.
4. Perform delayed hypersensitivity skin tests (see detailed description in anergy section). If nonreactive, consider immunizing with tetanus toxoid and re-evaluating in 1 month.
5. Do histologic examination of bone marrow or lymph node
6. Make in vitro measurement of function by assaying lymphocyte response to T cell mitogens or antigen.
7. Do in vitro co-culture experiments to assess function.
8. Make in vitro measurement of macrophage inhibiting factor (MIF) from lymphocytes exposed to an antigen.

should be examined for vaccination scars (indicating intact immunity at the time of vaccination), eczema, or Kaposi's sarcoma. The presence of lymph tissue, including tonsils, should be evaluated.

A complete blood count should be done to quantitate the number of lymphocytes. The total gamma globulin level should be checked, keeping in mind that a specific deficiency might not decrease the total amount of gamma globulin. Infections should be cultured to determine the responsible microbe.

If, after the above, an immunodeficiency is suspected, selected tests should be obtained (Table 3–35). Quantitation of individual immunoglobulins to rule out a specific deficiency, electrophoresis to look for a monoclonal protein, and reactivity to a screening panel of delayed hypersensitivity skin tests are easily determined and should be checked on all patients. Histologic examination of a lymph node biopsy is also helpful to check for depletion of the B- or T-cell areas.

Monoclonal antibodies that identify specific populations of B and T cells are widely available and provide valuable information about the number of cells, including the ratio of helper to suppressor T cells. Although these antibodies identify phenotypic markers on the cell surface, these generally correlate with function. For example, the monoclonal antibody OKT_4 binds to an antigen on the surface of T cells that generally have a helper or inducer function, while OKT_8 binds to those cells that generally have a suppressor function. If the helper-inducer subset is diminished, AIDS should be suspected. The presence of HIV-I virus infection should then be investigated by using the enzyme linked immunosorbent assay to look for antibody to the virus. Further confirmation of infection can be obtained by the Western blot technique, looking for viral encoded protein in cells.

Further tests to evaluate the function of the cells should also be done. All patients should have antibodies against typhoid, diphtheria, and tetanus.[122] If these are lacking, the patient can be immunized with tetanus and the specific antibody can be rechecked 1 month later.

Most other tests of immune function require a research laboratory. One of the most common and informative functional studies is assaying lymphocyte response in culture to a variety of mitogens and antigens. Co-culture experiments aid in defining helper- and suppressor-cell defects.

ANERGY

DEFINITION

Anergy is defined as nonreactivity at 48 to 72 hours to intradermal skin tests with a group of at least four antigens known to elicit a reaction in sensitized patients. It is a frequent finding in patients with disorders of cell mediated immunity but may also be encountered in a number of diverse diseases or incidentally during the course of a medical evaluation.

PATHOPHYSIOLOGIC CONSIDERATIONS

Because this delayed hypersensitivity reaction to an antigen is mediated by T cells, anergy suggests a deficiency of this T-cell system. This deficiency may involve an absolute decrease in the number of cells, a decrease in production of or reactivity to lymphokines, which are produced during the reaction, or an increase in suppression of the reaction by T suppressor cells. The latter is probably the most common mechanism.[123] Anergy may be associated with a decrease in humoral reactivity in certain diseases but most frequently is associated with intact antibody responses to the antigens.

DIFFERENTIAL DIAGNOSIS AND DIAGNOSTIC EVALUATION

Testing involves placing 0.1 ml of the antigen intradermally and reading the amount of induration at 48 to 72 hours. Unfortunately, there is no standard agreement on the exact criteria for a positive reaction. Most physicians accept 5 to 10 mm of induration. Likewise, there is no standard battery or concentrations of antigens to use. For example, mumps is not standardized for skin testing because there is a great deal of variation among different lots and debate whether induration or erythema should be considered positive. A good antigen, streptokinase-streptodornase, is no longer commercially available as a skin testing reagent.

Table 3–36 outlines the antigens most commonly used and the approximate percentage of individuals that reacts to them. There is limited data defining the expected rate of reactivity in different groups of individuals.[124–127] In general, approximately 90% of patients should react to at least one of these antigens, with the greatest percentage reacting to candida or tetanus. The degree of reactivity is strongly correlated to patient age for all antigens. Reactivity appears fairly steady until age 60, whereupon the reaction rate drops appreciably. The only exception to this is with purified protein derivative, with which the opposite occurs, the reaction rate increasing until about age 80.

To test reactivity in an anergic patient, i.e., one who is nonreactive to a panel of four to five antigens, a booster of tetanus toxoid can be administered (if the patient has not received one in the last 10 years) and the skin test reactivity checked again in one month. The majority of patients with intact delayed hypersensitivity should respond.[124] For research purposes only, an individual nonreactive to dinitrochlorobenzene or dinitrofluorobenzene can be immunized with one of these and have reactivity checked again in one month. This method is fraught with too many side effects, including the possibilities of severe reactions, to be used for routine diagnosis.

A number of clinical conditions can be associated with anergy (Table 3–37). In some cases the association is transient, as with a viral infection. In other cases, the clinical condition is evident, as in extreme age, malnutrition, or uremia. Sometimes the cause is iatrogenic, especially secondary to corticosteroid and cytotoxic drug use.

The greatest concern arises when anergy is shown to be present without an obvious cause. In such cases, the physician should evaluate the patient for an underlying immunodeficiency disease (e.g., AIDS) or lymphoproliferative disorder, especially Hodgkin's disease, granulomatous disease (notably sarcoidosis) and occult infection with mycobacteria. While it is commonly believed that anergy occurs only with miliary disease, occult infection should still be considered in the differential diagnosis of anergy. Interestingly, the anergy in tuberculosis may be specific only for PPD, with normal reactivity maintained towards the

Table 3–36. Antigens Most Commonly Employed to Test for Delayed Hypersensitivity and Expected Reaction Rates

Antigen and Concentration	Approximate Reaction Rate	Group Tested
Candida		
1:100 to 1:1000 w/v (weight/volume)	63 to 68%	Hospitalized adults
	92%	Nonhospitalized adults
Tetanus		
1:5 to 10 Lf/ml (limited flocculation units/ml)	28%	Hospitalized adults
	49 to 100%	Nonhospitalized adults
Mumps		
undiluted (standardized to 40 colony-forming units/ml)	59 to 68%	Hospitalized adults
Trichophyton		
1:100 to 1:1000 w/v (weight/volume)	62%	Hospitalized adults
	42%	Nonhospitalized adults
PPD		
5 to 250 TU (tuberculin units)	28 to 33%	Hospitalized adults
	30%	Nonhospitalized adults
Histoplasmin		
undiluted	26%	Nonhospitalized adults in Albuquerque, NM
Coccidioidin		
1:100 (Bioequivalent to US Ref. coccidioidin 1:100)	10 to 13%	Nonhospitalized adults in Albuquerque, NM and Los Angeles, CA

(Adapted from the literature.[124–127])

Table 3–37. Clinical Conditions Characterized by Anergy

Infections
  Viral
    Measles
    Hepatitis
    Infectious mononucleosis
  Mycobacterial
    Tuberculosis
    Leprosy
  Fungal
    Coccidioidomycosis
    Candidiasis
  Bacterial
    Brucellosis
    Salmonellosis
Neoplasms
  Lymphoidal
    Hodgkin's disease
    Non-Hodgkin's lymphoma
    Chronic lymphocytic leukemia
  Other neoplasms
Inflammatory diseases
  Sarcoidosis
  Granulomatous bowel disease
    (Crohn's disease)
  Granulomatous hepatitis
  Wegener's granulomatosis
  Lymphomatoid granulomatosis
Autoimmune diseases
  Lupus erythematosus
  Rheumatoid arthritis
  Hashimoto's thyroiditis
Other lymphopenic states
  Intestinal lymphangiectasia
  Chronic thoracic duct drainage
Malnutrition
Old age
Immunosuppressive therapy
  Corticosteroids
  Antilymphocyte sera
  Cytotoxic and
    chemotherapeutic agents
Antibiotics
Irradiation

(From Cooper, M.D., and Buckley, R.H.: Developmental immunology and the immunodeficiency diseases. JAMA *248:*2658. Copyright 1982, American Medical Association.)

other antigens.[128] Frequently the PPD reactivity returns as the patient is treated.[123]

PHAGOCYTIC SYSTEM DEFECTS

As discussed in the previous section, the phagocytic system, which includes polymorphonuclear cells (PMNs), eosinophils, macrophages, and dendritic cells, functions to phagocytize and kill invading mi-

crobes. Patients presenting with recurrent or severe

cific locations should be evaluated for a possible underlying immunodeficiency (Table 3–34). In the case of phagocytic defects, the presentation is similar to antibody deficiencies with recurrent bacterial infections.[129–131]

PATHOPHYSIOLOGIC CONSIDERATIONS AND DIFFERENTIAL DIAGNOSIS

Once a phagocytic defect is suspected, the difficulty arises in attempting to diagnose it specifically, primarily because the defect can be present at one of many points in the system, and because specific diagnostic tests are generally not available except in research laboratories. The phagocytic cells must be produced in the bone marrow, be released to the peripheral circulation, respond to chemotactic factors by migration to the affected area, opsonize microbes (in part by recognizing C3b, IgG, and fibronectin on their surfaces), ingest the organisms, and finally kill them intracellularly. Specific defects, both inherited and acquired, have been identified at almost all of these points. Some of the more common ones that are seen in adults are noted on Table 3–38. Most of the inherited disorders are present in childhood and are frequently fatal, although with good care some patients are surviving to adulthood. Very rarely a patient may present in adulthood with an undiagnosed inherited disorder.

Neutropenia, defined as less than 1500 neutrophils/mm³, is associated with a long list of medications and diseases. It is particularly notable with acute leukemias, severe infections, and Felty's syndrome. Susceptibility to a variety of bacterial and other infections increases dramatically when the total count is less than 500/mm³. Cyclic neutropenia is an uncommon disorder in which neutropenia occurs in a cyclic pattern approximately every 3 weeks. Chronic idiopathic neutropenia is of unknown cause, lasts months to years, and is usually asymptomatic or associated with only mild infections. The red cell and platelet counts are normal.

A long list of diseases is associated with defective function of the phagocytic system, classified according to type of defect (Table 3–38). A number of diseases, including diabetes mellitus, may be associated with multiple defects. Alcoholism is associated with an increased incidence of infections, in part because of defective adherence of neutrophils to vessel walls, a prelude to tissue migration.

An even longer list of diseases is associated with defects in chemotaxis, which can be a cellular defect, or a defect in chemotactic factor generation. Karta-

Table 3–38. Differential Diagnosis of Disorders of the Phagocytic System in Adults

Neutropenia
  Acquired (associated with drugs or diseases) cyclic neutropenia
  Chronic idiopathic neutropenia
Defective function
  Adherence
    Diabetes
    Alcohol
    Myelogenous leukemia
  Chemotaxis
    Diabetes
    Rheumatoid arthritis
    Systemic lupus erythematosus
    Severe infections
    Hypothermia
    Hypogammaglobulinemia or hypophosphatemia
    Down's syndrome
    Kartagener's syndrome
    Lazy leukocyte syndrome
    Hyper IgE syndrome
  Phagocytosis
    Cellular defect
      Diabetes
      Autoimmune disorders
      Hypophosphatemia
    Decreased opsonization
      Complement deficiencies
      Hypogammaglobulinemia
      Sickle cell disease
  Degranulation
    Chédiak-Higashi syndrome
  Intracellular killing
    Chronic granulomatous disease
    Familial lipochrome histocytosis
    Severe glucose-6-phosphate dehydrogenase deficiency
    Myeloperoxidase deficiency
    Malacoplakia
Other
  Hyposplenism
  Vitamin B$_{12}$ and folate deficiency
  Pulmonary alveolar proteinosis
  Idiopathic

gener's syndrome (sinusitis, bronchiectasis, and situs inversus) is marked by abnormal chemotaxis and random migration of neutrophils (chemokinesis). Definitive diagnosis is made by electron microscopy of the nasal mucosa or sperm showing the abnormal cilia structure. The same abnormal chemotaxis and random migration, along with impaired release of granulocytes from the bone marrow, is seen in lazy leukocyte syndrome. Clinically, patients present with low-grade fevers, recurrent gingivitis, stomatitis, otitis media, and neutropenia. Hyper IgE syndrome, discussed in detail in the section on IgE, is also associated with a cellular defect of chemotaxis. The clinical presentation is recurrent noninflamed (''cold'') staph skin infections, eczema, and elevated IgE. A number of case reports identify patients with comparable defects caused by a

wide range of mechanisms, such as lack of a membrane glycoprotein.[132–134]

As discussed in other sections, deficiencies in C3b and IgG lead to decreased opsonization.

Chédiak-Higashi is a severe disease inherited as autosomal recessive and usually fatal by age 20. Among the various defects associated with this disorder is failure of the neutrophils to degranulate and release lysosomal enzymes once phagocytosis has occurred.[135] Patients present with oculocutaneous albinism, photophobia, increased infections (especially Staphylococcus aureus), hepatosplenomegaly, and anemia. All leukocytes contain characteristic giant intracellular lysosome-like granules.

Chronic granulomatous disease, although primarily inherited as X-linked, has a more variable course then Chédiak-Higashi and occasionally may be first diagnosed in adulthood. Here neutrophils phagocytize and degranulate but are unable to generate H$_2$O$_2$ to kill the organisms.[136] Patients are characteristically infected with catalase-positive organisms (Staphylococcus aureus, most aerobic gram-negative enteric bacteria, candida, and aspergillus). This leads to chronic suppurative infections, especially of the skin, lymph nodes, lung, and bone marrow with atypical granuloma formation. Later there is a high incidence of pulmonary fibrosis and development of discoid lupus.[137] Diagnosis is made by testing for defective production of H$_2$O$_2$, most commonly by the nitroblue tetrazolium (NBT) reductase method (dye remains colorless) or by chemiluminescence. Carrier mothers have 50% of activity.

Severe glucose-6-phosphate dehydrogenase deficiency (less than 5 to 10% of activity) is associated with an increased susceptibility to infection because of neutrophil dysfunction.

Myeloperoxidase (MPD) deficiency may be the most common cause of phagocytic defects. Inherited as autosomal recessive, the increased incidence of bacterial and especially candida infections is due to lack of MPD in neutrophils. This can be evaluated by peroxidase stains. Chemiluminescence but not NBT is abnormal.

Unlike MPD deficiency, malacoplakia is an acquired monocyte disorder marked by an inability to digest certain gram-negative bacteria, leading to recurrent granulomata and chronic infections, especially of the urinary tract. Examination of the monocytes reveals large cytoplasmic inclusions (Michaelis-Gutmann bodies).

Hyposplenism, whether functional, as from sickle cell disease, or postsplenectomy, results in decreased clearance of invading organisms. Larger amounts of antibody are needed for efficient clearance.[138] Still, the

Table 3–39. Laboratory Evaluation of a Patient with a Suspected Disorder of the Phagocytic System

Complete blood count
Complete neutrophil count (every 3 days for 3 weeks if cyclic neutropenia is suspected)
Total and individual immunoglobulin levels
CH_{50}
Phosphate
B_{12}/folate levels
IgE if hyper IgE syndrome is suspected
ANA + RF if autoimmune disease is suspected
FBS/GTT if diabetes mellitus is suspected
Morphology of blood cells
    Chédiak-Higashi—giant lysosome-like granules in leukocytes
    Malacoplakia—large cytoplasmic inclusions in leukocytes
    Hyposplenism—poikilocytosis, target cells, spherocytes
    B_{12}/folate deficiency—large, hypersegmented polymorphonuclear cells
Evaluation of mobilization from marginated pools by epinephrine
Evaluation of mobilization from bone marrow by corticosteroids
Nitroblue tetrazolium dye reductase
Chemiluminescence
Glucose-6-phosphate dehydrogenase level
Peroxidase stain of leukocyte
Other
    Adherence to different surfaces
    Skin windows or Boydon Chamber to check migration/chemotaxis
    Time lapse cinematography of cells
    Other tests for defective H_2O_2 production
    Electron micrographs of cilia structure
    Quantitative killing assays
    Analysis of surface proteins or autoantibody production

overall incidence of fulminant sepsis is low—0.18/100 person years.[139] Deficiency of vitamin B_{12} and folate result in large hypersegmented neutrophils, which, at least in the case of B_{12} deficiency, may have decreased function.

Pulmonary alveolar proteinosis is a disorder of unclear origin associated with 1° or 2° defective alveolar macrophage function.

DIAGNOSTIC EVALUATION

The history is a vital part of the evaluation. The type and location of infections should be noted, along with associated diseases, drug use, or family history of comparable disorders. The physical exam should identify the location of infections and associated lymphadenopathy or hepatosplenomegaly. Down's syndrome should also be obvious from the physical exam.

A suggested laboratory evaluation is outlined on Table 3–39. Screening blood testing should be done to determine if there is neutropenia. If cyclic neutropenia is suspected the count should be checked every 3 days for 3 weeks. Immunoglobulin, complement, phosphate, B_{12}, and folate deficiencies should be

checked. Autoimmune disorders, hyper IgE syndrome, or diabetes mellitus should be screened for as well, if suspected.

Examination of the structure of blood cells is also helpful. Giant lysosome-like granules are seen in leukocytes in Chédiak-Higashi syndrome; large cytoplasmic inclusions are seen in leukocytes in malacoplakia. The neutrophils are large and hypersegmented in B_{12} and folate deficiency. The red cells show Howell-Jolly bodies, spherocytosis, poikilocytosis, and target cells in hyposplenism.

Mobilization of neutrophils from marginated pools can be tested by epinephrine and from the marrow by corticosteroids. Generation of H_2O_2 can be evaluated by a number of tests, most commonly reduction of NBT dye or chemiluminescence. In chronic granulomatous disease (CGD) both are abnormal; in myeloperoxidase deficiency only the latter is. Absence of G6PD in a cell will also not reduce NBT, leaving it colorless.

The G6PD level in the cells can be evaluated. Peroxidase staining will identify myeloperoxidase deficiency.

Other tests to determine the nature of a phagocytic defect are generally available only in research facilities. These include placement of skin windows to check migration; time lapse photography of cellular movement; Boyden chamber studies of migration/chemotaxis; quantitative killing assays; analysis of membrane proteins; and autoantibody formation, to name a few.

COMPLEMENT DEFICIENCIES

DEFINITION AND PATHOPHYSIOLOGIC CONSIDERATIONS

The complement system is a series of serum proteins that aids host defenses by acting as a nonspecific effector system for inflammation and the immune system.[140] Stimulation of this cascade of proteins by immune complexes (classic pathway) or by complex polysaccharides present in many bacterial and yeast cell walls (alternate pathway) leads to the production of a number of active components. The binding of these complement components to the large number of cells that have receptors for them results in a variety of changes that generally induce inflammation. For example, C3a and, to a greater extent, C5a, binding to specific receptors on a mast cell, can induce that cell to release its mediators, resulting in an immediate hypersensitivity reaction or inflammation. The binding of these same factors to a neutrophil can result in increased chemotaxis, whereas the binding of other complement components causes a respiratory burst or enhanced phagocytosis, enhancing the inflammatory reaction against a foreign substance. C3b and to a lessor extent, C5a can act as opsonins binding to a bacterium or other substance, enhancing its chance of being phagocytized. Activation of the complete complement cascade can lead to lysis of, for example, a red blood cell or a gram-negative bacterium.

DIFFERENTIAL DIAGNOSIS AND DIAGNOSTIC EVALUATION

If a patient relates a history of recurrent angioedema, of recurrent infections, especially pyogenic or with Neisseria, or of an autoimmune disease, a complement deficiency should be considered. The best screening test to obtain is a CH_{50}. Because the CH_{50} test measures the lysis of antibody-coated sheep red blood cells, it measures all the components indirectly, since the terminal components are responsible for the lysis. If one component is diminished, the cascade will slow and lysis of the cells will take longer. Complement is very temperature sensitive and will decay rapidly at room temperature. Therefore, a blood test drawn for determination of CH_{50} should be placed on ice and analyzed immediately. If there is a delay, the serum should be spun in the cold and stored at $-70°$ C. The CH_{50} will be prolonged if the specimen was not handled properly, probably the most common cause of an abnormal result. If the CH_{50} is normal it is unlikely that there is a significant defect of one of the individual components, and it is generally not necessary to pursue the investigation further. If it is abnormal, the individual components can be analyzed. Quantitation of C4, C3, and C1 esterase inhibitor is readily available, but analysis of most of the others requires a specialty laboratory. If C4 is low, the classic pathway is affected, as in immune complex mediated nephritis. If C4 is normal but C3 is low, the alternate pathway is being activated.

In the case of hereditary angioedema, C4, the substrate of the enzyme, is usually low. C2 is decreased during attacks. If the CH_{50} and C4 are low, a C1 esterase inhibitor level should be obtained. If this is normal and hereditary angioedema is still suspected clinically, a functional test of C1 esterase inhibitor should be performed, since this is abnormal in 15% of cases. If the C4 and C1 esterase inhibitor are low and the patient is elderly, angioedema associated with

malignancy should be considered. In this situation, Clq is usually decreased, in contrast to the normal levels in hereditary angioedema.

Understanding the function of the complement system, one can understand why deficiencies of various components are associated with an increased incidence of infections and an increased incidence of autoimmune-related diseases. This correlation may exist because, since complement helps in the clearance of immune complexes, a deficiency leads to an increased circulating number, or because, since the genes for complement may be related to immune response genes, an inherited disorder of one may be associated with deficiencies in the other.

Inherited deficiencies of the complement components are rare (Table 3–40),[141,142] and hence exact incidence figures are generally unknown. It is also unknown if a deficiency consistently results in disease. Patients have been described who lack C2 and Clq and yet are totally asymptomatic.

For those few patients well described in the literature who have a deficiency, it appears that lack of the early components of Clq, Clr, Cls, C2, C4, and C5 seems to be associated with an increased incidence of systemic lupus erythematosus-like disorders frequently associated with nephritis.

As discussed, deficiencies of other components are associated with an increased incidence of bacterial infections. Clq, C2,[143] and C3 deficiencies result in an increase in pyogenic infections, while deficiencies of C5, C6, C7, or C8 result specifically in an increase in Neisseria infections, especially recurrent ones.

An inherited deficiency of C1 esterase inhibitor is the cause of hereditary angioedema, discussed in the section on urticaria and angioedema. It appears that most patients have a relative deficiency of the enzyme and do not become symptomatic until it decreases substantially, perhaps by 25 to 50%. Of these patients, 85% have diminished enzyme levels; the remainder have a functionally inactive enzyme.

Certain disease states are associated with an acquired hypocomplementemia. The responsible mechanisms are generally hypercatabolism and production of antibody specific for individual components. There are many instances of complement utilization with normal serum levels locally, e.g., the kidney in nephritis or the synovium in rheumatoid arthritis. A decreased serum level suggests systemic immune complex mediated disease (e.g., SLE or vasculitis).

Decrease of Clq, C1, and C2 suggests activation of the classic pathway, whereas decrease of C3 with normal Clq, C4, and C2 suggests activation of the alternate pathway.

Acquired deficiency of C1 esterase inhibitor can

Table 3–40. Inherited Complement Deficiencies and Associated Diseases

Deficiency	Incidence (Where Known)	Associated Clinical Features
C1q		Systemic lupus erythematosis (SLE)-like syndrome Glomerulonephritis Combined immunodeficiency disease Hypogammaglobulinemia
C1r		SLE-like syndromes Glomerulonephritis
C1s		SLE
C2	0.01% 9 patients	None (common) Autoimmune disorders, especially lupus-like Recurrent pyogenic infections Juvenile rheumatoid arthritis
C3		Recurrent bacterial infections Nephritis
C4		SLE
C5	extremely rare	SLE-like syndrome Neisseria infections
C6		None Neisseria infections Raynaud's phenomenon
C7		None Neisseria infections Raynaud's phenomenon SLE-like syndromes
C8		None Neisseria infections SLE-like syndromes
C9		None
C1 esterase inhibitor		Hereditary angioedema
C3b inactivator		Recurrent bacterial infections

(Adapted from Fearon, D.T.: Complement. J Allergy Clin Immunol *71*:520, 1983; and Church, J.A., and Shlegel, R.J.: Immune Deficiency Disorders. *In* Immunology III. Edited by J.A. Bellanti. Philadelphia, W.B. Saunders, 1985.)

occur as a result of an underlying neoplasm, especially a lymphoproliferative malignancy presenting clinically as angioedema that may be difficult to differentiate from hereditary angioedema.[59a] In the former case, C1q is decreased, along with C4 and C2, unlike in hereditary angioedema.

REFERENCES

1. Smith, P.L., et al.: Physiologic manifestations of human anaphylaxis. J Clin Invest *66*:1072, 1980.
2. Silverman, H.J., Van Hook, C., and Haponik, E.F.: Hemodynamic changes in human anaphylaxis. Am J Med *77*:341, 1984.
3. Gleich, G.T., et al.: Cytotoxic properties of eosinophil major basic protein. J Immunol *123*:2925, 1979.
4. Erffmeyer, J.E.: Adverse reactions to penicillin. Ann Allergy *47*:288, 1981.
5. Sogn, D.D.: Penicillin allergy. J Allergy Clin Immunol *74*:589, 1984.
6. Levine, B.B., and Zolov, D.M.: Prediction of penicillin allergy by immunological tests. J Allergy *43*:231, 1969.
7. Sullivan, T.J., et al.: Skin testing to detect penicillin allergy. J Allergy Clin Immunol *68*:171, 1981.
8. DeSwarte, R.D.: Drug allergy—problems and strategies. J Allergy Clin Immunol *74*:209, 1984.
9. Reference 9 deleted.
10. Saxon, A.: Immediate hypersensitivity reactions to beta-lactase antibiotics. Rev Infect Dis *5*:S368, 1983.
11. Grieco, M.H.: Cross-allergenicity of the penicillins and the cephalosporins. Arch Intern Med *119*:141, 1967.
12. Petz, L.D.: Immunologic cross-reactivity between penicillins and cephalosporins: a review. J Infect Dis *137*(supp):374, 1978.
13. Delafuente, J.D., Panush, R.S., and Caldwell, J.R.: Penicillin and cephalosporins immunogenicity in man. Ann Allergy *43*:337, 1979.
14. Gordin, F.M., Simon, G.L., Wofsy, C.B., and Mills, J.: Adverse reactions to trimethoprim-sulfamethoxazole in patients with the acquired immune deficiency syndrome. Ann Intern Med *100*:495, 1984.
15. Garrelts, J.C., and Peterie, J.D.: Vancomycin and the "red man's syndrome." N Engl J Med *312*:245, 1985.
15a. Newfield, P., and Roizen, M.F.: Hazards of rapid administration of vancomycin. Ann Intern Med *91*:581, 1979.
15b. Pau, A.K., and Khakoo, R.: "Red-neck syndrome" with slow infusion of vancomycin. N Engl J Med *313*:756, 1985.
16. Schatz, M.: Skin testing and incremental challenge in the eval-

uation of adverse reactions to local anesthetics. J Allergy Clin Immunol 74:606, 1984.

17. Grammer, L.C., Chen, P.Y., and Patterson, R.: Evaluation and management of insulin allergy. J. Allergy Clin Immunol 71:250, 1983.

18. Grammer, L.C., and Patterson, R.: Proteins: Chymopapain and insulin. J. Allergy Clin Immunol 74:635, 1984.

18a. Fineberg, S.E., Galloway, J.A., Fineberg, N.S., and Goldman, J.: Effects of species of origin, purification levels, and formulation on insulin immunogenicity. Diabetes 32:7, 1983.

19. Kahn, C.R., and Rosenthal, A.S.: Immunologic reactions to insulin: Insulin allergy, insulin resistance, and the autoimmune insulin syndrome. Diabetes Care 2:283, 1979.

19a. Fineberg, S.E., et al.: Immunogenicity of recombinant DNA human insulin. Diabetologia 25:465, 1983.

20. Chamovitz, A., et al.: Human insulin in management of animal insulin allergy. J Allergy Clin Immunol 73 (Part 2):180, 1984 (abstr).

21. Bernstein, I.L.: Adverse effects of chemonucleolysis. JAMA 250:1167, 1983.

22. Grammar, L.C., and Patterson, R.: Proteins: Chymopapain and insulin. J Allergy Clin Immunol 74:635, 1984.

23. Medical News: Chymopapain injection—an often fruitless endeavor? JAMA 251:13, 1984.

24. Kapsalis, A.A., Sterne, J.J., and Bornstein, I.: Correlation between hypersensitivity to parenteral chymopapain and the presence of IgE anti-chymopapain antibody. Clin Exp Immunol 33:150, 1978.

25. Bernstein, D.J., Gallagher, J.S., Ulmer, A., and Bernstein, I.L.: Prospective evaluation of chymopapain sensitivity in patients undergoing chemonucleolysis. J Allergy Clin Immunol 73:458, 1985.

25a. Sagona, M.A., et al.: Evaluation of papain/chymopapain cross allergenicity. J Allergy Clin Immunol 76:776, 1985.

25b. Mansfield, L.E., Ting, S., Haverly, R.W., and Yoo, T.J.: The incidence and clinical implications of hypersensitivity to papain in an allergic population, confirmed by blinded oral challenge. Ann Allergy 55:541, 1985.

26. Caplan, S.N., and Berkman, E.M.: Letters to the Editor: Protamine Sulfate and Fish allergy. N Engl J Med 195:172, 1976.

27. Goldman, B.S., Joison, J., and Austen, W.G.: Cardiovascular effects of protamine sulfate. Ann Thor Surg 7:459, 1969.

28. Grant, J.A., et al.: Anaphylactic reactions to protamine on insulin-dependent diabetes after cardiovascular procedures. J Allergy Clin Immunol 73:180, 1984 (abstr.).

29. Knape, J.T., et al.: An anaphylactic reaction to protamine in a patient allergic to fish. Anesthesiology 55:324, 1981.

30. Simon, R.A.: Adverse reactions to drug additives. J Allergy Clin Immunol 74:623, 1984.

31. Wicher, K., and Reisman, R.E.: Anaphylactic reaction to penicillin (or penicillin like substance) in a soft drink. J Allergy Clin Immunol 66:155, 1980.

32. Nagel, J.E., Fuscaldo, J.T., and Freman, P.: Paraben allergy. JAMA 237:1594, 1977.

33. Schwartz, H.J.: Sensitivity to ingested metabisulfites. Variation in clinical presentation. J Allergy Clin Immunol 71:487, 1983.

34. Stevenson, D., and Simon, R.: Editorial: Sulfites and asthma. J Allergy Clin Immunol 74:469, 1984.

35. Sheppard, D., et al.: Lower threshold and greater bronchomotor responsiveness of asthmatic subjects to sulfur dioxide. Amer Rev Respir Dis 122:873, 1980.

36. Metcalfe, D.D.: Food hypersensitivity. J Allergy Clin Immunol 73:749, 1984.

37. Valentine, M.D.: Insect venom allergy: Diagnosis and treatment. J Allergy Clin Immunol 73:299, 1984.

38. Shepherd, G.: Update on Insect Allergy. Drug Therapy 13:147, 1983.

39. Mauriello, P.M., Barde, S.H., Georgitis, G.W., and Reisman, R.E.: Natural history of large local reactions from stinging insects. J Allergy Clin Immunol 74:494, 1984.

40. Greenberger, P.A.: Contrast Media Reactions. J Allergy Clin Immunol 74:600, 1984.

41. Greenberger, P.A., Patterson, R., and Radin, R.C.: Two pretreatment regimens for high risk patients receiving radiographic contrast media. J Allergy Clin Immunol 74:540, 1984.

42. Stevenson, D.D.: Diagnosis, prevention and treatment of adverse reactions to aspirin and non-steroidal anti-inflammatory drugs. J Allergy Clin Immunol 74:617, 1984.

43. Pleskow, W.W., et al.: Aspirin-sensitive rhinosinusitis asthma: Spectrum of adverse reactions to aspirin. J Allergy Clin Immunol 71:574, 1983.

44. VanArsdel, P.P.: Editorial: Aspirin idiosyncrasy and tolerance. J Allergy Clin Immunol 73:431, 1984.

45. Stevenson, D.D.: Diagnosis, prevention and treatment of adverse reactions to aspirin and non-steroidal anti-inflammatory drugs. J Allergy Clin Immunol 71:574, 1983.

46. Szczeklik, A., Gryglewski, R.J., and Czerniawska-Mysik, G.: Clinical patterns of hypersensitivity to nonsteroidal anti-inflammatory drugs and their pathogenesis. J Allergy Clin Immunol 60:276, 1977.

47. Sheffer, A.L., Soter, N.A., McFadden, E.R., and Austen, K.F.: Exercise induced anaphylaxis: a distinct form of physical allergy. J Allergy Clin Immunol 71:311, 1983.

48. Kidd, J.M., Cohen, S.H., Sosman, A.J., and Fink, J.N.: Food dependent exercise induced anaphylaxis. J Allergy Clin Immunol 71:407, 1983.

49. Sheffer, A.L.: Unraveling the mystery of idiopathic anaphylaxis. N Engl J Med 311:1248, 1984.

50. Sonon, L., Grammer, L.C., Greenberger, P.A., and Patterson, R.: Idiopathic anaphylaxis: A clinical Summary. Ann Intern Med 99:134, 1983.

51. Meggs, W.J., et al.: Progesterone sensitivity as a cause of recurrent anaphylaxis. N Engl J Med 311:1236, 1984.

52. Warin, R.P., and Champion, R.H.: Urticaria. Philadelphia, W.B. Saunders Co., 1974.

53. Mathews, K.P.: Urticaria and angioedema. J Allergy Clin Immunol 72:1, 1983.

54. Kaplan, A.P.: Angioedema. N Engl J Med 310:1662, 1984.

55. Vaida, G.A., Goldman, M.A., and Bloch, K.J.: Testing for hepatitis B virus in patients with chronic urticaria and angioedema. J Allergy Clin Immunol 72:193, 1983.

56. Phanuphak, P., et al.: Vasculitis in chronic urticaria. J Allergy Clin Immunol 65:436, 1980.

57. Soter, N.A.: Chronic urticaria as a manifestation of necrotizing venulitis. N Engl J Med 296:1440, 1977.

58. Zeiss, C.R., et al.: A Hypocomplementemic Vasculitis Urticarial Syndrome. Am J Med 68:867, 1980.

59. Sheffer, A.L., Austen, K.F., Rosen, F.S., and Fearon, D.T.: Acquired deficiency of the inhibitor of the first component of complement: Report of five additional cases with commentary on the syndrome. J Allergy Clin Immunol 75:640, 1985.

60. Meggs, W.J., et al.: Progesterone sensitivity as a cause of recurrent anaphylaxis. N Engl J Med 311:1236, 1984.

61. Kaplan, A.: Unusual cold-induced disorders: Cold-dependent dermatographism and systemic cold urticaria. J Allergy Clin Immunol 73:453, 1984.

62. Soter, N.A., et al.: Release of mast cell mediators and alterations in lung function in patients with cholinergic urticaria. N Engl J Med 302:604, 1980.

63. Gleich, G.J., et al.: Episodic angioedema associated with eosinophilia. N Engl J Med 310:1621, 1984.

64. Fields, T., Ghebrehiwet, B., and Kaplan, A.: Kinin formation in hereditary angioedema plasma: Evidence against kinin derivative from C2 and in support of ''spontaneous'' formation of bradykinin. J Allergy Clin Immunol 72:54, 1983.

65. Reed, C.E., and Friedlaender, M.: Immunological diseases of the eye. JAMA 248:2692, 1982.

65a. Lieberman, P., Crawford, L. and Drewry, R.D.: Allergic diseases of the eye and ear. In Allergic Diseases: Diagnosis and Management. Edited by R. Patterson. Philadelphia, J.B. Lippincott, 1980.

66. Zeiger, R.S., and Schatz, M.: Chronic rhinitis: A practical approach to diagnosis and treatment. Part I: Diagnosis. Immunol Allergy Practice 4:63, 1982.

66a. Mullarkey, M., Hill, J.S., and Webb, D.R.: Allergic and non allergic rhinitis: Their characterization with attention to the meaning of nasal eosinophilia. J Allergy Clin Immunol 65:122, 1980.

67. McFadden, E.R.: Pathogenesis of asthma. J Allergy Clin Immunol 73:413, 1984.

68. Szentivanyi, A.: The beta adrenergic theory of the atopic abnormality in bronchial asthma. J Allergy 42:203, 1968.

69. Venter, J.C., and Harrison, L.C.: Autoantibodies to B₂-adrenergic receptors: A possible cause of adrenergic hyperresponsiveness in allergic rhinitis and asthma. Science 207:1361, 1980.

70. Kaliner, M.: Hypotheses on the contribution of late-phase allergic responses to the understanding and treatment of allergic diseases. J Allergy Clin Immunol 73:311, 1984.

71. Cockcroft, D.: Hypothesis: mechanisms of perennial allergic asthma. Lancet July 30th, 1983, p. 253.

72. Bierman, C.W., Spiro, S.G., and Petheram, I.: Characterization of the late response in exercise induced asthma. J Allergy Clin Immunol 74:701, 1984.

73. Halwig, J.M., Greenberger, P.A., and Patterson, R.: Allergic bronchopulmonary aspergillosis. Immunol Allergy Practice 6:292, 1984.

74. Ricketti, A., et al.: Allergic bronchopulmonary aspergillosis. Arch Intern Med 143:1553, 1983.

75. Patterson, R., et al.: A radioimmunoassay index for allergic bronchopulmonary aspergillosis. Ann Intern Med 99:18, 1983.

76. Welliver, R.: Upper respiratory infections in asthma. J Allergy Clin Immunol 72:341, 1983.

77. Nelson, H.S.: Gastroesophageal reflux and pulmonary disease. J Allergy Clin Immunol 73:547, 1984.

78. Irwin, R.S., Correa, W.M., and Pratter, M.R.: Chronic persistent cough in the adult: the spectrum and frequency of causes and successful outcomes of specific therapy. Am Rev Respir Dis 123:413, 1981.

79. McFadden, E.R., Kiser, R., and Degroot, W.J.: Acute bronchial asthma. N Engl J Med 228:221, 1973.

80. Downing, E.T., et al.: Factitious Asthma: Physiologic approach to diagnosis. JAMA 248:2878, 1982.

81. Christopher, K.L. et al.: Vocal-cord dysfunction presenting as asthma. N Engl J Med 308:1566, 1983.

82. Fink, J.: Hypersensitivity pneumonitis. J Allergy Clin Immunol 74:1, 1984.

83. Pepys, J.: Occupational Respiratory Allergy: Clinics in Immunology and Asthma 4(1), 1984.

84. Salvaggio, J., and Kerr, R.M.: Hypersensitivity pneumonitis; state of the art. Chest 75:270, 1979 (Supplement).

85. Salvaggio, J.: Diagnosis and management of hypersensitivity pneumonitis. Hospital Practice 15:93, 1980.

86. Reynolds, H.Y., et al.: Analysis of cellular and protein content of bronchoalveolar lavage fluid from patients with idiopathic pulmonary fibrosis and chronic hypersensitivity pneumonitis. J Clin Invest 59:165, 1977.

87. Leatherman, J.W., Michael, A.F., Schwartz, B.A., and Hoidal, J.R.: Lung T cells in hypersensitivity pneumonitis. Ann Intern Med 100:390, 1984.

88. Gilchrest, B.: Pruritus: Pathogenesis, therapy and significance in systemic disease states. Arch Intern Med 142:101, 1982.

89. Weiszer, I.: Pruritis. In Allergic Diseases. Diagnosis and Management. Edited by R. Patterson. Philadelphia, J.B. Lippincott Co, 1980.

90. Beare, J.M.: Generalized pruritus. A study of 45 cases. Clin Exp Dermatol 1:343, 1976.

91. Winkleman, R.K., and Muller, S.A.: Pruritus. Annu Rev Med 15:53, 1964.

92. Cohen, S.G., and Ottesen, E.A.: The eosinophil, eosinophilia, and related disorders. In Allergy—Principles and Practice. Edited by E. Middleton Jr., C.E. Read, and E.F. Ellis. St. Louis, C.V. Mosby, 1983.

93. Kay, A.B.: The role of the eosinophil. J Allergy Clin Immunol 64:90, 1979.

94. Weller, P.: Eosinophilia. J Allergy Clin Immunol 73:1, 1984.

95. Beeson, P.B., and Bass, D.A.: The Eosinophil. Philadelphia, W.B. Saunders Co., 1977.

96. Gleich, G.T., et al.: Cytotoxic properties of eosinophil major basic protein. J Immunol 123:2925, 1979.

97. Shatz, M., Wasserman, S., and Patterson, R.: Eosinophils and immunologic lung disease. Med Clin North Am 65:1055, 1981.

98. Lynch, J.P., and Flint, A.: Sorting out the pulmonary eosinophilic syndromes. J Respiratory Diseases 5:61, 1984.

99. Fauci, A.S., et al.: The idiopathic hypereosinophilic syndrome. Ann Intern Med 97:78, 1982.

100. Gleich, G.J. et al.: Episodic angioedema associated with eosinophilia. N Engl J Med 310:1621, 1984.

101. Manuel, P.V., and Bahna, S.L.: Clinical aspects of serum total IgE level. Immunol Allergy Practice 5:212, 1983.

102. Geha, R.S.: Regulation of IgE synthesis in man. Current Concepts Allergy Immunol 15:1, 1984.

103. Geha, R.S.: Human IgE. J Allergy Clin Immunol 74:109, 1984.

104. Welliver, R.: Upper respiratory infections in asthma. J Allergy Clin Immunol 72:341, 1983.

105. Donabedian, H., and Gallin, J.I.: The hyperimmunoglobin E recurrent infection (Job's) syndrome. Medicine (Baltimore) 62:195, 1983.

106. Geha, R.S. et al.: Deficiency of suppressor T cells in the hyper-immunoglobulin E syndrome. J Clin Invest 68:783, 1983.

107. Buckley, R.H.: Immunodeficiency. J Allergy Clin Immunol 72:627, 1983.

108. Bretza, J.A., Chusid, M.J., Tencati, J.R., and Novey, H.: Adult immunodeficiency disorders. Immunol Allergy Practice 4:210, 1982.

109. Grieco, M.: Humoral and cellular responses to infections. In Infections in the Abnormal Host. Edited by M. Grieco. New York, Yorke Medical Books, 1980.

110. Seligman, S.J.: Pyogenic bacterial infections. In Infections in the Abnormal Host. Edited by M. Grieco. New York, Yorke Medical Books, 1980.

111. Kirpatrick, C.H.: Host defense against fungal infections. Am J Med 77:1, 1984 (Oct).

112. Cooper, M.D., and Buckley, R.H.: Developmental immunology and the immunodeficiency diseases. JAMA 248:2658, 1982.

113. Jacobson, K.W., and deShazo, R.D.: Selective immunoglobulin A deficiency associated with nodular lymphoid hyperplasia. J Allergy Clin Immunol 64:516, 1979.

114. Björkand, J., Bake, B., Oxelius, Y.-A., and Hanson, L.A.: Impaired lung function in patients with IgA deficiency and low levels of IgG2 or IgG3. N Engl J Med 313:720, 1985.

115. Beck, C.S., and Heiner, D.C.: Selective immunoglobulin G4 deficiency and recurrent infections of the respiratory tract. Am Rev Respir Dis 124:94, 1981.

116. Oxelius, V.: Immunoglobulin G (IgG) subclasses and human disease. Am J Medicine 77:7, 1984.

117. Ko, H.S., Chiorazzi, N., Waldman, T., and Rosen, F.: Evidence for a defect in "switch" T cells in patients with immunodeficiency and hyperimmunoglobulinemia M. N Engl J Med 314:409, 1986.

118. Sridama, V., et al.: Decreased levels of helper in T cells: A possible cause of immunodeficiency in pregnancy. N Engl J Med 307:352, 1982.

119. Fauci, A.S., moderator: The acquired immunodeficiency syndrome: an update. Ann Intern Med 102:800, 1985.

120. Reinherz, E.L., et al.: Immunodeficiency associated with loss of T4+ inducer T cell function. N Engl J Med 304:811, 1981.

121. Hermans, P.E., Diaz-Buxo, J.A., and Stobo, T.D.: Idiopathic late-onset immunoglobulin deficiency. Am J Med 61:221, 1976.

122. Podolsky, M.L.: Immune deficiency screening with the Schick test. Immunol Allergy Practice 4:45, 1982.

123. Cooper, M.D., and Buckley, R.H.: Developmental immunology and the immunodeficiency diseases. JAMA 248:2658, 1982.

124. Delafuente, J.C., Eisenberg, T.D., Hoelzer, D.R., and Slavin, R.: Tetanus toxoid as an antigen for delayed cutaneous hypersensitivity. JAMA 249:3209, 1983.

125. Palmer, D.L., and Reed, W.P.: Delayed hypersensitivity skin testing. 1. Response rates in a hospitalized population. J Infect Dis 130:132, 1974.

126. Fairshter, R.D., et al.: In vivo and in vitro cell mediated im-

munity to tetanus toxoid in adults. J Allergy Clin Immunol *66*:452, 1980.

127. Gordon, E.H., et al.: Delayed cutaneous hypersensitivity in normals: choice of antigens and comparison to in vitro assays of cell mediated immunity. J Allergy Clin Immunol *72*:487, 1983.

128. Nash, D.R., and Douglass, J.E.: Anergy in active pulmonary tuberculosis: a comparison between positive and negative reactors and an evaluation of STU and 250 TU skin test doses. Chest *77*:32, 1980.

129. Bretza, J.A., Chusid, M.J., Tencati, J.R., and Norey, A.: Adult immunodeficiency disorders. Immunol Allergy Practice *4*:210, 1982.

130. Cooper, M.D., and Buckley, R.H.: Developmental immunology and the immunodeficiency diseases. JAMA *248*:2658, 1982.

131. Klebanoff, S.J.: Neutrophil Dysfunction Syndromes. *In* Cecil. Textbook of Medicine. Edited by P.B. Beeson, W. McDermott, and J.B. Wyngoarden. Philadelphia, W.B. Saunders, 1979.

132. Crowley, C.A., et al.: An inherited abnormality of neutrophil adhesion. Its genetic transmission and its association with a missing protein. N Engl J Med *302*:1163, 1980.

133. Kramer, N., Perez, D., and Goldstein, I.M.: An immunoglobulin (IgG) inhibitor of polymorphonuclear leukocyte motility in a patient with recurrent infection. N Engl J Med *303*:1253, 1980.

134. Arnaout, M.A., et al.: Deficiency of a granulocyte-membrane glycoprotein (gp150) in a boy with recurrent bacterial infection. N Engl J Med *306*:693, 1982.

135. Root, R.K., Rosenthal, A.S., and Balesha, D.J.: Abnormal bactericidal, metabolic and lysosomal functions of Chediak-Higashi Syndrome leukocytes. J. Clin Invest *51*:649, 1972.

136. Johnston, R.B., Jr., Newman, S.L.: Chronic granulomatous disease. Pediatr Clin North Am *24*(2):365, 1977.

137. Dilworth, J.A., and Mandell, G.L.: Adults with chronic granulomatous disease of "childhood." Am J Med. *63*:233, 1977.

138. Hosea, S.W., Brown, E.J., Hamburger, M.I., and Frank, M.M.: Opsonic requirements for intravascular clearance after splenectomy. N Engl J Med *304*:245, 1981.

139. Schwartz, P.E., et al.: Postsplenectomy sepsis and mortality in adults. JAMA *248*:2279, 1982.

140. Fearon, D.T.: Complement. J Allergy Clin Immunol *71*:520, 1983.

141. Agnello, V.: Complement deficiency states. Medicine *57*:1, 1978.

142. Church, J.A., and Schlegel, R.J.: Immune Deficiency Disorders. *In* Immunology III. Edited by J.A. Bellanti. Philadelphia, W.B. Saunders, 1985.

143. Sampson, H.A., Walchner, A.M., and Baker, P.J.: Recurrent pyogenic infections in individuals with absence of the second component of complement. J Clin Immunol *2*:39, 1982.

CHAPTER **4**

HEMATOLOGIC AND
ONCOLOGIC PROBLEMS

Arnold Meisler, M.D. and Raj Mittal, M.D.

HEMATOLOGIC PROBLEMS

The key to the diagnosis of hematologic disease lies with simple diagnostic procedures, a history and physical examination, a complete blood count, and a careful scrutiny of the peripheral blood smear. Uncertainties that remain often can be resolved by the additional step of performing bone marrow aspiration and biopsy. On the basis of these simple tests, the general physician should be able to make a credible differential diagnosis and, in most cases, with the possible exception of the coagulopathies, a precise diagnosis. Often, more exotic laboratory techniques are available to delineate the disease, allow prognostication, and permit precise stratification for clinical trials. In most instances, however, these techniques are not required for the purpose of diagnosis.

At what point should the general physician seek the assistance of a hematologist? This distinction obviously cannot be made categorically; it depends on the physician's training and confidence in dealing with hematologic diseases. For instance, whereas the diagnosis and treatment of iron deficiency anemia is clearly within the scope of internal medicine, the physician may not feel knowledgeable enough to exclude sideroblastic anemia or a hemoglobinopathy. The material in this chapter facilitates at least a reasonable differential diagnosis. Even then, without familiarity in studying blood smears, the physician will surely overlook important diagnostic considerations. In fact, in order to properly use the text, the physician must be able to arrive at a diagnosis or at least recognize a major morphologic aberration. Only then will the appropriate differential diagnosis be suggested and the required supporting diagnostic tests obtained.

Detailed discussion of the entities considered here is clearly beyond the scope of this text, and the reader would do well to consult any of the standard textbooks available. We have sought, however, to make available the essential points of a disease entity in an easily assimilated form. Exigent situations arise so frequently in medicine that the busy practitioner is often denied the luxury of a leisurely perusal of pertinent literature. The format employed here allows the expeditious processing of a large body of information.

ABNORMAL PERIPHERAL BLOOD SMEAR

Careful examination of the peripheral blood smear can provide important information about the under-lying disease process. The blood smear should first be examined by a ×10 objective lens to find a "good area" where cells are evenly spread. Examination with a ×40 lens can be used for confirmation. Detailed examination of different cells is done with an oil immersion lens.

Red Cells

Normal red cells are normocytic normochromic, with a small area of central pallor that is about one fourth of the cell diameter. Macrocytosis (increase in cell size) and microcytosis (decrease in cell size) are discussed in another section. Anisocytosis (variation in red cell size) and poikilocytosis (variation in shapes of red cells) are seen in many hematologic disorders. Following are a few specific morphologic abnormalities of red cells.

SPHEROCYTES

Spherocytes are usually small, dense red cells with no area of central pallor. They are commonly seen in hereditary spherocytosis and immune hemolytic anemias. Other conditions associated with spherocytosis are extensive thermal burns, hypophosphatemia, Rh null disease, and many adverse nonimmune drug reactions.

STOMATOCYTES

Stomatocytes are red cells with a central slitlike area. They are associated with abnormalities of red-cell cation content and are seen in hereditary stomatocytosis, during bouts of acute alcoholism, in Rh null disease, and occasionally with neoplastic, cardiovascular, and hepatobiliary disorders.[1]

ELLIPTOCYTES

Elliptocytes are oval red cells typically seen in hereditary elliptocytosis (HE). Elliptocytes usually constitute more than 25% of circulating red cells in HE. They may be seen in smaller numbers in megaloblastic anemias (macro-ovalocytes), thalassemia, iron deficiency, sickle-cell diseases, and myelophthisic anemias.

ACANTHOCYTES

Acanthocytes are dense red cells with unevenly distributed thorny projections on their surfaces. They are related to alterations in membrane lipids and are seen in liver disease, in congenital abetalipoproteinemia, and after splenectomy. They should be differentiated from echinocytes or "spur" cells (seen in uremia), which have fairly regularly spaced and fewer projections.

TARGET CELLS

Red cells with a central spot of hemoglobin surrounded by a clear area that in turn is encircled by hemoglobin are called target cells because of their resemblance to a target. Target cells are seen in thalassemias, hemoglobin C disease, and obstructive jaundice, after splenectomy, and in lecithin-cholesterol acyltransferase (LCAT) deficiency. Occasional target cells may also be seen in iron deficiency anemias.

SCHISTOCYTES

Schistocytes are fragmented red cells that may take the shape of a helmet, crescent, triangle, etc. Fragmentation occurs secondary to direct physical trauma to the red cell, which reseals its membrane after losing part of the cell. Schistocytes are seen in disseminated intravascular coagulation, microangiopathic hemolytic anemia, and fragmentation secondary to malfunctioning prosthetic cardiac valves or severe valvular disease, especially aortic stenosis.

POIKILOCYTES

Tapered red cells with a droplike shape are called poikilocytes or teardrop cells. Prolonged trapping of the cells, probably in splenic sinusoids, produces this cell shape. Teardrop cells are seen commonly in myelofibrosis and myelophthisic anemias. They may also be noted in thalassemias and megaloblastic anemias.

RED CELL INCLUSIONS

Basophilic stippling is characterized by multiple fine, blue, or purple dispersed granules. The stippling results from the aggregation of ribosomes. It is noted in various anemias that involve impaired erythropoiesis with the exception of iron deficiency anemia. Stippling of the red cells is commonly seen in thalassemias, chronic lead poisoning (coarse stippling), and deficiency of pyrimidine 5'-nucleotidase.

Howell-Jolly bodies are round, dark purple nuclear remnants of about 1 μm in diameter that usually appear singly but occasionally in large numbers in young red cells, usually polychromatophilic erythroblasts. Howell-Jolly bodies are commonly seen after splenectomy and in thalassemias, severe hemolytic anemias, megaloblastic anemias, and myeloproliferative disorders.

Cabot rings are thin, blue or violet inclusions that may be in the shape of a ring, twisted loop, or figure eight. The mechanisms of their formation has not been agreed upon yet. Some postulate that they may be the remnants of the mitotic spindle, although others have found them to contain histone and iron. They may be seen in severe megaloblastic anemias, severe hypochromic anemias, myelofibrosis, and Di Guglielmo syndrome.[2]

Pappenheimer bodies are ferritin aggregates that stain off-blue on Wright's-Giemsa stain. They are distributed irregularly but usually close to the periphery of the cells. They occur singly or in pairs, tetrads or small clusters. They are common in anemias of poor iron utilization, such as thalassemias and chronic lead poisoning. They also appear secondary to severe alcoholism and after splenectomy.

White Cells

In addition to an increase or decrease in white cell count, abnormalities of white cells noted on blood smear include hyper- or hyposegmentation of neutrophils, leukocyte inclusions, and immature white cells.

HYPERSEGMENTATION

Hypersegmentation implies an increase in the segmentation of granulocytes, especially neutrophils. A single neutrophil with six or more lobes or three neutrophils with five lobes noted during a 100-cell differential count is considered hypersegmentation. Hypersegmentation to a lesser degree may be evident in other granulocytes. Hypersegmented granulocytes are usually seen in megaloblastic anemias.

PELGER-HUËT ANOMALY

Pelger-Huët anomaly of granulocytes may be inherited in an autosomal dominant fashion or it may be acquired. Pelger-Huët cells are characterized by reduced segmentation of nuclei, although chromatin appears mature. Bilobed cells may be "spectacle-like." In heterozygotes, about 30% of cells are unilobed, about 60% are bilobed, and usually 10% have three lobes; and rarely, a cell may have four lobes. The majority of the neutrophils in homozygotes are unilobed.

Acquired Pelger-Huët anomaly is commonly seen with myeloid leukemias and myeloid metaplasia. It may also be seen in multiple myeloma, chronic lymphocytic leukemia, leukemoid reactions, agranulocytosis, and myxedema.

GRANULOCYTE INCLUSIONS

In toxic granulation, the granules of neutrophils are larger than usual and stain darkly. These granules reflect the immaturity of the cytoplasm and the reduced number of cell divisions before the cells were released in the circulation. They are commonly seen in association with infections.

Döhle's bodies are blue-staining (Romanovsky's stain), discrete, oval or round inclusions in the peripheral cytoplasm of neutrophils. They consist of RNA and are considered to be lamellar aggregates of rough endoplasmic reticulum. They are commonly seen in association with infections and may also occur secondary to burns, cytotoxic drugs, and uncomplicated pregnancy.

May-Hegglin anomaly is characterized by large, basophilic, or pyroninophilic cytoplasmic inclusions in granulocytes. These inclusions resemble Döhle's bodies but are larger, more round and discrete, more numerous, and present in all granulocytes, including monocytes. These inclusions also consist of RNA of round endoplasmic reticulum but can be differentiated from Döhle's bodies ultrastructurally.[3] May-Hegglin anomaly is inherited in an autosomal dominant manner and is usually associated with variable thrombocytopenia and hypogranular giant platelets.

Alder-Reilly anomaly is characterized by large, numerous azurophilic or basophilic granules in granulocytes, monocytes, and lymphocytes. The granules can be differentiated from those of toxic granulations by the absence of Döhle's bodies, by large, abundant, purple-red granules in monocytes and lymphocytes, and by having more numerous inclusions in the bone marrow than in the peripheral blood. They are commonly seen in mucopolysaccharidoses.

Chédiak-Higashi anomaly is characterized by gigantic primary granules in granulocytes that stain intensely for peroxidase. Abnormal granules in lymphocytes are even larger. This autosomal recessive disorder is associated with partial oculocutaneous albinism, poor resistance to pyogenic infections, and increased tendency to bleed.

NEUTROPHILIA

Definition

Neutrophilia is defined as an increase in absolute neutrophil count (total white cell count × percentage neutrophils) above $7.5 \times 10^3/\mu l$. In the past, neutrophilia was incorrectly considered to be synonymous with leukocytosis, which refers to an increase in the total white cell count above $10.0 \times 10^3/\mu l$. Leukocytosis may also occur secondary to an increase in lymphocyte, eosinophil, monocyte, or basophil counts. Moderate or severe reactive leukocytosis, which may give the appearance of leukemia on the blood smear, has been termed a leukemoid reaction. Neutrophilia will be discussed in this section. Leukocytosis secondary to an increase in other white cells will be discussed in subsequent sections.

Pathophysiologic Considerations and Differential Diagnosis (Table 4–1)

Neutrophilia may occur because of demargination of cells from the marginated granulocyte pool to the

Table 4–1. Causes of Neutrophilia

Physiologic—exercise, stress, neonatal
Infections—usually caused by acute localized or systemic bacterial infections; may also occur secondary to fungal, rickettsial, spirochetal, parasitic, or certain viral infections
Inflammation—burns, tissue necrosis (e.g., myocardial infarction), pulmonary infarction, after surgery, collagen vascular disease, hypersensitivity reactions, other inflammatory disease
Metabolic disorders—diabetic ketoacidosis, uremia, eclampsia, acute poisoning (e.g., lead), digitalis
Acute hemorrhage
Acute hemolysis
Myeloproliferative disorders—myelocytic leukemias, myeloid metaplasia, polycythemia vera
Drugs—epinephrine, etiocholanolone, corticosteroids, lithium, etc.
Malignant neoplasms
Other causes—chronic idiopathic neutrophilia, hereditary neutrophilia

circulating granulocyte pool; increased release of cells from the marrow neutrophil storage reserve; increased neutrophil production; and decreased egress of neutrophils to the tissues or decreased neutrophil destruction.

Neutrophilia caused by marginal pool shift usually appears within minutes and may last for only minutes or for hours. It may occur following violent exercise, epinephrine injection, acute pain, marked changes in temperature, or emotional stress.

Neutrophilia caused by release of cells from the marrow storage compartment may occur secondary to various infections, inflammation, glucocorticoid, administration or injection of endotoxins, etiocholanolone, or corticosteroids. The increase in neutrophil count is usually modest. Release of neutrophils from the storage pool may be mediated by humoral factors. One such factor, neutrophil-releasing activity, may be secondary to activation of the complement system.

A complex series of maturational events follows a granulopoietic stimulus from infection or inflammation. Pleuripotent hematopoietic stem cells differentiate along the granulocytic line under the influence of growth factors termed colony stimulating activity (CSA).[4] In theory, disturbances in this complex regulatory system may cause an increase in neutrophil production even in the absence of a provocative stimulus. Malignant hematopoietic cells appear to proliferate autonomously without dependence on many of the normal regulators of growth.

Corticosteroids may decrease the movement of neutrophils from the vascular compartment to the tissues. Peripheral granulocytic survival may be prolonged in chronic myelogenous leukemia.

Diagnostic Evaluation

The diagnostic evaluation should include a complete history and physical examination, looking specifically for any evidence of common causes of neutrophilia such as infection, inflammation, and myeloproliferative syndromes. The clinician should perform a complete blood count, differential, and platelet count.

In addition, a critical review of the peripheral blood smear should be done. Acute neutrophilic response (e.g., in acute infection or acute hemorrhage) may be associated with a "shift to the left" in the granulocyte series, i.e., the appearance of bands or, occasionally, metamyelocytes. In chronic myeloid leukemia, granulocytes at different stages of maturation are noted. Metamyelocytes, bands, and mature neutrophils predominate, with a few myelocytes, promyelocytes, and occasionally a blast cell. Acute leukemias usually show blasts as the predominant white cell on peripheral smear. Neutrophils containing toxic granulations or Döhle's bodies suggest the presence of an infectious process. Chronic infections may have associated monocytosis. Immature red cells may be noted in myelofibrosis, acute hemorrhage, or hemolysis.

The patient's serum leukocyte alkaline phosphatase (LAP) score is decreased in chronic myelogenous leukemia (CML) and normal or elevated in leukemoid reaction. In a small number of cases in which the cause of neutrophilia is not evident, bone marrow aspiration and biopsy should be performed for morphology, cytogenetic analysis, and evidence of fibrosis. Cytogenetic analysis may be abnormal in leukemias and myeloproliferative disorders, with the characteristic Philadelphia chromosome in CML.

NEUTROPENIA

Definition

Neutropenia refers to a decrease in absolute neutrophil count (total white cell count per μl × percentage neutrophils) to less than 1500/μl for white adults. Average neutrophil counts may be lower in many blacks and Yemenite Jews.

Pathophysiologic Considerations and Differential Diagnosis (Table 4–2)

A decrease in the blood neutrophil count may occur without a decrease in the total blood granulocyte pool (pseudoneutropenia), e.g., acutely after injection of endotoxin, after dialysis, in certain chronic neutropenic states, as benign familial neutropenia, as the lazy leukocyte syndrome, and in malaria. More commonly, neutropenia is associated with a decrease in the total blood granulocyte pool (true neutropenia).

Neutropenia may occur secondary to decreased cell production, decreased release of cells from the marrow, increased cell destruction or sequestration, or a

Table 4–2. Causes of Neutropenia

Drugs, physical agents
  Antineoplastic chemotherapy
  Irradiation
  Aminopyrine
  Chloramphenicol
  Sulfonamides
  Antithyroid drugs
  Phenothiazines
  Anticonvulsants
  Phenylbutazone
  Meprobamate
Infections
  Bacterial
    Typhoid
    Paratyphoid
    Brucellosis
    Overwhelming sepsis
  Viral
    Measles
    Infectious hepatitis
    Influenza
    Rubella
  Protozoal
    Malaria
    Kala-azar
    Relapsing fever
  Rickettsial
    Rickettsial pox
    Typhus
    Rocky Mountain spotted fever
Hematologic diseases
  Leukemias
  Aplastic anemia
  Megaloblastic anemia
  Marrow infiltration by tumor
  Chronic idiopathic neutropenia
  Cyclic neutropenia
  Lazy leukocyte syndrome
  Chédiak-Higashi syndrome
Autoimmune disorders
  Systemic lupus erythematosus
  Felty's syndrome
Others
  Cirrhosis of liver with splenomegaly
  Banti's syndrome
  Gaucher's disease
  Hemodialysis

combination of these factors. Decreased production may occur predictably with certain agents, e.g., antineoplastic chemotherapeutic agents and irradiation, when a large enough dose is given. Drugs that only occasionally cause decreased production may be of the abrupt, hypersensitivity type, e.g., aminopyrine; of the slow, delayed type, e.g., phenothiazines; or a combination of both, e.g., antithyroid drugs and sulfonamides. Decreased or ineffective granulopoiesis may occur secondary to preleukemic states, in the myelophthisic process, and in megaloblastic anemia. Periodic marrow failure accounts for the decrease in neutrophil count in cyclic neutropenia. Decreased neutrophil survival may occur in autoimmune disorders, e.g., systemic lupus erythematosus, Felty's syndrome, cirrhosis with splenomegaly, and megaloblastic anemias.

Diagnostic Evaluation

A complete patient history including family history, information about drug and alcohol intake, and any history suggestive of infections should be obtained. A complete physical examination is essential in the diagnostic evaluation.

Important lab studies such as complete blood count, platelet count, and red cell indices should be performed initially. The peripheral blood smear should be carefully examined for any immature white cells. Atypical lymphocytes may be seen with neutropenia in viral infections. Patients with chronic neutropenia will need to have blood counts repeated two to three times per week for 5 to 6 weeks to evaluate the periodicity of neutropenia. Stains may be required in certain patients to exclude leukemic or other malignant processes. Antineutrophil antibodies may be looked for in patients with immune neutropenias.

In certain patients in whom the pathologic process may not be clinically evident, colony-forming unit–granulocyte macrophage and colony-stimulating activity (CSA) assay can be obtained to differentiate between stem cell and humoral disorders. A decrease in granulopoiesis secondary to cytotoxic suppressor cells or serum inhibitory factors can also be tested in vitro.

EOSINOPHILIA

Definition

Eosinophilia is defined as an increase in absolute eosinophil count (total white cell count × percentage eosinophils) to more than 700µl. The eosinophil count undergoes diurnal variation, with the highest count occurring in the morning and the lowest in the afternoon.

Pathophysiologic Considerations (Table 4–3)
(see Chapter 3)

Increased production of eosinophils occurs secondary to various factors released by T-lymphocytes sensitized by allergic reactions, parasitic disease, etc. Tissue eosinophilia may occur secondary to an eosinophil chemotactic factor released by stimulated lymphocytes or secondary to histamine and eosinophil chemotactic factor of anaphylaxis (ECF-A), which are released from mast cells during immediate hypersensitivity reactions.

Table 4–3. Causes of Eosinophilia

Parasitic infections
   Trichinosis
   Echinococcosis
   Strongyloides
   Hookworm disease
   Trichuriasis
   Toxocariasis
   Filariasis
   Schistosomiasis
   Cysticercosis
Allergic diseases
   Bronchial asthma
   Hay fever
   Urticaria
   Angioneurotic edema
   Serum sickness
   Allergic vasculitis
Skin diseases
   Dermatitis herpetiformis
   Pemphigus vulgaris
   Psoriasis
   Eczema
   Pityriasis rubra
   Icthyosis
   Prurigo
   Facial granulomas
Drug reactions
   Sulfonamides
   Nitrofurantoin
   Aspirin
   Iodides
Malignancy
   Hodgkin's disease
   Mycosis fungoides
   Chronic myelogenous leukemia
   Carcinomatosis (especially with necrosis)
   Polycythemia vera
Collagen vascular disorders
   Periarteritis nodosa
   Goodpasture's syndrome
   Rheumatoid arthritis
   Dermatomyositis
Hypereosinophilic syndromes
   Löffler's syndrome
   Pulmonary infiltration with eosinophilia (PIE) syndrome
   Löffler endocarditis
   Eosinophilic leukemia
Others
   Radiotherapy
   Peritoneal dialysis
   Splenectomy
   Hyperadrenocorticism
   Hereditary eosinophilia

Diagnostic Evaluation

A complete patient history with special emphasis on a history of allergies, drug intake, and pulmonary symptoms should be taken. Physical examination should be done with special emphasis on skin lesions, lymphadenopathy, or hepatosplenomegaly.

Initial laboratory tests should include CBC, differ-

Table 4–4. Causes of Basophilia

Neoplasia
  Myeloproliferative syndromes
    Chronic myelogenous leukemia
    Polycythemia vera
    Myelofibrosis
    Basophilic leukemia
    Mastocytosis
  Preleukemia
  Others
    Carcinoma
    Hodgkin's disease
Chronic hypersensitivity
  Drug, food, and inhalant hypersensitivity
  Injection of foreign protein
  Urticaria
  Hookworm infestation
Inflammatory conditions
  Ulcerative colitis
  Rheumatoid arthritis
Infections
  Smallpox
  Chickenpox
  Influenza
  Tuberculosis
Endocrine disorders
  Myxedema
  Diabetes mellitus
  Estrogens
  Antithyroid drugs
Others
  Following splenectomy
  Some chronic hemolytic anemias
  Sideroblastic anemia[5]

ential and platelet count, and evaluation of stool for ova and parasites. A peripheral blood smear should be screened for any immature white cells. The appearance of blasts indicates a rapid downhill course in patients with hypereosinophilic syndrome.

Finally, a biopsy of any significantly enlarged lymph node or skin lesions should be considered.

BASOPHILIA

Definition

Basophilia refers to an increase in absolute blood basophil count (total white cell count × percentage basophils above 150/μl).

Pathophysiologic Considerations (Table 4–4)

An increase in the basophil count may be reactive or neoplastic. Basophil numbers are commonly increased in myeloproliferative disorders; the highest numbers are seen in patients with chronic myelogenous leukemia in whom the basophil is neoplastic and who may possess Philadelphia chromosome. Reactive basophilia occurs in various inflammatory conditions and hypersensitivity reactions of the immediate type, which are usually accompanied by an increase in IgE.

Diagnostic Evaluation

The patient's workup should proceed based on the different causes (Table 4–4). Hepatosplenomegaly, lymphadenopathy, skin rash, and dermatographism should be looked for. A complete blood count and leukocyte alkaline phosphatase are helpful in diagnosing myeloproliferative syndromes. A peripheral blood smear showing immature white cells in various stages and decreased leukocyte alkaline phosphatase are noted in CML. Basophilia is usually modest in CML, but it may occasionally exceed 30% of the normal basophil count. Rarely, a basophil count of greater than 80% of peripheral blood leukocytes is noted early in the course of disease. Such patients are considered to have basophilic leukemia. Biopsy and bone marrow aspiration with cytogenetic analysis are helpful in patients suspected of having myeloproliferative and myelodysplastic syndromes. Red cell mass and plasma volume determinations are required in patients with high hematocrits. Additional workup depends on the physician's initial diagnosis in each individual case.

LYMPHOCYTOSIS

Definition

Lymphocytosis refers to an increase in the absolute lymphocyte count. Relative lymphocytosis refers to an increase in the percentage of lymphocytes without an increase in the total lymphocyte count, e.g., in conditions with neutropenia. An absolute lymphocytosis is said to exist when the number of lymphocytes exceeds 4000/μl.

Pathophysiologic Considerations and Differential Diagnosis (Table 4–5)

A discussion of lymphocyte development is beyond the scope of this section. It is clear, however, that the lymphopoiesis under normal circumstances is controlled by exposure to antigen, in keeping with the major function of these cells, which is to produce circulating antibodies (B cells) and express cellular immunity (T cells). The subject is complex and considerable interdependency of function is apparent, as, for example, the requirement of T cells for B-cell function. Modulating growth factors termed lymphokines are responsible for regulating the production and function of these cells. As with other hemopoietic cells, however, apparently autonomous proliferation may occur upon malignant transformation. Further, it has become apparent that viral genomes, on incor-

Table 4—5.   Causes of Lymphocytosis

Infections
  German measles
  Mumps
  Recovery from acute infections
Endocrine disorders
  Thyrotoxicosis
  Adrenal insufficiency
Acute infections
  Pertussis
  Infectious mononucleosis
  Acute infectious lymphocytosis
  Infectious hepatitis
  Cytomegalovirus infection
  Toxoplasmosis
Chronic infections
  Brucellosis
  Tuberculosis
  Secondary and congenital syphilis
Hematologic disorders
  Acute and chronic lymphocytic leukemia
  Lymphomas with a leukemic blood picture
  Heavy-chain disease
  Neutropenic conditions
Others
  Hypersensitivity reactions (occasionally)
  Post-transfusion syndrome

poration into lymphocyte DNA, can vastly modify and control these cells to the detriment of the host, e.g., in rubella, infectious mononucleosis, and AIDS.

Diagnostic Evaluation

It is essential to obtain a complete history and to perform a physical examination, looking particularly for splenomegaly, lymphadenopathy, or any evidence of an infection.

CBC, platelet count, and examination of a peripheral blood smear should be done initially. Study of structure of lymphocytes on blood smear evaluation provides important clues to the differential diagnosis of lymphocytosis. Small, mature-looking lymphocytes with a monotonous appearance are characteristic of chronic lymphocytic leukemia (CLL), whereas a predominance of immature blast cells is seen in acute lymphocytic leukemia, and relatively large cells with cleft nuclei are seen in certain lymphomas presenting with a leukemic blood picture.

An increase in atypical lymphocytes is noted in patients with infectious mononucleosis, cytomegalovirus infection, post-transfusion syndrome, toxoplasmosis, infectious hepatitis, and hypersensitivity reactions secondary to phenytoin and para-amino salicylic acid. In infectious mononucleosis usually more than 20% of the lymphocytes are atypical; the cells frequently are nongranular, with a vacuolated or foamy appearance.

Bone marrow aspiration and biopsy should be considered in patients with a clinical diagnosis of leukemia

or lymphoma to study structure, perform cytogenic analysis, and to stage lymphomas. In patients with marked lymphocytosis, cytogenetic analysis can be performed on lymphocytes obtained from the buffy coat. Cytogenetic analysis can provide prognostic information in patients with CLL.[6] Bone marrow cultures for acid-fast bacilli and fungi can be obtained in patients suspected of having disseminated tuberculosis or fungal infections.

Pertinent skin tests (purified protein derivative, fungal), serum titers (fungal, brucellar, toxoplasmal, and viral), and cultures in patients clinically suspected of having such infections are important additional diagnostic studies.

In patients with possible underlying lymphoma or undiagnosed chronic infection, e.g. tuberculosis, lymph node biopsy should be considered.

MONOCYTOSIS

Definition

Monocytosis refers to an increase in absolute monocyte count above $900/\mu l$ in adults.

Pathophysiologic Considerations and Differential Diagnosis (Table 4—6)

Circulating monocytes are cells in transit from bone marrow to tissues and body cavities, where they mature into macrophages. During their production they share with neutrophils a common progenitor cell, colony-forming unit–neutrophil-monocyte (CFU-NM), after which their maturation pathways diverge. Colony-stimulating activity (CSA) produced by monocytes as well as activated T-lymphocytes stimulates the proliferation of this common progenitor cell, and an inhibitor produced by neutrophils inhibits its proliferation. Prostaglandins and other inhibitory factors produced by monocytes inhibit the proliferation of monocyte precursors. In response to infection and immunologic reaction, monocytes and activated T-lymphocytes increase the production of CSF, leading to proliferation of monocyte precursors.

Diagnostic Evaluation

A complete history and a physical examination, looking specifically for causes like tuberculosis, chronic leukemias, and inflammatory disorders, provide important clues to diagnosis. A history of any recent antineoplastic chemotherapy or radiation therapy should be obtained, as the patient may be in the recovery phase from neutropenia. Monocytosis in disseminated tuberculosis may be severe enough to give a leukemoid picture. Serum leukocyte alkaline phos-

Table 4—6. Causes of Monocytosis

Hematologic disorders
  Myeloproliferative disorders
    Chronic myelomonocytic leukemia
    Chronic monocytic leukemia
    Polycythemia vera
    Idiopathic myelofibrosis
  Acute leukemias
    Acute myelomonocytic leukemia
    Acute monocytic leukemia
  Lymphomas
    Hodgkin's disease
    "True" histiocytic lymphoma
    Other lymphoma
  Miscellaneous
    Multiple myeloma
    Malignant histiocytosis
    Chronic neutropenias and during recovery from agranulocytosis
    Preleukemia
    Hemolytic anemias
    Lipid storage disorders
Nonhematologic malignancies
  Carcinoma of ovary, stomach, breast
Collagen vascular diseases
  Rheumatoid arthritis
  Systemic lupus erythematosus
  Temporal arteritis
  Myositis
  Polyarteritis nodosa
Granulomatous and inflammatory diseases
  Sarcoidosis
  Ulcerative colitis
  Regional enteritis
  Sprue
  Infections
    Tuberculosis
    Subacute bacterial endocarditis
    Syphilis
    Recovery from acute infections
  Drugs, toxins
    Tetrachlorethane poisoning
    Chronic high-dose steroid therapy

Table 4—7. Classification of Erythrocytosis

Relative erythrocytosis
  Decrease in plasma volume: burns, shock, severe diarrhea and vomiting, etc.
  Spurious (Gaisböck's syndrome)
Absolute erythrocytosis
  Myeloproliferative syndrome, e.g., polycythemia vera
  Secondary erythrocytosis
    Decreased tissue oxygenation with appropriate increase in erythropoietin production
      High altitude
      High-affinity hemoglobins
        Hemoglobin Chesapeake
        Congenital methemoglobinemia
      Carboxyhemoglobins secondary to smoke inhalation or drugs
      Hypoventilation syndromes
        Primary alveolar hypoventilation
        Pickwickian syndrome
      Chronic cor pulmonale
      Heart disease (right-to-left shunt)
      Intense cigarette smoking
    Increased erythropoietin production unrelated to hypoxia with aberrant or inappropriate erythropoietin production
      Malignancies
        Kidney
        Liver (hepatoma)
        Adrenal
        Lung
      Benign conditions
        Renal cysts, hydronephrosis
        Cerebellar hemangiomas
        Uterine myomata
        Pheochromocytoma
        Cushing's syndrome
        Aldosterone-producing adenomas
        Bartter's syndrome
      Renal transplantation
    Essential overproduction of erythropoietin

phatase and cytogenetic analysis should be obtained in patients suspected of having CML. In acute myelomonocytic or monocytic leukemia, serum and urinary lysozyme are often elevated, sometimes high enough to damage the renal tubules. Determination of this enzyme is useful in diagnosing this form of leukemia.

ERYTHROCYTOSIS

Definition

An increase in red cell count or hematocrit above normal is referred to as erythrocytosis.

Pathophysiologic Considerations (Table 4—7)

Erythrocytosis may be relative or absolute. Relative erythrocytosis is due to a decrease in plasma volume causing the red cell count and the hematocrit to appear increased, although the true red cell mass is normal. Absolute erythrocytocis refers to a true increase in red cell mass in the presence of a normal plasma volume. Absolute erythrocytosis may occur because of autonomous red cell proliferation in clonal stem cell disorders like polycythemia vera, or it may occur secondary to hypoxic stimulation of erythropoietin production or aberrant production of erythropoietin by tumor.

Differential Diagnosis (Table 4—8)

A patient with splenomegaly, thrombocytosis, leukocytosis, and polycythemia with no obvious cause will usually have polycythemia vera (Table 4—9).

Diagnostic Evaluation

The distinction between absolute and relative erythrocytosis may be made by determining the erythrocyte mass. This determination will not, however, differ-

Table 4—8. Differential Diagnosis of Erythrocytosis

	Relative	Absolute	
		Secondary	Polycythemia Vera
Splenomegaly	—	—	75–80%
Hepatomegaly	—	—	35%
Pruritus	—	—	+
Red cell mass	nl	+	+
White cell count	—	—	+ in 65%
Platelet count	—	—	+ in 50%
Absolute basophil count	—	—	+ in 65%
Peripheral blood smear	—	—	Occasional normoblast, "shift to the left" in myeloid series, abnormal platelet structure
Uric acid	—	—	+ in 40%
Leukocyte alkaline phosphatase	nl	nl	+ in 70%
Serum B$_{12}$	—	—	nl or +
Unsaturated B$_{12}$ binding capacity	—	—	+ in 75%
Bone marrow	—	Erythroid hyperplasia	Hyperplasia of all elements, absent iron in >90%
Serum erythropoietin (radioimmunoassay)	nl	>30 μ/ml in 94%	<30 μ/ml in 92%
Erythroid colonies on bone marrow culture	nl	nl	Growth of colonies in the absence of added erythropoietin

+ = Elevated

entiate secondary erythrocytosis and polycythemia vera. The fact that 20 to 25% of patients with polycythemia vera do not have splenomegaly further complicates distinguishing these disorders (Table 4–8). Cardiopulmonary disorders are suggested by a finding of significantly low arterial oxygen saturation. In erythrocytosis secondary to mutant hemoglobins with high oxygen affinity, the oxygen-dissociation curves are shifted to the left, reflected in a low P$_{50}$, the partial pressure of oxygen that gives 50% saturation of hemo-

Table 4—9. Diagnostic Criteria for Polycythemia Vera*

Major Criteria
    Increased red cell mass—males > 36 ml/kg, females > 32 ml/kg
    Normal oxygen saturation ≥ 92.1%
    Splenomegaly
Minor criteria
    Thrombocytosis > 400 × 10³/μl
    Leukocytosis > 12 × 10³/μl
    Leukocyte alkaline phosphatase score > 100
    Serum B$_{12}$ > 900 pg/ml or unsaturated B$_{12}$ binding capacity > 2200 pg/ml

*The presence of all three major criteria or the first two major criteria and any two minor criteria indicates a diagnosis of polycythemia vera.

Table 4—10. Causes of Microcytic Anemias

Iron deficiency anemia
  Decreased intake of iron (e.g., infancy)
  Decreased absorption of iron
    Malabsorption syndrome
    Gastric resection
  Increased iron requirement
    Pregnancy
    Intravascular hemolysis
  Blood loss
    Gastrointestinal: peptic ulcer, varices, malignancy, helminthiasis, etc.
    Genitourinary: excessive menstrual blood loss, uterine fibroids, malignant neoplasms
    Others: recurrent hemoptysis, trapping of blood in extracorporeal dialysis equipment, etc.
Thalassemias and hemoglobinopathies
  Beta-thalassemia minor and major
  Alpha-thalassemia minor
  Delta-beta-thalassemia
  Hemoglobin H disease
  Hemoglobin Lepore
  Hemoglobin E
Sideroblastic anemias
  Hereditary sideroblastic anemias
  Acquired sideroblastic anemias
    Idiopathic
    Drugs and chemicals: lead, ethanol, antituberculosis drugs (isoniazid, cycloserine, pyrazinamide), chloramphenicol, antineoplastic drugs
    Complicating other diseases
    Hematologic: chronic hemolytic anemias, myelofibrosis
      Neoplastic: lymphoma
      Inflammatory: rheumatoid arthritis
      Metabolic: uremia, myxedema
  Severe anemia associated with infection, inflammation, or malignancy

globin. These mutants are often electrophoretically silent. Erythrocytosis secondary to cysts or tumors should be specifically sought using appropriate radiologic techniques. In most if not all secondary polycythemia, the erythropoietin level in the blood will be elevated significantly.

MICROCYTIC ANEMIAS

Definition

Anemias with decreased mean corpuscular volume (MCV) of red cells are referred to as microcytic anemias. Iron deficiency is the most common example of microcytic hypochromic anemias. Mean corpuscular hemoglobin concentration (MCHC) is decreased in moderately severe or severe iron deficiency anemias.

Pathophysiologic Considerations (Table 4–10)

Impairment of hemoglobin synthesis results in microcytic hypochromic anemias. Deficiency of iron in iron deficiency anemias, defective heme synthesis in sideroblastic anemias, decreased or altered globin synthesis in thalassemias and hemoglobinopathies, and poor reutilization of iron in anemias of inflammation or malignancy result in poor hemoglobinization of red cells.

Diagnostic Evaluation and Differential Diagnosis

PATIENT HISTORY AND PHYSICAL EXAMINATION

Patients with iron deficiency anemia usually present with vague symptoms and signs of anemia. The site of blood loss may be evident in some cases. Glossitis, angular cheilitis, and koilonychia are encountered infrequently.

Patients with thalassemias are usually diagnosed during childhood. Classic clinical features include stunted growth, Down's syndrome facies, bony changes caused by expanded marrow cavities, hepatosplenomegaly, and hyperpigmentation. Complications of iron overload with endocrine and cardiac disturbances usually develop by the second or third decade.

Hereditary sideroblastic anemias may be X linked or autosomally inherited. The "classic" form usually occurs in young adults or early middle-aged males with a positive family history. Anemia usually tends to be quite severe. Acquired secondary sideroblastic anemias may be associated with various disorders and drugs (Table 4–10). Primary acquired sideroblastic anemia usually presents in patients over 50 years of age with symptoms of anemia. The spleen tip may be palpable in about half the patients. The presence of ringed sideroblasts in the bone marrow is required in order to make this diagnosis.

Anemia of chronic inflammation or malignancy is usually mild to moderate and is overshadowed by the clinical features of the underlying disease.

DIAGNOSTIC STUDIES

Laboratory values can be helpful in differentiating the major causes of microcytic anemias (Table 4–11).

Laboratory tests usually required in evaluation of a patient with microcytic anemias include complete blood count, platelet count, MCV, MCHC, reticulocyte count, and examination of the peripheral blood smear.

Red cells in early iron deficiency may be normocytic normochromic. MCV, however, is markedly reduced in severe iron deficiency anemias and thalassemias. The peripheral smear shows anisopoikilocytosis in both of these disorders, whereas in thalassemia, target cells and basophilic stippling may be prominent. Staining with supravital stains reveals inclusion bodies in thalassemic patients. Red cells in sideroblastic anemias show a dimorphic picture. Hypochromic microcytic cells with anisopoikilocytosis are noted with normocytic or slightly macrocytic cells. A few target cells, siderocytes, and occasional nucleated red cells may be present. Red cells in anemia of inflammation or malignancy are typically normocytic normochromic, but they may become slightly microcytic and hypochromic in severe anemias.

Mild thrombocytosis may occur with iron deficiency anemia. When iron deficiency is severe, thrombocytopenia may be noted instead of thrombocytosis. The reticulocyte count may be normal or slightly decreased in iron deficiency anemia, is usually elevated in thalassemias, and is normal or slightly elevated in sideroblastic anemias and anemia of inflammation or malignancy.

Evaluation of serum iron, iron binding capacity, and ferritin is also important (Table 4–11), as is examination of bone marrow. Erythroid hyperplasia is noted in iron deficiency anemia, thalassemia, and sideroblastic anemia, but not in the anemia of inflammation or malignancy. Marked basophilic stippling, inclusion bodies in erythroblasts on supravital stains, increased iron stores, and an increase in ringed sideroblasts in some cases are noted in thalassemic patients. Intense erythroid hyperplasia with an increase in abnormal ringed sideroblasts and iron stores and a shift to the left in the granulocytic line in some cases are noted in sideroblastic anemias. Sideroblasts and iron stores

Table 4–11. Differentiating Features of Microcytic Anemias

Tests	Iron Deficiency Anemia	Thalassemia	Sideroblastic Anemia	Anemia of Inflammation or Malignancy
Serum iron	Low	Normal	High	Low
Serum iron-binding capacity	High	Normal	Normal	Low
Serum ferritin	Low	Normal or high	High	Normal or high
Marrow iron stores	Low or absent	Normal or high	High	Normal or high
Marrow sideroblasts	Decreased or absent	Normal or increased	Increased	Decreased
Free erythrocyte protoporphyrin (FEP)	High	Normal	High	High
Hemoglobin A_2 or F	Normal	High	Normal	Normal

are absent in iron deficiency anemia. A normal-looking marrow with decreased serum iron, decreased marrow sideroblasts, and increased iron stores is quite typical of anemia of inflammation or malignancy.

Hemoglobin electrophoresis is obtained in patients suspected of having thalassemia. Elevated hemoglobin F and A_2 are noted in beta-thalassemias. Because of normal hemoglobin electrophoresis in adults with heterozygous thalassemia, this diagnosis is usually based on clinical suspicion and exclusion of other causes of microcytic anemias. Confirmation can be obtained by globin synthesis and gene mapping studies. In patients with alpha-thalassemia, Bart's hemoglobin is present at birth and disappears later in life. Occasionally, hemoglobin H inclusion bodies may be demonstrable on supravital staining in patients with alpha-thalassemic trait.

Obtaining a free erythrocyte protoporphyrin level is usually not required in clinical practice but may be useful in difficult cases (Table 4–11).

MACROCYTIC ANEMIAS

Definition

Anemias associated with increased red cell size are referred to as macrocytic anemias. The mean corpuscular volume (MCV) and the mean corpuscular hemoglobin (MCH) are increased, whereas the mean corpuscular hemoglobin concentration (MCHC) is normal.

Pathophysiologic Considerations (Table 4–12)

Megaloblastic anemias secondary to vitamin B_{12} or folic acid deficiency are the most common causes of macrocytic anemias. In macrocytic anemia, the primitive erythroid progenitor cells, termed megaloblasts,

Table 4–12. Classification of Macrocytic Anemias

Megaloblastic anemias
Increased membrane lipids
Hepatitis
Cirrhosis
Alcoholism
Obstructive jaundice
Postsplenectomy
Accelerated erythropoiesis
Hemolytic anemias
Hemorrhage
Endocrine disorders
Hypothyroidism
Miscellaneous
Preleukemia
5q⁻ syndrome
Acquired sideroblastic anemia
Myelophthisic anemia

are in a state of unbalanced cell growth with defective DNA synthesis and normal RNA and protein synthesis, resulting in a macrocyte with decreased survival.

In liver disease and in the postsplenectomy state, the red cell surface area is increased with an increase in membrane lipids. These cells are also called "thin leptocytes," as the red cells appear large on blood smear while their MCV is usually normal.

In states of accelerated erythropoiesis, there is an increase in the reticulocyte count, premature release of reticulocytes from the bone marrow, and accelerated hemoglobin synthesis without shortening of time between cell divisions. All of these factors contribute to increased red cell size.

Diagnostic Evaluation and Differential Diagnosis

PATIENT HISTORY AND PHYSICAL EXAMINATION

Different conditions are associated with megaloblastic anemias (Table 4–13). Symptoms of anemia are usually present with mild to severe pallor. Patients with pernicious anemia may present with paresthesias, sore tongue, and gastrointestinal complaints. The skin may have a lemon yellow tint because of pallor and mild icterus. Dorsolateral columns of spinal cord and the cerebral cortex may be involved in vitamin B_{12} deficiency but rarely so in folic acid deficiency. Congestive heart failure may occur in elderly patients with pernicious anemia.

DIAGNOSTIC STUDIES

Complete blood count, platelet count, MCV, MCH, MCHC, and examination of the peripheral blood smear are essential initial laboratory studies. In macrocytic anemias, hemoglobin and hematocrit are decreased, MCV and MCH are increased, MCHC is normal, the white cell count is normal or decreased. On evaluation of the blood smear, macro-ovalocytes and macrocytes are present in megaloblastic anemias, round macrocytes occur in states of accelerated erythropoiesis, and macrocytes with an increased area of central pallor and target cells are found in conditions associated with "thin" macrocytes. Hypersegmented polymorphs appear in megaloblastic anemias. A single polymorph with six or more lobes or more than three cells with five lobes constitutes hypersegmentation. In advanced anemia, punctate basophilia, Cabot's rings, Howell-Jolly bodies, and nucleated red cells may be noted.

The patient should be tested for serum and red cell folate and serum B_{12}. The serum folate level is sensitive to recent changes in dietary intake of folate, whereas red cell folate reflects tissue stores of folic acid. In patients with folic acid deficiency, serum and red cell folate levels are decreased. A modest reduction in

Table 4–13.   Classification of Megaloblastic Anemias

Vitamin B_{12} deficiency
  Decreased intake
    Poor diet
    Strict vegetarianism
  Decreased absorption
    Deficiency of intrinsic factor (IF)
      Pernicious anemia
      Gastrectomy (total or partial)
    Functionally abnormal intrinsic factor
    Defect in intrinsic factor–B_{12} complex absorption
      Familial selective vitamin B_{12}
      Malabsorption (Imerslund's syndrome)
    Competition for B_{12} by bacteria/parasites
      Bacterial overgrowth
        Blind loop syndrome
        Small-bowel diverticulosis
        Strictures
        Anastomosis and fistula
        Achlorhydria
      Parasites
        Fish tapeworm infestation (Diphyllobothrium latum)
    Ileal disorders
      Ileal resection
      Ileitis
      Infiltration by lymphoma
    Pancreatic disorders
      Chronic pancreatitis
    Zollinger-Ellison syndrome
    Drug-induced vitamin B_{12} malabsorption
      PAS
      Colchicine
      Neomycin
      Ethanol
      Potassium chloride
  Increased requirements
    Pregnancy (rare)
    Neoplasia; myeloproliferative syndromes
  Impaired utilization
    Transcobalamin II deficiency
    Abnormal transcobalamin II
    Nitrous oxide administration
  Miscellaneous
    Hemodialysis

Folate deficiency
  Decreased intake
    Poor diet
    Alcoholism

  Decreased absorption
    Tropical sprue
    Celiac disease
    Jejunal resection
    Intestinal short-circuits
    Intrinsic intestinal disease
    Congenital folate malabsorption
    Drug induced—anticonvulsants, oral contraceptives
  Increased requirements
    Pregnancy (common)
    Infancy
    Accelerated hematopoiesis
      Hemolytic anemias
      Hemorrhage
    Neoplastic disease
    Cirrhosis
  Impaired utilization
    Folic acid antagonists
      Methotrexate
      Trimethoprim
      Pyrimethamine
      Triampterine
      Pentamidine
    Alcohol
    Enzyme deficiencies
      Dihydrofolate reductase deficiency
      Foramininotransferase deficiency
      N^5 methyl-tetrahydrofolate reductase deficiency

Other causes of megaloblastic anemias
  Drugs that interfere with DNA metabolism
    Purine antagonists
      6-mercaptopurine
      6-thioguanine
      Azathioprine
    Pyrimidine antagonists
      6-azauridine
      5-fluorouracil
    Others
      Hydroxyurea
      Cytosine arabinoside
  Inborn metabolic disorders
    Lesch-Nyhan syndrome
    Orotic aciduria
  Unexplained origin
    Pyridoxine-responsive megaloblastic anemia
    Thiamine-responsive megaloblastic anemia
    Erythroleukemia

serum B_{12} level may occur in folate deficiency, but the decrease in folic acid levels is more severe.

The serum B_{12} level is decreased in vitamin B_{12} deficiency. As B_{12} appears to be required for the transfer of 5-methyl-tetrahydrofolate from plasma to red cells, red cell folate may be decreased and serum folate modestly increased in patients with vitamin B_{12} deficiency.

Bone marrow in macrocytic anemias is usually hypercellular with erythroid hyperplasia. Erythropoiesis is megaloblastic. Megaloblasts are large erythroid precursors with a delicate chromatin pattern and nuclear-cytoplasmic dissociation, i.e., mature-appearing cytoplasm with an immature nucleus. Giant metamyelocytes and myelocytes may be noted. Megakaryocytes may be reduced when anemia is severe.

The Schilling test is a test for absorption of vitamin B_{12} labeled with radioactive cobalt. After voiding, a fasting patient takes a 0.5- to 2-μg oral dose of labeled vitamin B_{12} and 24-hour urine collection is started. One to two hours later, a "flushing dose" of 1000 μg nonradioactive B_{12} is injected intramuscularly. The patient may eat after the flushing dose. Urinary excretion

Table 4—14. Causes of Normocytic Anemias

Anemia of chronic disorders, e.g., infection, inflammation, malignancy
Anemia of renal failure
Anemia of endocrine disorders
    Hypothyroidism (may be macrocytic or microcytic)
    Adrenal insufficiency
    Hypogonadism
Hypoplastic or aplastic anemia
Hemolytic anemias
Anemia of pregnancy (dilutional)
Anemia of bone marrow infiltration
Anemia of liver disease (may be macrocytic)
Recent blood loss
Early iron deficiency
Dyserythropoietic anemias

of the radioactive vitamin is measured. If urinary excretion of the radioactivity is reduced, intrinsic factor is given orally with the labeled vitamin (part II of the test), and urinary excretion of the absorbed labeled vitamin is measured.

In pernicious anemia and in conditions associated with intrinsic factor deficiency, absorption and urinary excretion of labeled vitamin B_{12} is decreased and then corrected when intrinsic factor is given with the labeled vitamin. In malabsorption syndromes, e.g., nontropical sprue, the addition of intrinsic factor does not improve the absorption of labeled B_{12}.

"Blocking" antibodies to intrinsic factor are present in 50 to 60% patients with pernicious anemia. Rare false positive tests may occur in patients with chronic gastritis. A combination of megaloblastic marrow, low serum B_{12}, and the presence of intrinsic factor antibodies is fairly diagnostic of pernicious anemia.

NORMOCYTIC NORMOCHROMIC ANEMIAS

Definition

Anemias with normal MCV and MCH are referred to as normocytic normochromic anemias.

Pathophysiologic Considerations and Differential Diagnosis

Many diverse disorders lead to the development of normocytic anemias (Table 4–14). Anemia of chronic disorders is usually mild, characterized by hypoferremia and increased iron stores. Red cell survival is decreased, with impaired marrow response and a block in the release of iron from macrophages to plasma. Anemia of renal failure is characterized by decreased red cell production, failure of the erythropoietin level to increase in response to anemia, and subnormal response of red cell precursors to erythropoietin. Red cell survival also is usually decreased. Anemias of

endocrine disorders are hypoproliferative anemias with normal red cell survival. Anemia of pregnancy is a dilutional anemia caused by increased plasma volume. It usually becomes manifest at about 8 weeks of pregnancy, progresses slowly to the 32nd to 34th week, and improves before delivery. Red cell survival is moderately shortened in liver disease, and cross-transfusion studies suggest the hemolytic factor to be extracorpuscular. Thin macrocytes and spur cells are noted in patients with liver disease caused by an increase in red cell membrane lipids.

Diagnostic Evaluation

In addition to a complete history and careful physical examination, several laboratory tests are important in the diagnostic evaluation of normocytic normochromic anemias. The physician should perform a CBC, differential count, reticulocyte count, and peripheral blood smear examination. Although these anemias are characteristically normocytic normochromic, anemia of chronic disorders may occasionally be hypochromic. Macrocytosis may occur in less than 10% of patients with hypothyroidism. Thin macrocytes and spur cells may be noted in anemia of liver disease. Teardrop red cells and immature red and white cell precursors in the blood smear are characteristic of myelophthisic anemia.

The reticulocyte count is increased in patients with hemolysis or recent blood loss. Increased basophilia of red cells, nucleated red cells, and microspherocytes indicate a hemolytic process. The reticulocyte count is normal or slightly decreased in other disorders producing normocytic anemias.

Serum hepatoglobin, Coombs', and urine hemosiderin tests are obtained to evaluate and confirm the diagnosis of hemolytic anemia in patients with an elevated reticulocyte count. If no evidence of hemolysis is detected, a source of recent bleeding should be looked for.

Serum iron, total iron-binding capacity (TIBC), and ferritin should be evaluated. Anemias of chronic disorders and other hypoproliferative anemias are characterized by hypoferremia, decreased total iron-binding capacity, and decreased, normal, or increased ferritin. Hypoferremia, increased TIBC, and decreased serum ferritin occur in patients with early iron deficiency who may still be normocytic normochromic.

Serum folate and vitamin B_{12} are usually obtained to exclude other contributory causes for anemia.

Bone marrow aspiration and biopsy are performed in patients with a decreased or normal reticulocyte count and in patients with an elevated reticulocyte count when the diagnosis is not evident by other laboratory tests. Marrow examination is useful in identifying hypoplasia and hyperplasia of hematopoietic cells, noting infiltration by carcinomas, lymphomas, myeloma, leukemia, etc., and assessing the status of iron stores. The bone marrow usually appears normal in anemias of chronic disorders, renal failure, and endocrine disorders; appears hypoplastic or aplastic in aplastic anemia and pure red cell aplasia; and appears hyperplastic in patients with hemolysis or recent blood loss. Increased iron stores and a decrease in sideroblasts is noted in anemias of chronic disorders. Binuclear or multinuclear normoblasts and other nuclear abnormalities are noted in congenital dyserythropoietic anemias. Often, ringed sideroblasts as well as an excess of blasts are seen.

Evaluation of endocrine, liver, and renal function should be performed when indicated by clinical impression.

DISORDERS OF HEMOGLOBIN SYNTHESIS

Disorders of hemoglobin synthesis can be divided into two major groups: disorders characterized by decreased synthesis of globin with normal structure (e.g., thalassemias), and hemoglobins with structural changes, usually a single amino acid substitution in a globin chain, that are synthesized at a normal rate (e.g., sickle-cell disease) (Table 4–15).

Thalassemias and sickle-cell disease are the most common genetically determined disorders of hemoglobin.

Thalassemias

PATHOPHYSIOLOGIC CONSIDERATIONS

Normal hemoglobins in an adult consist of Hb A ($\alpha_2 \beta_2$) 97%, Hb A_2 ($\alpha_2 \delta_2$) 2.5%, and Hb F ($\alpha_2 \gamma_2$) 0.5%. Alpha-thalassemias are characterized by lack of alpha-chain synthesis and an excess of beta and gamma chains that form relatively unstable tetramers, Hb H (β^4 and Bart's Hb (γ_4). Intracellular precipitation, inclusion body formation, and cell destruction occur in the bone marrow or peripheral blood. Beta-thalassemias are characterized by lack of beta-chain synthesis

Table 4–15. Disorders of Hemoglobin Synthesis

Decreased or absent synthesis of one of the subunits of globin
  Alpha-thalassemia
  Beta-thalassemia
Structural changes in globin (hemoglobinopathies)
  Hemoglobin with reduced solubility and gelation in deoxy form: sickle cell hemoglobin
  Hemoglobins with increased oxygen affinity, e.g., Hb Chesapeake
  Hemoglobins with decreased oxygen affinity, e.g., Hb Kansas
  Methemoglobinemia, e.g., Hb M
  Unstable hemoglobins, e.g., Hb Köln

and excess of γ-gamma-chains, which are very unstable. The anemia of thalassemias is the result of decreased globin production, ineffective erythropoiesis, and hemolysis. Compensatory bone marrow expansion occurs to increase red cell production.

Because the genes for hemoglobin synthesis are inherited autosomally patients may present in a heterozygous or homozygous state. Gene deletion is a common mechanism for alpha-thalassemia mutations, whereas single nucleotide substitutions account for a majority of beta-thalassemias.

DIAGNOSTIC EVALUATION

Patient History and Physical Examination. Clinically, the disease has been divided into three groups, thalassemia major corresponding to a homozygous state, thalassemia minor corresponding to a heterozygous state, and thalassemia intermedia, of intermediate severity, caused by partial suppression of genes. The disease is characterized by a chronic hemolytic state, splenomegaly, jaundice, gallstones, and skeletal changes.

A thalassemic patient may present to an internist with microcytic hypochromic anemia in the absence of iron deficiency or another obvious cause. Anemia may or may not be accompanied by splenomegaly and other evidence of hemolysis. A patient may also present with hemolysis during pregnancy, with intercurrent infections, or secondary to oxidant drugs (e.g., in hemoglobin H disease). These patients usually have a mild to moderate hemolytic anemia that is well tolerated; they present for the first time during exacerbation of hemolysis. Patients with thalassemia major who have survived into adulthood may present to the internist with problems of transfusional iron overload in addition to severe thalassemic changes.

Diagnostic Studies. Laboratory tests may reveal microcytic hypochromic anemia, mild reticulocytosis, low MCV, low MCH, and normal or low MCHC. The blood smear in addition shows anisopoikilocytosis, polychromasia, basophilic stippling, and target cells. Microcytosis is more prominent in thalassemias than in iron deficiency anemia. (For differential diagnosis from other microcytic anemias, see Table 4–11.)

Supravital staining with 1% cresyl blue may reveal inclusion bodies, e.g., in hemoglobin H disease. Increased Hb A_2 and Hb F in beta-thalassemias, and Hb H with low Hb A_2 and Bart's hemoglobin (about 10%) are noted in patients with Hb H disease. Serum iron is increased and serum transferrin is saturated. Serum unconjugated hyperbilirubinemia and increased urinary urobilinogen secondary to hemolysis are also found.

Bone marrow aspiration and biopsy show hypercellularity, normoblastic hyperplasia, defective hemoglobinization of normoblasts, and increased sideroblasts.

Globin chain synthesis can be measured in reticulocytes and in patients with normal hemoglobin electrophoresis who are suspected of having thalassemia.

Gene mapping with restriction endonuclease can detect gene deletions in alpha-thalassemias that indicate a carrier state.

Hemoglobinopathies

Sickle Cell Anemia. Hemoglobin S is characterized by substitution of valine for glutamic acid in the sixth position of the beta-chain. Polymerization of deoxygenated hemoglobin S is responsible for most of the symptoms of sickle-cell disease.

The clinical presentation of sickle cell anemia consists of vaso-occlusive crisis that occurs because of obstruction of microvasculature by sickled cells. Symptoms depend on the site of obstruction. Also, the patient may have aplastic crisis. A sudden increase in anemia is associated with reticulocytopenia and fever. A parvovirus-like agent (PVLA) has been detected in sera of patients with aplastic crisis.[8] PVLA suppresses erythropoiesis, probably by direct action on erythroid progenitors. Aplastic crises can also occur in association with bacterial infections, e.g., salmonella, pneumococci, and streptococci.

Sudden exacerbation of anemia may occur because of accelerated hemolysis or arrest of erythropoiesis caused by folate deficiency. Other features are impaired growth and development, and infections with Streptococcus pneumoniae, Hemophilus influenzae, and salmonella.

Laboratory studies that should be considered in the diagnostic evaluation include CBC and blood smear. Moderate degrees of normocytic normochromic anemia, leukocytosis, and mild thrombocytosis are usually present. The peripheral blood smear shows sickled red cells, target cells, polychromasia, basophilic stippling, nucleated red cells, and reticulocytosis. Howell-Jolly and Pappenheimer bodies reflect functional asplenia secondary to repeated splenic infarctions. Target cells are more prominent in patients with hemoglobin S/C-thalassemia disease and hemoglobin S/beta-thalassemia.

Hemoglobin electrophoresis should also be performed. Hemoglobin S is the major component, with some hemoglobin F. Hemoglobin A_2 is normal. There is no hemoglobin A present at alkaline pH, and hemoglobin D Punjabi occupies a position identical to hemoglobin S. Agar gel electrophoresis at acid pH will differentiate between hemoglobins D Punjabi and S.

Hemoglobin A_2 is increased in patients with Hemoglobin S/beta°-thalassemia disease.

Tests based on decreased solubility of hemoglobin S and sickling on deoxygenation are rarely used.

Hemoglobins with Increased Oxygen Affinity. These are present with erythrocytosis. (For differential diagnosis of erythrocytosis, see Table 4–8). Laboratory tests used for the diagnosis are hemoglobin electrophoresis and measurement of whole blood P_{50} in electrophoretically silent cases. Whole blood P_{50} (the oxygen pressure at which hemoglobin is 50% saturated) is decreased in high-affinity hemoglobins. Oxygen dissociation curve studies of purified hemoglobin to demonstrate a left shift of the curve may be required in difficult cases.

Hemoglobins with Decreased Oxygen Affinity (e.g., Hemoglobin Kansas). These are low-affinity hemoglobins present with cyanosis and normal oxygen tension. The diagnosis is usually made on starch gel electrophoresis of hemoglobin. In electrophoretically silent cases, a right shift of the oxygen dissociation curve needs to be demonstrated for diagnostic purposes.

Methemoglobinemia. There are M hemoglobins present with cyanosis and lack of exercise intolerance. The diagnosis can be made by spectroscopic examination and hemoglobin electrophoresis.

Unstable Hemoglobins (e.g., Hemoglobin Köln). This produces intracellular inclusions and hemolysis. Unstable hemoglobin disease is also known as congenital Heinz-body hemolytic anemia. Hemolytic episodes may occur secondary to infections or exposure to drugs like sulfonamides. Heinz bodies are noted during a hemolytic episode or after splenectomy.

Red cells may be slightly hypochromic, and reticulocytosis out of proportion to the degree of anemia may occur. Hemoglobin electrophoresis is often normal, so tests to demonstrate instability of hemoglobin are used for diagnostic purposes. The isopropranol stability test, the heat denaturation tests, and incubation of blood with brilliant cresyl blue to generate Heinz bodies are frequently used.

THROMBOCYTOSIS

Definition

An increase in the platelet count above normal (normal range, 150,000 to 450,000/μl) is referred to as thrombocytosis.

Pathophysiologic Considerations and Differential Diagnosis (Table 4–16)

Overproduction of platelets is the common underlying mechanism responsible for thrombocytosis.

Table 4–16.   Causes of Thrombocytosis

Physiologic: physical exercise, parturition, epinephrine
Primary thrombocytosis
   Essential thrombocythemia (ET)
   Polycythemia vera (PV)
   Agnogenic myeloid metaplasia (AMM)
   Chronic myelogenous leukemia (CML)
Secondary or reactive thrombocytosis
   Chronic inflammatory disorders and infections
      Rheumatoid arthritis
      Periarteritis nodosa
      Ulcerative colitis, regional enteritis
      Wegener's granulomatosis
      Sarcoidosis
      Osteomyelitis
      Tuberculosis
      Cirrhosis
      Acute rheumatic fever
   Acute inflammatory diseases and many acute infections
   Hematologic disorders
      Iron deficiency
      Hemolytic anemias
      Acute blood loss
      Recovery from a period of thrombocytopenia (rebound thrombocytosis)
      Hemophilia
      Tidal platelet dysgenesis
   Neoplasms
      Carcinomas, particularly lung and breast
      Hodgkin's disease, other lymphomas
      Multiple myeloma
   Postoperative
      Postsplenectomy, other surgical procedures
   Drugs
      Vincristine
   Miscellaneous
      Chronic renal disease
      Renal cysts
      Cushing's disease
      Glycogen storage disease
      Osteoporosis
      Trauma

Platelet survival is usually normal or slightly decreased. Thrombocytosis may also occur secondary to mobilization of extravascular platelet pools. Epinephrine releases the platelets from the splenic pool in the intravascular compartment. Physical exercise mobilizes nonsplenic platelet pools, and its effect is maintained in asplenic subjects.

Thrombocytosis is generally classified into two categories: reactive (or secondary) and autonomous (or primary) (Table 4–17). Reactive thrombocytosis is secondary to underlying primary conditions such as malignancy, inflammation, infection, and bleeding. Primary thrombocytosis is due to autonomous overproduction of platelets, e.g., in myeloproliferative disorders.

Reactive thrombocytosis may be acute or chronic. An elevated platelet count may be associated with ac-

celerated erythropoiesis, e.g., after acute hemorrhage or acute hemolytic anemias, suggesting an as yet unclear interrelationship between thrombopoietic and erythropoietic regulatory mechanisms. Platelet count may increase secondary to acute inflammation, tissue necrosis, and surgical procedures, and during recovery from an episode of thrombocytopenia. Postsplenectomy thrombocytosis occurs secondary to redistribution of the splenic platelet pool and an increase in platelet production. Platelet counts return to normal several weeks to months after splenectomy. Postsplenectomy thrombocytosis may persist, however, in patients with underlying myeloproliferative disorders or chronic anemia.

Chronic reactive thrombocytosis may occur secondary to chronic inflammatory disorders, some chronic infections, neoplasms, and iron deficiency anemia. Thrombocytosis has been commonly associated with carcinoma of the lung and breast and with Hodgkin's disease, but it may occur with any of the carcinomas or lymphomas. The reason for increased platelet production in patients with iron deficiency anemia and chronic blood loss is still unclear. Erythropoietin in large doses in vitro can increase the platelet count, but not in concentrations encountered in blood loss or iron deficiency.[9]

Primary thrombocytosis is secondary to autonomous proliferation of megakaryocytes and overproduction of platelets. Loss of regulatory control may be absolute or relative. Primary thrombocytosis commonly occurs with clonal stem cell disorders such as essential thrombocythemia, polycythemia vera, agnogenic myeloid metaplasia, and chronic myelogenous leukemia.

Diagnostic Evaluation

A complete history should be obtained and physical examination should be performed, looking particularly for splenomegaly and any evidence of bleeding or thrombosis or underlying primary disorders.

The following laboratory tests should be done in support of various diagnostic possibilities: CBC, differential count, and platelet count; critical evaluation of the peripheral blood smear; platelet aggregation studies with epinephrine, ADP, and collagen; and serum leukocyte alkaline phosphatase. If the diagnosis is still not evident, bone marrow aspiration and biopsy for morphology and cytogenetic analysis should be performed.

Differential Diagnosis

In patients with reactive thrombocytosis, the underlying primary condition, usually a malignancy, inflammatory disease, iron deficiency, or hemorrhage, is clinically evident. Occasionally, marked thrombo-

Table 4–17. Differences Between Primary and Reactive Thrombocytosis

	Autonomous (Primary) Thrombocytosis	Reactive (Secondary) Thrombocytosis
Duration	Persistent	Transient
Bleeding and thrombotic complications	Frequent	Rare
Splenomegaly	Common	Rare*
Platelet count	Frequently > 1000 × 10³/μl	Usually < 1000 × 10³/μl
Leukocyte count	May be elevated	Usually normal*
RBC count	May be elevated	Normal or decreased
Platelet structure	Usually abnormal	Usually normal
Bleeding time	Usually prolonged	Usually normal
Platelet aggregation studies	Usually abnormal	Normal
Marrow cytogenetics	Frequently abnormal	Normal

*Abnormal white count and splenomegaly may occur due to the underlying primary condition.

cytosis may be present with an occult malignancy. Bleeding and thrombotic complications are rare in reactive thrombocytosis but fairly common in primary thrombocytosis. Of the myeloproliferative disorders, bleeding and thrombotic complications are least frequent in CML in its stable phase. Patients with polycythemia vera are considered to be more prone to thrombotic complications, whereas patients with essential thrombocythemia and myeloid metaplasia are more prone to hemorrhagic complications.[10] Bleeding usually presents as bruising, ecchymosis, epistaxis, and mucosal hemorrhage.

Physical examination usually reveals splenomegaly in patients with myeloproliferative disorders. Of the patients with primary thrombocytosis, 80% are reported to have splenomegaly. Splenomegaly may be seen occasionally in patients with reactive thrombocytosis.

Elevated red and white cell count, nucleated red cells, teardrop cells, and immature white cells on peripheral blood smear suggest a myeloproliferative disorder (MPD). Abnormalities of platelet structure are common in MPD. Significant variations in the size of platelets, giant platelets, megakaryocyte fragments, and hypogranulated platelets are suggestive of MPD. Platelets in reactive thrombocytosis are more uniform in size and are usually small and fully granulated. Elevation in platelet count is usually transient in reactive thrombocytosis and returns to normal when the primary condition abates. The platelet count is usually less than $1 \times 10^6/\mu l$ in reactive thrombocytosis and frequently above that in primary thrombocytosis. The platelet count may go above $1 \times 10^6/\mu l$ after splenectomy and usually returns to normal in a few weeks to a few months unless the patient has an underlying myeloproliferative disorder or a persistent anemia. Patients with iron deficiency rarely may have a platelet count above $1 \times 10^6/\mu l$, particularly when associated with gastrointestinal hemorrhage.

Platelet aggregation studies are usually normal in reactive thrombocytosis and frequently abnormal in primary thrombocytosis. Lack of aggregation secondary to epinephrine is the most frequent abnormality.[11] Spontaneous aggregation of platelets may occur in myeloproliferative disorders and is reported to correlate with thrombotic complications.[12] Bleeding time is usually prolonged in primary thrombocytosis and normal in reactive thrombocytosis.

If the diagnosis is still not clear, bone marrow aspiration and biopsy should be performed for cytogenetic analysis. Abnormal cytogenetics suggests primary thrombocytosis. The Philadelphia chromosome is present in 90% of cases of CML. Bone marrow biopsy will frequently show panhyperplasia with prominent megakaryocytes in myeloproliferative disorders. A low serum leukocyte alkaline phosphatase score suggests CML.

THROMBOCYTOPENIA

Definition

Thrombocytopenia is defined as a decrease in the platelet count below normal (normal range, 150,000 to 450,000 μl).

Pathophysiologic Considerations and Differential Diagnosis

Thrombocytopenia may result from diminished production or ineffective thrombopoiesis, accelerated destruction of the platelets, or increased splenic pooling of the platelets. Thrombocytopenia is classified into hereditary and acquired thrombocytopenia (Table 4–18).

Whereas hereditary thrombocytopenias are very rare, acquired thrombocytopenias are common. Antineoplastic chemotherapy and radiation therapy, marrow infiltration, alcohol, and drugs are common causes of diminished platelet production. Idiopathic thrombocytopenic purpura (ITP), disseminated intravascular

Table 4—18. Classification and Causes of Thrombocytopenia

Hereditary thrombocytopenias
  Thrombocytopenia–absent radius (TAR) syndrome
  Constitutional (Fanconi's) aplastic anemia
  Wiskott-Aldrich syndrome
  Bernard-Soulier syndrome
  May-Hegglin anomaly
  Thrombopoietin deficiency
  Chédiak-Higashi syndrome
Acquired thrombocytopenia
  Diminished or defective thrombopoiesis
    Antineoplastic chemotherapy
    Radiation therapy
    Drugs—thiazide diuretics, alcohol, estrogens, interferon
    Aplastic anemia, megakaryocytic hypoplasia
    Vitamin B_{12} deficiency, folic acid deficiency
    Severe iron deficiency
    Marrow infiltration (myelophthisic): carcinomas, leukemias, para-proteinemias, histiocytosis, myelofibrosis, tuberculosis, osteopetrosis
    Myelodysplastic syndromes
    Uremia
    Viral infections: infectious mononucleosis, dengue fever, rubella, measles vaccine, AIDS
    Paroxysmal nocturnal hemoglobinuria
    Cyclic thrombocytopenia
    Hyperbaric exposure
  Increased destruction and/or sequestration of platelets
    Immune
      Idiopathic thrombocytopenic purpura
        Acute
        Chronic
      Post-transfusion purpura
      Isoimmune neonatal thrombocytopenic purpura
      Drug-induced: quinidine, sulfonamides, digitoxin, chlorothiazides, chlorpropamide, gold salts, methyldopa, p-amino salicylic acid (PAS), rifampin, carbamazepine, diphenyl-hydantoin, heparin
      Autoimmune disorders, e.g., systemic lupus erythematosus

    Lymphoproliferative disorders
    Acute autoimmune anemia with thrombocytopenia (Evan's syndrome)
    Antilymphocyte globulin
    Nonimmunologic
      Disseminated intravascular coagulation
      Thrombotic thrombocytopenic purpura
      Hemolytic uremic syndrome
      Infections
        Bacterial: septicemia, meningococcemia, subacute bacterial endocarditis, toxic shock syndrome, typhoid fever, scarlet fever, diphtheria, tuberculosis, brucellosis
        Rickettsial: typhus, Rocky Mountain spotted fever
        Fungal: disseminated histoplasmosis
        Protozoal: malaria, toxoplasmosis, trypanosomiasis
        Viral: mumps, varicella, disseminated herpes simplex, cytomegalovirus, infectious mononucleosis
      Snake bites
      Drugs directly toxic to circulating platelets: ristocetin, protamine, heparin
      Giant hemangioendotheliomas (Kasabach-Merritt syndrome)
      Peritoneal—venous shunting
      Prolonged Swan-Ganz catheterization
      Pre-eclampsia
      Massive burns
      Fat embolism
      Cyanotic congenital heart disease, aortic valvular disease
      Renal transplant rejection
      Renal vein thrombosis
    Increased sequestration of platelets
      Splenomegaly
      Hypothermia
  Dilutional effect
    Massive blood transfusion
    Exchange transfusion
  Miscellaneous
    Liver disease, hyperthyroidism

coagulation (DIC), drugs, and septicemias are common causes of accelerated destruction of platelets. Increased splenic pooling and destruction of platelets may occur in disorders associated with splenomegaly.

Diagnostic Evaluation

PATIENT HISTORY AND PHYSICAL EXAMINATION

A detailed history of drug intake, previous transfusion, malignancy, and infections should be obtained, and a past or family history of bleeding problems should be elicited. A detailed physical examination especially for evidence of bleeding into skin or mucosa (e.g., purpuric spots and ecchymoses), splenomegaly, and disseminated malignancy or infection, should be performed.

The age of the patient is important in the diagnosis. A young child with a recent history of upper respiratory infections is likely to have acute ITP. Hereditary thrombocytopenias, although rare, usually present in childhood. A young female with no obvious cause of thrombocytopenia is likely to have chronic ITP. Older thrombocytopenic male patients are more likely to have marrow infiltration by tumor, leukemias, myelodysplastic syndromes, pernicious anemia, or thrombocytopenia secondary to drugs like chlorothiazide, quinidine, methyldopa, chlorpropamide, or digitoxin.

The physical condition of the patient is important. Patients admitted to intensive care units or patients who are quite ill are likely to have thrombocytopenia from septicemia, disseminated intravascular coagulation, drugs and heparin used to flush various access lines.

DIAGNOSTIC STUDIES

CBC, differential and platelet count should be done. Platelets in ITP are usually larger than normal. Giant platelets with hypogranular forms may be seen in smoldering leukemia or preleukemia. Platelets that are gigantic are seen in Bernard-Soulier syndrome and May-Hegglin anomaly. A leukoerythroblastic picture suggests a myelophthisic process. Fragmented red cells (schistocytes) may be seen in disseminated intravascular coagulation in other microangiopathic conditions, and in patients with prosthetic cardiac valves.

If the peripheral blood smear suggests DIC, prothrombin time (PT) test, a partial thromboplastin time (PTT) test, and a thrombin time test should be performed, and serum fibrin degradation products (FDP) should be obtained.

If the diagnosis is still not evident, bone marrow aspiration and biopsy are performed, to assist in differentiating between disorders of decreased production and disorders of accelerated peripheral destruction or sequestration, and in identifying a myelophthisic process.

In a patient suspected of having ITP, platelet-associated IgG (PA IgG) levels can be obtained. A positive result adds little to the diagnosis, but a negative result makes diagnosis of ITP unlikely.[13,14] In patients with post-transfusion purpura, platelet-specific antibodies, commonly anti-Pl[A1], may be detected.

QUALITATIVE DISORDERS OF PLATELET FUNCTION

Definition

In a patient with a normal platelet count and prolonged bleeding time, qualitative disorders of platelet function should be suspected.

Pathophysiologic Considerations (Table 4–19)

Primary hemostasis is characterized by vascular contractility and a platelet phase of hemostasis. The platelet phase, for the sake of simplicity, is divided into three phases:

1. Platelet adhesions (platelet–vessel wall interaction): On vascular injury, platelets adhere to subendothelium (e.g., collagen). Such adhesion requires the presence of von Willebrand's factor in the plasma and specific platelet receptors (von Willebrand's receptor or platelet glycoprotein I). Platelet glycoprotein I is absent in Bernard-Soulier syndrome.

2. Platelet release reaction: Platelets release contents of their granules, e.g., ADP and fibrinogen, and other factors that mediate platelet aggregation. Deficiency of platelet granules is known as storage pool deficiency. Abnormal release in the presence of normal granule contents is known as an abnormal release mechanism.

3. Platelet aggregation (platelet to platelet interac-

tion): Close reversible apposition of platelets, called primary aggregation, in vitro precedes platelet release reaction. Secondary irreversible aggregation occurs in response to released granule contents. Fibrinogen and fibrinogen receptors on platelets are required for platelet aggregation. Fibrinogen receptors are absent in Glanzmann's thrombasthenia. In conjunction with primary hemostasis, the coagulation system is activated to produce fibrin.

Differential Diagnosis

A combination of prolonged bleeding time with a normal platelet count may be noted in von Willebrand's disease and vascular purpuras, in addition to platelet disorders. Inherited disorders of platelet function are rare, whereas acquired disorders are quite common. Drugs, myeloproliferative disorders, use of extracorporeal circulation, and elevated FDP levels are common causes of platelet dysfunction.

Evaluation

In the evaluation of these patients, the severity of the bleeding should be assessed. Generally defects of platelet adhesion and platelet aggregation are associated with more severe bleeding than defects of release mechanism.

Family history and a detailed history of drug and alcohol intake should be obtained.

CBC, platelet count, and bleeding time are essential initial laboratory tests. PT and PTT are usually obtained in a bleeding patient to make sure that coagulation system is normal. In platelet aggregation studies, platelet aggregation secondary to ADP and epinephrine in concentrations of 5 μM or higher normally shows both primary and secondary aggregation patterns. Collagen and thrombin act by stimulating the release reaction. Some drugs inhibit the aggregation by specific agonists (Table 4–20.).

Based on the clinical evaluation and preliminary studies listed above, a diagnosis can be made in most acquired disorders of platelet function. If a patient has prolonged PTT with normal platelet count and prolonged bleeding time with no obvious cause, a diagnosis of von Willebrand's disease should be considered and specific tests performed. If the patient has a history of bleeding problems since early age, an inherited disorder should be considered. Complete testing for these disorders can be performed only in referral coagulation labs.

SPLENOMEGALY

Definition

Splenomegaly refers to enlargement of the spleen. Generally a palpable spleen is considered to be en-

Table 4–19. Classification of Qualitative Disorders of Platelet Function

Inherited
  Defects of platelet adhesion
    Bernard-Soulier syndrome
  Defects of primary aggregation
    Glanzmann's thrombasthenia
  Defects of platelet secretion
    Storage pool deficiency
    Abnormal release mechanism
      Cyclo-oxygenase deficiency
      Defects in thromboxane A_2 and calcium mobilization
  Defects of platelet secretion in association with other congenital abnormalities
    Hermansky-Pudlak syndrome
    Chëdiak-Higashi syndrome
    Thrombocytopenia—absent radius (TAR) syndrome
    Wiskott-Aldrich syndrome
    Heritable disorders of connective tissue
    May-Hegglin anomaly
    Allport's syndrome
  Disorders of platelet secretion in association with disorders of factor VIII complex
    Hemophilia A
    Von Willebrand's disease
  Abnormalities of platelet procoagulant (PF-3) activity
Acquired
  Hematologic disorders
    Myeloproliferative syndromes
      Essential thrombocythemia
      Polycythemia vera
      Agnogenic myeloid metaplasia
      Chronic myelogenous leukemia
    Dysproteinemias
      Macroglobulinemia

      Multiple myeloma
    Disorders with increased levels of serum fibrin degradation products (FDP)
      Disseminated intravascular coagulation
      Liver disease
      Fibrogenolysis
    Dysfibrinogenemia, afibrinogenemia
    Immune thrombocytopenia
    Others
      Acute and chronic leukemias
      Leukemic reticuloendotheliosis
      Pernicious anemia
      Glucose-6-phosphate dehydrogenase deficiency
      Thalassemias
      Sickle cell anemia
  Uremia
  Drugs
    Anti-inflammatory drugs: aspirin, sulfinpyrazone, indomethacin, phenylbutazone, ibuprofen
    Plasma expanders: dextran and similar polymers
    Antibiotics: carbenicillin, ticarcillin, methicillin, ampicillin, penicillin G, amantadine, nitrofurantoin
    Antidepressants: tricyclic antidepressants, phenothiazines
    Antihistamines: diphenhydramine
    Adrenergic blockers: phentolamine, propranolol
    Local and general anesthetics
    Vasodilators: hydralazine, nitroprusside
    Others: dipyridamole, furosemide, ethanol, vitamin E, clofibrate, tolbutamide
    Miscellaneous: following extracorporeal circulation or renal transplantation, and with infectious mononucleosis, congenital heart disease, Bartter's syndrome

Table 4–20. Drugs Inhibiting Platelet Aggregation

Collagen
Arachidonic acid
ADP
Epinephrine
Serotonin
Thrombin
Ristocetin
Aspirin, amitriptyline
Aspirin
Furosemide
Phentolamine
Cyprohepatidine
Heparin

larged, although a spleen tip may be palpable in 3% of normal young adults.

Pathophysiologic Considerations and Differential Diagnosis (Table 4–21)

Because the spleen consists of T- and B-lymphocytes, plasma cells, and phagocytic cells, it enlarges as a result of reactive proliferation in various infections and inflammatory disorders. Splenomegaly may also occur from infiltration by neoplastic cells (e.g., leu-

kemias), tumors, or lipid-laden macrophages, as in Gaucher's disease. Because the spleen is a scavenger of physically or immunologically altered red cells, it enlarges in hereditary hemolytic anemias (e.g., hereditary spherocytosis) and acquired hemolytic anemias (e.g., autoimmune hemolysis). The spleen may act as a site of hematopoiesis in myeloid metaplasia and severe hemolytic anemias. The spleen may be passively congested in portal hypertension and severe congestive heart failure.

Diagnostic Evaluation

Splenomegaly is commonly associated with hematologic abnormalities, lymphadenopathy, or both. A complete history and physical examination usually provide clues to the possible cause.

Complete blood count and peripheral blood smear findings may be diagnostic of chronic and acute leukemias. Atypical lymphocytes are seen in infectious mononucleosis, lymphocytes with hairy projections are found in hairy-cell leukemia, and immature red and white cells are noted in myeloid metaplasia and myelofibrosis. Increased reticulocyte count and spherocytes may be noted in hemolytic anemias.

Table 4–21.   Causes of Splenomegaly

Infections
  Subacute bacterial endocarditis
  Infectious mononucleosis
  Typhoid fever
  Tuberculosis
  Brucellosis
  Malaria
  Kala-azar
  Schistosomiasis
  Histoplasmosis
  Syphilis
  Splenic abscess
Inflammatory disorders
  Rheumatoid arthritis
  Felty's syndrome
  Systemic lupus erythematosus
  Sarcoidosis
Congestive splenomegaly
  Portal hypertension due to cirrhosis of liver
  Portal or splenic vein thrombosis or stenosis
  Severe congestive heart failure
Infiltrative splenomegaly
  Gaucher's disease
  Niemann-Pick disease
  Amyloidosis
  Hurler's syndrome
Neoplastic
  Myeloproliferative syndromes
    Chronic granulocytic leukemia
    Polycythemia vera
    Essential thrombocythemia
    Myelofibrosis
    Agnogenic myeloid metaplasia
  Lymphomas
  Hairy-cell leukemia
  Chronic and acute leukemias
  Histiocytosis X (Hand-Schüller-Christian and Letterer-Siewe diseases)
  Metastatic tumors
Hematologic disorders
  Hemolytic anemias, e.g., hereditary spherocytosis, autoimmune hemolytic anemias, hemoglobinopathies, pernicious anemia, severe iron deficiency anemia
Miscellaneous
  Splenic cysts
  Cavernous hemangioma

On chemistry profile, abnormal liver function tests may be noted in patients with cirrhosis and portal hypertension, and infiltration of the liver may be seen in metabolic and neoplastic disorders. Patients with hemolytic anemias may have indirect hyperbilirubinemia.

Chest x-ray provides information about the presence and extent of any mediastinal and hilar adenopathy that may occur in lymphomas, leukemias, tumors, sarcoidosis, tuberculosis, and chronic fungal infections; it may show parenchymal cavitary lesions in tuberculosis and pulmonary infiltrates. Computed tomog-

raphy of both the chest and abdomen may be required to demonstrate nodal enlargement.

Bone marrow aspiration and biopsy is usually diagnostic in patients with acute leukemias and myelofibrosis. Bone marrow biopsy may show involvement by lymphoma, tumors, lipid-laden macrophages in Gaucher's disease, noncaseating granulomas in sarcoidosis, and caseating granulomas in tuberculosis and fungal infections. Bone marrow cultures may occasionally be positive in tuberculosis and fungal infections.

Specific serologic studies may be useful in ruling out infectious mononucleosis, malaria, typhoid fever, disseminated histoplasmosis, rheumatoid arthritis, and systemic lupus erythematosus. A serum haptoglobin test and Coombs' test, in addition to reticulocyte count and evaluation of serum bilirubin, should be performed in patients suspected of having hemolytic anemias.

In patients with lymphadenopathy, if the diagnosis is not reached after routine and pertinent laboratory tests, a lymph node biopsy is obtained. Inguinal lymph nodes should be avoided as a site of biopsy. Excisional lymph node biopsy should be obtained to provide adequate tissue for special studies and details of node architecture.

Watchful waiting is sometimes the most prudent approach to the asymptomatic patient with splenomegaly who has no other signs of disease.

PROLONGED PROTHROMBIN TIME (PT) AND PARTIAL THROMBOPLASTIN TIME (PTT)

Prothrombin Time

DEFINITION

Prothrombin time measures the extrinsic (factor VII) and common (factors X and V, prothrombin, fibrinogen) pathways of coagulation.

PRINCIPLE OF THE PT TEST

This test measures the production of fibrin by plasma after the addition of calcium and excess tissue thromboplastin. Factor VII in the plasma is activated by tissue factor in the presence of calcium (extrinsic pathway). Factor VIIa tissue factor complex activates factor X, which begins the common pathway. The interaction of factor Xa with factor V, calcium, and plasma factor 3 leads to the formation of prothrombinase, which converts prothrombin to thrombin. Thrombin in turn converts fibrinogen to fibrin. The normal range of prothrombin time is 10.5 to 12.5 seconds, but the actual value varies in different laboratories. Results are interpreted in relation to simultaneously run prothrombin time tests on normal plasma. Prothrombin

Table 4–22. Causes of Prolonged PT

Hereditary deficiencies of factors VII, X, and V, prothrombin, and
   fibrinogen
Vitamin K deficiency (decreased factors II, VII, IX, X)
Oral anticoagulants, e.g., warfarin
Liver disease
Disseminated intravascular coagulation
Hypofibrinogenemia and dysfibrinogenemia
Therapeutic fibrinolysis
Heparin
Factor inhibitors
Artifactual (in patients with elevated hematocrit)

Table 4–23. Causes of Prolonged PTT

Deficiency of one or more factors involved in intrinsic and common
   pathway, i.e., prekallikrein, HMW kininogen, factors XII, XI, X, IX,
   VIII, and V, prothrombin, and fibrinogen
Coagulation factor inhibitors, lupus anticoagulant
Fibrin-split products
Heparin administration

time will be prolonged if the level of any of the factors assayed by this system is less then 10% of normal plasma. Prothrombin time is more sensitive to deficiencies of factors VII and X than to prothrombin and fibrinogen.

CAUSES AND INTERPRETATION OF PROLONGED PT
(Table 4–22)

Prothrombin time may be prolonged artifactually in patients with polycythemia because of the higher concentration of citrate obtained in the plasma. This artifact can be corrected by preparing special tubes with amounts of citrate adjusted for different hematocrits. Prothrombin time may be artifactually shortened by storage of citrated plasma, by about 2 seconds for every 3 or 4 hours of storage. This is particularly so in women taking oral contraceptives or in pregnant women.

Prolonged PT is commonly seen in acquired disorders; abnormal PTT is more often associated with hereditary factor deficiencies. An isolated prolongation of PT with normal PTT is an unusual finding and is seen with congenital deficiency of factor VII. Abnormalities of PT in combination with prolonged PTT are more common and are usually seen in vitamin K deficiency, warfarin therapy, disseminated intravascular coagulation, and liver disease. Disseminated intravascular coagulation is associated with prolonged thrombin time and elevated fibrin-split products. Abnormal thrombin time may also be noted in liver disease, hypofibrinogenemia, dysfibrinogenemia, and heparin use.

Partial Thromboplastin Time

DEFINITION

Partial thromboplastin time measures the intrinsic pathway (prekallikrein, HMW kininogen, factors XII, XI, IX, and VIII) and the common pathway (factors X and V, prothrombin, fibrinogen).

PRINCIPLE OF THE PTT TEST

Activated PTT (APTT) is generally preferred to the nonactivated PTT. Optimum activation of the intrinsic

pathway is obtained by the presence of surface reagents, e.g. kaolin in APTT reagent, whereas in the nonactivated procedure, activation is provided by glassware, syringe, etc. 0.1 ml of citrated plasma is incubated with 0.1 ml of APTT reagent (surface agent + phospholipid) at 37° C for 5 minutes. 0.1 ml of 0.025M calcium chloride is added and clotting time is recorded. Contact activation of the intrinsic system occurs because of the surface agent present in the APTT reagent, which results in the formation of IXa–PF-3–Ca–VIII complex. This complex acts on factor X, which activates the common pathway system resulting in fibrin formation. The normal APTT range is 26 to 36 seconds, but it varies with the equipment and the reagent used. PTT will be prolonged if any of the essential factor levels are less than 20% of normal. The PTT determined by the standard methods is prolonged in the deficiency of prekallikrein (Fletcher factor), but the abnormality is markedly decreased if contact activation is allowed for a longer time, e.g., 15 minutes, instead of the usual 5 minutes.

CAUSES AND INTERPRETATION OF PROLONGED PTT
(Table 4–23)

PTT, like PT, may be artifactually prolonged in patients with elevated hematocrit because of the relatively higher concentration of citrate in the plasma. PTT may be shorter than normal following a poor venipuncture.

In evaluating a patient with prolonged PTT, the physician should establish any history of abnormal bleeding and determine its severity. Prolonged PTT in the absence of any bleeding symptoms is present in deficiencies of prekallikrein, HMW kininogen, or factor XII, or in the presence of a lupus anticoagulant. Patients with a lupus anticoagulant usually do not have any bleeding problems but may rarely have thrombotic episodes. Lupus anticoagulant is a common cause of prolonged PTT and can be tested by mixing half of normal plasma with half of test plasma and performing an APTT on the mixture. PTT will almost always be correctable by normal plasma in the presence of factor deficiencies but not when a lupus anticoagulant is present.

Prolonged APTT in the presence of a bleeding diathesis is usually secondary to deficiencies of factors VIII, IX, and XI. Bleeding disorder is usually severe in patients with factor VIII (hemophilia A) or IX (hemophilia B) deficiency. Factor XI deficiency is usually a clinically mild disorder. Prolonged APTT in association with abnormal bleeding time is typically seen in von Willebrand's disease. Small amounts of heparin present in the intravenous catheters used to draw blood may be an unsuspected cause of prolonged PTT.

APTT may be shortened in the presence of high levels of any single factor, commonly factor VIII, or in disseminated intravascular coagulation when activated factors are present in the test plasma.

MYELODYSPLASTIC SYNDROMES

Definition

Myelodysplastic syndromes are a group of poorly defined hematopoietic disorders with an increased propensity to develop into acute nonlymphocytic leukemia. They are characterized by ineffective erythropoiesis, peripheral blood cytopenias, and hypercellular or normocellular bone marrow. These disorders have also been referred to as preleukemia, smoldering leukemias, and oligoblastic leukemias.

Pathophysiologic Considerations (Table 4–24)

Myelodysplastic syndromes may be idiopathic or secondary to known carcinogens like radiation, antineoplastic chemotherapy (e.g., alkylating agents), and chemical agents (e.g., benzene).

Primary myelodysplastic syndromes are clonal disorders of pluripotent stem cells and are of unknown cause. The clonal nature of the defect was demonstrated in a woman heterozygous for glucose-6-phosphate dehydrogenase and a myelodysplastic syndrome.[15] The abnormal clone appears to have a growth advantage over normal hematopoietic precursors, which results in cytopenias and an increase in blasts.

Differential Diagnosis

When an elderly patient develops unexplained cytopenia with a cellular marrow, a diagnosis of acute leukemia or a myelodysplastic syndrome should be suspected. Megaloblastic anemias and paroxysmal nocturnal hemoglobinuria in the cytopenic phase should be considered in the differential diagnosis.

Therapy-related myelodysplastic syndromes are often associated with hypocellular marrow or marrow fibrosis with a cellular marrow and ringed sideroblasts.

Differentiating features of primary myelodysplastic syndromes on peripheral blood smear and bone marrow are presented in Table 4–25. According to FAB classification, over 30% of blasts in bone marrow will suffice for the diagnosis of acute myelogenous leukemia.[16] Marrow blasts in myelodysplastic syndromes are less than 30%.

5q-syndrome is characterized by the changes as noted in refractory anemia (RA) with 5q-chromosomal abnormality (q 15; q 31) and increased numbers of small atypical mononuclear or bilobed megakaryocytes.

Diagnostic Evaluation

PATIENT HISTORY AND PHYSICAL EXAMINATION

Patients with primary myelodysplastic syndromes are elderly (50% are greater than 60 years old) with a male predominance (65%). Patients generally present with weakness and pallor and occasionally with easy bruising or bleeding manifestations. About 10 to 30% will develop overt leukemia. Some of the patients may go for 10 or more years before developing acute myelogenous leukemia. Survival is usually short, with a median of 27 months.[17] Death may be due to acute leukemia, hemorrhage or infection secondary to cytopenias, or unrelated causes.

DIAGNOSTIC STUDIES

These patients in general show evidence of ineffective hematopoiesis characterized by refractory cytopenias despite hypercellular or normocellular bone marrow.

On peripheral blood smear, red cells may be slightly macrocytic or normocytic normochromic. Anisocytosis, poikilocytosis, polychromasia, basophilic stippling, and reticulocytopenia are commonly present. Neutropenia with an absolute neutrophil count less than 2000/µl is noted in about 50% of cases. Hyposegmented (acquired Pelger-Huët anomaly) or hypersegmented neutrophils may be noted. Neutrophils may have abnormally large granules or poor granule formation. Abnormalities of platelets include thrombocytopenia, abnormalities of size and shape, and hypogranular forms.

Bone marrow is hypercellular or normocellular and generally shows abnormalities of all three cell lines.

Table 4–24. Classification of Myelodysplastic Syndrome

Primary myelodysplastic syndromes (French-American-British (FAB) cooperative group classification)
Refractory anemia (RA)
  Refractory anemia with ringed sideroblasts (RARS) or idiopathic acquired sideroblastic anemia (IASA)
  Refractory anemia with excess blasts (RAEB)
  Chronic myelomonocytic leukemias (CMML)
  Refractory anemia with excess blasts in transformation (RAEB-IT)
Secondary myelodysplastic syndromes
  Therapy-related (radiation therapy, alkylating agents, etc.)
  Chemical agents: benzene
  Drugs: chloramphenicol

Table 4–25. Differentiating Features of Myelodysplastic Syndromes

	Peripheral Blood	Bone Marrow
Refractory anemia (RA)	Anemia, reticulocytopenia blasts ≤1%	Hypercellular or normocellular Variable dyserythropoiesis granulocytes and megakaryocytes usually normal Blasts ≤5%
Refractory anemia with ringed sidero-blasts (RARS)	As above; RBCs may have dimorphic picture	Ringed sideroblasts >15%
Refractory anemia with excess blasts (RAEB)	Abnormalities usually present in all 3 cell lines Blasts <5% Monocytes <1000/ml	Hypercellular, dysgranulopoiesis, dyse-rythropoiesis, and/or dysmegakary-opoiesis Ringed sideroblasts ±, blasts >5% but <20%
Chronic myelomonocytic leukemia (CMML)	RAEB + monocytes >1000/µl	As in RAEB with increase in monocyte precursors Blasts often <5% but may have up to 20%
Refractory anemia with excess blasts in transformation (RAEB-IT)	Blast ≥5%	Blasts >20% but <30% Auer rods ±

Red cell precursors show hyperplasia, megaloblastoid features, multinuclearity, and ringed sideroblasts. White cell precursors may show an increase in myeloblasts and monoblasts, acquired Pelger-Huët anomaly, abnormal granulation, and Auer rods. Megakaryocytes are normal or increased in number. Micromegakaryocytes with one or two nuclei, hypogranulated forms, or large mononuclear megakaryocytes may be noted.

Cytogenetic abnormalities resemble those noted in acute myelogenous leukemia. Chromosome abnormalities frequently noted are monosomy for 7, trisomy for 8, 9, and 21, deletion of 5 and 20 (5q- or 20q-) and 17q isochromosome.

Marrow in vitro culture studies may show decreased colony-forming ability of CFU-GM, abortive "clusters," and an increase in the proportion of clusters to colonies.

On flow cytometry studies, patients with a stable clinical course have been reported to have higher fractions of proliferating cells than those who developed acute leukemia or died early in the course of disease.[18]

MYELOPROLIFERATIVE DISORDERS

Definition

The myeloproliferative disorders are a group of clonal stem cell disorders characterized by proliferation of red cells, granulocytes, or platelets. There is no clear consensus on which conditions should be included, and frequently a precise distinction cannot be made among them. Most hematologists would probably include chronic myelogenous leukemia (CML), polycythemia vera (PV), idiopathic myelofibrosis (IMF) (often called agnogenic myeloid metaplasia), and essential thrombocythemia (ET). While one particular cell type may predominate, hyperplasia of the other cell types will occur almost invariably and their bone marrows may be virtually indistinguishable. Moreover, transitions of one disease to another have been documented. With the exception of the unique occurrence of the Philadelphia chromosome in CML, no other clinical or laboratory feature can be said to occur exclusively in any one of these diseases.

Pathophysiologic Considerations

The myeloproliferative disorders are clonal neoplasms arising at the level of the pluripotent myeloid stem cell or the totipotent myeloid stem cell. Isoenzyme studies in glucose-6-phosphate dehydrogenase heterozygotes and chromosomal studies have revealed the monoclonality of the lesion in CML.[19] The Philadelphia chromosome (Ph[1]), an abnormal chromosome 22, results from a translocation between chromosome 22 and 9, t (9; 22) and is present in 90% of patients with CML. It can be detected in erythrocytes, granulocytes, and megakaryocytic cells. Lymphocytes may or may not be part of the clone. Recent studies have revealed that oncogene c-abl is translocated from chromosome 9 to 22, resulting in expression of a hybrid protein abl-bcr.[20,21]

In the development of CML, the leukemic clone gains growth advantage over normal hematopoietic stem cells. Virtually all the pluripotent myeloid stem cells, erythrocytes, granulocytes, and platelets are derived from this leukemic clone.

Increased marrow fibrosis in IMF is possibly explained by stimulation of fibroblast growth by an excess of platelet-derived growth factor (PDGF) released by abnormal hematopoietic cells.

Differential Diagnosis (Table 4–26)

CML should be differentiated from granulocytic leukemoid reactions. Leukemoid reactions are usually secondary to an infection or tumor, though cells less mature than metamyelocytes are uncommon in a blood smear. The leukocyte alkaline phosphatase score is high or normal and Philadelphia chromosome is absent in a leukemoid reaction. In about half of the patients with CML, a white cell count greater than 100,000/μl is present, whereas a white cell count is usually less than 100,000/μl in leukemoid reactions. Polycythemia vera can be differentiated from other causes of polycythemia based on guidelines detailed in the section on erythrocytosis. The differential diagnosis of ET is discussed in the section on thrombocytosis.

Idiopathic myelofibrosis may be confused with hairy-cell leukemia presenting with splenomegaly, pancytopenia, and marrow fibrosis. Teardrop poikilocytosis, a leukoerythroblastic reaction in myelofibrosis, and characteristic "hairy" lymphocytes that stain for tartarate-resistant acid phosphatase (TRAP), as well as the characteristic bone marrow biopsy in hairy-cell leukemia, should help differentiate these two disorders. Myelofibrosis may also occur secondary to granulomatous disorders, chronic infections (tubercular, fungal), and tumors. The diagnosis depends on identifying the underlying primary condition. Increased marrow fibrosis may also develop in later stages of CML and polycythemia vera.

Diagnostic Evaluation

PATIENT HISTORY AND PHYSICAL EXAMINATION

Patients with polycythemia vera usually present with symptoms caused by circulatory disturbances in the central nervous system, e.g., headache, dizziness, vertigo, and tinnitus. Facial plethora and conjunctival injection are usually evident on presentation. Bleeding and thrombotic complications are frequent in polycythemia vera and essential thrombocythemia. Patients with CML or IMF usually present with generalized weakness, pallor, or a dragging sensation in left upper quadrant of the abdomen.

Splenomegaly is common in all chronic myeloproliferative syndromes but is more pronounced in patients with CML or IMF.

DIAGNOSTIC STUDIES

The physician should obtain a CBC, differential count, platelet count, and peripheral blood smear. Table 4–26 gives the comparative features of the chronic myeloproliferative syndromes. Careful scrutiny of peripheral blood smear is essential. The blood smear in IMF reveals teardrop poikilocytosis and a leukoerythroblastic reaction, i.e., immature granulocytes, erythroblasts, and nucleated red cells. The blood smear in CML reveals mature and immature granulocytes at various stages, predominately myelocytes, metamyelocytes, mature neutrophils, and a variable increase in eosinophils and basophils. Promyelocytes and blast cells are usually less than 10% of the nucleated leukocytes in the peripheral smear. A few erythroid precursors may also be noted, and the platelet count is normal or increased. The platelet count in essential thrombocythemia is frequently above $1 \times 10^6/\mu l$, and the blood smear may show variations in

Table 4–26. Comparative Features of Chronic Myeloproliferative Syndromes

	Chronic Myelogenous Leukemia	Polycythemia Vera	Idiopathic Myelofibrosis	Essential Thrombocythemia
Splenomegaly	Moderate to massive	Moderate	Massive in 33% >5 cm in 33% <5 cm in 33%	Mild
Hepatomegaly	Common	In 33% of patients	Common	Present in 40% of patients
Sternal tenderness	Common	Rare	Rare	Rare
Neutrophils	↑↑↑	↑↑, N	↑, N, ↓	↑, N
Red cells	↓, N	↑↑↑	↓, ↑	N, ↑
Platelets	↑↑, N	↑↑, N	↑, N, ↓	↑↑↑
Marrow fibrosis	± (late)	± (late)	+, +++	± (late)
Leukocyte alkaline phosphatase	↓ in 90%	↑ (70%), N	N, ↑	N, ↑
Philadelphia chromosome	+ in 90%	Absent	Absent	Absent
Transformation into acute leukemia	100%	10%–20%	10%	5%–10%

platelet size, giant platelets, and megakaryocyte fragments. In early stages of polycythemia vera, the blood smear may be normal or may show signs of iron deficiency. Anisocytosis, poikilocytosis, polychromatophilia, and occasional nucleated red cells appear as the disease progresses.

In patients suspected of having polycythemia vera, red cell mass should be determined. For further discussion on polycythemia vera, refer to the section on erythrocytosis.

The physician should also establish the presence of leukocyte alkaline phosphatase (LAP) (Table 4–26). In addition, he should perform bone marrow aspiration and biopsy, and iron and reticulin stain. Bone marrow biopsy is required to properly assess the marrow cellularity. Bone marrow is hypercellular in PV, CML, and ET. Bone marrow aspiration may yield a "dry tap" in myelofibrosis. Reticulin stain reveals increased fibrosis in IMF. Increased marrow fibrosis may develop late in the course of the disease in other chronic myeloproliferative syndromes, as well. Marked granulocytic hyperplasia is noted in CML with an increase in the ratio of myeloid to erythroid from a normal of 2-5:1 to 10-50:1. Panhyperplasia of all three elements, particularly of red cell precursors, and decreased or absent stainable iron are noted in polycythemia vera. In ET, large megakaryocytes with multiple lobes, as well as hyperplasia of red and white cell precursors, are seen. Megakaryocytic hyperplasia may be noted in IMF also.

Marrow cytogenetics reveals Philadelphia chromosome in 90% of patients with CML. Various nonspecific chromosome abnormalities are noted in other chronic myeloproliferative disorders.

Platelet aggregation studies may be obtained in patients with bleeding complications. For further discussion of ET, see the section on thrombocytosis.

MONOCLONAL GAMMOPATHIES

Definition

The appearance of a monoclonal immunoglobulin or a light-chain spike on serum or urine electrophoresis is referred to as monoclonal gammopathy.

Pathophysiologic Considerations (Table 4–27)

Monoclonal immunoglobulins are produced by abnormal clones of immunoglobulin-secreting lymphocytes or plasma cells that may be neoplastic or benign. Neoplastic proliferations are associated with B-lymphocyte malignancies, e.g., multiple myeloma and lymphomas.

Benign proliferation of immunoglobulin-secreting

Table 4–27. Classification of Monoclonal Gammopathies

Monoclonal gammopathies associated with B-lymphocyte or plasma cell neoplasms
  Multiple myeloma
  Waldenström's macroglobulinemia
  Lymphomas
  Chronic lymphatic leukemia
  Heavy-chain diseases
Secondary monoclonal gammopathy
  Sepsis
    Tuberculosis
    Osteomyelitis
    Cytomegalovirus infections
    Mycoplasma pneumonia
    Viral hepatitis
  Neoplasms of cells not secreting immunoglobulins
    Various carcinomas
    Malignant melanoma
    Angiosarcoma
    Oligodendroglioma
  Autoimmune disorders
    Systemic lupus erythematosus
    Rheumatoid arthritis
    Periarteritis nodosa
    Scleroderma
    Necrotizing vasculitis
    Myasthenia gravis
    Pernicious anemia
    Pemphigus
  Hepatobiliary disease
    Cirrhosis
    Hepatitis
    Methotrexate hepatotoxicity
    Biliary tract disease
  Immune deficiency syndromes
  Miscellaneous
    Gaucher's disease
    Acute porphyria
    Sarcoidosis
    Pyoderma gangrenosum
    Parathyroid adenoma
    Paget's disease of bone
Benign monoclonal gammopathy

cells may occur in infections, inflammatory disorders, and carcinomas, especially in the colon and rectum. Such monoclonal spikes are usually transient and disappear on recovery from the primary disorder. When a monoclonal spike is persistent and not associated with other disorders, it is known as benign monoclonal gammopathy (BMG). The abnormal clone of B-lymphocytes or plasma cells proliferates to reach a steady-state level and usually remains at that level for many years. These cells, unlike those in multiple myeloma, do not produce osteoclast-activating factor (OAF), which has been implicated in causing the bone lesions and hypercalcemia seen in multiple myeloma. A small proportion of patients with BMG develop overt myeloma after a variable time period.

Differential Diagnosis

It is of paramount importance to differentiate between benign monoclonal gammopathy and malignant plasma cell dyscrasias. Malignant plasma cell dyscrasia should be suspected if the patient has osteolytic bone lesions, hepatosplenomegaly, extraskeletal plasmacytoma, anemia or pancytopenia, hypercalcemia, marrow plasmacytosis greater than 15%, abnormal plasma cell morphology (immature, multinucleated plasma cells), serum M component (IgG > 3.0 gm/dl, or IgA or IgM > 1.5 gm/dl), high urinary light-chain concentration, rising M component, or decrease in polyclonal immunoglobulins.

Benign monoclonal gammopathy is the most common immunoglobulin disorder. It can usually be diagnosed by using the above-mentioned criteria. In a few cases, however, one may be certain of correct diagnosis only on prolonged follow-up.

Diagnostic Evaluation

PATIENT HISTORY AND PHYSICAL EXAMINATION

Multiple myeloma is characterized by osteolytic bone lesions, hypercalcemia, anemia, and bone marrow infiltration by plasma cells. Waldenström's macroglobulinemia is associated with hepatosplenomegaly and the hyperviscosity syndromes. Lytic bone lesions and hypercalcemia are usually not seen.

Secondary monoclonal gammopathies are associated with clinical features of the underlying disease. Benign monoclonal gammopathy is characterized by the lack of osteolytic bone lesions and no apparent underlying disorder. It is usually discovered incidentally.

DIAGNOSTIC STUDIES

CBC and platelet count are related to the underlying disorder. Anemia is common in multiple myeloma, and the severity of anemia correlates with the tumor burden. Urine analysis may reveal proteinuria, and a chemistry profile may show hypercalcemia or azotemia. The physician should perform a serum and 24-hour urine protein electrophoresis. In benign monoclonal gammopathy of IgG type, the serum M component is usually less than 3.0 gm/dl; in IgA or IgM types, the serum M component is usually less than 1.5 gm/dl.

Qualitative and quantitative serum and urine protein immunoelectrophoresis should be obtained for characterization of abnormal immunoglobulin or light-chain type. The serum M component is an IgM in Waldenström's macroglobulinemia. Serum immunoglobulins other than the M component are normal in BMG and decreased in malignant plasma cell dyscrasias.

Table 4–28. Causes of Hyperviscosity Syndrome

Disorders involving plasma proteins
  Lymphoplasmacytic dyscrasias
    Waldenström's macroglobulinemia
    Multiple myeloma
    Extramedullary plasmacytoma
  Lymphocytic malignances
    Chronic lymphocytic leukemia
    Diffuse lymphomas
  Others: cryoglobulinemia, rheumatoid arthritis
Disorders of formed elements of blood
  Myeloproliferative syndrmes—polycythemia vera

On bone marrow examination, marrow plasma cells are within normal limits or less than 10% in BMG. Marrow plasmacytosis of 15%, immature or multinucleated plasma cells, and plasma cells in sheets are noted in multiple myeloma. In Waldenström's macroglobulinemia, the predominant abnormal cell is a plasmacytoid lymphocyte in association with small lymphocytes and plasma cells.

A skeletal survey should be obtained in patients suspected of having malignant plasma cell dyscrasias. Bone scans are less sensitive in multiple myeloma and are frequently negative.

HYPERVISCOSITY SYNDROMES

Definition

Hyperviscosity syndromes refer to the effects of increased viscosity or increased resistance of blood to flow in the circulation. Patients often present complaining of fatigue with various neurologic and visual disturbances and bleeding manifestations.

Pathophysiologic Considerations (Table 4–28)

Hyperviscosity of the blood may occur because of increased concentration or structural abnormalities, of formed elements of blood, particularly red cells, or plasma proteins.

Monoclonal macroglobulinemia (increase in IgM) is the most common cause of hyperviscosity syndromes. The high molecular weight of IgM (850,000) and the unusual configuration of IgM pentamer make it prone to increasing the viscosity of blood. IgA M components are the second most common cause of hyperviscosity. Hyperviscosity is unusual with IgG M components, and it occurs only occasionally with very high concentrations of IgG or with IgG molecules that have increased tendency to aggregate. IgG 3 is the most common subtype that tends to aggregate.

Disorders associated with the formation of circulating immune complexes, e.g., cryoglobulinemias, may also rarely produce hyperviscosity. Increased concentration of red cells in myeloproliferative syndromes, particularly polycythemia vera, can also produce a clinical picture of hyperviscosity syndromes. In addition, because of increased resistance of blood to flow, vascular occlusions occur in microvasculature, accounting for the clinical symptoms.

Differential Diagnosis

Waldenström's macroglobulinemia is characterized by hepatosplenomegaly, lymphadenopathy, anemia, absent or minimal bone lesions, and absence of hypercalcemia.

Patients with IgM myeloma have more pronounced punched-out bone lesions, hypercalcemia, and absence of hepatosplenomegaly and lymphadenopathy. Patients with chronic lymphocytic leukemia or diffuse lymphomas are characterized by their usual clinical findings.

Diagnostic Evaluation

PATIENT HISTORY AND PHYSICAL EXAMINATION

The patient may present with such general signs and symptoms as weakness, fatigue, anorexia, and dilated tortuous veins. He may have clinical features of underlying disorders such as hepatosplenomegaly, lymphadenopathy, and absent or minimal bone lesions in Waldenström's macroglobulinemia or chronic lymphocytic leukemia. Multiple skeletal lytic lesions may be present in myeloma. Among the possible visual disturbances are visual impairment, dilated tortuous retinal veins, alternating constrictions and distensions of retinal veins (link-sausage effect), retinal hemorrhages and exudates. The patient may have neurologic and central features such as headache, vertigo, confusion, stupor, seizures, coma, cerebrovascular occlusions and hemorrhages, myelopathies, peripheral neuropathies (Bing-Neel syndrome), and deafness. He may have manifestations of cryoglobulins, such as cold hypersensitivity, Raynaud's phenomenon, and peripheral vascular occlusions. Bleeding manifestations may include purpura, epistaxis, and gastrointestinal bleeding. Also, the patient may have congestive heart failure.

DIAGNOSTIC STUDIES

Diagnostic studies include CBC and platelet count; serum calcium, BUN, and creatinine; serum protein electrophoresis and urine protein electrophoresis; immunoelectrophoresis (for positive identification of the M component); relative serum viscosity (patients are rarely symptomatic with relative serum viscosity of less than 4 centipoise), skeletal survey; and bone marrow examination, which may show infiltration by plasma cells in multiple myeloma, plasmacytoid lymphocytes in Waldenström's macroglobulinemia, and mature, small lymphocytes in CLL.

In patients with bleeding manifestations the physician should assess bleeding time and perform platelet function studies, thrombin time, PT and PTT tests. Serum cryoglobulins should be ascertained in patients with cold hypersensitivity or Raynaud's phenomenon.

ONCOLOGIC PROBLEMS

In no field of medicine is the physician called upon to blend his art and science so skillfully as in oncology. For many patients, it is almost gratuitous to assert that the diagnosis of cancer is equated to a sentence of death. That the emotional consequences are often devastating to the patient as well as the family has been treated in detail in many monographs devoted to the subject. What, then, do we hope to communicate in this brief chapter on aspects of neoplastic disease in a textbook of medicine?

While it is evident that many of the major neoplastic diseases are not curable, the view that there is no treatment should be abandoned. Above all, the physician must see to it that reasonable hope be sustained and the patient's needs and comforts be met. Clearly, the gravity of the illness cannot be denied, nor should unreasonable expectations be engendered; such encouragement is unwise and, indeed, harmful. A positive attitude among professional personnel dealing with the patient and the family will do much to dispel the anger, desperation, and air of grim resignation that often take hold. The family requires direction that the physician is uniquely able to provide. His consistency and availability, with a proper mixture of gentle firmness, do much to mitigate what otherwise might be a catastrophic depression.

Although definitive treatment for a neoplasm might be lacking, many complications that may occur during the course of the disease may be prevented. In recent years, oncologists have become concerned as much with the quality of life of the patient as with its prolongation. Life-sustaining measures are of arguable value to the patient if, for example, he becomes paraplegic as a result of a preventable spinal cord lesion. The thrust of this chapter is to identify medical problems that may arise during the course of a malignant disease. Some of these are completely preventable if recognized in time. Others can be effectively palliated if the process is recognized and its pathogenesis understood. Still others might be allowed to provide a humane mode of death to a terminally ill patient. Hence, the wisdom of vigorously treating hypercalcemia in a patient with a far-advanced neoplasm can be seriously questioned. These diagnostic problems and subsequent decisions can be resolved only by the well-informed and compassionate physician.

CENTRAL NERVOUS SYSTEM INVOLVEMENT IN NEOPLASTIC DISEASES

Definition

Involvement of the nervous system in the course of cancer is exceedingly common. Early diagnosis obviates the necessity for emergency intervention and in many cases results in very satisfactory palliation. Several large series indicate that fully 25% of patients with cancer demonstrate intracranial metastases, and 5% show evidence of spinal extradural masses at the time of autopsy. These figures will be very much higher if only lung, breast, and prostate tumors are considered.

Pathophysiologic Considerations (Table 4—29)

The specific causes of neurologic syndromes will vary greatly with the type of neoplasm. Thus, metastases from solid tumors will cause CNS symptoms due largely to mass effects, while leukemia and lymphomas commonly cause hemorrhage, infarction, and infections. Table 4—29 lists some of the common causes of nervous system syndromes.

Differential Diagnosis

The earliest symptoms of a cerebral mass and leptomeningeal diseases may be persistent headache, a change in cognition, which the patient often volunteers, and, later, depression of the sensorium. An early seizure can be due to the production by leptomeningeal metastases of a carcinomatous meningitis. Diagnosis of leptomeningeal disease is favored by the presence

Table 4—29. Causes of CNS Disease in Cancer

Mass effect of metastatic tumor
Leptomeningeal metastases
Cerebrovascular disorders
Infections
Side effects of chemotherapy
Paraneoplastic syndromes

of signs of meningeal irritations and cranial nerve deficits, which are separate anatomically. Severe obtundation, headache, and objective neurologic findings constitute a true medical emergency, and cerebral herniation may be imminent or may have already occurred. The presence of fever with any of the above signs or symptoms requires that a pyogenic meningitis or brain abscess be considered.

Among the most prevalent of the CNS lesions producing extensive morbidity and anguish in a patient with cancer is spinal cord compression caused by tumor in the epidural space. Virtually all of these patients will have complained of back pain for weeks or months preceding presentation. A majority will show evidence of tumor in the vertebral body by x-ray of the spine. The pain will be local or radicular and corresponds to the level of the tumor. The pain will be local or radicular and corresponds to the level of the tumor. It is often intensified by percussion over the spine or by a Valsalva maneuver. Full recovery of functions is unlikely if diagnosis and treatment are delayed until paralysis supervenes.

Vascular disease of the central nervous system is a relatively common cause of symptoms in cancer patients. Cerebral hemorrhage may occur secondary to a lowered platelet count or as a manifestation of disseminated intravascular coagulations (DIC). Leukostasis with hemorrhagic infarction of the brain is seen in acute myeloblastic leukemia or the accelerative phase of chronic myelogenous leukemia. The peripheral blood blast count is usually in excess of 50,000/μl. Bleeding into a hemorrhagic metastasis is most common with melanoma or a germ cell tumor. Symptomatic thrombotic or embolic cerebral infarcts are seen most commonly in patients with DIC and nonbacterial thrombotic endocarditis. A syndrome recognized relatively recently that may or may not be associated with tumor infiltration of the dura is sagittal sinus thrombosis. Patients may present with headache, seizures, obtundations, and hemiparesis.

A variety of metabolic disturbances may give rise to changes in cognition and even obtundation with or without motor-sensory findings. Hypercalcemia will be considered below. Severe hyponatremia occurring as the hallmark of the syndrome of inappropriate antidiuretic hormone secretion (SIADH) may cause lethargy, confusion, seizures, or coma. SIADH is seen commonly with small-cell carcinoma of the lung. These abnormalities will be discussed in more detail under metabolic abnormalities.

Although it is not commonly recognized, chemotherapeutic agents cause a variety of signs and symptoms referable to the nervous system, especially in elderly patients. While most of these reactions are rare,

Table 4–30. Common Paraneoplastic Syndromes of the Nervous System

Syndrome	Clinical Features	Associated Neoplasms
Subacute cerebellar degeneration	Symmetrical cerebellar signs, dementia, CSF pleocytosis, protein elevation	Lung, colorectal, ovary, prostate
Dementia	Slowly progressive, occasionally acute; may be accompanied by other neurologic findings	Lung
Sensorimotor peripheral neuropathy	Rarely may be pure motor or sensory elevated CSF protein	Lung, lymphoma, breast, colorectal
Dermatomyositis	Gradual development of muscle weakness, elevated CPK, skin rash	Lung, ovary, stomach
Eaton-Lambert syndrome	Weakness and easy fatigability of proximal muscles, diplopia, dysarthria, poor response to Tensilon, facilitated muscle response to repeated stimulus by EMG	Lung, ovary, stomach

some, such as the peripheral neuropathy caused by vincristine, the lethargy and somnolence associated with asparaginase and interferon, and the ototoxicity of cis-platinum, are relatively common. Fluorouracil and procarbazine may rarely cause a neurologic syndrome indistinguishable from that of a mass lesion in the brain.

Finally, the physician must be aware that a bewildering array of signs and symptoms in the nervous system and elsewhere may occur in the course of cancer unrelated to tumor deposits. These are collectively called the paraneoplastic syndromes and will be considered in more detail in a later section (Table 4–30). In at least one of these syndromes, the Eaton-Lambert syndrome, an autoantibody to the presynaptic membrane active zone has been demonstrated, which results in decreased acetylcholine secretion. The paraneoplastic syndromes are relatively uncommon and diagnosis is one of exclusion. These neurologic syndromes may not remit even when the tumor is removed. Moreover, they may appear months before the associated neoplasm has manifested itself.

Diagnostic Evaluation

A complete history and physical examination often will allow the physician to assess the role of vascular complications in the causation of the syndrome being observed. Blood chemical determinations including electrolytes, creatinine, and calcium will suggest metabolic causes for disturbances in the nervous system.

A CT or MRI scan is essential for the diagnosis of lesions in the cranium and in the substance of the brain. If meningitis is suspected or a lumbar puncture required for any reason, a CT scan must be obtained to ascertain evidence of increased intracranial pressure. The CT scan may also allow visualization of vertebral lesions that are not visible by x-rays.

Lumbar puncture is necessary to confirm the presence of meningitis. The procedure should always be preceded by a CT scan and should probably not be performed unless the platelet count is greater than 30,000/μl. Platelet transfusions may be required.

In certain tumors such as small-cell carcinoma of the lung, multiple lesions in the central nervous system are present concomitantly. For example, in a National Cancer Institute study, 25% of the patients with intracranial metastases also had carcinomatous leptomeningitis, and 20% of patients with carcinomatous leptomeningitis had intracranial metastasis. Of the patients with spinal cord compression, 50% had a simultaneous intracranial metastasis. The appropriate x-ray studies should be performed to rule out metastases in all parts of the neuraxis even if only a single site appears to be involved.

Myelography should be performed in all patients with persistent local or radicular pain whether or not neurologic findings are present. The presence of a vertebral lesion and pain makes myelography imperative.

CARDIOVASCULAR INVOLVEMENT IN NEOPLASTIC DISEASES

Superior Vena Cava (SVC) Syndrome

DEFINITION

The superior vena cava is the ultimate venous channel for the return of blood from the head, upper extremities, and upper thorax. Occlusion of the vessel results in a distinctive syndrome that requires early treatment but is usually not a true medical emergency.

PATHOPHYSIOLOGIC CONSIDERATIONS

In the current era, virtually all SVC syndromes result from neoplastic involvement of the mediastinum. The SVC may be compressed externally by tumor masses, or the wall of the vessel may be involved by the tumor, causing thrombosis. Most commonly the tumors arise in the lung (especially small-cell carcinoma) or are lymphomas arising in the mediastinal lymph nodes.

DIFFERENTIAL DIAGNOSIS

The superior vena cava syndrome is sufficiently distinctive to offer no problem with recognition when it is fully developed and caused by venous hypertension.

Its severity depends on the rapidity of development, the degree of obstruction, and the extent of collateral circulation.

Symptoms include headache, dizziness, hoarseness, visual changes, stridor, respiratory distress, syncopal episodes, and even seizures. Most patients will have had these symptoms for less than a month.

The physical signs of SVC syndrome may include thoracic venous distension, edema of the face, neck vein distension, tachypnea, cyanosis, edema of the upper extremities, paralysis of the true vocal cord, and occasionally Horner's syndrome. Patients having back pain should be evaluated by myelography for associated spinal cord compression.

DIAGNOSTIC EVALUATION

In most cases the diagnosis is clear from the clinical picture and is confirmed by a chest x-ray showing a widened superior mediastinum and often a hilar mass. About 25% of patients will also have a pleural effusion, from which a cytologic diagnosis can be made in a majority of cases.

Since immediate treatment is rarely necessary, 4 or 5 days can be spent profitably attempting to make a precise diagnosis. Because small-cell carcinoma of the lung and lymphoma are the usual causes of the syndrome, biopsy of a superficial lymph node will often give the diagnosis. Bronchoscopy may be performed if the patient is able to assume the supine position, allowing the procedure to be done. In general, surgical procedures such as mediastinoscopy or thoracotomy should be avoided if at all possible.

If immediate treatment is required before the diagnosis is established 2000 to 3000 rads of radiation may be administered without substantially altering the histopathology. A diagnosis must ultimately be established because virtually all of these patients will require systemic therapy.

Cardiac Tamponade

DEFINITION

Tamponade of the heart secondary to tumor involvement of the pericardium with the formation of a pericardial effusion is a frequently overlooked diagnosis that may result in death. Nevertheless, less than 30% of the patients with neoplastic pericarditis have symptoms.

PATHOPHYSIOLOGIC CONSIDERATIONS

A wide variety of tumors may produce pericardial metastases that ultimately result in tamponade. These include metastases from lung, lymphoma, breast, melanoma, and sarcoma. The mechanism by which fluid in the pericardial space limits diastolic filling and reduces stroke volume is similar to the mechanism produced by other causes of pericarditis and will not be discussed here. As with SVC syndrome, the symptoms observed depend on the rapidity with which the fluid accumulates and the total amount of fluid. The fluid itself is usually bloody, has a high protein content, and usually will not clot.

Patients who receive radiation to the mediastinum, especially if it exceeds 4000 rads, may develop pericarditis. Usually pericarditis occurs during the first year after the completion of radiation, but many years may elapse before it becomes manifest. Initially, acute pericarditis may not be clinically evident. Ultimately, the patient may demonstrate the syndrome of constrictive pericarditis.

DIFFERENTIAL DIAGNOSIS

The clinical picture is indistinguishable from other forms of pericardial effusion. Often, pleural effusions may also be present. The majority of patients with malignant pericardial effusions will be relatively asymptomatic, and the diagnosis is suggested by only the cardiac configuration in the chest x-ray.

DIAGNOSTIC EVALUATION

Apart from the chest x-ray, the simplest, most consistently helpful diagnostic modality is echocardiography. The effusion resulting from radiation pericarditis is often not distinguishable from that of neoplastic pericarditis. In both cases the fluid may be bloody and contains no malignant cells. In radiation pericarditis, however, there may be other signs of radiation-induced injury in the surrounding lung.

Nonbacterial Thrombotic Endocarditis (NBTE)

This syndrome is usually considered a part of the spectrum of the paraneoplastic diseases. The patient's signs and symptoms stem from the presence of sterile, verrucous, bland, fibrinous lesions on the left-sided heart valves. The clinical manifestations in patients, who are usually afebrile, relate to embolic episodes usually involving the brain but also the spleen and other peripheral sites. These vegetations are often smaller than 2 mm and therefore may not produce a loud heart murmur or even be detectable by echocardiography. Usually the underlying malignancy is far advanced.

Thrombophlebitis, Migratory Thrombophlebitis, and Trousseau's Syndrome

The syndrome of migratory, superficial thrombophlebitis occurring with a malignancy, usually mucin-secreting adenocarcinomas, was described over a century ago. Most frequently it occurs with pancreatic or lung cancer. No specific cause can be identified in the majority of these patients to explain their hypercoagulable state, but the most frequently identifiable etiologic factor is the presence of disseminated intravascular coagulation (DIC), which was discussed in a previous section.

HYPERCALCEMIA

Definition

This discussion could reasonably be included in the section that follows on metabolic abnormalities in malignancy. However, because it is such a common abnormality and may be life threatening but is reversible if recognized, it is discussed separately. In excess of 10% of patients with cancer will develop hypercalcemia during the course of their disease. Hypercalcemia associated with malignancy is now the most common cause of elevated serum calcium in hospitalized patients. Since patients with neoplasm often have a decrease in serum albumin, allowance must be made for the fact that the major fraction of serum calcium is protein bound. A useful formula to make this correction is: corrected calcium (mg/dl) = measured calcium + (4-albumin g/dl) $\times$ 0.8.

Pathophysiologic Considerations

Hypercalcemia in neoplastic disease is usually considered to be one of the paraneoplastic syndromes because, whether or not actual bone lesions are present, the disruption in calcium homeostasis appears to be due to excessive or de novo secretion of humoral substances that favor bone resorption and, at least in some cases, decreased bone formation. Two major groups of patients may be distinguished, those with bone metastases and those with no evidence of metastatic disease in bone. In the former group, the most common solid tumors producing hypercalcemia are breast, lung, and kidney. Carcinoma of the thyroid, ovary, and colon are less common causes. Of the hematopoietic malignancies associated with lytic bone lesions and hypercalcemia, multiple myeloma is the most frequent. Hypercalcemia with bone lesions may be a prominent feature of large-cell lymphomas, Burkitt's lymphoma, and T-cell leukemia or lymphoma. In T-cell lymphoma, lytic lesions may or may not be seen. In some cases, when biopsy is performed on a lytic lesion, increased osteoclastic activity but no tumor may be present.

More than 20% of patients with tumor-associated hypercalcemia have no metastases demonstrable by either x-rays or bone scan. Most commonly, hypercalcemia is associated with head and neck tumors and with cancer of the lung (squamous or large-cell) or kidney. Tumors diagnosed as squamous cell carcinoma seem especially prevalent in this category. Among the hematopoietic neoplasms, T-cell leukemia or lymphoma and large-cell lymphoma are relatively frequent causes of the syndrome.

In recent years, a variety of humoral substances has been implicated in the cause of hypercalcemic syndromes. Not only do these substances appear to play a role in hypercalcemia occurring in the absence of bone disease, but some, such as the prostaglandins, appear to mediate bone resorption at the site of local tumor deposits. For example, although breast cancer cells in vitro can destroy bone directly, Mundy and co-workers have found that studies by electron microscopy suggest that osteoclast activation is the major mechanism of bone destruction.[22,23] A variety of humoral factors including the prostaglandins (PGE$_2$) may be released either by the tumor itself or by the tumor's stimulation of surrounding mononuclear cells to release the factor, which in turn stimulates the activity of osteoclasts.

Table 4–31 indicates that the osteoclast-activating factor is responsible for bone lysis in hematopoietic neoplasms such as multiple myeloma. Mundy has recently pointed out that this entity is comprised of a family of bone-resorbing cytokines secreted by lymphocytes. These include colony-stimulating factors of the granulocyte-macrophage series (CSF-GM) and CSF-1, a macrophage stimulator that also stimulates proliferation of osteoclasts. Other factors such as lymphotoxin and interleukin-1 also cause increased bone-resorbing activity.

It should be emphasized that ectopic parathormone has only rarely been implicated in paraneoplastic hypercalcemia. Many of the growth factors such as those shown in Table 4–31 have parathormone-like effects, as indicated by elevated levels of cyclic AMP in the urine, and a decreased renal threshold for phosphorus. Unlike PTH, however, they do not cause renal bicarbonate wasting and subsequent hyperchloremic acidosis seen in primary hyperparathyroidism, nor are they associated with increased serum 1,25-(OH)$_2$ vitamin D concentrations, increased gut absorption of calcium, or increased bone formations. These latter are all seen association with primary hyperparathroidism.

Differential Diagnosis

The clinical manifestations are varied and depend a great deal on the duration and magnitude of the hypercalcemia. The majority of patients seen with hypercalcemia are virtually asymptomatic and have only

Table 4–31. Putative Humoral Mediators of Bone Resorption and Hypercalcemia in Cancer*

Tumor Group	Type of Tumor	Humoral Factor	Local or Systemic
Hematopoietic tumors	Myeloma, lymphoma, T-cell lymphoma	Osteoclast-activating factor (OAF)	Local
		1,25 (OH_2) vitamin D	Systemic
Solid tumors with bone metastases	Breast, lung, kidney	Prostaglandin (PGE_2)?	Local
Solid tumors without bone metastases	Lung, kidney, head, and neck	Transforming growth factor (TGF), factors interacting with PTH receptor†, colony-stimulating activity	Systemic

*Table modified from Mundy, G.R., et al.: The hypercalcemia of cancer. N Engl J Med *310*:1718, 1984, with permission.
†PTH parathormone

a minimal elevation in calcium. Nevertheless, treatment must be instituted because in just a short period of time, as little as a week or two, the serum calcium may elevate to dangerous levels. The clinical picture is summarized in Table 4–32.

While the causes of hypercalcemia are legion, only a few other entities deserve serious consideration in the differential diagnosis. In a patient with an obvious neoplasm, especially one involving the lung or breast, there usually is not much doubt as to the cause. Among the important entities that need to be considered in an older patient are primary hyperparathyroidism, hyperthyroidism, adrenal insufficiency, immobilization, medication with thiazides or lithium, and granulomatous diseases such as sarcoidosis and tuberculosis.

Finally, it should be appreciated that a diagnosis of primary hyperparathyroidism, especially when it occurs in a familial setting, requires that the patient be investigated further for one of the multiple endocrine neoplasia syndromes. Diagnosis of familial hyperparathyroidism, depending on the particular syndrome, makes testing for an islet-cell tumor of pancreas, pheochromocytoma, and medullary carcinoma of the thyroid mandatory.

Diagnostic Evaluation

Serum calcium in excess of 14.5 mg/dl is commonly associated with malignant disease. Specific tests are required, depending upon what other diagnosis is being entertained. Hyperparathyroidism is associated with an elevated serum chloride concentration and an elevation of immunoreactive PTH in serum (see Chapter 11).

METABOLIC ABNORMALITIES

While hypercalcemia, discussed in the previous section, is one of the most frequent metabolic abnormalities associated with malignant disease, other exigent metabolic abnormalities occur with sufficient frequency to require consideration.

Tumor Lysis Syndrome

DEFINITION

Dramatic and life threatening electrolyte abnormalities may supervene when a large mass of tissue is destroyed following chemotherapy or radiation exposure.

PATHOPHYSIOLOGIC CONSIDERATIONS

This syndrome has been reported following treatment of certain rapidly proliferating hematopoietic neoplasms including undifferentiated lymphomas, such as Burkitt's, and acute lymphoblastic leukemia. It is a rare complication of treatment of small-cell carcinoma of the lung. The destruction of a large mass of tissue results in the release of intracellular potassium, phosphate, and nucleic acid constituents, including purines. Metabolism of the latter produces uric acid, which is only sparingly soluble at acid pH. Maximum urine concentration and uric acid precipitation occurs in the collecting ducts causing subsequent blockage.

Hyperphosphatemia has been associated with acute renal failure, presumably secondary to precipitation of calcium phosphate in the kidney. Moreover, hypocalcemia may occur in this syndrome, even to the extent of producing tetany.

Table 4–32. Clinical Summary of Hypercalcemia in Neoplasia

Neurologic	Renal	Gastrointestinal	Cardiac
Fatigue, apathy muscle weakness, behavioral disturbances, stupor, coma	Polyuria, polydipsia, renal insufficiency	Anorexia, nausea, vomiting, constipation, abdominal pain, peptic ulcer	Arrhythmias, digitalis sensitivity, hypertension

DIAGNOSTIC EVALUATION

The diagnosis is confirmed by finding azotemia, hyperuricemia, hyperphosphatemia, hypocalcemia, and hyperkalemia. The latter may be responsible for serious arrhythmias and sudden death. Generally the syndrome develops 1 to 5 days after starting therapy, and its occurrence correlates with the mass of the tumor and level of serum LDH activity. Patients at greatest risk of developing the syndrome are those who have electrolyte and uric acid abnormalities before the start of therapy; hence every effort should be made to correct hyperuricemia, azotemia, and hyperphosphatemia before embarking on a therapeutic regimen, and hydration, allopurinol, and cautious alkalinization should precede therapy when abnormalities are detected. If hypocalcemia is detected, alkalinization should be avoided because of the danger of tetany.

Syndrome of Inappropriate Secretion of Antidiuretic Hormone (SIADH)

DEFINITION AND PATHOPHYSIOLOGIC CONSIDERATIONS

Dilutional hyponatremia secondary to tumor secretion of arginine vasopressin (AVP) is relatively common in the course of lung cancer, particularly small-cell carcinoma of the lung (about 10% of patients). In addition, radioimmunoassay demonstrates that these tumors also secrete oxytocin and neurophysins (proteins that bind the two hormones). A variety of other neoplasms are also associated with this syndrome, presumably by the same mechanism, including leukemias, lymphomas, and carcinoma of the pancreas. SIADH is also seen accompanying intrathoracic infections such as tuberculosis and may occur in the course of diseases of the central nervous system, including trauma, tumors, and infections. Two chemotherapeutic agents, vincristine and cyclophosphamide, may also cause dilutional hyponatremia. These drugs may cause SIADH by a direct nephrotoxic effect.

DIFFERENTIAL DIAGNOSIS AND DIAGNOSTIC EVALUATION

The continuous production of AVP results in hypo-osmolality of extracellular fluid and high urinary sodium excretion in the presence of serum hyponatremia (Table 4–33).

The clinical picture of SIADH is that of water intoxication and hyponatremia (the cause of the excessive urinary loss of sodium is unclear). Lethargy and weakness are virtually always present. Patients may be confused and stuporous and may even show focal neurologic signs and have seizures. If these criteria are fully met, it is unlikely that an error in diagnosis can be made. Although volume depletion secondary to intense diuretic therapy also could be responsible

Table 4–33. Criteria for SIADH*

Hypo-osmolality of extracellular fluid (less than 280 mOsm/kg H_2O)
Hyponatremia and continued urinary excretion of sodium in the absence of diuretics
Urine less than maximally diluted (usually greater than 500 mOsm/kg H_2O)
No evidence of volume depletion
Normal renal and adrenal function

*Adapted from Bunn, P.A., and Minna, J.D.: Paraneoplastic syndromes. In Cancer Principles and Practice of Oncology. Edited by V. DeVita, S. Rosenberg, and S. Hellman. Philadelphia, J.B. Lippincott Co., 1985. Also from Bartter, F.C., and Schwartz, W.B.: Am J Med 42:790, 1967.

for such a picture, the diagnosis would not readily be missed after a careful history and physical examination. A helpful clue suggesting previous diuretic therapy would be the presence of hypochloremia and elevated serum bicarbonate. Difficulties may arise in determining the precise cause, as, for example, in small-cell carcinoma of the lung with brain metastases treated with cyclophosphamide and vincristine. Each of these, the primary tumor, the metastases in the brain, and the therapy may be responsible for the syndrome. On occasion, patients will present with severe hyponatremia and no evidence of tumor. Again, provided that volume depletion can be ruled out, the most likely cause is an occult carcinoma, usually small-cell.

In evaluating the patient with SIADH, the physician should determine electrolytes and osmolality of the serum and urine. In general, determination of serum AVP is neither available nor necessary for the diagnosis.

Hypokalemic Syndromes

A variety of tumors may be associated with hypokalemia. In some of these conditions such as small-cell carcinoma of the lung, which produces ACTH ectopically, the resultant hypokalemia may clearly be designated part of a paraneoplastic syndrome. In others, such as certain endocrine tumors of the pancreas, the distinction is not nearly as clear. For example, the WDHA syndrome, characterized by watery diarrhea, hypokalemia, and achlorhydria, appears to be associated in at least one third of cases with a noninsulin-secreting adenoma of the pancreas producing VIP (vasoactive intestinal polypeptide). A number of cells comprising the islets of the pancreas appear to produce this polypeptide in small quantities normally. If this production is substantiated, one could no more designate the syndrome as paraneoplastic than designate Cushing's syndrome caused by adrenocortical carcinoma as paraneoplastic. The hallmark of paraneoplastic syndromes is ectopic production of the humoral mediator.

ECTOPIC ACTH SYNDROME

About 15% of all cases of overt Cushing's syndrome are due to ectopic production of ACTH. Most commonly the syndrome of hypokalemia, alkalosis, hypertension, muscle weakness, glucose intolerance, and mental changes is produced by small-cell carcinoma of the lung or by pancreatic or thymic tumors. Carcinoids are also capable of producing the syndrome, and the concept has arisen that no matter which organ contains the malignant tumor responsible for ACTH production, the basic cell type is of either small-cell or carcinoid structure; a consensus on this point has not been reached. Within the last decade, the concept has been further expanded such that the cells responsible for ACTH production are all of neural crest origin and include a carcinoid–oat cell variety and a pheochromocytoma-neuroblastoma group. Not unexpectedly, tumors in a large number of organs have been associated with Cushing's syndrome. The diagnosis is suggested by high levels of plasma ACTH (in excess of 200 pg/ml), loss of normal diurnal variation, and lack of suppression by dexamethasone.

HORMONE-PRODUCING ENDOCRINE TUMORS

The syndromes of multiple endocrine neoplasia have already been discussed. Thorough discussion of these entities is beyond the scope of this section (see Chapter 11). A variety of tumors of the gastrointestinal tract may be associated with massive diarrhea and hypokalemia.

In the WDHA syndrome, which is associated with pancreatic adenomas and other GI tumors, the putative mediator, vasoactive intestinal polypeptide (VIP), is responsible for stool volumes that may be as large as 8 L/day. Other gastrointestinal hormones may also play a role.

The Zollinger-Ellison syndrome (ZES), characterized by severe peptic ulcer disease with multiple ulceration, frequently is associated with diarrhea, which may be the predominant presenting feature in 15 to 20% of cases. While ZES is usually associated with a gastrin-producing non-β cell adenoma of the pancreatic islets, other polypeptide hormones, including VIP, may be involved in producing diarrhea. Up to 75% of these adenomas are malignant, and up to 50% of the patients may have multiple endocrine neoplasia syndrome. The diagnosis is suspected in patients who have particularly intractable peptic ulcer disease with multiple ulcers, pain, and quick recurrence after treatment. A definitive diagnosis of a gastrinoma is made by a radioimmunoassay for gastrin in the serum.

Malignant carcinoid, an uncommon tumor of the gastrointestinal tract arising in the argentaffin cells in the base of the intestinal crypts as well as in the lung

and ovary, may in about 15% of cases produce a distinctive clinical picture called carcinoid syndrome, characterized by flushing, telangiectasis, diarrhea, bronchospasm, endocardial fibrosis, glucose intolerance, arthropathy, and hypotension. Most of these features are related to the production by the tumor of serotonin, but some are related to other mediators, including prostaglandin, bradykinin, and histamine. The diarrhea and resultant hypokalemia appear to be due to serotonin's effects on GI motility. The diagnosis is confirmed by finding elevated levels of 5-OH-indoleacetic acid in the urine.

Lactic Acidosis

Metabolic acidosis caused by the accumulation of lactic acid in the blood may be associated with impaired oxygen delivery to the tissues resulting from circulatory insufficiency. It may also occur during the course of neoplastic diseases, as well as during other illnesses such as liver disease, infection, and pancreatitis in which circulatory factors do not appear to play a role. Among malignant diseases lactic acidosis is especially prevalent in leukemia and lymphoma but may occur in solid tumors as well. The common factor appears to be extensive involvement of the liver by tumor, which may compromise the liver's ability to extract lactic acid from the blood.

The clinical picture is one of metabolic acidosis that ultimately may cause circulatory collapse and death. In the presence of an anion gap that is otherwise unexplained, the serum lactic acid, which is normally less than 2 mOsm/kg H_2O, should be measured. Blood pH may be near normal or even high in the early stage of the disorder because of a compensating respiratory alkalosis.

Hypoglycemia

Hypoglycemia caused by insulin overproduction by the cells of the pancreatic islets is not considered a paraneoplastic syndrome. An increase in the number of cells (an insulinoma), though they be neoplastic, might reasonably be associated with increased insulin production. Nevertheless, because the cells are transformed, they do not respond to the usual regulatory mechanisms controlling the normal cell. About 25% of the patients with multiple endocrine neoplasia type I have insulinoma.

A variety of other tumors may uncommonly be associated with hypoglycemia. Odell and Wolfsen estimate that 65% of these are mesenchymal tumors.[24] Most occur in the abdomen and are either retroperitoneal or occur within the peritoneal cavity. These tumors are generally very large, weighing an average of 2.5 kg but perhaps as much as 10 kg. Current thought suggests that the humoral substances involved are the somatomedins that are normally produced by the liver. Their hypoglycemic action resembles that of insulin in various bioassays and they bind to the insulin receptor. However, they are not reactive in the insulin radioimmunoassay. Their activity is sometimes refined to an nonsuppressible, insulin-like activity (NSILA). Patients presenting with hypoglycemia often have attacks of hypoglycemia prior to evidence of the tumor's presence. These attacks are brought on by physical exertion and fasting.

PULMONARY INVOLVEMENT IN NEOPLASTIC DISEASE

Pleural Effusion

The occurrence of a pleural effusion in the course of malignant disease is so common that detailed discussion is hardly warranted. A few important aspects should be reviewed for the sake of emphasis, however.

The most common mechanism involved in producing the effusion is obstruction of the pleural lymphatics by cords of tumor cells. In neoplasms such as lymphomas that cause significant mediastinal lymphadenopathy, transudative effusion may form without involvement of the pleural lymphatics. Treatment of the mediastinum alone may result in resolution of the effusion.

In patients complaining of dyspnea, cough, and, occasionally, chest pain, distinguishing a simple effusion from a pulmonary embolus may be difficult. The dyspnea in both conditions may be out of proportion to the amount of fluid accumulated. Even without an embolic event, a patient with as little as 300 cc of fluid may be dyspneic, with a normal Po_2, presumably because of neurogenic reflexes originating in the pleura. A pulmonary embolus would be more likely to produce a lowering of the Po_2 and an abnormal ventilation perfusion scan.

Pleural effusions secondary to pleural metastases are usually exudative and often bloody. The criteria of Light and Ball are used to distinguish a transudate from an exudate.[25] Any one of the following suggests an exudate: (1) an LDH in the fluid greater than 200; (2) a ratio of fluid protein to serum protein greater than 0.5; (3) a ratio of the LDH in the fluid to that in the serum of greater than 0.6. Cytological studies of the fluid usually will reveal malignant cells.

Pulmonary Leukostasis

Pulmonary complications should be anticipated during the course of leukemia when the blast count exceeds 50,000/μl, most commonly in the course of acute myeloblastic leukemia and in the accelerated phase of chronic myelogenous leukemia. Its occurrence in other phases of chronic myelogenous leukemia and in acute lymphoblastic leukemia is uncommon. In essence, the syndrome results from plugging of the capillaries in the lung and brain with masses of aggregated blast cells. The pathogenesis of these lesions stems from the physical characteristics of the myeloblast, its large size and its lack of deformability.

The syndrome is characterized by dyspnea, hypoxia, and tachypnea. Nervous system signs include stupor, delirium, dizziness, tinnitus, ataxia, visual blurring, and papilledema. Measurement of the Po_2 is inaccurate in the presence of hyperleukocytosis and should not be used. These signs and symptoms constitute a true emergency that may result in circulatory collapse and intracranial hemorrhage if leukapheresis is not undertaken immediately.

Pulmonary Hemorrhage

Massive pulmonary hemorrhage, though not encountered frequently, is frightening and dramatic. Generally, such a diagnosis is considered if more than 200 cc of blood are expectorated at one time or over a 24-hour period. Its occurrence secondary to a blood dyscrasia such as disseminated intravascular coagulation or thrombocytopenia has been considered in another chapter. Hemorrhage resulting from tumor necrosis or erosion of a blood vessel is considered here.

Following a hemorrhage, the patient is often dyspneic, tachypneic, and very anxious. Within hours, radiographs may show a diffuse bilateral infiltrate resembling pulmonary edema. Consolidation of a single lobe, unilateral pulmonary infiltrates, or nodular densities may be seen. No matter how far advanced the patient's disease, efforts to arrest bleeding must be made or the patient will literally drown in his own blood.

Pulmonary Metastases

Surgical extirpation of pulmonary metastases remains an area of controversy in oncology. In a patient who has no evidence of tumor elsewhere, and whose tumor is responsive to chemotherapy, surgery may constitute a curative procedure. More commonly, it prolongs life significantly when performed on suitable adult patients. In patients who are otherwise healthy and have no underlying pulmonary disease, surgical removal of multiple and bilateral lung nodules is well tolerated.

Patients with long disease-free intervals (greater than 12 months) prior to the appearance of metastases tend to survive significantly longer after surgery. Most of this experience has been verified in patients with soft-tissue sarcomas, osteoblastic sarcomas, and renal cell carcinoma, but we have certainly seen this success in colon carcinoma. The latter patients are unusual in that they tended to be free of liver metastases, while most patients with metastatic neoplasms in the lung also have liver involvement.

The volume doubling time of the tumor also seems to predict patients who will do well following surgery for metastatic disease. Recall that the volume doubling time is not the same as the diameter doubling time, but rather is the time it takes for the diameter to increase by a factor of 1.26. A series of reports has indicated that patients whose tumor doubling time is longer than 40 days tend to survive more than 2 years. We tend to feel this doubling time is too short and favor a volume doubling time of greater than 60 days before seriously considering surgery. Moreover, while it appears that multiple nodules, if within reason, do not adversely affect survival other than by making surgery more extensive, the detection of many small nodules (less than 5 mm in diameter) by CT scan would preclude a surgical procedure. We have seen such small nodules begin to grow very rapidly once the great bulk of tumor has been removed. Again, the physician should not proceed with resection if tumor exists in a location other than the lung. The aim is to ensure at least one year of high-quality survival after surgery.

Osteoblastic sarcoma and testicular tumors are special cases for which resection is not considered in the above discussion. These and other tumors that are relatively sensitive to chemotherapeutic agents may be cured by regimens that include surgical removal of metastatic disease. Such decisions require considerable experience and should be made by an oncologist.

Pulmonary Toxicity of Cancer Drugs (Table 4–34)

A relatively large number of active chemotherapeutic agents associated with pulmonary toxicity will, if unrecognized, lead to pulmonary insufficiency and death. Unfortunately, no distinctive clinical picture is evident; most of the affected patients complain of dyspnea and nonproductive cough, and fine rales are often detected at the lung bases. Early chest x-rays may not show evidence of disease, but with time, most will show an increase in interstitial markings. Late in the course, fibrosis will appear. A gallium scan may be useful in detecting diffuse bilateral disease, but it may not be more helpful than a reduced P_{O_2} and P_{CO_2}. The diffusing capacity of the lung will be reduced early in the course of chemotherapy, and later pulmonary function studies will show evidence of restrictive disease. None of these manifestations is absolutely characteristic, and pulmonary infections caused by cytomegalovirus and pneumocystis carinii must be excluded from the diagnosis.

Radiation Pneumonitis

No more than 5% of patients receiving radiation to the chest show evidence of significant radiation pneumonitis. On the other hand, certain high-risk groups will show a much higher incidence, such as patients with mediastinal Hodgkin's disease or carcinoma of the lung in whom a considerable amount of lung tissue is irradiated with doses in excess of 4000 rads. For example, patients with massive mediastinal Hodgkin's disease involving more than one third of the thoracic diameter will have an incidence of 20 to 30%.

The determining factors in the development of lung damage are the dose of radiation delivered, over what time interval it is delivered, and the volume of the lung irradiated. Previous irradiation and prior or simultaneous administration of radiation-sensitizing chemotherapeutic agents such as Adriamycin will also play a role. Current therapy of bulky mediastinal Hodgkin's disease calls for initial chemotherapy to reduce the mediastinal bulk and then radiation therapy. Although this approach does not eliminate lung injury, it appears to minimize it.

Many patients with radiation pneumonitis are completely asymptomatic, and chest x-rays months later show only dense fibrotic bands outlining the radiation ports. On the other hand, patients with a relatively small area of irradiated lung will show cough, some dyspnea, and a low-grade fever. With more of the lung field irradiated the symptoms become progressively worse, requiring prednisone for control. The areas of infiltration should correspond to the radiation port films. There should not be a lobar distribution, and lymph node involvement does not occur. Moreover, the symptoms are remarkably well suppressed by prednisone. Often the pneumonitis will take many months to subside.

The differential diagnosis includes infection and recurrence of the primary disease. There is no clear method for ruling these out except by doing the appropriate cultures and evaluating the patient for signs of active disease elsewhere if a lymphoma is involved.

MISCELLANEOUS PARANEOPLASTIC SYNDROMES

Fever

Fever not caused by infection occurs infrequently in solid tumors but is more prevalent in lymphomas and leukemia. Petersdorf found that 5% of 351 cancer patients developed fever that could be ascribed only

Table 4–34. Pulmonary Toxicity of Cancer Drugs*

Drug	Incidence	Disorder	Clinical Course	Treatment
Bleomycin	5% in patients <70 yrs 15% in patients >70 yrs Increased with emphysema and previous radiation	Interstitial pneumonitis, fibrosis	Toxicity may develop following one to two courses but usually >450 mg/m$_2$; not reversible after fibrosis	d.c. drug prednisone
Alkylating agents (busulfan, nitrosourea, cyclophosphamide, chlorambucil)	Busulfan 2–11% (pathologic findings in up to 45%); nitrosourea 15%; >50% for BCNU > 1500 mg/mg$_2$	Interstitial pneumonitis, fibrosis	Toxicity may occur 1 to 3 years after drug is started or stopped; once process starts it is usually irreversible and progressive	No treatment
Mitomycin	5–12% Not clearly dose related	Interstitial pneumonitis, fibrosis	Onset of toxicity within 6 months of starting therapy; resolves rapidly after stopping drug	Discontinue drug
Procarbazine	Rare	Eosinophilia, interstitial pneumonitis	Allergic reaction, fever, chills, arthralgia, urticaria, eosinophilia	Discontinue drug
Methotrexate	Rare	Interstitial and alveolar infiltration, multinucleated giant cells	Toxicity begins days to months after starting drug, associated with fever, cough, hypoxia, and dyspnea; bilateral pulmonary infiltrates	Discontinue drug
Cytosine arabinoside	Unknown	Proteinaceous alveolar exudates, interstitial infiltrate	Pulmonary edema-like picture coming on within one month of last drug ingestion	Unknown

*From Weiss, R.B., and Muggia, F.M.: Cytotoxic drug-induced pulmonary disease. Am J Med 68:259–266, 1980, with permission.

to their tumors. The diagnosis is one of exclusion and therefore falls into the category of "fever of unknown origin" as described by Petersdorf and Beeson, i.e., temperature elevation exceeding 101° F fever on several occasions; during an illness lasting at least 3 weeks; and fever for which no diagnosis is apparent after a week's study in the hospital (see Chapter 5).[26] In 1961, of 100 such patients studied, 19 had fever caused by malignancies, of which seven were solid tumors. Among the more common solid tumors producing this syndrome were melanoma and carcinomas in the pancreas, stomach, esophagus, and kidney. Evidence of significant liver involvement is characteristic. Petersdorf and Beeson described a leukemoid reaction in their two patients with pancreatic carcinoma, and we have seen this association on several occasions.

Hypernephroma of the kidney is a tumor notorious for producing pyrexia without other visible signs of its presence. The only other evidence supporting such a diagnosis may be the discovery in the urine of red blood cells, which may be few in number and only intermittently present.

A description of the variety of pyrogenic humoral mediators is beyond the scope of this discussion. To date, no one mediator has been implicated in the cause of fever in malignant disease.

Weight Loss

Patients with neoplastic disease are characteristically anorectic and have lost weight, often to a degree disproportionate to the amount of discernible disease and unexplainable by obstructive phenomena, pain, or evidence of encroachment on normal structures. Moreover, the weight loss and anorexia may occur prior to the discovery of the tumor. This phenomenon is entirely dissimilar to simple starvation, in which the subject reduces his caloric expenditure and ceases using amino acids for gluconeogenesis. The patient with a neoplasm continues to expend calories and maintains a high basal metabolic rate in the face of reduced intake. Gustatory sensation is perverted with marked aversion to meat and protein and diminished appreciation of sweetness. Physicians speculate that patients experience humoral resetting of the "satiety" and "appetite" center in the hypothalamus. Recent evidence has suggested that a monokine produced from endotoxin-stimulated macrophages is responsible for dramatically decreasing the activity of key lipogenic enzymes. This factor is either identical or closely homologous to tumor necrosis factor.

Nephrotic Syndrome

The nephrotic syndrome occurring just prior to or during the course of neoplastic disease has been rec-

Table 4–35. Dermatologic Signs of Malignancy

Lesion	Description	Associated Malignancy
Dermatomyositis (>40 yrs)	Heliotrope erythema on upper cheeks, eyelids, temples; edema of hands and arms; erythema of scalp and alopecia; calcification usually precedes signs of neoplasm	Breast, lung, GI, GU, lymphoma
Hypertrichosis lanuginous	Long, fine, silky hair on face and other sites usually hairless	Lung, rectum, bladder
Pachydermoperiostosis	Skin of forehead and scalp thickened and thrown into folds; skin of hands and feet thickened; increased sebum on face and scalp	Lung, stomach, esophagus, thymus
Amyloid deposits	Small, glistening, yellow and pink papules on eyelids and central areas of face, lips; macroglossia	Myeloma, macroglobulinemia
Acanthosis nigricans	Confluent hyperpigmented, hyperkeratotic verrucosities in body folds, axilla, areola, umbilicus; keratoderma of palms and soles	GI, lung, ovary
Flushing (episodic)	Telangiectasia on face or upper trunk; hyperpigmentation on legs, forearms, and trunk with hyperkeratosis	Carcinoid
Erythema gyratum repens	Gyrate, wavy bands that change rapidly with marginal desquamation and pruritus on trunk, neck, and extremities	Very high incidence of malignancy, especially breast and lung.
Necrotic migratory erythema	Generalized symmetrical dermatitis over perineum, buttocks, and extremities, or circinate areas of blistering followed by hyperpigmentation in some areas.	Glucagonoma
Exfoliative dermatitis (associated with malignancy in 10–20% of cases)	Erythema followed by scaling	Lymphoma

ognized for the past 20 years. Hodgkin's disease has been the tumor most frequently associated with the syndrome. The pathologic findings are most consistent with those of lipoid nephrosis. Only minimal abnormalities of the glomeruli are seen, and no deposits containing immunoglobulin are detected. About 20% of the cases of nephrotic syndrome in Hodgkin's disease have pathologic evidence of nephritis of varying sorts. Patients with non-Hodgkin's lymphoma will also demonstrate the nephrotic syndrome, but less frequently than in Hodgkin's disease. Usually, immunoglobulin deposits are detectable in their glomeruli.

In carcinomas of the lung, colon, and stomach, immune complexes appear to play a role in producing a membranous glomerulonephritis, which is the most common pathologic lesion found. The prevalence of carcinoma in all patients with nephrotic syndrome and a membranous lesion of their glomeruli is said to be 5 to 10%.

The activity of nephrosis is related to the activity of the tumor. When the neoplasm is in remission, the renal disease will disappear or be ameliorated. Conversely, the renal disease will be exacerbated when the tumor is active. Considering the tumor's conjunction with the immunopathologic findings, physicians conclude that tumor antigens play a crucial role in the development of the glomerular disorder.

Pulmonary Hypertrophic Osteoarthropathy

Pulmonary hypertrophic osteoarthropathy (PHO) is a paraneoplastic syndrome that is often associated with lung cancer (usually not small-cell) but that may be caused by metastatic tumor in the chest from any primary site. As with others of these syndromes already discussed, signs and symptoms may appear before the patient is aware of the malignant neoplasm.

The syndrome consists of clubbing of the fingers and toes, periostitis of the long bones, and sometimes a polyarthritis that may resemble rheumatoid arthritis. The hands, feet, and joints may be hyperemic. Patients may occasionally present without clubbing but with periostitis or polyarthritis. Usually, periostitis is seen in the distal ends of the tibia, fibula, humerus, radius, or ulna. The joints usually involved are the wrists, knees, and ankles, and effusions may be present. Bone scan over the affected areas may be positive even before signs of periostitis are seen in the x-ray. Removal of the tumor does not always result in remission of symptoms.

Dermatologic Syndromes

With no manifestations can the astute physician demonstrate his knowledge, powers of observation, and acumen to better advantage than with the dermatologic manifestations of systemic disease. Neoplasms present such a wide variety of dermatologic lesions that discussing them in a few paragraphs is an impossible task. (See Chapter 18.) In this section we deal in an abbreviated form with lesions that are surrogates for the malignant tumor rather than lesions that are themselves composed of malignant cells. In most cases the humoral link between the tumor and the skin lesion is unknown, although one can reasonably speculate that tumor-engendered antibodies or growth factors produced by the tumor are implicated. Some of the hereditarily determined lesions will be discussed in a later section.

Table 4–35 presents an incomplete survey of dermatologic signs of malignancy. The rule must be that if the nature of a nodule or plaque is obscure, biopsy must be performed. Many lesions appear well in advance of symptoms and signs of the neoplasm.

REFERENCES

1. Davidson, R.J., How, J., and Leisels, S.: Acquired stomatocytosis: Its prevalence and significance in routine hematology. Scand J Haematol 19:47, 1977.
2. Kass, L.: Origin and composition of Cabot rings in pernicious anemia. Am J Clin Pathol 64:53, 1975.
3. Cawley, J.C., and Hayhoe, F.G.: The inclusions of the May-Hegglin anomaly and Dohle bodies of infection: an ultrastructural comparison. Br J Haematol 22:491, 1972.
4. Chikkapa, G., Chanana, A.D., Chandra, P. and Cronkite, E.P.: Kinetics and regulation of granulocyte precursors during a granulopoietic stress. Blood 50:1099, 1977.
5. May, M.E., and Waddell, C.C.: Basophils in peripheral blood and bone marrow. A retrospective review. Am J Med 76:509–511, 1984.
6. Han, T, et al.: Prognostic importance of cytogenetic abnormalities in patients with chronic lymphocytic leukemia. 310:288–92, 1984.
7. Nienhuis, A.W., Anagnou, N.P., and Ley, T.J.: Advances in thalassemia research. Blood 63:738–758, 1984.
8. Davis, L.R.: Aplastic crises in haemolytic anemias: The role of a parvovirus-like agent. Br J. Haematol 55:391–393, 1983.
9. Evatt, B.L., Spivak, J.L., and Levin, J.: Relationships between thrombopoiesis and erythropoiesis: with studies of the effects of preparations of thrombopoietin and erythropoietin. Blood 48:547–558, 1976.
10. Walsh, P.N., Murphy, S., and Barry, W.E.: The role of platelets in the pathogenesis of thrombosis and hemorrhage in patients with thrombocytosis. Thromb Haemost 38:1085, 1977.
11. Schafer, A.I.: Bleeding and thrombosis in the myeloproliferative disorders. Blood 64:1–12, 1984.
12. Wu, K.K.: Platelet hyperaggregability and thrombosis in patients with thrombocythemia. Ann Intern Med 88:7, 1978.
13. Kelton, J.G., Powers, P.J., and Carter, C.J.: A prospective study of the usefulness of the measurement of platelet-associated IgG for the diagnosis of idiopathic thrombocytopenic purpura. Blood 60:1050–1053, 1982.
14. Burns, T.R., and Saleem, A.: Idiopathic thrombocytopenic purpura. Am J Med 75:1001–1007, 1983.
15. Raskind, W.H., et al.: Evidence for a multistep pathogenesis of a myelodysplastic syndrome. Blood 63:1318–1323, 1984.
16. Bennet, J.M., et al.: The French-American-British (FAB) cooperative group. Proposals for the classification of the myelodysplastic syndromes. Br J Haematol 51:189–199, 1982.
17. Weisdorf, D.J., Oken, M.A., Johnson, G.H., and Rydell, R.E.: Chronic myelodysplastic syndrome: short survival with or without evolution to acute leukemia. Br J Haematol 55:691–700, 1983.
18. Montecuco, C., et al.: Flow cytometric DNA content in myelodysplastic syndromes. Cytometry 4:238–243, 1983.
19. Fialkow, P.J.: Chronic myelogenous leukemia: clonal origin in a stem cell common to granulocyte, erythrocyte, platelet and monocyte and macrophage. Am J Med 63:125, 1977.
20. Koeffler, P.H., and Golde, D.W.: Chronic myelogenous leukemia—New Concepts. N Engl J Med 304:1201–1209, 1981.
21. DeKlein, A., van Kessel, A.G., and Grosveld, G.: A cellular oncogene is translocated to the Philadelphia chromosome in chronic myelocytic leukemia. Nature 300:765–767, 1982.
22. Mundy, G.R., et al.: The hypercalcemia of cancer. N Engl J Med 310:1718–1727, 1984.
23. Mundy, G.R., Ibbotson, K.J., and D'Souza, S.M.: Tumor products and the hypercalcemia of malignancy. J Clin Invest 76:391–394, 1985.
24. Odell, W.D., and Wolfson, A.R. Humoral syndromes associated with cancer. Ann Rev Med 29:379–406, 1978.
25. Light, R.W., and Ball, W.C.: Pleural effusions: the diagnostic separation of transudates and exudates. Ann Intern Med 77:507–513, 1972.
26. Petersdorf, R.G., and Beeson, P.B.: Fever of unexplained origin: report on 100 cases. Medicine 40:1–30, 1961.

GENERAL REFERENCES

Balcerzak, S.P., and Bromberg, P.A.: Secondary polycythemia. Semin Hematol 12:353, 1975.
Berlin, N.I.: Diagnosis and classification of the polycythemias. Semin Hematol 12:339, 1975.
Boggs, D.R.: Physiology of neutrophil proliferation, maturation and circulation. Clin Haematol 4:535, 1975.
Bunn, P.A., and Minna, J.D.: Paraneoplastic syndromes. In Cancer, Principles and Practice of Oncology. Edited by V. DeVita, S. Rosenberg, and S. Hellman. Philadelphia, J.B. Lippincott Co., 1985, pp. 1803–1806.
Cartwright, G.E., and Deiss, A.: Sideroblast, siderosites and sideroblastic anemia. N Engl J Med 292:185, 1975.
Clark, R.A.F., and Kaplan, A.P.: Eosinophil leukocytes: structure and function. Clin Haematol 4:635, 1975.
Crocco, J.A., et al.: Massive hemoptysis. Arch Intern Med 121:494–498, 1968.
Douglas, S.W., and Adamson, J.W.: The anemia of chronic disorders: studies of marrow regulation and iron metabolism. Blood 45:55, 1975.
Fauci, A.S., et al.: The idiopathic hypereosinophilic syndrome: clinical, pathophysiologic, and therapeutic consideration. Ann Intern Med 97:78, 1982.
Gross, N.J.: Pulmonary effects of radiation therapy. Ann Intern Med 86:81–92, 1977.

Helm, F., and Helm, J.: Cutaneous markers of internal malignancies. *In* Cancer Dermatology. Edited by F. Helm. Philadelphia, Lea & Febiger, 1979, pp. 242–283.

Hoffbrand, A.V.: The megaloblastic anemias. Clin Haematol *5*:471, 1976.

Kane, M.G., O'Dorsio, T.M., and Krijs, G.J.: Production of secretory diarrhea by intravenous infusions of vasoactive intestinal polypeptide. N Engl J Med *309*:1482–1485, 1983.

Krieger, D.T.: Brain peptides. What, where and why? Science *222*:975–985, 1983.

Levin, W.C.: Symposium on Myeloma. Arch Intern Med *135*:27, 1975.

Lichtman, M.A.: Granulocyte and monocyte abnormalities. Clin Haematol *4*:483, 1975.

Lichtman, M.A., and Rowe, J.M.: Hyperleukocytic leukemias: rheological, clinical, and therapeutic considerations. Blood *60*:279–283, 1982.

Linstedt, G., et al.: Serum ferritin and iron deficiency anemia in hospital patients. Lancet *1*:205, 1980.

Maldonado, G.E., and Hanlon, D.G.: Monocytosis. Mayo Clin Proc *40*:248, 1965.

Marks, C.: Carcinoid Tumors: A Clinicopathologic Study. Boston, G.K. Hall, 1979.

McGrath, M.A., and Penny, R.: Paraproteinemia: blood hyperviscosity and clinical manifestations. J Clin Invest *58*:1115, 1976.

McIntyre, O.R., and Ebaugh, F.G., Jr.: Palpable spleens in college freshmen. Ann Intern Med *66*:301, 1967.

Mills, J.A.: A spectrum of organ systems that respond to cancer. The joints and connective tissue. Ann NY Acad Sci *230*:443–447, 1974.

Murano, G.: A basic outline of blood coagulation. Semin Thromb Hemost *6*:140, 1980.

Park, R., and Arieff, A.I.: Lactic acidosis. Adv Intern Med *25*:33–68, 1980.

Plum, F., and Posner, J.: Diagnosis of stupor and coma. Philadelphia, Davis Co., 1972, pp. 63–139.

Putnam, J.B., et al.: Analysis of prognostic factors in patients undergoing resection of pulmonary metastases from soft tissue sarcomas. J Thorac Cardiovasc Surg *87*:260–268, 1984.

Rodicho, L.D., et al.: Early diagnosis of spinal epidural metastases. Am J Med *70*:1181–1189, 1981.

Rosen, P., and Armstrong, D.: Nonbacterial thrombotic endocarditis in patients with malignant neoplastic disease. Am J Med *54*:23–29, 1973.

Row, P.G., et al.: Membranous nephropathy: long term follow-up and association with neoplasia. Q J Med *44*:207–239, 1975.

Sack, G.H., Levin, J., and Bell, W.R.: Trousseau's syndrome and other manifestations of chronic disseminated coagulopathy in patients with neoplasms. Medicine *56*:1–37, 1977.

Schloesser, L.: The diagnostic significance of splenomegaly. Am J Med Sci *245*:118, 1963.

Schneider, B.S., and Manulo, A.: Paraneoplastic syndromes. Unusual manifestations of malignant disease. Disease-a-Month, February, 1979.

Shimm, D.S., Logus, G.L., and Rigsby, L.C.: Evaluating the superior vena cava syndrome. JAMA *245*:951–953, 1981.

Solomon, A.: Homogenous (monoclonal) immunoglobulins in cancer (editorial). Am J Med *63*:169, 1977.

Takita, H., et al.: Surgical management of metastases to the lung. Surg Gynecol Obstet *152*:191–194, 1981.

Theologides, A.: The anorexia-cachexia syndrome. Ann NY Acad Sci *230*:14–22, 1974.

Theologides, A.: Neoplastic cardiac tamponade. Semin Oncol *5*:181–189, 1978.

Thompson, J.C., et al.: Natural history and experience with diagnosis and treatment of the Zollinger-Ellison syndrome. Surg Gynecol Obstet *140*:721, 1975.

Torti, F.M., et al.: A macrophage factor inhibits adipocyte gene expression: an *in vitro* model of cachexia. Science *229*:867–869, 1985.

Tsokos, G.C., Balow, J.E., and Spiegel, R.J.: Renal and metabolic complications of undifferentiated and lymphoblastic lymphomas. Medicine *60*:218–229, 1981.

Turitto, V.T., Weiss, H.J., and Baumgartner, H.R.: Decreased platelet adhesion on vessel segments in von Willebrand's disease: a defect in initial platelet attachment. J Lab Clin Med *102*:551, 1983.

Van Furth, R.: Origin and genetics of monocyte macrophages. Semin Hematol *7*:125, 1970.

Weiss, H.: Platelet physiology and abnormalities of platelet function (Parts I and II). N Engl J Med *293*:531, 580, 1975.

Zaino, E.C.: Pathophysiology of thalassemia. Fourth Cooley's Anemia Symposium. Ann NY Acad Sci *344*:284, 1980.

CHAPTER **5**

INFECTIOUS DISEASES
Burke A. Cunha, M.D.

APPROACH TO THE PATIENT WITH FEVER

DEFINITION AND PATHOPHYSIOLOGIC CONSIDERATIONS

The majority of patients with infectious diseases have fever, an elevation in body temperature. Accordingly, fevers are regarded as a cardinal sign of infectious disease. Not all infectious diseases are associated with fever, however, and many noninfectious disease entities are accompanied by fever. The approach to the patient with fever is therefore concerned with two fundamental problems; first, the clinician must differentiate the infectious from the noninfectious causes of fever, and second, he must determine the specific infectious disease entity associated with the fever.

The relationship of the fever to diagnostic procedures or surgery, recent travel, pets, or exposure to other infected individuals is extremely important. The temporal relationships of the fever as well as the analysis of the fever pattern is extremely helpful in diagnosing many infectious diseases. Unfortunately, classic fever patterns are not uniformly associated with specific disease entities, and the majority of infectious disease processes have no particular fever pattern associated with them.

The magnitude of the fever may have great diagnostic significance. Very high fevers ($\geq106°$ F) are usually not associated with infectious disease processes and may be due to a variety of noninfectious disease entities, i.e., central fever, heatstroke, malignant hyperthermia, drug fever, etc. Minimal or absent febrile response may be present in patients with infectious diseases, in uremic patients, in elderly patients, or those with overwhelming sepsis.

In immunocompetent hosts, use of the "102° F rule" conveniently separates many benign causes of fever from their infectious counterparts. For example, acute cholecystitis without complications is usually associated with fevers of less than 102° F. In contradistinction, cholangitis is regularly associated with fevers in excess of 102° F. Acute myocardial infarctions that are not massive are associated with fevers less than 102° F, whereas patients with pericarditis not infrequently have fevers in excess of 102° F. Patients with uncomplicated thrombophlebitis usually do not have fevers in excess of 102° F, whereas those with suppurative phlebitis usually do. Septic pulmonary emboli may be distinguished from bland pulmonary emboli by fevers in excess of 102° F. Acute uncomplicated pancreatitis is associated with fevers of less than 102° F, but patients with pancreatic abscess regularly have elevations in excess of 102° F. Viral hepatitis caused by HAV, HBV, or NANB does not produce fever in excess of 102° F. However, other viral diseases of the liver, for example, cytomegalovirus (CMV) or infectious mononucleosis, may be associated with fevers in excess of 102° F, as may hypersensitivity reactions involving the liver.

Fever patterns of themselves are helpful in certain situations. A "hectic, septic fever" pattern though the least specific and therefore the least useful fever pattern, usually suggests a septic process, especially an abscess (usually intra-abdominal, renal, or pelvic). "Hectic, septic fevers" may also be found in association with a variety of other infectious disease entities, e.g., endocarditis, malaria, kala-azar, etc.

A "sustained fever" pattern provides much more diagnostic information, provided that the fever is not artificially modified by antipyretic maneuvers or medications. "Sustained fever" patterns are classically associated with brucellosis, typhoid fever, or psittacosis but may be found in central nervous system infections, scarlet fever, tularemia, or Rocky Mountain spotted fever.

"Remittent" fevers are usually caused by Mycoplasma, Legionella, tuberculosis, or falciparum malaria infections. "Relapsing fevers" are uncommon, but the fever pattern when present is of considerable diagnostic importance. "Relapsing fevers" may be seen with suppurative cholangitis, malaria, relapsing fever, rat-bite fever, brucellosis, yellow fever, dengue fever, etc.

Specific fever patterns such as a "camel-back" fever curve provide highly specific and useful information. The camel-back fever pattern is associated with only two specific infectious disease entities, Colorado tick fever and dengue fever. Similarly, a "double quotidian" fever, defined as two fever spikes within 24 hours (not induced by antipyretic medication), limits differential diagnostic possibilities to relatively few diseases. Double quotidian fevers are classically associated with right-sided gonococcal endocarditis, kala-azar, adult Still's disease, or mixed malarial infections. This fever pattern may also be seen in miliary tuberculosis and legionnaires' disease.

Of critical importance in analyzing fever patterns in patients is the relationship between the pulse and the temperatures. Every degree of fever over 102° F results in an increase in the pulse rate of 10 beats per minute. Hence, the patient with 102° F should have a pulse of 130 beats per minute; the patient with 103° F should have a pulse of 140 beats per minute, etc. A discrepancy in pulse rate increase in relation to the degree of fever is termed "relative bradycardia." Relative bradycardia is a common and extremely useful feature in the analysis of complex fevers in ambulatory patients and especially in hospitalized patients. Relative bradycardia is particularly useful in the diagnosis of typhoid fever, malaria, legionnaires' disease, psittacosis, and drug fever.

An excessive increase in the pulse rate relative to the temperature is termed "relative tachycardia." Relative tachycardia occurs less frequently and is therefore less useful than relative bradycardia, but it is associated with two important infectious disease entities, diphtheria and clostridial infections. Relative tachycardia may also provide the only clue to multiple small, "clinically silent" pulmonary emboli.

Fever patterns are also important in assessing the efficacy of antimicrobial therapy. Frequently, the retrospective response of a patient to a particular antibiotic given as a therapeutic trial may suggest the diagnosis of a particular infectious disease entity. For example, a bacterial pneumonia not responding to beta-lactam antibiotics but responding to a trial of erythromycin or doxycycline may retrospectively suggest atypical pneumonia caused by Mycoplasma, Legionella, psittacosis, etc.

The febrile response is commonly misperceived as "bad." Though clinicians and the public commonly believe that the higher the fever, the more sick the patient or the worse the prognosis, quite the opposite is true. Patients with overwhelming sepsis or a poor prognosis usually present with subnormal temperatures. The absence of an appropriate febrile response is the harbinger of a stormy course or a fatal outcome. The patient's febrile response should be regarded as an adaptive host defense mechanism that should be preserved, if not augmented. Antipyretics or fever-lowering procedures should be avoided, if at all possible, to provide the patient with the "benefit of fever" to maximize the host defense response, to accurately characterize the fever pattern, and to monitor therapeutic efficacy of antimicrobial therapy. In general, fevers above 106° F should be lowered to avoid neuronal damage. In addition, patients with serious cardiopulmonary disease should not be permitted to have temperatures in excess of 102° F because of the strain that such an elevated temperature places upon the heart and the lungs (Table 5–1).

DIAGNOSTIC EVALUATION

The general approach to the patient with fever (possibly caused by infectious disease) is the same as for the patient with other medical problems. The infectious disease clinician uses the information obtained in the history, physical examination, and routine laboratory tests to suggest one or more "syndromes" and form a working diagnosis. The clinician then uses further laboratory tests, which are usually more sophisticated, to arrive at a specific diagnosis. The importance of the syndromic approach in infectious disease cannot be overemphasized (see Chapter 4). The application of known basic principles as "aphorisms" best explains the approach to the patient with an infectious disease. For example, if the patient presents as an atypical pneumonia, the infectious disease clinician must apply historical and laboratory information to differentiate viral, mycoplasmal, Legionella, tularemia, Q fever, and psittacosis pneumonias.

Patient History

That "the history is the diagnosis," true in general internal medicine, is also true in infectious diseases. The infectious disease clinician is particularly interested in identifying other infected individuals with whom the patient may have been in contact. A history of recent travel in an underdeveloped area greatly limits diagnostic possibilities in an acutely ill patient. Acutely ill patients returning from abroad usually have common, as opposed to exotic, infectious diseases, e.g., tuberculosis, typhoid fever, malaria, or one of the infectious dysenteries (Table 5–2). A history of pet or animal contact is extremely important in identifying the infectious zoonoses. Young patients who have hamsters at home as pets and present with a flulike illness and aseptic meningitis should immediately raise the possibility of lymphocytic choriomeningitis (LCM). Many disease and animal "associations" are classic, e.g., salmonellosis with turtles, bubonic plague with prairie dogs, or typhus with flying squirrels. Few confirmatory tests are needed to make the diagnosis. In other situations, the number of diseases associated with certain animals, i.e., dogs and cats, is very great, and therefore such a history is less helpful and requires many additional diagnostic tests for final diagnosis (Table 5–3).

Physical Examination

The physical examination of the patient with an infectious disease is largely unrewarding unless the patient has adenopathy or splenomegaly or skin lesions. Physical findings of a general nature, i.e., costovertebral angle tenderness, lobar consolidation, heart murmur, etc., do not usually provide specific diagnostic information and are usually readily identified by the house officer or internist.

Patients presenting with lymphadenopathy present

Table 5—1. Diagnostic Fever Patterns in Infectious Diseases

≥ 106° F	*≤ 98° F*
Central fevers (hemorrhage, trauma, infection, malignancy)	Elderly patients
Infusion-related sepsis (contaminated infusate)	Uremia
Heat stroke	Overwhelming infection
Malignant hyperthermia	Hypothyroidism
Bacterial Infections (rare)	Cold exposure
Acquired Immune Deficiency Syndrome (AIDS)	
Drug fever (usually 102°–105°F)	

The 102° F Rule in Differential Diagnosis

≤ 102° F	*≥ 102° F*
Acute cholecystitis	Cholangitis
Acute myocardial infarct	Pericarditis
Thrombophlebitis	Suppurative phlebitis
Pulmonary emboli-infarction	Septic pulmonary emboli
Acute pancreatitis	Pancreatic abscess
Viral hepatitis	Nonviral liver disease, drug fever, leptospirosis

Hectic, Septic Fevers

Abscess (especially intra-abdominal, renal, pelvic)
Frequent use of antipyretics
Kawasaki's disease
Miliary tuberculosis
Subacute bacterial endocarditis
Malaria
Kala-azar

Sustained Fevers

Scarlet fever
Brucellosis
Central nervous system infections
Rocky Mountain spotted fever
Tularemia
Typhoid fever
Psittacosis

Relative Bradycardia

Dengue fever
Typhoid fever
Typhus (epidemic)
Malaria
Leptospirosis
Yellow fever
Legionnaires' disease
Psittacosis
Lymphomas (occasionally)
Central nervous system lesions (occasionally)
Drug fever

Relative Tachycardia

Supraventricular arrhythmias
Hyperthyroidism
Pulmonary emboli
Clostridial sepsis
Diphtheria

Remittent Fevers

Mycoplasma
Legionella?
Falciparum malaria
Tuberculosis

Relapsing Fevers

Dengue
Yellow fever
Brucellosis
Suppurative cholangitis
Malaria
Rat-bite fever
Relapsing fever (B. recurrentis)

Camel-back Fevers

Colorado tick fever
Dengue fever

Double Quotidian Fevers

Right sided gonococcal endocarditis
Kala-azar
Adult Still's disease (JRA)
Mixed malarial infections
Miliary tuberculosis
Legionnaires' disease

Table 5–2.   Common Illnesses in Patients Returning from Recent Foreign Travel

Typhoid fever
Malaria
Pulmonary tuberculosis
Viral hepatitis
  Hepatitis A (HAV)
  Hepatitis B (HBV)
Infectious diarrheas
  Toxigenic E. coli
  Cholera
  Amebic dysentery
  Shigella dysentery
  Campylobacter
  Giardiasis
  Yersinia

with either regional or generalized lymph node involvement (Table 5–4). Regional adenopathy most commonly suggests a local bacterial infection, but it is frequently associated with tularemia, primary syphilis, cutaneous tuberculosis, sporotrichosis, cat-scratch fever, chancroid, lymphogranuloma venereum, rat-bite fever (S. minus), lymphoma, or plague. Generalized adenopathy suggests the possibility of a wide variety of disorders that usually present with other associated symptoms, thereby limiting diagnostic possibilities. Generalized adenopathy is a feature of histoplasmosis, infectious mononucleosis, secondary syphilis, dengue fever, toxoplasmosis, rubella, lymphoma, serum sickness, systemic lupus erythematosus (SLE), rheumatoid arthritis, and myeloid metaplasia.

If splenomegaly is found in association with node involvement, diagnostic possibilities may become readily apparent (Table 5–5). For example, a young patient with generalized adenopathy and splenomegaly may well have infectious mononucleosis, SLE, etc., but is not likely to have cytomegalovirus or subacute bacterial endocarditis, which are not usually associated with generalized adenopathy. In contrast, patients presenting with splenomegaly in the absence of regional or generalized adenopathy may have a wide variety of infectious and noninfectious diagnostic possibilities. As in general medicine, disease entities that occur frequently should be considered first, and the least likely diagnostic possibilities should be considered later in the patient's workup.

Skin lesions are of great diagnostic significance in the study of infectious disease, as well as in dermatology. A discussion of all of the noninfectious disease processes that may mimic an infectious disease cutaneously is beyond the scope of this section and constitutes a major portion of the speciality of dermatology (see Chapter 18). However, an acutely ill patient presenting with a rash and fever is properly the domain of the infectious disease clinician. Diagnostic possibilities are immediately narrowed because the patient is febrile and acutely ill, and the problem may be approached according to the kind of rash that the patient manifests. An acutely ill patient with a petechial or hemorrhagic rash may have meningococcemia, disseminated intravascular coagulation (DIC), overwhelming staphylococcal and pneumococcal sepsis, epidemic typhus, Rocky Mountain spotted fever, one of the viral hemorrhagic fevers, or toxic shock syndrome. It is important to determine whether the rash is primarily central with a peripheal component or primarily peripheral with a central component. Involvement of the palms and soles with the rash also yields important diagnostic information (Table 5–6).

Frequently, it is the noncutaneous manifestations associated with the underlying disease entity that provide the most important diagnostic information. For example, an acutely ill patient with a petechial rash and bilateral conjunctivitis could have either meningococcemia or toxic shock syndrome. If the patient has relative bradycardia, then epidemic typhus or one of the viral hemorrhagic fevers would be the primary diagnostic possibility. Diagnoses of acutely ill patients presenting with vesicular rashes are really limited to two possibilities, i.e., disseminated varicella-zoster or a severe Stevens-Johnson syndrome (Table 5–7). Once again, the application of the same principles of rash distribution, palm and sole involvement, and associated features should make the diagnosis relatively straightforward.

The most difficult patient is one that is acutely ill and febrile with a maculopapular rash (Table 5–8). Maculopapular rashes are the least specific and therefore least diagnostically helpful eruption. Maculopapular rash may be associated with scarlet fever, measles, atypical measles, rubella, enteroviral infections, Kawasaki disease, or drug fevers. Relative bradycardia in such patients would immediately suggest the possibility of drug fever, as sore throat, diarrhea, or aseptic meningitis would suggest an enteroviral cause. Atypical measles would be suggested by pulmonary involvement and a rash with urticaria or a petechial component. As with all rashes, the most important feature is the location of the lesion rather than its particular appearance. The second most important feature is its distribution. Lastly, as has been mentioned, the associated features are frequently helpful in making a specific etiologic diagnosis in the acutely ill patient with a fever and a rash.

Diagnostic Studies

LABORATORY TESTS

The basic laboratory tests obtained in the office or hospital may provide important diagnostic information

Table 5–3.　Infectious Diseases Associated with Animal Contact

Animal	Disease	Exposure	Animal	Disease	Exposure
Cats	Cat-scratch fever*	Contact	Sheep, Goats	Q fever*	Inhalation
	Cutaneous larval migrans (Ancylostoma)*	Contact		Brucellosis*	Ingestion
				Campylobacter	Ingestion
	Pasteurella multocida*	Contact		Rift Valley fever	Bite
	Toxoplasmosis*	Ingestion		Orf	Contact
	Giardiasis	Ingestion		Foot and mouth disease	Contact
	Campylobacter	Ingestion		Leptospirosis	Contact
	Plague	Flea bite		Pneumocystis carinii	Inhalation
	Strongyloidiasis	Ingestion		Echinococcosis*	Ingestion
	Paragonimiasis*	Ingestion		Tuberculosis	Inhalation
	Visceral larval migrans*	Ingestion		Anthrax	Contact
	Rabies*	Bite		Tularemia	Contact
	Yersinia	Ingestion		Salmonella	Ingestion
	Leishmaniasis	Contact		Pasteurella	Bite
	Trypanosomiasis	Bite		Yersinia	Ingestion
Dogs	Echinococcosis*	Ingestion		Listeria	Ingestion, contact
	Giardiasis	Ingestion	Swine	Anthrax	Contact
	Dirofilaria immitis	Mosquito bites		Brucellosis*	Ingestion
	Visceral larval migrans (toxocariasis)*	Ingestion		Salmonellosis*	Ingestion
				Erysipeloid*	Contact
	Pasteurella multocida*	Contact, bites		Trichinosis*	Ingestion
	Salmonella*	Ingestion		Tapeworm (T. solium)*	Ingestion
	Boutonneuse fever	Bite		Campylobacter	Ingestion
	Paragonimiasis*	Ingestion		Fasciolopsis*	Ingestion
	Plague	Flea bite		Echinococcosis*	Ingestion
	Campylobacter	Ingestion		Rabies	Bite
	Leptospirosis*	Contact		Foot and mouth disease	Contact
	Brucellosis	Ingestion		Leptospirosis*	Contact
	Rabies	Bite		Listeria	Ingestion, contact
	Cutaneous larval migrans (Ancylostoma)*	Contact	Horses	Anthrax	Contact
				Meliodosis	Contact, ingestion
	Pneumocystis carinii	Inhalation		Maduromycosis	Contact
	Anthrax	Contact		Campylobacter	Ingestion
	Listeria	Ingestion		Tuberculosis	Inhalation
	Trypanosomiasis	Bite		Tularemia	Contact
	Leishmaniasis	Bite		Yersinia	Ingestion
Birds	Psittacosis*	Contact		Leptospirosis	Contact
	Cryptococcosis*	Inhalation		Foot and mouth disease	Contact
	Blastomycosis	Ingestion		Listeria	Ingestion, contact
	Histoplasmosis	Inhalation		Rabies*	Bite
	Q fever	Inhalation		Japanese B encephalitis	Bite
Rodents	Leptospirosis*	Contact		Eastern equine encephalitis	Bite
	Plague*	Flea bite		Venezuelan equine encephalitis	Bite
	Rat-bite fever	Bite		Pasteurella multocida	Bite
	Relapsing fever	Tick bite	Cattle	Milker's nodule (pseudocowpox)	Contact
	Tapeworm (Hymenolepsis)	Ingestion		Campylobacter	Ingestion
	Leishmaniasis	Flea bite		Q fever*	Inhalation
	Trypanosomiasis	Bug bite		Brucellosis*	Ingestion
	Typhus (murine or scrub)	Flea or mite bite		Tuberculosis*	Ingestion
	Typhus (Queensland tick typhus, North Asian tick typhus)	Tick bite		Anthrax*	Contact
				Leptospirosis*	Contact
	Lymphocytic choriomeningitis*	Contact		African trypanosomiasis	Bite
	Erysipeloid	Contact		Rabies	Bite
	Rocky Mountain spotted fever*	Bite		Listeria	Ingestion, contact
	Boutonneuse fever	Bite		Salmonella*	Ingestion
	Salmonella	Ingestion		Echinococcosis*	Ingestion
	Schistosomiasis	Contact		Tapeworm (beef)	Ingestion
	Pneumocystis	Inhalation		Foot and mouth disease	Contact
Prairie dogs	Plague*	Flea bite	Monkeys	Tuberculosis	Inhalation
Bats, Raccoons, Foxes, Skunks	Rabies*	Bite		Melioidosis	Contact
				Amebiasis	Ingestion
Rabbits, Muskrat	Plague	Flea bite		Malaria (Simian)	Mosquito bite
	Tularemia*	Contact		Sparganosis	Ingestion
	Rocky Mountain spotted fever	Tick bite		Filariasis	Mosquito bite
	Brucellosis	Ingestion		Arboviruses	Mosquito bite
				Herpes (Simian)	Bite
Turtles	Salmonella*	Ingestion		Hepatitis	Contact
				AIDS (African Green Monkey)	Contact

* = Most important zoonoses

Table 5–4.   Differential Diagnosis of Lymphadenopathy

Regional Adenopathy	Generalized Adenopathy
Any local bacterial infection	Brucellosis
Tularemia	Leptospirosis
Syphilis (primary)	Miliary tuberculosis
Tuberculosis (typical/atypical)	Histoplasmosis
Sporotrichosis	Infectious mononucleosis
Herpes zoster, herpes simplex	Dengue fever
Cat-scratch fever	Syphilis
Leishmaniasis	Scrub typhus
Scrub typhus	Toxoplasmosis
Chancroid	Rubella
Lymphogranuloma venereum	Waldenström's
Rat-bite fever (S. minus)	macroglobulinemia
Metastatic carcinoma	Lymphoma
Lymphoma	Serum sickness
Plague	Pseudolymphoma (phenytoin)
Kawasaki's disease	Hyperthyroidism
	Systemic lupus erythematosus
	Rheumatoid arthritis
	Sarcoidosis
	Myeloid metaplasia
	Immunoblastic
	lymphadenopathy
	AIDS (HIV-I)

Table 5–5.   Differential Diagnosis of Splenomegaly

Typhoid fever	Lymphoma
Tularemia	Leukemia
Subacute bacterial endocarditis	Myeloid metaplasia
Brucellosis	Polycythemia vera
Miliary tuberculosis	Rheumatoid arthritis
Infectious mononucleosis	Felty's syndrome
Cytomegalovirus	Systemic lupus erythematosus
Toxoplasmosis	Serum sickness
Rocky Mountain spotted fever	Sarcoidosis
Murine typhus	Amyloidosis
Histoplasmosis	Gaucher's disease
Secondary syphilis	Splenic hemorrhage
Malaria	Splenic infarct
Schistosomiasis	Splenic artery aneurysm
Leishmaniasis	Splenic cyst
Kala-azar	Splenic abscess
Portal hypertension (2° any	Splenic tumor
cause)	
Cirrhosis	
Portal or splenic vein	
thrombosis	
Anemia	
Thrombotic thrombocytopenic	
purpura	
Pseudolymphoma	

in a variety of infectious diseases. In general, the most helpful nonspecific tests are the hemogram, the erythrocyte sedimentation rate (ESR), urinalysis, and liver function tests. In addition, any lesion or fluid that is available should be cultured for organisms appropriate to the diagnosis.

The least specific and least helpful laboratory finding among the routine tests is the peripheral white count. A peripheral white count may be elevated as a result of any process that causes demargination of white blood cells from blood vessels and therefore is not indicative of an infectious disease process. The elevation of the peripheral white count provides little meaningful diagnostic or prognostic information and should not be relied upon to distinguish infection from noninfection or viral from bacterial infection.

Similarly, a "shift to the left" indicating immature forms in the periphery is also not specific and does not always indicate an infectious cause.

Of much greater diagnostic significance is the finding of leukopenia, which may provide the clue to overwhelming sepsis, a viral infection, malaria, kala-azar, lupus, hypersplenism, or drug fever (Table 5–9). Lymphocytosis is a much more specific finding than leukocytosis and may suggest a wide variety of diagnostic possibilities, such as viral infections, tuberculosis, Rocky Mountain spotted fever, syphilis, toxoplasmosis, brucellosis, pertussis, histoplasmosis, tularemia, or kala-azar. Monocytosis is an infrequent finding but is very helpful when present and may suggest the possibility of brucellosis, sarcoidosis, lupus, tuberculosis, malignancy, or recovery from acute infection.

Eosinophilia has great diagnostic importance in infectious as well as noninfectious disease. Alone it is a nonspecific finding, but when paired with other diagnostic tests, historical information, or physical findings it may provide a clue to the diagnosis. "Low-grade eosinophilia" may be found in a variety of conditions, including leukemias, lymphomas, drug fever, scarlet fever, adrenal insufficiency, and inflammatory bowel disease, etc. "High-grade eosinophilia" is associated with the tissue phase of parasite migration, pulmonary infiltrates with eosinophilia (PIE) syndrome, etc. (see Chapters 3 and 4). Basophilia suggests smallpox, chickenpox, lymphoma, leukemia, or a myeloproliferative disorder. An increase in platelets usually suggests tuberculosis or malignancy but may be seen after splenectomy or in Kawasaki disease or hemorrhage, as well as in rheumatoid arthritis or cirrhosis. A decrease in platelets is less helpful and is not usually associated with infectious diseases unless the patient is septic with DIC. Atypical lymphocytes are a very important finding and may be associated with any viral infection, but particularly with infec-

Table 5–6.   Differential Diagnosis of Petechial/Hemorrhagic Rashes in the Acutely Ill Patient

Disease	Distribution of Rash		Palm/Sole Rash	Appearance of Rash After Fever	Associated Features
	Central > Peripheral	Peripheral > Central			
Meningococcemia	+	+	+	1–2 hours	Bilateral conjunctivitis Irregular lesions/distribution Late winter/early spring Severe headache (especially with meningitis) Herpes labialis (if meningitis) History of mild recent upper respiratory tract infection
Disseminating intravascular coagulation	+	+	+	V	Secondary to sepsis from obvious source Thrombocytopenia Microangiopathic hemolytic anemia Bleeding from venipuncture sites Renal insufficiency
Overwhelming staphylococcal sepsis	−	+	+	V	Usually obvious staphylococcal focus or staph acute bacterial endocarditis Distal extremity hemorrhagic nodules/infarcts (asymmetrical)
Overwhelming pneumococcal sepsis	−	+	+	1–2 days	Asplenic patients (trauma, staging procedures for lymphoma, sickle cell anemia) Hypotension/shock despite adequate antibiotic/fluid therapy
Epidemic typhus	+	−	−	3–6 days	Summer months Begins in axilla Severe headache, dry cough Relative bradycardia Gangrene of nose, earlobes, scrotum, vulva, fingers, toes Occasionally splenomegaly
Rocky Mountain spotted fever	−	+	+	2–3 days	Late spring/early fall Begins in wrists/ankles Severe headache, splenomegaly Periorbital/peripheral edema No lung involvement Positive OX-2, OX-19 serology
Dengue/viral hemorrhagic fevers	+	−	+	3–4 days	Appropriate travel history Begins in thorax/axilla "Camel-back fever" curve Severe headache/severe myalgias "Palpable pinpoint petechiae" Relative bradycardia
Toxic shock syndrome	+	+	+	1–2 days	Persistent hypotension despite fluid replacement Conjunctivitis Tampon user/surgical wound/menses Liver/renal dysfunction Maculopapular rash Periorbital/facial/extremity edema Sore throat/vagina (oral/vaginal erythema) Watery diarrhea Nausea/vomiting Headache/myalgias

V = variable

Table 5–7. Differential Diagnosis of Vesicular Rashes in the Acutely Ill Patient

| Disease | Distribution of Rash | | Palm/Sole Rash | Appearance of Rash after Fever | Associated Features |
	Central > Peripheral	Peripheral > Central			
Disseminated vari-cella zoster	+	+	+	V	Immunocompromised hosts Lesions of mouth/vulva Pneumonia Painful lesions all in *different* stages of development Vesicles "drop of dew" on skin appear with "red halo" Pustules late
Erythema multi-forme/Stevens Johnson syndrome	+	–	–	V	"Iris/target" lesions associated with herpes, myco-plasma, drugs Perioral lesions/conjunctivitis with Stevens Johnson syndrome

V = variable

tious mononucleosis. Atypical lymphocytes are also seen in patients with malaria, toxoplasmosis, syphilis, pertussis, or brucellosis.

The erythrocyte sedimentation rate is a very sensitive but not very specific test (Table 5–10). Diagnostic specificity may be increased by pairing the ESR with another finding. For example, a patient with proximal muscle aches without frank weakness and a very elevated ESR is likely to have giant cell arteritis. Either the finding of proximal muscle aches or an isolated ESR elevation would be unhelpful if considered alone. Other causes of a very highly elevated ESR include drug fever, gonococcal arthritis, osteomyelitis, malignancy, subacute bacterial endocarditis, abscess, and multiple myeloma. A normal ESR is frequently associated with typhoid fever, malaria, or brucellosis, as well as a variety of other disorders. A very low ESR may be an important clue to trichinosis, especially if associated with eosinophilia. Polycythemia vera or severe anemia also may lower the ESR.

Abnormal liver function tests, i.e., an elevation of the alkaline phosphatase and serum transaminases, is an extremely helpful finding in approaching a patient with fever and the possibility of an infectious disorder (Table 5–11). Passive congestion of the liver or infiltrative disease of the liver (especially granulomatous liver diseases) causes abnormal liver function tests. Viral hepatitis (caused by hepatitis A, B, non A, or non B) is associated with extreme elevations in the serum transaminases ≥1000 units. Other viral infections affecting the liver, such as CMV, infectious mononucleosis, etc., usually result in modest elevations of the serum transaminases in the 200- to 300-unit range. Other diseases associated with more modest abnormalities of liver function include Legionella, psitta-

cosis, Q fever, brucellosis, leptospirosis, toxoplasmosis, and yellow fever. Drug fever is an important cause of mild elevation of the serum transaminases in hospitalized patients with fever.

In addition to culture of the urine, the finding of sterile pyuria is important in a patient with infectious disease (Table 11–12). Sterile pyuria suggests interstitial nephritis, any inflammatory disease of the lower genitourinary tract (trichomoniasis), brucellosis, leptospirosis, or tuberculosis. Sterile pyuria is also frequently a feature of toxic shock syndrome. Microscopic hematuria suggests an inflammatory or neoplastic process in the genitourinary tract, adenoviral infection, tuberculosis, or Staphylococcus saprophyticus infection.

In summary, the approach to a patient with an infectious disease involves finding appropriate clues in the history, physical examination, and laboratory tests that suggest a particular syndrome. The constellation of signs and symptoms suggesting a particular syndrome determines the diagnostic possibilities, which are further narrowed by re-evaluating the patient for more specific historical and laboratory clues that will suggest a particular diagnosis. The temporal relationship of the disease to the fever, as well as the way the disease is "behaving" in a patient, may suggest that the process is autoimmune, neoplastic, or infectious in nature. With the majority of patients, if the clinician can characterize a disorder as a particular syndrome, specific or definitive diagnostic tests may be ordered to confirm the definitive diagnosis. Situations that present particular diagnostic difficulty and are confusing, i.e., fever in the compromised host, fever in the hospitalized patient, or fever of undetermined origin, require a different diagnostic approach and are discussed separately later in this section.

Table 5–8. Differential Diaganosis of Maculopapular Rashes in the Acutely Ill Patient

Disease	Distribution of Rash		Palm/Sole Rash	Appearance of Rash after Fever	Associated Features
	Central > Peripheral	Peripheral > Central			
Scarlet fever	+	−	+	1–2 days	Nausea/vomiting Circumoral pallor "Strawberry" tongue Pastia's lines "Sandpaper skin" Pseudoappendicitis Abdominal pain Eosinophilia Wound/sore throat 2° group A Strep. Palatal petechiae
Measles	+	−	+	2–3 days	Toxic appearance Deep red/purple/brown rash begins on face Cough Conjunctivitis Pneumonia (giant cell) Encephalitis Pseudoappendicitis Koplik's spots Desquamation late
Atypical measles	−	+	+	2–3 days	History of "killed" measles vaccine Begins on extremities, may have urticarial or petechial component Always pneumonia/pulmonary infiltrate Elevated erythrocyte sedimentation rate Eosinophilia Rheumatoid factor
Rubella	+	−	+	1–7 days	Postcervical/occipital adenopathy Palatal petechiae No upper respiratory tract infection Face to feet in 3 days Conjunctivitis
Enteroviruses	+	−	+	5–7 days	Predilection for face Maculopapular component Diarrhea/sore throat Hepatitis/aseptic meningitis
Kawasaki's disease	+	−	+	V	Conjunctivitis Edema of hands/feet Meatal inflammation Erythema tongue/mouth sometimes with E. multiform-like lesions Thrombocytosis Nonspecific ECG changes Less than 5 years of age More than one week of prolonged fever (unresponsive to ASA therapy) Negative streptococcal cultures/serology
Drug fever	+	−	+	V	Negative blood cultures Looks "relatively well" unless coexistent infection Elevated liver function tests, erythrocyte sedimentation rate, eosinophilia Relative bradycardia

V = variable

Table 5–9. Laboratory Tests in Infectious Diseases—Hemogram

Leukocytosis

Any stress
Acute infection
Intoxications
Myeloproliferative diseases
Tissue inflammation/injury

Leukopenia

Overwhelming sepsis
Viral hepatitis
Malaria
Kala-azar
Infectious mononucleosis
Rubella
Measles
Psittacosis
Gaucher's disease
Systemic lupus erythematosus
Hypersplenism
Drug fever

Lymphocytosis

Tuberculosis
Infectious mononucleosis
Cytomegalovirus
Rocky Mountain spotted fever
Syphilis
Toxoplasmosis
Rubella
Brucellosis
Acute lymphatic leukemia
Pertussis
Kala-azar
Histoplasmosis
Tularemia
Mumps

Monocytosis

Brucellosis
Sarcoidosis
Systemic lupus erythematosus
Rheumatoid arthritis
Gaucher's disease
Tuberculosis
Malignancy
Rocky Mountain spotted fever
Inflammatory bowel disease
Recovery from acute infection

Thrombocytosis

Tuberculosis
Malignancy
Kawasaki's disease
Hemorrhage
Postsplenectomy
Rheumatoid arthritis
Cirrhosis

Thrombocytopenia

Disseminated intravascular coagulation (DIC)
Thrombotic thrombocytopenic purpura (TTP)
Idiopathic thrombocytopenic purpura (ITP)
Myelophthisic anemia
Toxic shock syndrome (TSS)

Atypical lymphocytes

Malaria
Toxoplasmosis
Syphilis
Pertussis
Brucellosis
Viral infection
Infectious mononucleosis (>15%)

Eosinophilia

Proximal gastrointestinal parasites (except Giardia)
Leukemias/lymphomas
Trichinosis
Periarteritis nodosa
Sarcoidosis
Adrenal insufficiency
Scarlet fever
Drug fever
Myeloproliferative diseases
Infectious bowel diseases
Tissue phase of parasite migration*
Tropical eosinophilia*
Löffler's syndrome*
Pulmonary infiltration eosinophilia syndromes*
Pernicious anemia
Chlamydia

Basophilia

Smallpox
Chickenpox
Lymphomas/leukemias
Myeloproliferative diseases

* = over 10% eosinophils

Table 5–10. Laboratory Tests in Infectious Diseases—Erythrocyte Sedimentation Rate (ESR)

Highly Elevated ESR (≥ 100 mm/hour)	*Normal ESR*	*Low ESR (≤ 10 mm/hour)*
Drug fever	Typhoid fever	Trichinosis
Gonococcal arthritis	Early pregnancy	Polycythemia vera
Osteomyelitis	Osteoarthritis	Severe anemia
Malignancy	Most viral diseases	
Subacute bacterial endocarditis	Malaria	
Abscess	Brucellosis	
Multiple myeloma		
Giant cell arteritis		

Table 5–11.   Laboratory Tests in Infectious Diseases—Abnormal Liver Function Tests

Passive liver congestion	Viral hepatitis
Infiltrative liver disease	Hepatitis A
Drug fever	Hepatitis B
Legionella	Hepatitis non A, non B
Psittacosis	Cytomegalovirus
Q fever	Infectious mononucleosis
Brucellosis	Yellow fever
Leptospirosis	Liver abscess
Toxoplasmosis	Liver metastases

Table 5–12.   Urinalysis in Infectious Diseases

Sterile Pyuria
    Any inflammatory process in the genitourinary tract
    Any cause of interstitial nephritis
    Brucellosis
    Leptospirosis
    Toxic shock syndrome
    Tuberculosis
    Renal abscess (cortical)
    Enterovirus
    Diphtheria
Microscopic Hematuria
    Glomerulonephritis
    Genitourinary malignancy
    Adenoviral cystitis
    S. saprophyticus

FEVER OF UNKNOWN ORIGIN (FUO)

DEFINITION

A fever of unknown origin is defined as an illness characterized by a temperature greater than 101° F on one or more occasions over at least a 3-week period that remains undiagnosed after 1 week of in-hospital evaluation.

PATHOPHYSIOLOGIC CONSIDERATIONS

A variety of noninfectious and infectious stimuli act through a single mechanism to produce fever. Low molecular weight proteins called endogenous pyrogens (EP) stimulate the thermoregulatory center of the hypothalamus to produce the febrile response. Viruses, rickettsia, bacteria, antigen-antibody complexes, etc. cause the release of endogenous pyrogen from a variety of cells, especially polymorphonuclear leukocytes (PMNs) circulating monocytes, tissue macrophages, and Kupffer's cells in the liver. Additionally, certain malignant cells may produce endogenous pyrogens or endogenous pyrogen-like substances that stimulate the hypothalamus to produce fever.

DIFFERENTIAL DIAGNOSIS

Most fevers of unknown origin (FUO) are caused by treatable diseases (Table 5–13). Infections are the most frequent and important cause of fever of unknown origin. The most important causes of infection in a patient with FUO are endocarditis, tuberculosis, or intrahepatic infection or abscess. The second most important cause of FUO is malignant disease. In this category, lymphomas and to a lesser extent hypernephromas (renal cell carcinomas) are the most frequent cause of fever on a neoplastic basis. Connective tissue diseases constitute the third most frequent cause of FUO and are important because the majority of these disease entities are treatable. Giant cell arteritis (GCA), systemic lupus erythematosus, and generalized vasculitis are the most important disease entities to be considerered in this category. Lastly, a variety of miscellaneous conditions may present as FUO, including multiple pulmonary emboli, inflammatory bowel disease, and drug fever. In approximately 10% of patients, no cause is found for prolonged fevers after extensive hospital workups.

DIAGNOSTIC EVALUATION

Patient History

A number of clues from the patient's history suggest causes of fever of unknown origin. Endocarditis is suggested by a history of periodontal disease, dental manipulation, or GI/GU manipulation in a patient with a history of rheumatic fever or heart murmur. Endocarditis should also be suspected in patients with a history of prosthetic heart valves or parenteral drug abuse. Unexplained renal insufficiency, left ventricular failure, blindness, stroke, or meningitis should suggest the diagnosis of endocarditis. Similarly, unexplained changes in mental status or unexplained low back pain with fever suggests endocarditis. Patients presenting as FUO with a heart murmur and history of severe headache or myalgias have endocarditis resulting from psittacosis, brucellosis, or leptospirosis.

A previous history of or contact with a patient with tuberculosis strongly suggests the possibility that the patient may have nonrenal tuberculosis or miliary tuberculosis as the cause of the FUO. While most patients with pulmonary tuberculosis present with fever and a nonproductive cough, patients having an FUO caused by tuberculosis give little or no history referable to the respiratory tract. Patients with disseminated or

Table 5–13.   Causes of Fever of Unknown Origin

Infections	Neoplasms
Infective endocarditis	Hodgkin's/nonHodgkin's lymphoma
Tuberculosis	Hypernephroma (renal cell carcinoma)
Intra-abdominal/pelvic abscess (splenic, subphrenic, subhepatic,	Atrial myxoma
hepatobiliary, pancreatic, colon, appendix)	Hepatoma
Genitourinary abscess (intrarenal, perinephric, prostatic)	Liver metastases
Dental infection/abscess	Collagen vascular diseases
Typhoid fever	Giant cell arteritis
Brucellosis	Periarteritis nodosa
Syphilis	Systemic lupus erythematosus
Leptospirosis	Rheumatoid arthritis
Histoplasmosis	Miscellaneous disorders
Malaria	Granulomatous hepatitis
Toxoplasmosis	Alcoholic liver disease
Cytomegalovirus	Inflammatory bowel disease
Infectious mononucleosis	Whipple's disease
Trichinosis	Familial Mediterranean fever
Legionella	Cyclic neutropenia
	Drug fever
	Recurrent pulmonary emboli

miliary tuberculosis have few, if any, historical clues to suggest the diagnosis. The only clue to tuberculous meningitis complicating miliary tuberculosis may be the subacute onset of mental confusion or dementia. A history of unexplained hematuria or flank pain in a patient presenting with FUO suggests the possibility of renal tuberculosis. Weakness and weight loss may be found in a variety of diseases, including tuberculosis, and are of little diagnostic significance. However, weight loss without diminished appetite suggests tuberculosis rather than malignancy in the patient presenting with FUO. The diagnosis of disseminated tuberculosis should be considered in any patient without a history suggesting any specific disorder, especially if the patient is known to have had a positive PPD reaction in the past, has come from an area where tuberculosis is endemic, or has had a history of contact with infected individuals.

Patients with intra-abdominal abscesses as a cause of FUO usually give a history of weight loss with or without abdominal pain. A previous history of GI/GU surgery with abdominal pain strongly suggests the possibility of an intra-abdominal abscess as the cause of fever. The pain is usually located in the area of the previous surgery and is invariably present over the area of the underlying abscess. In a patient with a previous history of hepatobiliary surgery, pleuritic chest pain suggests the presence of cholangitis or liver abscess. A history of right lower quadrant pain would suggest abscess caused by a perforated appendix or a perforated cecal diverticulum. A history of left lower quadrant pain suggests ruptured diverticuli, pericolonic or intra-abdominal abscess secondary to a previous surgical procedure, or abscess secondary to perforation caused by a colonic malignancy. Of these, right upper quadrant pain caused by a hepatobiliary abscess and right lower quadrant pain caused by a perforated appendix are the most frequent historical clues to an abscess.

A variety of other uncommon or unusual infectious diseases may present as a FUO (Table 5–14). A history of contact with animals or animal-contaminated food products suggests the possibility of psittacosis, leptospirosis, brucellosis, or Q fever. Severe headache in the absence of meningitis or other associated symptoms suggests the presence of malaria or brucellosis in the FUO patient. In addition to tuberculous meningitis, mental confusion in the FUO patient in the absence of other historical clues suggests typhoid fever, brucellosis, or cryptococcal meningitis. FUO patients with severe myalgias may have gonococcal arthritis, trichinosis, or toxoplasmosis. Fatigue or malaise in the FUO setting suggests typhoid fever, cytomegalovirus (CMV), or infectious mononucleosis. The history of a rat bite suggests infection caused by S. minus if the febrile illness began within a month after the rat bite. Chronic pharyngitis suggests a viral cause on the basis of CMV, infectious mononucleosis, or respiratory viruses.

The majority of patients presenting as FUOs with malignancy have Hodgkin's disease or non-Hodgkin's lymphoma. These patients usually complain of night sweats, malaise, weight loss with decreased appetite, or pruritus. Frequently, fever is the only clue to the presence of a retroperitoneal lymphoma. Patients with leukemia or preleukemia may complain of bone pain (sternal pain) and low-grade fevers.

Fever and hematuria in association with early fatigability and weight loss suggest renal cell carcinoma

Table 5–14. Historical Clues to FUO

Animal Contact
Psittacosis
Leptospirosis
Brucellosis
Cat-scratch fever
Q fever

Headache
Malaria
Brucellosis

Mental Confusion
Sarcoidosis
Tuberculosis
Metastatic carcinoma
Cryptococcal meningitis
Brucellosis
Typhoid fever

Myalgias
Gonococcal arthritis
Trichinosis
Endocarditis
Adult juvenile rheumatoid arthritis
Toxoplasmosis
Systemic lupus erythematosus
Periarteritis nodosa
Rheumatoid arthritis
Familial Mediterranean fever

Headache/Myalgias
Psittacosis
Q fever
Brucellosis
Streptobacillary fever
Leptospirosis

Medication/Toxic Substance Exposure
Drug fever

Nonproductive Cough
Tuberculosis
Q fever
Typhoid fever
Legionnaires' disease

Fatigue
Carcinoma
Lymphoma
Viral hepatitis
Cytomegalovirus
Infectious mononucleosis
Typhoid fever
Systemic lupus erythematosus
Rheumatoid arthritis
Toxoplasmosis

Back Pain
Brucellosis
Endocarditis

Neck Pain
Subacute thyroiditis
Adult juvenile rheumatoid arthritis
Giant cell arthritis (angle of jaw)

(hypernephroma). Hypernephroma may present as flank tenderness or a sensation of fullness in the flank. Often called the "internist tumor," hypernephromas may present with evidence of distant metastasis to brain and bone. A history referable to distant organ involvement and fever in the absence of liver metastasis suggest the diagnosis of renal cell carcinoma.

The patient with left atrial myxoma may give a history compatible with emboli phenomona to the central nervous system or to the peripheral vessels. A history of changing heart murmur in the absence of endocarditis suggests the presence of left atrial myxoma. Fever associated with right upper quadrant fullness or pain may suggest the presence of a hepatoma, but often a history of fever is all that is elicited in patients with hepatomas as well as those with liver metastasis. Other tumors that are associated with low-grade fevers that may present as FUOs include bronchogenic carcinoma and adenocarcinoma of the colon. Patients with solid tumor malignancies do not usually give a history of sustained fever. Fever in the presence

of headache/mental confusion suggests the possibility of brain metastasis from lung, breast, colon, prostate, etc.

Visual disturbances, proximal muscle weakness, jaw pain, or headache in an elderly patient suggests giant cell arteritis.

Physical Examination

Examination of the patient with fever of unknown origin for physical clues is extremely important (Table 5–15). Concentrating first upon the infectious causes of FUOs, the clinician should examine the patient for evidence of heart murmur, which suggests endocarditis or atrial myxoma. Liver enlargement suggests alcoholic liver disease, lymphoma, or metastatic carcinoma. Splenomegaly, if present, is an extremely important clue pointing to the diagnosis of lymphoma, Hodgkin's lymphoma or non-Hodgkin's lymphoma, chronic myelogenous leukemia, disseminated tuberculosis, brucellosis, infectious mononucleosis, cytomegalovirus, systemic lupus erythematosus, toxoplas-

Table 5–15. Physical Clues to FUO

Eye—Orbital Involvement

Lymphoma
Metastatic carcinoma

Band Keratopathy

Adult juvenile rheumatoid arthritis
Sarcoidosis

Dry Eyes

Rheumatoid arthritis
Systemic lupus erythematosus
Periarteritis nodosa

Conjunctivitis

Chlamydia
Tuberculosis
Histoplasmosis
Cat-scratch fever

Conjunctival Suffusion

Leptospirosis
Relapsing fever

Subconjunctival Hemorrhage

Endocarditis
Trichinosis

Uveitis

Tuberculosis
Adult juvenile rheumatoid arthritis
Toxoplasmosis
Sarcoidosis
Systemic lupus erythematosus

Lymphadenopathy

Lymphoma
Rheumatoid arthritis
Systemic lupus erythematosus
Tuberculosis
Infectious mononucleosis
Cytomegalovirus
Toxoplasmosis

Sternal Tenderness

Myeloproliferative diseases
Metastatic carcinoma
Brucellosis
Leukemia

Heart Murmur

Endocarditis
Atrial myxoma

Hepatomegaly

Lymphoma
Metastic carcinoma
Alcoholic liver disease

Splenomegaly

Leukemia
Lymphoma
Tuberculosis
Brucellosis
Endocarditis
Cytomegalovirus
Infectious mononucleosis
Malaria
Toxoplasmosis
Systemic lupus erythematosus
Rheumatoid arthritis
Sarcoidosis
Psittacosis
Relapsing fever
Alcoholic liver disease

Splenic Abscess

Endocarditis
Typhoid fever
Brucellosis

Epididymo-orchitis

Tuberculosis
Lymphoma
Brucellosis
Leptospirosis
Periarteritis nodosa
Blastomycosis
Infectious mononucleosis

Spinal Tenderness

Vertebral osteomyelitis
Subacute bacterial endocarditis
Brucellosis
Typhoid fever

Tenderness of the Costovertebral Angle

Perinephric abscess
Chronic pyelonephritis

Arthritis

Familial Mediterranean fever
Lymphogranuloma venereum
Tuberculosis
Streptobacillary fever
Rheumatoid arthritis
Systemic lupus erythematosus

mosis, rheumatoid arthritis, sarcoidosis, psittacosis, relapsing fever, malaria, or endocarditis. Clearly, hepatosplenomegaly would suggest lymphoma or alcoholic liver disease as the most frequent cause of combined organ enlargement. Tender splenomegaly suggesting a splenic abscess raises the possibility of brucellosis, typhoid fever, or endocarditis.

Bony tenderness suggests a variety of causes of FUO; sternal tenderness suggests brucellosis, myeloproliferative disease, or neoplastic involvement of the marrow of the sternum. Spinal tenderness suggests vertebral osteomyelitis, brucellosis, or typhoid fever. CVA tenderness suggests chronic pyelonephritis or perinephric abscess.

Physical examination of the eyes is also rewarding. Proptosis of the eyes suggests retro-orbital carcinoma or lymphoma. "Dry eyes" suggests rheumatoid ar-

thritis, SLE, or periarteritis nodosa alone or in association with Sjörgen's syndrome. Conjunctival suffusion in an FUO patient suggests relapsing fever or leptospirosis. The impressive conjunctival suffusion or hemorrhage seen with trichinosis is not usually present in patients with trichinosis presenting as FUOs. Subjunctival hemorrhages suggest endocarditis and are rarely present in prolonged trichinosis. Sarcoidosis or adult Still's disease as suggested by band keratopathy is found with examination of the eyes. Conjunctivitis suggests Chlamydiae, tuberculosis, histoplasmosis, or cat-scratch fever as a cause of FUO. The presence of uveitis suggests tuberculosis, adult Still's disease, toxoplasmosis, sarcoidosis, or SLE. Obscure, nondeforming arthritis in a patient with FUO suggests the possibility of familial Mediterranean fever, lymphogranuloma venereum, tuberculosis, streptobacillary fever, rheumatoid arthritis, or SLE. Diffuse symmetrical involvement of lymph glands suggests lymphoma, rheumatoid arthritis, SLE, infectious mononucleosis, cytomegalovirus, or toxoplasmosis. Abdominal tenderness in an FUO patient, however subtle, may suggest the presence of an occult intraabdominal abscess.

Diagnostic Studies

LABORATORY TESTS

Physicians commonly order a variety of sophisticated serologic tests in patients with FUO to try to make the diagnosis. While serologic tests for rare diseases, e.g., serology for Q fever, are indicated in rare cases when the history, physical examination, and other laboratory tests point to the disease, ordering such specific tests for everyone is not cost effective and has a very low diagnostic yield.

More importantly, routine laboratory tests may provide important clues to support the working differential diagnosis established by the history and the physical examination (Table 5–16). The hemogram provides a variety of interesting parameters that may suggest the diagnosis. Since anemia is a nonspecific finding, usually representing the anemia of chronic disease, it is nonspecific and of no value in the diagnosis of FUO.

Leukopenia suggests disseminated or miliary tuberculosis, brucellosis, SLE, lymphoma, or leukemia. A monocytosis greater than 10% suggests CMV, tuberculosis, brucellosis, lymphoma, endocarditis, carcinoma, or Crohn's disease.

Eosinophilia is uncommon in patients with FUO but if present quickly limits diagnostic possibilities to trichinosis, lymphoma, a Chlamydial infection, drug fever, or periarteritis nodosa. Patients with trichinosis and FUO usually have no eosinophilia apparent at the time of presentation; evidence of eosinophilia must be sought from previous office or hospital records.

Basophilia, the most unusual hematologic abnormality, is at the same time the most specific, suggesting carcinoma or lymphoma in patients with FUO. Chronic lymphocytosis suggests tuberculosis, infectious mononucleosis, or CMV. The presence of atypical lymphocytes suggests CMV, toxoplasmosis, or viral hepatitis. High-grade atypical lymphocytes, i.e., greater than 20%, limit diagnostic possibilities to infectious mononucleosis.

Thrombocytosis suggests chronic bone marrow stimulation caused by any chronic disease, infectious or noninfectious, but particularly suggests tuberculosis or carcinoma. Similarly, thrombocytopenia is associated with viral diseases as well as a variety of neoplastic disorders.

The erythrocyte sedimentation rate is a useful test, especially when elevated to very high levels, i.e., greater than 100 mm/hour. In the patient with FUO, such high ESRs suggest carcinoma, lymphoma, familial Mediterranean fever, endocarditis, giant cell arteritis, hypernephroma, adult Still's disease, or drug fever. Rarely, such high sedimentation rates are seen in other diseases, such as infectious mononucleosis, CMV, toxoplasmosis, etc. An extremely low sedimentation rate approaching 0 in a patient with FUO strongly suggests the possibility of trichinosis.

Chronic liver disease, specifically chronic hepatitis, is the most frequent cause of IgM rheumatoid factor elevation in FUO patients. An increase in rheumatoid factors is also seen in rheumatoid arthritis, as well as subacute bacterial endocarditis.

Increased serum transaminases suggest diffuse liver involvement characteristic of infectious mononucleosis, CMV, Q fever, psittacosis, leptospirosis, toxoplasmosis, brucellosis, or drug fever.

Elevation of the alkaline phosphatase alone or greatly in excess of serum transaminase elevations suggests an infiltrative or obstructive pattern in the liver from a variety of causes. In the FUO patient, an elevated alkaline phosphatase suggests miliary tuberculosis, lymphomatous involvement of the liver, infectious mononucleosis (particularly of the typhoidal variety), CMV, adult juvenile rheumatoid arthritis (Still's disease), subacute thyroiditis, giant cell arteritis, liver metastases, biliary tract obstruction, hypernephroma, or periarteritis nodosa.

RADIOLOGIC STUDIES

Radiologic and other imaging techniques have been useful in defining disorders suggested by the history or laboratory tests. Abdominal ultrasonography is most useful for the detection of bile duct dilatation in the presence of an obstructing lesion and is an insensitive way of detecting intra-abdominal abscesses. A negative ultrasonic examination of the abdomen rules out an intra-abdominal abscess. Abdominal ultrasonography is also useful in detecting intrahepatic, intrasplenic, intrahepatic/perinephric-occupying lesions.

A two-dimensional echocardiography of the heart is useful in detecting vegetations that would suggest the presence of endocarditis and in detecting a mass suggesting a left atrial myxoma. Echocardiology results must be interpreted with caution; a negative report does not rule out endocarditis, the presence of vegetations does not necessarily mean that the vegetations are infected. Right sided cardiac lesions are not well visualized on two-dimensional echocardiography.

The CT scan has been widely used to detect occult abdominal abscesses and, to a lesser extent, periaortic/

Table 5-16.   Laboratory Clues to FUO

Monocytosis Cytomegalovirus Tuberculosis Brucellosis Endocarditis Lymphoma Carcinoma Crohn's disease	*Rheumatoid Factor* Subacute bacterial endocarditis Chronic active hepatitis Rheumatoid arthritis Malaria
Eosinophilia Trichinosis Lymphoma Chlamydia Drug fever Periarteritis nodosa	*Erythrocyte Sedimentation Rate (>100 mm/hr)* Adult juvenile rheumatoid arthritis Giant cell arteritis Hypernephroma Endocarditis Drug fever Familial Mediterranean fever Carcinoma Lymphoma Abscess
Leukopenia Miliary tuberculosis Brucellosis Systemic lupus erythematosus Lymphoma Leukemia	
Basophilia Carcinoma Lymphoma	*Alkaline Phosphatase* Miliary tuberculosis Lymphoma Mononucleosis (typhoidal) Cytomegalovirus Adult juvenile rheumatoid arthritis Subacute thyroiditis Giant cell arteritis Infiltrative liver disease Biliary obstruction Hypernephroma Periarteritis nodosa Liver metastases
Lymphocytosis Tuberculosis Infectious mononucleosis Cytomegalovirus	
Atypical Lymphocytes Infectious mononucleosis Cytomegalovirus Toxoplasmosis Viral hepatitis	*Serum Transaminases* Infectious mononucleosis Cytomegalovirus Q fever Psittacosis Drug fever Leptospirosis Toxoplasmosis Brucellosis Legionella
Thrombocytosis Chronic diseases (e.g., tuberculosis) Carcinoma/lymphoma	
Thrombocytopenia Viral diseases Carcinoma	

retroperitoneal node involvement suggesting lymphoma. Positive CT scan results for nodes or a mass lesion may be extremely helpful in directing further diagnostic attention to a particular area for subsequent invasive procedures. As with ultrasonography, a negative CT scan does not rule out small abscesses in the liver or elsewhere within the abdominal cavity.

Gallium scans have been used to detect obscure infectious disease processes, abscesses, or neoplastic diseases. Gallium scans are particularly useful in detecting occult abscesses or lymphomas. Unfortunately, gallium scans may be falsely positive or falsely negative, misleading the clinician in his diagnostic approach. Importantly, gallium scans may be falsely negative if performed when the patient is on steroids or

certain antibiotics, e.g., chloramphenicol. As with all radiologic investigative techniques, these tests should be regarded as most useful in localizing or characterizing suspected disorder; they are less sensitive as a screening procedure.

Diagnostic Approach

A clinical approach to the patient with a FUO may be straightforward or fairly complex, depending upon the cause of the prolonged fever. The great majority of patients will have clues obtained from the history, physical examination, or selected laboratory tests that point to the diagnosis or at least limit differential diagnostic possibilities. Diagnostic tests should not be ordered indiscriminately, but should be used to make a diagnosis suggested by diagnostic clues. Blood tests covering a variety of diagnostic possibilities should not be ordered at the outset, but rather should be ordered selectively as the diagnostic workup proceeds and specific disease entities need to be considered. Most patients will have one or more diagnostic clues that provide the bases for a direct diagnostic approach.

Of the infectious disease entities, tuberculosis and endocarditis continue to be the most important disease entities to consider, regardless of the initial presentation. These entities should be ruled out with certainty. Occult intra-abdominal sepsis is the next most important diagnostic possibility to be considered. Usually the patient has vague tenderness, abnormal liver function tests, or questionable findings in one or more radiologic tests that will suggest an occult abscess in the abdomen.

Of the neoplastic disorders, hypernephroma (renal cell carcinoma) as well as occult lymphomas should be particularly looked for. Occult lymphomas are usually retroperitoneal, and hypernephromas may present as a manifestation of distant metastases.

In the collagen vascular group, giant cell arteritis in particular should not be overlooked as a cause of FUO in the elderly patient. A very highly elevated erythrocyte sedimentation rate in association with proximal limb girdle soreness or stiffness should alert the clinician to the presence of giant cell arteritis. Although the diagnosis of adult giant cell arteritis, atypical rheumatoid arthritis, or systemic lupus may be difficult, usually one or more clues are provided in the course of the patient's evaluation that should lead to the correct diagnosis. Drug fevers may be particularly baffling, especially if due to chronic exposure to nonmedicinal fumes or chemicals. A careful history of drug exposure should be taken in all cases of FUOs when there are no diagnostic clues to suggest a diagnosis.

Approximately 10% of patients will have no diagnosis after a thorough and extensive FUO evaluation and workup. Many of these patients will remain undiagnosed, and their readmission at a later time for further diagnostic evaluation should be strongly considered. The importance of time should be emphasized in patients with a negative initial FUO workup. Some febrile conditions will resolve spontaneously with time and other diseases such as occult lymphomas will manifest themselves over time. Tests that were initially negative should be repeated since they may become positive later.

Most diagnoses may be established without the use of invasive techniques, using instead appropriate laboratory tests based upon the diagnostic clues presented by the patient. However, a small number of patients

Table 5–17. Invasive Diagnostic Procedures in FUO

Small-bowel Biopsy	*Bone Marrow Biopsy*
Whipple's disease	Lymphoma
Lymphoma	Histoplasmosis
	Miliary tuberculosis
Liver Biopsy	Brucellosis
Cirrhosis	Sarcoidosis
Granulomatous hepatitis	Toxoplasmosis
Alcoholic hepatitis	Typhoid fever
Chronic active hepatitis	Giant cell arteritis
Hepatoma	
Metastatic carcinoma	
Sarcoidosis	
Miliary tuberculosis	
Brucellosis	
Toxoplasmosis	
Leptospirosis	

will require invasive procedures to make the diagnosis (Table 5–17). Small-bowel biopsy will confirm the diagnosis of Whipple's disease or confirm the presence of a lymphoma of the small bowel. Liver biopsy should be performed if liver function tests are abnormal or if a systemic disease, e.g., miliary tuberculosis, is suspected. Liver biopsy is particularly important in diagnosing the granulomatous hepatitides and may also point to the presence of primary liver cancer or metastatic liver carcinoma. Bone marrow biopsy, similarly, is useful in diseases that are generalized and may involve the bone marrow. Miliary tuberculosis, as well as histoplasmosis, brucellosis, toxoplasmosis, and typhoid fever, may be diagnosed by bone marrow biopsy. The diagnosis of giant cell arteritis and lymphoma may also be made by bone marrow biopsy. Exploratory laparotomy should be entertained as a diagnostic procedure only if there are definite signs and symptoms pointing to the abdomen or if liver function tests are abnormal and liver biopsy is negative. By combining noninvasive and invasive tests, based upon specific diagnostic clues, the cause of prolonged fevers can be determined in the great majority of patients.

HOSPITAL-ACQUIRED FEVER

DEFINITION

Any patient developing a significant temperature that was not present on his admission to the hospital is said to have a hospital-acquired fever. Hospital-acquired fevers occur in medical and surgical patients and may have a noninfectious or an infectious cause.

Because fever frequently suggests infection, temperature elevation is an important diagnostic clue alerting the clinician to the possibility of a large number of infectious and noninfectious diseases.

PATHOPHYSIOLOGIC CONSIDERATIONS

Fever is a host's nonspecific response to a variety of stimuli. Temperature elevation may be produced by virtually any inflammatory process, regardless of whether the inciting agent is infectious or noninfectious. The infectious causes of fever are usually mediated by the production of endogenous pyrogen from white blood cells or from a variety of microorganisms. Fever from a noninfectious cause is not as well understood. In general, fever is associated with the release of the chemical mediators of inflammation, which are released by a variety of stimuli when the inflammatory response is evoked.

DIFFERENTIAL DIAGNOSIS (Table 5–18)

Fever developing during hospitalization will usually have an infectious origin. The differential diagnosis of the infectious causes of hospital-acquired fever includes bacterial or viral pharyngitis, nosocomial pneumonias, IV line or device-associated infections, infectious diarrhea, pyelonephritis or bacteremia, transient bacteremias resulting from tissue manipulation during procedures, osteomyelitis, and endocarditis. If the patient has had surgery, febrile conditions associated with surgery need to be considered as well. Wound infections are a common cause of postoperative fever in the surgical patient. Occasionally, acute sinusitis, postperfusion syndrome caused by cytomegalovirus (CMV), or viral hepatitis caused by hepatitis B virus or non A non B (NANB) virus may be responsible for fever in the postoperative surgical patient. In the postpartum patient the differential diagnostic possibilities are the same as for medical or surgical patients, with the added consideration of pelvic septic thrombophlebitis.

All hospitalized patients may have a variety of noninfectious diseases that present with febrile manifestations. In the elderly debilitated bedridden medical patient, phlebothrombosis or thrombophlebitis with or without pulmonary emboli or infarction may be associated with fever. Such patients may also experience myocardial infarction during their hospitalization. Previously quiescent gout may flare during any stressful episode during hospitalization but in particular may follow silent myocardial infarction. Fever 24 to 48 hours following infusion of blood or blood products is frequently associated with fever; the transfusion re-

Table 5–18. Causes of Hospital-acquired Fever

Nonsurgical Causes of Fever
  Infectious causes
    Pharyngitis
    Pneumonia
    IV line infections
    Diarrhea
    Pyelonephritis
    Transient bacteremia
    Endocarditis
    Osteomyelitis
  Noninfectious causes
    Pulmonary emboli/infarction
    Adrenal insufficiency
    Myocardial infarction
    Transfusion reaction
    Acute gout
    Drug fever
Postoperative Causes of Fever
  Infectious causes
    Pharyngitis
    Pneumonia
    IV line infections
    Diarrhea
    Pyelonephritis
    Transient bacteremia
    Endocarditis
    Osteomyelitis
    Wound infections
    Acute sinusitis
    Postperfusion syndrome
    Viral hepatitis (HBV, NANB)
  Noninfectious causes
    Pulmonary emboli/infarction
    Adrenal insufficiency
    Myocardial infarction
    Transfusion reaction
    Acute gout
    Drug fever
    Anesthetic-induced fever
    Postpericardiotomy syndrome
    Post-thoracotomy/pericardiotomy syndrome
Postpartum Causes of Fever
  Infectious causes
    Pharyngitis
    Pneumonia
    IV line infections
    Diarrhea
    Pyelonephritis
    Transient bacteremia
    Endocarditis
    Osteomyelitis
    Pelvic thrombophlebitis
    Septic abortion
  Noninfectious causes
    Pulmonary embolic/infarction
    Adrenal insufficiency
    Myocardial infarction
    Transfusion reaction
    Acute gout
    Drug fever

action may be mild or severe. Patients on steroids may develop acute adrenal insufficiency if the steroid dose is not increased to meet the additional stress of illness or if the steroid dose on admission was tapered too quickly during hospitalization. The most common cause of fever of noninfectious origin in the generalized hospital population, both medical and surgical, is drug fever. Drug fevers account for approximately 10% of all febrile cases in the hospitalized patient. As a diagnosis it is frequently overlooked because it is suspected infrequently and because it often mimics an infectious process.

Surgical patients may have any one of the many noninfectious causes of fever that the medical patient may have but in addition may have anesthetic-induced fever or, following thoracotomy, may develop post-thoracotomy/pericardiotomy syndrome. In neurosurgical patients, posterior fossa syndrome frequently is associated with fever and may be confused with bacterial meningitis.

The noninfectious causes of fever in the postpartum patient are the same as for the medical and surgical patient. The cause of hospital-acquired fever may be relatively obvious, e.g., osteomyelitis underlying a decubitis ulcer, or may be relatively obscure, e.g., relative adrenal insufficiency. The diagnostic evaluation of the patient will, in the majority of the cases, determine the cause of hospital-acquired fever.

DIAGNOSTIC EVALUATION

Patient History

In the medical patient, a history of chronic congestive heart failure, chronic obstructive pulmonary disease, alcoholism, and similar diseases may suggest the presence of a nosocomial pneumonia. Patients with a history of inflammatory bowel disease may be particularly prone to develop antibiotic-associated colitis while on antimicrobial therapy. Patients with a history of chronic pyelonephritis may develop acute exacerbations of pyelonephritis if catheterized with an indwelling Foley catheter. A history of an invasive diagnostic procedure or tissue manipulation earlier in the patient's hospital stay may suggest subsequent endocarditis. A previous injury, e.g., an old war wound with or without sinus tract formation, may suggest the presence of osteomyelitis.

In the surgical patient, acute sinusitis may accompany prolonged nasotracheal intubation. A history of having received a large volume of blood during the previous 3 weeks may suggest the possibility of postperfusion syndrome caused by CMV. A history of blood transfusions may also suggest the possibility of

NANB hepatitis or, less frequently, hepatitis B virus infection. Postpartum patients receiving large volumes of blood may also develop viral hepatitis or postperfusion syndrome, but these diseases are infrequent causes of fever in obstetrics and gynecology because the volume of blood needed for obstetric and gynecologic procedures is usually less than that for surgical procedures, e.g., open heart surgery. In all other respects postpartum patients resemble young medical patients in terms of the infectious causes of fever in the postpartum period.

The history may be of assistance in pointing to the noninfectious cause of fever in both medical and surgical patients. A history of tuberculosis or histoplasmosis, in addition to chronic steroid dependence, may suggest the presence of adrenal insufficiency. Silent myocardial infarction is particularly associated with alcoholic, diabetic, and uremic patients. Silent myocardial infarction is particularly common after abdominal or genitourinary procedures and should be considered in these patients as a source of fever; appropriate tests should be ordered to make the diagnosis.

A history of gout may presage an acute gouty attack during any acute illness or stress. Patients with drug fever may give an atopic history but usually give no history of hypersensitivity reactions to allergens or medications. The patient does, however, provide a history during hospitalization of being on one or more "sensitizing" medications frequently associated with drug fevers.

In the patient undergoing surgery, anesthetic-induced fever may be suggested by a history of the use of halothane in previous surgical procedures. Characteristically the illness produced by subsequent exposures to halothane is more dramatic and occurs sooner after the surgical procedure with each exposure. Postpericardiotomy syndrome should be entertained as a diagnosis in patients undergoing surgery with a history of thoracotomy 3 or more weeks prior to the onset of the hospital-acquired fever. These patients frequently complain of pleuritic chest pain, which in the appropriate setting should also suggest the diagnosis.

Physical Examination

A physical examination may be very helpful in pinpointing the cause of hospital-acquired fever in both medical and surgical patients. Hospitalized patients with pharyngitis complain of pharyngeal soreness. Examination of the oropharynx reveals an erythematous pharynx usually without exudates. Pneumonia may be suggested by adventitious sounds over the involved areas in the lung, especially in patients using respiratory support equipment. Patients with diarrhea have generalized colicky abdominal pain with or without associated tenesmus. Pyelonephritis is almost invariably associated with unilateral CVA tenderness and a temperature $\leq 102°$ F in patients with indwelling Foley catheters. Patients with transient bacteremias resulting from invasive procedures have little in the way of physical findings except for fever and chills. Endocarditis is classically associated with a new or changing heart murmur in the presence of fever. Hospital-acquired endocarditis is invariably associated with invasive diagnostic procedures or open heart surgery. Osteomyelitis of the foot, especially in diabetic patients, may be the cause of fever, a chronic draining sinus tract located in the webbed spaces between the toes is particularly easy to miss.

Surgical patients having postperfusion syndrome or NANB or NBV viral hepatitis will have tenderness over the liver to deep percussion. Patients with postperfusion syndrome caused by CMV in addition may have mild pharyngitis, splenomegaly, or posterior cervical or generalized adenopathy. The liver may be enlarged in CMV, HBV, or NANB hepatitis. Additionally, patients with hepatitis induced by an anesthetic (e.g., halothane) may have liver tenderness and/or enlargement. Patients with postpericardiotomy syndrome may have the unilateral pleural effusion and/or splinter hemorrhages on physical examination. Following any neurosurgical procedure, the presence of a stiff neck with fever suggests the possibility of posterior fossa syndrome. The fever is caused by the inflammatory response of blood in the cerebrospinal fluid. Fever resolves temporarily as the red cells are cleared by normal mechanisms by the CSF. In the postpartum patient septic pelvic thrombophlebitis is suggested by fevers in excess of 102° F with an auscultatory finding in the chest suggesting septic pulmonary emboli.

Physical findings in noninfectious fever relate to organ system involvement. Pulmonary emboli with infarction may be suggested by the finding of lower extremity tenderness over the deep veins of the foot or calves. Dullness to percussion over the involved area of the chest may be present in such cases. Patients with myocardial infarction may manifest a new S_4 or S_3 gallop and/or changes in S_1 or S_2 suggesting myocardial infarction. Intense pain involving a joint, particularly the first metatarsal joint, suggests an exacerbation of gout in the patient with a predisposition or history of gout. Patients with adrenal insufficiency usually have no specific signs associated with chronic Addison's disease and may present only with unexplained hypotension and fever not responsive to volume replacement. Similarly, drug fever is not usually associated with specific findings unless rash is present. The rash associated with drug fevers is usually maculopapular but may be petechial, is usually trunkal, and may involve the palms and the soles. The rash may or may not be pruritic and resolves upon discontinuation of the offending "sensitizing" medication. In severe reactions to drugs, other cutaneous manifestations may be present, i.e., erythema nodosum, erythema multiforme, or Stevens-Johnson syndrome. However, in most cases of hospital-acquired fever caused by medications the physical findings are conspicuously absent.

Diagnostic Studies

LABORATORY TESTS

The history and physical examination point to the diagnosis in some cases of hospital-acquired fever, but the majority of infectious and noninfectious cases are dependent upon laboratory tests for a precise diagnosis. General screening laboratory tests are of little help in the diagnosis of hospital-acquired fever. Specific abnormalities of the hemogram that may be useful include the finding of leukopenia, which suggests the presence of a viral cause especially if found in association with atypical lymphocytes, i.e., HBV, NANB, or CMV.

An increase in the white blood cell count is a nonspecific finding and is of little diagnostic usefulness. Importantly, noninfectious disease, e.g., drug fever, may be associated with an increase in white count with a shift to the left, thereby mimicking an infectious process.

Routine urinalysis would be expected to be abnormal in cases of pyelonephritis, in which bacteriuria and pyuria are invariably present.

Abnormal liver function tests, i.e., slightly elevated transaminases and/or alkaline phosphatase, suggest the presence of drug fever or postperfusion syndrome caused by CMV, Legionella pneumophilia or Legionella-like organisms. Profound elevations of liver enzymes suggest halothane-associated hepatitis or viral hepatitis caused by HPV or NANB.

More specific tests, if ordered, may point to a specific etiologic diagnosis. For example, the finding of a depressed serum phosphorus in a patient with nosocomial pneumonia should immediately suggest Legionella pneumophilia or a Legionella-like organism (in the absence of other causes of hypophosphatemia). An elevated serum calcium associated with eosinophilia in a patient who was hypotensive would suggest adrenal insufficiency. An elevated serum uric acid level may suggest acute gout or myocardial infarction (serum uric acid levels are usually normal or depressed in acute gouty attacks).

The presence of fibrin split products (FSP) with an

elevated ESR suggests occult pulmonary microemboli. A very high elevation of the ESR would suggest pneumonia, pyelonephritis, endocarditis, osteomyelitis, pulmonary emboli, postpericardiotomy syndrome, or drug fever. To increase its diagnostic specificity, the ESR must be paired with other diagnostic findings. For example, an ESR of greater than 100 mm/hour associated with eosinophilia strongly suggests the presence of drug fever. A very high ESR in association with abnormal liver function tests suggests postperfusion syndrome or viral hepatitis. Clearly, adrenal function tests will be needed to confirm or rule out adrenal insufficiency; ECG and cardiac enzymes are needed to rule out myocardial infarction; a greatly elevated ESR with splinter hemorrhages suggests postpericardiotomy syndrome or endocarditis.

Examination of the stool for fecal leukocytes in a patient with diarrhea acquired in the hospital suggests C. difficile colitis that may or may not be associated with the use of antibiotics. C. difficile toxin titers confirm the diagnosis of antibiotic-associated colitis.

Throat culture for bacteria/viruses confirms the presence of pharyngitis as the cause of fever. Culture of sputum from patients on respiratory support equipment or with tracheostomies reflects colonization of the upper respiratory tract infection rather than of lower respiratory tract pathogens. Culture of purulent drainage from a wound confirms the diagnosis of wound infection. Culture of a draining sinus tract from chronic osteomyelitis reflects skin flora, and culture of bone biopsy material is usually required to determine the pathogen involved in chronic osteomyelitis. Culture of the urine for bacteria and association with the appropriate clinical syndrome makes the diagnosis of pyelonephritis. Negative culture of the cerebrospinal fluid following craniotomy with the presence of red blood cells in the cerebrospinal fluid makes the diagnosis of posterior fossa syndrome.

Positive blood cultures usually signify bacteremia. The clinician must first differentiate false positive blood cultures caused by contamination of the needle, syringe, or blood culture bottle during the blood culture drawing process. Also, the clinician should suspect the diagnosis of pseudobacteremia if the patient's clinical syndrome is inconsistent with the disease caused by the blood culture isolates.

Excluding contaminates and pseudobacteremia, positive blood cultures, by isolating the organism, may provide assistance in localizing the origin of the infection. Aerobic gram-negative rods are frequently recovered in the blood in hospital-acquired pneumonia, pyelonephritis, or IV line infections. Transient bacteremia accompanied by a single temperature spike may follow invasive diagnostic procedures, especially those of the abdominal or GU tract. Persistent high-grade bacteremia suggests endocarditis or IV line infection. Negative blood cultures in a patient with relative bradycardia and abnormal liver function tests limit diagnostic possibilities to Legionella infection and drug fever. Gram-positive bacteremia caused by Staphylococci suggests IV line infection, osteomyelitis, or acute endocarditis. Enterococcal bacteremia points to the biliary tract or urinary tract and to a lesser extent to the abdomen or pelvis. Enterococcal bacteremia in the absence of other organisms usually suggests a urinary tract source. Polymicrobial bacteremia including enterococci usually suggests a biliary or intra-abdominal or pelvic focus of infection.

Device-associated bacteremia is an important cause of hospital-acquired fever (Table 5–19). Intravenous catheter sepsis is suggested by recovery of Staphylococci, gram-negative bacilli, aerobic bacilli, enterococci, or Candida from the blood and by semiquantitative catheter tip cultures. The recovery of unusual organisms in blood culture in one or more patients suggests infusion-related sepsis. Culture of the infusion fluid suggests intrinsic infusion-related sepsis. Importantly, such contaminated fluids are not turbid, and those particularly suspect are glucose-containing fluids or fat emulsions used in hyperalimentation. Extrinsic-related sepsis is suggested by negative catheter tip and infusate cultures. All line-related medications, disinfectants, and flushing solutions and the hands of intensive care personnel should be cultured for the pathogens isolated from the blood.

RADIOLOGIC STUDIES

Radiological tests are helpful in relatively few causes of hospital-acquired fever. The chest x-ray is essential in the diagnosis of nosocomial pneumonias. Unfortunately, most hematogenously acquired gram-negative nosocomial pneumonias have a nonspecific x-ray appearance. These pneumonias are usually symmetrical lower lobe processes with or without cavitation or other distinguishing features. Legionella pneumonia is characterized by some degree of asymmetry and rapid progression, usually without cavitation. Blunting of the costophrenic angle may suggest pulmonary infarction, heart failure secondary to myocardial infarction, or postpericardiotomy syndrome. Bone x-rays may reveal the presence of long-standing osteomyelitis but are unhelpful in acute osteomyelitis of less than 2 weeks' duration. Plane film of the abdomen may reveal impending toxic megacolon from antibiotic-associated diarrhea or show small shrunken kidneys caused by pre-existing chronic pyelonephritis. Echocardiography of the heart may reveal vegetation suggesting endocarditis. Intra-abdominal or pelvic ab-

Table 5–19. Device-associated Sepsis

Type of Line Infection	Lab/Clinical Clues
Pseudobacteremia	Clustering of unusual organisms in blood culture Patient not clinically bacteremic Blood culture isolates don't match clinical setting
Intravenous/intra-arterial line sepsis	Patient clinically bacteremic without source of bacteremia Recovery of staphylococci, aerobic gram-negative bacilli, enterococci, or Candida from blood Blood culture isolate same as semiquantitative catheter tip culture Access site inflamed/infected or may be infected
Infusion-related sepsis (intrinsic)	Patient bacteremic without another source of bacteremia Semiquantitative catheter tip culture negative No associated phlebitis/cellulitis at access site Infusion fluid not turbid Glucose-containing fluids/fat emulsions particularly suspect Infusate isolates same as blood isolates Clustering of "unusual organisms" in blood culture
Infusion-related sepsis (extrinsic)	Same as intrinsic infusion-related sepsis except culture of infusate fluid negative Culture all line-related disinfectants, medications, flushing solutions, etc., and hands of appropriate ICU personnel

(Adapted from Cunha, B.A.: Intravascular line infections. Infec Dis Pract 8:1–7, 1985.)

scess may be localized with ultrasonography, gallium scan, or CT scan.

Diagnostic Approach

Some causes of hospital-acquired fever are obvious from the history and physical examination; hospital-acquired pharyngitis, diarrhea, transfusion reaction, acute gouty attack, or wound infection are all relatively straightforward. The cause of hospital-acquired fever can usually be determined by focusing diagnostic attention on the most frequent disease entities, i.e., IV line infections, nosocomial pneumonias, wound infections or abscesses, and drug fevers. Other diagnoses should be suspected when the obvious causes are not found; usually there are specific clues to both the infectious and noninfectious causes of fever from the history, physical examination, and laboratory tests.

The clinician should look at the most frequent sites of possible infection as a cause for the hospital-acquired fever. The use of intravenous lines, especially if in place longer than 72 hours, suggests device-associated infection as the cause of fever. CVA tenderness points immediately to pyelonephritis, whereas pleuritic chest pain suggests nosocomial pneumonia, pulmonary infarction, or postpericardiotomy syndrome.

The diagnosis of hosspital-acquired pneumonia depends upon the demonstration of an infiltrate compatible with a bacterial pneumonia and the presence of fever. Such patients typically develop their infiltrates after a week or more in the hospital. Although sputum cultures are notoriously unreliable in the diagnosis of pneumonia, blood cultures may be positive in a mi-

nority of patients and may provide important bacteriologic information, albeit retrospectively. A chest x-ray should be obtained to confirm or rule out nosocomial pneumonia.

The postpartum patient with B. fragilis bacteremia and nodular densities on chest x-ray and a fever in excess of 102° F is likely to have pelvic septic thrombophlebitis. Bland pulmonary emboli from the lower extremities are associated with fevers of less than 102° F. Painless myocardial infarction may be suspected from a rise in fever to less than 102° F accompanied by a simultaneous increase in white count and ESR. Persistent bacteremia in the absence of an explainable source suggests an intravascular infection, e.g., endocarditis, until proven otherwise. Wound infections rarely cause high-grade fevers and usually do not exceed 102° F. Intra-abdominal abscess may be suggested by the occurrence of a fever 1 to 2 weeks following surgery with an increase in the ESR. Any intrathoracic abdominal or pelvic procedure will transiently raise the ESR, which promptly falls following the surgical procedure but may not become entirely normal for weeks or months. Therefore, the abrupt increase in the ESR following serially declining sedimentation rates postoperatively suggests abscess or drug fever. Patients with pelvic abscesses may look particularly "well," as do patients with drug fever. Localization of intra-abdominal abscesses is usually confirmed by indirect radiologic means, e.g., CT scan or ultrasonography.

Drug fever is a common cause of hospital-acquired fever and is suggested by the presence of negative blood cultures (excluding contaminates or pseudobac-

Table 5–20. Clinical Features of Drug Fevers

History

Some individuals are atopic
May have been on "sensitivity medication" for days/years

Physical Exam

Low- to high-grade fevers
Relative bradycardia with temperature greater than 102° F
Look "inappropriately well" for degree of fever
Rash (uncommon), usually maculopapular (occasionally with a
  petechial component); central, and may involve the palms/soles

Laboratory Tests

Elevated WBC count (usually with left shift)
Eosinophilia (low-grade) uncommon (less than 20%)
Elevated erythrocyte sedimentation rate in majority of cases (may
  be very rapid 60 to greater than 100 mm/hour)
Elevated IgE levels (transiently)
Mild elevation of alkaline phosphatase/serum transaminases (greater
  than 90%)

teremias) in a patient looking inappropriately "well" for the degree of fever (Table 5–20). If the temperature is ≤102° F, relative bradycardia is nearly always present and strongly suggests the diagnosis. The presence of abnormal liver function tests in such a patient is further evidence for a diagnosis of drug fever. Only 20% of patients with drug fever will have a low-grade eosinophilia (less than 5% of total WBC). However, the presence of low-grade eosinophilia associated with abnormal liver function tests and an elevated sedimentation rate provides the basis for making the presumptive diagnosis of drug fever. IgE levels may be transiently elevated in patients with drug fever. The diagnosis may be confirmed by sensitizing medications; the fever promptly disappears within 72 hours unless a rash is present. A hospital-acquired fever and rash almost invariably suggests a drug fever. The clinician may be further confused by hypersensitivity

reactions caused by drugs, since an increase in the white count with a shift to a left frequently accompanies drug reactions. The clinician is further misled by not appreciating that practically all medications may be associated with drug hypersensitivity reactions. Easily overlooked as a cause of drug fever are sleep medications, pain medications, diuretics, antiarrhythmics, and stool softeners, which have all been implicated in hypersensitivity reactions (Table 5–21) The only medications not associated with drug fever include parenteral multivitamin preparations, steroids, digoxin, and birth control pills. All antibiotics may cause hypersensitivity reactions, but particularly sulfonamides, penicillin derivatives, and cephalosporins are associated with drug fevers. Antibiotics not associated with drug fevers include aminoglycosides, erythromycin, the tetracyclines, clindamycin, chloramphenicol, and vancomycin.

Postperfusion syndrome, mild hepatitis, and postpericardiotomy syndrome are frequent diagnostic considerations in patients who had thoracotomy or open heart surgery. Postperfusion syndrome caused by CMV usually occurs 30 to 40 days following a surgical procedure and is characterized by a mild mononucleosis-like illness with atypical lymphocytes, abnormal liver function tests, mild pharyngitis, posterior cervical adenopathy, or splenomegaly.

Patients with transient bacteremias usually have a single temperature spike from 103 to 105° F, with shaking chills but no other localizing signs or symptoms.

In addition to obtaining blood cultures, a careful search should be made for the event associated with the bacteremia. For example, manipulation or irrigation of a Foley catheter, a wound, or nasotracheal suction or irrigation may all be associated with single fever spikes and may be difficult to analyze unless the

Table 5–21. Sensitizing Medications

Common Sensitizers	Uncommon Sensitizers	Very Rare Sensitizers
Antibiotics*	All others	Digoxin
Sleep medications		Steroids
Antiseizure medications		Diphenhydramine
Stool softeners		(Benadryl)
Diuretics		Aspirin
Antihypertensives		Vitamins
Antidepressants/tranquilizers		Aminoglycosides
Antiarrhythmics		Tetracycline
Nonsteroidal anti-inflammatory drugs		Erythromycin
		Clindamycin
		Chloramphenicol
		Vancomycin

*Exceptions are listed under "Very Rare"
(Adapted from Cunha, B.A.: Fever: Significance in the Hospital Setting. *In* The Theory and Practice of Infection Control. Edited by I. Gurevich, P. Tafuro, and B.A. Cunha. New York, Praeger Publishing, 1984, p. 173.)

chart is carefully read for documentation of these procedures. The patient with an indwelling Foley catheter who is febrile presents a difficult diagnostic problem for the clinician. The problem is compounded when culture of the urine reveals a microorganism known to be a uropathogen, e.g., one of the gram-negative aerobic bacilli. Fever in a catheterized patient who is a normal host should not be ascribed to urinary catheterization, because catheter-associated bacteriuria results in pyelonephritis, bacteremia, or fever in excess of 102° F only if the patient is an immunocompromised host, has pre-existing renal disease, or has partial or total obstruction. Compromised hosts with diabetes or SLE or on steroids may develop pyelonephritis or bacteremia from cystitis with little or no febrile response. The source of bacteremia is correctly traced to the urinary tract in these patients predisposed to urosepsis.

FEVER IN THE COMPROMISED HOST

DEFINITION

The term "compromised host" is used to describe patients with a qualitative or quantitative defect in one or more defense mechanisms. Defects in the immune system may be either congenital or, more frequently, acquired. When clinicians use the term "compromised hosts," they are usually referring to the subset of patients that are febrile and leukopenic. Chronic lymphatic leukemia, the lymphomas, Acquired Immune Deficiency Syndrome, and the acute leukemias are all associated with specific immune defects. When such patients are treated with chemotherapeutic agents, the diseases associated with neutropenia are superimposed on the underlying host defense defects. For this reason, patients with these disorders usually encountered in the hospital setting receiving chemotherapy are referred to as "leukopenic compromised hosts."

Patients with neoplastic and non-neoplastic conditions that are associated with non-specific immune defects may be referred to as "nonleukopenic compromised hosts." Such patients are those with diabetes, patients with SLE, those on steroid therapy, alcoholic patients, patients with uremia, asplenic individuals, patients with sarcoidosis, patients of advanced age, and patients with multiple myeloma. (Although a multiple myeloma is a neoplastic disease, it has been grouped with the other benign entities because it shares similar defects in host defense mechanisms.)

PATHOPHYSIOLOGIC CONSIDERATIONS

The majority of compromised patients become infected from their endogenous flora. The clinical presentation of the infectious disease process is predictable based upon specific immune defects. Exogenous introduction of organisms acquired in the hospital as the result of invasive devices or procedures also frequently occurs in the compromised hosts.

Understanding the underlying immune defects is critical to predicting the likely infecting organisms and their clinical expression (Table 5–22). For instance, a decrease in neutrophils to less than 1000 cells cu/mm (leukopenia) is associated with infections caused by Staphylococcus aureus, enteric bacilli, Pseudomonas aeruginosa, or fungi (Candida, Aspergillus, etc.). Defects in the T-lymphocytes/macrophage axis are associated with infections caused by intracellular pathogens, such as Listeria, Salmonella, Nocardia, Mycobacteria, and Legionella. Patients with this defect are also frequently infected by obligate intracellular microorganisms—(Cryptococcus, Candida, Histoplasma, etc.), parasites (Pneumocystis, Toxoplasma, or Strongyloides), or viruses (herpes simplex, varicella-zoster, or cytomegalovirus).

In contradistinction, patients with hypogammaglobulinemia secondary to B-lymphocyte defects have difficulty eliminating encapsulated pathogens, i.e., the pneumococci, Hemophilus influenzae, etc. Congenitally acquired complement deficiencies are associated with recurrent or disseminated neisserial infections. Asplenic individuals are particularly prone to infections by pneumonococci, Hemophilus influenzae, or meningococcus. Nonleukopenic compromised hosts usually have a qualitative defect in some phase of neutrophil function, i.e., chemotaxis, opsonization, or phagocytosis, and are particularly susceptible to infection by pneumococci, Hemophilus influenzae, and, to a lesser extent, enteric gram-negative bacilli.

Conversely, by knowing which diseases are associated with which immune defects, the clinician can anticipate the usual pathogens in a given situation (Table 5–22). A patient with acute myelogenous leukemia (AML) rendered leukopenic by chemotherapy is predisposed to infections caused by an inadequate number of neutrophils. Patients with lymphomas, sarcoidosis, or AIDS have defects in T-lymphocyte and macrophage function and are predictably susceptible to intracellular pathogens. Multiple myeloma (MM) is classically associated with defects in B-lymphocyte function, and chronic lymphatic leukemia (CLL) is

Table 5–22. Immune Defects Associated with Microorganisms and Diseases

Immune Defect	Diseases	Bacteria	Fungi	Microorganisms Parasites	Viruses
Neutrophil (PMN)	Acute myelogenous leukemia	S. aureus Enteric bacilli Pseudomonas aeruginosa	Candida Aspergillus Mucor		
T-lymphocyte/ macrophage	Hodgkin's/ non-Hodgkin's lymphoma AIDS Sarcoidosis	Listeria Salmonella Nocardia Mycobacteria Legionella pneumophilia Corynebacteria	Cryptococcus Candida Histoplasma Coccidioides	Pneumocystis Toxoplasma Strongyloides	Herpes simplex Herpes zoster varicella Cytomegalovirus Adenovirus
B-lymphocyte	Multiple myeloma Chronic lymphatic leukemia	S. pneumoniae H. influenzae Enteric bacilli		Pneumocystis Giardia	Echovirus
Complement	Congenital defects	Neisseria			
Asplenia		S. pneumoniae H. influenzae Neisseria			

associated with a combined B-lymphocyte/T-lymphocyte defect, with T-lymphocyte dysfunction usually more severely depressed than B-lymphocyte function. Patients with sickle cell anemia, those staging laparotomies for lymphoma, or those who have had traumatic loss of the spleen all suffer from anatomic or functional asplenia.

Similarly, the physician must consider the clinical expression of the microorganism based on the association between the microorganism and a specific immune defect (Table 5–22). For example, patients with B-lymphocyte defects are predisposed to infections by pneumococcus or Hemophilus influenzae, which usually manifest clinically as bacteremia, pneumonia, or meningitis. Hence, patients presenting with B-lymphocyte defects should be carefully evaluated for these infections. In contrast, gastroenteritis developing in such patients should not be ascribed to B-lymphocyte dysfunction because neither pneumococcus nor Hemophilus influenzae causes gastroenteritis; a careful search should be made for Giardia, however (Table 5–22).

DIFFERENTIAL DIAGNOSIS

Nonleukopenic Compromised Hosts. Specific organ involvement in patients with predictable immune defects quickly limits diagnostic possibilities to a limited number of microorganisms (Table 5–23). Most nonleukopenic compromised hosts present with evidence of bacteremia, pneumonia, meningitis, or urosepsis. Skin infections caused by Candida may occur

Table 5–23. Infection in Nonleukopenic Compromised Hosts with Diminished Neutrophil Function

Bacterial infections
  Organisms
    S. pneumoniae
    H. influenzae
    Enteric bacilli (especially Klebsiella)
  Type of infections
    Bacteremias
    Pneumonias
    Meningitis
    Urinary tract infections
Fungal infections
  Organisms
    Candida
    Mucor
  Type of infections
    Candida (fungemias, urinary tract infections, skin infections)
    Mucor (rhinocerebral mucormycosis, pneumonia)

fairly frequently in such patients, especially in patients with diabetes or on steroids.

Patients with alcoholic liver disease and cirrhosis usually present with bacteremia secondary to neutrophil dysfunction, as well as with a decrease in the "filter function" of the reticuloendothelial system of the liver. Alcoholic patients with ascites may present with abdominal tenderness resulting from spontaneous bacterial peritonitis caused by common aerobic gram-negative bacilli or pneumococci.

Patients with SLE are predisposed to eye infections (panophthalmitis), pneumonia, or urosepsis. The febrile patient with SLE may be particularly difficult to evaluate since lupus cerebritis may mimic bacterial meningitis, lupus pneumonitis may mimic bacterial pneumonia, vasculitic involvement of the right upper quadrant commonly may mimic cholecystitis, and attacks of acute abdominal pain may suggest a surgical abdomen with bacterial peritonitis.

Diabetic patients are particularly prone to skin infections of the lower extremities and to urinary tract infections, but these usually present no diagnostic difficulties.

Sepsis in a patient with uremia may be particularly difficult to assess because these patients are often afebrile or hypothermic and infrequently have positive blood cultures. However, until proven otherwise, urosepsis should be the presumptive working diagnosis in all uremic patients.

Sarcoidosis is, in general, an afebrile disease. Fever in a patient with sarcoidosis suggests meningeal sarcoidosis, extensive granulomatous involvement of the liver, or uveal/parotoid involvement (Heerfordt's syndrome). If the patient has none of these variants of sarcoidosis associated with fever, a careful search should be made for tuberculosis, which frequently occurs in these patients. Patients with sarcoidosis not infrequently have Nocardia infections, which are frequently manifest as a pulmonary infiltrate or a CNS mass lesion. Asplenic patients frequently die of overwhelming sepsis; death may occur within hours after the infection is clinically manifested. Less frequently pneumonitis or meningitis may be the presenting manifestation of infection in asplenic individuals.

Patients with multiple myeloma usually present with urinary tract infections, pneumonitis, or bacteremia. Renal dysfunction secondary to "myeloma kidney" anatomically predisposes such patients to the usual uropathogens. Occasionally, patients with multiple myeloma may present with gastroenteritis secondary to giardiasis or echovirus infection.

Leukopenic Compromised Hosts. Leukopenic compromised hosts in the traditional sense include infected patients already affected by the acute leukemias, CLL, the lymphomas, and AIDS. The immune defects in any of these patients may be compounded or extended by chemotherapy. The most frequent infectious diseases occurring in this group are bacteremia, pneumonitis, meningitis, and intra-abdominal sepsis. History, physical examination, and laboratory tests should seek to identify infection in the appropriate anatomic areas.

No meaningful diagnostic information may be obtained by the disease presentation of bacteremias because all bacteremias present in the same fashion. If a compromised host presents with meningitis, a careful analysis of the host defense defects would be helpful in the differential diagnosis (Table 5–24). Compromised hosts with defects in neutrophil numbers or function having meningitis will most likely have the common enteric gram-negative bacilli, Pseudomonas, or Bacillus species in their CSF. Fungal meningitis caused by Aspergillus, Mucor, or Candida is, unfortunately, quite common in such patients and usually occurs after weeks of hospitalization.

A compromised host with meningitis with depressed T-lymphocyte/macrophage function would be expected to have any one of the intracellular pathogens present in the cerebrospinal fluid or brain. Such individuals are frequently infected with Listeria, Nocardia, Mycobacterium avium intracellulare, Cryptococcus, Toxoplasma, Strongyloides, herpes varicella-zoster, or CMV. Nocardia and Toxoplasma characteristically present as mass lesions, e.g., brain abscess. Varicella-zoster, CMV, or toxoplasmosis may cause meningoencephalitis. B-lymphocyte dysfunction predisposes to meningitis caused by pneumococcus or Hemophilus influenzae. Patients with recurrent meningococcemia or disseminated meningococcal disease should be considered to have defects in the terminal components of complement (C6, C7, C8).

Similar analysis may be applied in compromised hosts presenting with pulmonary infiltrates (Table

Table 5–24. Meningitis in the Compromised Host

Immune Defect	Bacteria	Fungi	Parasites	Viruses
Neutrophil (PMN)	Enteric bacilli Pseudomonas Bacillus	Aspergillus Mucor Candida		
T-lymphocyte/macrophage	Listeria Nocardia* Mycobacterium avium intracellulare	Cryptococcus	Toxoplasma* Strongyloides	Varicella zoster† Cytomegalovirus‡
B-lymphocyte	S. pneumoniae H. influenzae			Echovirus
Complement	Neisseria			
Asplenia	S. pneumoniae H. influenzae			Echovirus

* = abscess; † = meningoencephalitis; ‡ = encephalitis

Table 5–25. Pneumonia in the Compromised Host

Immune Defect	Bacteria	Fungi	Parasites	Viruses
Neutrophil (PMN)	S. pneumoniae S. aureus Klebsiella E. coli Pseudomonas Bacillus	Aspergillus Candida Mucor		
T-lymphocyte/macrophage	Nocardia Legionella pneumophilia Mycobacteria Corynebacteria Chlamydia	Cryptococcus Histoplasma Coccidioides Blastomyces	Pneumocystis Toxoplasma Strongyloides	Cytomegalovirus Varicella-zoster Adenovirus
B-lymphocyte	S. pneumoniae H. influenzae Neisseria			
Complement	S. pneumoniae H. influenzae Neisseria			
Asplenia	S. pneumoniae H. influenzae Neisseria			

5–25). Diseases associated with leukopenia are manifest as pneumonia secondary to gram-negative bacilli, Aspergillus, Candida, or Mucor. Pneumonia in a patient with T-lymphocyte/macrophage dysfunction may occur from infection by Nocardia, Legionella pneumophilia, Mycobacteria, Chlamydia, Cryptococcus, Histoplasma, Coccidioides, Blastomyces, Pneumocystis, Toxoplasma, Strongyloides, CMV, or varicella-zoster. Patients with B-lymphocyte dysfunction have no difficulties with intracellular pathogens, but are predisposed to pneumococcal or Hemophilus influenzae pneumonia. Similar pathogens are present in asplenic patients presenting with pneumonitis.

Any compromised host presenting with intra-abdominal sepsis usually has the infection as a result of perforation secondary to endogenous organisms (Table 5–26). Chemotherapy frequently causes multiple ulcers of the gastrointestinal tract that may be manifest as bacteremia or fungemia. If these ulcerations progress in the presence of thrombocytopenia to perforation, the presentation is that of intra-abdominal in-

fection. In patients with neutrophil dysfunction presenting with intra-abdominal infection, gram-negative organisms, including Pseudomonas and Aeromonas hydrophilia, are frequently responsible for the intra-abdominal infection. Perforation of a necrotic tumor may result in localized or generalized Clostridial sepsis. Fungi normally residing in the gastrointestinal tract, usually Candida or Aspergillus may cause intra-abdominal infection. Intra-abdominal infection in a patient with T-lymphocyte/macrophage dysfunction may be due to Salmonella, Mycobacterium avium intracellulare, Strongyloides, Cryptospordia, Isospora, or CMV. Patients with B-lymphocyte dysfunction frequently have gastroenteritis caused by giardiasis or echoviruses.

Compromised hosts occasionally present with skin manifestations of disease. Skin lesions in all compromised hosts should be aspirated and a biopsy for Gram's stain and culture performed. Such lesions may provide the only information to make an etiologic diagnosis. Ecthyma gangrenosum usually found on the

Table 5–26. Sepsis in the Compromised Host

Immune Defect	Bacteria	Fungi	Parasites	Viruses
Neutrophil (PMN)	Enteric bacilli Pseudomonas Aeromonas hydrophila Clostridium	Candida Aspergillus Mucor		
T-lymphocyte/macrophage	Salmonella Mycobacterium avium intracellulare		Strongyloides Cryptosporidia Isospora	Cytomegalovirus Adenovirus
B-lymphocyte		Giardia		Echovirus

axilla or groin is usually associated with Pseudomonas but also may be due to Serratia or Aeromonas hydrophilia bacteremia. A nodular lesion in a leukemic patient should always, especially in AML, suggest the possibility of disseminated fungal disease, particularly disseminated Candidiasis. In general, in the compromised host, nodular or ulcerative lesions that contain fungi on microscopic examination always suggest a disseminated rather than a localized disease. Furthermore, severely neutropenic patients frequently present with polymicrobial infections of the mouth or perianal area. In the presence of neutropenia, signs of inflammation are subtle or nonexistent, and evidence of peritonitis as well as ischiorectal or perirectal abscess should be carefully sought.

In the leukopenic compromised host, the clinical manifestation of infection is frequently subtle or atypical, and the clinician must be extremely careful in assessing relatively minor changes in features such as mental status, the chest x-ray, temperature, skin lesions, abdominal pain, and sore throat that would be of little significance in a noncompromised individual but may be of great significance in a leukopenic compromised host.

DIAGNOSTIC EVALUATION

Patient History

Patients that are nonleukopenic compromised hosts, i.e., those that are elderly or on steroids or have cirrhosis, uremia, diabetes, SLE, or sarcoidosis, usually report some history of organ dysfunction associated with the disease or report that they had a particular disorder in the past. It is important to determine if the patient has a particular disease entity associated with qualitative immune defects so that clinical presentation may be predicted on the basis of the host defense defect.

Patients with diabetes, elderly patients, or those on steroids usually have few complaints revealed in the history, whereas patients with uremia, SLE, multiple myeloma, asplenia, or recurrent Neisserial infections usually provide historical clues to their illness. Patients with previously undiagnosed uremia may complain of paresthesias in the "stocking/glove" distribution of the extremities, a metallic taste in the mouth, unexplained abdominal pain, or general malaise. Patients with SLE usually give a complex history of poorly localized bouts of pain in various organ systems reflecting multisystem vasculitic involvement of the disease. The patient may complain of sensitivity to light, hair loss, rash, arthralgias or myalgias, mouth ulcers, or numbness in the extremities. A patient with pre-

viously undiagnosed sarcoidosis may present with an acute febrile illness and may complain of parotid swelling or eye pain or dryness. Shortness of breath, with or without a nonproductive cough, and persistent nasal stuffiness may suggest the diagnosis. Bone pain, fatigue, or uremic symptoms may be experienced by the patient with undiagnosed multiple myeloma. Patients with chronic meningococcemia or gonococcemia complain of periodic attacks of fever associated with arthralgias or myalgias and have pustular skin lesions on the extremities. Asplenic individuals give a history of surgical removal of the spleen or a disease that results in functional asplenia, e.g., sickle cell anemia.

Leukopenic compromised hosts presenting with an undiagnosed malignancy and fever provide few, if any, historical clues. Patients with acute leukemia may complain of easy fatigability or tendency to bruise, bone pain, or a history of bleeding following a minor dental or surgical procedure. Patients with a chronic lymphatic leukemia may notice diffuse adenopathy or complain of early satiety resulting from massive splenomegaly. Patients with lymphoma may have noticed a previously unrecognized "lump" and may complain of night sweats, weight loss, easy fatigability, or pruritus following a hot bath. The AIDS patient may provide a history of homosexual or bisexual behavior, intravenous drug abuse, close contact with an AIDS patient, or exposure to the secretions of a patient with AIDS, i.e., health care work (for example, from needle stick exposure). Skin lesions (Kaposi's sarcoma) may be reported as the initial manifestations of AIDS in some patients, while others will report a history of severe oral or genital Candida or herpes infection that is resistant to the usual therapeutic modalities. A patient with AIDS may also complain of profound weight loss and profuse diarrhea, as well as shortness of breath or mental status changes.

In summary, most compromised hosts present with an unknown disease with fever. The historical clues may be useful in diagnosing the disease in the patient on initial presentation. However, once the patient has been diagnosed, for example, as having AML, there are usually few clues from the history to assist in narrowing diagnostic possibilities.

Physical Examination

Nonleukopenic compromised hosts usually present with fairly predictable pathogens based on their immune defect. Usually the clinician's attention is directed to the lungs or the CNS as the focus of the infectious process.

Bacteremias or urinary tract infections usually present with nonspecific features, i.e., shaking chills or dysuria. Cultures of the blood and urine are taken to provide precise etiologic information regarding the infecting organism.

Pneumonias are usually due to pneumococcus or Hemophilus influenzae but may also be caused by a variety of gram-negative organisms. Both pneumococcus and Hemophilus influenzae present most frequently as right lower lobe infiltrates or segmental defects. Although neither organism frequently produces cavitation, Hemophilus influenzae is associated with a small pleural effusion. Enteric gram-negative organisms are frequently associated with cavitation or empyema and begin primarily as unilateral or bilateral lower lobe pneumonias.

Legionella or Legionella-like organisms may occur in any patient but are present particularly in nonleukopenic compromised hosts. Infection with Legionella may mimic the usual bacterial pneumonias, but is characterized by extrapulmonary manifestations and rapid progression on the chest x-ray. Patients with Legionella infections usually complain of nonspecific abdominal pain or headache; mental confusion may be noticed by a friend or relative. Relative bradycardia is a reliable finding, and usually liver function tests are abnormal, the CPK is elevated, and the serum phosphorus is depressed.

Meningitis in compromised, nonleukopenic patients may be produced by the same pathogens causing pneumonitis. Pneumococcal meningitis tends to be more fulminant than Hemophilus influenzae meningitis, but otherwise the presentations are clinically indistinguishable. A definitive diagnosis may be made by analysis of CSF fluid obtained by lumbar puncture. Gram's stain and culture is the preferred technique, but CIE of the cerebrospinal fluid, blood cultures, or urinary antigen tests may provide additional useful information.

Physical findings in the nonleukopenic compromised host group relate to organ system involvement associated with the underlying disease. Since such patients present primarily with bacteremia, meningitis, pneumonia, or urosepsis, they have central nervous system or pulmonary symptoms.

Patients with sarcoidosis may have evidence of uveitis, parotid gland enlargement, skin changes (erythema nodosum), or cranial nerve abnormalities (CN VII palsy). Massive bilateral hilar adenopathy on physical examination may be manifested as a positive d'Espine's sign, but otherwise signs of consolidation or fluid in the chest are absent, though dry crackling rales may be heard on auscultation.

Patients with SLE are particularly difficult to diagnose because on physical examination they have few signs referable to organ system involvement. Manifestations are usually those of SLE and may readily be confused with superimposed infection. On physical examination, there is no way to determine if the lupus patient with cerebritis, acute abdominal pain, or chest pain truly has a superimposed infectious disease process.

Patients with cirrhosis usually have the stigmata of alcohol-induced liver disease and may have ascites. The presence of ascites and fever in a patient with cirrhosis suggests primary peritonitis in the absence of other diagnostic possibilities. Patients with asplenia have evidence of sickle-cell disease or a surgical scar. Patients with myeloma may have tenderness over areas of involved bone. Patients with recurrent neisserial infections will have a few pustular lesions located in the periarticular areas on the extremities. In contrast, in patients with chronic gonococcemia the lesions are asymmetrically distributed in the extremities with no particular relationship to joints.

Diabetic patients with ketoacidosis may present with rhinocerebral mucormycosis and altered mental status. Usually the patient has some degree of ophthalmoplegia and a "black patch" in the nose or oropharynx. Sinus films reveal partial or total opacity of one or more sinuses. Diagnosis is made by a punch biopsy of one of the "black patch" areas revealing invasive nonseptate hyphae in the tissue sample. Diabetic patients, as well as other nonleukopenic compromised hosts, are frequently troubled with Candida urinary tract infections, skin infections, or disseminated candidiasis. Fortunately, Candida is easily cultured from the blood, skin, and urine, and the organism is readily detected in these locations. Disseminated candidiasis may be difficult to diagnose but should be suspected in immunosuppressed hosts, particularly those on steroids or those receiving a long course of antibiotic therapy. Disseminated candidiasis is suggested by the finding of candidal enophthalmitis on retinal examination, candidal pyelonephritis, candidal skin rash, or nodules. Primary candidal pneumonia or meningitis is distinctly unusual.

The leukopenic compromised host has minimal physical findings, especially in the presence of neutropenia. Patients without few white cells have minimal evidence of inflammation on physical examination; cellulitis may appear to be particularly unimpressive but may represent life threatening infection in such patients. Ecthyma gangrenosum is usually observed in the axilla or groin but may occur anywhere, such as in the chest. Such lesions initially are reddish papules and evolve into necrotic black eschars. Ecthyma gangrenosum on physical examination suggests bacteremia by Pseudomonas, Serratia, Aeromonas, or other gram-negative organisms. Splenomegaly suggests ALL, CLL, or Hodgkin's lymphoma.

Table 5–27. Infection in Patients with Multiple Myeloma/Asplenia with Diminished B-Lymphocytic/Complement Function

Bacterial infections
  Organisms
    S. pneumoniae
    H. influenzae
    N. meningitis
  Type of infection
    Bacteremias
    Meningitis
    Pneumonias
Parasitic infections
  Organisms
    Giardia
  Type of infection
    Gastroenteritis
Viral infections
  Organisms
    Echoviruses
  Type of infection
    Gastroenteritis

Table 5–28. Infection in Patients with Acute Myelogenous Leukemia with Diminished Neutrophil Number/Function

Bacterial infections (50%)
  Organisms
    Pseudomonas, S. aureus, Klebsiella, E. coli
    JK diphtheroids, S. epidermidis
    Anaerobes not important in febrile leukopenic compromised hosts
  Type of infections common during induction of chemotherapy
    Bacteremias
    Pneumonias
Fungal infections (50%)
  Organisms
    Candida (60%)
    Aspergillus (30%)
    Mucor (10%)
  Type of infections
    Fungemias—Candida, Torula
    Esophagitis—Candida, Aspergillus
    Pneumonias—Aspergillus, Mucor, Candida
      Aspergillus (80%)
        Lung initial site (90%)
        Dissemination to any organ (50%)
        Associated sinusitis (5%)
        Aspergillus pneumonia
          Wedged shaped pulmonary infiltrate
          Pleuritic chest pain, infarction
          Nasal culture positive for Aspergillus
      Mucor (5%)
        Mimics Aspergillus (invades blood vessels)
        Lung initial site (unlike in diabetes mellitus)
        Mimics Allescheria boydii and pseudo-Allescheria boydii
          (Both resistant to amphotericin B)

On physical examination, patients with AIDS usually have evidence of oral or genital herpes or candida infection. Evidence of Kaposi's sarcoma must be looked for carefully in the physical examination, since in the mouth or between the toes, the purple papule suggestive of the disease may escape notice. Chorioretinitis caused by CMV, toxoplasmosis, or disseminated tuberculosis must also be carefully sought in the AIDS patient. Diffuse adenopathy in a febrile compromised host may suggest the presence of Waldenström's macroglobulinemia, miliary tuberculosis, SLE, or lymphoma.

With the exception of skin findings or splenomegaly/adenopathy, physical examination is infrequently helpful in determining the cause of fever in AIDS patients.

In the leukopenic compromised host the clinician is faced with the same clinical presentations as in nonleukopenic compromised individuals, but the number of diagnostic possibilities is greatly increased.

Patients with multiple myeloma or without a spleen also present with bacteremias, meningitis, or pneumonia (Table 5–27). The same general approach as described for nonleukopenic patients is useful in these patients. In addition, myeloma patients are particularly predisposed to gastroenteritis, which may be due to Giardia or one of the enteroviruses, usually echovirus. Giardiasis is suggested by the presence of belching or flatulence associated with a chronic or subacute diarrheal illness. Weight loss, malaise, and low-grade fever may accompany giardiasis. Echoviral infections may be associated with headache, aseptic meningitis, or rash, but only rarely with pneumonitis.

A patient with acute myelogenous leukemia usually presents with a bacterial or fungal infection (Table 5–28). Most patients will present with a bacteremia or fungemia or with pneumonitis. Patients with Aspergillus or Candida may present with fungal esophagitis. The general approach is to culture the blood for bacteria and fungi and to look for signs of pulmonary involvement. The patient usually presents with a diffuse, nondescript, symmetrical lower lobe pulmonary infiltrate not suggestive of any particular pathogen. As mentioned previously, both the noninfectious causes of infiltrates in these patients, i.e., leukostasis, pulmonary drug reactions, noncardiac pulmonary edema, etc., and infectious causes should be carefully considered in all such patients.

Few general statements can be made because of the wide variety of pathogens encountered, but pneumonia caused by Pseudomonas aeruginosa and Aspergillus are two of the most frequent lethal problems in patients with AML. Pseudomonas pneumonia when acquired by the hematogenous route has no distinguishing clinical features, but early and rapid cavitation may provide a clue to the diagnosis. Patients with Aspergillus pneumonitis usually have some degree of pleuritic chest pain and a pleural based, wedge shaped pulmonary infiltrate. Disseminated aspergillosis occurs in

50% of patients with aspergillus pneumonia, and the clinician should search for signs of Aspergillus infection in the CNS, skin, gastrointestinal tract, and kidneys. Nasal cultures are positive for Aspergillus in many of these patients and may provide a clue to the cause of the fungal pneumonitis.

Although Mucor occurs much less frequently than Aspergillus it invades blood vessels and mimics Aspergillus pneumonia by mimicking a pulmonary infarction. In patients with acute myelogenous leukemia, pulmonary mucor is the most frequent manifestation of mucormycosis. Rhinocerebral mucor, though associated with patients with diabetic ketoacidosis, is not seen in patients with AML. Other unusual organisms such as Allescheria or pseudo-Allescheria infections may mimic mucoid pneumonitis in these patients. Therefore, if an AML patient presents with a pulmonary infarct-like picture, fungal pneumonia caused by Aspergillus, Mucor or Allescheria should be seriously considered.

The definitive diagnosis of fungal pneumonia is made by demonstrating on biopsy tissue invasion by the fungus. The mere recovery of the organism by transbronchial biopsy, even with specially shielded catheter tips, does not provide definitive diagnostic information and usually indicates oropharyngeal or bronchial colonization. Open lung biopsy remains the preferred procedure for characterizing profuse pulmonary infiltrates in the patient with AML. Patients with acute lymphatic leukemia have many of the same problems with bacterial pathogens as the patients with AML have, but in addition have particular difficulties with viral and parasitic microorganisms. Pneumocystis carinii pneumonia is frequent in the patient with ALL, in contrast to the patient with AML (Table 5–29). The presentation may be an acute mimicking of bacterial pneumonia but more commonly presents as a weaker or slowly worsening shortness of breath, eventuating in a diffuse perihilar infiltrate on admission to the hospital. Patients with pneumocystis pneumonia have no distinguishing clinical characteristics, and the chest x-ray is unhelpful. Because Pneumocystis carinii pneumonia is not associated with localized infiltrates, pleural effusions, or cavitation, the presence of these findings with Pneumocystis carinii pneumonia indicates the presence of another organism alone or superimposed upon pneumocysitis pneumonia. Cryptococci, Legionella pneumophilia, or CMV frequently are copathogens with pneumocystis pneumonia; therefore, a localized infiltrate in a Pneumocystis patient with ALL should immediately suggest the possibility of superimposed cryptococcus. Localized herpes zoster or disseminated varicella zoster frequently complicates ALL. Diagnosis is not usually a problem, how-

Table 5–29. Infection in Patients with Acute Lymphatic Leukemia with Diminished T-Lymphocyte/Macrophage Function

Bacterial infections (50%)
  Organisms
    Pseudomonas, S. aureus, Klebsiella, E. coli
    Legionella/Legionella-like organisms
  Type of infections
    Bacteremias
    Pneumonias
Parasitic infections (25%)
  Organisms
    Pneumocystis carinii
  Type of infections
    Acute Pneumocystis pneumonia
    Subacute Pneumocystis pneumonia
Viral infections (25%)
  Organisms
    Herpes zoster, varicella zoster, (cytomegalovirus)
  Type of infections
    Herpes zoster (localized in 5%)
    Varicella zoster
      Leukopenia is a risk factor
      Bacterial suprainfection (10%)
      30% disseminate to liver, brain
    Herpes simplex virus
      Esophagitis
      Encephalitis
      Both disseminated to lungs
    Cytomegalovirus
      No distinguishing features on chest x-ray
      Always found with P. carinii
      Large intranuclear inclusions in alveolar cells

ever, because the skin is involved in both of these disorders and hence material is readily available for biopsy. It should be remembered that patients with disseminated varicella zoster not infrequently have disseminated infection involving the liver or brain. ALL patients presenting with mental confusion may have Legionella pneumophilia, hypoxemia secondary to Pneumocystis carinii, or herpes simplex encephalitis. Standard blood tests as well as analysis of the CSF fluid should clarify diagnostic possibilities. Patients with CLL may present with mass lesions of the brain caused by Nocardia, Histoplasma, or Cryptococcus. CT scan localization will be of assistance in indicating the preferred biopsy procedure for definitive diagnosis. Patients with disseminated histoplasmosis may present with tongue lesions. Patients with Nocardia or Cryptococcus may present with simultaneous involvement of the lungs and brain that may provide a clue to the diagnosis.

Abnormal liver function tests in a CLL patient with pulmonary infiltrates suggest Legionella pneumophilia, Nocardia, Histoplasma, or CMV (Table 5–30). It is worthwhile to make such assumptions to limit di-

Table 5–30.   Infection in Patients with Chronic Lymphatic Leukemia with Diminished T-Lymphocyte/Macrophage Greater than B-Lymphocyte Function

Bacterial infections
  Organisms
    Pseudomonas, S. aureus, Klebsiella, E. coli
    Hemophilus influenzae
    Nocardia
    Legionella/Legionella-like organisms
  Type of infections
    Bacteremias
    Pneumonias
    Meningitis/brain abscess
Fungal infections
  Organisms
    Histoplasma
    Cryptococcus
  Type of infections
    Pneumonia
    Meningitis
Viral infections
  Organisms
    Herpes zoster
  Type of infections
    10% disseminated disease

agnostic possibilities until a definitive diagnosis can be made by a tissue biopsy.

Patients with lymphoma, sarcoidosis, or AIDS also have a wide variety of possible presentations and pathogens. These patients represent a continuum ranging from sarcoidosis, in which the defect in T-lymphocyte macrophage function is relatively mild, to AIDS, in which T-lymphocyte function is essentially nonexistent. Patients with sarcoidosis classically have Nocardia infections involving the lung, brain, or both (Table 5–31). Such patients may also be infected with a variety of other common bacterial pathogens but are not troubled with many other infectious disorders. Patients with lymphomas are frequently infected with

Table 5–31.   Infection in Patients with Sarcoidosis with Mild T-Lymphocyte/Macrophage Dysfunction

Bacterial infections
  Organisms
    Listeria
    Legionella/Legionella-like organisms
    Nocardia
    Pneumococcus
    M. tuberculosis
  Type of infections
    Bacteremias
    Pneumonias
    Meningitis
Fungal infections
  Organisms
    Cryptococcus
  Type of infection
    Meningitis/brain abscess
    Pneumonia

Table 5–32.   Infection in Patients with Hodgkin's Lymphoma/Non-Hodgkin's Lymphoma with Moderate T-Lymphocyte/Macrophage Dysfunction

Bacterial infections (60%)
  Organisms
    Pseudomonas, S. aureus, Klebsiella, E. coli
    Listeria, Legionella/Legionella-like organisms, Nocardia
    Pneumococcus important in non-Hodgkin's lymphoma
  Type of infections
    Bacteremias
    Pneumonias
    Meningitis
Parasitic infections
  Organisms
    Toxoplasmosis
    Pneumocystis
    Babesia
    Strongyloides
  Type of infections
    Pneumonia
    Central nervous system toxoplasmosis
    Babesiosis
    "Hyperinfection syndrome" (polymicrobial bacteremias)
Fungal infections
  Organisms
    Cryptococcus
  Type of infection
    Meningitis/brain abscess
    Pneumonia
Viral infections
  Organisms
    Herpes simplex
    Cytomegalovirus
  Type of infections
    Disseminated herpes zoster
      Late in disease
      Diminished incidence of dissemination
      With non-Hodgkin's lymphoma

Listeria, Nocardia, herpes simplex, or Cryptococcus (Table 5–32). Because the association between lymphomas and the microorganism responsible is well established, it is relatively apparent where to look and on what to perform a biopsy to make a definitive diagnosis.

In contradistinction, AIDS patients may have one or more organisms or groups of organisms that may be classified as pathogens or nonpathogens (Table 5–33). AIDS patients usually present with an encephalopathic picture, pneumonitis, intractable diarrhea, skin lesions, oropharyngeal or perianal Candida or herpes infections, or high spiking fevers with diffuse adenopathy. Lesions in the area of the oropharynx are fairly straightforward and easily confirmed by culture techniques or direct immunofluorescent techniques.

Esophagitis may be due to herpes or Candida and is usually secondary to distal extension from an oropharyngeal focus. Abdominal pain suggesting peritonitis may be the result of Strongyloides bile perforation

Table 5–33. Infection in Patients with AIDS with Severe T-Lymphocyte/Macrophage Dysfunction

Bacterial infections (60%)
 Organisms
  Pseudomonas, S. aureus, Klebsiella, E. coli
  Listeria, Legionella/Legionella-like organisms, Nocardia
  Pneumococcus
  Mycobacterium avium-intracellulare, Mycobacterium
   tuberculosis
 Type of infections
  Bacteremias
  Pneumonias
  Meningitis
Parasitic infections
 Organisms
  Toxoplasmosis
  Pneumocystis
  Babesia
  Strongyloides
  Cryptosporidia/Isospora
 Type of infections
  Pneumonia
  Central nervous system toxoplasmosis
  Babesiosis
  "Hyperinfection syndrome" (polymicrobial bacteremias)
  Diarrhea
Fungal infections
 Organisms
  Cryptococcus
 Type of infection
  Meningitis/brain abscess
  Pneumonia
Viral infections
 Organisms
  Herpes simplex
  Cytomegalovirus
 Type of infection
  Disseminated herpes zoster
  Cytomegalovirus (chorioretinitis, pneumonitis, adrenalitis)

in hyperinfection syndrome, the clue to which is the association between polymicrobial bacteremia or polymicrobial meningitis and abdominal pain in an immunosuppressed patient previously harboring Strongyloides stercoralis. Since enteric organisms are so infrequently associated with meningitis, their presence in an immunosuppressed patient with AIDS should suggest disseminated strongyloidiasis until proven otherwise. Severe and protracted diarrhea in an AIDS patient suggests infection caused by Cryptosporidia, Isospora, Entamoeba histolytica, or a combination of all three. Fecal leukocytes are usually present, and except for Cryptosporidia, which requires special techniques, the organisms may be identified by standard stool parasite procedures.

Pneumonia in the AIDS patient is almost invariably due to Pneumocystis carinii. CMV usually accompanies pneumocystis in the lungs and may be associated with chorioretinitis, cerebritis, or adrenalitis in the

AIDS patient. Chorioretinitis in the AIDS patient may also be due to tuberculosis, toxoplasmosis, or fungi.

Because the laboratory tests associated with HIV-I infection do not provide information regarding opportunistic pathogens in AIDS patients, tissue biopsy is the only way to make a definitive diagnosis in AIDS patients with diffuse pulmonary infiltrates. Though CMV or herpes may be readily cultured from AIDS patients, doing so does not indicate or localize their pathogenic role in the individual patient. AIDS patients presenting with encephalitis may have meningitis caused by a variety of pathogens, meningoencephalitis, or mass lesions of an infectious or neoplastic origin. CT scans may be useful in localization of lesions for biopsy and may be of some assistance in differentiating neoplasms from brain abscess.

Analysis of cerebrospinal fluid from lumbar puncture is useful in AIDS patients with common neuropathogens, Listeria, or Cryptococcus but is unhelpful in diagnosing other organisms. Unusual primary lymphomas and tumors of the CSF are common in AIDS patients and must be differentiated from tuberculosis, toxoplasmosis, Nocardia, etc., which are frequently seen in AIDS patients. Once again, definitive diagnosis is possible only by brain biopsy in the majority of cases.

Noninfectious diseases occur in the compromised host and mimic infectious complications. Such problems are often difficult to identify particularly in patients with pulmonary infiltrates. ARDS, leukostasis, drug reaction, radiation pneumonitis, left ventricular failure, or intrapulmonary hemorrhage may all mimic an infectious pneumonia. Usually there are sufficient clues from the history, physical examination, and laboratory tests to permit an accurate diagnosis, although invasive procedures may occasionally be necessary to rule out an infectious cause.

Diagnostic Studies

LABORATORY TESTS

In nonleukopenic compromised hosts, routine laboratory tests often provide important diagnostic information to the nature of the disorder and its severity. Abnormal urinalysis may suggest the diagnosis of sarcoidosis, SLE, diabetes mellitus, or uremia. A white blood cell count may reveal leukopenia, which is frequently associated with SLE or alcoholic liver disease. Leukocytosis is a nonspecific finding and provides little diagnostic information. Eosinophilia or basophilia may be associated with sarcoidosis. Thrombocytopenia frequently occurs in association with alcoholic liver disease or SLE. Thrombocytosis suggests a variety of chronic diseases but may provide a useful clue pointing to the presence of occult bleeding, asplenia, or tuberculosis. Protein electrophoresis may reveal hypergammaglobulinemia in sarcoidosis and AIDS. Polyclonal gammopathies may occur in chronic liver disease as well.

In febrile leukopenic compromised hosts, routine diagnostic tests are rarely helpful. Hemogram may suggest the presence of a hematologic malignancy. Eosinophilia or basophilia may be associated with myeloproliferative diseases, the chronic leukemias, or the lymphomas. Thrombocytosis without another cause, such as a chronic infection, suggests a malignancy until proven otherwise. T_4/T_8 helper/suppressor ratios will be depressed in many acute infectious disease processes and are permanently depressed in patients with AIDS.

In all febrile leukopenic compromised hosts, blood cultures for bacteria and fungi should be carried out. Skin lesion, e.g., nodules or ecthyma gangrenosum, should be aspirated and a biopsy performed for Gram's stain, special stains, and culture. The finding of pseudohyphes in the aspirate of a nodule in a patient with AML may be the only clue suggesting disseminated candidiasis. Urosepsis in such patients is easily diagnosed by culture of the urine for the usual aerobic gram-negative pathogens or gram-positive cocci.

If the patient presents with meningitis, lumbar puncture should be performed unless specifically contraindicated. The CSF should be cultured for bacteria and fungi, and the latex agglutination tests for cryptococci should be carried out on all patients. Culture of the sputum is rarely helpful in such patients with pneumonitis, since cultures frequently reveal colonizing organisms rather than true pathogens. Diarrhea in such patients suggests Clostridium difficile mediated colitis. C difficile colitis, which may be diagnosed by toxin assay of the stool, may occur in cancer patients receiving chemotherapy or, more frequently, in patients receiving antibiotics. In patients with AIDS, the clinician should carefully search for Isospora and Cryptosporidia.

RADIOLOGIC STUDIES

A nonleukopenic compromised host usually has pulmonary infiltrates through an infectious origin that can be predicted from the specific immune defect associated with the underlying disease. In contradistinction, febrile leukopenic compromised hosts with pulmonary infiltrates are a difficult diagnostic challenge. Many noninfectious and infectious diseases produce nonspecific patterns on conventional chest x-ray, and noninfectious diseases mimic infectious complications. Such problems are often difficult to perceive, particularly in patients with pulmonary infiltrates. ARDS,

leukostasis, drug reactions, radiation pneumonitis, left ventricular failure, or intrapulmonary hemorrhage may all mimic an infectious pneumonia. Usually there are sufficient clues from the history, physical examination, and laboratory tests to permit an accurate diagnosis, but occasionally invasive procedures may be necessary to rule out an infectious origin. Leukopenic compromised hosts may have an infiltrate caused by a drug reaction, further proliferation of the underlying malignancy, secondary malignancy, metastasis to the lung, or infections caused by opportunistic organisms. Multiple immune defects in such patients predisposed to a wide variety of organisms makes the diagnosis by chest x-ray virtually impossible.

In general, localized pulmonary infiltrates are more likely than diffuse infiltrates to be infected. Localized infiltrates may be due to pulmonary hemorrhage or infarction or more commonly to some infectious disease process. Diffuse infiltrates are the most difficult to diagnosis because of the many noninfectious diseases that they mimic.

Drug reactions produce bilateral symmetrical infiltrates, as do cardiac-pulmonary edema, leukemic infiltration or lymphangiectatic spread of carcinoma, or adult respiratory distress syndrome. Intracellular pathogens such as Pneumocystis carinii, CMV, miliary tuberculosis, and invasive fungi (particularly Aspergillus or Candida) also usually present as bilateral symmetrical infiltrates.

The presence of a pleural effusion in the compromised host suggests Legionella pneumophilia, Nocardia, or actinomycosis. In general, viral and parasitic diseases in compromised hosts are not associated with pleural effusions. Pleural effusion may also be secondary to a subdiaphragmatic process, pulmonary infarction, pancreatitis, or congestive heart failure. The common bacterial pneumonias associated with pleural effusion, such as Hemophilus influenzae and Group A Streptococci, may also be seen in immunocompromised hosts. If there are no contraindications, pleural effusions should be tapped for pleuritic fluid analysis, special stains, and culture in compromised hosts as well as in normal patients.

Compromised hosts presenting with a cavitary lesion will usually have Aspergillus, Nocardia, Cryptococcus, or Staphylococcus aureus. Other causes of cavitary lesions such as pulmonary infarction, bronchogenic carcinoma (squamous cell carcinoma), or lung abscess should also be considered as diagnostic possibilities in such patients. CT scanning may be of use in differentiating cavitary lesions from solid lesions but is used primarily to provide localizing rather than diagnostic information. If not contraindicated, a cavity lying close to the surface should be aspirated percutaneously by the skinny needle technique. Transbronchial biopsy via bronchoscopy may be the preferred procedure in patients with cavitary lesions lying near accessible bronchi.

The choice of an invasive procedure for a compromised host with diffuse pulmonary infiltrates depends upon the clinician's expertise and experience. Transbronchial biopsy, bronchial lavage, percutaneous needle aspiration, biopsy by limited thoracotomy, or biopsy by full open thoracotomy have all been used successfully in various centers. Open lung biopsy is preferred by many specialists in the field because it offers abundant tissue for analysis and is not associated with a high morbidity. Special stains and culture techniques should be applied to tissue specimens by any or all of the diagnostic procedures.

GENERAL REFERENCES

Alexander, H.L.: Reactions with Drug Therapy. Philadelphia, W.B. Saunders, 1955, pp. 49–65.

Altemeier, W.A., Culbertson, W.R., Fuller, W.D., and Shook, C.D.: Intra-abdominal abscesses. Am J Surg *125*:70, 1973.

Baker, R.R., Tumulty, P.A., and Shelley, W.M.: Topics in clinical medicine. The value of exploratory laparotomy in fever of undetermined etiology. Johns Hopkins Med J *125*:159, 1969.

Barbour, G., and Juniper, K.: A clinical comparison of amebic and pyrogenic abscesses of the liver in 66 patients. Am J Med *53*:323, 1972.

Braude, A.I. (ed.): Medical Microbiology and Infectious Diseases. 2nd Ed. Philadelphia, W.B. Saunders, 1985.

Cluff, L.E., and Johnson, J.E. (eds.): Clinical Concepts of Infectious Diseases. 3rd Ed. Baltimore, Williams and Wilkins, 1982.

Christie, A.B.: Infectious Diseases: Epidemiology and Clinical Practice. 3rd Ed. New York, Churchill Livingston, 1980.

Greico, M.H. (ed.): Infections in the Abnormal Host. New York, Yorke Medical Books, 1980.

Gurevich, I., Tafuro, P., and Cunha, B.A. (eds.): The Theory and Practice of Infection Control. New York, Praeger Scientific, 1984.

Hoeprich, P.D. (ed.): Infectious Diseases. 3rd Ed. Philadelphia, Harper & Row, 1983.

Kluger, M.J.: Fever: Its Biology, Evolution, and Function. Princeton, Princeton University Press, 1979.

Lawson, J.H.: A Synopsis of Fevers and their Treatment. 12th Ed. London, Lloyd-Luke (Medical Books), 1977.

Mandel, G.L., Douglas, R.G. Jr., and Bennett, J.E. (eds.): Principles and Practice of Infectious Diseases. 2nd Ed. New York, John Wiley & Sons, 1985.

Petersdorf, R.G., et al. (eds.): Harrison's Principles of Internal Medicine. 10th Ed. New York, McGraw-Hill, 1983).

Prentice, H.G. (ed.): Clinics in Haematology. Philadelphia, W.B. Saunders, 1984.

Reese, R.E., and Douglas, R.G. Jr., (eds.): A Practical Approach to Infectious Diseases. 1st Ed. Boston, Little Brown & Co., 1983.

Rubn, R.H., and Young, L.S. (eds.): Clinical Approach to Infection in the Compromised Host. New York, PLenum Medical Book Co., 1981.

Sanford, J.P., and Luby, J.P. (eds.): Infectious Diseases. New York, Grune and Stratton, 1981.

Simmons, R.L., and Howard, R.J. (eds.): Surgical Infectious Diseases. New York, Appleton-Century-Crofts, 1982.

Waldman, R.H., and Kluger, R.M. (eds.): Textbook of Infectious Diseases. New Hyde Park, NY, Medical Examination Publishing Co., 1985.

Wyngaarden, J.B., and Smith, L.H. Jr. (eds.): Cecil Textbook of Medicine. 17th Ed. Philadelphia, W.B. Saunders, 1985.

Yoshikawa, T.T., Chow, A.W., and Guze, L.B. (eds.): Infectious Diseases: Diagnosis and Management. Boston, Houghton-Mifflin, 1980.

CHAPTER 6

PULMONARY PROBLEMS

B. Taylor Thompson, M.D. and Homayoun Kazemi, M.D.

COUGH

DEFINITION

Cough is one of the most common respiratory symptoms and is defined as a forceful and explosive expiration that functions to remove secretions, foreign bodies, and other irritants from the respiratory tract.

PATHOPHYSIOLOGIC CONSIDERATIONS

Each cough involves a complex reflex arc that begins with mechanical or chemical stimulation of cough receptors, which are located in the tracheobronchial tree and the upper respiratory tract (nasopharynx, paranasal sinuses, pharynx, auditory canals, and tympanic membranes). Cough receptors are also found in the pleura, the pericardium, the diaphragm, and the stomach. Afferent impulses are carried over the vagus, trigeminal, glossopharyngeal, and phrenic nerves to the "cough center" located diffusely in the medulla. Efferent pathways include the vagus, recurrent laryngeal, phrenic, and spinal motor nerves.

The cough mechanism has three phases. After an initial inspiratory phase, the second or compressive phase begins with glottic closure, relaxation of the diaphragm, and contraction of expiratory muscles. The expiratory or explosive phase follows when the glottis opens. Contraction of expiratory muscles persists during this phase. High intrathoracic pressures produce dynamic compression of airways, reduce their cross-sectional area, and maintain the high flow rates necessary to clear secretions and foreign bodies.

Cough can be produced by inflammatory, mechanical, chemical, or thermal stimulation of cough receptors or by irritation of afferent pathways anywhere in the cough reflex arc. Hence, a large number of conditions can produce cough.

Cough as a prominent symptom of an acute illness suggests infection of the upper or lower respiratory tracts, such as laryngitis, tracheobronchitis, or pneumonia. Asthma, pulmonary emboli, pulmonary edema, and aspiration of foreign material or inhalation of noxious gases can all produce acute cough. Additional causes are listed in Table 6–1.

Many chronic diseases may produce cough as a prominent symptom. Differential diagnosis is generally more complex. The most common causes of chronic cough are chronic bronchitis, asthma, and postnasal drip. Causes of chronic cough, some of which may also present as acute cough, are listed in Table 6–2.

DIAGNOSTIC EVALUATION

Patient History

The history will help suggest the diagnosis in the majority of patients. A history of acute upper respiratory tract illness followed by hoarseness suggests acute laryngitis. A nonproductive cough of sudden onset is common in early tracheobronchitis, pneumonia, or pulmonary embolism, or after acute inhalation injury or aspiration. Purulent sputum usually signifies infection in the tracheobronchial tree, usually tracheobronchitis or pneumonia.

Physical Examination

The character of the sputum is often helpful in determining the diagnosis. Purulent sputum suggests pneumonia. Copious, foul-smelling, purulent sputum whose production may be influenced by posture suggests lung abscess, bronchiectasis, or empyema with bronchopleural fistula. Pink, frothy sputum suggests pulmonary edema, and thick, bloody sputum in an alcoholic suggests Klebsiella pneumonia. Thick, tenacious sputum, occasionally with mucus plugs, suggests asthma, cystic fibrosis, or allergic bronchopulmonary aspergillosis.

The timing of the cough may also provide a useful clue. Postprandial cough suggests reflux esophagitis with or without aspiration. Esophageal diverticulum and tracheoesophageal fistula should also be considered. Nocturnal cough may be caused by congestive heart failure or asthma or may result from aspiration from the above-mentioned esophageal diseases.

Table 6–1. Causes of Cough

Most Common	Common	Rare
Tracheobronchitis	Pulmonary edema	External or middle ear disease
Asthma	Pulmonary embolism	Epiglottitis
Pneumonia	Aspiration (liquid or solid)	Pertussis
Inhalation of noxious fumes (cigarette smoke)	Anxiety	Typhoid fever
		Paratyphoid fever
		Rubeola

Table 6–2. Causes of Chronic Cough*

Most Common	Common	Rare
Chronic bronchitis	Gastroesophageal reflux	Mediastinal disease (neoplasm, aortic aneurysm)
Asthma	Neoplasm (particularly bronchogenic carcinoma)	Nasal polyps
Postnasal drip	Bronchiectasis	Osteophytes of cervical spine
Chronic inhalation of noxious fumes (smokers' cough)	Lung abscess	Transvenous pacemaker
	Chronic pneumonia (fungi, tuberculosis)	External or middle ear disease
	Chronic pulmonary edema	Esophageal cyst
	Mitral stenosis	Pharyngeal diverticulum
	Cystic fibrosis	
	Diffuse interstitial lung disease	

*Virtually any disorder that stimulates cough receptors or afferent nerve pathways can cause cough.

The character of the cough may suggest the site of anatomic involvement. A "brassy" cough suggests tracheal involvement; a "barking" cough suggests epiglottic involvement. Chronic cough with hoarseness should suggest laryngeal neoplasm or involvement of the recurrent laryngeal nerve by mediastinal tumor or by aortic aneurysm of the transverse aorta. A cough described as "throat clearing" suggests postnasal drip. Chronic cough is common in cigarette smokers and usually disappears with cessation of smoking. The appearance in a cigarette smoker of a new cough that lasts for more than a few weeks or a change in the character of a longstanding cough should raise the question of bronchogenic carcinoma.

Diagnostic Studies

The cause of acute cough can usually be diagnosed after taking a careful history and performing a physical examination of the upper and lower respiratory tracts. Patients suspected of having pneumonia should have a chest x-ray, and their sputum should be examined microscopically and bacteriologically.

In determining the cause of chronic cough, although the history, physical examination, and chest x-ray are extremely useful, confirmation often requires additional tests. When history, physical examination, and chest x-rays are unremarkable, pulmonary function testing should be the next step. An obstructive defect that improves significantly with bronchodilators suggests asthma. In some patients with asthma, however, cough is the sole presenting symptom and pulmonary function tests may be normal. Methacholine challenge is then used to diagnose the increased airway responsiveness characteristic of cough-variant asthma. If history and physical examination, chest x-ray, and pulmonary function tests with methacholine provocation are unremarkable, fiberoptic bronchoscopy is often the next step, particularly in patients over the age of 45 with a significant smoking history.

In other patients, the symptoms and signs will suggest esophageal disease and the appropriate workup may include a barium swallow, an upper gastrointestinal series, esophageal pH testing, or esophageal manometry. In other patients, the history will suggest cardiovascular disease and the appropriate workup may include ventilation/perfusion lung scanning, pulmonary angiography, or cardiac catheterization. In other patients, the history will suggest disease of the upper respiratory tract, and sinus films may be helpful in confirming the diagnosis.

DYSPNEA

DEFINITION

Dyspnea may be defined as an undue awareness of respiratory effort. The subject often refers to "breathlessness" or "shortness of breath" that results in discomfort or distress. Dyspnea may be associated with a wide variety of diseases, including emphysema, asthma, pulmonary fibrosis, pulmonary embolism, congestive heart failure, and acute anemia. It may also be described by a normal individual during strenuous exercise (Table 6–3).

PATHOPHYSIOLOGIC CONSIDERATIONS

Dyspnea is one of the more difficult symptoms to ascribe to a specific pathophysiologic abnormality. The sensation of breathlessness probably originates in the respiratory apparatus, involving a number of sensory receptors. Juxtacapillary receptors (J. receptors) located in the lung interstitium sense increases in pulmonary interstitial pressure that can occur with pulmonary congestion or infiltration. Other parenchymal receptors, as well as receptors in the diaphragm, pleura, and mediastinum, may sense changes in lung

Table 6–3. Causes of Dyspnea

Most Common	Common	Uncommon
Chronic bronchitis	Diffuse interstitial lung disease	Arteriovenous shunt
Emphysema	Pulmonary vascular disease (including pulmonary emboli; pulmonary hypertension)	Abnormal hemoglobin
Asthma	Anemia (particularly acute)	Hyperthyroidism
Pulmonary congestion or edema (i.e., left heart failure, mitral stenosis)	Obesity	Congenital heart disease (tetralogy of Fallot, pulmonic stenosis)
Psychogenic or functional	Ascites	
	Chest wall abnormalities (including kyphoscoliosis)	
	Pleural disease (including pleural effusion, fibrosis, and tumor)	
	Neuromuscular disease	
	Metabolic acidosis	
	Pneumonia	
	Upper airway obstruction	
	High altitude	

volume and tension. The carotid body stimulation from arterial hypoxemia, hypercapnia, or acidosis increases minute ventilation and can be important in causing the sensation of dyspnea in some patients, but in the majority arterial blood gases bear little relationship to the presence of dyspnea. Cardiovascular stretch receptors and tissue receptors may be important in monitoring the circulatory and metabolic changes of exercise. These diverse sensory impulses are integrated in the central nervous system. Dyspnea results when the sensory input reaches the consciousness level and causes discomfort, anxiety, or distress.

Dyspnea is an early feature in chronic bronchitis and emphysema, associated with a reduced maximum breathing capacity and correlating to the degree of airway obstruction. Increased resistance to airflow and altered chest wall mechanics increase the work of breathing that is thought to contribute to dyspnea in these patients.

Dyspnea is a frequent complaint in patients with interstitial lung disease of any cause. In this group of disorders, reduced lung compliance results in greater work of breathing and dyspnea. In addition, J. receptors sensing interstitial inflammation may also contribute to dyspnea. Dyspnea is a common finding in cardiac disease and relates to pulmonary congestion resulting in reduced lung compliance, increased work of breathing, and J. receptor activation. Modest arterial hypoxemia and impaired cardiac output combine to reduce oxygen delivery to respiratory muscles and may also contribute to dyspnea. Impaired oxygen delivery secondary to reduced hemoglobin is also important in the dyspnea associated with anemia.

DIAGNOSTIC EVALUATION

Patient History and Physical Examination

When assessing the significance of dyspnea it is essential to determine its mode of onset and severity. The severity is determined by the minimal level of activity that is associated with breathlessness, such as breathlessness while climbing a flight of stairs, breathlessness while walking a short distance on level ground, breathlessness while talking, dressing, washing, etc., and breathlessness at rest.

Dyspnea in chronic bronchitis and emphysema usually begins as breathlessness on exertion and progresses to breathlessness at rest. Dyspnea that is present only at rest or that is described as "inability to take a deep breath" and characterized by deep sighs is characteristic of psychogenic or functional dyspnea. An exception to this characterization is asthma, which may produce severe dyspnea at rest occasionally following periods of strenuous exercise. Nocturnal dyspnea that awakens the patient from sleep almost always indicates organic disease and is very suggestive of congestive heart failure. Asthma, however, may also be associated with nocturnal cough and dyspnea.

In contrast to patients with chronic bronchitis and emphysema, who experience a gradual increase in dyspnea over months to years, patients with acute onset of shortness of breath often have asthma, pneumothorax, or pulmonary embolism. Acute dyspnea may also complicate acute myocardial infarction, pneumonia, or bronchiolitis.

Physical examination in the dyspneic patient is focused on the chest. In addition to careful examination for signs of acute and chronic lung disease, particular attention must be paid to the cardiac examination. An S_3 gallop suggesting left heart failure, a diastolic rumble suggesting mitral stenosis, and an accentuated pulmonic closure sound and right ventricular lift suggesting pulmonary hypertension are all valuable clues.

Diagnostic Studies

History and physical examination supplemented by chest x-ray, hematocrit, and pulmonary function tests will suggest the diagnosis in a great majority of patients. Resting arterial blood gases are seldom helpful. In some patients, primarily those with cardiovascular and pulmonary diseases, the organ system most responsible for dyspnea may not be clear. In this setting, exercise testing not only serves to quantitate dyspnea but also may be able to differentiate a cardiac from a pulmonary cause and is often helpful in directing further diagnostic and therapeutic efforts.

ABNORMAL BREATHING PATTERNS

Clinically useful information can often be gained by observing the pattern of breathing. Respiratory rate, depth, and regularity should be noted, along with the apparent effort required to breathe. Normally, a subject breathes 8 to 16 times per minute with a regular rate and a relatively constant tidal volume of 400 to 800 cc. Occasional deep inspirations, or sighs, occur about three times every hour.

Obstructed Breathing. In the presence of airway obstruction, the pattern of respiration is often characterized by a slow rate and an increased tidal volume. This pattern of breathing decreases turbulent airflow and reduces work of breathing. With severe obstruction the rate is increased and the increased effort to breathe may be manifest by the use of accessory muscles of inspiration and the appearance of intercostal and supraclavicular retractions.

Restrictive Breathing. With reduced compliance of the lungs, pleura, or chest wall, a restricted breathing pattern emerges characterized by a small tidal volume and a rapid respiratory rate. This reduces the work required to distend the abnormally stiffened respiratory apparatus with each breath.

Kussmaul Breathing. This breathing pattern is characterized by regular deep respirations with a slightly rapid rate. It is normally seen in exercise and is characteristic of the respiratory response to metabolic acidosis.

Cheyne-Stokes Respiration. This particularly striking breathing pattern consists of periods of gradually increasing tidal volume followed by periods of decreasing tidal volume and apnea. Apnea is characteristically of 15 to 20 seconds' duration. Cheyne-Stokes respirations are seen in patients with cerebral damage, particularly with bilateral cortical and diencephalic lesions and with increased intracranial pressure. Cheyne-Stokes respirations are also seen in congestive heart failure and uremia and following administration of respiratory depressants (i.e., morphine). Cheyne-Stokes breathing can also be seen in normal infants, sleeping adults, and in normal individuals at high altitude.

Biot's Breathing. Biot's breathing, or atactic breathing, is a form of periodic breathing characterized by one or more respiratory efforts of varying depth following periods of apnea of unequal length. Biot's breathing is seen in central nervous system lesions involving the brain stem, including infarction or hemorrhage, medullary tumors, and expanding lesions of the posterior cranial fossa. Biot's breathing may also be seen in bulbar poliomyelitis.

Gasping Respiration. Gasping respiration is characteristic of severe cerebral hypoxia and is often seen shortly before death. The respiratory rate is often only 1 to 5 breaths per minute, and during inspirations all accessory muscles contract. Expiration is completely passive. It is rare for adults to recover after this pattern of breathing is established.

PLEURITIC CHEST PAIN

DEFINITION

Pleuritic pain is defined as pain that is accentuated by breathing, coughing, or sneezing. Pleuritic pain is often described as sharp, "knifelike," or stabbing and is localized in the chest, back, or shoulder. Other causes of thoracic pain include the deep, squeezing exertional chest pain of angina pectoris, the substernal burning of peptic esophagitis, and the severe central chest pain, often with radiation to the back, of aortic dissection (Table 6-4). Pulmonary pain syndromes also include the searing post-tussive substernal pain of tracheobronchitis and the substernal, occasionally exertional pain of pulmonary hypertension that is often mistaken for angina. In general these patterns of thoracic pain are not greatly influenced by breathing and will not be discussed further here.

Table 6–4. Thoracic Pain

Pleuritic pain
    Pleural and pericardial inflammation
    Diseases of the chest wall and spine
Pulmonary pain
    Tracheobronchial inflammation
    Distension of pulmonary arteries (pulmonary hypertension)
Cardiac pain
    Myocardial ischemia or infarction
    Pericarditis
Esophageal pain
    Esophageal irritation, distension, spasm
Aortic pain
    Aortic adventitial disruption (aortic dissection)

Table 6–5. Causes of Pleuritic Chest Pain

Pleural disease
    Pneumothorax
    Infectious pleuritis
    Systemic disorders
        Rheumatoid arthritis
        Systemic lupus erythematosus
        Uremia
        Vasculitis
    Neoplasm
        Primary
        Metastatic
    Dressler's syndrome
    Diaphragmatic irritation
    Idiopathic pleuritis
Pulmonary disease with pleural extension
    Pneumonia
    Neoplasm
        Primary
        Metastatic
    Pulmonary embolism or infarction
    Mediastinal disease with pleural-pericardial extension
        Pericarditis
        Mediastinitis
        Pneumomediastinum
        Neoplasm
Chest wall disease
    Costochondritis
    Rib fracture or periosteal hematoma
    Periostitis
    Muscle spasm or myositis
    Herpes zoster
    Thoracic osteoarthritis, spondylitis
    Arthritis of shoulder
    Subacromial bursitis

PATHOPHYSIOLOGIC CONSIDERATIONS

Pleuritic pain results from the stimulation of pain receptors located in the parietal pleura, the inferior pericardium, and the bone and soft tissues of the chest wall. The visceral pleura and lung parenchyma are devoid of pain fibers. The parietal pleura covers the inner surface of the chest wall, the diaphragm, the mediastinum, and the pulmonary hilum. Inflammation or stretching of the parietal pleura produces a highly painful response. The parietal pericardium, on the other hand, is relatively insensitive to pain except in its inferior aspect, where a few pain fibers are present. Pericardial inflammation often causes pain by irritation of adjacent mediastinal and diaphragmatic parietal pleural reflections.

Chest wall structures sensitive to pain include the costochondral and costovertebral joints, the periosteum of the ribs and sternum, the chest wall muscles including intercostals and pectorals, and the overlying skin and soft tissues. Diseases in the thoracic spine and shoulder joints may also result in pain accentuated by respiratory movements. Some of the causes of pleuritic chest pain are listed in Table 6–5.

DIAGNOSTIC EVALUATION

Patient History

The history is often helpful in suggesting the cause of pleuritic pain. The acute onset of severe pleuritic pain suggests pneumothorax or pulmonary embolism. Pleuritic pain often of sudden onset and frequently with shifting foci may be seen in epidemic or viral pleuritis (Bornholm disease), which often follows an acute febrile illness with prominent myalgias. Pleuritic pain, fever, and purulent sputum suggest pleural extension from bacterial pneumonia, and pleuritic pain with hemoptysis and dyspnea suggest pulmonary embolism with infarction. Positional pleuritic pain, particularly if pain increases while lying flat and is relieved by

sitting upright, suggests pericarditis. Pleuritic pain referred to the shoulder suggests irritation of the pericardium or of the central parietal pleural reflections of the diaphragm. Pain caused by inflammation of the peripheral aspects of the diaphragm is referred to the T_6 dermatome. Subphrenic abscess, splenic infarction, or extension of a pulmonary parenchymal process may all result in diaphragmatic irritation and diaphragmatic pleurisy. Pleuritic pain may also occur days to weeks after myocardial infarction or after thoracotomy, as in Dressler's syndrome. Pleuritis may also complicate systemic disease, including systemic lupus erythematosus, rheumatoid arthritis, and some systemic vasculititides, all of which indicate some involvement of the pleura.

Physical Examination

Physical examination begins with a careful search for localized tenderness characteristic of costochondritis, rib fracture, periosteal hematoma, and inflammation of the soft tissues, breasts, or shoulders. Subcutaneous crepitus on palpation and a "crunching" sound over the precordium on auscultation suggest pneumomediastinum. A coarse "leathery" sound at end inspiration and early expiration typifies a pleural rub and is due to the apposition of roughened pleural surfaces often found in patients with fibrinous pleuritis.

Diagnostic Studies

A chest x-ray should be performed in patients with pleuritic pain without obvious chest wall tenderness to suggest a diagnosis. A careful examination of peripheral lung markings may reveal a pneumothorax. A peripheral-based infiltrate suggests either pulmonary infarction or pneumonia. The lateral film should be closely examined for evidence of pleural fluid, and a pericardial fat pad sign should be sought as evidence of pericardial effusion. The mediastinum should be carefully examined for evidence of pneumomediastinum. Special views to evaluate rib fractures are only occasionally helpful. Electrocardiogram in acute pericarditis characteristically shows diffuse ST-segment elevation, and low voltage may be seen in large pericardial effusions. Examination of pleural fluid, serologic tests for immunologic disease, ventilation perfusion lung scanning, or pulmonary arteriography are required in some patients. Detailed neurologic testing including myelography may be needed in patients with suspected thoracic disc disease or spondylitis.

WHEEZE

DEFINITION

Wheezes are musical lung sounds that are characteristic of airway obstruction. Wheezes may be present during inspiration or expiration and may be heard at a distance from the patient or with only a stethoscope. Wheezing should be distinguished from stridor, which is a harsh noise produced during respiration in patients with obstructing lesions of the upper airways and is best heard by placing the stethoscope over the anterior trachea.

PATHOPHYSIOLOGIC CONSIDERATIONS

Wheezing is produced when airway narrowing and high airflow combine to produce vibration or flutter of the bronchial walls or of an obstructing airway lesion. In diffuse airway narrowing, wheezing probably originates in the first five to seven airway divisions, where

Table 6–6. Causes of Wheezing

Peripheral airway obstruction
  Asthma
    Extrinsic
    Intrinsic
    Exercise- and cold-induced
    Drug-induced
      Aspirin, tartrazine, Indomethacin
      Beta blockers
      N-acetyl-L-cystein
  Cardiac asthma
  Pulmonary embolism
  Aspiration
  Bronchiolitis
  Cystic fibrosis
  Carcinoid syndrome
  Environmental and occupational exposure
    (i.e., SO_2, toluene diisocyanate)
Upper airway obstruction
  Intrinsic lesions
    Tumors
    Stricture
    Angioedema
    Foreign body
    Epiglottitis
  Extrinsic compression
    Retropharyngeal abscess or hematoma
    Thyroid hemorrhage, carcinoma
    Aortic arch aneurysm
    Mediastinal tumors
    Esophageal carcinoma
  Functional
Pulmonary infiltrates with eosinophilia
  Acute (Löffler's) and chronic
  Tropical eosinophilia
  Bronchopulmonary aspergillosis
  Vasculitis

flow velocities are high. Extensive narrowing of small airways (those less than 2 mm in diameter) does not result in wheezing because the flow velocities in this region of the tracheobronchial tree are low. In diffuse intrathoracic airway narrowing such as that seen in asthma, wheezing is often most pronounced during expiration. Intrathoracic pressures combine with airway edema, increased secretions, and bronchospasm to further reduce bronchial caliber. Conversely, in extrathoracic obstruction, such as that seen in laryngeal carcinoma, wheezing is often most pronounced during inspiration.

DIAGNOSTIC EVALUATION

Patient History and Physical Examination

Many diseases may result in wheezing (Table 6–6). Wheezes should be characterized as focal or diffuse and as inspiratory or expiratory. Wheezing in asthma is diffuse and characteristically polyphonic. Patients with asthma may report wheezing after exercise, after exposure to cold air, following aspirin ingestion, or after exposure to known or suspected allergens or non-specific airway irritants. Many patients with asthma have increased wheezing after respiratory infections. The intensity and duration of wheezing bear little relationship to the degree of physiologic obstruction and may be absent in patients with severe obstruction and extremely low flow rates. Better indicators of the severity of airway obstruction in asthma are the use of accessory muscles of respiration and the presence of a pulsus paradoxus, both of which indicate that flow rates may be less than 25% of normal. The absence of wheezes may also be misleading during recovery from a severe asthmatic attack. Small airway abnormalities and mild obstruction may persist for 2 to 3 weeks in the absence of wheezing and may predispose the individual to further attacks if treatment is not continued. Finally, patients with asthma may present with cough or episodic dyspnea without wheezing. Examination may reveal clear lung fields, and pulmonary function tests may be normal.

Wheezing may also occur in some patients with left heart failure (cardiac asthma). Diagnosis can be difficult as diffuse wheezing may obscure the detection of rales, a gallop rhythm, or murmurs. Distended neck veins, peripheral edema, and hepatic congestion are helpful clues in diagnosing left heart failure. Paroxysms of nocturnal wheezing and dyspnea also suggest left heart failure. Dyspnea characteristically improves slowly after the patient assumes an upright position. Nocturnal cough, dyspnea, and wheezing are also common in asthma and in chronic bronchitis, but dyspnea often improves after expectorating airway secretions or after use of an inhaled bronchodilator. Nocturnal wheezing in asthmatic patients and in patients with chronic obstructive pulmonary disease should also raise the question of gastroesophageal reflux with or without aspiration.

Diffuse wheezing may be seen in pulmonary thromboembolism. Wheezing occurring with gastrointestinal disturbances and flushing suggests the diagnosis of carcinoid. Focal wheezing always suggests the presence of an endobronchial lesion, primarily tumors or foreign bodies. History of aspiration, loss of consciousness, a seizure disorder, or wheezing after dental manipulation are all clues to a possible aspirated foreign body. Inspiratory wheezing, particularly if associated with stridor, should suggest upper airway obstruction. Angioedema, tracheal or laryngeal tumors, and foreign bodies are major concerns.

Diagnostic Studies

Laboratory workup is directed toward confirming a diagnosis suspected after examination. Sputum or blood eosinophilia, elevated IgE, and positive skin tests characterize extrinsic or allergic asthma. Bronchial provocation testing (methacholine challenge) may be necessary to diagnose cough-variant asthma in patients with otherwise normal pulmonary function studies or in those who have failed an empiric trial of bronchodilator therapy. In selected cases a detailed cardiovascular workup, ENT examination, or esophageal testing is indicated. Many patients with focal wheezing require fiberoptic bronchoscopy to search for a possible foreign body or a tumor.

CYANOSIS

DEFINITION

Cyanosis, the presence of a bluish tinge to the mucous membranes and the nailbeds, is a common manifestation of pulmonary or cardiac disease and implies the presence of a significant amount of unsaturated hemoglobin in the blood. In order to recognize cyanosis clinically, it is best to look at the nailbeds or the mucous membranes in good natural light. It is also helpful to look for cyanosis when the hands are warm and well perfused.

PATHOPHYSIOLOGIC CONSIDERATIONS

Cyanosis is clinically appreciated when there is approximately 5 g of unsaturated hemoglobin in the blood. In most instances, this implies an oxygen saturation of 85% or less in the blood.

DIAGNOSTIC EVALUATION

Physical Examination

Most clinical observers will see cyanosis at the level of 85% oxyhemoglobin desaturation. However, cyanosis may not always accompany desaturation; in other words, there can be significant hypoxemia without observation of cyanosis by the clinician at the bedside. Clinical perception of cyanosis is also affected by the hemoglobin concentration; the lower the hemoglobin, the more difficult it is to appreciate cyanosis. Cyanosis can also be present with low cardiac output secondary to peripheral stasis. In an individual with a normal hemoglobin concentration, if cyanosis is noticed clinically, chances are that the arterial P_{O_2}

is approximately 50 mm Hg or less. When there is hypoxemia and cyanosis, there may be also associated clinical signs and symptoms reflecting oxygen lack, which could include fatigue and lassitude, headaches, poor judgment, restlessness, and some increase in heart rate. Cyanosis can also be present when there is methemoglobinemia, whether it is of toxic or congenital origin, as well as sulfhemoglobinemia, in which part of the hemoglobin molecule is occupied by these substances instead of oxygen.

Causes of cyanosis are many, but can be divided into those resulting from pulmonary disease and those resulting from cardiac disease. Pulmonary insufficiency is associated with hypoxemia in a variety of pulmonary disorders involving airways, pulmonary parenchyma, and the pulmonary vascular bed. Physiologically, cyanosis and hypoxemia in pulmonary disease are most commonly due to $\dot{V}/\dot{Q}$ imbalance, followed in frequency by alveolar hypoventilation and then by right-to-left shunt. In cardiac disease, cyanosis and hypoxemia are due to congenital anomalies of the heart (right-to-left shunt), and, in severe heart failure, to peripheral circulatory stasis.

Diagnostic Studies

Cyanosis observed at the bedside or in the office is best verified by measurement of arterial oxygen tension and saturation. This can be done by obtaining an arterial blood sample while the patient is breathing room air. Once the presence of hypoxemia is ascertained, careful evaluation of the cardiac and pulmonary systems is mandatory and can begin with a careful history and physical examination. Diagnosis may require evaluation of the chest x-ray and electrocardiographic abnormalities, and performance of lung function tests and, as needed, invasive or noninvasive diagnostic cardiac tests, such as echocardiography, cardiac catheterization, and various forms of nuclear scanning.

Again, it is important to emphasize that cyanosis is associated with hypoxemia but that there can be significant hypoxemia without clinically detectable cyanosis.

HEMOPTYSIS

DEFINITION AND PATHOPHYSIOLOGIC CONSIDERATIONS

Hemoptysis, or the expectoration of blood, is a significant event and causes apprehension and concern in the patient.

Table 6–7. Causes of Hemoptysis

Infections
  Bronchitis (acute and chronic)
  Bronchiectasis
  Pneumonia
  Lung abscess
  Tuberculosis
  Fungal infections
  Parasitic infections
Neoplasms
  Bronchogenic carcinoma
  Bronchial adenoma
Cardiovascular disorders
  Pulmonary infarction
  Pulmonary venous hypertension; mitral stenosis, left heart failure
  Primary pulmonary hypertension
  Pulmonary arteriovenous malformations (e.g., hereditary hemorrhagic telangiectasis)
  Eisenmenger's syndrome
  Pulmonary vasculitis; Wegener's granulomatosis, Goodpasture's syndrome; Behçet's syndrome
  Idiopathic pulmonary hemosiderosis
Trauma
  Pulmonary contusion
Hematologic disorders
  Anticoagulant therapy
  Blood dyscrasia
Pseudohemoptysis
  Aspirated blood from upper gastrointestinal hemorrhage
  Bleeding from upper airway lesions: oropharyngeal and laryngeal carcinoma, epistaxis
  Serratia marcescens infection

The causes of hemoptysis are many (Table 6–7). It is important to remember that the commonest cause of hemoptysis is infection, which is associated with bronchitis. Many other serious and potentially life threatening conditions, however, may be associated with hemoptysis. Furthermore, hemoptysis can also be part of the bleeding diathesis associated with certain malignancies or coagulation defects (Table 6–7).

DIFFERENTIAL DIAGNOSIS AND DIAGNOSTIC EVALUATION

It is important to establish whether blood is actually being coughed up and mixed with bronchial secretions or whether it is actually being vomited, implying some problem in the gastrointestinal tract. In addition, it is important to differentiate bleeding from the gums or the oral area from bleeding in the lower respiratory tract. Furthermore, it is important to know whether the bleeding is from the nasopharynx or simply from the nose. Asking a few questions on initial examination will allow the physician to establish whether the blood is truly coming from the respiratory tract, the GI tract, or the nasopharynx. For example, in hemoptysis blood is usually fresh and red and there is some blood streaking of sputum for some period of time afterwards. This is not the case with hematemesis, in which the vomited blood is more likely to be dark brown; blood originating from the upper nasopharynx is not associated with subsequent streaking of sputum with blood. Establishing whether the bleeding is from the nasopharynx or mouth can be done relatively easily on the first encounter with patient.

Because pulmonary causes of hemoptysis are usually associated with some abnormality on the chest x-ray, a chest x-ray must be obtained and carefully evaluated in all cases. If the chest x-ray looks normal, however, a careful examination of the heart is necessary to rule out the presence of mitral stenosis or some other cardiac lesion that might cause pulmonary venous hypertension.

The sputum should be examined for the presence of malignant cells, as well as for infectious organisms such as tuberculosis, or pyogenic infections such as pneumococcal pneumonia. Sputum culture for fungi and mycobacteria is essential. Complete blood count, including platelet count, is important in identifying the cause of hemoptysis and thus establishing whether hemoptysis is due to a generalized bleeding diathesis.

Bronchoscopy is also important in establishing the cause of hemoptysis. In many instances it can be the diagnostic procedure of choice, particularly in establishing the presence of a bronchial adenoma or bronchogenic carcinoma. Furthermore, bronchoscopy allows the physician to know the possible site of bleeding within the lung at which point further diagnostic procedures can be concentrated. At the time of bronchoscopy, the physician can look for possible malignant cells in bronchial washings obtained from each lobe and segment of the lung.

At times in a limited number of cases, it may be important to perform bronchography to identify special areas of bronchiectasis that may have caused the bleeding. CT scan of the chest can also be of help in identifying specific lesions within the lung that may be associated with hemoptysis. If hemoptysis persists and no obvious diagnosis can be made from the prior studies, in unusual circumstances the physician might consider pulmonary angiography, particularly to look for AV malformations that may not be readily visible on regular chest x-ray examination. In rare instances, when the hemoptysis persists and the chest x-ray shows abnormalities indicating interstitial fibrotic changes, a lung biopsy may be necessary to establish a definitive diagnosis in diseases such as idiopathic pulmonary hemosiderosis.

In a significant group of patients, no specific cause for recurrent hemoptysis can be identified after all diagnostic tests have been exhausted. These patients need to be followed carefully and over long periods of time. More often than not, however, no specific diagnosis can ever be made; these patients require a significant amount of reassurance based on the evaluation by the physician and the results of negative tests.

CLUBBING AND HYPERTROPHIC PULMONARY OSTEOARTHROPATHY

Definition

Clubbing is enlargement of the terminal phalanges of the fingers and toes, usually involving all or most of the digits, and can be seen in association with a large number of disorders. Clubbing is a painless condition marked by thickening and hypertrophy of the soft tissues underneath the nail and becomes apparent in its early phases by the changing angle formed by the root of the nail with the nailbed. This angle becomes enlarged and exceeds 180°. As clubbing progresses, the nail gradually thickens, bends, and develops longitudinal ridges, and eventually a bulbous appearance is given to the terminal phalanges. This hypertrophy of the soft tissue and enlargement of the tip of the finger or toe creates a classic drumstick appearance. On examination, there is sponginess to the root of the nail on gentle pressure; the skin is stretched and glistening and somewhat red. Clubbing usually develops slowly over many months or years. Occasionally, in association with a suppurative condition in the thorax, it can occur within a week or so. Regression and complete disappearance of clubbing can also occur but usually follows correction of the associated lesion, such as an intrathoracic malignancy.

PATHOPHYSIOLOGIC CONSIDERATIONS

Causes of clubbing are many (Table 6–8). The exact mechanism of clubbing is unknown, but morphologically the flow of blood to the tips of the fingers and toes increases, as does the number of capillaries in these areas. How these changes are brought about is unclear in relation to the primary lesion. Both malignant and nonmalignant conditions are associated with clubbing, and the primary disease process can involve many different systems (Table 6–8). In addition to its involvement with the cardiorespiratory system, club-

Table 6–8.   Causes of Clubbing

Pulmonary
  Malignant
    Bronchogenic carcinoma
    Pleural mesothelioma
    Metastatic malignancies to the lung
  Infections
    Lung abscess
    Empyema
    Bronchiectasis
    Pulmonary tuberculosis (rare)
    Fungal infections (rare)
  Interstitial lung disease—pulmonary fibrosis of any origin
  Obstructive lung disease—emphysema and bronchitis (rare)
  Miscellaneous
    Fibrous tumors of the pleura
    Pulmonary arteriovenous malformations
Cardiac
  Congenital cyanotic heart disease
  Subacute bacterial endocarditis
  Atrial myxoma
Gastrointestinal tract
  Biliary cirrhosis
  Ulcerative colitis
  Regional ileitis (Crohn's disease)
  Chronic bacterial diarrhea
  Steatorrhea
  Peptic ulceration of the esophagus
Malignancies other than primary thoracic malignancies
  Chronic myelocytic leukemia
  Thymoma
  Hodgkin's disease
Familial or congenital clubbing

Table 6–9.   Causes of Hypertrophic Pulmonary Osteoarthropathy

Bronchogenic carcinoma—usually adenocarcinoma
  or squamous cell
Pleural mesothelioma
Metastatic tumors to the lung
Hematologic malignancies
Very severe and sustained hypoxemia

bing is associated with diseases of the GI tract and other malignancies. Benign or "familial" clubbing can occur when there is a significant family history of clubbing.

DIAGNOSTIC EVALUATION

When a patient presents with clubbing, a history must be obtained specifically to rule out the various causal disorders, after which the workup can be directed to the organ at fault. A chest x-ray should be obtained in every instance, since the overwhelming majority of patients with clubbing have disease of the respiratory or cardiac system for which a chest x-ray can identify the primary associated lesion.

In many of the disorders of the cardiorespiratory system in which clubbing is present, there may also be concurrent cyanosis; certainly in many of the pulmonary and congenital cardiac disorders, cyanosis and clubbing are seen together.

Another condition seen in association with clubbing is hypertrophic pulmonary osteoarthropathy. In almost 90% of the cases this condition occurs with concurrent malignancies of the respiratory tract. Hypertrophic

pulmonary osteoarthropathy is characterized by tenderness of wrists and ankles, for which the basic pathologic process is a subperiostitis with subperiosteal new bone formation. Usually there is symmetrical involvement of the distal segments of the long bones of the arms and legs. Furthermore, there could be associated effusion in wrists, knees, and ankles. The patient may complain of joint pain and stiffness initially. On examination, pressure on the distal end of the long bones is very painful, particularly around wrists and ankles. An x-ray examination usually shows the new subperiosteal bone formation, and, pathologically, periostitis is present and there is infiltration of the periosteum with round cells. The specific cause of hypertrophic pulmonary osteoarthropathy is unknown, but it is of interest that in many instances the symptoms of hypertrophic pulmonary osteoarthropathy, namely, painful long bones and joints, can disappear soon after a vagotomy or thoracotomy or following resection of the primary tumor. Causes of hypertrophic pulmonary osteoarthropathy are shown in Table 6–9. Since in a large number of cases the condition is seen in association with pulmonary malignancies, it is essential that a chest x-ray be obtained as a first test to see if the lesion can be identified, and the workup should concentrate on identifying the source of the primary site of the tumor.

SOLITARY PULMONARY NODULE

DEFINITION

A solitary pulmonary nodule is a round or oval roentgenographic shadow that varies in size from 1 to 6 cm. The lesion must be surrounded by air-containing lung and must be fairly well circumscribed.

PATHOPHYSIOLOGIC CONSIDERATIONS

Over 45 malignant and benign conditions may result in the development of a solitary pulmonary nodule

Table 6–10. Solitary Pulmonary Nodules

Neoplastic
  Bronchogenic carcinoma
  Metastatic neoplasm
  Bronchioloalveolar carcinoma
  Bronchial adenoma
  Hamartoma
  Lymphoma
Infectious
  Tuberculosis
  Histoplasmosis
  Coccidioidomycosis
  Cryptococcosis
  Hydatid cyst
  Dirofilaria
Developmental
  Bronchogenic cyst
  Pulmonary arteriovenous fistula
Miscellaneous
  Rheumatoid nodule
  Pulmonary hematoma
  Lipoid pneumonia
  Pulmonary infarct
  Wegener's granulomatosis
"Pseudonodules"
  Nipple shadows
  Interlobar pleural effusion
  Pleural nodules, plaques, or neoplasms
  Skin and chest wall tumors

(Table 6–10). Because many solitary pulmonary nodules, particularly in older patients, represent primary bronchogenic carcinoma, and because lesions detected in this stage are potentially surgically curable, a thorough and careful evaluation of all pulmonary nodules must be undertaken. The thrust of the evaluation process is thus to classify the lesion as malignant or benign.

DIAGNOSTIC EVALUATION

Patient History and Physical Examination

Clinical and x-ray criteria are helpful in the differentiation of malignant and benign solitary nodules (Table 6–11). Malignancy becomes a greater concern with increasing age. Less than 1% of solitary nodules in patients less than 35 years of age are malignant, but over 50% are malignant in those over the age of 50. Symptoms compatible with a lung neoplasm in an older cigarette smoker or symptoms present with a potential extrathoracic neoplasm suggest a relationship to malignancy. The absence of such symptoms, a history of residence in an area to which granulomatous disease is endemic, or a history of exposure to tuberculosis is helpful in suggesting a benign diagnosis but, particularly in the older patient, cannot be relied upon to preclude malignancy.

The appearance on x-ray of a solitary pulmonary nodule may suggest a benign diagnosis, particularly if the lesion is calcified. If the pattern of calcification is lamellar, diffusely stippled, dense central, or "popcorn," the nodule is most likely benign. Eccentric calcification, however, cannot be used to rule out malignancy and may be seen in scar carcinoma.

Diagnostic Studies

Examination of a prior chest x-ray is the single most important step in the evaluation of a solitary pulmonary nodule, and a thorough search for all previous chest x-rays is mandatory. If a lesion was present on a previous film and has not changed in size for over 2 years, a benign diagnosis is likely and the patient may be followed with serial chest x-rays. In lesions that have changed in size, the rate of change is often helpful in evaluating possible malignancy. Lesions that have doubled in volume in less than 1 month are often inflammatory, with the exception of rapidly growing metastatic choriocarcinoma, testicular carcinoma, and osteogenic sarcoma. The primary tumor, however, is usually apparent by the time the pulmonary metastases appear. A long doubling time, one exceeding 18 months, also suggests a benign diagnosis, particularly hamartoma or histoplasmoma. An intermediate doubling time suggests malignancy, particularly broncho-

Table 6–11.   Benign and Malignant Solitary Pulmonary Nodules—Clinical and Roentgenographic Characteristics

		Benign	Malignant
Clinical	Age	< 40	> 45
	History	Tuberculosis and histoplasmosis exposure; mineral oil use	Known extrathoracic primary
	Symptoms	Absent	Present
X-ray	Size	< 2 cm	> 2 cm
	Border	Smooth, well circumscribed	Ill-defined, spiculated
	Calcification	Central, laminated, multiple punctate, "popcorn"	Rare; peripheral calcification in "scar carcinoma"
	Satellite lesion	More common	Less common
	Doubling time < 1 month or > 18 months	Usual	Unusual

genic carcinoma. Most bronchogenic carcinomas have a doubling time from 1 to 18 months, with a median of 120 days.

If an old chest x-ray is not available, tomography or CT scanning may be required to determine the presence of calcium and the pattern of calcification. Sputum cultures and sputum cytology are usually of little value, and an extensive search for an extrathoracic malignancy is fruitless in the absence of suggestive symptoms or signs. Skin tests and serologic tests may be of value in some cases. Percutaneous transthoracic needle aspiration biopsy is effective in establishing a malignant diagnosis in 90% of selected cases, though a negative result does not preclude malignancy.

The management of each case must be individualized. If a solitary pulmonary nodule is stable (no change for 2 years) or possesses central or "popcorn calcification," it can be presumed benign and the patient can be followed by serial chest x-rays. A search for an extrathoracic malignancy that may have metastasized to the lung is indicated if the patient has suggestive symptoms or signs or abnormal routine laboratory tests. In the remaining patients over the age of 35 years, the lesion should be resected, particularly in the cigarette smoker.

PLEURAL EFFUSION

DEFINITION

The pleura is a serous membrane that lines the chest wall, diaphragm, and mediastinum (parietal pleura) and the lung parenchyma and interlobular fissures (visceral pleura). Normally a thin, clinically undetectable film of pleural fluid is present in this potential space. Excess accumulation of pleural fluid is referred to as pleural effusion. Other fluid collections in the pleural space include hemorrhagic pleural effusions (resulting in hemothorax), purulent pleural effusions (empyema), or chylous pleural effusions (chylothorax). Fluid collections in the pleural space must be distinguished from pleural thickening or fibrosis and pleural tumors.

PATHOPHYSIOLOGIC CONSIDERATIONS

Fluid in the pleural space (approximately 10 cc per hemithorax) is constantly being formed from the systemic capillaries of the parietal pleura where Starling's forces (Fig. 6–1) favor the formation of approximately

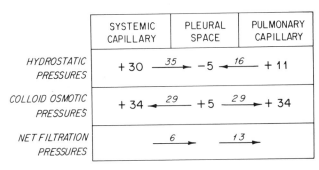

Fig. 6–1. Normal hydrostatic and colloid osmotic pressures (in cm H$_2$O) are shown for the systemic capillaries of the parietal pleura, for the pulmonary capillaries of the visceral pleura, and for the pleural space. Net pressures are indicated above the arrows. Arrows indicate the direction of net hydrostatic and osmotic forces. The net gradient is greater for fluid resorption (13 cm) than for fluid formation (6 cm), and excess pleural fluid does not accumulate.

100 cc of pleural fluid/hour. A small amount of protein also leaks into the pleural space, so that, normally, pleural fluid protein concentration is 1.5 g/dl or lower. Low hydrostatic pressure in the pulmonary capillaries of the visceral pleura favors fluid movement from the pleural space at an estimated capacity of 300 ml/hour. Visceral pleural lymphatics remove protein and fluid at a rate of approximately 20 ml/hour, the net effect is constant flow of pleural fluid across the pleural space with a considerable reserve to prevent fluid accumulation.

An alteration in the above forces can lead to development of pleural effusion. When the accumulation of pleural fluid results from alterations in hydrostatic or oncotic pressure, the effusion is referred to as a transudate. The pleural surfaces are not involved by a primary disease process. Causes of transudative pleural effusions are listed in Table 6–12.

Exudative pleural effusions occur when the pleura or the pleural lymphatics are diseased. This can result in either increased permeability of the pleura to protein, as in parapneumonic effusions, or decreased lymphatic clearance, as in some malignancies. Causes of exudative pleural effusions are listed in Table 6–13.

Table 6–12.   Causes of Transudative Pleural Effusions

Congestive heart failure
Nephrotic syndrome
Hepatic cirrhosis
Peritoneal dialysis
Myxedema
Pulmonary emboli
Sarcoidosis
Glomerulonephritis

Table 6–13. Causes of Exudative Pleural Effusions

Malignancy
  Metastatic neoplasm
  Mesothelioma
Infections
  Bacterial
    Tuberculous
  Fungal
  Mycoplasmal
  Parasitic
  Viral
Subphrenic inflammation
  Pancreatitis
  Abscess (splenic, intrahepatic)
  Postoperative
  Dialysis
Pulmonary embolism
Immunologic disease
  Rheumatoid pleuritis
  Systemic lupus erythematosus (including drug-induced)
  Sjögren's syndrome
  Angioimmunoblastic lymphadenopathy
  Dressler's syndrome
  Familial Mediterranean fever
Drug-induced pleuritis
  Nitrofurantoin
  Methylseroside
  Dantrolene
  Procarbazine
  Bromocriptine
Miscellaneous
  Asbestos exposure
  Meigs' syndrome
  Esophageal perforation
  Yellow nail syndrome
  Urinary tract obstruction
  Trauma (hemothorax)
Chylothorax

DIAGNOSTIC EVALUATION

Patient History and Physical Examination

The symptoms of a patient with a pleural effusion are dictated by the underlying process causing the effusion. Symptoms resulting from the effusion itself include chest pain, cough, and dyspnea. Chest pain results from inflammation of the parietal pleura, since only the parietal pleura has pain fibers. Cough is often dry and nonproductive. Dyspnea is also relatively common and is often out of proportion to the size of the pleural effusion.

The physical examination often shows the presence of an effusion. On inspection, the hemithorax may be larger and the intercostal spaces blunted if the pleural effusion is large and the pressure increased. Shifting dullness on percussion is the hallmark of an effusion. Other findings include diminished breath sounds and reduced tactile fremitus. Egophony is often heard just above the effusion because of compression of the ad-

jacent lung. Pleural rubs, caused by the apposition of inflamed pleural surfaces, are characterized by coarse, leathery sounds that are most often heard in late inspiration and early expiration. Pleural rubs are often associated with local pain.

Other physical findings may suggest the cause of the effusion. Cardiomegaly, jugular venous distension, and peripheral edema suggest congestive heart failure. Ascites and jaundice suggest cirrhosis. Polyarthritis and subcutaneous nodules suggest rheumatoid effusion, and hypertrophic osteoarthropathy suggests metastatic carcinoma. Upper abdominal tenderness suggests subphrenic abscess or pancreatitis.

Diagnostic Studies

The chest x-ray confirms the presence of pleural fluid. The fluid, if free flowing, accumulates in the dependent portion of the pleural space. The earliest sign of excess pleural fluid, obliteration of the posterior costophrenic angle from the lateral projection, occurs when an excess of 75 cc of pleural fluid is present. With approximately 175 cc of fluid, the lateral costophrenic sulcus on the posterolateral x-ray becomes blunted. However, up to 500 cc of pleural fluid may accumulate before this angle is obscured. Occasionally as much as 1000 cc of pleural fluid accumulates in an intrapulmonary location without obliteration of the costophrenic sulcus. These subpulmonic effusions are suspected if the hemidiaphragm is elevated, if the apex of the apparent hemidiaphragm is shifted laterally, or if the tip of the gastric bubble is greater than 2 cm below the left hemidiaphragm.

Interlobar tracking of fluid is especially common in patients with congestive heart failure. These fluid collections simulate parenchymal mass lesions and, since they disappear with resolution of the pleural effusion, are referred to as "vanishing" tumors or "pseudo" tumors.

Whenever an abnormal chest x-ray suggests the diagnosis of pleural effusion, a decubitus view should be obtained to ascertain if the fluid is free flowing. If free pleural fluid is present, one should consider performing thoracentesis. The main purpose is to determine if the fluid is an exudate or a transudate. This distinction is made by analysis of the pleural fluid and serum LDH and protein. Using criteria established by Light, an exudate is present if any one of the following three criteria are met: pleural fluid LDH is greater than two thirds of the upper limit of the normal serum value, the pleural fluid to serum LDH ratio is greater than 0.6, or the pleural fluid to serum protein ratio is greater than 0.5. If none of the criteria are met, the fluid is a transudate and attention is turned to the diagnosis and treatment of what in the vast majority of cases is congestive heart failure, cirrhosis, or nephrosis.

The major challenge lies in differentiating the many causes of an exudative effusion. Pleural fluid appearance should be noted and the following tests should be performed on the pleural fluid: glucose, white blood cell count and differential, amylase, cytology, and routine bacteriologic culture in febrile patients or in those with suspected parapneumonic effusions.

Most effusions are yellow and, if transudative, clear. True bloody effusions signify greater than 5000 red blood cells per mm³ and fail to clear during the thoracentesis. Bloody effusions with a hematocrit greater than 1% suggest malignant pleural disease, pulmonary embolus, or trauma. Cloudy pleural effusions should be centrifuged and the supernatant examined. A cloudy supernatant suggests chylous effusion or pseudochylous effusion. A triglyceride level should then be determined. Values greater than 110 mg/dl signify a chylothorax and imply interruption of the thoracic duct. Triglyceride values less than 50 mg/dl indicate a pseudochylous effusion, usually in the setting of longstanding pleural inflammation such as that seen in rheumatoid or tuberculous pleuritis. Intermediate triglyceride values require lipoprotein electrophoresis and the demonstration of chylomicrons for the diagnosis of chylous effusion.

The pleural fluid glucose offers a valuable differential point. If the glucose is less than 60 mg/dl, bacterial infection, malignancy, tuberculosis, and rheumatoid arthritis are suggested. Extremely low glucose values (less than 10 mg/dl) suggest rheumatoid pleuritis. An elevated amylase suggests pancreatitis, esophageal perforation, or malignancy.

The pleural fluid white count is of limited use. Most transudates have less than 1000 cells per mm³. Parapneumonic effusions often have more than 10,000 cells per mm³, but substantial overlap occurs among the various causes of exudative effusions. The differential count is of much greater diagnostic use. Neutrophil predominance suggests a parapneumonic effusion, pulmonary embolism, subphrenic abscess, early tuberculous effusion, or pancreatitis. Lymphocyte predominance suggests malignancy or tuberculosis. Mesothelial cells are rarely seen in tuberculous effusions. Eosinophils suggest air in the pleural space, hemothorax, pleural effusion secondary to parasites or fungal diseases, Hodgkin's disease, or bronchogenic carcinoma. Cytologic examination of the pleura is very useful, and malignant cells are identified from over 50% of patients with malignant effusion.

After these initial studies, some additional tests of the pleural fluid may be helpful in selected patients. Pleural fluid complement levels are low in pleural effusions complicating systemic lupus erythematosus (SLE) and rheumatoid arthritis. LE cells in the pleural fluid are virtually diagnostic of systemic lupus. Rheumatoid factor titers greater than serum values suggest rheumatoid pleuritis. A low pleural fluid pH (less than 7.20) suggests one of seven conditions: parapneumonic effusion requiring chest tube, esophageal rupture, rheumatoid arthritis, tuberculous pleuritis, malignancy, systemic acidosis, and hemothorax.

Other tests, including carcinoembryonic antigen (CEA), fibrinogen degradation products, LDH isoenzymes, and lysozyme are of little diagnostic value. Chromosome analysis (for the differentiation of malignant from benign effusions), hyaluronidase (increased in mesothelioma), and lymphocyte subset analysis by monoclonal antibody staining (for a diagnosis of lymphoma) are useful diagnostic procedures but not widely available.

If malignancy or tuberculosis is suspected but not confirmed by the above tests, a closed pleural biopsy is indicated. The combination of a pleural biopsy and culture of pleural tissue is successful in a diagnosis of 50 to 80% of tuberculous effusions. Pleural biopsy also complements pleural fluid cytology in the diagnosis of malignant effusions, with the combination yielding a positive test in 60 to 70% of malignant effusions. In both tuberculous and malignant effusions, a repeat pleural biopsy will yield a diagnosis in an additional 10 to 20%.

Fiberoptic bronchoscopy is indicated for those with an underlying parenchymal abnormality; it is important to remove as much fluid from the pleural space as possible so that the underlying lung can be examined radiographically. CT scanning of the thorax is also helpful in evaluating the underlying pulmonary parenchyma. Ventilation/perfusion lung scanning for the diagnosis of pulmonary emboli is often difficult to interpret in large pleural effusions, and pulmonary arteriography or lower extremity studies for deep venous thrombosis may be necessary in patients suspected of having pulmonary emboli. Pleuroscopy or open pleural biopsy may be required in selected patients when less invasive procedures have failed to yield a positive diagnosis.

MEDIASTINAL MASSES

DEFINITION

The mediastinum is an anatomic division of the thorax bounded superiorly by the thoracic inlet, inferiorly by the diaphragm, posteriorly by the thoracic vertebra, and anteriorly by the sternum. The mediastinum is further subdivided into three compartments. The anterior mediastinum is bounded anteriorly by the sternum and posteriorly by the pericardium, aorta, and bracheocephalic vessels. The posterior mediastinum is located between the pericardium and the anterior aspect of the vertebral column. The middle mediastinum, containing pericardium, heart, and great vessels, lies in between.

The mediastinum is the site of a number of mass lesions, including benign and malignant neoplasms and cysts. Anatomic subdivisions of the mediastinum contain structures that are often unique to it; hence, differential diagnosis begins with knowledge of the structures present in each compartment (Table 6–14). The anterior compartment contains the thymus gland, the anterior mediastinal lymph nodes, and the internal mammary arteries and veins. Lesions in the anterior mediastinum include thymomas, substernal goiters and parathyroid tumors, lymphomas, and germinal cell neoplasms. The middle mediastinum contains the pericardium, heart, ascending and transverse aorta, trachea, and main bronchi with their contiguous nodes, and the pulmonary artery and veins. The middle mediastinum is a common site of lymph node involvement by lymphoma, Hodgkin's disease, metastatic neoplasms, or infectious mononucleosis, or by involvement secondary to granulomatous mediastinitis. In addition, bronchogenic and pleuropericardial cysts, as well as aortic arch aneurysms and vascular dilatation of the pulmonary arteries, result in middle mediastinal masses. Posterior mediastinum contains the sympa-

thetic chains and is the site of all neurogenic tumors found in the thorax. Other structures include the esophagus, the descending aorta, the thoracic duct, and the posterior mediastinal lymph nodes. Esophageal neoplasm, hiatal hernia, esophageal diverticulum, and descending thoracic aortic aneurysm are other lesions encountered in the posterior mediastinum. Neurogenic, neuroenteric, and gastroenteric cysts may also be found in the posterior compartment.

DIAGNOSTIC EVALUATION

Patient History and Physical Examination

Approximately one-third of patients with mediastinal masses are asymptomatic, with diagnosis first suspected from a routine chest x-ray. The remaining patients complain most commonly of cough, chest pain, and dyspnea. Malignant mediastinal lesions are more often symptomatic, usually with chest pain and cough.

A number of assorted symptoms and signs may assist in the diagnosis of mediastinal lesions. Thymomas are common mediastinal lesions and may be associated with symptoms of myasthenia gravis. Neurogenic tumors may be associated with hypertrophic osteoarthropathy and may also occur as part of von Recklinghausen's neurofibromatosis. Hormonal activity of some neurogenic tumors, particularly ganglioneuromas and neuroblastomas, may result in diarrhea, flushing, hypertension, and sweating. Large teratomas and mesotheliomas may produce hypoglycemia. Lymphoma or Hodgkin's disease may be associated with

Table 6–14. Mediastinal Masses by Predominant Compartment

Anterior Compartment	Middle Compartment	Posterior Compartment
Thymoma	Lymph node enlargement	Neurogenic neoplasms
Germinal cell neoplasm (i.e., teratoma)	Malignant	Meningocele
Thyroid masses	Lymphoma	Esophageal lesion
Parathyroid masses	Hodgkin's disease	Neoplasm
Lymphoma	Metastatic neoplasm (pulmonary or	Diverticulum
Mesenchymal neoplasms (i.e., lipoma,	extrapulmonary)	Megaesophagus
lymphangioma)	Inflammatory	Hiatal hernia
	Sarcoidosis	Bochdalek's hernia
	Granulomatous mediastinitis	Thoracic spine lesions
	Infectious mononucleosis	Metastatic neoplasm
	Beryllium disease	Infectious spondylitis
	Dilantin-induced	Fracture with hematoma
	Bronchogenic cyst	Extramedullary hematopoiesis
	Aortic arch aneurysm	Descending aortic aneurysm
	Pulmonary artery dilatation	Neurenteric cyst
	Pleuropericardial cyst	Gastroenteric cyst
	Tracheal tumors	
	Cardiac aneurysm	
	Foramen of Morgagni hernia	

(From Fraser, R.G., and Pare, J.A.P. (eds): Diagnosis of Diseases of the Chest. 2nd Ed. Philadelphia, W.B. Saunders, 1978, p. 1819–1870.)

peripheral lymphadenopathy (especially supraclavicular) or splenomegaly. Mediastinal and systemic adenopathy as part of an acute febrile illness with sore throat or splenomegaly suggests mononucleosis.

Other mediastinal lesions produce symptoms by local compression of mediastinal structures. Cough from tracheal compression or infiltration may be seen in aortic dissection, malignant neoplasms, and infected bronchial cysts. Compression of the left recurrent laryngeal nerve from middle mediastinal tumors produces hoarseness. Pressure symptoms may also be seen with encroachment of esophagus, heart, and great veins.

Diagnostic Studies

Localization of a lesion on a routine chest x-ray allows for a preliminary differential diagnosis. CT scanning of the thorax with contrast enhancement establishes the precise anatomic localization and characterizes the lesion as vascular, cystic, calcified, or fat-containing in the vast majority of cases. Further testing is then directed by these findings.

REFERENCES

Corraro, W., Braman, S.S., and Irwin, R.S.: Chronic cough as the sole presenting manifestation of bronchial asthma. N Eng J Med *300*:633–637, 1979.

Fishman, A.P. (ed.): Pulmonary Diseases and Disorders. New York, McGraw-Hill, 1980.

Fraser, R.G., and Pare, J.A.P.: Diagnosis of Diseases of the Chest. 2nd Ed. Volume I–IV. Philadelphia, W.B. Saunders, 1979.

Irwin, R.S., Corraro, W., and Pratte, M.R.: Chronic cough in the adult: The spectrum and frequency of causes and successful outcome of specific therapy. Am Rev Respir Dis *123*:413–417, 1981.

Irwin, R.S., Rosen, M.J., and Braman, S.S.: Cough. A comprehensive review. Arch Intern Med *137*:1186–1191, 1977.

Kazemi, H.: Disorders of the Respiratory System. Volume II. The Science and Practice of Medicine. New York, Grune and Stratton, 1976.

GENERAL REFERENCES

DYSPNEA

Shore, N.S., and Kazemi, H.: Examination of the patient with respiratory disease. *In* Disorders of the Respiratory System. Volume II. The Science and Practice of Medicine. Edited by H. Kazemi. New York, Grune and Stratton, 1976, pp. 56–58.

ABNORMAL BREATHING PATTERNS

Smalhout, B.: Central respiratory disorders. *In* Handbook of Clinical Neurology. Volume I. Edited by P.J. Vinken and G.W. Bruga. Amsterdam, North Holland Publishing Co., 1969.

WHEEZE

McDonnell, K.F.: Differential diagnosis of asthma. *In* Bronchial Asthma: Mechanisms and Therapeutics. Edited by E.B. Weiss and A.S. Segon. Boston, Little, Brown and Co., 1976.

CYANOSIS

Shore, N.S., and Kazemi, H.: Examination of the patients with respiratory disease. *In* Disorders of the Respiratory System. Volume II. The Science and Practice of Medicine. Edited by H. Kazemi. New York, Grune and Stratton, 1976, pp. 61–62.

HEMOPTYSIS

Weaver, L.J., Solliday, N.H., and Cugell, D.W.: Selection of patients with hemoptysis for fiberoptic bronchoscopy. Chest *76*:7–10, 1979.

CLUBBING

Fischer, D.S., Singer, D.H., Feldman, S.M.: Clubbing, a review, with emphasis on hereditary acropachy. Medicine *43*:459–479, 1964.

Lonken, P.N., and Fishman, A.P.: Clubbing and hypertrophic osteoarthropathy. *In* Pulmonary Diseases and Disorders. Edited by A.P. Fishman. New York, McGraw-Hill, 1980, pp. 84–91.

SOLITARY PULMONARY NODULE

Fraser, R.G., and Pare, J.A.P.: Neoplastic diseases of the lungs. *In* Diagnosis of Diseases of the Chest. 2nd Ed. Volume II. Philadelphia, W.B. Saunders, 1978, pp. 1049–1055.

PLEURAL EFFUSION

Light, R.W.: Pleural Diseases. Philadelphia, Lea & Febiger. 1983.

MEDIASTINAL MASS

Fraser, R.G., and Pare, J.A.P.: Diseases of the mediastinum. *In* Diagnosis of Diseases of the Chest. 2nd Ed. Volume III. Philadelphia, W.B. Saunders, 1979, pp. 1798–1870.

CHAPTER 7

CARDIOVASCULAR PROBLEMS

Robert E. Whalen, M.D.

This section is designed to provide a logic tree for the clinician who is presented with a patient with a potential cardiovascular problem. It moves from a list of the most common presenting symptoms to the physical signs associated with various cardiovascular diseases. Finally, the various historical and physical features of specific disease entities are summarized briefly under specific headings with an analysis of laboratory approaches to diagnosis. A patient's presenting complaint may be general, seemingly nonspecific and unfocused. It may call many diagnoses to the mind of the clinician with broad experience with many forms of cardiovascular disease. This broad unfocused complaint must initially be further defined by a careful delineation of the details of the symptoms, thus eliminating a host of potential diagnoses. A knowledge of the details of the symptoms should enable the clinician to target the physical examination so as to elicit the presence of or ascertain the absence of the physical signs that will suggest a small number of potential or actual diagnoses.

Table 7–1 outlines the content of the chapter, beginning with symptoms that will be used as a broad introduction to potential diagnoses.

Table 7–1. Cardinal Manifestations of Cardiovascular Diseases

Symptoms
Fatigue
Chest pain
Dyspnea
Palpitations
Syncope
Swelling
Claudication
Raynaud's phenomenon
Physical signs
Arterial pulses
Venous pulses
Cyanosis
Clubbing
Heart sounds
Murmurs
Bruits
Clicks and snaps
Extracardiac sounds
Filling sounds and gallops
Arrhythmias
Cardiomegaly
Prominent syndromes
Ischemic heart disease
Congenital heart disease in the adult
Mitral valve prolapse
Myocarditis and cardiomyopathies
Pericardial effusion and cardiac tamponade
Constrictive pericarditis
Acute and chronic congestive heart failure
Cardiogenic shock
Pulmonary hypertension
Cardiac arrest and sudden death

FATIGUE

DEFINITION

Fatigue is an almost ubiquitous symptom in our society today. In simplest terms it can be defined as a sensation of excessive tiredness while performing activities that previously had not induced this sensation. The definition is couched in terms such that the patient uses himself as his own control; that is, the patient will be able to look back to some standard of his normal sense of well-being and be able to compare his present inability to perform specific tasks to his previous ability. Using the patient as his own control in this way obviates the problem of wide discrepancies in personal activity levels of individual patients. In essence, the individual patient should be able to know with clear detail what activities he now cannot perform or what work schedules he now cannot meet as compared to what he could have done 6 to 12 months previously (see Chapter 14).

Fatigue is one of the most frequent chief complaints that the patient with cardiovascular disease may bring to the physician, and even if it is not the most prom-inent complaint it is almost always a feature of the patient's illness. Often it is recognized only in retrospect by the patient after some more dramatic sign of cardiovascular disease has manifested itself. For instance, it is not at all rare for the patient who has developed angina or had an acute myocardial infarction to recall in retrospect that he really had not been feeling well and had definitely noted excessive fatigue for months prior to the initial dramatic clinical event such as the onset of angina or infarction.

Table 7–2 provides a broad frame of reference for the clinician as he attempts to focus on the potential causes for fatigue in a patient. Though the table is focused on cardiovascular problems, there are many other diseases or syndromes that may bring the patient to the clinician with a complaint of fatigue. Perhaps the most common cause of fatigue other than a cardiovascular disease or defect is the deconditioning process resulting from our sedentary society with its automobiles, elevators, and work-saving devices in the home. Fatigue also is often the first manifestation of depression; again, other historical features elicited from the patient should rapidly move the clinician's

Table 7–2. Causes of Fatigue

General Physiologic Problems	Specific Clinical Entities
Inadequate cardiac output	Left ventricular dysfunction
	Ischemic heart disease
	Cardiomyopathy
	Myocarditis
	Valvular defects
	Obstructed cardiac valve
	Valvular defect
	Intracardiac tumors or thrombi
	Insufficiency or regurgitation of cardiac valves
	Pulmonary-vascular cause
	Primary or secondary pulmonary hypertension
	Congenital cardiac lesions
	Intracardiac shunts
	Pericardial disease
	Constriction
	Effusion
	Rhythm disturbances
	Complete heart block
	Prolonged tachycardia
Excessive demand for cardiac output	Hypermetabolic states
	Fever, septicemia
	Hyperthyroidism
	AV fistula
Inadequate tissue oxygenation	Anemia
	Carbon monoxide intoxication
	Congenital heart disease with right-to-left shunt

attention away from the cardiovascular system and toward his emotional status. Fatigue may also be one of the earliest recognized complaints of patients with Cushing's syndrome. Certainly lupus erythematosus may have a long background of fatigue as an underlying complaint before the disease becomes overtly manifest. In general, then, specific symptoms of a noncardiac nature accompanying fatigue draw the clinician's attention away from merely the cardiovascular system.

PATHOPHYSIOLOGIC CONSIDERATIONS AND DIFFERENTIAL DIAGNOSIS

Lacking overt signs or symptoms pointing him away from the cardiovascular system, the clinician must entertain the possibility that the complaint of fatigue is in fact related to something wrong in the cardiovascular system. Table 7–2 provides a general differential framework from which to begin to arrive at a specific etiologic diagnosis from the symptom of fatigue. Fatigue can be considered the result of three possible problems involving the cardiovascular system.

Cardiac Output Inadequacy. The first is simply that the patient does not have the ability to generate a cardiac output adequate to support the tissues' oxygen requirements for the activity the patient is performing.

The simplest approach to further categorizing the

possible sources of cardiac output inadequacy is to review what can go wrong with the various components of the heart that participate in the maintenance of an adequate cardiac output.

Left Ventricular Myocardial Dysfunction. Perhaps the most frequent cause for decreased left ventricular function leading to fatigue is the presence of ischemic heart disease that has not yet manifested itself by angina or infarction. Although there may be no overt physical signs of ischemic heart disease discernible at rest, examination after exercise may demonstrate transient rales and an S3 gallop. Moreover, evidence of significant arteriosclerotic cardiovascular disease in other parts of the body manifested by bruits over major vessels or claudication should be given great weight in considering the possibility of the presence of "silent ischemic heart disease" in the patient who presents with fatigue.

Just as there may be no cardiac physical findings to substantiate the diagnosis, routine laboratory measurements such as the electrocardiogram and the chest x-ray may be entirely normal. It is only with the recent advent of radionuclide imaging that it has become clear that patients with "silent ischemic heart disease" may have perfectly normal left ventricular function at rest. The presence of the ischemic process becomes manifest only with exercise, during which the left ventricular ejection fraction falls precipitously from a normal level of above 55% to below 40% and left ventricular wall motion abnormalities develop. It is presumed that the patient who presents with fatigue resulting from the ischemic heart disease is unable to maintain an adequate cardiac output with physical activity simply because his ventricle is not able to maintain an effective ejection fraction when stressed. The decreased oxygenation and nutrition of the myocardium is due to inadequate blood flow to the myocardium caused by obstruction of coronary arteries.

Left ventricular dysfunction may also result from a variety of forms of cardiomyopathy, which will be reviewed later; suffice it to say that decreased left ventricular ejection fraction and decreased cardiac output are almost inevitably associated with chronic hypertrophy and eventually dilatation associated with a cardiomyopathy.

While ischemic heart disease and cardiomyopathy may present with a slowly progressive course, acute myocarditis usually presents suddenly and is associated with not only fatigue but often florid heart failure.

Valvular Defects. Although the myocardium may be able to contract vigorously, it does little good if the valves that control inflow and outflow from the ventricular cavities are either obstructed or incompetent. Certainly two of the most common causes for progressive fatigue are mitral and aortic stenosis. Indeed, fatigue is frequently the first symptom of mitral stenosis. While reduction in previous physical activity may also occur in the patient with aortic stenosis, physical activities more frequently may be limited by the development of anginal-type chest pain or presyncope.

Stenosis of the pulmonic and tricuspid valves may also be associated with fatigue, though fatigue is rarely the first presenting complaint of these disorders. Because tricuspid stenosis is almost always associated with advanced rheumatic involvement of the mitral or aortic valve, signs of left ventricular dysfunction or mitral valve dysfunction become overt before the tricuspid stenosis is detected, frequently as a surprising hemodynamic finding at catheterization. Pulmonic stenosis in the adult rarely causes fatigue as a primary complaint. When it reaches the point at which the adult is limited by the severity of the pulmonic stenosis, there are almost always signs of severe right ventricular hypertension and frequently signs of tricuspid regurgitation or shunting from right to left across a probe-patent foramen ovale.

To deliver normal cardiac output the left ventricle must receive adequate amounts of blood from the right heart. Disease of the mitral valve may either prevent the arrival of appropriate amounts of blood into the left ventricle, as in the case of mitral stenosis, or pro-

duce regurgitation backward across the mitral valve, thus preventing adequate delivery of blood from the left ventricle into the aorta and the systemic circulation, as in the case of mitral insufficiency. It should be recognized, however, that since the blood being transferred from the right heart to the left heart must traverse the pulmonary circuit, any obstruction to flow in the pulmonary circuit may lead to an inadequate cardiac output.

Pulmonary-Vascular Cause. Primary pulmonary hypertension, which is most frequently seen in young females, often presents as progressive fatigue and can be diagnosed by physical and laboratory evaluation. On physical examination the patient will usually have a distinct right ventricular lift caused by compensatory right ventricular hypertrophy, and a loud palpable pulmonic closure sound indicative of pulmonary hypertension. Such patients will frequently have tricuspid regurgitation and cyanosis, because the elevated right sided pressures leading to a right-to-left shunt at the atrial level across a probe-patent foramen ovale allow delivery of unoxygenated blood into the left heart and its distribution to the periphery, where cyanosis is noted. Pulmonary hypertension may also result from secondary causes such as advanced parenchymal disease or chronic obstructive lung disease. The fatigue seen in these patients may be due not so much to the decreased cardiac output associated with pulmonary arteriolar obstruction as to the inability of the lungs to completely oxygenate blood as a result of the underlying lung disease.

Congenital Cardiac Lesions. Although a structural abnormality of a cardiac valve is the most common cause for symptoms of stenosis and regurgitation, similar complaints, particularly of fatigue, are encountered in the rare patient with a cardiac tumor. The vast majority of these arise in the atria, particularly the left atrium. These produce decreased cardiac output by obstructing flow from atrium to ventricle and by valvular regurgitation.

Although the adult who presents with congenital heart disease, particularly with an intracardiac shunt, may not complain initially of fatigue, it is not at all rare to have the patient note, after he has recovered from repair of the congenital intracardiac lesion, that he had never realized what normal exercise tolerance was until the defect was repaired. Indeed, chronic fatigue may occur over such a long period of time and with such a slow and progressive course that the patient himself does not recognize that his exercise tolerance has declined until late in the course of the congenital heart disease. The physical signs in such patients will be reviewed below.

Pericardial Disease. Patients with diseases of the

pericardium, particularly those with constrictive pericarditis, may present with a complaint of fatigue. Constrictive pericarditis may be an extremely slowly evolving process unassociated with symptoms other than increasing fatigue. Pericardial effusion, frequently seen in acute pericarditis, will usually present with symptoms other than just fatigue. However, in some patients the pericardial effusion may develop over a very long period of time and indeed may be associated with limited cardiac output during exercise. The most frequent cause for such a pericardial effusion is myxedema. However, in patients with myxedema it is often difficult to tell whether the pericardial effusion, which may be massive, is the cause of the fatigue or whether the general fatigue is actually related more to the hypometabolic state caused by the hypothyroidism.

Rhythmic Disturbances. Finally, cardiac output may be significantly limited by a small number of rhythm disturbances. It is clear from animal studies and clinical experience that a normal cardiac output can be maintained with heart rates as low as approximately 60, but that as the heart rate falls below 60 and is limited to a level of 40 or below, many patients will be unable to generate greater cardiac output with activity and thus will begin to complain of fatigue. In the elderly age group fatigue may be the first manifestation of complete heart block, with rates in the thirties or low forties, if the patient has not had a more catastrophic manifestation such as syncope or cardiac arrest. Similar to inadequate cardiac output with bradycardia, tachycardia, which decreases time for diastolic filling, may lead to a decreased cardiac output and thus provoke fatigue. The most frequent clinical situation in which this is encountered is atrial fibrillation. The fatigue and decreased cardiac output may be due not only to the rapid ventricular rate but also to the loss of the "atrial kick" or augmentation that increases ventricular filling prior to each ventricular contraction. The patient may complain of fatigue before he recognizes a rapid irregular heartbeat with a sensation of palpitations. Patients with paroxysmal atrial tachycardia or atrial flutter seldom come to the physician with a chief complaint of fatigue because these rhythms are usually relatively self-limited and, when they do occur, provoke symptoms of their own, such as palpitations, rather than fatigue. Similarly, ventricular tachycardia seldom presents with a complaint of fatigue since it usually is of such a rapid rate that there are other initial manifestations, such as syncope or subsequent ventricular fibrillation.

Excessive Demand for Cardiac Output. While the heart for the variety of reasons listed above may find itself unable to maintain a cardiac output to meet usual needs and thus provoke fatigue as a symptom, the heart itself may actually be performing optimally but the systemic metabolic demands imposed on the heart may be so excessive that there is inadequate tissue oxygenation. This can be seen in the case of fever and septicemia. Hyperthyroidism may also produce an excessive demand for cardiac output by increasing the metabolic demand of all the organs of the body and at the same time increasing the heart rate. Under these circumstances the heart may be structurally sound and performing far above its resting capabilities but just cannot meet the body's metabolic demand.

Another cause for excessive demand for cardiac output is the presence of an arteriovenous fistula. Under these circumstances the major portion of the blood ejected by the heart is committed to moving directly from the arterial to the venous system, so that the actual percentage of the cardiac output that is effective in providing oxygen and metabolic products to peripheral tissues is far less than under normal circumstances. Left-to-right shunt flow from an arterial to a venous bed under these circumstances may be so great as to actually exceed the amount of flow to the entire rest of the body. A history of a penetrating wound and the observation that one limb is actually larger than the contralateral limb with a continuous bruit over some portion of the enlarged limb is sufficient evidence to strongly raise the possibility of an arteriovenous fistula. The presence of the fistula can be confirmed clinically by eliciting Branham's sign, which is an almost immediate decline in heart rate during the occlusion of the arteriovenous fistula and the sudden increase in heart rate when the occlusion of the arteriovenous fistula is relieved.

Inadequate Tissue Oxygenation. Finally, fatigue, can be provoked, not because of inadequate cardiac output resulting from a cardiac defect or because of excessive demand for cardiac output owing to metabolic states, but rather because of inadequate tissue oxygenation produced by noncardiac problems. Inadequate tissue oxygenation can be caused by anemia. Despite the high flow to vascular beds, the number of oxygenated red cells is relatively inadequate to deliver enough oxygen to meet tissue needs. In the case of carbon monoxide intoxication there may be an adequate number of red cells delivered to peripheral vascular beds, but carbon monoxide tightly bound to the hemoglobin displaces the normally carried oxygen. Thus, the red cells may arrive at the right vascular bed in adequate numbers but they do not carry with them the necessary oxygen. Also, certain forms of congenital heart disease, particularly with right-to-left shunts in which the patient has a relatively large amount of unoxygenated blood in the arterial system, may lead

190 CARDIOVASCULAR PROBLEMS

Table 7–3. Classification of Chest Pain

Cardiac
    Typical Heberden's angina
    Atypical angina, anginal equivalent
    Variant Prinzmetal angina
    Unstable angina, accelerating angina
    Coronary insufficiency, preinfarction angina, intermediate
        syndrome
    Myocardial infarction
    Nonanginal myocardial ischemia
    Nonobstructive, nonspastic angina
    Mitral valve prolapse
Aortic pain
    Aortic dissection
Musculoskeletal
    Cervical radiculopathy
    Joint pain
        Shoulder pain (bursitis, rotator cuff injury, biceps tendinitis)
        Costochondrodynia, xyphoidynia
Pleuropericardial pain
    Pericarditis
    Pleuritis
    Pneumothorax
    Mediastinal emphysema
Gastrointestinal disease
    Hiatal hernia with reflux esophagitis, esophageal spasm
    Cholecystitis with or without gallstones
    Peptic ulcer disease
    Pancreatitis
Pulmonary disease
    Pulmonary hypertension
    Pneumonia
    Pulmonary embolus

to inadequate tissue oxygenation and thus a sense of fatigue, as noted above. However, these are almost inevitably associated with obvious signs such as cyanosis and clubbing.

CHEST PAIN

While the complaint of chest pain inevitably raises the question of cardiac disease, there are obviously many noncardiac causes for chest pain. When the chest pain is cardiac, a variety of syndromes with different historical features help establish a diagnosis and point toward appropriate diagnostic and therapeutic maneuvers. Table 7–3 itemizes the various pathophysiologic considerations of patients complaining of chest pain.

Cardiac. Definition and Differential Diagnosis. The most frequently encountered form of cardiac chest pain is typical angina pectoris, as described and named by Heberden.[1] A review of the Greek and Latin origins of the word "angina" emphasizes the very specific nature of the chest discomfort, which the patient frequently identifies spontaneously and almost diagnostically. The word "angina" is derived from the Latin word "angere," that is, to choke or smother. Thus, the patient who complains of a choking or smothering sensation and has some difficulty getting his breath during heavy activity is describing angina pectoris in its most classic form. Heberden in his description in 1772 described the salient features of angina. Classic Heberden's angina is a sensation of choking or pressure, usually located in the substernal area or low in the neck; it is precipitated by heavy physical activity, particularly after a meal or in cold weather, and is typically relieved within a matter of minutes after cessation of physical activity or the application of sublingual nitroglycerin. Emotional stimulation, particularly accompanied by physical activity such as occurs during sexual intercourse, commonly provokes classic angina. The discomfort originating in the substernal area may radiate, usually to the left arm but occasionally to the right arm as well as up the neck and jaw.

Many patients present with what we would term "atypical angina," which is in general produced by the same factors that provoke Heberden's typical angina but is associated with a different location or radiation of discomfort. It is not rare for a patient with angina to complain primarily of an aching sensation on exertion in the wrists, elbows, or shoulders. Prompt relief by cessation of the exertion or by nitroglycerin suggest that this is indeed atypical angina or an anginal equivalent. There are occasionally almost bizarre presentations of this atypical angina. For instance, there are well-documented cases of exertion-induced headaches caused by coronary insufficiency. Occasionally the site of previous trauma, such as the site of a previously extracted tooth or a traumatic wound in the head and neck region, may be the focal point for the atypical angina or anginal equivalent.

An initial complaint of dyspnea on exertion can after further questioning be found, like atypical angina, to be precipitated by factors other than simply exertion. This sensation of dyspnea with activity or emotion is promptly relieved by cessation of whatever activity provoked it. The diagnostic hint that points toward myocardial ischemia as the cause of the patient's unusual complaint is that the dyspnea is quite reproducible in terms of precipitating factors, location, and prompt relief by either cessation of the activity or by nitroglycerin.

While Heberden gained recognition in 1772 for the description of classic angina pectoris, Prinzmetal gained equal recognition in 1960 for defining another symptom complex caused by coronary insufficiency, which he entitled variant angina.[2] He described a form of chest pain that had many of the qualities of the chest pain described by Heberden but was rarely associated with exertion, frequently occurred at rest without obvious provocation, and often developed at a specific time in the day or night with an unusual reproducibility. Patients with Prinzmetal's, or variant angina, frequently note that they will awaken at the same time at night with the chest discomfort, which is promptly relieved with nitroglycerin. Such patients will frequently deny any exertional component and indeed will be able to go to their physiologic limit on the treadmill without showing electrocardiographic changes of myocardial ischemia. The chest discomfort is frequently accompanied by premature ventricular contractions and even transient ventricular tachycardia or ventricular fibrillation, all of which are promptly eliminated by sublingual nitroglycerin.

Pathophysiologic Considerations and Diagnostic Evaluation. There has been a tendency to attribute Heberden's typical angina to the presence of occlusive atherosclerotic lesions in the major coronary arteries, while Prinzmetal's variant angina has been attributed to spasm of the coronary arteries. In recent years it has become evident that this explanation is too simplistic. It is clear that patients with subtotal occlusive lesions of the major coronary arteries may indeed have an element of spasm superimposed on the occlusive lesions, provoking the symptoms of angina. It is also clear that some patients with rest angina alone and many of the features of Prinzmetal's angina may have significant occlusive lesions without evidence of spasm. The majority of patients with Prinzmetal's variant angina will have evidence of atherosclerotic changes even if only minor. In such patients it is presumed that the decreased coronary blood flow and thus angina is due to the combined effect of spasm of a normal portion of the coronary artery wall over or around a partial or nonobstructive atherosclerotic plaque.

Patients with typical Heberden's angina, atypical angina or anginal equivalent, and Prinzmetal's variant angina may have perfectly normal ECGs at rest or during periods of remission from their symptoms. During an acute episode, however, the electrocardiogram will show characteristic changes in the majority of cases. During typical angina there will usually be ST-segment depression or, less frequently, ST-segment elevation in the electrocardiographic leads appropriate to the area where coronary blood flow is decreased. During episodes of Prinzmetal or variant angina the electrocardiogram typically shows ST-segment elevation, often with ectopic ventricular activity. These electrocardiographic changes may be detected by Holter monitoring, during which the patient is careful to indicate by signaling the tape recorder that he is having symptoms. The characteristic ST-segment elevation may occur frequently in the patient with Prinzmetal's variant angina while the patient is totally asymptomatic.

The specificity of Holter monitoring to establish a diagnosis of either typical or variant angina has been limited by artifactual changes in the ST-segment produced by change in the relation of the electrodes to the heart with movement or respiration. Furthermore, the lead configuration of the Holter monitoring system may not detect certain ST-segment changes. It should be noted that the damping circuits installed in hard wire electrocardiographic monitoring systems to maintain effective baseline stability may mask the ST-segment changes that occur during either one of these forms of angina.

While angina has been categorized as typical, atypical, or variant, it may also be considered in terms of its pattern. Thus, it can be labeled stable, which indicates that its frequency, precipitating factors, length, severity of symptoms, and response to medication remain the same over a defined period of time; or it can be alternatively categorized as unstable or accelerating, if the frequency and severity of the angina is increased despite little change in the frequency of precipitating activities. When the angina becomes prolonged to perhaps as long as 10 minutes, frequently occurs at rest or awakens the patient at night, and is unrelieved by 3 sublingual nitroglycerin tablets given 5 minutes apart, the condition is often termed coronary insufficiency, preinfarction angina, or the intermediate syndrome. For all practical purposes these terms have been used to describe the set of circumstances and symptoms that taken alone are compatible with acute myocardial infarction but upon further laboratory study show no evidence of myocardial damage.

The pain of myocardial infarction is a further intensification of the pain described with angina pectoris. It is usually more severe and more prolonged and is often associated with diaphoresis, nausea, and even vomiting. While it may be difficult to determine specific criteria of duration, frequency, and severity, the patient himself is often able to recognize that this particular pain is different from his previous episodes of chest pain and, indeed, is a myocardial infarction. The diagnosis may be confirmed with the development of diagnostic Q waves and elevations in cardiac isoenzymes, the typical constellation of clinical symptoms and laboratory findings seen in transmural myocardial infarction. There can, however, be significant myocardial necrosis with a similar severity of chest pain and enzyme increase in patients who have sustained a subendocardial myocardial infarction. In such patients, though there may be no diagnostic Q waves in the electrocardiogram, almost inevitably there are transient ST-segment depressions or elevations, often followed by T-wave inversion.

Not all myocardial infarctions, neither transmural nor subendocardial, necessarily present with these dramatic symptoms or laboratory findings. Careful longitudinal follow-up of a group of citizens of Framingham, Massachusetts would indicate that approximately 25% of myocardial infarctions occur so quietly that the patient cannot recall any clinical event that he or a practiced physician can recognize in retrospect as a myocardial infarction, despite the fact that the patient has recently acquired ECG changes of myocardial infarction. It should also be recognized that patients undergoing the pain of myocardial infarction may have electrocardiograms that can easily be read as normal when they are initially seen in the emergency room or even in retrospect, although subsequent ECGs obtained hours later may well demonstrate the evolution of a myocardial infarction. This observation has led to the dictum in many emergency rooms that the electrocardiogram should not be used to rule out the diagnosis of myocardial infarction, but rather to confirm it in the patient who has been admitted for treatment of infarction or to detect a myocardial infarction in a patient in whom it was not even suspected because of the atypical nature of the symptoms. In short, if a patient with a classic history of acute myocardial infarction presents with prolonged, severe chest pain, diaphoresis, nausea, and shortness of breath, he should be admitted for observation with the presumptive diagnosis of myocardial infarction regardless of the electrocardiographic findings.

It is probably more important to obtain an electrocardiogram on the patient who presents to the emergency room with totally atypical chest pain that is not thought to be due to coronary insufficiency than it is to obtain one in a patient with a classic history for myocardial infarction.

There are patients who may have prolonged, rather severe substernal chest pain with many of the features of myocardial ischemia but who do not have the classic features of angina in terms of precipitating or relieving factors. These patients frequently have pain that would be labeled coronary insufficiency, preinfarction angina, or the intermediate syndrome except that on further laboratory investigation these patients do not have occlusive disease of their coronary arteries. This finding is classic in patients with hypertrophic cardiomyopathies with or without obstruction to the outflow tract of the left ventricle. Typically, the pain is not precipitated by any specific factor, nor is it relieved by the usual measures that relieve angina, such as sublingual nitroglycerin. The pain is almost undoubtedly myocardial in origin and presumably, particularly in the case of hypertrophic cardiomyopathies, is due to an inadequate delivery of oxygen to the hypertrophied myocardium, despite anatomically normal coronary arteries. Apparently the demand for myocardial oxygen consumption related to the hypertrophic process exceeds the coronary blood flow available from the normal coronary distribution.

While we have discussed the genesis of angina and coronary insufficiency in terms of atherosclerotic obstructive lesions or spasm, it seems clear that there is a group of patients who have anginal-type pain but cannot be demonstrated in the catheterization laboratory to have any obstructive lesions in their coronary arteries, nor do they develop coronary artery spasm after challenge with ergonovine. Such patients have typical angina pectoris and otherwise negative catheterization findings until their coronary blood flow is measured after stress. In this group of patients it would appear that the ability of the microcirculation in the myocardium to vasodilate or develop a hyperemic response is severely limited. Thus, the patients develop an anginal-type syndrome without obstruction or spasm in their major coronary arteries. The frequency of this phenomena is not known because the techniques for measuring coronary blood flow in the human are so complex that it is not the normal practice of the standard cardiac catheterization laboratory to test individuals for the presence of this abnormality. It is not a rare phenomenon in medical centers that catheterize a large number of patients to have an occasional patient who has what is felt to be a classic history for angina pectoris return from the catheter laboratory with absolutely normal findings in terms of the coronary anatomy and the absence of spasm.

Finally, patients with mitral valve prolapse frequently present with chest pain. The chest pain characteristically has features that are the opposite of those noted in patients with typical Heberden's angina. The chest pain is usually nonexertional, prolonged, nonradiating, and unresponsive to nitroglycerin. It may be associated with areas of localized tenderness over the chest wall, particularly the costochondral junctions. The pain is frequently located beneath the left breast. The source or cause of the pain is unknown.

Aortic Pain. Definition. Trauma to the aorta may provoke severe chest pain that is indistinguishable from that of myocardial infarction. The prototype is the pain of aortic dissecting aneurysm. Perhaps its greatest distinguishing feature is that it is often reported as a sudden, tearing, sharp pain that is unremitting and almost unresponsive to large doses of morphine or its derivatives. The pain frequently originates in the intrascapular area rather than in the anterior precordium, although its origin from the anterior precordium does not preclude the diagnosis.

Differential Diagnosis. The features of the pain, in addition to the absence of a major peripheral pulse that had previously been noted, should be an important indication for the diagnosis of aortic dissection. Electrocardiographic changes are not rare in aortic dissection because frequently severe hypertension is associated with dissection and acute ST-segment depressions are compatible with subendocardial ischemia.

Typically, chest x-ray shows widening of the mediastinum with a roughening of the edge of the descending thoracic aorta as it appears along the left cardiac border. Unfortunately these x-ray findings are sometimes difficult to elicit because the patient is so ill that the only way to obtain a chest film is to use a portable chest x-ray technique, which, because of the short focal distnce, distorts the mediastinal shadow and frequently makes it appear larger than it would if the standard standing six-foot chest film were obtained. In the past it has frequently been necessary to perform retrograde aortography to establish the diagnosis. This procedure in itself carries certain risks because of the chance of entering the false channel and even perforating the aorta, which is already weakened by the process of dissection and the inflammation that follows shortly thereafter. More recently the development of digital subtraction techniques has allowed the intravenous injection of a large bolus of contrast media for well-detailed imaging of the aorta.

In our experience an even less traumatic approach has been successful. Thoracic CT scans of the aorta will usually demonstrate not only the origin but the eventual re-entry of the channel of dissection. This can all be accomplished without contrast media, although on occasion it is necessary to highlight the main channel and the false channel by obtaining a CT scan after enhancement with intravenous injection of contrast material. In isolated cases it is possible to demonstrate the dissection by echocardiography. This technique is less valuable as it may not give a full range of the extent, origin, or termination of the dissection.

Musculoskeletal Pain. *Definition.* Not all chest pain is cardiac in origin, and certainly many patients considered to have angina pectoris may in reality have pain arising from the musculoskeletal system of the chest. Such pain may be fleeting, cramping, or dull and prolonged. It frequently occurs at rest and seldom is consistently associated with a particular activity.

Pathophysiologic Considerations and Differential Diagnosis. The relative frequence of angina occurring in shoulders or upper arms may lead one to overlook the possibility of a cervical radiculopathy as the source for the presumed anginal pain. The discomfort in the arm, shoulder, or neck caused by cervical radiculopathy may be related to exertion in the sense that a specific form of activity may provoke the discomfort, but rarely is the discomfort promptly eliminated when the precipitating activity is stopped. The pain of cervical radiculopathy is usually prolonged, relatively unremitting, and unresponsive to nitroglycerin. In addition to chest, neck, and arm pain related to pressure on the cervical nerves, chest pain may arise from disease in the shoulders or possibly in the costochondral joints and the xyphoid process. The pain of bursitis may be severe and almost debilitating, but it is rarely exertion induced or relieved by rest.

On physical examination, areas of point tenderness are easily elicited. Rotator cuff injuries to the shoulder may also be associated with pain that can frequently be confused with cardiac pain and falsely attributed to exertion, since specific forms of physical activity involving the shoulder, such as putting washing on the clothes line or lifting heavy objects, may initially appear to be the precipitating factors. It is not exertion per se, but rather stress on the shoulder joint that is precipitating the pain. The same observations are equally true for such localized problems as biceps tendinitis. Some patients presenting with chest pain will have obvious tenderness along the sternal border, particularly on the left side in the region of the costochondral junctions. Whether this tenderness is actually due to an inflammatory process in the joint between the cartilage and the rib end is questionable, but it has been treated with anti-inflammatory agents as well as radiation therapy with occasional dramatic results. After careful questioning and on physical examination it is clear that this pain is not cardiac because it does not have the classic features of angina and can easily be precipitated by palpation over the costochondral junctions. Similar pain can be elicited in many patients by palpation over the xyphoid process. Again, this so-called xyphoidynia does not have the hallmarks for cardiac pain. However, it should arouse the suspicion of underlying peptic ulcer disease, hiatal hernia, or gallbladder disease, since a high incidence of these gastrointestinal disorders has been noted with xyphoidynia.

Pleuropericardial Pain. *Definition.* Irritation of both the pleura and the pericardium can produce chest pain that is at times indistinguishable from pain of cardiac origin. The hallmark of this form of pain is its close correlation with respiration or movement of the torso. Typical pleural or pericardial pain may be as severe as the pain associated with myocardial infarction. It is classically described as gripping, grating, or knifelike and is accentuated by inspiration and partially relieved by purposeful splinting of the chest wall. This pain may be more severe with the patient in different positions. Some patients may find it impossible to lie flat; others will find it impossible to sit up; some patients may find relief by lying on either side. It is worth recognizing that pleuritis and pericarditis frequently coexist, since the same pathologic process may involve both the pleura and the pericardium simultaneously.

Differential Diagnosis. The differential diagnosis is made much easier when either a pleural or pericardial rub elicited in several body positions can be heard. It is not rare for the physician to be unable to hear a rub with a patient sitting upright but to hear it with the patient lying flat, and vice versa. The absence of the rub does not imply the absence of underlying inflammation in the pleura or the pericardium, because the severity of the pain may prevent the patient from producing enough respiratory excursion to produce the rub (see Chapter 6).

A pericardial rub can frequently be differentiated from a pleural rub because of its constancy despite respiration and its easy timing with the cardiac cycle. A pericardial rub may have one, two, or three components. To detect more than one component it may be necessary to listen for these components with varying degrees of inspiration and expiration. The first component, the systolic pericardial rub, is presumably due to primary inflammatory involvement of the pericardium overlying the contracting ventricles that produced the rub with ventricular systole. If the pericardium is more extensively involved than in the region of the ventricles, there may also be a diastolic component to the rub. Involvement of the pericardium overlying the atrial appendages frequently results in a third component, which occurs in presystole coincident with atrial contraction. The presence of this presystolic component in the rub is virtually diagnostic of a pericardial rub; this component, in addition to the relationship to cardiac contraction and the presence of such a rub in the absence of respiratory movement, serves to separate it from a pleural rub.

Much of the pain of pleuritis or even pericarditis may be attributed to the involuntary contraction of the intercostal muscles, which occurs in an effort to prevent excursion that would lead to irritation of the pleura and the pericardium. Thus, other conditions that may provoke spasm of the intercostal muscles may also be associated with chest pain mimicking cardiac pain. Spontaneous pneumothorax, which almost inevitably carries with it pleural inflammation, may thus produce the intercostal splinting and pain that is mistaken for myocardial pain.

Mediastinal emphysema, or collecting of air in the mediastinum, represents a rare but important cause for chest pain, usually in young patients, that may totally simulate the chest pain of myocardial infarction but that can be differentiated by its historical setting and certain classic physical findings. In the case of mediastinal emphysema, an alveolus or a group of alveoli rupture deep within the lung and air dissects back along the pulmonary vessels, allowing the collection of a small amount of air in the mediastinum between the pleural reflection and the pericardium. Gross examples of this are seen occasionally in the recovery room after thoracic procedures.

Mediastinal emphysema can also occur spontaneously in a healthy patient, although the air in the mediastinum is of such a small amount that routine chest x-rays will not demonstrate the air, as they normally do in overt cases. Patients with spontaneous mediastinal emphysema are frequently young (below age 30) and present to the emergency room with oppressive substernal chest pain with occasional radiation to the shoulder and the arm and with a history quite compatible with myocardial infarction. On careful questioning the patient may volunteer that when he lies in a particular position, especially the left lateral position, he may be able to hear a ticking or dripping sound within his chest. This presumably is due to the crepitation created by the air in the pleuropericardial reflexion as the heart contracts and relaxes, redistributing the bubbles of air in the pleuropericardial space. These patients may also have the same complaints as the patient with pericarditis; namely, there are certain positions they cannot tolerate because of the exacerbation of the chest pain.

On physical exam, there can often be heard a crunching sound during systole along the left sternal border. This so-called Hamman's sign may be elicited only in a specific position, such as sitting forward or lying in the left lateral position. It is frequently heard only during certain phases of respiration, usually during mid inspiration and not at end expiration or end inspiration. In addition to Hamman's sign, these patients will frequently have a popping or scratching midinspiratory sound heard in systole along the left sternal border that does not have the harsh quality of Hamman's crunch. Chest x-ray will rarely show air in the mediastinum but will frequently show a small pneumothorax, usually on the left.

Gastrointestinal Disease. *Differential Diagnosis.* Many disease processes arising in the gastrointestinal system may simulate cardiovascular chest pain. A large portion of the adult population, particularly obese individuals, has a high incidence of hiatal hernia, which of itself probably does not provoke chest pain similar to cardiac pain but when associated with reflux esophagitis may cause the esophagus to become irritated and develop spasm. Such spasm can certainly simulate the pain of cardiac origin, and the full gamut of cardiovascular studies may be required to rule out the presence of coincident cardiac disease. It should be emphasized that esophageal spasm seldom radiates in the fashion that the pain of coronary insufficiency does, but it can radiate even to the jaws and teeth in unusual circumstances. The development of pain after large meals, present particularly after lying down and often associated with waterbrash, should alert the clinician to the possibility that he is dealing with esophageal pain rather than cardiac pain. It should be emphasized that the demonstration of a hiatal hernia with or without esophageal spasm should not preclude further investigation to rule out a myocardial source for chest pain, since the two disease processes occur with such a high frequency in the middle-aged population that there are inevitably combinations of both conditions in many patients.

Pain originating from peptic ulcer disease is less frequently confused with pain of cardiac origin, although when the pain is localized high in the epigastrium it is sometimes difficult to separate the two by only the history. The pain of cholecystitis with or without gallstones may be so variable that it can easily be mistaken for cardiac pain, and vice versa. It is well recognized that pain from the gallbladder bed can be reflected, particularly to the right shoulder and even to the right arm. Less frequently it is noted in the left shoulder. Pancreatitis may pose a more difficult differential diagnosis than would immediately be supposed. In acute extensive pancreatitis there actually is irritation of the retroperitoneal diaphragmatic area, which in turn may be associated with pleural and pericardial inflammation, which is presumably the cause of the small pleural effusion occasionally seen in the pancreatitis and of the T-wave changes in ECG that may lead to strong suspicions that a cardiac event is occurring. The T-wave changes may be due to either pericarditis or electrolyte imbalances.

Pulmonary Disease. Differential Diagnosis. Intrinsic diseases within the lung other than pneumonia and pulmonary embolus with infarction and coincident pleuritis are a rare cause for chest pain simulating cardiac pain. In both pneumonia and pulmonary embolus with infarction the pain is usually due to pleural irritation, frequently resulting in detection of a pleural rub and rales. In the case of massive pulmonary embolism, severe right ventricular hypertension may develop, producing right ventricular ischemia and chest pain that may be indistinguishable from that of myocardial infarction.

Patients with pulmonary hypertension frequently have pressing, prolonged, oppressive substernal chest pain that may be misinterpreted as being due to coronary insufficiency. It has been attributed to right ventricular ischemia secondary to the right ventricular hypertension and increased myocardial oxygen demand of the hypertrophied right ventricle. This pain is usually slow in onset, dull, nonradiating, and slow in offset. On rare occasions it may be relieved by nitroglycerin, perhaps because of the venous pooling produced by the nitroglycerin and thus the decreased right ventricular volume and right ventricular wall stress.

DYSPNEA

DEFINITION

Dyspnea may be broadly defined as an abnormal, uncomfortable awareness of breathing. It is strictly a subjective sensation. It may be accompanied by hyperpnea, an increased depth and rate of respiration, by tachypnea, an increased respiratory rate with usually shallow respirations, or by trepopnea, a preference for sleeping on one particular side in the recumbent position. However, patients with dyspnea may have none of these abnormal breathing patterns and still complain of a sensation of difficulty obtaining satisfactory ventilation (see also Chapter 6).

PATHOPHYSIOLOGIC CONSIDERATIONS

The mechanism for dyspnea has not been well defined. It has been hypothesized that the misalignment of muscle spindles in the respiratory musculature is detected by receptors in the musculature and conveyed to the central nervous system via the vagus nerve. It has also been postulated that distension of pulmonary veins may act in a similar manner. Whether the dyspnea in the cardiac patient is accounted for by alterations in respiratory mechanical factors resulting from fluid retention or by distension of pulmonary veins secondary to an elevated left atrial or left ventricular end-diastolic pressure is conjectural.

DIFFERENTIAL DIAGNOSIS

Patients with cardiac disease may have different clinical settings for the development of dyspnea. Dyspnea on exertion is a classic form seen in the cardiac patient, as is paroxysmal nocturnal dyspnea, which may be so severe as to awaken the patient from sleep and force him to sit bolt upright in bed in order to regain a sense of normal respiration. Many patients with cardiac disease will develop Cheyne-Stokes respirations, particularly at rest or while asleep. While some patients may be awakened at night during the rapid inspiratory phase of Cheyne-Stokes respiration, many cardiac patients with Cheyne-Stokes respirations do not recognize the altered respiratory pattern or dyspnea and do not awaken during the night. Wood coined the term trepopnea and in a series of classic studies demonstrated that cardiac patients almost inevitably have a side they prefer to sleep on.[3] If they are moved without being awakened to the opposite side they will rapidly awaken and turn to the side of preference. Cardiac patients usually prefer to sleep on their right side.

The most obvious decision a physician must make when faced with the complaint of dyspnea is whether it is due to cardiac or respiratory causes. In some cases in which the cardiac condition has led to secondary pulmonary ventilatory deficiencies, assignment of the cause of dyspnea may be all but impossible.

Dyspnea is often the first manifestation of cardiac failure or inadequate cardiac output. Thus the same factors listed under fatigue that are considered in reviewing the causes of inadequate cardiac output (Table 7–2) should be reviewed when a patient presents with dyspnea.

PALPITATIONS

DEFINITION

Palpitations represent the subjective awareness of the heart beating. In general the awake adult is seldom aware of his or her heartbeat, although the more forceful or presumably larger ejection fractions associated with anxiety or excitement may be felt in unusual circumstances. Either slow or fixed heart rates with normal electrical conduction are seldom perceived.

Many patients complaining of palpitations who undergo ambulatory ECG monitoring will fail to detect premature beats or will label normal beats palpitations as often as they will correctly detect abnormally conducted or premature beats. Thus, the complaint of palpitations does not necessarily mean that the patient is having a cardiac arrhythmia. The patient may simply

Table 7–4. Classification of Palpitations

Normal sinus rhythm
Single or sporadic palpitations
   Premature atrial or ventricular contractions
Rapid palpitations
   Sinus tachycardia
   Paroxysmal atrial or ventricular tachycardia
   Paroxysmal atrial flutter or fibrillation
Slow palpitations
   Sinus bradycardia
   Junctional rhythm
   Complete heart block
Regular vs irregular palpitations
   Sinus tachycardia, paroxysmal atrial tachycardia, paroxysmal atrial flutter, and paroxysmal ventricular tachycardia (regular) versus multiple premature atrial or ventricular beats, paroxysmal atrial fibrillation (irregular)

be in a heightened state of awareness and thus feels normally conducted heartbeats.

DIFFERENTIAL DIAGNOSIS

Table 7–4 provides an outline for attempting to differentiate potential forms of palpitations. As previously stated, normal sinus rhythm usually is not associated with palpitations, but during periods of physical or emotional stress the normal adult can frequently perceive the heartbeat. Single or sporadic palpitations are almost inevitably due to premature atrial or ventricular contractions. Auscultation of the patient who frequently has this complaint will usually indicate that there are relatively long periods of normal sinus rhythm interspersed with a series of premature beats usually followed by a compensatory pause. It is not possible by auscultation to determine if the premature beat is arising from the atrium or the ventricle; auscultation serves only to confirm the presence of premature beats and also to confirm that the patient has the symptoms at the same time he has the premature beat. Electrocardiography, performed even on a random basis, will frequently confirm the presence and the nature of the premature beat associated with the palpitations. In more complex and confusing situations 24-hour ambulatory electrocardiographic monitoring with a tape recorder (Holter monitoring) may be necessary to better define the arrhythmia associated with the symptom.

Rapid palpitations may occur with sinus tachycardia, paroxysmal atrial or ventricular tachycardia, and paroxysmal atrial flutter or fibrillation. Slow palpitations may occur in the patient who develops transient sinus bradycardia, junctional rhythm, or complete heart block. Whether the palpitations are slow or fast, it is helpful to know if they are regular. If the palpitations are rapid and regular one must determine whether one is dealing with sinus tachycardia, paroxysmal atrial tachycardia, paroxysmal atrial flutter, or, less likely, paroxysmal ventricular tachycardia. If the palpitations are reported as rapid and irregular one must distinguish between premature atrial or ventricular beats occurring in salvos and paroxysmal atrial fibrillation. The differentiation of atrial fibrillation from multiple premature beats occurring in an irregular fashion cannot always be ascertained by auscultation alone; again, the electrocardiogram settles the issue.

Patients who complain of the sudden onset of rapid regular palpitations usually are describing paroxysmal atrial tachycardia, particularly if the termination of the palpitations is as sudden as the onset. The less frequent cause for this pattern of sudden onset, sudden offset is paroxysmal atrial flutter. Paroxysmal ventricular tachycardia may also have the same features of sudden onset and offset, but because of its usually rapid rate and its tendency to degenerate into ventricular fibrillation, syncope becomes a more overriding complaint from the patient.

Some patients with paroxysmal atrial tachycardia and paroxysmal atrial flutter may develop presyncope with the arrhythmia, particularly if they have valvular heart disease, which further compromises cardiac output during the period of tachycardia; as a general rule, however, these forms of paroxysmal tachycardia are not associated with syncope. It also should be recognized that, although the hallmark of paroxysmal atrial tachycardia or atrial flutter is sudden termination of the rhythm, the patient himself may not feel that the rhythm is terminated so suddenly because the rhythm does not always immediately revert from its paroxysmal form to normal sinus rhythm, instead passing through a transient period of irregular premature atrial contractions, in the case of paroxysmal atrial tachycardia, or a transient period of irregular atrial fibrillation, in the case of the termination of paroxysmal atrial flutter.

SYNCOPE

DEFINITION

Syncope is best defined as a transient sudden loss of consciousness. It should be carefully differentiated from what might better be called presyncope, which is the sudden sensation of near fainting, lightheadedness, or dizziness. While presyncope may be anteced-

Table 7–5. Classification of Syncope

Cardiac syncope
  Outflow tract obstruction
    Aortic stenosis
    Idiopathic hypertrophic subaortic stenosis
    Pulmonary embolus
    Primary pulmonary hypertension
  Inflow tract obstruction
    Cardiac tumors
    Pericardial effusion with tamponade
  Acute myocardial damage
    Massive myocardial infarction
    Cardiac rupture
  Cardiac arrhythmias
    Tachycardia
    Ventricular tachycardia and fibrillation
      "Quinidine syncope" or "Torsades des Pointes"
      Prolonged QT syndrome
    Bradycardia
      Sinus arrest or sinoatrial block
        Carotid sinus syncope
      Complete heart block
      Deglutition (glossopharyngeal) syncope
Peripheral vascular syncope
  Orthostatic hypotension
  Vasovagal syncope
Central nervous system syncope
  Central seizures
  Narcolepsy with or without cataplexy
  Micturition syncope
  Cough syncope
  Vertebrobasilar insufficiency
  "Drop attacks"
Other noncardiovascular causes of syncope
  Hypoglycemia
  Hyperventilation
  Hysteria

ent to a true syncopal episode, it never involves true loss of consciousness, and it is frequently difficult to demonstrate any cardiovascular abnormality during the period of presyncope. The term black-out, which is frequently used as a synonym for syncope, is casually used to include such situations as transient loss of memory, transient weakness or lightheadedness, or true syncope with loss of consciousness (see Chapter 15).

PATHOPHYSIOLOGIC CONSIDERATIONS AND DIFFERENTIAL DIAGNOSIS

Table 7–5 gives a classification and a differential diagnosis for syncope. Cardiac syncope can be conceptualized into factors that either prevent adequate outflow from the heart or eliminate adequate inflow to the heart. Outflow from the left ventricle of the heart is typically limited by the presence of severe aortic stenosis or idiopathic hypertrophic subaortic stenosis. Syncope under these circumstances may actually be due to a ventricular arrhythmia such as ventricular tachycardia. Obstruction to outflow from the right heart, whether due to hypertrophic subpulmonic stenosis, pulmonary valvular stenosis, pulmonary embolus, or pulmonary hypertension, may also provoke syncope since this obstruction quickly eliminates any venous return to the left heart and therefore prevents adequate cardiac output even though left ventricular function may be normal. Massive pulmonary embolus, particularly a saddle embolus obstructing both pulmonary arteries, may be associated with syncope. Primary pulmonary hypertension may also be associated with syncope.

Although pulmonary embolus and primary pulmonary hypertension, which prevent transfer of blood from the right heart to the left heart, have been considered examples of outflow obstruction of the right ventricle, they might also well be considered examples of factors that prevent inflow of blood to the left ventricle. There are other factors, such as cardiac tumors and pericardial effusion with tamponade, that may lead to obstruction of inflow into the ventricles and hence may provoke syncope.

Acute severe myocardial damage may lead to sudden loss of left ventricular ejection, as is seen in massive myocardial infarction or in cardiac rupture associated with myocardial infarction. Here again, classification comes into play, because in the case of cardiac rupture the mechanism of loss of cardiac output may actually result from acute pericardial tamponade rather than loss of left ventricular function alone.

One of the most common causes for syncope is the presence of cardiac arrhythmias, which include ventricular tachycardia and ventricular fibrillation. These are most frequently seen as the consequence of ischemic heart disease but may occur in other conditions such as the prolonged QT syndrome and hypertrophic cardiomyopathies, and as an unforeseen and unwelcome consequence of antiarrhythmic therapy for cardiac arrhythmias.

For many years isolated cases of "quinidine syncope" have been recognized by clinicians, but only recently has the genesis of this unhappy event become clear. Some patients, particularly those with prolonged QT intervals and hypokalemia who are exposed to antiarrhythmic agents such as quinidine or procaine amide, may develop ventricular tachycardia with a distinctive pattern. This ventricular tachycardia frequently degenerates into ventricular fibrillation, which may then spontaneously revert to normal sinus rhythm. The distinctive electrocardiographic pattern of this ventricular tachycardia has been labeled "Torsades des Pointes"[4,5]; that is, turning around a point. In essence, there is a series of rapid, somewhat irregular, broad

QRS complexes, initially upright and then seeming to twist to become inverted over the course of one or two beats. This arrhythmia was thought to be rare, but it is now apparent from frequent electrocardiographic monitoring that a much larger number of patients who are placed on antiarrhythmic agents may develop this arrhythmia than had previously been thought. The fact that a patient has regained consciousness without apparent long-term damage does not mean that he had a benign faint; it may indeed indicate he had an episode of ventricular tachycardia that degenerated to ventricular fibrillation, which then reverted spontaneously to normal sinus rhythm, particularly if the patient is taking antiarrhythmic agents.

Several families were initially identified as having a combination of deafness and a prolonged QT interval by electrocardiogram. These families were noted to have a high incidence of spontaneous ventricular fibrillation frequently induced by exercise. It has now become apparent that deafness does not have to be a feature of this syndrome; there are well-documented families with the syndrome in whom children experience sudden death.

Atrial tachycardia and atrial fibrillation may on rare occasion be associated with syncope, usually in the elderly patient, who develops a rapid ventricular rate in excess of 160 beats per minute. Many times there will be coincident cerebrovascular disease.

Just as too rapid a ventricular rate will decrease overall cardiac output to the point at which cerebral blood flow is inadequate to maintain consciousness, so too a slow heart rate may produce inadequate cardiac output with the same consequences. Severe sinus bradycardia or sinus exit block may provoke syncope. Stimulating the carotid sinus, which elicits the carotid sinus reflex with consequent vagal stimulation, may provoke bradycardia and syncope. In the days of the high starched collar this stimulation was a more readily recognized cause for syncope. Indentation of the high starched collar into the neck—and thus inadvertent carotid massage—while the head was twisted would involve the appropriate reflex to produce severe bradycardia and syncope.

Complete heart block is associated with syncope in connection with several possible arrhythmias, including profound bradycardia, asystole, ventricular tachycardia, and ventricular fibrillation, all of which prevent adequate cardiac output and blood flow to the brain and thus produce syncope.

On rare occasions the act of swallowing may provoke syncope, known thus as deglutition or glossopharyngeal syncope. For reasons not clear, in susceptible individuals the act of swallowing apparently stimulates the vagus nerve and provokes transient asystole.

Abnormalities of the peripheral vascular system may provoke syncope by lowering effective circulating blood volume and effective perfusion pressure and by decreasing flow to the brain. When patients with orthostatic hypotension arise to a sitting or standing position, the arterial system does not constrict rapidly enough to prevent pooling of blood in the periphery, and consequently cardiac output and cerebral blood flow are decreased. The sudden loss of peripheral vascular tone is compounded by the fact that the loss is frequently associated with an absence of a normal tachycardic response to maintain cardiac output. This constellation of events is frequently seen in the diabetic patient.

Vasovagal syncope, which is known as a common faint, is frequently encountered in the patient who is presented with a life situation from which he would just as soon flee, such as the sight of blood or the anticipation of venesection. As the term implies, there are essentially two components to the syncopal episode. One is bradycardia caused by vagal stimulation and the other is transient loss of vascular tone. Thus, just as in the case of orthostatic hypotension, there is peripheral pooling of the circulating blood volume and inappropriate bradycardia, limiting the amount of cardiac output and cerebral blood flow and hence precipitating loss of consciousness and syncope. The dual mechanism of this syndrome has been graphically demonstrated with the advent of implantable pacemakers. Many patients who have had pacemakers implanted because of severe bradycardia still continue to have syncope because, although the bradycardia has been eliminated by the pacemaker, the loss of peripheral vascular tone and subsequent pooling of the blood volume in the extremities still occurs.

While problems with the cardiovascular system are responsible for the majority of causes for syncope, the central nervous system without provocation from cardiovascular deficits may still provoke syncope. Diseases of the central nervous system, whether they be grand mal seizures or petit mal seizures, may produce transient syncope. With petit mal seizures there is seldom loss of muscle tone and falling. Such patients appear to have only a sudden loss of awareness of what is going on around them. Narcolepsy, which is the sudden onset of a sleeplike trance, also produces transient loss of consciousness. It may also be accompanied by cataplexy, the involuntary shaking of large muscle groups.

One of the more common causes for central nervous system syncope is micturition syncope. The classic appearance is in the elderly patient with prostatic obstruction who arises from sleep to urinate. He is found unconscious in the bathroom, urination completed. This syncope probably results from a combination of reflexes, one of which is vagal stimulation as he strains to urinate; another is due to a reflex arc in which sudden decompression of the bladder provokes a poorly defined reflex that in turn provokes syncope.

One of the most interesting forms of syncope is cough syncope. This, too, has a fairly typical clinical setting. The usual patient with cough syncope is a short, squat male with chronic obstructive lung disease or chronic bronchitis who in the midst of a barrage of coughs suddenly loses consciousness. This syncope is caused by cerebral ischemia. The increase in venous hydrostatic pressure during the cough is so great that it raises the venous pressure in the central nervous system to above the arterial pressure; the brain can actually be seen to blanch as arterial inflow is halted.

Another cause of central nervous system syncope is compromise to the vertebral basilar system. Also sudden lifting of the head or turning of the neck may occlude the vertebral arteries as they run through the transverse processes of the cervical vertebrae. This leads to transient ischemia of the brain stem, producing "drop attacks." This complaint is not uncommon among elderly patients who travel to Europe to admire cathedral ceilings.

There are other noncardiovascular causes for syncope, although the speed of the onset of syncope is less dramatic than that seen in situations in which the cardiovascular or central nervous system is immediately involved. These include hypoglycemia, hyperventilation, and hysteria. So-called hysterical faints may have a large vasovagal component; whether they are truly different in mechanism from vasovagal syncope is debatable. There are also patients who have so-called myoclonic attacks, in which they suddenly fall to the ground and just as suddenly quickly arise to resume their normal activity. These are not accompanied by loss of consciousness.

SWELLING

DEFINITION

The general term "swelling" has been used to indicate the accumulation of extracellular fluids in a variety of available spaces, including the skin, pleural cavity, peritoneal cavity, and extremities.

Table 7–6. Differential Diagnosis of Swelling

Cardiac causes
  Congestive heart failure
  Cardiac tumors
  Tricuspid stenosis or regurgitation
  Constrictive pericarditis or pericardial effusion
Pulmonary causes
  Cor pulmonale
Hepatic causes
  Cirrhosis
  Chiari's syndrome
  Portal vein thrombosis
Abdominal tumors
Renal causes
  Nephrotic syndrome
  Chronic renal insufficiency resulting from diverse causes
  Renal vein thrombosis
Stasis
  Venous
    "Physiologic" or postural
    Secondary to chronic thrombophlebitis
    Pregnancy
  Lymphatic
    Obstruction of lymphatics
    Milroy's disease, Noonan's syndrome, lymphedema praecox
    Elephantiasis
Microvascular
  Angioneurotic edema
  Inflammatory lesions
Hormonal imbalance
  Menstrual, pregnancy
  Myxedema
  Cushing's disease or therapeutic steroid therapy

PATHOPHYSIOLOGIC CONSIDERATIONS AND DIFFERENTIAL DIAGNOSIS

Table 7–6 lists a simple differential diagnosis for accumulation of such fluids in these compartments. With regard to the cardiovascular system, the most common cause of swelling is congestive heart failure, usually caused by left ventricular failure or a valvular abnormality, both of which decrease cardiac output and thus decrease renal blood flow and consequently lead to accumulation of sodium and water. Under these circumstances the plasma volume expands and eventually fluid accumulates in the tissues. When the congested organs can no longer contain the excess fluid, it is released from these capillary networks within the organ and accumulates in compartments surrounding the organ.

Obstructive or constrictive phenomena that limit inflow into the heart may lead to elevated venous pressures and subsequent extravasation of fluid into various body compartments. Thus, swelling is frequently seen with constrictive pericarditis and pericardial effusion, both of which limit inflow to the heart. Cardiac tumors that obstruct inflow, particularly right atrial myxomas, may be associated with edema formation without

pleural effusion. Tricuspid valvular disease may lead to the same type of elevated venous pressure and the same phenomenon. In the carcinoid syndrome there may be marked fibrous thickening of the subendocardial portion of the right ventricle, as well as tricuspid stenosis, which has similar manifestations.

Changes in the pulmonary circulation do not produce fluid accumulation directly but do so secondarily by causing right ventricular hypertrophy, decreased right ventricular compliance, and frequently, tricuspid regurgitation. Under these circumstances not only is there increased venous pressure and congestion because of the elevated venous pressure, but almost always there is decreased cardiac output with decreased sodium and water clearance from the kidney, which leads to edema formation and the clinical syndrome of cor pulmonale.

Diseases of the liver, particularly cirrhosis, and, less frequently, obstruction of hepatic veins (Chiari's syndrome), and portal vein thrombosis, may lead to ascites. Abdominal swelling may be due to abdominal tumors, whether they be primary isolated tumors or metastatic tumors. The differential diagnosis of abdominal swelling or ascites may be complex in women who may have carcinoma of the ovary or in cirrhotic patients who have functional murmurs on the basis of their anemia.

Malfunction of the kidney with subsequent accumulation of sodium and water, for whatever renal cause, may produce the same swelling as seen in patients with cardiovascular disease. The absence of obvious cardiac causes for the swelling and a careful laboratory analysis of renal function should serve to incriminate the kidney rather than the heart.

Probably the most frequent cause of swelling, particularly of the feet and ankles, is stasis. These stasic causes are usually the consequence of deep venous disease, often chronic or recurrent deep venous thrombosis. However, they can be seen in healthy normal patients under specific circumstances. Patients who assume an upright position, whether sitting or standing for long periods of time, may develop edema of the ankles without any obvious venous disease. This is a frequent phenomenon following long trips in automobiles or airplanes, during which the subject places prolonged orthostatic pressure on the venous system in the legs and does not maintain a normal circulatory pattern by moving about periodically. Pregnancy may also provoke edema without overt venous disease, although during the pregnant state venous compliance is increased. This increase in venous compliance and venous congestion with increased circulating volume is not the only cause for the edema seen in pregnancy. It is believed that the gravid uterus may produce occlusion of the inferior vena cava and its branches returning from the lower extremities to the extent that the hydrostatic pressure in the venous system of the legs is markedly increased and there is effusion of fluid into the subcutaneous tissues of the feet and ankles.

Obstruction of the lymphatic system, particularly from the legs, may be precipitated by radical dissection of the groin or radiation therapy during which the normal lymphatic channels are disrupted, thus increasing lymphatic pressure and creating effusion into the subcutaneous tissues. Various hereditary diseases such as Milroy's disease, Noonan's syndrome, or lymphedema praecox may be associated with disruption of lymphatic channels in the legs and thus with edema of the legs. This edema is usually long standing and the swelling does not have the pitting character that other forms of edema of the legs have. Elephantiasis, which is massive swelling of an extremity caused by damage to lymphatics following filarial infestation, is a rare cause of lymphedema in the Western world.

Conditions that affect the integrity of the capillary wall may also lead to swelling. Various inflammatory lesions may be associated with peripheral edema. Allergic reactions also may cause peripheral edema. Angioneurotic edema may be associated with swelling in a variety of compartments, including the feet, hands, and arms.

Hormonal imbalances, particularly in females, are associated with swelling. It is common for women to have a transient 3- to 4-pound weight gain preceding the menstrual cycle, manifested by swelling not only of the feet but also of the hands. This swelling is frequently seen in pregnancy. There are also women who have a remarkable tendency to suddenly retain fluids, probably as a result of a hormonal imbalance not yet well defined. Patients with myxedema may also develop swelling, but this swelling is usually not pitting, as is seen in patients with cardiovascular disease. Furthermore, the weight gain usually seen when swelling occurs in the patient with cardiac disease is unlikely to occur in the patient with myxedema because the majority of such patients maintain or lose total body weight while still developing the brawny edema of myxedema. Patients with Cushing's disease also may develop peripheral swelling, as do patients on therapeutic steroid therapy.

CLAUDICATION

DEFINITION

Claudication refers to the cramplike pain that arises in muscle groups because of decreased blood flow to the muscle group and presumably because of ischemia. Claudication almost always occurs in the lower extremities after exercise. Typically the patient complains of a cramplike calf pain after walking a limited distance that is promptly relieved when the patient stops and rest for a minute or so.

PATHOPHYSIOLOGIC CONSIDERATIONS AND DIFFERENTIAL DIAGNOSIS

Claudication is almost always due to atherosclerotic narrowing of the vessels supplying the legs, whether it be at the level of the aorta, the common iliacs, or the more distal femoral circulation. Although the process is almost inevitably due to atherosclerosis, it should be recognized that homocystinuria, a genetic condition in which medium-sized arteries may become occluded at a relatively early age, may provoke claudication. Other genetic diseases such as pseudoxanthoma elasticum are associated with claudication at an early age. On rare occasions peripheral arterial emboli from the heart or atheromatous plaques in proximal arteries may occlude distal arteries and provoke claudication.

Claudication may develop in the upper extremities as well as the lower extremities if the same atherosclerotic process involves the blood supply to the upper extremities. Atherosclerotic obstruction of the innominate artery or the subclavian arteries and their branches may produce the same symptoms in the arms as are felt in the legs. Circulation to the upper extremities may be maintained by collateral circulation, including collaterals from the vertebral basilar system. In an obstructed subclavian artery, flow may actually move from the cerebral circulation through the circle of Willis to the vertebral artery, entering the subclavian artery just beyond the obstruction of the subclavian artery and producing the subclavian steel syndrome. Thus, the patient's complaint of arm pain or fatigue while exercising the arm and the simultaneous development of neurologic symptoms should alert the physician to the possibility that there is indeed a subclavian steel and that the increased demand for blood flow in the arm is producing a decrease in basilar-vertebral blood flow, with consequent ischemia in the brain.

The vast majority of patients with claudication, particularly of the legs, can be detected by careful palpation of the peripheral pulses. A small percentage of patients may have a congenital absent dorsalis pedis pulse or such a small vessel that the pulse cannot be felt, but in these patients there will be a bounding posterior tibial pulse since the blood supply to the foot is carried by the large posterior tibial artery. Thus, absence of dorsalis pedis pulses does not necessarily indicate atherosclerotic obstruction some place higher in the femoral system.

Hair growth is frequently compromised in patients with claudication, particularly claudication of the legs, and such patients frequently will not have hair on the dorsum of the foot or on the upper portion of the shins of the legs. After the careful palpation of the pulses at the sites of major arterial inflow to the affected extremity, auscultation over the pulse should be carefully performed. A bruit over the femoral artery of the leg that has claudication will further confirm the presence of a probable atherosclerotic lesion. The presence of a continuous bruit over an artery will indicate that the obstruction is so severe that the diastolic pressure in the artery proximal to the obstruction remains higher than the systolic pressure distal to the obstruction, thus producing a gradient throughout systole and diastole such that there is continuous flow over the obstructed area of the artery. Palpation and auscultation of pertinent arteries should be done not only at rest but after exercise, since on many occasions flow to the extremity at rest is adequate. It is only with increasing demands for greater blood flow with exercise that the velocity of flow increases to the point at which it will provoke a bruit. Blood flow in an extremity may be adequate to produce a pulse at rest, but once an extremity is exercised and peripheral vasodilatation occurs, flow through the proximal artery may not be adequate to maintain a pulse; thus, the disappearance with exercise of a pulse in an extremity and the appearance of a bruit over a large artery supplying that extremity is clear evidence of an obstructive process in the proximal artery. It is not rare to encounter a patient with a complete obstruction of the distal abdominal aorta, usually proximal to the bifurcation, who may have palpable pedal pulses at rest but who will lose these pulses very quickly once the extremity is exercised. When palpation of the pulse is difficult, such as in cases in which there is excessive fat or perhaps even peripheral edema, the use of a Doppler flow detector may be very useful. Occasionally patients with coarctation of the aorta may complain of claudication, but this is unusual because collateral arterial channels have usually formed in such profusion that blood supply to the legs remains adequate even with exercise.

RAYNAUD'S PHENOMENON

DEFINITION

In 1862, Raynaud, a French physician, described the sudden onset of blanching of the digits of an ex-

tremity associated with dull aching pain and eventually followed by a rubor-like discoloration of the digits.[6] This syndrome is usually precipitated by exposure to cold, but it is not rare for emotional upsets to produce the same constellation of symptoms. When the condition occurs without any seeming associated disease, it is called Raynaud's disease. When, frequently, it is an accompaniment or a precursor to a systemic disease, it is called Raynaud's phenomenon or syndrome, indicating that it is just one feature of another more significant illness.

In Raynaud's syndrome or phenomenon, the most common accompanying disease is scleroderma or its variants, such as CREST syndrome. CREST syndrome consists of subcutaneous calcifications, Raynaud's phenomenon, esophageal dysfunction, sclerodactyly, and telangiectasia. Raynaud's syndrome may also be associated with certain specific occupations that have as a common feature both exposure to cold and the use of vibratory tools. Thus, the syndrome has been recognized for many years among miners who work in cold, damp environments using drills. More recently it has been recognized in gas station attendants who are frequently exposed to cold and also use vibratory tools in the repair of automobiles in inclement weather. Workers in chemical plants using vinyl chloride also have a higher incidence of Raynaud's syndrome for reasons that are not clear.

In some patients, the appearance of Raynaud's syndrome may be extremely rapid and attributable to one single event, such as sudden exposure to extreme cold. In these patients there may be a rapid deterioration of circulation to an extremity and ulcers may form on the fingertips.

PATHOPHYSIOLOGIC CONSIDERATIONS

The exact pathogenesis of Raynaud's disease or syndrome has not been completely elucidated, but is presumed that the fundamental problem is inappropriate and prolonged vasospasm of the small digital arteries. If the spasm is prolonged enough it may be associated with fibrinoid degeneration of these digital arteries with subsequent permanent occlusion of the arteries. Decreased flow to the digital subcutaneous tissue over a long period of time may produce ulcers. The ulcers may simulate felons or other digital infected foci, but the primary problem is not involvement with bacteria, but rather ischemia to the subcutaneous tissues and subsequent secondary infection. Extensive attempts to treat the infection alone seldom eliminate the ulcer or preserve subcutaneous tissue in the digits. Thus, while infection should be treated with appropriate antibiotics and any local measures that appear necessary, the primary aim should be to eliminate the vasospasm with drugs such as calcium-channel blocking agents or intra-arterial reserpine. On rare occasions, repeated stellate ganglion blocks may be necessary to prevent recurrent spasm of the digital arteries. Raynaud's syndrome is usually self-limited; it may be relatively severe for one or several winter seasons, but the majority of patients will note a gradual lessening of symptoms over the course of time, unless the Raynaud's phenomenon was a precursor to a more serious systemic illness such as scleroderma.

Raynaud's disease is most frequently encountered in young healthy females. It is usually precipitated by the patient's encountering sudden changes in temperature. While it usually occurs when the patient is suddenly chilled in the fall or winter, it may also occur when the patient is suddenly chilled when leaving a warm room and entering a cold one or when a patient exposes the extremities to cold while searching in the freezer for an item. Primarily it is the hands that are usually involved, but some patients have equal problems with blanching and pain in the toes. Rare patients may complain of the same phenomena in the nose and ears.

ARTERIAL PULSE ABNORMALITIES

INTRODUCTION

The arterial pulse is a product not only of forces generated in the left ventricle but also of factors occurring in the peripheral arterial system. The more peripheral the arterial pulse where measured or palpated the more significant the properties of the arterial system in determining the characteristics of the arterial pulse wave form. Such factors as the distensibility of the arterial wall and the presence of standing waves may work against the distinctive features of the central aortic pulse that are of diagnostic value, so it is important to choose for examination an arterial pulse that is relatively close to the heart. In most cases, this will be the carotid artery. The arterial pulsations felt beneath the fingertips placed over peripheral arteries is commonly thought to be due to systolic expansion of the vessel as it is filled with ejected blood from the left ventricle. In actuality, there is really extremely little expansion (probably less than 2% of the radius) of a peripheral artery such as the radial artery during

Table 7–7. Arterial Pulses

Mechanism of arterial pulses
Where to palpate
Different arterial pulse forms
Normal arterial pulse
Hyperkinetic arterial pulse
Water hammer pulse
Collapsing pulse
Pulsus bisferiens
Bigeminal pulse
Dicrotic arterial pulse
Pulsus alternans
Pulsus paradoxus
Hypokinetic pulse
Severe left ventricular dysfunction
Pulsus parvus et tardus

systole. This degree of expansion associated with the increase in systolic volume of the pulse is not detectable by the palpating finger. The systolic pulsation felt beneath the palpating finger over a peripheral pulse is actually due to lateral or twisting movement of the tethered peripheral artery in response to the percussion wave generated from the heart.

Arterial pulses should be palpated bilaterally in order to detect any difference in amplitude of comparable pulses. For instance, a difference in amplitude between the two brachial arteries would suggest a partial occlusion of a proximal portion of the subclavian artery, arousing the suspicion of the subclavian steal syndrome in a patient with syncope or presyncope. Peripheral pulses from different extremities should also be palpated simultaneously, particularly in the case of the hypertensive patient. In patients with coarctation of the aorta the arrival of the systolic pulsation in the carotids will be distinctly earlier than the arrival of the systolic pulse wave in the femoral arteries because flow to the femoral arteries is interrupted by the coarctation and is dependent on flow from collateral channels. This discrepancy in the timing of the arterial pulse between the carotids and the femoral arteries, along with a higher blood pressure in the upper compared to lower extremities, is virtually diagnostic of coarctation of the aorta.

DIFFERENT PULSE FORMS

The normal pulse is initiated by ejection of blood into the aorta and is characterized by a rapid upstroke, or the so-called anacrotic limb of the arterial pulse. Under normal circumstances this is the only portion of the arterial pulse wave that is felt. Under abnormal conditions there can be other components of the palpated arterial pulse. Table 7–7 lists various forms of abnormal or unusual arterial pulses.

Hyperkinetic Arterial Pulses. Bounding arterial

pulses associated with large stroke volumes and accompanied by a rapid large-amplitude upstroke and usually a rapid downstroke of the arterial pulse have been grouped under the general term hyperkinetic arterial pulses.[7] The hemodynamic hallmark of all these types of pulses is a large stroke volume. Large stroke volumes may be encountered in young people with hyperdynamic circulation, in pregnant women, or in patients with fever, thyrotoxicosis or anemia. Patients with profound bradycardia, whether it be due to sinus bradycardia or complete heart block, may also have bounding pulses as they generate large stroke volumes in an effort to maintain a normal cardiac output. Patients with large stroke volumes with relatively rapid runoff into low resistance circulatory beds may also present with bounding pulses, as is seen in patients with patent ductus arteriosus and large arteriovenous fistula.

The most common abnormality of the cardiovascular system associated with bounding or hyperkinetic pulse is aortic regurgitation. Here again, there is a large stroke volume that is delivered to a relatively dilated periphery. The large stroke volume accounts for the rapid forceful upstroke of the arterial pulse. The rapid decline in the arterial pulse wave is primarily due to the dilated periphery and is compounded by the reflux of blood back into the ventricle across the incompetent aortic valve. The rapid delivery and rapid egress of blood from the arterial system can be noted not only by palpation but also by visualization of the fundi where the retinal arteries can actually be seen to pulsate, which does not occur in normal patients. A peripheral manifestation of this phenomena is Quincke's pulse, in which small systolic pulsations are noted in the nail beds.

Other terms have been loosely used to apply to the hyperkinetic pulse, although they really have a narrower meaning. The term ''water hammer pulse'' was actually derived from a Victorian vessel toy that was a sealed tube containing water in a vacuum. When it was turned upside down the water struck the lower end of the tube, producing a hammerlike sound. Water hammer pulse thus refers to the extremely rapid forceful upstroke of the limb of the arterial pulse wave. The term ''collapsing pulse'' has also been used to indicate a bounding pulse, but in actuality it describes the very rapid decline in the downslope of the arterial pulse, which more appropriately can result from a rapid decline in peripheral resistance rather than necessarily from a large stroke volume.

Finally, this group of hyperkinetic arterial pulses has occasionally been termed a Corrigan's pulse. This appellation also has minor historical deficiencies in that Corrigan in 1832 actually referred to visual pulses in the neck and upper extremities, not the palpable pulses. Thus, Corrigan was visualizing what can be palpated in situations in which hyperkinetic arterial pulses are present.

Pulsus Bisferiens. Pulsus bisferiens refers to an arterial pulse during which there is a rapid early rise in pressure followed by a brief decline in the pressure wave, then a second systolic peak in arterial pressure with a somewhat slower decline. This second peak has been termed the tidal wave. This phenomenon is due not only to alterations in left ventricular contraction pattern but also to changing factors in peripheral arterial resistance patterns. It can be noted in patients with combined aortic stenosis and aortic regurgitation as well as in other states associated with increased left ventricular stroke volume, such as exercise, fever, and a patent ductus arteriosus. However, it has come to be known as a hallmark in the diagnosis of hypertrophic subaortic stenosis. In this condition the initial rapid upstroke is created by early rapid emptying of the hypertrophied left ventricle. The second upstroke or tidal wave is probably a manifestation of reflected waves from the periphery, since this phenomenon can be obliterated by paralysis of the nerves supplying the peripheral arterial system. While pulsus bisferiens is striking when intra-arterial pressure tracings are obtained in patients with hypertrophic subaortic stenosis, it is frequently difficult to detect by physical examination alone.

Bigeminal Pulse. Bigeminal pulse refers to the pulse encountered in patients with ventricular bigeminy. In this disorder the premature ventricular beat occurs slightly earlier than the normal beat would, thus decreasing the amount of time for ventricular filling and consequently decreasing the volume of left ventricular ejection, producing a situation in which there appears to be a strong beat followed by a somewhat weaker beat followed again by a strong beat and then a weak beat. The premature ventricular beat may be so premature that there is little, if any, blood ejected from the ventricle; this can produce a situation in which palpation of the peripheral pulse appears to demonstrate bradycardia but auscultation of the heart reveals twice as many beats than are palpated peripherally.

Dicrotic Arterial Pulse. Bigeminal pulse must be differentiated from the dicrotic arterial pulse, in which two arterial pulse beats can be palpated, one of which is in systole and the other in diastole. The diastolic component is due to an accentuation of the normally appearing dicrotic wave in the arterial pulse. This dicrotic arterial pulse is usually encountered in situations in which there is left ventricular dysfunction with decreased left ventricular stroke volume and, presumably, compensatory elevated systemic arterial resistance.

Pulsus Alterans. Pulsus alternans must be distinguished from pulsus bisferiens, bigeminal pulse, and dicrotic arterial pulse. In pulsus alternans the amplitude of every other beat is less than the preceding beat. The beat with the diminished amplitude is clearly systolic, as determined by simultaneous auscultation while palpating a peripheral arterial pulse. It can be differentiated from bigeminal pulse by determining during simultaneous cardiac auscultation and palpation of an arterial pulse that there is not a premature beat associated with the diminished palpated arterial pulse. It can be differentiated from the dicrotic arterial pulse in that the second pulse of the dicrotic phenomenon occurs in diastole, not systole. Pulsus alternans can best be demonstrated by having the patient arise from the supine position to a standing position, a position change frequently marked by a brief run of pulsus alternans. Pulsus alternans is almost inevitably evidence of severe left ventricular dysfunction.

Pulsus Paradoxus. Pulsus paradoxus is detected by determining the systolic blood pressure while observing the patient's respiratory cycle. It consists of a fall in systolic pressure during inspiration of greater than 10 mm Hg. In cases of marked paradoxus the decline in systolic pressure during inspiration can actually be detected by palpating a peripheral artery.

Pulsus paradoxus is not truly paradoxical since it is an accentuation of a normal physiologic phenomenon. During normal inspiration there is an increase in the venous capacitance of the lungs, leading to a small decrease in filling of the left heart that in turn leads to a decreased stroke volume and therefore a decline in systolic pressure. In certain pathologic conditions, however, such as pericardial effusion with tamponade, this normal physiologic phenomenon is accentuated. During pericardial tamponade the venous return to the right heart is still increased by inspiration. This produces engorgement of the right ventricle and shifting of the ventricular septum toward the left ventricle; thus, left ventricular diastolic volume is decreased and left ventricular stroke volume even more decreased than it would be by the normal pooling of blood in the pulmonary venous system. Thus, this accentuated decline in left ventricular filling and stroke volume during inspiration is detected by a decline of greater than 10 mm Hg in the systolic pressure. Pulsus paradoxus is also encountered in disorders such as asthma or chronic obstructive lung disease in which there is maximum inspiratory effort. Though the exact cause is not defined, it is reasonable to presume that, just as happens in pericardial tamponade, the increase in negative intrathoracic pressure produced during the maximum inspiratory effort actually increases venous inflow to the right ventricle to the point at which it can shift the ventricular septum toward the left ventricle, thus decreasing left ventricular filling.

Hypokinetic Arterial Pulse. Just as the arterial pulse can be characterized as hyperkinetic, it also can be considered in terms of being hypokinetic. This weak low-amplitude pulse is produced by a decreased rate and duration of ejection of the left ventricle almost inevitably associated with severe left ventricular dysfunction. It is encountered clinically in patients with left ventricular failure and mitral or aortic stenosis.

The pulse in patients with aortic valvular stenosis is very hypokinetic and has been termed "pulsus parvus et tardus" from the Latin, meaning "small and delayed." This abnormal pulse form is detected in the carotids, where not only is the pulse difficult to palpate because of its decreased amplitude but also it appears to be delayed because of the prolonged upstroke of the pulse wave. It is frequently accompanied by a detectable impulse on the upstroke of the ejection wave, which is analogous to the early anacrotic limb seen in aortic valvular stenosis. In addition to this impulse there are frequently vibrations along the upstroke of the pulse wave that are detected by the fingertips as a shuddering sensation. This sign of aortic stenosis may be masked in the elderly patient because of decreased distensibility in the peripheral arteries, which tends to mask the delay in the upstroke of the arterial pulse.

VENOUS PULSE ABNORMALITIES

INTRODUCTION

Observation and analysis of the venous pulse wave may provide helpful clues to the underlying cardiac disorder. The right internal jugular vein is best chosen for observation since it most closely reflects right atrial pressure. This pulse can be best seen at the base of the neck just lateral to the sternocleidomastoid muscle. It is frequently easier to observe if light is shone tangentially across the base of the neck, thus providing a shadow effect that allows perception of the movement of the venous pulse. The relationship of the various components of the venous pulse to cardiac events can best be correlated by simultaneously observing the right internal jugular vein and palpating the left carotid artery and/or listening to the heart. The neck should be positioned upright at any angle necessary to be able to discern the top or meniscus of the venous column in the right internal jugular vein. The pulse should be examined not only for its elevation above the angle of Louis of the sternum, but also for various waves and troughs, or descents.

Traditionally, the height of the venous column in the internal jugular vein has been used to determine the general status of the volume of blood available to the heart. In an extrapolation of this concept, the observation of the height of the venous column has been used as a component in the process of making a diagnosis of congestive heart failure. Under normal circumstances, the height of the column in the right internal jugular vein will not exceed a position 3 cm above the angle of Louis of the sternum. The angle of Louis is taken as a reference point since it lies 5 cm above the floor of the right atrium and serves as a fixed distance away from the atrium regardless of what position the patient assumes, providing the patient is not recumbent. It should be emphasized that the prominence of the venous pulse in the neck is a function not only of the blood volume occupying the venous system, but also of the tone of the veins. Under circumstances in which there is marked decrease in venous tone there may actually be marked increases in blood volume without the expected elevation in the column of the jugular venous pulse. Conversely, under circumstances in which there is marked venoconstriction, the column of blood in the right internal jugular vein may exceed 3 cm above the angle of Louis without there being an increased volume in the venous system.

Table 7–8 lists the components of the normal jugular venous pulse. Initially there is an upward deflection, labeled the *a* wave. This deflection occurs with atrial contraction during late-diastolic filling of the right ven-

tricle. It is frequently difficult to separate this atrial contraction wave from the underlying carotid systolic pulsation that occurs very shortly after atrial contraction. The *a* wave is followed by a decline in pressure that is associated with a fall in the column of blood in the jugular vein, labeled the *x* descent. The decline is due to downward displacement of the tricuspid valve as systole is initiated in the right ventricle. The *x* descent is transiently interrupted by a small, usually indiscernible *c* wave, which is due to backward bulging of the tricuspid valve leaflets up into the atrium during ventricular systole. Following this transient *c* wave, the *x* descent continues until a new wave, the *v* wave, starts its ascent. The *v* wave is due to atrial filling. The *v* wave continues until the atrium is filled and is followed by a rapid descending wave termed the *y* descent, which corresponds to simultaneous ventricular filling and atrial emptying. At slow rates there is frequently a small hump on the venous wave as it ascends to form the *a* wave. This *h* wave may be only a reflection of maximum filling of the atrium, thus leaving no further filling force to continue the pressure rise within the atrium. In any case, the *h* wave is seldom detectable by the naked eye and is very shortly followed by the *a* wave of atrial contraction.

PATHOPHYSIOLOGIC CONSIDERATIONS AND DIFFERENTIAL DIAGNOSIS

Table 7–8 lists some of the clinical abnormalities associated with changes in the components of the jugular venous pressure wave. Anything producing resistance to ejection of blood from the atrium will increase the *a* wave; thus, tricuspid stenosis, because it obstructs outflow from the right atrium, is associated

Table 7–8. Venous Pulse Waves and Descents

Component	Hemodynamic Event	Clinical Abnormality	
		Increased or Prolonged	Decreased or Absent
a wave	Atrial contraction	Tricuspid stenosis Pulmonic stenosis Pulmonary hypertension AV dissociation (Cannon *a* wave)	Atrial fibrillation
x descent	Downward displacement of tricuspid valve	Pericardial constriction or tamponade	Tricuspid regurgitation
c wave	Backward bulge of tricuspid valve during ventricular systole		
v wave	Atrial filling	Tricuspid regurgitation Atrial septal defect	
y descent	Atrial emptying and ventricular filling	Tricuspid regurgitation Pericardial constriction Severe RV failure	Tricuspid stenosis Atrial myxoma
h wave	Prolonged atrial filling		

with a large *a* wave. Disorders that stiffen the right ventricle and make it more difficult to fill will also make necessary greater atrial contraction and a larger *a* wave. Such disorders include pulmonic stenosis and pulmonary hypertension. During atrioventricular dissociation, whether it is due to varying degrees of heart block or even ventricular tachycardia, the atrium may be forced to contract against a closed tricuspid valve, which produces large *a* waves, called cannon *a* waves. Needless to say, if there is no effective atrial contraction, as occurs in atrial fibrillation, there is no discernible *a* wave.

The *x* descent is most frequently altered by the presence of tricuspid regurgitation. Indeed, it may be obliterated by the regurgitant flow from the right ventricle across the incompetent tricuspid valve. In pericardial constriction or tamponade, the *x* descent may occasionally be precipitous (Gibson's Sign[8]). This rapid *x* descent, followed by a prominent *v* wave or atrial filling wave, followed again by a rapid *y* descent (Freidreich's Sign[9]), may produce a W shaped venous pulse. A sharp *x* descent may help separate constriction from heart failure and tricuspid stenosis, since these latter two conditions do not have rapid *x* descents.

The classic sign of pericardial constriction is Kussmaul's sign, which is the loss of the normal decrease in the height of the jugular venous pulse with inspiration. Indeed, there may even be an increase in the jugular venous distension during inspiration, rather than the decrease expected from inspiration. In constriction, venous filling is limited by the rigid pericardium, which prevents inflow from neck veins into the heart. This is not true in tamponade with pericardial effusion; venous inflow is not impaired during inspiration, and hence flow increases and pressure declines in the neck veins during inspiration. If Kussmaul's sign is present with a pericardial effusion it indicates the presence of constriction in addition to effusion, a clinical entity called constrictive-effusive pericarditis.

The *c* wave, caused by the backward bulging of the tricuspid valve, which very transiently interrupts the *x* descent, is seldom observed at the bedside and does not produce significant clinical information. The atrial filling wave, or the *v* wave, will be markedly increased by tricuspid regurgitation and may be increased in the presence of an atrial septal defect. The *v* wave in an atrial septal defect may reach the same height as the *a* wave because the right atrium is filled not only from the venae cavae, but also from the left atrium. The *y* descent, or ventricular filling wave, will be increased or prolonged by tricuspid regurgitation because of the increased volume in the right atrium from the normal venous return and the regurgitant flow from the right ventricle. The *y* descent may also be increased in the

case of pericardial constriction or severe right ventricular failure, in which the distended or constricted right ventricle can only briefly initially accept the increased venous blood volume from the contracting right atrium. The *y* descent will be decreased or prolonged by the presence of tricuspid stenosis or a right atrial myxoma.

CYANOSIS

DEFINITION AND PATHOPHYSIOLOGIC CONSIDERATIONS

Cyanosis can be broadly defined as the bluish discoloration seen in the skin and mucous membranes resulting from excessive amounts of reduced hemoglobin. It has been traditionally separated into *peripheral* and *central* cyanosis (see also Chapter 6).

In *peripheral* cyanosis there is excessive extraction of oxygen from peripheral tissues, leaving markedly desaturated venous blood returning from the periphery. It can be seen in patients who have markedly low cardiac outputs and therefore extract more than normal amounts of oxygen from the capillary networks; cyanosis can also be seen in situations in which arterial flow to the periphery, particularly in an extremity, is decreased, necessitating excessive oxygen extraction. This situation occurs in normal patients who may become chilled, producing a compensatory arterial vasospasm in the extremities followed by compensatory increased oxygen extraction from blood being delivered to the extremities. Cyanosis seen in patients with Raynaud's phenomenon appears to result from this process. In addition to this mechanism, there is undoubtedly some venous spasm that produces distension of venous tufts in the skin, thus allowing increased collections of desaturated blood to become more apparent beneath the skin surface.

Central cyanosis has been ascribed to decreased oxygenation of blood being ejected from the heart. It is most commonly seen in mucous membranes. In the adult, the most frequent cause lies in the lungs. Patients with intrinsic parenchymal disease of the lungs are unable to oxygenate blood being transferred from the right to the left heart. A less common cause in the adult, but a source of major concern in the infant or child, is the presence of a right-to-left shunt allowing relatively unoxygenated venous blood to pass from chambers of the right heart directly to the left heart, thus preventing normal oxygenation in the lungs. Patients with methemoglobinemia, who have no intracardiac shunt or intrinsic lung disease, may present with central cyanosis because of decreased amounts of oxygenated hemoglobin.

Differential cyanosis, i.e., the presence of more or less cyanosis in the toes than in fingers, may be seen rarely in the adult with congenital heart disease. Blue fingers and pink toes suggest the presence of complete transposition of the great vessels, with preductal coarctation of the aorta and pulmonary hypertension leading to delivery of oxygenated blood to the toes through a patent ductus arteriosus with a reversed shunt. The more common situation is to see the adult patient with pink hands and blue toes, a result of pulmonary hypertension and a right-to-left shunt through a patent ductus arteriosus, which allows preferential shunting of unoxygenated blood to the toes via the patent ductus arteriosus while the hands receive oxygenated blood that has managed to traverse the lungs and be ejected from the left ventricle.

CLUBBING

DEFINITION AND PATHOPHYSIOLOGIC CONSIDERATIONS

Clubbing of either the fingers or the toes can best be defined as a bulbous enlargement of the distal portion of the digit. The first sign of clubbing is a spongy softening of the tissue at the base of the nail plate when the area is gently squeezed. Under normal circumstances the angle between the nail skin fold and the nail plate (Lovibond's angle) should not exceed 180°. The first sign of clubbing even before the distal portion of the digit becomes bulbous is an increase in this angle to greater than 180°. Clubbing is thought to be due to the development of multiple small arteriovenous fistulas in the region of the base of the nail plate.

DIFFERENTIAL DIAGNOSIS

Table 7–9 lists the diagnostic considerations to be entertained when clubbing presents as a physical sign. The most common cardiovascular cause for clubbing is congenital cyanotic heart disease, but it is also seen in cor pulmonale and bacterial endocarditis. It is less frequently noted in pulmonary AV fistula.

Clubbing results less commonly from a cardiovas-

Table 7–9. Causes of Clubbing

Cardiovascular causes
　Congenital cyanotic heart disease
　Bacterial endocarditis
　Cor pulmonale
　Pulmonary AV fistula
Pulmonary causes
　Inflammatory (bronchiectasis, lung abscess)
　Pneumoconiosis, cystic fibrosis, idiopathic interstitial fibrosis
　Neoplasm
Extrathoracic disease
　Gastrointestinal (sprue, ulcerative colitis, regional enteritis)
　Hepatic (biliary cirrhosis, liver abscess, amyloidosis)
　Toxic (arsenic, phosphorus, alcohol, beryllium)
　Familial
　Miscellaneous (pyelonephritis, syringomyelia, chronic granulocytic leukemia, hyperparathyroidism)

cular abnormality than from lesions in the pulmonary system. Patients with inflammatory responses such as bronchiectasis and lung abscesses may present with clubbing. Parenchymal lung disease including pneumoconiosis, cystic fibrosis, and idiopathic interstitial fibrosis also may be accompanied by clubbing. Clubbing may be the first sign of the development of a pulmonary neoplasm preceding all other symptoms. Various other diseases listed as extrathoracic diseases may be associated with clubbing (Table 7–9).

It is worth noting that clubbing may occur in families and is thus not necessarily evidence of underlying disease. The clubbing seen in pyelonephritis and hyperparathyroidism is often a result of resorption of the bone of the distal phalanges but maintenance of normal soft tissue content, leaving a foreshortened, soft, bulbous distal digit (see also Chapter 6).

HEART SOUNDS

INTRODUCTION

Any analysis of the clinical meaning of variations in heart sounds and the presence of different murmurs requires an understanding of events occurring within the heart during the cardiac cycle.[10] Valve closing and opening sounds result from the sudden cessation of movement of valve cusps previously moving at high velocity. Starting with systole, the first mechanical event in the cardiac cycle is contraction of the left ventricle, followed shortly by contraction of the right ventricle. As the ventricular pressure rises to exceed the atrial pressures, first the mitral, then the tricuspid valve leaflets close. The slight asynchrony of the contraction of the two ventricles accounts for the difference in timing of the closure of the mitral and tricuspid valves and thus the normal physiologic splitting of the first heart sound. The pressure in the ventricles eventually rises to the point at which it exceeds the pressures in the aorta and pulmonary artery, and the aortic and pulmonary valves open. As ventricular ejection ceases and ventricular pressure falls, the pressure within the pulmonary artery and aorta eventually exceeds the pressure in the ventricles, and the pulmonic and aortic valves close, creating the second heart sound. Because the velocity of contraction is greater in the left ventricle than in the right ventricle and because left ventricular emptying precedes that of the right ventricle, aortic closure normally will occur before pulmonic valvular closure.

PATHOPHYSIOLOGIC CONSIDERATIONS

Alterations in electrical activation, in the volume of blood to be ejected, or in the resistance to ejection may significantly alter these relationships among cardiac events. For instance, right bundle branch block produces a wider-than-expected splitting of the first heart sound. A simplistic explanation of this would be that the delayed electrical activation of the right ventricle leads to delay in right ventricular contraction, therefore delaying closure of the tricuspid valve. However, in some cases of right bundle branch block there is no audible or measureable delay of closure of the tricuspid valve, that is, no widely split first heart sound. The intensity of the valve closure sounds is most closely correlated with the distance the valve leaflets have to move from their open to their closed position. In cases of right bundle branch block in which there is no increased splitting of the first heart sound it has been shown by echocardiography that there was no delay in closure of the tricuspid valve. It is presumed that time during diastole had been sufficient for right ventricular filling so that the valve leaflets are very closely aligned in the closed position and thus have very little distance to travel once the ventricle initiates contraction. Reverse splitting of the first heart sound, in which the mitral valve closure sound occurs before that of the tricuspid valve, may occur in cases of elevated left atrial pressure such as mitral stenosis and atrial myxoma.

Observations concerning variations in timing and intensity of the components of the second heart sound are of much greater clinical significance that those of the first heart sound. As was reviewed above, the second heart sound is normally split. The initial component of the second heart sound is the aortic closure

sound, which is shortly followed by a softer pulmonic closure sound. This is best heard during mid inspiration when right ventricular filling is normally augmented by the negative intrathoracic pressure that produces increased venous inflow. The increased right ventricular filling requires more prolonged right ventricular ejection and therefore causes a delay in the pulmonic closure sound. In addition, there may be a component of increased pulmonary venous capacitance leading to decreased return of blood to the left ventricle and a decreased left ventricular ejection with consequent earlier aortic valve closure. This wider physiologic splitting during inspiration is eliminated during expiration, partly because there is decreased venous return of the right heart, thus shortening right ventricular ejection time, and perhaps partly because there is increased left ventricular filling and slight prolongation of left ventricular ejection time leading to almost superimposition of the pulmonic and the aortic closure sounds upon each other. This physiologic splitting, namely, a wide separation between the aortic and pulmonic closure sounds during inspiration and superimposition of the two valve closure sounds during expiration, does not occur in the case of an atrial septal defect because during expiration the right ventricle is not being deprived of venous filling. The normal decrease of right ventricular filling during expiration is essentially cancelled by the flow of blood across the atrial septal defect into the right atrium and thence to the right ventricle, thus providing the right ventricle with an ample stroke volume so that the pulmonic closure still occurs after aortic closure.

Paradoxical or reverse splitting of the second heart sound occurs when the pulmonic closure sound precedes the aortic closure sound; thus, splitting of the two sounds will actually be maximal during expiration and minimal during inspiration. The most frequent cause for this phenomenon is left bundle branch block. In this setting the left ventricle is activated late, allowing the right ventricle to complete its ejection and the pulmonic valve to close before the aortic valve closes. This may also occur in Wolff-Parkinson-White syndrome, in which a major portion of the right ventricle is activated early because of the accessory pathway and thus right ventricular ejection proceeds before left ventricular ejection. Delay of left ventricular ejection because of aortic stenosis will delay aortic closure and therefore superimpose it on the pulmonic closure sound. Severe left ventricular failure or ischemia may so decrease the rate of left ventricular ejection that aortic closure is relatively late in relation to pulmonic closure.

MURMURS

PATHOPHYSIOLOGIC CONSIDERATIONS AND DIFFERENTIAL DIAGNOSIS

A murmur is an auscultatory sound of cardiac or vascular origin. It is distinguished from brief sounds such as heart sounds, clicks, snaps, and gallops by its significant duration. Murmurs are created by excessive turbulence or the formation of vortices that produce sound. An understanding of the sequence of cardiac events also allows a clear understanding of the causes and characteristics of various murmurs, particularly of systolic murmurs. Table 7–10 provides a classification for murmurs.

Systolic Murmurs. Ejection Murmurs. Ejection murmurs are generated in the outflow tract of either ventricle, whether the obstruction is at the subvalvular, valvular, or supravalvular position. Typically called crescendo-decrescendo or diamond-shaped murmurs, they start shortly after but not with the first heart sound and end shortly before but not with the second heart sound. The murmur does not occur immediately after the first heart sound because the flow across the pulmonic and aortic valves that results in the murmur is not produced during isovolumic contraction of the ventricles, when the pressure has risen to a point high enough to close either the tricuspid or mitral valve (creating the first heart sound) but not to the point at which it will open the aortic or pulmonic valve and produce flow across the valves. A period of silence immediately follows the second heart sound because the diastolic closing of the pulmonic or aortic valve has occurred and there is no further forward flow across these valves. Ejection murmurs are characteristic of obstruction to outflow from either the left or right ventricle.

Under certain circumstances there may be a systolic murmur, termed the murmur of relative stenosis, with the diamond pattern frequently attributed to valvular stenosis without anatomic narrowing of semilunar valves or obstruction beneath the valve in the outflow tract of the ventricles. This murmur does not result from any structural defect in the heart or in the semilunar valves, but from excessive flow and presumed turbulence during the coursing of the blood through

Table 7–10. Classification of Murmurs

Timing and Type	Abnormality
Systolic	
Ejection	Valvular pulmonic and aortic stenosis
	Subvalvular pulmonic and aortic stenosis
	Supravalvular aortic stenosis
	"Relative" stenosis
Pan or holosystolic	Mitral and tricuspid regurgitation
	Ventricular septal defect
Late systolic	Mitral valve prolapse
	Myxoma
Whoop or honk	Mitral valve prolapse
Cardiopulmonary	Murmur during inspiration or expiration producing alterations in lung volume and therefore increased transmission of heart sounds
Diastolic	
Regurgitant	Aortic and pulmonic regurgitation
Rumble	Mitral stenosis, myxoma
	Austin Flint murmur
	"Relative" mitral or tricuspid stenosis
Throughout systole and diastole (Continuous)	Venous hum
	Patent ductus arteriosus
	Coronary arteriovenous fistula
	Ruptured sinus of Valsalva aneurysm
	Coarctation of aorta with collaterals
	Pulmonary arteriovenous fistula
	Multiple peripheral pulmonary artery stenoses
	Mammary souffle
	Aortic regurgitation with ventricular septal defect
To-and-fro	Aortic regurgitation and stenosis

the ventricular outflow tracts. It is frequently heard in patients with hyperdynamic circulatory states with high stroke volumes and is presumably generated because of high flow across an outflow tract and a semilunar valve that was not built to handle such high flows. These conditions are probably the genesis of the functional systolic ejection murmur heard so often in young patients and are also the cause of the murmur heard in atrial septal defect. In an atrial septal defect the outflow tract of the right ventricle and the pulmonic valve must accommodate not only the normal venous return from the vena cavae but also the excessive venous return coming from the atrial septal defect. Thus, right ventricular stroke volume may be several times normal values.

Pan or Holosystolic Murmurs. A pan or holosystolic murmur, as its name would imply, is a murmur that occurs throughout systole starting with the first heart sound and ending with the second heart sound. It usually has the same intensity throughout systole and does not have the typical diamond shape or crescendo-decrescendo character of the ejection murmur. These murmurs occur under circumstances in which, because of minimal increases, ventricular systolic pressure exceeds the pressure in the atria or in one of the two communicating ventricles so that either flow will start into the atria as a result of insufficiency of either the mitral or tricuspid valve, or flow will start from one ventricle to the other because of the presence of a ventricular septal defect. Under these circumstances, shortly after the increase in normal ventricular pressure associated with early systole, flow will begin and a murmur occur as a regurgitant fraction of the ventricle is forced into either the atria or the opposite ventricle. This flow will continue throughout ventricular systole and will actually go on beyond the closure of the aortic and pulmonic valve, which coincides with the second heart sound. This continued flow right up to and sometimes through the second heart sound occurs because the systolic pressure in the ventricle continues to exceed the pressure in either one of the atria or in the opposite ventricle after ejection into the aorta or pulmonary artery has ceased. When the left ventricular pressure falls to its normal end-diastolic level, which is less than the atrial filling pressure, regurgitant flow from the ventricle will cease as normal flow from the atria to the ventricles begins.

Late Systolic Murmurs. Whereas the most common murmur encountered with mitral or tricuspid regurgitation is a holosystolic murmur, a so-called late-systolic murmur may be associated with mitral regurgitation, in particular, and tricuspid regurgitation, less frequently. This murmur is characterized by onset during mid-to-late systole, usually with a gradual increase

in intensity until the second sound is encountered. The murmur may occur so late in systole that it may be misconstrued as a diastolic murmur. The vast majority of patients with late-systolic murmur have mitral or, less frequently, tricuspid valve prolapse. The regurgitation across the valve occurs in late systole; there is no regurgitation during early systole. It should be pointed out that this regurgitant murmur also can happen in the case of atrial myxoma.

Systolic Whoop or Honk. There is one systolic murmur, called the precordial whoop or honk, that is so distinctive that once it is heard it will never be forgotten by the observer and is easily recognized the next time it is encountered. It sounds much like the high-pitched, almost musical whooping sound of a child with classic whooping cough, or like the sound of geese. The systolic whoop is quite variable and may appear and then disappear from beat to beat. Usually initiated by a systolic click, it frequently occurs in the latter part of systole. It may be so loud that not only the patient but also other observers may hear it without the use of a stethoscope. The murmur may be associated with particular body positions and is heard most frequently with the patient sitting while leaning forward and somewhat to the left. Initially it was thought to be an extra cardiac sound, but from cineangiographic and echocardiographic studies it has become clear that it is almost inevitably associated with, and thus almost pathognomonic of, mitral valve prolapse.

Diastolic Murmurs. In general, diastolic murmurs are due to either retrograde flow across an insufficient semilunar valve or antegrade flow across a stenosed atrioventricular valve. The diastolic murmur of semilunar valve insufficiency is a high-pitched murmur starting immediately with valve closure or the second heart sound. The murmur is best heard in the early part of diastole and only in the case of massive regurgitation across a semilunar valve is it heard throughout diastole.

Regurgitant Murmurs. The murmur of aortic regurgitation can be easily recognized as a high-pitched diastolic murmur starting with the aortic closure sound.

The murmur of pulmonic insufficiency starts with the pulmonic closure sound and is also heard in early diastole. However, this murmur is frequently heard to begin slightly after the aortic closure sound and is thus perceived to have been displaced more toward mid diastole. This distortion occurs because the right ventricular stroke volume is increased by the pulmonic regurgitation and because right ventricular ejection time is prolonged, thus delaying the pulmonic closure sound even more than it normally is delayed after aortic closure. The pulmonic closure sound may be difficult to hear, leaving just the murmur of pulmonic insufficiency, which seems to start well after the second heart sound, caused by the single aortic closure. The murmur of pulmonic insufficiency may be indistinguishable from that of aortic insufficiency. This is the case when pulmonary hypertension is associated with pulmonic insufficiency, producing the so-called Graham Steell murmur.

Rumbles. Diastolic murmurs caused by antegrade flow across atrioventricular valves produce a lower-frequency rumbling sound. The classic cause for a diastolic rumble is mitral stenosis. The diastolic rumble of mitral stenosis goes through phases of loudness during diastole in a patient with normal sinus rhythm. The murmur will be loud early in diastole when the gradient between the left atrium and left ventricle is greatest. During mid diastole as the gradient between the left atrium and left ventricle narrows with left atrial emptying, the intensity of the murmur will decline. Late in diastole the murmur will again become louder, producing so-called late-diastolic accentuation as a result of left atrial contraction and increased flow across the stenotic mitral valve. During atrial fibrillation, the late-diastolic accentuation will be lost because there is no coordinated atrial contraction to increase flow across the mitral valve as normally occurs late in diastole. Thus, in patients with atrial fibrillation, the mitral diastolic rumble frequently seems to have the same intensity throughout diastole.

Aortic regurgitation with its high-frequency diastolic component may also be associated with a low-frequency diastolic rumble at the apex, the so-called Austin Flint murmur. The murmur results from partial closure of the mitral valve, as left ventricular pressure is increased rapidly by left atrial emptying and aortic regurgitation, with a consequent increase in the velocity of flow across the mitral valve from left atrium to left ventricle. Further velocity of flow across the mitral valve is supplied by atrial systole, leading to presystolic accentuation of the murmur. In cases of severe aortic regurgitation with rapid ventricular filling and pressure rise, the mitral valve closes prematurely and does not open during atrial systole. Thus, in severe aortic regurgitation the presystolic component of the Austin Flint murmur is lost.

The murmur of tricuspid stenosis may have the same characteristics as that of mitral stenosis, although it is usually of lower frequency because it is generated by a much lower pressure gradient between the right atrium and right ventricle. It is frequently difficult to differentiate this murmur from a mitral diastolic rumble of mitral stenosis, which is usually present. In this situation, recognition that the rumble close to the left sternal border becomes louder with inspiration as flow across the stenotic tricuspid valve increases may help to distinguish this murmur from that of mitral stenosis.

Murmurs can be generated from the mitral and tricuspid regions even when the structure of the valves is normal if flow across these valves is increased. This relative stenosis accounts for the low-pitched rumbling sound that may be heard in the case of an atrial septal defect, tricuspid and mitral regurgitation, and various congenital lesions that lead to increased flow across the mitral valve, such as atrial and ventricular septal defects and patent ductus arteriosus. A rumbling, low-pitched murmur can also be heard across the tricuspid or mitral valve during the acute phase of rheumatic fever, when the valve leaflets have been thickened by the inflammatory process (Carey-Coombs murmur).

Continuous Murmurs. *Pathophysiologic Considerations.* Continuous murmurs occur when there is a constant gradient between a relatively high-pressure chamber and a lower-pressure chamber. These murmurs are therefore often heard throughout systole and diastole and typically have their peak intensity close to or superimposed on the second heart sound. Not all continuous murmurs are heard throughout the cardiac cycle, however.

Intrathoracic continuous murmurs must be differentiated from venous hums. The venous hum is a continuous murmur originating in the jugular venous system, usually in hypermetabolic or hyperdynamic states. The hum may actually be transmitted down along the left sternal border and may mimic the continuous murmur of patent ductus arteriosus. The presence of a venous hum can be confirmed by elimination of the hum by occluding the right internal jugular vein with a finger while auscultating either the base of the neck or the base of the heart.

The murmur of patent ductus arteriosus occurs throughout systole and diastole because the systolic and diastolic pressures of the aorta always exceed the same pressures in the pulmonary artery, allowing continued flow across the patent ductus arteriosus during both systole and diastole. The murmur may have a high-pitched whirring sound, particularly in cases of a small patent ductus arteriosus. If a ductus is large and flow is great, the murmur may take on a more rumbling quality with increased intensity and is known as a "machinery-like" murmur. The murmur of a coronary arteriovenous fistula, which typically has the high-pitched whirring, almost hum-like quality, may be difficult to differentiate from a murmur of a patent ductus arteriosus because both murmurs are often heard loudest high along the left sternal border. If the murmur radiates well out along the left clavicle, it is almost certainly due to a patent ductus arteriosus rather than a coronary arteriovenous fistula.

Aneurysms of the sinus of Valsalva may rupture into the right ventricle, right atrium, or less frequently into the left atrium. Under all these circumstances, the pressure in the aortic sinus will exceed the pressure in these chambers and thus flow will be continuous during systole and diastole. Prior to the rupture of sinus of Valsalva aneurysm there may be a systolic ejection murmur caused by a partial obstruction of the right ventricle's outflow tract resulting from the impingement of the dilated sinus of Valsalva aneurysm on the outflow tract; once rupture occurs, the murmur becomes continuous.

Coarctation of the aorta is typically associated with a prolonged systolic ejection-type murmur often best heard between the scapulae. There may be a continuous murmur, however, when there are large collateral channels, particularly those involving the intercostal arteries, which are frequently seen as visible pulsations. This continuous murmur may be due to the phase lag of flow through the collateral channels and the flow through the tight coarctation, thus producing a murmur in diastole arising from the excessive delayed flow in the intercostal arteries.

Abnormalities in the pulmonary circulation may also be associated with continuous murmurs. Pulmonary arteriovenous fistulas, which are a component of Osler-Weber-Rendu disease, have been associated with continuous murmurs. One of the features of postrubella syndrome in the fetus is the development of multiple stenoses of the branches of the pulmonary artery. Here again, because of the stenotic lesions, the systolic and diastolic pressure in the pulmonary artery exceeds that in the venous and capillary beds distal to the point of obstruction, allowing for continued flow during systole and diastole.

In a small percentage of pregnant and lactating women, a high-pitched continuous murmur may be heard along the left sternal border and may be confused with a small patent ductus arteriosus. This so-called mammary souffle is due to increased flow in the superficial arteries supplying flow to the hypermetabolic breast. This murmur can be distinguished from that of patent ductus arteriosus by pressing the finger on breast tissue and applying occlusive pressure lateral to the stethoscope, thus temporarily occluding flow through the superficial mammary arteries.

It is often difficult to decide whether the murmur of aortic regurgitation with a ventricular septal defect is truly a continuous murmur. It occurs throughout systole because of the high left-ventricular stroke volume and continues throughout diastole because a portion of the regurgitant flow continues throughout diastole from the aorta into the left ventricle and the relatively low-pressure right ventricle. It may have the same features of accentuation around the second heart sound that the typical continuous murmur has because there is continuous flow during systole into the right ventricle across the ventricular septal defect and during diastole across the incompetent aortic valve.

To-and-fro Murmurs. To-and-fro murmurs may be confused with continuous murmurs. This confusion is classically seen in the case of combined aortic stenosis and aortic regurgitation. Under these circumstances, there is a prolonged systolic ejection murmur because of aortic stenosis and there is a loud prolonged diastolic murmur because of aortic regurgitation. This murmur can best be differentiated from a continuous murmur because of a biphasic increase in intensity in the murmur. The first portion of increased intensity is the systolic ejection portion of the aortic stenotic murmur. The second component is the diastolic component of aortic regurgitation. This so-called to-and-fro variation in the intensity of the murmur differentiates it from the continuous murmur, which usually has a single peak intensity in the region of the second heart sound. It should be noted that such a to-and-fro murmur may be present only when aortic regurgitation is present. Under these circumstances, the systolic ejection murmur is a murmur of "relative" aortic stenosis in which the large amount of blood that is refluxed back into the left ventricle during diastole is again ejected across a nonstenotic aortic valve. The increased flow across the valve produces turbulence and a systolic murmur.

Cardiopulmonary Murmurs. On rare occasions, the clinician may hear a systolic ejection murmur-type sound occurring only during systole and almost always with inspiration and, less frequently, with expiration. The sound does not have the characteristics of a pericardial rub, nor is it always reproducible in the same patient. It is not present at end inspiration nor end expiration and can be completely eliminated by having the patient hold his breath. It is thought that this so-called murmur is actually a variation in the intensity of breath sounds produced by transient compression of pulmonary parenchymal tissues during systole. In short, it is thought to be due to increased transmission of breath sounds through lung tissue compressed by the heart during systole. It is most often heard over the base of the left lung posteriorly in patients with thin chest walls and narrow AP diameters. The most frequent accompanying cardiac abnormality, if there is one, is mitral valve prolapse.

Eponymic Murmurs. Throughout the course of history of auscultation, various physicians have noted murmurs or unusual cardiac sounds that occur in specific clinical situations. These observations have led to the naming of the murmur or the physical sign after the clinician who popularized the observation. Table

7–11 lists the most common of these murmurs or cardiac sounds. McKusick has described the characteristics of these murmurs or cardiac sounds and has provided thumbnail sketches of their namesakes.[11] An awareness of these eponyms not only serves to enliven insight during teaching rounds but also sharpens the clinician's observational skills when he encounters a particular cardiac abnormality.

BRUITS

DEFINITION AND PATHOPHYSIOLOGIC CONSIDERATIONS

A bruit is a murmur that is heard over a peripheral vessel. Its genesis is essentially the same as that of cardiac murmurs, namely, sound generated in the vessel because of turbulence or the formation of vortices. The turbulence or vortices are generated because of either excessive flow in a normal vessel or normal flow in a partially obstructed vessel. Turbulence and hence bruits may also be generated in vessels with normal circumference and normal flows if the vessels themselves are tortuous, presumably interrupting the velocity profile of blood flow. Furthermore, it is possible to hear bruits in normal patients with normal vessels and normal flows if the examining stethoscope is pressed too firmly against the artery under investigation. Pressure of the stethoscope produces narrowing of the internal diameter of the artery and thus some obstruction to flow. These "iatrogenic" bruits are more frequently encountered in young healthy patients, particularly if they have a hyperdynamic circulation.

DIFFERENTIAL DIAGNOSIS AND DIAGNOSTIC EVALUATION

The most common sites for bruits in the patient with cardiovascular disease, and the areas that should be checked in every physical examination, are the carotid arteries at the angle of the jaw, the abdominal aorta, the femoral arteries, and the upper quadrants of the abdomen, particularly in cases of hypertension. Less common sites for auscultation, whose examination would presuppose some specific clue from the history, would be over the head, seeking evidence of an arteriovenous fistula, over the eyeball, seeking the presence of a cerebral aneurysm, and over the popliteal arteries, if a popliteal aneurysm is suspected.

An arterial bruit must be separated from a venous hum, particularly when auscultation is performed in the region of the carotids. A venous hum is usually continuous throughout systole and diastole and can be obliterated by occlusion of the jugular venous system at the base of the neck with pressure applied by a finger. Most arterial bruits are systolic. In the adult they usually indicate obstruction resulting from an atherosclerotic process. In some adults with extremely tortuous external carotid systems, there may be a bruit heard behind the ear by both the patient and the physician. Arteriography will demonstrate that there is no true obstruction, just increased tortuosity.

When a bruit over a peripheral artery is both systolic and diastolic, having the qualities of a continuous murmur, there is usually severe obstruction. The marked obstruction produces such a low pressure distal to the area of obstruction that the pressure during diastole, distal to the obstruction, is less than that encountered proximal to the obstruction. Thus, a systolic bruit results from the narrowing as blood is projected through the area of obstruction; further flow occurs during diastole across the obstruction because the diastolic pressure is greater proximal to the obstruction than distal to the obstruction. Certain maneuvers may convert a

Table 7–11. "Eponymic" Murmurs

Eponym	Murmurs and the Lesion
Hodgkin-Key murmur	Purring murmur of aortic regurgitation caused by retroversion of a cusp
Cole-Cecil murmur	Murmur of aortic regurgitation heard best in left axilla
Duroziez's murmur	To-and-fro murmur over femoral artery in aortic regurgitation
Carey-Coombs murmur	Soft diastolic murmur in acute rheumatic fever or relative AV valve stenosis
Austin Flint murmur	Presystolic murmur simulating mitral stenosis in aortic regurgitation
Gibson murmur	Continuous murmur of patent ductus arteriosus
Lerman-Means scratch	Scratchy systolic sound over pulmonic area in thyrotoxicosis
Roger's murmur	Prolonged murmur of uncomplicated ventricular septal defect
Graham Steell's murmur	Diastolic murmur caused by pulmonary hypertension
Still's murmur	Musical, presumably functional systolic murmur in children
Hamman's sign	Crunching or scratchy sound along left sternal border in mediastinal emphysema
Gallavardin phenomenon	Musical murmur loudest at apex in aortic stenosis

Table 7–12.   Classification of Clicks and Snaps

Ejection clicks
    Normal
    Aortic outflow tract abnormality
        Aortic valvular stenosis
        Bicuspid aortic valve
        Aortic dilatation
    Pulmonary outflow tract abnormality
        Pulmonary valvular stenosis
        Idiopathic dilatation of the pulmonary artery
        Pulmonary hypertension
Nonejection clicks
    Mitral or tricuspid valve prolapse
Opening snaps
    Mitral and tricuspid stenosis
    Ebstein's anomaly
    Atrial septal defect, ventricular septal defect, patent ductus
        arteriosus

systolic bruit into a continuous bruit, particularly in the legs. At rest there may be only a systolic bruit over the femoral artery, but with exercise of the legs, which lowers peripheral resistance in the distal arterial system in the muscle beds of the legs, a diastolic gradient can occur across the obstructed femoral artery, leading to continued flow through diastole and conversion of the systolic bruit into a continuous bruit.

The abdomen should be examined carefully for bruits since these may indicate the presence of obstructive disease in the aorta, an abdominal aortic aneurysm, or, on rare occasions, isolated renal artery obstruction. The presence of a unilateral bruit in the upper quadrant of the abdomen is suggestive of but certainly not diagnostic of unilateral renal artery obstruction.

CLICKS AND SNAPS

DEFINITION

In addition to relatively high-pitched normal heart sounds whose components vary with respiration, there are a variety of high-pitched sounds termed clicks and snaps that have come to have clinical meaning. Table 7–12 categorizes these different types of clicks and opening snaps.

PATHOPHYSIOLOGIC CONSIDERATIONS AND DIFFERENTIAL DIAGNOSIS

The ejection click is a sharp, high-pitched early-systolic sound that is associated with the sudden halt in the upward movement of the cusps of either the aortic or the pulmonary valve, or with dilatation of the aorta or the pulmonary artery. It is thought that such sounds can be detected in patients with normal hearts and normal valves, though in many cases long-term follow-up studies of these patients have eventually demonstrated the presence of an abnormality of the aortic valve. The ejection click is commonly seen in aortic valvular stenosis, particularly early in the course before the valve becomes severely fibrosed and calcified. At that point, the click may be lost, presumably because of immobility of the valve cusps. The ejection click is also heard with a bicuspid aortic valve. Indeed, it is not rare for patients who have had only ejection clicks early in life to develop the murmur of aortic stenosis as the presence of a bicuspid aortic valve with gradual stenosis becomes more apparent.

An ejection click is heard for similar reasons in the case of pulmonary valvular stenosis and is frequently heard in idiopathic dilatation of the pulmonary artery, just as it is heard in aortic dilatation. The cause of the ejection click in the case of dilatation of either the aorta or the pulmonary artery is not known, but Leatham suggests that the dilated vessels may serve to accentuate normal ejection vibrations.[10]

Nonejection clicks, which consist of one or more high-pitched, sharp sounds occurring usually in early-to-mid systole well after the normal position for an ejection click, have in the past been attributed to extracardiac sources such as pleuropericardial adhesions. With the advent of modern phonocardiography and echocardiography, it has become apparent that these nonejection clicks are almost inevitably associated with mitral or tricuspid valve prolapse.

Opening snaps are high-pitched, brief sounds occurring early in diastole shortly after the second heart sound in association with opening of the atrioventricular valves in the presence of either mitral or tricuspid valve stenosis. The opening snap is thought to be due to sudden movement of the cusps of the AV valve, accelerated by the high filling pressure in the atrium, downward toward the ventricle during diastole. In general, the greater the degree of stenosis, the closer the opening snap is to the second heart sound. This reasoning stems from the fact that the tighter the valve, the greater the diastolic filling gradient between the atrium and the ventricle and vice versa; hence, a high gradient will produce early rapid movement of the cusps of the valve into the ventricle. The opening snap may disappear as the valve becomes fibrosed and calcified.

The opening snap of either AV valve may be confused with the split second heart sound. In the case of mitral stenosis, the distinction can be made between

Table 7–13. Extracardiac Sounds

Pleuropericardial
    Rubs
    Pericardial knock
    Pleuropericardial adhesions
    Mediastinal emphysema (Hamman's sign)
    ? Pneumothorax
Other sounds
    Lerman-Means scratch
    Diaphragmatic flutter
    Sounds of gastrointestinal origin

an opening snap and a split second heart sound by listening over the suprasternal notch, since the sound of the opening snap is reflected back into the left atrium and up the left main-stem bronchus to the trachea whereas the pulmonic closure sound that is a component of the split second sound will not be heard in the suprasternal notch. Separation of a mitral opening snap and a tricuspid opening snap may be difficult but frequently can be accomplished by listening carefully during inspiration, for then the right atrial pressure is further elevated by venous inflow and thus the gradient between the right atrium and right ventricle is accentuated, producing a snapping sound arising from the tricuspid valve before the snap arising from the stenotic mitral valve.

The large anterior cusp associated with Ebstein's anomaly may cause a diastolic opening snap. Increased flow across the atrioventricular valves, as is seen in the case of the tricuspid valve with an atrial septal defect and the case of the mitral valve with large left-to-right shunts resulting from ventricular septal defects and patent ductus arteriosus, may occur, but these snaps are seldom audible clinically and are more frequently determined by careful phonocardiography.

EXTRACARDIAC SOUNDS

DEFINITION AND PATHOPHYSIOLOGIC CONSIDERATIONS

Extracardiac sounds may best be defined as those sounds noted during auscultation that do not emanate directly from cardiac chambers or cardiac valves. Table 7–13 lists the most frequently encountered extracardiac sounds. They may be associated with movement of the chambers of the heart during systole and diastole because cardiac movement may involve distortion of structures close to the heart. In the past,

many clicks and murmurs that we now know are related to valvular defects such as a prolapsing mitral valve had been attributed to extracardiac sources such as pleuropericardial adhesions. The extensive knowledge about valvular prolapse gained using phonocardiography and echocardiography has served to show that most of these presumed extracardiac sounds are actually related to abnormal movement of usually the mitral and occasionally the tricuspid valve.

DIFFERENTIAL DIAGNOSIS

Inflammation of either the pleural or pericardial surface may be associated with a rub. Pleural rubs are clearly associated with the respiratory cycle. Pericardial rubs are associated with the cardiac cycle. Some confusion may arise when the rub is heard only during one phase of the respiratory cycle. Under these circumstances a pericardial rub can be properly differentiated from a pleural rub by carefully noting that even though the rub may be heard only in mid inspiration, it is consistently associated with systole and/or diastole. As previously mentioned, since rubs can frequently be heard only in certain body positions, detection of a rub requires listening to patients while they are sitting and lying, both flat and in the lateral positions.

A pericardial knock might best be considered as originating from the left ventricle because it is generally acknowledged to be analogous to the filling sound of the left ventricle noted in normal young patients, in patients with marked mitral regurgitation, or in patients with congestive heart failure. It differs from the so-called third heart sound, or S_3 gallop, in such patients by appearing earlier in diastole than sounds associated with these conditions. Pericardial knock is thought to occur when left ventricular filling is restricted, not so much by a thickened indistensible left ventricular muscle, but by a thickened pericardium that prevents normal distension of the left ventricle during early diastole. The knock does not require the presence of calcium in the pericardium and may persist after a pericardiectomy, perhaps because of residual left ventricular myocardial disease, which frequently occurs in long-standing constrictive pericarditis.

Pleuropericardial adhesions have been noted in patients who have systolic clicks. Though in the past these clicks have been attributed to the pleuropericardial adhesion, which association is undoubtedly true in some cases, many times these systolic clicks are probably more likely to be associated with mitral or tricuspid valve prolapse.

As mentioned previously, mediastinal emphysema may be associated with Hamman's sign, a crunching or multicomponent scratchy sound heard along the left sternal border during systole, usually during mid inspiration.

Scratching, crunching sounds such as described by Hamman have also been described in cases of pneumothorax. It seems likely, however, that these sounds are actually due to the coincident mediastinal emphysema rather than simply the presence of the pneumothorax, because these sounds are most frequently seen in patients with small left pneumothoraces such as are seen in patients with recognized mediastinal emphysema. They are seldom noted in patients with a right pneumothorax.

A host of other sounds associated with noncardiac causes has been noted while auscultating the heart. The Lerman-Means scratch is a scratchy sound heard over the pulmonic area during systole, particularly in patients with thyrotoxicosis, and has been thought to be due to systolic distension of the pulmonary artery resulting from a hyperdynamic state associated with thyrotoxicosis. Diaphragmatic flutter may sound like a to-and-fro shuffle similar to a pericardial friction rub or a tic-toc tapping, swishing, or churning sound. It may be associated with pain reminiscent of angina pectoris and may be differentiated from a cardiac sound by the fact that its rhythm is totally distinct from that of the heart and because it can be heard well away from the precordium. Diaphragmatic flutter is rare and occurs in paroxysms. Finally, sounds arising in the gastrointestinal tract may be noted while auscultating the heart. In the presence of a hiatal hernia with reflux or in the case of a distended stomach with air fluid level, there may be a sloshing sound that may be synchronous with the heartbeat. Sounds arising from the gastrointestinal tract have also been reported when large amounts of air distend the splenic flexure of the colon, producing a metallic knocking noise. The origin of these sounds can be presumed when they disappear with elimination of air from the upper or lower gastrointestinal tract. They will frequently disappear when the patient assumes a standing position, as well.

FILLING SOUNDS AND GALLOPS

DEFINITION

Filling sounds are usually low-pitched diastolic sounds associated with rapid ventricular filling or filling of the ventricles with an excessive volume.

Table 7–14. Classification of Filling Sounds and Gallops

Filling sounds
  Normal
  Mitral or tricuspid regurgitation
  Tumor "plops"
S_3 or ventricular gallop
S_4 or atrial gallop
Summation gallop

PATHOPHYSIOLOGIC CONSIDERATIONS AND DIFFERENTIAL DIAGNOSIS

Table 7–14 classifies filling sounds and gallops. They have been attributed to the final halt of the distended ventricular wall and are thus a function not only of the degree of flow into the ventricle but also of the state of the left ventricular musculature. Filling and gallop sounds occur only in diastole, and while so-called systolic gallops have been described in the past literature, these were most probably systolic clicks.

A filling sound is difficult to differentiate from an S_3 gallop because both have the same auscultatory qualities and occur at the same time in the cardiac cycle. In general, "filling sound" has been attributed to the sound heard in young normal patients as well as in those who have increased volumes returning to the ventricles, such as is seen in mitral regurgitation. In this context, it does not carry the connotation of left ventricular dysfunction. Filling sounds are heard almost universally in children and in a progressively decreasing percentage of adults in each progressively older age group, such that it is rarely heard beyond the age of 40. A filling sound is frequently heard in mitral, and, less frequently, tricuspid regurgitation. A separate and distinct type of early diastolic filling sound is the so-called tumor "plop." This sound is the hallmark of an atrial myxoma. It occupies essentially the same part of the cardiac cycle as a filling sound or S_3 gallop. Its distinguishing feature is that the timing of its onset after the second heart sound is variable, whereas the other two sounds have a uniform occurrence in relation to the second heart sound. Documentation of this distinction often requires phonocardiography.

Gallop rhythm is the term applied when there is a tripling or quadrupling of the heart sounds in such a manner as to simulate the hoof beat of a galloping horse. It was first defined by Potain[12] and has since been extensively described with clinical correlations by Warren and many others.[13,14] A gallop sound is indistinguishable from the previously noted filling sound, and, indeed, whether the sound is labeled a gallop or a filling sound is usually a reflection of the observer's belief as to whether it is a normal physio-

Table 7–15. Conditions Associated with Gallops

S₄ (Atrial gallop)
  Hypertension (systemic and pulmonary)
  Aortic and pulmonic stenosis
  Ischemic heart disease
  Cardiomyopathy
  Hyperdynamic states (anemia, thyrotoxicosis, arteriovenous
    fistula)
  Prolonged PR interval
S₃ (Ventricular gallop)
  Congestive heart failure
Summation gallop
  Usually congestive heart failure

logic phenomenon or evidence of underlying myocardial disease. These low-pitched sounds are basically related to ventricular filling and occur at the two times in diastole when there is maximum ventricular filling, namely, early in diastole when the ventricular or S₃ gallop is noted, and late in diastole when the atrial or S₄ gallop is noted. The S₃ gallop occurs approximately 0.15 seconds after the second heart sound and is associated with the early rapid ventricular filling phase of the cardiac cycle. It is usually low-pitched and frequently difficult to hear. Left ventricular gallop is best heard at the apex with the patient lying in the left lateral position. It frequently disappears when the patient stands and can be accentuated by elevating the patient's legs when he lies flat. Right ventricular gallop frequently can be heard better low along the left sternal border. It is the hallmark and often the first sign of ventricular failure. It may come and go as ventricular failure worsens or improves.

The S₄ or atrial gallop occurs in association with atrial contraction and thus occurs in presystole during the final filling phase of the ventricle. While it is associated temporally with atrial contraction, its genesis, again, is the state of the ventricular myocardium. Thus, any process that leads to hypertrophy, decreased viscosity, or stiffening of the left ventricle may be associated with an S₄ gallop (Table 7–15). Again, conditions that will markedly increase ventricular filling during atrial contraction, such as anemia, thyrotoxicosis, or arteriovenous fistula, may also be associated with S₄ gallops. A prolonged PR interval with associated early atrial contraction in relation to closure of the AV valves may produce an S₄ gallop as the atrial contraction wave is superimposed on the earlier rapid ventricular filling wave.

When both an S₄ and S₃ gallop are present and if the heart rate is appropriate and (usually) rapid, they may be superimposed one on the other, producing a summation gallop. When the heart rate is slow and the two gallops are easily separated by auscultation, a quadruple sound may occur. This is created by the

sequence of the initial S₄ gallop followed by the first heart sound, then the second heart sound followed by the S₃ gallop.

ARRHYTHMIAS

INTRODUCTION

An understanding and categorization of the myriad arrhythmias that may occur in patients requires some definition of terms and concepts.[15]

Certain specialized tissues in the heart are endowed with a characteristic known as automaticity, meaning that excitation may be initiated in the absence of an outside stimulus. The primary site of such automaticity is the sinoatrial (SA) node, from which the initial stimulus for muscle contraction spreads through the atrial musculature and the specialized atrial conduction tracts to the atrioventricular (AV) node. After some delay in conduction in the AV node, the electrical stimulus passes into the His system, which gives rise to the right and left bundles. From there the stimulus travels to the Purkinje system, which distributes it to the ventricular musculature. The electrical stimulus, termed a transmembrane action potential, when recorded electrically has a sharp upstroke followed by a delayed shoulder and then a rapid downstroke. This rapid downstroke is followed by a relatively flat phase, called the diastolic phase of the transmembrane action potential. In tissues with automaticity, the diastolic wave of the transmembrane potential gradually rises to a point at which a threshold is reached and a new action potential is initiated. This gradual increase in the diastolic portion of the transmembrane action potential is the source of normal automaticity seen in pacemaker tissues in the heart. Under certain circumstances, the diastolic portion of the transmembrane potential may be interrupted by sharp upstrokes that reach the threshold level and thus provoke depolarization. These "afterpotentials" are considered an abnormal form of automaticity and may actually provoke cardiac arrhythmias.

While automaticity occurring in pacemaker tissue is the usual source of stimulus for cardiac contraction, another mechanism, re-entry, may cause abnormalities in cardiac stimulation. In a broad sense, the re-entrant mechanism requires areas in the conducting system of the heart or in the myocardium where there may be slowing of the transmission of the action potential. If

Table 7–16. Classification of Atrial Arrhythmias

Atrial bradyarrhythmias
   Sinus arrhythmia
   Sinus bradycardia
   Sinus node arrest
   Sinoatrial block
Atrial tachyarrhythmias
   Due to automaticity
      Sinus tachycardia
      Atrial tachycardia
         Digitalis excess
      Multifocal atrial tachycardia
      Nonparoxysmal AV junctional tachycardia with AV dissociation
   Due to re-entry
      Sinus node re-entry
      Paroxysmal atrial, junctional, nodal, supraventricular,
        reciprocal, reciprocating, re-entrant tachycardia
      Atrial flutter
      Atrial fibrillation
Syndromes
   With bradycardia
      Sick sinus syndrome or brady-tachy syndrome
   With tachycardia
      Wolff-Parkinson-White syndrome (Kent bundle)
      Lown-Ganong-Levine syndrome (James fibers)

the slowing of the action potential is sufficiently long to extend throughout the normal repolarization of neighboring conduction tissue or ventricular myocardium, the action potential that was slowed may emerge from the area of slowing to depolarize tissue that had previously been depolarized and then repolarized by the normal initial action potential traveling through more rapid circuits. Thus, it is possible for one action potential to be split into a rapid component that produces relatively earlier depolarization and repolarization, and into a component that, after being delayed in tissue, emerges and reprovokes depolarization in the previously depolarized tissue.

Thus, there are at least three mechanisms to explain depolarization of conducting tissue and myocardium, namely, normal automaticity, abnormal automaticity with afterpotentials, and re-entrant mechanisms. Regardless of what mechanism is operational, the transmission of the electrical signal may be affected by so-called blocks as it travels from its site of origin into the periphery. Block of transmission may be complete, partial, or unidirectional; that is, in conducting tissue there may be no antegrade block but there may be retrograde block, and vice versa.

DIFFERENT FORMS OF ARRHYTHMIAS

Atrial Arrhythmias. Table 7–16 provides a classification and framework for thinking of various atrial arrhythmias. The most common cause for an atrial bradyarrhythmia is sinus arrhythmia, which is the normal slowing of the SA node and thus heart rate seen during inspiration, most frequently in children and young adults. This slowing is thought to be due to the Bainbridge reflex, during which increased atrial filling stimulates the vagus nerve, thus slowing SA nodal discharge. It may not necessarily be associated with slow heart rates, and while it is common in young people, it can occasionally be seen in elderly patients. Sinus arrhythmia may also occur without relationship to the respiratory cycle.

Other causes of atrial bradyarrhythmia include sinus bradycardia, which is seen in patients with high degrees of vagal tone and is common in well-trained athletes. Both arrhythmias are usually asymptomatic. Sinus node arrest is failure of the sinus node to provoke a stimulus or an action potential. In sinoatrial exit block, the action potential is generated within the sinus node, but because of structural or physiologic defects in tissue surrounding the sinus node, the signal is never conducted to the atrial musculature. Both sinus node arrest and sinoatrial exit block are frequently asymptomatic. When they provide a prolonged period of time for ventricular filling, however, the subsequent increased stroke volume may be perceived by the patient as a palpitation.

Atrial tachyarrhythmias may be separated into those caused by automaticity and those caused by re-entry.

Sinus tachycardia does not represent an abnormality of the sinus node, but rather a response of the sinus node to variations in tone of the autonomic nervous system and increases in circulating catecholamines. It is usually relatively slow in onset and offset but it may be rapid enough to be confused with various forms of paroxysmal atrial tachycardia. Valsalva's maneuver or carotid massage, which provoke vagal stimulation, will produce a gradual slowing of sinus tachycardia, whereas in the case of paroxysmal atrial tachycardias, if these maneuvers produce any change, it is a sudden abrupt return to a slower sinus rhythm.

Atrial tachycardias are generally thought to be due to automaticity if 1) P-wave morphology during the tachycardia is different from that during normal sinus rhythm; 2) there is a gradual increase in the rate of the tachycardia, or a so-called warm-up period, during which a premature atrial contraction occurs during the tachycardia; and 3) the tachycardia cannot be terminated by pacing.

Atrial tachycardia resulting from automaticity is a relatively uncommon form of atrial tachyarrhythmia. One of the more common causes is thought to be digitalis excess. Multifocal atrial tachycardia is an arrhythmia characterized by an atrial rate greater than 110, at least three different P-wave morphologies, and variable PR intervals. It is most frequently seen in patients with chronic obstructive lung disease, and its appearance can be precipitated and its frequency increased by theophylline. Of major importance in recognizing the arrhythmia is differentiating it from atrial fibrillation. The multiforme P waves may be confused with atrial fibrillation waves, and the varying conduction of the abnormal P waves may produce grossly irregular R waves on the ECG, thus leading to confusion with atrial fibrillation. The arrhythmia does not respond to the usual treatment of atrial fibrillation with digitalis and quinidine. Indeed, these drugs may lead to further clinical deterioration in a patient, since many times the arrhythmia was provoked by a combination of chronic obstructive lung disease and digitalis excess.

Nonparoxysmal AV junctional tachycardia with AV dissociation or so-called accelerated junctional rhythm is thought to be due to automaticity. It usually occurs at slow heart rates and has a gradual onset and offset. It is most frequently seen in the setting of an acute diaphragmatic myocardial infarction or digitalis toxicity.

Re-entry is probably the most frequent mechanism for the development of atrial tachyarrhythmias. Sinus node re-entry characterized by an atrial tachycardia with P-wave morphology identical to that seen in normal sinus rhythm is an infrequent arrhythmia. It is rarely sustained and rarely requires treatment.

Classic paroxysmal atrial tachycardia, with its sudden onset and sudden offset as well as termination by vagal maneuvers or catecholamine injection, is a re-entrant atrial tachyarrhythmia that has acquired a variety of new names, including junctional, nodal, reciprocal, reciprocating, and re-entrant tachycardia. This plethora of new names stems from studies in the electrophysiology laboratory that have demonstrated that re-entry mechanisms may occur not only in the atrium but in the AV node, through accessory pathways around the AV node and even possibly in an accessory AV node. These arrhythmias cannot be differentiated clinically, and electrophysiologic studies are necessary if the cause is not obvious from surface electrocardiography.

It now seems probable that the vast majority of cases of atrial flutter are due to a re-entrant mechanism. The majority of current evidence would also suggest that the maintenance of atrial fibrillation is due to a re-entrant mechanism.

Several syndromes, because of their unique features, have been identified with atrial arrhythmias. The sick sinus syndrome, or brady-tachy syndrome, has become increasingly more recognized since the advent of cardiac pacemakers. Although the term "sick sinus syndrome" implicates primarily the sinus node, there

is also evidence of conduction abnormalities in the rest of the conducting system. It is characterized by periods of normal sinus rhythm punctuated by episodes of a variety of atrial arrhythmias, including sinus arrest, severe sinus bradycardia, atrial fibrillation, atrial tachycardia, and atrial flutter. It is most common in elderly individuals and is rarely seen before middle age.

Pre-Excitation and Arrhythmias. *Pathophysiologic Considerations.* Recurrent episodes of supraventricular tachycardia may indicate an underlying anomaly of the conducting system. In 1893, Kent described the presence of bundles of tissue connecting the atria to the ventricles.[16] Ferrer carefully reviewed the evolution of ideas and observations following Kent's work that have culminated in our understanding of the variety of forms of pre-excitation, many of which are associated with tachyarrhythmias.[17] Ferrer succinctly outlined the premise that during embryologic development of the heart, faulty development of the atrioventricular rings may lead to incomplete separation of the atria from the ventricles, thus leaving holes or clefts in the AV ring where connections between the atria and ventricles may persist. Furthermore, there may be projections of conducting tissue upward from the right and left bundles as well as the His bundle into the lower portion of the AV node. Because of these embryologic phenomena, accessory pathways for conduction may persist between the atria and the ventricles and from the lower regions of the AV node or His bundle to distant portions of the ventricular conducting system. These connections may lead to accessory conduction pathways that participate in re-entrant arrhythmias.

In 1930, Wolff, Parkinson, and White described an electrocardiographic pattern characterized by a short PR interval with what appeared to be a bundle branch block pattern that was associated with paroxysmal tachycardia.[18] While describing a syndrome that won them medical immortality, these authors did not understand the full anatomic and physiologic implications of their observation. In the Wolff-Parkinson-White (WPW) syndrome there is an accessory pathway connecting the atrium to the ventricle that allows a portion of the normal electrical signal generated in the SA node to travel from the atrium directly to the ventricle, bypassing the atrioventricular node. Thus, early depolarization of the ventricle results because this signal does not have to pass through the relatively slowly conducting AV node. This premature ventricular depolarization produces the slurring of the upstroke of the QRS complex, termed a delta wave, which provokes an electrocardiographic pattern suggestive of bundle branch block. The PR interval, which traditionally had been felt to be due to the normal delay in transit through the AV node, appears shortened because ventricular depolarization and the early portion of the QRS was initiated by the signal's traveling down the accessory pathway rather than solely by the signal's passing down the slower atrioventricular node. Thus, the Wolff-Parkinson-White syndrome is due not to accelerated atrioventricular conduction in the AV node nor to bundle branch block, but rather to the presence of an accessory pathway that produces premature depolarization of the ventricle with a prolonged QRS complex simulating bundle branch block.

Through more recent electrophysiologic studies it is clear that there are three general types of accessory pathways.[19] The original accessory pathway from atria to ventricles passing through the atrioventricular ring around its outer margins described by Kent accounts for the Wolff-Parkinson-White syndrome. While this syndrome was initially thought to be due solely to an accessory pathway between the anterolateral portion of the right atrium and the upper portion of the right ventricle, it was quickly recognized that there were other loci for such accessory pathways between the atria and the ventricles. Ohnell described the posterior pathway between the left atrium and the left ventricle,[17] and it is now recognized that there can be pathways at any point along the rim of the atrioventricular ring. Under all these circumstances there will be premature depolarization of the portion of the ventricle with early distortion of the QRS complex leading to a delta wave, if the accessory pathway conducts antegrade.

It was later discovered that there are also conducting pathways in the region of the AV node that allow direct communication between the atria and the bundle of His. These have been termed James fibers. Under these anatomic circumstances the electrical impulse from the atrium will bypass the AV node but will enter the normal His Purkinje system, producing a normal depolarization pattern in the ventricles. Since it bypasses the AV node the PR interval will be short, but since they do not provoke premature ventricular depolarization as they enter the normal His Purkinje system there will be no distortion of the QRS complex. The combination of a short PR interval with a normal QRS complex in association with atrial tachyarrhythmias is known as the Lown-Ganong-Levine syndrome.

The third type of accessory pathway consists of connections between the lower portion of the atrioventricular node, the upper part of the bundle of His, the ventricular septum, or the upper part of the right or left bundle branches. These accessory pathways described by Mahaim are associated with a normal PR interval because the atrioventricular node is traversed in a normal fashion by the signal from the atria, but delta wave or prolonged QRS is present because there

is premature depolarization of the ventricle as the electrical signal travels down the Mahaim fiber before the normal impulse reaches the ventricular musculature through the His-Purkinje system.

Wolff-Parkinson-White syndrome provides the prototype for understanding tachycardias associated with pre-excitation and accessory pathways. The most common tachyarrhythmia associated with the Wolff-Parkinson-White syndrome is a supraventricular tachycardia in which a premature beat initiates a re-entrant arrhythmia during which the electrical impulse travels downward through the normal atrioventricular node and then rapidly retrograde back up to the atrium through the accessory pathway. Many patients with recurrent atrial tachyarrhythmias on this basis may never show the typical short PR interval and delta wave in the QRS pathognomonic of the Wolff-Parkinson-White syndrome because there is antegrade or forward block in the accessory pathway without retrograde block. Thus, there is no conduction from atrium to ventricle that would lead to the short PR and delta wave, yet there is the possibility of rapid retrograde or backward conduction up the accessory pathway from ventricle to atrium. This absence of evidence of Wolff-Parkinson-White syndrome during the routine ECG in spite of the recurrence of atrial tachyarrhythmias caused by an accessory pathway has been termed concealed Wolff-Parkinson-White syndrome. Its presence can be confirmed by careful electrophysiologic study, which should be initiated if the tachyarrhythmias are recurrent, poorly controlled by drugs, or associated with syncope.

Syncope in Wolff-Parkinson-White syndrome might be due to an inordinately rapid tachyarrhythmia resulting from the re-entrant mechanism described above, or it might have a far more ominous cause. If antegrade or forward conduction is possible in the accessory pathway and the patient with such a pathway develops atrial flutter or atrial fibrillation, there will be no delay or decrease in the number of electrical signals entering the ventricle, as should happen if all the impulses from the fibrillating or fluttering atrium were to enter the AV node. Under these circumstances the ventricle receives anywhere from 300 to 600 impulses per minute, which may eventually provoke ventricular fibrillation. Syncope in a patient with an electrocardiographic pattern of the Wolff-Parkinson-White Syndrome calls for appropriate electrophysiologic studies, since the likelihood is that the syncope is due to ventricular fibrillation.

Patients with the Lown-Ganong-Levine syndrome (short PR interval, normal QRS) with James fibers that short-circuit the atrioventricular node and travel directly from the atria to the His bundle are also fre-

Table 7–17.　Ventricular Arrhythmias

Premature ventricular beats
　　Simple premature ventricular beat
　　Bigeminy, trigeminy, etc.
　　Parasystole
Ventricular tachycardia
　　Accelerated idioventricular rhythm
　　Torsades des Pointes
Ventricular fibrillation

Table 7–18.　Diseases Associated with Ventricular Tachycardia

Ischemic heart disease
Cardiomyopathies
　　Myocarditis
　　Hypertrophic obstruction cardiomyopathy (IHSS)
Sarcoid heart disease
Mitral valve prolapse
Complete heart block with Stokes-Adams attacks
Prolonged QT syndrome

quently afflicted with tachyarrhythmias. They may have recurrent episodes of re-entrant or reciprocating tachycardia as described above with the Wolff-Parkinson-White syndrome. In addition, they may be associated with an extremely rapid ventricular response to atrial flutter or fibrillation, since, again, the normal, slowly conducting atrioventricular node is bypassed and the ventricle is exposed to rapid stimuli arising from the atria. The exact role that Mahaim fibers may play in the role of atrial tachycardias is not clear. They may have a more important role in the genesis of ventricular tachycardia than in atrial tachycardia.

Ventricular Arrhythmias. Table 7–17 lists the various common ventricular arrhythmias.

While the past decade has seen a remarkable elucidation of the mechanisms of atrial and nodal arrhythmias, we are still in the infancy of our understanding of the mechanism of ventricular arrhythmias. For example, the mechanism for the production of a simple premature ventricular beat has not been defined. Premature ventricular contractions (PVCs) are probably the most common arrhythmia encountered in man and the most frequent cause for the complaint of palpitations. In different studies they have been reported in as little as 0.8 to as much as 62% of presumably healthy adults. Their incidence increases in healthy adults who take in excessive amounts of caffeine, nicotine, or alcohol. PVCs may be provoked by stimuli from the central nervous system, including strong emotions and intracerebral injuries such as head trauma, with or without subarachnoid or intracerebral hemorrhage. Because of the high incidence of premature ventricular beats among a presumably healthy population, this arrhythmia has been considered essentially benign. However, in the setting of organic heart disease, premature ventricular beats may indicate a poor prognosis. They are seen in almost every patient undergoing acute myocardial infarction who has continuous electrocardiographic monitoring. In the postinfarction period, patients with premature ventricular contractions have a poorer long-term prognosis than those without premature ventricular beats.

Although premature ventricular beats may often occur singly and in a seemingly isolated fashion, they

may also frequently occur with a fixed coupling interval after a normal ventricular beat, termed bigeminy. When the premature ventricular beat follows with a fixed coupling interval after every second normal beat it has been termed trigeminy; when it occurs after every third normal beat it has been termed quadrigeminy. In general, it has been felt that the presence of a fixed coupling interval indicates that the premature beat arises because of re-entry, although there is some experimental evidence to indicate that it can occur with triggered activity in the ventricle. When PVCs occur at a fixed interval but without relation to normally conducted beats and thus without a fixed coupling interval, they have been presumed to arise from a parasystolic focus. True parasystole is uncommon and is presumed to be due to the presence of an automatic focus in the ventricle, which is presumably protected from depolarization by the normally conducted ventricular depolarization wave.

The mechanism for the development of ventricular tachycardia is still a matter for debate. Ventricular tachycardia has been defined as 3 or more ectopic ventricular beats occurring at a rate of 100 beats per minute or more. Most episodes of ventricular tachycardia are initiated by a relatively late-occurring coupled ectopic beat from a ventricular focus. It has been attributed to automaticity, triggered activity, micro reentry circuits within the ventricle, and macro re-entry circuits involving the specialized conduction systems such as Mahaim fibers. A re-entry mechanism has been demonstrated in the majority of patients with sustained ventricular tachycardia who have been studied electrophysiologically.

Ventricular tachycardia usually occurs in a diseased heart. Table 7–18 lists the most commonly encountered forms of heart disease associated with ventricular tachycardia, the most frequent of which by far is ischemic heart disease. Brief runs of ventricular tachycardia are frequently seen during the acute phase of a myocardial infarction and may be documented during the late phase of myocardial infarction using Holter monitoring. Ventricular tachycardia is frequently associated with left ventricular aneurysm formation following a myocardial infarction.

Various cardiomyopathies are frequently associated with ventricular tachycardia. Ventricular tachycardia may be the first sign of acute myocarditis. Patients with hypertrophic obstructive cardiomyopathy, or idiopathic hypertrophic subaortic stenosis (IHSS), have a significant incidence of ventricular tachycardia, which frequently accounts for the syncopal episodes described by such patients.

While patients with sarcoid involvement of the heart usually develop forms of heart block, they may manifest themselves by ventricular tachycardia. Patients with mitral valve prolapse have a high incidence of premature ventricular beats, and a small number of these patients will have ventricular tachycardia as a complicating feature of their anomaly. In addition, approximately one third of the patients with complete heart block who develop syncope or Stokes-Adams attacks will have ventricular tachycardia as the primary arrhythmia provoking the syncope. Families have been reported in whom members have prolonged QT intervals and experience sudden death. Initially sudden death was thought to be associated with congenital deaf-mutism, but it is clear that it can occur without deafness.

An accelerated idioventricular rhythm, which is characterized by a wide QRS arrhythmia at a rate varying from 50 to 100, has been given a variety of names, including idioventricular tachycardia, nonparoxysmal ventricular tachycardia, and slow ventricular tachycardia. It is frequently noted in patients with an acute myocardial infarction, particularly those with diaphragmatic myocardial infarctions. These rhythms are usually benign and do not respond to antiarrhythmic therapy.

There is one pattern of ventricular tachycardia, Torsades des Pointes, that has a particular clinical and therapeutic implication.[4,5] It is a form of ventricular tachycardia in which the polarity of the initially positive or negative QRS reverses as the arrhythmia proceeds, becoming opposite to its initial direction and thus appearing to produce a twisting of the points of the QRS complexes. This ventricular tachycardia was thought to be a rare arrhythmia, but it has become clear with more frequent continuous electrocardiographic monitoring that it is a relatively common arrhythmia, particularly in association with a prolonged QT interval and the use of Type I antiarrhythmic drugs. It is undoubtedly the cause of the previously infrequently reported cases of "quinidine syncope."

The exact mechanism of the development and maintenance of ventricular fibrillation has not been defined with a unifying theory. It would appear that the underlying mechanism is probably related to the presence of multiple re-entry circuits within the ventricle; during ventricular fibrillation there is a random distribution of electrical impulses so that many areas of the muscle are being depolarized while other areas are being repolarized, provoking the uncoordinated contractile pattern seen in the ventricle. An electrical impulse delivered during the "vulnerable period" presumably finds the ventricle in varying states of repolarization and thus allows the development of multiple, uncoordinated re-entry circuits. This process can be enhanced by ischemia, accounting for the higher frequency of ventricular fibrillation during acute myocardial infarction.

Although ventricular tachycardia is commonly recognized because of rapid wide QRS complexes, it should be recognized that a wide QRS alone does not indicate that the arrhythmia is originating from the ventricle. The widened QRS may be due to so-called aberrancy, which is a temporary abnormally prolonged intraventricular conduction delay associated with impulses arising above the ventricle. Marriott and Myerburg summarized the three forms that can be noted with aberration.[20] The first and most common form is seen when a supraventricular impulse enters the ventricular conduction system while the ventricle is still refractory. It usually occurs with a premature beat and is associated with a right bundle branch block-type pattern. The second form is the widened QRS seen when an accessory pathway is active, such as in the Wolff-Parkinson-White syndrome. In essence, a portion of the ventricle is depolarized prematurely through the accessory pathway before the remainder of the ventricle is depolarized using the normal nodal-His-Purkinje system. The third form of aberration is due to a lengthening of the ventricular cycle. Under these circumstances, only late-arriving supraventricular beats are aberrant, and the term brady-dependent bundle branch block has been used.

BLOCKS AND THE CONDUCTION SYSTEM

DEFINITION

Formation and conduction of a normal electrical signal may occur at various sites in the specialized

Table 7–19. Blocks in Conduction System

Sinoatrial block
 Sinus node arrest
 Sinus node exit block
Atrioventricular (AV) block
 First degree
 Second degree
  Mobitz Type I (Wenkebach)
  Mobitz Type II
 Third degree (complete heart block vs AV dissociation)
Bundle branch block

conduction system of the heart. Lack of this formation or conduction of the electrical signal has generally been termed a block.

PATHOPHYSIOLOGIC CONSIDERATIONS AND DIFFERENTIAL DIAGNOSIS

Table 7–19 provides a simplified outline of various blocks encountered in the electrocardiogram. A block may be due to anatomic causes, such as is seen with severing of the His bundle in cases of severe calcific aortic stenosis, or it may be due to physiologic causes, such as are seen where varying degrees of refractoriness are encountered. Sinoatrial block may be due either to complete failure of the sinus node to generate a stimulus, called sinus node arrest, to prevention of conduction of the normal sinus signal through surrounding atrial tissue because of physiologic or anatomic limitations in the tissue surrounding the sinoatrial node.

Atrioventricular (AV) block is delay or absence of conduction through the atrioventricular node. Classically it has been divided into first degree, second degree, and third degree block. First degree block is characterized by a prolongation of the PR interval to greater than 0.21 seconds. Prolongation is due to delay of conduction through the AV node. All signals arriving from the atrium are conducted in a one-to-one fashion through the AV node to the His-Purkinje system. First degree AV block may be a normal variant and is frequently seen in digitalized patients without evidence of digitalis toxicity. It has been reported in highly conditioned athletes, who regain a normal PR interval when they become deconditioned.

Second degree AV block indicates that a variable number of electrical signals entering the AV node will not emerge to produce depolarization of the His-Purkinje system. Thus, there may be 2:1, 3:1, 4:1, or more complex variations, such as 3:2, 4:3, etc., of the ratio of atrial signals to an eventual ventricular conduction. Second degree AV block has been divided into Type I and Type II. This classification was pop-

ularized by Mobitz, who emphasized the difference between the two forms of AV block. Mobitz Type I block, which was actually initially described by Wenckebach, is characterized by excessive delay of conduction in the AV node to the point where one or more signals may actually be lost, leading to the absence of ventricular stimulation and a QRS complex. In a typical Mobitz Type I or Wenckebach phenomenon, there is progressive prolongation of the PR interval until eventually a P wave is not followed by a ventricular response, producing a dropped beat. While the PR interval progressively elongates, the PP interval stays constant but the RR interval shortens. This phenomenon may be seen in normal patients and in patients with digitalis excess or acute myocardial infarction.

Mobitz Type II block, which incidently was also described by Wenckebach, is characterized by the loss or dropping of a QRS complex in the setting of a normal PR interval and normal PP interval. Whereas Mobitz Type I block has been attributed to a physiologic block within the AV node, Mobitz Type II block is thought to be due to either a physiologic or an anatomical block in the His bundle. Mobitz Type I and II blocks cannot be differentiated from each other if the AV block is 2:1 with a normal P-QRS conduction pattern followed by a P wave with a dropped QRS because there are insufficient cycles to be able to discern a difference between a PR interval and an RR interval. Differentiation of these two forms of block is clinically important, since Mobitz Type I phenomenon is in most cases a benign arrhythmia that seldom leads to consideration for pacemaker implantation, whereas Mobitz Type II block may be a harbinger of complete heart block or cardiac arrest.

Third degree block indicates that there is no relationship between atrial activity and ventricular activity. This block has been termed complete heart block, which indicates that there is complete block of antegrade signals traveling from the atrium to the ventricle, but it does not necessarily mean that there cannot be conduction from ventricle to atrium. Thus, the activity of the atria and the ventricles is dissociated, at least in terms of antegrade or forward conduction. This dissociation between atria and ventricles has lead to significant confusion between the terms complete heart block and AV dissociation. "Complete heart block" should be reserved for those situations in which there is a reasonably normal atrial activity and rate but no appropriate response in the ventricle because of block in the atrioventricular node or the His bundle. AV dissociation is seen when the atrial rate is so slow that a lower pacemaker in the His system or in the ventricles may actually exceed the atrial rate, and thus signals arriving from the atrium find the ventricle refractory; or a focus in the His system or ventricles may become so rapid that the normally formed atrial signals find the ventricles refractory, as is seen in ventricular tachycardia.

Bundle branch block may occur either because of isolated blocks in the ventricle or as a result of prolonged ventricular depolarization caused by diffuse or localized disease in the ventricular musculature. Isolated blocks usually occur in the right bundle rather than the left bundle because the left bundle arborizes very shortly after its origins from the His bundle, leading to many pathways for ventricular depolarization. Anatomic blocks in the conduction system without necessary involvement of the myocardium may occur in the case of Lenegre's disease or Lev's disease. Lenegre's disease is a degenerative process involving the conduction system that frequently causes right bundle branch block and left anterior hemiblock. Many patients who eventually develop complete heart block will first have this combination of right bundle branch block and left anterior hemiblock; however, many patients may maintain this pattern throughout life without ever developing heart block. Lev's disease is due to interruption of the conducting system by outside processes such as a fibrosis or calcification that arise in areas close to the conducting system. The association of calcific aortic stenosis with complete heart block is a manifestation of this process. The fibrosis and calcification associated with the calcific aortic stenotic process occur in close proximity to the His bundle and indeed may invade the His bundle, producing a mechanical separation of the conduction system from the atrium to the ventricle. Excessive fibrosis of the central fibrous body, through which courses the His bundle, may also lead to disruption of the His bundle and the development of complete heart block.

CARDIOMEGALY

DEFINITION

In general, the term cardiomegaly simply means an enlarged heart. While observation that the heart is enlarged is useful to the clinician as he tries to focus his differential diagnosis, the recognition of specific chamber enlargement is even more helpful in refining the reason for the patient's cardiac complaints. It should be emphasized that while the heart may appear enlarged by physical examination or chest x-ray, there are variations in normal heart size that do not necessarily indicate organic heart disease. The heart of a trained athlete, for instance, may be enlarged as a compensatory mechanism developed to allow the athlete to generate the greater than normal cardiac output necessary to achieve supranormal physical feats. On the other hand, the heart may appear to be inordinately small in cases of emphysema and Addison's disease. The presence of such conditions in a patient with organic heart disease may thus lead the clinician astray if he demands cardiomegaly as a sine qua non for making a specific cardiac diagnosis.

DIAGNOSTIC EVALUATION

Physical Examination

Prior to laboratory evaluation of heart size, physical examination with an emphasis on inspection and palpation of the precordium may provide valuable clues as to not only general cardiomegaly but also specific chamber enlargement that may not be evident even on chest x-ray. Inspection of the precordium may provide evidence of left ventricular enlargement or hypertrophy in the region of the left fourth and fifth interspace; a prominent pulsation close to the lower left sternal border or in the epigastrium may indicate right ventricular enlargement.

Palpation of the point of maximal impulse (PMI) in the left fourth, fifth, or sixth interspace at the point of maximal cardiac impulse provides useful information concerning the status not only of the left ventricle but occasionally of the left atrium. In the case of hypertension with left ventricular hypertrophy, the PMI is usually discrete, brisk, and relatively brief. On the other hand, in the case of aortic or mitral regurgitation, the PMI is usually diffuse, heaving, or rolling and is usually displaced downward toward the left, thus lying in the left sixth interspace beyond the midclavicular line and often in the anterior axillary line. In ischemic heart disease, there is often a distinctive bulge during systole in the left third and fourth interspace somewhat closer to the left sternal border than the usual PMI. This bulge may be noted in the case of a left ventricular aneurysm and also during episodes of angina, presumably because of transient dyskinesia of the left ventricular myocardium. In mitral stenosis, the PMI may be normally located in the left fifth interspace along the midclavicular line, but this impulse has a distinctive snapping quality rather than the somewhat diffuse quality of the PMI noted with valvular regurgitation or left ventricular dysfunction. A combination of such a distinctive snapping, short, discrete PMI and a right ventricular lift strongly suggests the presence of mitral stenosis. Other unusual impulses palpated during physical examination may carry some specific hints as to the presence of cardiovascular lesions. Pulsations in the region of the left sternoclavicular joint have been noted in cases of aortic dissection.

Diagnostic Studies

RADIOLOGIC STUDIES

While newer laboratory modalities and physical examination may provide evidence of cardiomegaly and selective cardiac chamber enlargement, by far the most useful and ubiquitous technique for determining cardiomegaly is the chest x-ray. Standard posterior-anterior (PA) and lateral views of the chest provide a wealth of information about cardiac chamber size. These views can be supplemented with oblique views, particularly incorporating a barium swallow to provide even more information. Table 7–20 lists various diagnoses associated with selective chamber enlargement by chest x-ray. Once again, it should be noted that generalized cardiac enlargement as defined by the simple cardiothoracic ratio, in which the silhouette of the heart exceeds 50% of the total width of the thoracic cage at its maximum, does not automatically imply cardiac disease in the healthy individual who has engaged in vigorous conditioning sports. It should be recognized also that an enlarged silhouette, which is presumed to be the cardiac shadow, may not always be just the cardiac shadow; there are circumstances in which the cardiac shadow appears enlarged not because of actual cardiac chamber enlargement but rather because of lesions that are extracardiac. In children, particularly in infancy, the thymus may remain enlarged, producing an impression of cardiomegaly by chest x-ray. Various mediastinal tumors may simulate enlargement of either the heart or the great vessels. Thickening of the pericardium from pericardial disease may also simulate cardiomegaly, as does a large pericardial effusion. Finally, patients who have prominent pectus excavatum may have a chest x-ray strongly suggesting cardiomegaly, presumably because of inward crowding of the heart, which produces a ''pancaking'' effect that results in an enlarged cardiac silhouette.

The standard PA view provides the most useful information concerning the presence of cardiomegaly and selective chamber enlargement. It not only provides an overall view of total cardiac size but also enables one to recognize which particular chambers of the heart are involved. In left ventricular enlargement, not only will the total cardiac size be increased, but the point of maximum lateral displacement of the left

Table 7–20.   Differential Diagnosis of Cardiomegaly

Pseudocardiomegaly
  Thymic enlargement
  Mediastinal tumors
  Pericardial disease
  Skeletal abnormalities (pectus excavatum)
Specific chamber enlargement
  Right atrium
    Tricuspid stenosis and regurgitation
    Myxoma
    Ebstein's anomaly
    Pulmonic stenosis
    Pulmonary hypertension
    Atrial septal defect
    Anomalous venous drainage
    Cardiomyopathy
  Right ventricle
    Pulmonary stenosis
    Pulmonary hypertension
      Primary
      Secondary to pulmonary causes
      Secondary to left heart disease
        Congestive heart failure
        Mitral valve disease
    Increased flow
      Atrial septal defect
      Anomalous pulmonary venous drainage
      Ventricular septal defect
    Congestive heart failure secondary to left heart disease
  Left atrium
    Mitral stenosis
    Atrial myxoma
    Mitral regurgitation
    Ventricular septal defect
    Patent ductus arteriosus
    Left ventricular disease
      Cardiomyopathy
      Hypertrophy secondary to hypertension or left ventricular outflow obstruction, aortic stenosis
      Cardiomyopathy
  Left ventricle
    Left ventricular outflow obstruction
    Aortic regurgitation
    Mitral regurgitation
    Ventricular septal defect
    Patent ductus arteriosus
    Cardiomyopathy
  Aorta
    Tortuous aorta
    Aortic stenosis
    Aortic regurgitation
    Cystic medial necrosis (Marfans)
    Aortic aneurysm
    Dissection
    Saccular aneurysm (syphilitic)

ventricle, which conforms to the PMI on physical examination, will be displaced beyond the mid-clavicular line and downward toward lower intercostal spaces such as the left sixth and seventh intercostal space. A line drawn from a point in the midcardiac shadow to this most lateral displacement of the left cardiac border will be displaced downward from a horizontal line. This radiographic vector indicates left ventricular enlargement. An increase in left atrial size is indicated by the presence of a "double density" in the upper portions of the cardiac shadow. This double density is due to increased size of the left atrium, which sits somewhat higher than the more anterior and lower right atrium. Left atrial enlargement is also indicated by a widening of the normal angle between the left and right main-stem bronchi, since the enlarged left atrium displaces the left main-stem bronchus upward. As the left atrium enlarges, the left atrial appendage, lying along the left heart border just below the pulmonary artery, also enlarges, producing straightening of the left heart border. When the PA chest film is accompanied by a barium swallow, the barium column can be seen to be displaced laterally to the right as a result of the encroachment of the enlarged left atrium on the esophagus. Right atrial enlargement is indicated by prominence of the lower right cardiac border.

The lateral view of the chest x-ray may also provide evidence of left ventricular enlargement. Rigler's sign, which is a sign of left ventricular enlargement, is determined by choosing a point 2 cm above the place where the inferior vena cava enters the cardiac shadow and by measuring the distance from that point to the posterior cardiac border along a line parallel to an intervertebral interspace. If this distance exceeds 1.7 cm, left ventricular enlargement is present, presuming there is not evidence of right ventricular enlargement as well. Right ventricular enlargement is detected when the retrosternal cardiac shadow occupies more than two thirds of the retrosternal length. Left atrial enlargement is present when the left main-stem bronchus is noted to be displaced superiorly. Again, a barium swallow will demonstrate left atrial enlargement in this view when the barium-filled esophagus is displaced posteriorly by the enlarged left atrium.

The right anterior oblique view will demonstrate enlargement of the outflow tract to the right ventricle and the pulmonary artery. A barium swallow in this view, again, will demonstrate posterior displacement by the enlarged left atrium of the barium-filled esophagus.

LABORATORY TESTS

Although the primary tool in making the observation of cardiomegaly has been the standard chest x-ray, there are now other laboratory modalities available to indicate cardiac enlargement, particularly of specific chambers. Careful correlation of electrocardiographic findings with the status of various cardiac chambers has led to a well-defined series of criteria for evaluating cardiac chamber enlargement. The echocardiogram is

going through much the same evolution of correlation of echocardiographic findings with pathologic findings, so that there is also a gradually accumulating series of criteria for evaluating selective chamber enlargement. Radionuclide studies that allow visualization of internal chamber size have also enlarged our understanding of signs of selective cardiac chamber enlargement. Magnetic resonance imaging (MRI) offers a new tool to define not only the external cardiac enlargement but also selective internal chamber enlargement, as well as enlargement of different segments of cardiac chambers.[21]

ISCHEMIC HEART DISEASE

DEFINITION AND PATHOPHYSIOLOGIC CONSIDERATIONS

Ischemic heart disease is a term applied to indicate left ventricular dysfunction caused by decreased oxygenation in myocardial tissue. Decreased oxygenation is almost always associated with deposition of atheromatous material in coronary arteries leading to decreased coronary blood flow and therefore decreased oxygen delivery to the myocardium. Because of this almost inevitable incidence of atheromatous obstruction of coronary arteries, ischemic heart disease has also been termed arteriosclerotic heart disease. However, because flow to the myocardium may be compromised by other processes, such as the spasm that occurs in Prinzmetal's variant angina, which may produce the same symptoms as atheromatous obstruction of the coronary arteries, the term ischemic heart disease has been preferred. The myocardium may receive inadequate oxygen either because there is an excessive demand for oxygen or because there is a decreased supply. Excessive demand is created by conditions that require increased work of the myocardium, such as aortic stenosis or severe hypertension. Decreased supply is almost inevitably due to atheromatous obstruction of one or more coronary arteries but may also be seen in the case of severe anemia. Even in the severely anemic patient who develops angina pectoris there is almost always a component of atheromatous obstruction in addition to the anemia to account for the development of angina. On the other hand, classic angina may develop in patients with aortic stenosis or aortic regurgitation without any obstruction to the coronary arteries.

DIAGNOSTIC EVALUATION

Ischemic heart disease resulting from atherosclerosis of the coronary arteries may present in several ways: 1) as classic angina pectoris (described previously), 2) as acute myocardial infarction with or without preceding angina pectoris, or 3) as acute or chronic congestive heart failure without preceding infarction or angina. This latter presentation has also been termed arteriosclerotic or ischemic cardiomyopathy. By far the most frequent manifestations of ischemic heart disease in the general population are either angina pectoris or acute myocardial infarction.

Patient History

The presence of certain risk factors lends weight to the possible diagnosis of ischemic heart disease. A strong family history of premature ischemic heart disease, and hypertension, hypercholesterolemia, and cigarette smoking should focus suspicion on the diagnosis of ischemic heart disease in a patient presenting with chest pain or unexplained heart failure. With a strong family history of premature ischemic heart disease, the likelihood is even greater if the patient in addition has a history of cigarette smoking.

Physical Examination

Aside from a careful evaluation of a patient's symptoms (see Chest Pain) there are remarkably few physical signs of ischemic heart disease. Cardiac examination is usually normal except in the case of arteriosclerotic cardiomyopathy, in which there may be all the signs expected in severe left ventricular dysfunction. The presence of bruits over large arteries in patients who are suspected of having ischemic heart disease strongly increases the possibility of ischemic heart disease. Much debate has been raised over whether diagonal clefts in the earlobes and the presence of hair in the auditory canal may be a strong predictor of underlying ischemic heart disease. While these are frequent findings in patients with heart disease, their sensitivity and specificity as predictors are still being argued.

Diagnostic Studies

Because of the paucity of physical findings available to corroborate a suspected diagnosis of ischemic heart disease, a battery of laboratory studies have been developed to try to establish the diagnosis. A variety of blood lipid studies have been used in attempting to identify patients with ischemic heart disease, but the sensitivity and specificity of these studies are not adequate to be used for diagnostic purposes when encountering the individual patient.

LABORATORY TESTS

The resting electrocardiogram was the first laboratory test to gain wide usage in making a diagnosis of ischemic heart disease. In general, a resting electrocardiogram may provide information of varying certitude in establishing a diagnosis of ischemic heart disease. Q waves of at least .04 seconds in duration in the standard limb leads or absent R waves in the first three precordial leads are usually indicative of previous myocardial infarction. These findings may be noted in an asymptomatic patient (particularly one with left ventricular hypertrophy), and although they may lead to the false impression that the patient has undergone a myocardial infarction in the past, the absence of symptoms does not preclude the possibility that the patient has had a previous silent myocardial infarction. Serial electrocardiograms obtained on a group of patients during the Framingham study would indicate that greater than 25% of patients who do indeed develop electrocardiographic signs of myocardial infarction can recall no symptoms in a preceding 6 months before the development of electrocardiographic signs of infarction. Ischemic patterns on the ECG characterized by hyperacute peaking of T waves, ST-segment elevation, and T-wave inversion all point to a diagnosis of ischemic heart disease, particularly when they are obtained in an acute situation.

Because all these electrocardiographic signs may occur under other circumstances, they are not diagnostic. The pain of acute pericarditis may mimic that of myocardial infarction or severe coronary insufficiency. Under these circumstances there will be prominent ST-segment elevation usually without T-wave inversion. In the acute situation, however, who is to say whether the ST-segment changes are due to pericarditis or due to early myocardial injury? In the case of pericarditis, subsequent serial electrocardiograms may show a delayed T-wave inversion and a persistence of ST-segment elevation over a relatively long period of time, indicating that the acute chest pain was most likely due to pericarditis rather than to myocardial damage. Only on very rare occasions will pericarditis produce QRS changes suggestive of myocardial infarction. In addition to the fact that there are a variety of causes for changes in the QRS, ST segment, and T wave that may simulate ischemic heart disease, there are many situations in which ischemic heart disease is present but the electrocardiogram is entirely normal. In fact, approximately 20% of patients who have undergone documented myocardial infarctions with QRS changes may, over the course of time, lose these QRS changes and appear to have normal electrocardiograms.

Because of these vagaries of the resting electrocardiogram with regard to its diagnostic utility, various protocols have been developed to document the electrocardiogram during and immediately after exercise-induced stress. The fundamental premise underlying these studies is that while myocardial blood flow adequate for myocardial oxygenation at rest shows a normal resting electrocardiogram, the imposition of new demands for oxygen delivery to the tissues and thus increased myocardial blood flow will result in ischemic changes on the electrocardiogram. The classic ischemic response sought in these studies is ST-segment depression of at least 1 mv lasting for .08 seconds. Terminal deflection of the ST segment lower than its initial starting point is felt to further heighten the possibility of an ischemic response on the electrocardiogram. ST-segment elevation of greater than 1 mv may also be seen occasionally during exercise testing and carries the same connotation.

Master was the first investigator to popularize an attempt to evoke an ischemic electrocardiographic response with exercise. He obtained a resting electrocardiogram and then had his patients walk back and forth over two steps. The Master "two-step" exercise test suffered from lack of sensitivity and specificity. The effort demanded of the patient was often too little to provoke an ischemic response, and Master's criteria for positivity were so broad that a large number of patients who did not have ischemic heart disease were falsely labeled as having the disease.

Since Master's pioneering work, exercise testing has been repeatedly modified and its accuracy tested against epidemiologic criteria as well as anatomic studies obtained from coronary arteriography. The most frequently used technique involves the continuous electrocardiographic monitoring of a patient as he walks on a treadmill until his so-called target heart rate, which is determined by his age, is reached. The most common protocol currently used is the Bruce protocol, in which every 3 minutes the speed and grade of the patient's walk are rapidly increased. The Bruce protocol has the virtue of getting the patient to a rapid heart rate relatively quickly. On the other hand, it has the disadvantage of imposing a fairly high degree of physical stress rapidly. Deconditioned patients and patients in the elderly age group frequently have difficulty, if not great anxiety, attempting to keep up with the treadmill even in its early stages. The Balke-Ware protocol eliminates some of the problems of the Bruce protocol because it entails walking at a constant speed of approximately 2 to 3.3 miles per hour with 2 to 5% increases in grade every 2 to 3 minutes. The patient is thus able to become accustomed to a walking pace and the only new stress he faces is the change in the

grade every 3 minutes. Results from the Bruce and the Balke-Ware protocols can easily be correlated.

Exercise electrocardiography is contraindicated in patients who have either acute myocardial infarction, recent changes in ECG suggestive of acute ischemia, unstable angina pectoris, significant aortic stenosis, digitalis therapy, and left bundle branch block. Such exercise electrocardiography is contraindicated in situations in which there is evidence of unstable coronary blood flow, such as recent ischemic ECG changes and unstable angina, because of the fear of provoking an acute myocardial infarction. It is contraindicated in aortic stenosis because these patients may develop effort-induced arrhythmias and cardiovascular collapse. It is contraindicated in digitalis therapy because patients taking digitalis, even if they have normal resting ST segments, may with exercise develop what would appear to be diagnostic ST-segment changes yet have no evidence of coronary artery disease. Finally, the exercise electrocardiogram is not helpful in patients with left bundle branch block because these patients already have a distortion of the ST segment, making interpretation of exercise-induced ST-segment changes impossible.

The accuracy of exercise testing in predicting whether a patient does or does not have ischemic heart disease has been a point of debate for many years. The sensitivity of the test, that is, the test's ability to detect patients with ischemic heart disease, and the specificity of the test, that is, the test's ability to identify only patients who have ischemic heart disease, are basically dependent on the incidence of ischemic heart disease among a population similar to the patient being tested. The ultimate meaning of this to the clinician is that an exercise tolerance test should not be interpreted in a vacuum. For instance, women below the age of 40 may have positive stress tests, but because there are very few women in this group who have ischemic heart disease, there is a very high likelihood, approaching 40%, that a positive test in a woman under 40 will be a false positive test. On the other hand, a male over the age of 50 with a history compatible with angina pectoris and a positive exercise stress test will have a very high likelihood of having ischemic heart disease. Thus, interpretation of the electrocardiographic changes must be integrated with consideration of the patient's age, sex, and clinical history.

RADIOLOGIC STUDIES

Because of these problems of specificity and sensitivity with exercise electrocardiography, investigators have turned to newer techniques to attempt to document the presence of ischemic heart disease. These have included techniques to identify the presence and location of an acute myocardial infarction (^{99m}Tc stannous pyrophosphate uptake), flow determinations to an infarcted and ischemic myocardium using ^{201}Tl and left ventricular function studies using ^{99m}Tc. The technetium stannous pyrophosphate study identifying the presence of an acute myocardial infarction is based on the knowledge that calcium rapidly accumulates in the area of infarction and that technetium complexes with the calcium, providing an area of relatively high radioactivity, or a "hot spot." This physical/chemical reaction occurs between 48 and 72 hours after the infarction and gradually declines over the following 7 days. Because of difficulties in interpreting the results of these studies and the development of newer, more precise enzyme techniques for detecting myocardial infarction, this particular form of radionuclide scanning is seldom indicated. Perhaps its most important indication is to document a possible myocardial infarction that may have occurred 3 to 4 days before the patient's entry into the hospital, during which time his enzyme levels for myocardial damage may have disappeared.

Thallium scanning is based on the premise that thallium acts hemodynamically and biologically much as potassium does and thus will traverse the myocardial microcirculation like normal blood. Absence of evidence of thallium in images obtained with an Anger camera indicates an occlusion of flow to a portion of the myocardium. Absence of thallium noted at rest presumably implies infarction and subsequent fibrosis. On the other hand, an area of the myocardial image that is not detectable after exercise but that had been present at rest presumably implies exercise-induced ischemia. Thus, thallium is used as an attempt to determine patterns of myocardial blood flow at the microcirculatory level.

Several techniques have been developed to test the functional integrity of the left ventricle on the presumption that if the left ventricle does not perform normally, as evidenced by a decrease in ejection fraction with exercise, or by the detection of wall motion abnormalities at rest or during exercise, these abnormalities must be due to decreased nourishment or ischemia of the myocardium. First-pass radionuclide angiography, which consists of a bolus injection of ^{99}Tc, provides a brief image with an Anger camera of the radioactive bolus disbursed in the cardiac chambers. Sequential images obtained from the Anger camera allows for determination of left ventricular end-diastolic and end-systolic volumes and thus a calculation of ejection fraction.

Similar information may be obtained using a technique termed equilibrium gated blood pool imaging or multigated acquisition scans (MUGA). In this technique, ^{99}Tc is used to label the blood pool passing through the heart, not by allowing imaging of the disbursement of the ^{99}Tc bolus, as in the case of the first-pass technique, but by labeling the red blood cells with the technetium. Multiple images of the blood pool in the cardiac chambers are obtained at precise, consistent intervals after the QRS complex. These images are added together to obtain cleaner images. These end-systolic and end-diastolic images are obtained in order to calculate an ejection fraction and also to provide a picture of regional wall motion both at rest and with exercise.

The first-pass technique has the advantage of allowing data acquisition relatively rapidly so that observations can be made at peak exercise. The disadvantage is that repeated injections of radioactive material are required if several observations must be made. The advantage of the MUGA technique is that once the blood pool is labeled, multiple observations may be made over the course of several hours without repeat injections of radioactive material. This also allows multiple views of the myocardial cavity and thus possibly a better understanding of potential wall motion abnormalities. The disadvantage is that adequate data acquisition may be impossible because acquisition time may be so long that the patient cannot continue peak physical exercise long enough to obtain peak exercise values.

Though newer radionuclide procedures have a significantly higher level of sensitivity and specificity than the exercise electrocardiogram does, they are not free of the same problems. For instance, while normal men will almost consistently increase their left ventricular ejection fractions with exercise, normal women will frequently decrease their ejection fractions with exercise. Furthermore, women may develop wall motion abnormalities that further confound the diagnosis. Thallium imaging has been extremely successful in certain laboratories, but its lack of reproducibility across the country has limited its diagnostic value.

Because of its simplicity, echocardiography has been recruited to attempt to define left ventricular function and wall motion abnormalities in patients with presumed or suspected ischemic heart disease. The advent of two-dimensional echocardiography has encouraged even further exploration of these methods. The problem of quantifying these observations is just beginning to be approached; its solution will be a necessary culmination of efforts to use echocardiography in the diagnosis of ischemic heart disease.

Prolonged ambulatory recording of the electrocardiogram using a tape recorder system (Holter monitoring) may provide useful information in selected patients with ischemic heart disease. Documenting ischemic ST-segment changes during normal daily activity in the patient with suspected ischemic heart disease would be extremely useful, but current instrumentation is inadequate. Earlier recording systems made evaluation of ST-segment changes difficult to detect and evaluate because, in attempting to eliminate artifacts, these systems were designed to eliminate events of low frequency, such as are ST-segment changes. The opportunity to record from only one and even two electrode sites also limited the detection of ST-segment changes. Furthermore, normal physical activity such as hyperventilation, changes in body position, and situations provoking tachycardia or anxiety may provoke ST-segment changes that are not due to ischemic heart disease. Some of these technical problems in earlier recording systems may well be eliminated by computerized digital recording systems using microprocessors.

Despite all these limitations, prolonged ambulatory electrocardiographic recording may be helpful in establishing a diagnosis of ischemic heart disease in selected patients. For instance, demonstrating that there are repetitive episodes of ST-segment elevation, some of which are accompanied by angina, can be vital in diagnosing Prinzmetal's variant angina. Such patients classically have negative treadmill electrocardiograms, and approximately 10% of these patients will have a negative or nonspastic response to ergonovine administration during cardiac catheterization. It has now become clear that patients with classic angina pectoris may have frequent episodes of ischemic ST-segment changes without anginal symptoms. These may be detected by prolonged ambulatory electrocardiographic monitoring, but, again, the separation of true ST-segment depression and artifacts poses a problem.

Because of the problems with specificity and sensitivity for all the methods for diagnosing ischemic heart disease, cardiac catheterization with coronary arteriography has remained the standard. During cardiac catheterization, a left ventricular cineangiogram will demonstrate the dimensions of the ventricle in systole and diastole and thus allow a calculation of ejection fraction. More importantly, left ventricular cineangiography will allow documentation of wall motion abnormalities that are secondary to ischemia. Coronary arteriography with multiple views of the opacified coronary tree will demonstrate partial or total occlusive lesions caused by atheromatous plaquing. Coronary arteriography should be performed not only "at rest" but also after ergonovine stimulation in order to detect the possibility of coronary artery spasm as a cause for the patient's complaint of angina.

CONGENITAL HEART DISEASE IN THE ADULT

DEFINITION

The term "congenital" is derived from the Latin, meaning "born with." While the vast majority of forms of congenital heart disease make themselves manifest in infancy or early childhood, some forms of congenital heart disease become obvious only in early or middle adult life. The presentation of a patient with congenital heart disease, particularly with a significant intracardiac shunt is almost a rare phenomenon now because of remarkable advances in pediatric cardiology. Even so, some rudimentary understanding and classification of congenital heart disease is worth retaining, even if only to know where to start investigation of the potential problem.

PATHOPHYSIOLOGIC CONSIDERATIONS AND DIFFERENTIAL DIAGNOSIS

Perloff pointed out that a classification of all potential lesions should have some logic in order to make sense of the myriad of potential congenital lesions involving the heart. Table 7-21 is derived from Perloff's all-encompassing classification of congenital heart disease. It is less detailed than his original but provides a useful logic tree to begin to sort out the location and types of congenital lesions that may be present.

The first question to be answered when a patient appears to have congenital heart disease is whether the patient is cyanotic. If the patient is acyanotic, the next

Table 7-21. Classification of Congenital Heart Disease

Acyanotic
  Without a shunt
    Malformation in the left heart
    Malformation in the right heart
  With a left-to-right shunt
    Atrial level
    Ventricular level
    Between aorta and right heart
    Between aorta and pulmonary artery
    Multiple shunts
Cyanotic
  With increased pulmonary blood flow
  With normal or decreased pulmonary blood flow
    Dominant left ventricle
    Dominant right ventricle

Table 7–22.   Congenital Heart Disease in the Adult

Obstructive or regurgitant lesions
    Aortic valvular and subvalvular lesions
    Pulmonary valvular or subvalvular lesions
    Mitral regurgitation
    Coarctation of the aorta
Shunts
    Left-to-right
        Atrial septal defect
        Ventricular septal defect
        Patent ductus arteriosus
        Multiple shunts
        Atrioventricular canal defects
    Right-to-left
        Tetralogy of Fallot
        Eisenmenger complex
Electrocardiographic lesions
    Congenital complete heart block
    Congenital junctional rhythm
    Pre-excitation syndromes
    Prolonged QT syndromes

question is whether there is evidence of a shunt, which in the absence of cyanosis would be from left to right rather than right to left. In the acyanotic patient, the presence of a shunt is best determined by an examination of the chest film, which in the case of a left-to-right shunt will show evidence of increased pulmonary blood flow. If there is no evidence of a shunt, the next question regards whether the malformation is in the left heart or in the right heart. This determination inevitably involves establishing whether there are valvular or subvalvular lesions. If there is increased pulmonary blood flow indicating a left-to-right shunt, the level of the shunt must be determined: is it atrial, ventricular, or above the level of aortic valve, involving a communication between either the aorta and the heart or the aorta and the pulmonary circulation.

If the patient is cyanotic it is important to determine if pulmonary blood flow is increased, which would indicate the presence of a left-to-right shunt in addition to the right-to-left shunt evident from cyanosis. For a more detailed classification, the reader is referred to Perloff's excellent book.[22]

Aortic Stenosis or Regurgitation. It is now clear that congenital malformation of either the pulmonic or the aortic valve and lesions beneath these valves may become hemodynamically evident only in adult life (Table 7–22). For many years it was felt that isolated aortic stenosis or regurgitation, which were encountered relatively late in adult life, were due to rheumatic fever. It is now clear that isolated aortic stenosis and regurgitation are more likely to be due to gradually evolving destruction of the aortic valve resulting from an underlying congenital anomaly in the valve. Alterations in flow patterns and demands for increased ve-

locity of flow across a mildly narrowed aortic valve eventually lead to fibrosis and calcification and all the hemodynamic signs and consequences of aortic stenosis. The systolic ejection murmur heard in a child and presumed to be an innocent murmur may actually be the murmur of aortic stenosis that is hemodynamically insignificant in childhood but that is the harbinger of hemodynamically significant aortic stenosis in the adult. It is not rare for the adult who presents with all the hemodynamic signs and symptoms of severe aortic stenosis to casually recall that he was almost deferred for military service in World War II because of a murmur noted during his preinduction physical examination. In extremely rare cases there may be outflow obstruction from the left ventricle, not at the valvular level but at the supravalvular level. It is also rare to encounter isolated membranous subvalvular stenosis in the adult, but it occurs more frequently than supravalvular aortic stenosis. It is frequently associated with aortic regurgitation and a variable degree of aortic valvular stenosis because the high-velocity eccentrically directed jet from the outflow tract to the left ventricle leads to fibrosis and calcification of what may have been a normal aortic valve.

Mitral Regurgitation. Just as isolated aortic valvular disease had been attributed primarily to rheumatic fever, isolated mitral regurgitation previously also had been attributed to earlier rheumatic fever. It is now apparent that many, if not the majority, of cases of isolated mitral regurgitation are due to a congenital lesion of the mitral valve, usually mitral valve prolapse, which will be discussed at greater length later in this chapter. Suffice it to say that there are well-documented cases of mid-systolic clicks and innocuous mitral murmurs early in life with gradual progression of signs of an increasing mitral regurgitation that eventually requires mitral valve replacement.

Coarctation of the Aorta. Patients with coarctation of the aorta are usually diagnosed in childhood, but it is not rare to have an occasional patient appearing for hypertensive evaluation who turns out to have coarctation of the aorta. The diagnosis is indicated by the near absence of femoral pulses in the young patient, the phase lag of the systolic pulse between the carotids and the femoral artery, and palpable if not visible arterial collaterals high on the thoracic cage. The diagnosis is further corroborated by the presence of rib notching on chest x-ray, as well as the reversed E sign in the thoracic aorta. This sign is created by dilatation of the aorta adjacent to the area of narrowing caused by the coarctation, which in turn is adjacent to resumption of, or an increase in, the normal descending thoracic aortic shadow.

Atrial Septal Defects. Although it is unusual for

patients with complex intracardiac shunts to present in adult life, it is not rare to see a patient with a left-to-right shunt. The most frequent form of congenital heart disease, if mitral valve prolapse is not considered, is an atrial septal defect. Such patients may not have been diagnosed early in life because the systolic murmur, caused by increased flow across the outflow tract of the right ventricle, had been diagnosed as an innocent flow murmur. These patients are frequently asymptomatic by their testimony, but once the atrial septal defect is repaired they clearly recognize that they had lived their entire lives with decreased exercise tolerance compared to their contemporaries. In the adult, physical examination will demonstrate a right ventricular lift, a systolic ejection murmur along the left sternal border often with a mid-systolic scratching sound similar to multiple systolic ejection clicks, and a persistently split second heart sound during inspiration and expiration. The electrocardiogram will show an incomplete right bundle branch block-type pattern in the majority of these patients. The chest x-ray will show a marked increase in pulmonary blood flow with plethoric lung fields and prominent pulmonary veins. Patients will usually have cardiomegaly with right ventricular enlargement easily detectable on the lateral chest x-ray. The aortic knob is typically small as compared to the generalized cardiomegaly that appears on the PA film.

Atrial septal defects may generally be classified into two groups: ostium primum defects and secundum defects. Secundum defects arise high in the atrial septum (sinus venosus defects), in the central portion of the atrial septum (fossa ovalis defects), or low in the right atrium close to the entrance of the inferior vena cava (inferior vena caval defects). Ostium primum atrial septal defects are a manifestation of a defect in development of the atrioventricular cushions. As such, they lie low and medial in the atrial septum, frequently close to the atrioventricular node. They may be associated with defects in the formation of the ventricular septum and in the cusps of the mitral and tricuspid valve because all these structures are dependent on normal development of the atrioventricular cushions in early embryologic life.

Ventricular Septal Defects. Adults are less likely to present with ventricular septal defects than with atrial septal defects since ventricular septal defects have loud holosystolic murmurs that are seldom confused with the innocent flow murmurs heard frequently in youth. On physical examination, patients with ventricular septal defects frequently have evidence of left ventricular enlargement, a systolic thrill low along the left sternal border, and a loud holosystolic murmur heard over the entire precordium but particularly well low along the left sternal border, and they will have normal physiologic splitting of the second heart sound. The presence of normal physiologic splitting of the second heart sound and the fact that the murmur is holosystolic rather than ejection help to separate the ventricular septal defect from an atrial septal defect. The electrocardiogram will frequently show left and right ventricular hypertrophy. Chest x-ray will demonstrate cardiomegaly with both right and left ventricular enlargement, as well as increased pulmonary blood flow.

Patent Ductus Arteriosus. Patent ductus arteriosus may carry few, if any, symptoms into adult life. The diastolic component of the continuous murmur may be so soft and high pitched that it may be missed during childhood. Occasionally the first manifestation of a patent ductus is the realization that the patient has bacterial endocarditis; only after this diagnosis is established does it become apparent that the patient has a patent ductus arteriosus with a barely audible continuous murmur. If the ductus is small with low shunt flow the precordium will feel normal, although with high shunt flows there is often a palpable thrill high along the left sternal border radiating slightly out beneath the left clavicle. With a large ductus, there will be both a left and a right ventricular heave and a continuous murmur heard best high along the left sternal border with radiation beneath the left clavicle. The electrocardiogram may show right and left ventricular hypertrophy and the chest x-ray will show increased pulmonary blood flow.

Shunts. The presence of one left-to-right shunt does not preclude the possibility that there may be other left-to-right shunts. For instance, it is not rare to have the combination of a ventricular septal defect and a patent ductus arteriosus, and atrial septal defects may accompany ventricular septal defects, particularly in the case of atrioventricular cushion lesions.

It is relatively rare for an adult to present with a right-to-left shunt because this shunt usually produces cyanosis that would have alerted the patient's family and pediatrician to seek further investigation before the patient reached adult life. However, if the shunt is relatively small and the cyanosis therefore relatively mild, the diagnosis may not be made before adult life. Probably the most common cause for cyanosis in right-to-left shunts seen in adult life is the presence of pulmonary stenosis and a ventricular septal defect, that is, tetralogy of Fallot or one of its variants. When there is mild stenosis, such patients have been called "pink tetrads" or "pink tetralogies." Such patients have so-called bidirectional shunting, meaning they have both left-to-right and right-to-left shunts. On physical examination, they frequently will have evidence of left ventricular and right ventricular hypertrophy, and because they have a ventricular septal defect they may have a systolic thrill and a holosystolic murmur low along the left sternal border. They have pulmonic stenosis and thus should have a systolic ejection murmur along the left sternal border, although it is frequently difficult to separate this murmur from the holosystolic murmur accompanying the ventricular septal defect. Careful auscultation high along the left sternal border over the pulmonic area may allow detection of systolic ejection murmur separate from the holosystolic murmur. The second heart sound is single because the pulmonic closure sound is almost inaudible as a result of the presence of pulmonic stenosis.

The adult with cyanosis need not have tetralogy of Fallot or one of its variants. The adult may present with a history of gradually increasing cyanosis and decreasing exercise tolerance caused by the reversal of a previous left-to-right shunt to a right-to-left shunt. This so-called Eisenmenger complex may start off as an atrial septal defect, a ventricular septal defect or a patent ductus arteriosus with a left-to-right-shunt, and thus with no evidence of cyanosis. As the increased pulmonary blood flow provokes pulmonary hypertension in a pulmonary arterial bed that is probably hyperreactive, however, pulmonary resistance increases, thus decreasing pulmonary flow and reversing the shunt so that unoxygenated venous blood moves right to left across the defect previously associated with the left-to-right shunt.

While patients with the Eisenmenger complex will be cyanotic, indicating a right-to-left shunt, they also may have small degrees of left-to-right shunt. The patient may present with cyanosis but no heart murmur because, since the shunt flow is relatively small, as pressures become balanced in the right and left ventricles a murmur that had previously been heard may disappear. The predominant finding on palpation of the chest is right ventricular enlargement with a palpable pulmonary closure sound. If there is no murmur, as is frequently the case, the patient will have a loud snapping pulmonary closure sound as a result of the pulmonary hypertension. The electrocardiogram may show either right or left ventricular hypertrophy or it may be normal.

Conduction System Abnormalities. Traditionally, discussions of congenital heart disease have been limited to structural defects of cardiac chambers and variations in the normal direction of blood flow within the heart and its great vessels. However, it is now clear that there are numerous congenital anomalies of the formation of the conduction system of the heart. It has long been known that congenital heart block may be familial, and numerous studies of the hearts in such

patients have demonstrated abnormalities in the development of the His bundle, the AV node, or the connections between the lower atrial musculature and the AV node. Families with congenital junctional rhythm have been reported by Bacos, et al.[23] Pre-excitation syndromes with accessory pathways, such as the Wolff-Parkinson-White syndrome, are clearly congenital and many times familial. A group of families with a prolonged QT interval and sudden death has been reported.

MITRAL VALVE PROLAPSE

DEFINITION

Mitral valve prolapse (MVP) is a clinical condition in which one or both mitral leaflets are noted to protrude backward into the atrium during ventricular systole. It has been given a variety of names, including floppy valve syndrome, ballooning mitral valve, click murmur syndrome, and Barlow's syndrome. A review of the older literature indicates that it has been recognized for over a century,[24] but it has received widespread recognition only recently, since the frequent use of echocardiography and cardiac catheterization for chest pain of unknown cause.

PATHOPHYSIOLOGIC CONSIDERATIONS

The primary pathologic defect is myxomatous degeneration of valvular tissue. This degenerative process may involve not only the mitral but also the tricuspid valve, and it is not rare for a patient to have both mitral and tricuspid valve prolapse. It is familial and congenital and thus probably represents the most common form of congenital heart disease in the adult. The exact incidence of the defect is not clear because different definitions of the syndrome vary from requiring all the overt clinical manifestations of the syndrome to accepting only an echocardiographic demonstration of prolapse. The defect has been reported in from 1 to 17% of the general population. A reasonable estimate would be approximately 10%, with slightly higher incidence in females and lower incidence in males. The genetic defect, whatever it may be, involves not only the heart, but undoubtedly the skeletal system as well, because there is a relatively high incidence of pectus excavatum and the so-called straight back syndrome in patients with mitral valve prolapse. It has been suggested that the central nervous system may also be involved as there appears to be a higher-than-expected incidence of psychiatric disorders and symptoms of neurasthenia.

Although attention has been focused on the mitral leaflets, the syndrome involves all the components of the mitral apparatus. Patients with MVP have an enlarged atrioventricular ring diameter, such that the diameter usually exceeds the maximum diastolic diameter of the left ventricle. The mitral leaflets are thin and often voluminous and the chordae may be thin and enlongated. Contraction of the papillary muscle may be abnormal, and there are a variety of abnormalities of localized left ventricular contraction patterns. MVP may be associated with mitral regurgitation of massive amounts, eventually requiring mitral valve replacement.

DIFFERENTIAL DIAGNOSIS

Mitral valve prolapse with mitral regurgitation has to be differentiated from rheumatic heart disease with mitral regurgitation. This differentiation is relatively easy when there is a mid-systolic click and a late-systolic murmur, but when the mitral regurgitation becomes very prominent, the click is lost and the murmur becomes holosystolic without necessarily late-systolic accentuation. The differentiation can usually be made by echocardiography. Patients with hypertrophic subaortic stenosis may have auscultatory findings mimicking those of mitral valve prolapse except that there is no mid-systolic click and usually no late-systolic accentuation of the murmur. Patients with left atrial myxomas may also have the late-systolic murmur associated with mitral valve prolapse, but, here again, they do not have the multicomponent mid-systolic click associated with the syndrome.

DIAGNOSTIC EVALUATION

Patient History

The signs and symptoms of the syndrome usually become manifest between late adolescent years and middle age. The patient frequently presents with a complaint of palpitations that are due to premature atrial or premature ventricular contractions. Approximately 10% of such patients will have documented paroxysmal atrial tachycardia or paroxysmal atrial fibrillation. In fact, probably the majority of patients previously designated as having lone atrial fibrillation of unknown origin actually had, or have, mitral valve prolapse as the underlying problem.

Chest pain is a frequent symptom that precipitates medical evaluation. It has been considered atypical because it is not typical of the classic pain of coronary insufficiency. However, the pain is so typical for mitral valve prolapse that the diagnosis can almost be made from listening to the patient's history. The pain is usually dull and aching and may involve the entire precordium but is frequently located beneath the left breast. It may radiate to the arms but rarely to the throat or jaw and unlike angina is seldom associated with shortness of breath during exertion. It is usually nonexertional and can be prolonged anywhere from hours to almost days, and it is seldom relieved consistently by any medication, although occasional patients will obtain relief with sublingual nitroglycerin.

In addition to the prolonged episodes of chest pain, patients frequently complain of a generalized, diffuse fatigue and a chronic sensation of dyspnea. A small number of patients will have syncope of unknown cause. Cerebrovascular accidents, particularly those compatible with embolic phenomena in the young, have been attributed to MVP. The symptoms are often episodic, with periods of several weeks to months of remission and then a recurrence lasting weeks at a time.

Physical Examination

Physical examination often demonstrates asthenia, especially in female patients. The patient has pectus excavatum and a straightened dorsal spinal column without the usual lordotic curve. A cardiopulmonary murmur may be heard particularly over the left base of the lung posteriorly. Cardiac examination may demonstrate a more prominent point of maximal impulse than would be expected. There may be frequent premature beats. Between the apex and the left sternal border there is usually a mid- to late-systolic click, which may have several components. Because the click may be present only in one particular position, the patient must be examined while sitting, standing, and lying on the back, as well as lying in the left lateral position. At the apex and along the lower portion of the left sternal border there may be a soft systolic ejection murmur or, more specifically, a systolic murmur that begins in early to mid systole and is accentuated in late systole. The murmur may become late systolic in only one body position, particularly the left lateral decubitus position. In a very small percentage of these patients, there will be an intermittent systolic whoop or honk that also is heard in only one particular body position. The presence of the mid- to late-systolic click and the late-systolic murmur as well as the honk may be variable from day to day.

Diagnostic Studies

The electrocardiogram may confirm the presence of premature atrial or premature ventricular contractions and may show T-wave inversion, primarily in the inferior leads but also occasionally in several of the precordial leads. If significant mitral regurgitation has been present long enough, there will be signs of left ventricular hypertrophy and strain. The chest x-ray may demonstrate pectus excavatum and a straightened dorsal spinal column, as was noted on physical examination. The heart itself is usually normal in size unless the pectus excavatum is pronounced or mitral regurgitation has been present long enough to produce left ventricular and left atrial enlargement. M-mode echocardiography will demonstrate prolapse of the posterior leaflet into the left atrium during systole. With the widespread use of two-dimensional echocardiography, it has become apparent that not only the posterior leaflet is involved, but frequently the anterior mitral leaflet as well. Left ventricular cineangiography will demonstrate bulging of the mitral leaflets back into the left atrium during systole, particularly in the right anterior oblique view.

It is now clear that the course of mitral valve prolapse is quite variable. The vast majority of individuals with the syndrome will remain asymptomatic and be recognized only during routine health examinations. In a small number of patients this syndrome may not be so benign. As the patient ages, the mitral regurgitation may become severe enough to require mitral valve replacement. Mitral regurgitation may arise acutely because of rupture of a chordae. The deformed valve may become the site of bacterial endocarditis. The arrhythmias may not remain benign. Recurrent paroxysmal atrial tachycardia and atrial fibrillation become more prominent as the patient ages and eventually the patient may develop chronic atrial fibrillation, even though there may be no mitral regurgitation. Sudden death from ventricular arrhythmias has been reported in a small number of patients with mitral valve prolapse. Since the syndrome is so ubiquitous and the number of cases of sudden death so small, it is clear that this is a very rare complication. There is some evidence to suggest that this complication is more likely to be familial.

MYOCARDITIS AND CARDIOMYOPATHIES

DEFINITION

Myocarditis is an inflammatory response involving the ventricular musculature. Such a response may be

Table 7–23. Pathophysiologic Agents of Myocarditis

Viral
  Coxsackie B, echoviruses, poliomyelitis, etc.
Bacterial
  Diphtheria, tuberculosis, infective endocarditis, etc.
Rheumatic
Spirochetes
  Syphilis, leptospirosis, etc.
Rickettsia
  Typhus, Rocky Mountain spotted fever, Q fever
Mycotic organisms
  Blastomycosis, candidiasis, aspergillosis, etc.
Helminthic organisms
  Trichinosis, echinococcus, ascaris, etc.
Protozoal organisms
  Chagas' disease, toxoplasmosis, malaria, etc.

provoked by virtually any organism that can infect man. Because the infecting agent may cause nonspecific and transient symptoms and because the inflammatory effects of such agents may be manifest long after the agents may have been present in the myocardium, the incidence of myocarditis is not known. It is undoubtedly far more common than is usually surmised. Acute florid myocarditis is recognized when the patient presents with signs of acute congestive heart failure, fever, disproportionate tachycardia in relation to fever, and unexplained prolonged fatigue. Acute myocarditis may be accompanied by nonspecific T-wave changes and cardiac arrhythmias, which serve as clues to the involvement of the myocardium. There may be transient cardiomegaly with pulmonary congestion by chest x-ray. The recent development of endomyocardial biopsy techniques has allowed further documentation of the presence of an inflammatory response in the myocardium. However, the specificity and the sensitivity of findings obtained from endomyocardial biopsies are still a matter of debate because pathologic criteria for making a diagnosis of myocarditis are still ill defined.

PATHOPHYSIOLOGIC CONSIDERATIONS AND DIFFERENTIAL DIAGNOSIS

Wenger et al. have provided an extensive description of various infective agents that have been associated with myocarditis.[25] Table 7–23 outlines the general group of organisms with pertinent examples. Probably the most common cause for acute myocarditis in the U.S. is involvement of the myocardium by viral agents, most commonly Coxsackie B enterovirus. Echoviruses have also been implicated in the development of myocarditis. There is seldom pathologic material to establish involvement of the myocardium because patients with Coxsackie B or echovirus infections are frequently not diagnosed, and, even when the diagnosis is made, they rarely die. Although poliomyelitis is a rare disease today in developed countries, its prevalence and relatively acute mortality in past decades provided singular proof that the myocardium can be the site of viral infestation and inflammation.

Bacterial infections may also provoke myocarditis. The majority of patients dying of diphtheria are noted to have signs of acute myocarditis. Patients with disseminated tuberculosis have been noted to have involvement with the myocardium, particularly with tuberculomas involving the conduction system. Patients with bacterial or infective endocarditis will have signs of myocarditis, particularly if the illness has been unrecognized and untreated for a long period of time. Rheumatic fever caused by streptococcal pharyngitis is associated with myocarditis, not because of actual infection of the myocardium with the streptococcal organism, but rather because of some inflammatory mechanism that is still poorly understood. The myocardium may become involved with spirochetes associated with syphilis and leptospirosis. Various rickettsial diseases such as typhus and Rocky Mountain spotted fever are associated with myocarditis. A variety of mycotic organisms are also associated with myocarditis. Helminthic organisms, such as trichinosis and the echinococcus organism, may involve the myocardium. Trypanosoma cruzi is a protozoal organism common in areas of South America that not only produces acute myocarditis, but also may produce lasting myocardial damage. The manifestation of the infection with the protozoal organism may initially be so slight that the patient does not even recognize he had been ill. The ultimate manifestation of previous infection may be delayed for several decades, at which time signs of congestive heart failure appear. Thus, acute Chagas' disease may be so subtle as to be unrecognized, but the eventual outcome is chronic Chagas' disease manifested by unremitting congestive heart failure in middle age.

It seems fitting to follow a discussion of myocarditis with a discussion of the cardiomyopathies, because there is a gradually accumulating body of information to suggest that at least some of the cardiomyopathies eventuate from prior myocarditis. The term cardiomyopathy is used generally to indicate a structural, and therefore functional, abnormality of the left and/or right ventricle. Table 7–24 provides a classification of cardiomyopathies modified from a concept popularized by Goodwin.[26] In general, the cardiomyopathies may be considered under three broad headings, namely those that present primarily as *dilated cardiomyopathies;* those that present primarily with *hypertrophic cardiomyopathies;* and those that present

Table 7–24. Classification of Cardiomyopathies

Dilated cardiomyopathies
  Viral
  Idiopathic
  Familial
  Ischemic
Hypertrophic cardiomyopathies
  Nonobstructive
  Obstructive
Restrictive cardiomyopathies
  Endomyocardial fibrosis
  Carcinoid syndrome
  Sarcoidosis
  Amyloidosis
Other forms of cardiomyopathies
  Hemochromatosis
  Glycogen, lipid, and mucopolysaccharide storage disorders
  Neurologic and neuromuscular diseases
  Chemically induced cardiomyopathies
  Radiation induced cardiomyopathies
  Nutritional disorders

primarily as *restrictive cardiomyopathies* in which diastolic filling is severely limited. Finally, a fourth category has been added to Table 7–24: *other forms of cardiomyopathies* encompasses diverse conditions that may adversely affect ventricular function.

A unified etiology for these different cardiomyopathies is still not elucidated. There is strong circumstantial evidence to indicate that dilated cardiomyopathies frequently are related to previous viral myocarditis. There are several lines of observations that would point in this direction. Cases of dilated cardiomyopathy have been noted to evolve following acute myocarditis. There is a high incidence of cardiac abnormalities after recovery from acute viral myocarditis. High viral antibody titers have been noted in patients with dilated cardiomyopathy. A less than universal observation has been that biopsy-proven myocarditis may be found in some patients with dilated cardiomyopathy.[27] Finally, there are immunoregulatory defects in patients with cardiomyopathy. A possible unifying hypothesis to these observations is that a prior viral infection precipitates an immunologic reaction that leads to damage to the myocardium. It is strongly suspected that cases of dilated cardiomyopathies that have been termed idiopathic are probably postviral cardiomyopathies.

It has been noted that there are well-documented families with a high incidence of dilated cardiomyopathies. Whether this incidence is due to a congenital abnormality in the formation of the myocardium or to a congenital susceptibility to viral infection and thus to postviral cardiomyopathy is a matter of conjecture.

The question of whether ischemic cardiomyopathy is truly a cardiomyopathy is more of a nosologic argument than a clinical one. Many cases of unremitting congestive heart failure and cardiomegaly with markedly dilated ventricular chambers are due to progressive destruction of myocardial tissue secondary to decreased myocardial blood flow. The most common cause for this decreased myocardial blood flow is obviously atherosclerotic obstruction of major coronary arteries. Because this process of myocardial destruction, caused by ischemia, may occur without overt signs of ischemic heart disease such as recurrent myocardial infarction or angina, ischemic cardiomyopathy has been included under the classification of dilated cardiomyopathies.

The hypertrophic cardiomyopathies are characterized by markedly thickened ventricular walls and normal or small ventricular cavities, usually in both systole and diastole. They have generally been divided into nonobstructive and obstructive forms of hypertrophic cardiomyopathy. The primary site of thickening of the myocardium is the ventricular septum. Although the free wall of either ventricle may also be hypertrophied, it is less thick than the septum. The fundamental structural abnormality in hypertrophic cardiomyopathy appears to be a basic disarray of the orientation of muscle bundles. In nonobstructive hypertrophic cardiomyopathies, there is no obstruction to flow in the outflow tract of the ventricles and thus there is no systolic pressure gradient in the ventricle.

In the case of obstructive cardiomyopathy, the hypertrophy becomes so prominent in the septum and high posterolateral wall of the ventricle that there is obstruction to outflow from the ventricle, whether it be right or left, during systole. Thus, during the early descriptive period hypertrophic obstructive cardiomyopathy was called idiopathic hypertrophic subaortic or subpulmonic stenosis. In some patients, the hypertrophy of the upper portion of the ventricular septum is so great that there is systolic obstruction to outflow in both the right and left ventricles, leading to gradients between the cavity of each ventricle and the region beneath the semilunar valves of each ventricle.

Patients with hypertrophic cardiomyopathy will generally have physical, electrocardiographic, and x-ray findings compatible with left ventricular enlargement. The echocardiogram has been invaluable in establishing this diagnosis in many patients who are asymptomatic. The echocardiographic hallmark of hypertrophic cardiomyopathy is the demonstration of an asymmetrically thickened ventricular septum that is significantly thicker than the free wall of the ventricle. In the case of hypertrophic obstructive cardiomyopathy, in addition to this disproportionate thickening of the ventricular septum, there will also be systolic anterior motion of the anterior leaflet of the mitral valve.

Furthermore, during diastole, the anterior leaflet of the mitral valve will frequently appear to touch the septum, probably because of the small size of the ventricular cavity during diastole. Whether the nonobstructive and the obstructive forms of hypertrophic cardiomyopathy are truly distinct is debatable, because there are families in which both forms can be detected by echocardiography and because patients with hypertrophic nonobstructive cardiomyopathy have been noted to progress to the stage at which there is evidence at catetheterization of obstruction in the outflow tract to the left ventricle. This progression from the nonobstructive to the obstructive form may be associated with the development of a fibrotic plaque on the mural endocardium of the outflow tract of the septum. The fibrotic plaque occurs at the level of the distal margin of the anterior leaflet of the mitral valve and may be a consequence of systolic anterior motion of the mitral valve.

The differential diagnosis of hypertrophic obstructive cardiomyopathy includes calcific aortic stenosis, mitral regurgitation, ventricular septal defect, and mitral valve prolapse. In all these conditions there may be a prolonged systolic murmur that may be interpreted as being holosystolic, although phonocardiography will demonstrate that the murmur is actually ejection in quality.

Typically, in aortic stenosis there is a systolic thrill over the aortic area, the murmur radiates well to the suprasternal notch and to the carotid arteries, the aortic closure sound is absent, the carotid upstroke is parvus et tardus in character, the aortic root will appear dilated on chest x-ray, and there will be calcium in the aortic valve leaflets on lateral chest x-ray or by fluoroscopy. In general, none of these characteristics are true in the case of hypertrophic obstructive cardiomyopathy.

Classically, the murmur is heard low along the left sternal border and is certainly more intense there than over the aortic area. The murmur seldom radiates well to the carotids, the aortic closure sound is preserved, the carotid pulse has a bisferiens rather than pulsus parvus et tardus quality, and dilatation of the aortic root as well as calcification of the aortic valve are absent. Though these distinctions may be helpful, they are not universal because there are well-documented cases of combined aortic valvular stenosis and hypertrophic obstructive cardiomyopathy.

The differentiation of hypertrophic obstructive cardiomyopathy from mitral regurgitation would appear to be easy because the murmur of mitral regurgitation is holosystolic, whereas the murmur of hypertrophic cardiomyopathy is ejection in quality. However, because mitral regurgitation is one of the lesions encountered with hypertrophic obstructive cardiomyopathy, both lesions are frequently present. Many patients who were diagnosed as having the loud murmur of mitral regurgitation have been demonstrated by cardiac catheterization and echocardiography to have hypertrophic obstructive cardiomyopathy. Because patients with ventricular septal defects usually have holosystolic murmurs rather than ejection-type murmurs, the correct diagnosis should be determined by auscultation. However, it is recognized that a small number of patients with ventricular septal defects may have ejection systolic murmurs, thus confounding the differential diagnosis.

The third and least common major category of cardiomyopathies has been termed restrictive cardiomyopathies, indicating that the primary problem is one of ventricular filling during diastole. Such patients, while having difficulty with ventricular filling, have no difficulty with left ventricular ejection and actually may have hypercontractile ventricles. Early during the description of various forms of cardiomyopathies, these patients were designated as having the empty ventricle syndrome, because at cardiac catheterization they were noted to eject almost all the contrast media injected in the ventricle. In the tropical zones of the world, the most common cause for this syndrome is endomyocardial fibrosis, but amyloidosis is probably a more common cause in more temperate zones. Goodwin has proposed that endomyocardial fibrosis, hypereosinophilic syndrome, Löffler's endocarditis, and eosinophilic leukemia all are manifestations of the same disease process that eventuates in extensive endocardial scarring and thus decreased diastolic filling of the ventricle. Endomyocardial fibrosis may involve either or both ventricles. In the case of predominant right ventricular involvement, which is less frequent than left ventricular involvement, the patient will have many of the features suggestive of constrictive pericarditis such as distended neck veins and ascites. In predominant left ventricular involvement there will be symptoms of decreased cardiac output, particularly with exertion, and frequently the murmur of mitral regurgitation will be present.

Other infiltrative processes may produce restrictive cardiomyopathy. Metastatic carcinoid is associated with increased subendocardial fibrosis, particularly involving the right ventricle. It may also be associated with tricuspid and pulmonic stenoses. It rarely involves the left side of the heart. Amyloidosis may involve any level of the ventricle and thus impede diastolic filling. Sarcoidosis, while presenting primarily with cardiac arrhythmias, may so infiltrate and involve the ventricular myocardium that the first symptoms may be identical to those of restrictive cardiomyopathy.

There are other forms and sources of cardiomyopathy listed in Table 7–24. Goodwin has provided a more detailed and descriptive outline of these entities.[26] Some of these might be subcategorized under dilated or restrictive cardiomyopathies. For instance, in hemochromatosis, deposition of iron in myocardial cells leads to a dilated cardiomyopathy and eventual congestive heart failure. Deposition of glycogen, lipids, and mucopolysaccharides, on the other hand, limits diastolic filling of the ventricles, which acts more like restrictive cardiomyopathies. A host of neurologic and neuromuscular diseases, including Duchenne's muscular dystrophy, are associated with cardiomyopathies. Exposure to various chemicals and drugs may also provoke cardiomyopathies. It has long been suspected that lead, which frequently contaminates moonshine liquor, may provoke a cardiomyopathy. Excessive amounts of cobalt once used as a defoaming agent in the manufacture of certain beers is thought to have led to a congestive-type cardiomyopathy. There is a gradually increasing body of clinical and laboratory evidence to indicate that alcohol abuse may lead to myocardial dysfunction and a cardiomyopathy. Also, various drugs used to treat specific diseases are known to be associated with the development of cardiomyopathies. Emetine and chloroquine, used in the treatment of amebiasis, may produce myocardial degeneration. Methysergide (Sansert) may produce endocardial fibroelastosis similar to that seen in carcinoid syndrome, except that in carcinoid syndrome the primary lesions are usually in the right heart, whereas in methysergide-induced endocardial fibroelastosis the primary lesions are usually in the left side of the heart. Currently popular agents in the treatment of neoplastic disease such as cyclophosphamide and adriamycin are known to produce myocardial damage eventuating in heart failure. Radiation therapy for neoplastic diseases is also known to affect not only the pericardium and myocardium but also the coronary arteries. The combination of radiation therapy and use of a chemotherapeutic agent that is toxic to the myocardium appears additive in terms of the development of myocardial damage. Various nutritional disorders including beriberi, pellagra, and kwashiorkor also have been identified with left ventricular muscular damage and are therefore considered potential causes for cardiomyopathy.

PERICARDIAL EFFUSION AND CARDIAC TAMPONADE

DEFINITION

The normal pericardial space contains up to approximately 30 ml of lymphatic fluid. Accumulation of greater than this amount of fluid constitutes a pericardial effusion. If the fluid accumulates slowly in the pericardial space there may be enough time for the normally stiff pericardium to stretch and thus accommodate increased fluid volumes without any hemodynamic consequences. Under these circumstances, which constitute the development of a chronic pericardial effusion, the patient will frequently be asymptomatic and not show any hemodynamic signs of cardiac tamponade. If the accumulation of fluid in the pericardial space is rapid, thus not affording time for the pericardium to stretch, the patient may present with overt signs of cardiac tamponade.

PATHOPHYSIOLOGIC CONSIDERATIONS AND DIFFERENTIAL DIAGNOSIS

Table 7–25 provides a classification for pericardial effusion on the basis of the acute or chronic process. The most common causes for acute effusions are trauma, acute pericarditis, metastatic pericardial involvement, and aortic dissection. It should be emphasized that trauma may provoke a pericardial effusion without necessarily perforation of a cardiac chamber. This kind of trauma is seen frequently after automobile accidents involving steering wheel injuries. Pericardial effusion is not rare after cardiac surgery. Ensuing cardiac tamponade may be difficult to separate from a low cardiac output state during the early recovery period from the cardiac surgery. Perforation of the heart and, therefore, acute pericardial effusion may occur during routine cardiac catheterization, during placement of transvenous pacemaker electrodes, and also during placement of Swan-Ganz catheters for hemodynamic monitoring on the Cardiac Care Unit. Acute pericarditis, whether it be due to viral or bacterial infections, may be associated with pericardial effusions. Collagen diseases, particularly lupus erythematosus, may first present as acute pericarditis or even acute pericardial effusion. Involvement of the pericardium with metastatic implants may be associated with acute pericardial effusion, due to either a transudative phenomenon or bleeding from the implants. Dissection of the proximal aorta with perforation of the aorta into the pericardial space may also provoke acute pericardial effusion.

Chronic pericardial effusions may occur as manifestations of metabolic and systemic disorders. Advanced hypothyroidism is frequently associated with a pericardial effusion. The relatively long latent period between the onset of decreased thyroid function and overt signs of hypothyroidism provides ample time for the pericardium to stretch, so pericardial effusions under these circumstances rarely provoke serious hemodynamic consequences. While collagen diseases may present with acute pericardial effusion, they are also often associated with a chronic hemodynamically insignificant pericardial effusion. At autopsy, approximately 6 to 10% of patients with rheumatoid arthritis show significant pericardial effusions, but echocardiography would indicate that up to 30% of patients with active rheumatoid arthritis have measurable increases in fluid in the pericardial space. Effusions under these circumstances are almost always associated with high rheumatoid factor titers and rheumatoid nodules. Sarcoidosis is usually considered to involve the myocardium and the conduction system, but it also may involve the pericardium and produce a chronic pericardial effusion.

Infectious diseases may be associated with chronic pericardial effusions, but the most frequent organisms are tuberculosis and various fungal infections. Slowly accumulating chronic pericardial effusions have been seen following a myocardial infarction as described by Dressler. Primary malignancies involving the pericardium, particularly mesothelioma, not only may produce a picture of constrictive pericarditis because of the thickening and stiffening of the invaded pericardium, but also may produce pericardial effusion. While metastatic pericardial involvement may provoke acute pericardial effusions, particularly because of

Table 7–25. Classification of Pericardial Effusions

Acute effusions
  Trauma
    Injury with or without cardiac perforation
    Postoperative
    Associated with catheterization
  Acute pericarditis
    Viral
    Bacterial
    Collagen diseases
  Metastatic pericardial involvement
  Aortic dissection
Chronic effusions
  Metabolic and systemic disorders
    Hypothyroidism
    Collagen diseases
    Sarcoidosis
  Infectious diseases
    Tuberculosis
    Fungal infections
  Postmyocardial infarction (Dressler's syndrome)
  Primary malignancy
    Mesothelioma
  Metastatic pericardial involvement
  Drug induced
    Anticoagulant therapy
    Procainamide
    Hydralazine

bleeding from the metastatic implants, the effusion frequently develops slowly because of transudation of fluid from the metastatic implants. Finally, drugs currently used in clinical practice may provoke chronic pericardial effusion. A sudden change in heart size or early signs of cardiac tamponade in a patient on anticoagulant therapy should alert the clinician to the possibility of pericardial effusion. Usually the anticoagulant therapy is an additive factor to some underlying cause for the development of the effusion. This appears to be the case in many cases of postmyocardial infarction syndrome with pericardial effusion. The relative decline in the incidence of postmyocardial infarction pericardial effusion, or Dressler's syndrome, may well be due to the decline in the use of anticoagulants after myocardial infarction. Procainamide frequently produces a pleural and pericardial inflammatory response, which may in turn provoke a chronic pericardial effusion. High-dose hydralazine as used in earlier days of drug management of hypertension may produce a lupus-like syndrome with an associated pericarditis and pericardial effusion.

As a pericardial effusion increases in amount, a point will be reached at which diastolic filling of the ventricles will be limited, producing cardiac tamponade. If the accumulation is not halted or if the effusion is not drained, the patient will eventually die. Accumulation of fluid in the relatively nondistensible pericardium initially limits cardiac filling and, therefore, cardiac output. As cardiac output declines, arterial pressure and coronary artery filling decrease. Coronary blood flow and thus myocardial function are further compromised by tachycardia and, perhaps, by external pressure on the superficially lying coronary arteries. Eventually, this decline in cardiac filling, decrease in cardiac output, falling arterial and coronary artery filling pressures, and decreased coronary flow lead to severe myocardial ischemia, which further limits cardiac output and intensifies the above-mentioned compensatory physiologic responses to the pericardial effusion.

DIAGNOSTIC EVALUATION

As mentioned above, a pericardial effusion may be essentially silent unless there are the beginning signs of cardiac tamponade. If, however, there is sufficient pericardial effusion to significantly compromise ventricular filling, the compromised ventricular filling can be detected usually on physical examination. The patient with overt cardiac tamponade will appear dyspneic and often diaphoretic and will have a varying state of consciousness. He will have tachycardia, usu-

ally hypotension, a narrow pulse pressure, and pulsus paradoxus. The neck veins will be distended but he will not have Kussmaul's sign, which is the decline in jugular venous distension associated with inspiration. Kussmaul's sign is absent in pericardial effusion because even though there is decreased diastolic filling of the heart, there is still an increase in venous filling and thus a decrease in jugular venous distension during inspiration. Presence of Kussmaul's sign in the setting of a pericardial effusion is evidence of an underlying constrictive pericarditis. Cardiac examination may or may not reveal absence of a cardiac impulse at the usual point of maximal impulse. A pericardial rub may or may not be heard. Ewart's (or Pins') sign may be noted during examination of the base of the left lung posteriorly. This sign, which consists of dullness to percussion and increased breath sounds over this region, is thought to be due to compression of the lower lobe of the left lung by the distended pericardium.

Laboratory diagnosis provides evidence leading to suspicion or confirmation of pericardial effusion, depending on the modality chosen. The electrocardiogram may show signs of pericarditis and, in addition, show electrical alternans in which the amplitude of the P, QRS, and T may fluctuate significantly in height. A chest x-ray will frequently show an enlarged cardiac silhouette with a water bottle–shaped heart. It should be emphasized, however, that in the case of an acute effusion the cardiac silhouette may appear normal in size, and only if a chest film prior to the illness is available for comparison will it become obvious that the size of the cardiac silhouette has, indeed, increased. Whereas in the past invasive techniques such as cardiac catheterization and angiography had been used to confirm the diagnosis, echocardiography has now assumed primacy in establishing the diagnosis of pericardial effusion, even in situations in which there is no evidence of cardiac tamponade. In the past, when only M-mode echocardiography was available, there were still problems in establishing a diagnosis of pericardial effusion, particularly when there was a loculated effusion. However, with the advent of sophisticated two-dimensional echocardiography, this diagnosis is rarely, if ever, missed. With two-dimensional echocardiography, the pericardial effusion, whether it be loculated or not, is apparent. There is frequently right ventricular compression as well as congestion of the superior and inferior venae cavae. The interventricular septum may be seen to move toward the left ventricular cavity during inspiration as the right heart fills with a greater volume of blood during inspiration.

CONSTRICTIVE PERICARDITIS

DEFINITION

Constrictive pericarditis is a fibrous thickening of either or both the parietal and the visceral (epicardium) layers of the pericardium. It is frequently accompanied by calcification in the pericardium. When present with pericardial effusion, constrictive pericarditis is termed effusive constrictive pericarditis. Often the constrictive element becomes apparent only when the pericardial effusion has been eliminated and the patient is still left with signs of decreased ventricular filling.

PATHOPHYSIOLOGIC CONSIDERATIONS

Table 7–26 outlines potential causes for the development of constrictive pericarditis. The vast majority of cases of constrictive pericarditis are idiopathic. It is strongly suspected that these cases are the residual effects of previous subclinical acute pericarditis probably caused by viral agents. Since there is no good laboratory marker for mild cases of pericarditis, there has been no way to identify patients with mild pericarditis and thus to determine the actual incidence of the eventual development of constrictive pericarditis following various forms of pericarditis.

Many infective agents have been reported to produce constrictive pericarditis. The most frequently cited agent is tuberculosis, although viral, fungal, and bacterial agents have also been known to produce constrictive pericarditis. All the collagen diseases have been associated with occasional cases of constrictive pericarditis, although it is relatively rare in lupus erythematosus.

Just as certain drugs may provoke a pericardial effusion, so too they may they provoke constrictive pericarditis. Invasion of the pericardium by primary tumors such as mesothelioma or metastatic tumors such

Table 7–26. Causes of Constrictive Pericarditis

Idiopathic
Infectious agents
  Tuberculosis, viral, fungal, echinococcus, amoebic, pyogenic
Collagen diseases
Drugs—procainamide, methysergide, hydralazine
Neoplasms
  Primary
  Metastatic
Post-traumatic with hemopericardium
Following cardiac surgery

as carcinoma of the lung or breast also may produce the hemodynamic findings of constrictive pericarditis. Trauma to the pericardium, particularly followed by significant hemopericardium is known to encourage the development of constrictive pericarditis.

Perhaps the most frequently identified cause of constrictive pericarditis in the U.S. is previous open heart surgery. Although constrictive pericarditis was almost unheard of following "closed" valvular procedures such as closed mitral valvulotomy, it is not a rare phenomenon following procedures using cardiopulmonary bypass, particularly coronary artery bypass graft surgery. The constrictive pericarditis following coronary artery bypass graft procedures is distinctive in that the visceral pericardium or epicardium is so severely involved that it is often difficult to free the underlying entrapped ventricular musculature.

The primary physiologic problem in constrictive pericarditis is that the fibrosed, thickened, stiff pericardial sac prevents normal filling of the heart. This problem usually involves all chambers of the heart, although there are well-recognized cases of involvement of only a small portion of the pericardium, leading to isolated restriction of filling of a particular cardiac chamber, usually the left ventricle. A band of constriction may be so discrete as to produce a hemodynamic picture of subpulmonic stenosis with normal function of all other chambers.

Because ventricular filling is restricted, central venous pressure as well as jugular venous pressure is elevated. Inspiration does not alter this rigid restriction of cardiac filling. Thus, there is no increased venous filling during inspiration, nor is there a decrease in jugular venous distension during inspiration. Hence, Kussmaul's sign, which is the persistence of jugular venous distension or an increase in jugular venous distension during inspiration, is present with constrictive pericarditis. Because there is little variation in the degree of ventricular filling, pulsus paradoxus, frequently seen in pericardial effusion, is rarely seen in constrictive pericarditis.

DIFFERENTIAL DIAGNOSIS

The major problem in differential diagnosis is to separate constrictive pericarditis from chronic pericardial effusion and congestive heart failure, which are usually caused by a cardiomyopathy. Physical examination, which demonstrates the presence of Kussmaul's sign and the absence of pulsus paradoxus, will frequently serve to differentiate constrictive pericarditis from pericardial effusion. In the case of effusive constrictive pericarditis, this differentiation cannot be made until the pericardial effusion is eliminated. While it is relatively easy to separate constrictive pericarditis from pericardial effusion on the basis of physical findings and cardiac catheterization, such is not the case when there is a possibility of a cardiomyopathy. Restrictive cardiomyopathies, which have as one of their characteristics stiffened inelastic ventricular walls and thus decreased ventricular filling, act hemodynamically almost the same as constrictive pericarditis. Dilated cardiomyopathies may be difficult to separate from constrictive pericarditis with cardiac catheterization alone, because in these circumstances even the normal pericardium may serve to restrict filling of the dilated cardiac chambers. Even evidence by catheterization, echocardiography, or radionuclide scanning of a poorly contracting ventricle, which would point toward congestive heart failure rather than constriction, may not be diagnostic, because end-stage constriction is associated with myocardial atrophy. On rare occasions, because of this difficulty in separating constrictive pericarditis from cardiomyopathies, and because of the devastating consequences of missing a treatable condition such as constrictive pericarditis, exploratory thoracotomy may be necessary.

DIAGNOSTIC EVALUATION

Patient History

Recognition of this basic underlying physiology explains the typical historical and physical findings in patients with constrictive pericarditis. The patient usually complains of gradually increasing easy fatigability and eventually of marked dyspnea on exertion. He rarely complains of orthopnea or paroxysmal nocturnal dyspnea. The typical end-stage appearance of a patient with constrictive pericarditis is that of a wasted, pot-bellied, edematous, dyspneic male. The wasting may be due to a protein-losing enteropathy, which frequently accompanies the condition, to chronic renal insufficiency, or to cardiac cachexia related to decreased cardiac output. The pot-belly, which is evidence of ascites, and the peripheral edema are consequences of persistently elevated venous pressures resulting from the constrictive process.

Physical Examination

On physical examination, the patient is noted to have jugular venous distension with a sharp x and y descent of the jugular venous impulse, a positive Kussmaul's sign, and a prominent third heart sound or pericardial knock that is sharper in quality and occurs somewhat earlier in diastole than the usual S_3 ventricular gallop. One third of patients presenting with the signs of constrictive pericarditis will be in atrial fibrillation. There

is almost inevitably hepatomegaly and ascites, as well peripheral edema.

Diagnostic Studies

The electrocardiogram is nonspecific, although it will almost always show abnormal T waves. The chest x-ray typically shows a normal-sized or only moderately enlarged heart, although one third of the patients with constrictive pericarditis will present with frank cardiomegaly. This cardiomegaly is due to either marked thickening of the pericardium related to the underlying disease process or to a coexistent pericardial effusion. An over-penetrated chest x-ray or cardiac fluoroscopy will usually demonstrate calcium in the pericardium. The echocardiogram rarely shows a thickened pericardium because the true dimensions of the pericardium are difficult to separate from other mediastinal echoes. The presence of relatively small ventricular cavities and relatively large atrial cavities created by elevated venous pressures should raise the possibility of constrictive pericarditis, particularly in the patient who is initially suspected of having congestive heart failure. Cardiac catheterization demonstrates a series of findings that when taken in their entirety usually establish the diagnosis of constriction. The sharp x and y descent of the jugular venous pulse is seen in right atrial pressure tracings, producing a so-called M sign; early diastolic filling of the ventricle is rapid but ceases abruptly as the stiffened pericardium prevents further filling. This effect produces a "dip and shoulder" sign or a "square root" sign in ventricular pressure tracings. Since distension of all chambers is limited by the rigid pericardium, diastolic pressures will be equal in all the chambers, including the pulmonary artery. All of these hemodynamic findings may be masked if the total venous volume has been decreased by diuretic therapy; they may be revealed by a rapid infusion of saline that restores or increases venous volume.

ACUTE AND CHRONIC CONGESTIVE HEART FAILURE

DEFINITION

The term heart failure in a broad context indicates a situation in which the heart cannot provide enough cardiac output to meet the metabolic demands of the body. The addition of the term congestive connotes

Table 7–27.   Classification of Heart Failure

Acute (pulmonary edema)
  Increased pulmonary capillary wedge pressure
    With left ventricular failure
      Infarction, acute valve damage, acute shunt
    Without left ventricular failure
      Mitral stenosis, left atrial or ventricular myxoma
      ? acute hypervolemia
  Due to alteration of alveolar capillary membranes (Acute
      Respiratory Distress Syndrome [ARDS])
    Infection
    Inhaled toxins
    Aspiration pneumonia
    Radiation pneumonia
    Hypersensitivity pneumonias
  Lymphatic dysfunction
    After lung transplantation
    Lymphangitic carcinomatosis
    Fibrosing lymphangitis
  Unknown causes
    High altitude pulmonary edema
    Neurogenic pulmonary edema
    Narcotic overdose
    Pulmonary embolism
    Eclampsia
    After cardioversion, anesthesia, cardiopulmonary bypass
Chronic heart failure
  Myocardial dysfunction
    Ischemia
    Cardiomyopathies
    Hypertension
    Cor pulmonale
  Valvular dysfunction
    Stenosis
    Regurgitation
  Increased demand
    Thyrotoxicosis
    Anemia
    Fever with or without septicemia
    Hypervolemia
    AV fistula
    Left-to-right shunt

the development of edema, either in the lungs or in the periphery. The primary cause for edema formation is inadequate renal blood flow and consequent inadequate elimination of sodium and water. Elevated venous pressure per se, which itself is due to inadequate cardiac output, plays a lesser role in the formation of edema than do problems in renal blood flow. Heart failure has been arbitrarily separated into acute and chronic heart failure, primarily based on the course of the development of symptoms (Table 7–27). Acute congestive heart failure indicates the relatively sudden onset of symptoms related to inadequate cardiac performance. Pulmonary congestion is a feature of both categories of heart failure, though the patient who presents with acute heart failure is more likely to present with acute pulmonary edema. Some patients who present with pulmonary edema will, in retrospect, have

had a relatively prolonged period of low-grade, almost unrecognized chronic congestive heart failure.

PATHOPHYSIOLOGIC CONSIDERATIONS

Acute. The classification of acute heart failure in Table 7–27 is modified from Ingram and Braunwald's.[28] Acute congestive heart failure with pulmonary edema occurs when there is an increased pulmonary capillary wedge pressure with subsequent extravasation of fluid into the pulmonary alveoli. The most common precipitating factor is acute left ventricular failure, which is frequently seen with myocardial infarction. However, dramatic examples of left ventricular failure can be seen when there is acute valvular damage such as a ruptured papillary muscle or chordae tendinae and the development of an acute left-to-right shunt. Increased pulmonary capillary wedge pressure may occur when there is actually obstruction to outflow from the pulmonary venous bed. Such obstruction is most frequently seen in mitral stenosis and can also occur with left atrial or left ventricular myxomas. Under these circumstances, pulmonary capillary wedge pressure is elevated because of the obstructive phenomenon, while the left ventricular end-diastolic pressure remains normal and, indeed, left ventricular function is normal. Under very unusual circumstances, normal left ventricular function may be overwhelmed by acute hypervolemia. Left ventricular failure is rare in the normal heart, which has a tremendous capacity to pump large volumes. Acute congestive heart failure induced by excessive intravenous infusions is almost always associated with underlying left ventricular disease.

Extravasation of fluid into the alveoli may be due also to a loss in the integrity of the alveolar capillary membrane. Under these circumstances, pulmonary capillary wedge pressure will be normal, but the patient will have an excessive amount of fluid in the alveoli and thus acute pulmonary edema. This acute respiratory distress syndrome (ARDS) has long been recognized in premature infants, but only recently has it become well recognized in the mature lungs of the adult. It has been associated with pulmonary infections, particularly viral, and inhalation of toxins. Aspiration pneumonia may destroy the integrity of the alveolar capillary membrane and present a radiologic picture suggestive of pulmonary edema. Radiation pneumonia has been recognized when massive doses of radiation have been used to treat neoplasms. Hypersensitivity pneumonias, particularly resulting from drugs such as nitrofurantoin, are not rare. Disruption or dysfunction of the normal lymphatic drainage of the lungs may also lead to extravasation of fluid into the alveoli.

High-altitude pulmonary edema is frequently seen in young, otherwise healthy persons who suddenly ascend to high altitudes. It is also usually associated with excessive physical activity such as skiing. It rapidly responds to an elevation in the inspired oxygen content or to a return to a more normal altitude.

Neurogenic pulmonary edema may be induced in laboratory animals by injection of fibrin products into the ventricles of the brain. It is thought to occur occasionally in humans after trauma to the brain and even after central seizures.

Pulmonary edema associated with narcotic overdose was originally thought to be due to impurities in the intravenously injected narcotic mixture. Now, however, because of well-documented cases of pulmonary edema after the oral ingestion of narcotics, the role of impurities in the intravenous, street-obtained narcotic mixture is not so clear.

Acute pulmonary edema occasionally occurs with an acute pulmonary embolus. The reasons for this association are not clear, although one explanation is the possibility that hyperperfusion of unobstructed pulmonary vascular beds and thus extravasation of fluid into the alveoli may occur in the perfused lung with intact circulation. Eclampsia may also be associated with pulmonary edema, though it is often difficult to attribute edema solely to the eclampsia because most such patients have relatively acute hypertension, decreased renal function, and perhaps left ventricular dysfunction.

There are rare cases of acute pulmonary edema reported following cardioversion, anesthesia, and cardiopulmonary bypass. In many of these cases, it is difficult to separate the possibility of underlying left ventricular dysfunction.

Chronic. Chronic congestive heart failure may be separated into three categories according to genesis. One form, myocardial dysfunction, caused by ischemia, cardiomyopathies, or hypertension, is readily recognized. Cor pulmonale, another cause, basically implies that the primary source of difficulty is the lung, with subsequent pulmonary hypertension and right ventricular failure.

The second form, chronic valvular dysfunction caused by either stenosis or regurgitation of a valve, may lead to decreased cardiac output and chronic congestive heart failure.

Finally, the heart may fail to meet the metabolic demands of the body if there are increased demands made on it. Thyrotoxicosis, anemia, fever, or hypervolemia are frequently an underlying cause for left ventricular dysfunction when associated with conges-

tive heart failure, emphasizing that the normal heart can meet almost all demands impressed upon it. The flow in an arterial venous fistula may so monopolize the cardiac output that the heart may not be able to generate sufficient cardiac output to meet the demands of peripheral tissues and may thus produce heart failure. Large left-to-right cardiac shunts may eventuate in congestive heart failure for the same reasons.

CARDIOGENIC SHOCK

DEFINITION AND PATHOPHYSIOLOGIC CONSIDERATIONS

The term "shock" has had many connotations, ranging from an acute withdrawal state seen in the patient who has experienced emotional trauma to the profound hemodynamic derangement seen after physical trauma or cardiac damage. The fundamental lesion in shock is inadequate perfusion of vital organs, eventually leading to cellular damage and death. In cardiogenic shock, such derangement of tissue nourishment may result from collapse of the driving force for perfusion, namely the heart. Shock may in other cases result from collapse of the multitudinous peripheral reflexes and mechanisms that maintain appropriate organ flow. Table 7–28 separates various categories

Table 7–28. Classification of Shock

Cardiogenic
  Myocardial infarction
  Myocarditis
  Myocardial depression
    Hypoxia and acidosis
    Depressant factors
  Cardiac compression or obstruction
    Cardiac tamponade
    Constrictive pericarditis
    Cardiac myxomas
    Pulmonary embolus
  Cardiac arrhythmias
Noncardiogenic
  Hypovolemia
  Trauma
  Sepsis
  Vasodilatation
  Anaphylaxis
  Metabolic causes
    Adrenal insufficiency
    Hypoglycemia
    Poisons
  Prolonged hypoxia

of shock into cardiogenic and noncardiogenic causes. Since all the categories are frequently associated with hypotension, there is a tendency to cite a specific blood pressure in the definition of shock. However, as we have said, the critical issue is the state of perfusion of vital organs. Remarkably low arterial pressure may maintain adequate tissue nutrition if appropriate peripheral reflexes are acting in tandem.

Cardiogenic shock refers to a condition in which the heart cannot generate adequate flow to meet peripheral tissue demands. In keeping with the concept of the primacy of the perfusion of peripheral tissues in defining shock, the clinical requirements for a diagnosis of cardiogenic shock have generally included systolic blood pressure less than 90 mm Hg; cold, clammy, or diaphoretic skin; altered mental status; and urinary output of less than 30 ml/hour. This set of clinical circumstances is most frequently encountered with acute myocardial infarction. It is less frequently encountered with myocarditis, which usually presents with acute pulmonary edema. Hypoxia, acidosis, and other depressive factors such as drugs may produce such myocardial depression that adequate tissue perfusion cannot be maintained.

As noted in previous sections, cardiac compression caused by tamponade or constriction may severely limit adequate tissue flow. Indeed, the problem of separating cardiac tamponade from cardiogenic shock resulting from myocardial infarction is one of the more difficult differential diagnoses encountered in clinical medicine. Cardiac myxomas may produce cardiogenic shock by occupying large volumes of the cardiac chamber and obstructing outflow from the heart. Large pulmonary emboli, particularly a so-called saddle embolus, which lodges in the main pulmonary artery and obstructs flow to the left and right pulmonary arteries, may so limit transfer of blood from the right heart to the left heart that cardiac output is severely limited. Profound bradycardia and tachycardia may also limit cardiac output and thus adequate tissue perfusion.

DIAGNOSTIC EVALUATION

When evaluating the patient in shock, the physician must consider the possibility of a noncardiogenic cause. Hypovolemia, due to hemorrhage, dehydration, or a loss of plasma from the effective circulating blood volume, may produce shock mimicking cardiogenic shock. Trauma might be best subtitled under this category, as crush injuries may lead to loss of capillary integrity and collection of fluid in the injured portion of the body. Burns may lead to massive loss of circulating blood volume. Sepsis may produce a shocklike condition because of vasodilation. Under these

circumstances the patient may not appear cold or clammy, leading to the slang expression "warm shock." Anaphylaxis may lead to cataclysmic loss of all peripheral vascular tone and profound hypotension as well as shock. Metabolic causes such as adrenal insufficiency, hypoglycemia, and various poisons produce a shocklike picture, as does prolonged hypoxia.

Cardiogenic shock may best be differentiated from noncardiogenic shock by estimating or determining central venous pressure, for usually cardiogenic shock will be associated with a markedly elevated central venous pressure and noncardiogenic shock will be associated with a low or normal central venous pressure. Careful examination of the jugular venous pulse may clarify the situation because an elevated central venous pressure should be associated with increased jugular venous distension. However, it should be recognized that in profound cardiogenic shock, venous spasm may be so severe that the jugular veins may not appear distended. When there is any doubt as to the pathogenesis of the shocklike condition, central venous pressure monitoring by a Swan-Ganz catheter is of great help.

Even when it is obvious that there has been a myocardial infarction, knowledge of the right-sided pressures versus left-sided pressures may be essential in determining whether to use volume augmentation to treat the cardiogenic shock or to rely on other measures such as ionotropic agents, afterload reduction, or vasoconstrictors. Infarction primarily involving the right ventricle is associated with an elevated right atrial and right ventricular end-diastolic pressures, while the pulmonary capillary wedge pressure, which is a reflection of the function of the left ventricle, may be normal. Under these circumstances, there may have to be a period of volume expansion to maintain cardiac output. On the other hand, a primary insult to the left ventricle is associated with an elevated pulmonary capillary wedge pressure, which may well be reflected backward to the right ventricle and right atrium. Addition of volume under these circumstances would be unlikely to enhance cardiac output and more likely to hasten pulmonary edema.

PULMONARY HYPERTENSION

DEFINITION AND PATHOPHYSIOLOGIC CONSIDERATIONS

Pulmonary hypertension is generally defined as a pulmonary arterial pressure of greater than 25/15 mm

Table 7–29. Causes of Pulmonary Hypertension

Primary pulmonary hypertension
   Vasoconstrictive pulmonary hypertension
   Multiple silent pulmonary thromboembolism
   Pulmonary veno-occlusive disease
Secondary pulmonary hypertension
   Pulmonary hypertension secondary to lung destruction
     Chronic obstructive lung disease
     Diffuse interstitial disease
       Fibrosis
       Granulomatous disease
       Multiple pulmonary emboli
   Pulmonary hypertension without lung destruction
     Thoracic deformities
     Neuromuscular diseases
     Obesity
     Sleep apnea
     Primary alveolar hypoventilation
   Cardiac causes for pulmonary hypertension
     Chronic congestive heart failure
     Left-sided valvular stenosis or regurgitation
     Left-sided cardiac tumors
     Large left-to-right shunts

Hg. There are many potential causes for pulmonary hypertension (Table 7–29). In the past, it was relatively easy to outline a conceptual classification for pulmonary hypertension.

There is a vast group of patients with underlying pulmonary or cardiac disease that leads to a secondary elevation in pulmonary arterial pressure. These patients have thus been considered as having secondary pulmonary hypertension. When no pulmonary or other cause for the documented pulmonary hypertension is determined, the patient is considered to have primary pulmonary hypertension.

More recent scrutiny of patients with primary pulmonary hypertension, particularly with autopsy studies, has served to separate a group of patients that share the same clinical picture but some of whose members do not have what appears to be a primary vasoconstrictive process in the pulmonary arteries to account for their pulmonary hypertension. This group of patients includes those who have multiple silent pulmonary thromboembolic disease and patients with veno-occlusive disease of the lungs, who only at autopsy can be distinguished from patients with venoconstrictive pulmonary hypertension, for whose pulmonary hypertension there is no other discernible cause.

For all practical purposes, patients with pulmonary hypertension demonstrated by cardiac catheterization without any obvious pulmonary or cardiac cause may be labeled clinically as having primary pulmonary hypertension. There are certain clinical features in patients with vasoconstrictive pulmonary hypertension that tend to separate them from patients with pulmo-

nary thromboembolism and pulmonary veno-occlusive disease. In almost all series of vasoconstrictive pulmonary hypertension, females predominate over males, pregnancy tends to provoke or aggravate this syndrome, and Raynaud's phenomenon occurs frequently. A familial incidence of vasoconstrictive pulmonary hypertension has been reported. Also, vasoconstrictive pulmonary hypertension may occur in children, a group that infrequently has thromboembolism.

DIAGNOSTIC EVALUATION

Whether the pulmonary hypertension is due to vasoconstrictive pulmonary hypertension or to veno-occlusive disease or thromboembolism, the symptoms and physical findings are essentially the same. The primary and most dramatic symptom is repetitive episodes of syncope. Dyspnea on exertion and easy fatigability are almost constantly present. These patients may have a dull, nondescript, nonanginal-type, aching substernal discomfort that is prolonged in comparison to that of angina pectoris. This discomfort is thought to be due to right ventricular ischemia, although the possibility that dilatation of the main pulmonary artery and its major branches might produce such pain still exists. Physical examination reveals a right ventricular lift. On auscultation there is frequently a short systolic ejection murmur, a loud pulmonic closure sound (P2), and an early diastolic blowing murmur of pulmonary regurgitation. In addition, if the pulmonary hypertension and right ventricular hypertension have been prolonged, there may be signs of tricuspid regurgitation with a holosystolic blowing murmur somewhat louder on inspiration, as well as prominent jugular venous distension and hepatic enlargement.

Laboratory examination demonstrates ECG changes of right ventricular hypertrophy as well as right atrial enlargement. Echocardiography demonstrates signs of right ventricular enlargement and usually evidence of tricuspid regurgitation. The E to F slope of the anterior leaflet of the mitral valve may be decreased, suggesting the presence of mitral stenosis, but movement of the posterior leaflet is normal. Cardiac catheterization remains the primary tool for establishing a diagnosis of primary pulmonary hypertension. Determining whether the pulmonary hypertension is due to a vasospastic element or to thromboembolism or veno-occlusive disease is a function of the pathologist. Ventilation perfusion scans of the lung are seldom definitive in establishing a diagnosis of multiple small pulmonary emboli and thus are not diagnostic. Pulmonary angiography, while carrying a somewhat higher risk in these patients, may demonstrate the presence of multiple, relatively large, asymmetrical perfusion defects, which would lead to the impression that the patient has multiple pulmonary emboli. However, once again, in the situation in which there are multiple small pulmonary emboli, vasoconstrictive pulmonary hypertension cannot be differentiated from pulmonary veno-occlusive disease or multiple pulmonary thromboembolism.

While there are many forms of secondary pulmonary hypertension (Table 7–29), the critical lesions (those that are potentially correctable) involve problems in the left side of the heart. Cardiac catheterization, with determination of cardiac output, allows the determination of the total pulmonary resistance and pulmonary vascular resistance, thus defining whether the pulmonary hypertension is simply a reflection of elevated left-sided cardiac pressures or whether there is, indeed, a vasoconstrictive element in the pulmonary circulation. Stenosis or regurgitation of the mitral or aortic valve may produce secondary pulmonary hypertension, which is corrected when the valvular lesion is repaired. Thus, patients who present with signs of pulmonary hypertension of unknown origin, after a careful pulmonary evaluation, should undergo cardiac catheterization.

CARDIAC ARREST AND SUDDEN DEATH

DEFINITION

Cardiac arrest has been broadly defined as sudden cessation of cardiac function. In its narrowest sense, the term connotes cessation of an effective cardiac contraction caused by either asystole or ventricular fibrillation. In a broader and more clinical sense, it may include profound bradycardia and rapid tachycardias that, while having a recognizable cardiac contraction, still produce the clinical picture of unconsciousness, agonal breathing, and possibly seizure activity. The physician called to the bedside of a patient with a cardiac arrest is unlikely to define the mechanism for the inadequate cardiac function until resuscitative efforts have begun and an electrocardiogram has been obtained.

Sudden death may be broadly defined as a clinically unexplained rapid cessation of cardiac action in a previously healthy individual. Recognizing that the terms ''rapid'' and ''sudden'' are relative, sudden cardiac

Table 7–30. Cardiac Causes for Sudden Death

Coronary artery abnormalities
  Congenital anomalies
    Single coronary artery
    Anomalous origin of left coronary artery from anterior sinus of Valsalva
  Coronary arteritis
    Periarteritis nodosa, Kawasaki disease
    Luetic arteritis with osteal stenosis
  Coronary embolism
    Paradoxical embolus
    Bacterial endocarditis
    Embolus from left atrium or ventricle
    Calcific embolus from mitral or aortic valve
    Coronary artery ectasia
  Arteriosclerotic coronary artery disease
  Coronary spasm
Myocardial abnormalities
  Myocarditis
  Hypertrophic cardiomyopathy
  Cardiac tumors
  Cardiac or aortic rupture producing cardiac tamponade
Valvular disease
  Aortic stenosis
  Aortic regurgitation
  Valvular rupture
  Mitral valve prolapse
Conduction abnormalities
  Prolonged QT syndromes
  Accessory pathways
  Recurrent ventricular tachycardia
  Complete heart block

death can more precisely be defined as an unexpected cardiac death occurring without preceding symptoms or with symptoms occuring less than an hour before the death. This event occurs over 400,000 times a year in the U.S. In the relatively few situations in which the exact mechanism of cardiac arrest has been defined, ventricular fibrillation is almost inevitably documented as a cause.

PATHOPHYSIOLOGIC CONSIDERATIONS

While arteriosclerotic coronary artery disease is found in approximately 80% of patients dying with sudden death, there are other cardiovascular causes that must be considered (Table 7–30).

Congenital anomalies of the coronary arteries are now recognized with increasing frequency during cardiac catheterization. Sudden death has on rare occasions been associated with such anomalies. There are isolated cases of sudden death reported in patients with either a single coronary artery or a vestigial right coronary artery. In addition, there is some evidence to suggest that origination of the left coronary artery from the anterior sinus of Valsalva, in which the left coronary artery travels between the anteriorly positioned pulmonary artery and the posteriorly positioned aorta, may be associated with sudden death. These deaths have usually occurred during heavy physical activity, and it has been hypothesized that the distended aorta and main pulmonary artery may occlude the elongated left coronary artery as it passes between these two vessels.

An inflammatory response in and around the coronary arteries has been noted in various collagen diseases, but in periarteritis nodosa there is aneurysm formation, leading to the potential rupture of such aneurysms. Coronary artery aneurysms are also noted in Kawasaki disease. This syndrome is characterized by fever, mucocutaneous lesion, lymphadenopathy, and coronary arteritis, usually occurring in children. In the past, when syphilis presented major cardiovascular problems, luetic arteritis with osteal stenosis was a recognized cause of sudden death.

Coronary embolization may produce myocardial infarction but sudden death less frequently. Paradoxical embolization across an atrial or ventricular septal defect or even embolization from the venous system across a probe patent foramen ovale may occur. More frequently, embolization from the dilated fibrillating left atrium or from a mural thrombus in the left ventricle is a source for embolic occlusion of a coronary artery. Occasionally, bits of calcium from the diseased mitral or aortic valve may provoke occlusion of a coronary artery. A small number of patients may have marked ectasia of the coronary arteries, producing a picture much like multiple aneurysms of the coronary arteries. Thrombus formation may occur in these ectatic areas of the coronary arteries, leading to distal embolization of the coronary tree.

While arteriosclerotic coronary artery disease is found in 80% of patients dying a sudden cardiac death, the exact cause and effect relationship between the arteriosclerotic process and the sudden death is not always clear. It may well be that thrombi or platelet aggregates form in regions of significant stenosis in the coronary tree and lead to acute ischemia and electrical instability, which eventuates in sudden death. It is not always possible to detect this train of events at autopsy because of the thrombolytic process that may occur between the time of sudden death and the postmortem examination. Finally, coronary artery spasm, which is now recognized clinically, may provoke prolonged ischemia and therefore arrhythmias or may encourage the formation of thrombosis, thus leading to infarction and sudden death.

Abnormalities in the myocardium may be associated with sudden death. Acute myocarditis, particularly occurring in children, has been thought to be a cause for sudden death. In many adults dying with sudden death there are inflammatory changes within the myocardium, but the exact relationship of these changes to sudden death is clouded by the fact that similar changes have also been found in patients who have not died of sudden death. The most frequent myocardial lesion associated with sudden death is hypertrophic cardiomyopathy. Approximately 15% of patients with this lesion will eventually die with sudden death. Cardiac tumors may produce sudden death by occluding flow through or out of the heart. Cardiac rupture following a silent myocardial infarction or, less frequently, following mitral valve replacement may produce cardiac tamponade and sudden death.

The most common valvular disease associated with sudden death has been aortic stenosis, but this may also occur in approximately 9% of patients with aortic regurgitation. Sudden rupture of a cardiac valve may produce sudden severe pulmonary edema and rapid death. As indicated previously, mitral valve prolapse has been associated with sudden death, presumably on the basis of a ventricular arrhythmia precipitated by the frequent premature ventricular beats noted in many of these patients. Considering the frequency of mitral valve prolapse in the general population, its precipitation of sudden death is rare.

It is now recognized that conduction abnormalities are associated with sudden death. Prolonged QT syndromes, particularly in children, are associated with sudden death. In the adult with a tendency toward a prolonged QT interval, hypokalemia and/or the addition of Type I antiarrhythmic agent such as quinidine and procainamide may provoke Torsades des Pointes with eventual deterioration of the ventricular flutter-type pattern to ventricular fibrillation. Accessory pathways with rapid antegrade conduction in combination with atrial fibrillation may provoke ventricular fibrillation. Finally, there are patients who have recurrent episodes of ventricular tachycardia of unknown cause. Many such patients have underlying arteriosclerotic coronary artery disease with or without a ventricular aneurysm. Some may have an underlying unrecognized myocarditis, but, excluding this group of patients, there is still a large group of patients with recurrent ventricular tachycardia, the cause of which is unknown. Complete heart block may be associated with ventricular arrest, profound bradycardia, or ventricular fibrillation.

The above classification emphasizes structural abnormalities that may lead to sudden cardiac death, but it does not address the role of the central nervous system in provoking sudden death. Profound, prolonged vasovagal responses may be associated with severe bradycardia, anoxia, and subsequent ventricular arrhythmias and sudden death. Sudden emotional stimuli have been documented to provoke ventricular fibrillation. Thus, sudden death may be provoked by abnormal function of higher centers in the central nervous system, the only manifestation of which is cardiac arrest.

REFERENCES

1. Heberden, W.: Some account of a disorder in the breast. Med Trans Roy Coll Phys 2:59, 1772.
2. Prinzmetal, M., et al.: Variant form of angina pectoris: Previously undelineated syndrome. JAMA 174:1794, 1960.
3. Wood, F.C.: Trepopnea. Arch Intern Med 104:966–973, 1959.
4. Kossman, C.E.: Torsades des Pointes: An addition to the nosography of ventricular tachycardia. Am J Cardiol 42:1054, 1978.
5. Smith, W.M., and Gallagher, J.J.: Les Torsades des Pointes. Ann Intern Med 93:578, 1980.
6. Raynaud, A.G.M.: Del' Asphyxie Locale et de la Gangrene Symetrique des Extremites. Paris, Rignoux, 1862, p. 6.
7. O'Rourke, R.A.: Physical examination of the arteries and veins. In The Heart. Edited by J.W. Hurst. 5th Ed. New York, McGraw-Hill Book Company, 1982, p. 188.
8. Gibson, R.: Atypical constrictive pericarditis. Br Heart J 14:53, 1959.
9. Freidreich, N.: Krankheiten des Herzens. Handb. d. spec. Path. v. Therap. Edited by Virchow. 2:262, 1855.
10. Leatham, A.: Auscultation of the Heart and Phonocardiography. 2nd Ed. Edinburgh, Churchill Livingstone, 1975.
11. McKusick, V.A.: Cardiovascular Sound in Health and Disease. Baltimore, The Williams and Wilkins Co., 1958, p. 27.
12. Potain, P.C.: Du rhythme cardiaque appele' bruit gallop. In Classics in Arterial Hypertension. Edited by A. Ruskin. Springfield, Ill., Charles C Thomas, Publisher, 1956.
13. Warren, J.V.: Editorial. Gallop rhythm. Circulation 15:321, 1957.
14. Warren, J.V., Leonard, J.J., and Weissler, A.M.: Gallop rhythm. Ann Intern Med 48:580, 1958.
15. Gallagher, J.J.: Mechanisms of arrhythmias and conduction abnormalities. In The Heart. 5th Ed. Edited by J.W. Hurst. New York, McGraw-Hill Book Company, 1982, p. 489.
16. Kent, A.F.S.: Researches on structure and function of mammalian heart. J Physiol 14:233, 1893.
17. Ferrer, M.I.: Preexcitation Including the Wolff-Parkinson-White and Other Related Syndromes. Mount Kisco, N.Y., Futura Publishing Company, Inc., 1976.
18. Wolff, L., Parkinson, J., and White, P.D.: Bundle branch block with short P-R interval in healthy young people prone to paroxysmal tachycardia. Am Heart J 5:685, 1930.
19. Gallagher, J.J., et al.: Wolff-Parkinson-White Syndrome: The problem, evaluation, and surgical correction. Circulation 51:767, 1975.
20. Marriott, H.J.L., and Myerburg, R.J.: Recognition of arrhythmias and conduction abnormalities. In The Heart. 5th Ed. Edited by J.W. Hurst. New York, McGraw-Hill Book Company, 1982, p. 519.
21. Higgins, C.B., et al.: Magnetic resonance imaging in hypertrophic cardiomyopathy. Am J Cardiol 55:1121, 1985.
22. Perloff, J.K.: The Clinical Recognition of Congenital Heart Disease. 2nd Ed. Philadelphia, W.B. Saunders, 1978.
23. Bacos, J., Eagan, J., and Orgain, E.S.: Congenital familial nodal rhythm. Circulation 22:887, 1960.
24. Jeresaty, R.M.: Mitral Valve Prolapse. New York, Raven Press, 1979.
25. Wenger, N.K., Abelman, W.H., and Roberts, W.C.: Myocarditis. In The Heart. 5th Ed. Edited by J.W. Hurst. New York, McGraw-Hill Book Company, 1982, p. 1278.
26. Goodwin, J.F., Roberts, W.C., and Wenger, N.K.: Cardiomyopathy. In The Heart. 5th Ed. Edited by J.W. Hurst. New York, McGraw-Hill Book Company, 1982, p. 1299.
27. Robinson, J.A., and O'Connell, J.B. (eds.): Myocarditis: Precursor of Cardiomyopathy. Lexington, MA. The Collamore Press, D.C. Heath and Company, 1983.
28. Ingram, R.H., Jr., and Braunwald, E.: Pulmonary edema: Cardiogenic and non-cardiogenic. In Heart Disease: A Textbook of Cardiovascular Medicine. 2nd Ed. Edited by: E. Braunwald. Philadelphia, W.B. Saunders Co., 1984, p. 560.

CHAPTER 8

HYPERTENSION

Thomas G. Pickering, M.D., D.Phil.

DEFINITION

There is no universally agreed upon definition of hypertension because blood pressure, like body weight and height, has a continuous distribution within the population, and because in any one individual blood pressure varies greatly from moment to moment, depending on the circumstances in which it is measured.[1] Any definition of hypertension is thus arbitrary and should be operational.[2]

The risks associated with high blood pressure increase progressively as blood pressure increases (Fig. 8–1). Only a relatively small number of patients have severe hypertension and are at very high risk individually. The majority of hypertensive patients have only a mild elevation of pressure and risk but because of their greater numbers actually account for the bulk of blood pressure-related morbidity.

While the risks associated with hypertension are quantitative rather than qualitative, the decision to treat—should the patient be given medication or not— is a qualitative one.

The following general guidelines for evaluating patients with high blood pressure are suggested, using a triage system based on the height of the blood pressure and related complications (Fig. 8–2). It should be emphasized that, because of the variability of blood pressure, high blood pressure should not be defined on the basis of a single reading. Also, since the risks associated with high blood pressure occur equally for elevations of systolic and diastolic pressures, both readings should be taken into account when evaluating individual patients. The following strategy for evaluating patients' blood pressure is recommended.

1. Observe only:
   a. when diastolic blood pressure is below 95 mm Hg
   b. when systolic blood pressure is below 145 mm Hg

   At this level of blood pressure the increased risk is very small, and blood pressure measurement on different occasions will frequently show a reduction of blood pressure without any intervention. Further investigations of underlying causes is not warranted in adults, although this level of blood pressure may definitely be abnormal in children. In pregnant women, a blood pressure of more than 140/90 mm Hg is considered abnormal.

2. Investigate cause and then treat:
   a. when diastolic blood pressure is above 95 mm Hg
   b. when systolic blood pressure is above 145 mm Hg

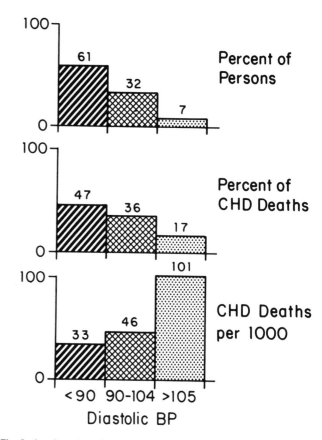

Fig. 8–1. Data from Framingham Pooling Project showing incidence of coronary heart disease (CHD) in relation to different levels of diastolic pressure.

c. in the absence of acute complications

In such patients the risk associated with the hypertension can normally be considered to outweigh the side effects of treatment. If treatment is contemplated, it is logical before beginning treatment to investigate the underlying cause of the hypertension so that the 5 or 10% of patients with secondary or curable forms of hypertension can be identified, since in many cases the treatment may itself make the diagnosis more difficult.

In patients with diastolic pressures between 95 and 104 mm Hg the decision to treat should be based not only on the height of the blood pressure, but also on the presence or absence of other cardiovascular risk factors.

3. Treat immediately and investigate cause later:
   a. when diastolic blood pressure is above 130 mm Hg

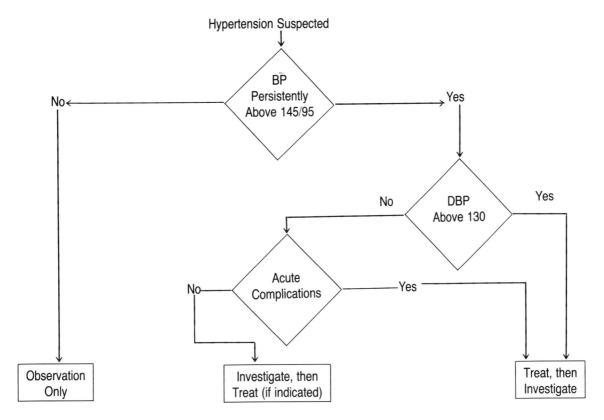

Fig. 8–2. Triage system for initial management of hypertension.

b. when systolic blood pressure is above 220 mm Hg

c. in the presence of any of the following associated findings:

pulmonary edema

coronary ischemia

cerebrovascular ischemia or hemorrhage

hypertensive encephalopathy

dissecting aneurysm

toxemia of pregnancy

In such patients, many of whom have malignant or accelerated hypertension, the acute risk is sufficiently high to warrant immediate treatment, with investigation of the underlying cause beginning later. In some of these patients such as those with acute pulmonary edema, the blood pressure elevation is not necessarily sustained, but in those in whom it is, secondary forms of hypertension are relatively common.

PATHOPHYSIOLOGIC CONSIDERATIONS AND DIFFERENTIAL DIAGNOSIS

In general, hypertensive patients can be classified in two ways: first, according to the severity of hypertension, and second, according to the underlying pathophysiologic considerations (Table 8–1).

Some commonly used terms are described below.

Classification Based on Severity and Type

Borderline Hypertension. This is usually defined as a diastolic blood pressure between 90 and 100 mm Hg. The term mild hypertension is also used and has been defined as diastolic blood pressure between 90 and 104 mm Hg.

Moderate Hypertension. As defined by the Joint National Commission,[4] moderate hypertension refers to patients with diastolic pressures between 105 and 114 mm Hg.

Accelerated Hypertension. This is another poorly defined term, usually taken to indicate severe hypertension that is progressing to the malignant phase (e.g., with hemorrhages and exudates in the fundi, but no papilledema).

Malignant Hypertension. Malignant hypertension is not defined simply on the basis of severe elevation of blood pressure but is a distinct clinical and pathologic entity.[4] Left untreated, it progresses rapidly to renal failure, cerebral hemorrhage, and death. Experimentally it is characterized by acute vascular damage and high plasma renin activity; clinically, by the presence of papilledema, hemorrhages, and exudates in the optic fundi, and usually by azotemia and proteinuria. Secondary causes of hypertension are relatively common, although malignant hypertension is uncom-

Table 8–1. Classification of Hypertension

Based on Pathophysiology	Based on Severity and Type
Primary	Borderline
Essential	Moderate
High renin	Systolic
Normal renin	Accelerated
Low renin	Malignant
Secondary	Hypertensive encephalopathy
Renal	
Renovascular	
Fibromuscular	
Atheroma	
Other	
Renal parenchymal disease	
Pyelonephritis	
Glomerulonephritis	
Polycystic kidneys	
Analgesic nephropathy	
Renin-secreting tumor	
Adrenal	
Aldosterone-secreting tumor	
Pseudoprimary hyperaldosteronism	
Dexamethasone-suppressible aldosteronism	
Cushing's syndrome	
Congenital adrenal hyperplasia	
Pheochromocytoma	
Coarctation of the aorta	
Liddle's syndrome	
Iatrogenic	
Oral contraceptives	
Nasal decongestants	
Nonsteroidal anti-inflammatory drugs	
Monoamine oxidase inhibitors	

mon in primary aldosteronism (a low-renin form of hypertension) and possibly does not occur in coarctation of the aorta (perhaps because in this condition the kidneys are protected from the effects of the hypertension).

Labile Hypertension. This term was used to describe the "labile" phase hypertension was thought to go through before becoming "fixed" or "established." The term is a misnomer, however, because in general blood pressure variability increases with the severity of hypertension.

Paroxysmal Hypertension. A minority of patients do not show a generally increased variability of blood pressure, but rather have normal levels interspersed with episodes of severely elevated blood pressure. This is characteristic of a number of conditions, including:

1. Pheochromocytoma.
2. Spinal cord transection, in which patients have low blood pressure most of the time but demonstrate paroxysmal reflex elevation of blood pressure during bladder distension or muscle spasm, probably caused by disinhibition of spinal autonomic centers.[5]
3. Posterior fossa tumors, in which increased pres-

sure in the region of the area postrema of the brain stem can cause sympathetically mediated elevation of blood pressure.[6]

4. Acute pulmonary edema. Systolic blood pressure may rise rapidly to near 300 mm Hg and is accompanied by sweating, dyspnea, rales, and rhonchi. If blood pressure returns to normal when the acute episode resolves, cardiac conditions such as aortic stenosis and myocardial ischemia should be suspected. If pulmonary edema occurs in the setting of chronic hypertension, renovascular hypertension should be suspected.
5. Pseudopheochromocytoma, a poorly defined entity, in which patients show a pheochromocytoma-like picture clinically and biochemically but lack a tumor; their principal abnormality may be a failure to conjugate plasma catecholamines.[7]
6. Hypertensive crisis with monoamine oxidase inhibitors.
7. Clonidine withdrawal. Sudden cessation of clonidine or guanabenz therapy may cause an acute sympathetic discharge.

Systolic Hypertension. This is a raised systolic pressure (e.g., above 170 mm Hg) with a normal diastolic pressure (e.g., below 90 mm Hg) that may be characteristic of several conditions, such as systolic hypertension of the elderly. Systolic blood pressure increases more than diastolic, probably reflecting a decreased arterial distensibility. The prognosis is as bad as for diastolic hypertension, but conclusive evidence that treating such patients reduces their risk is currently lacking.

There may also be a moderate elevation of systolic pressure in bradycardia, when bradycardia is extreme and stroke volume is increased (e.g., from heart block, or from sinus bradycardia as occurs in athletes).

Also, pulse pressure may be increased as a result of both a high forward stroke volume and diastolic regurgitation in aortic regurgitation.

Finally, a widened pulse pressure is associated with an increased cardiac output and vasodilation in hyperthyroidism.

Hypertensive Encephalopathy. Hypertensive encephalopathy is severe hypertension with central nervous system changes such as headache, alteration of consciousness, visual loss, and seizures. It is thought to be due to a failure of cerebral autoregulation, with disruption of the blood-brain barrier leading to cerebral edema.[9] It is important to distinguish hypertensive encephalopathy from stroke, because the condition is reversible if the pressure is lowered.

Classification Based on Pathophysiologic Considerations

Primary (Essential) Hypertension. Although often regarded as a single entity, essential hypertension is more probably the end result of several different mechanisms. It is defined only in the negative sense, i.e., by the absence of any identifiable secondary cause (Table 8–1). A useful classification, from the point of view of both the underlying etiology and selection of antihypertensive therapy, is to subdivide it into high-renin, normal-renin, and low-renin subtypes.[10]

Secondary Hypertension. Less than 10% of all hypertensive patients have secondary forms of hypertension. High blood pressure can result from a variety of primary renal diseases, endocrine disorders, systemic diseases, and the intake of medications (Table 8–1).

Renovascular Hypertension. The most common cause of secondary hypertension is renal artery stenosis.[11] Three major entities of renovascular hypertensions are encountered. Fibromuscular dysplasia typically occurs in young white women and is rare in blacks. Onset of hypertension is acute. Physical examination usually reveals the presence of an abdominal bruit. In 80% of these patients, plasma renin activity is high.

Atheroma of the renal artery can also cause reno-

vascular hypertension. The atheromatous form of renovascular hypertension is seen more commonly in middle-aged smokers and should be suspected after acute onset or exacerbation of pre-existing hypertension. Abdominal or other sites for vascular bruit are common. These patients may also have clinical evidence of other atheromatous lesions. As with fibromuscular dysplasia, plasma renin activity is high in the majority of patients.

Arteritis is an uncommon cause of renovascular hypertension. The sedimentation rate may be high.

Renal Parenchymal Diseases. Parenchymal diseases of the kidneys are commonly associated with hypertension.[12] The most frequent causes are pyelonephritis, glomerulonephritis, polycystic kidneys, and analgesic nephropathy. Patients with parenchymal renal disease frequently complain of nocturia. Loin pains and palpable kidneys are suggestive of polycystic kidney disease. Azotemia is frequently present, though its absence does not preclude a renal origin for hypertension. Proteinuria is also common, although it is not specific for parenchymal renal disease. It may occur either as a result of primary renal disease or secondarily in any form of severe hypertension.

Aldosterone-Secreting Tumor. This is a rare cause of secondary hypertension.[13,14] A long history of severe hypertension is typical but not invariable. Hypertension in aldosterone-secreting tumor rarely becomes malignant. There are usually no specific signs or symptoms. Unexplained hypokalemia and hypernatremia is the hallmark of this condition. Very low plasma renin and high aldosterone are typical laboratory findings.

Other Types of Hypertension Associated with Hypokalemia. Dexamethasone-suppressible hyperaldosteronism is a rare form of hypertension associated with hypokalemia.[13,14] This rare disorder is associated commonly with hypokalemia, low renin, and high aldosterone, as in aldosterone-secreting tumor. This entity, however, unlike aldosterone-secreting tumor, is familial and occurs mainly in young men. Biochemical abnormalities are reversed by a 1- to 2-mg daily dose of dexamethasone. In dexamethasone-suppressible hyperaldosteronism both adrenal glands are enlarged.

In idiopathic (pseudoprimary) hyperaldosteronism, biochemical abnormalities resemble those of aldosteronoma but are less marked. Usually both adrenals, or only one in exceptional cases, are mildly enlarged.

Liddle's Syndrome. Liddle's syndrome is a very rare form of hypokalemia associated with hypertension, but the level of aldosterone is low.[15] This entity is a familial disorder of an inherited defect in sodium transport.

Pheochromocytoma. Pheochromocytoma is also a rare cause of hypertension.[16] Hypertension may be pa-

Table 8–2.   Conditions in Which Hypertension is Usually an Incidental Finding

Cushing's syndrome
Acromegaly
Hyperparathyroidism
Hyperthyroidism
Congenital adrenal hyperplasia
Scleroderma
Polyarteritis nodosa
Systemic lupus erythematosus
Diabetes mellitus

roxysmal or sustained. Presenting symptoms of pheochromocytoma can be described as the "five Ps"—paroxysms, pain, pallor, palpitations, and perspiration. High urine and plasma catecholamines are diagnostic for pheochromocytoma. Hypermetabolism occurs secondary to the increased levels of circulating catecholamines. Orthostatic hypotension may occur because of contracted blood volume.

Coarctation of the Aorta. This type of hypertension mostly occurs in young patients.[17] There is usually severe hypertension with wide pulse pressure in the arms, but not in the legs (thigh cuff should be used to confirm blood pressure). Weak femoral pulses are characteristic. A bruit in the interscapular area is virtually pathognomonic.

Renin-Secreting Tumor. Renin-secreting tumor is a rare cause of secondary hypertension.[18] Plasma renin activity is very high—usually above 50 ng/ml/hour. Renal function is normal. Low serum potassium and sodium occur secondary to the overactive renin-angiotensin-aldosterone system. There may be evidence of an extrarenal or intrarenal tumor.

Hypertension as an Incidental Finding

A number of clinical entities may be associated with hypertension[19] (Table 8–2). The clinical features of these entities will not be discussed here. However, several relevant clinical clues will be briefly mentioned.

Cushing's syndrome must be distinguished from hypertension accompanying simple obesity. Useful features favoring a diagnosis of Cushing's syndrome include central distribution of obesity, weakness, plethora, and ecchymoses. The diagnosis is confirmed by a high 24-hour urine cortisol level and dexamethasone suppression test with 1 mg at bedtime. Plasma cortisol remains high (above 7 μg/100 ml) in the following day's 8 A.M. sample.

Hypertension is present in about 30% of patients with acromegaly. Hyperparathyroidism should be suspected if serum calcium rises following start of diuretic therapy. Patients with hyperthyroidism have a high

cardiac output with systolic but not diastolic hypertension as a result of the hypermetabolic state.

Hypertension can also be associated with scleroderma.[20] As a result of thrombotic microangiopathy in the kidney there may be azotemia, high renin, and malignant hypertension.

As a result of focal renal ischemia, patients with polyarteritis nodosa may have a high-renin form of hypertension.[21] Patients with systemic lupus erythematosus (SLE) may develop hypertension with renal damage and lupus nephritis. Also, the prevalence of hypertension is doubled in patients with diabetes mellitus as compared to normal subjects. The development of hypertension is often associated with renal damage.[22]

Hypertension may be detected in children with congenital adrenal hyperplasia. The condition is discussed in more detail below (see Hypertension in children).

DIAGNOSTIC EVALUATION

Patient History

Taking a careful history may provide additional clues to the existence of hypertension and its possible cause. A positive family history of hypertension suggests essential rather than secondary hypertension. A family history of medullary carcinoma of the thyroid or hyperparathyroidism may indicate coexistence of pheochromocytoma.

Excessive intake of alcohol may be associated with hypertension,[23] and heavy smoking may be associated with malignant or renovascular hypertension.[24] In addition, a number of drugs can raise blood pressure. Drug-induced hypertension is observed most commonly with the chronic use of oral contraceptives, nasal decongestants, nonsteroidal anti-inflammatory drugs, and monoamine oxidase inhibitors.

Probably more than 90% of hypertensive patients have essential hypertension. Secondary forms of hypertension, however, are relatively common in patients with severe hypertension and in younger age groups. In general, secondary forms of hypertension should be suspected under circumstances of young age, documented recent onset of hypertension, severe hypertension, bruits, unexpected hypokalemia, renal disease, or paroxysmal symptoms.

Physical Examination

Symptoms and physical signs are usually few or nonspecific in hypertensive patients but when they occur are of value for establishing both the severity of the hypertension and its underlying cause.

SIGNS

In addition to an elevated blood pressure, a number of helpful signs may provide clinical clues to the cause of hypertension.

Mild orthostatic hypotension, if not secondary to medication, should arouse suspicion of pheochromocytoma. With idiopathic orthostatic hypotension, there may be hypertension when the patient is supine and hypotension when he is upright. In addition, pulsus alternans suggests left ventricular failure, and a silent period is often heard in systolic hypertension of the elderly.

Left ventricular hypertrophy (sustained LV impulse) suggests sustained hypertension and is itself a significant risk factor.[25]

Fundal changes are helpful in evaluating the severity of hypertension rather than the underlying cause.[26] The earliest change to occur in hypertension is thickening of the arteriolar wall, which results in an increased reflection of light, giving the appearance of ''copper wiring'' or ''silver wiring.'' Arteriovenous nicking is seen where the veins cross behind the arteries and is due to partial obstruction or kinking of the vein by the thickened artery. These changes correspond to stages I and II of the Keith-Wagener grading system.

In more severe hypertension, hemorrhages, exudates, cotton-wool spots, and papilledema may occur. Hypertensive hemorrhages are typically flame shaped, in contrast to the dot shaped hemorrhages of diabetes. Cotton-wool spots are areas of whitish discoloration near the optic disk and are thought to be caused by ischemic infarction of nerve fibers. They are common in accelerated or malignant hypertension but can occur in other conditions. Hypertensive exudates are whitish or yellowish areas with irregular but sharply defined borders and are made of aggregations of fibrin and other plasma constituents. These changes constitute stage III of the Keith-Wagener classification.

Papilledema (stage IV of Keith-Wagener) is due to swelling of the optic disk, which is at least in part the result of raised intracranial pressure, and is characteristic of but not specific to malignant hypertension.

Another sign of hypertension is diminished femoral pulses, which suggest arteriosclerosis or, in young patients, coarctation of the aorta.

When bruits are detected, certain areas should be examined. Bruits over the carotid artery are nearly always due to arteriosclerosis. Interscapular bruits suggest coarctation of the aorta; with abdominal bruits, arteriosclerosis or fibromuscular dysplasia of renal arteries are likely. Femoral bruits usually signify arteriosclerosis.

Finally, simple obesity is associated with increased blood pressure, even after adjusting for cuff size.[27]

SYMPTOMS

Although the majority of patients with essential hypertension have no symptoms that can clearly be related to the hypertension itself,[28] a number of nonspecific symptoms may be seen in patients with severe hypertension. Because both headache and hypertension are common problems, it is only to be expected that they coincide in many people. A causal connection is unusual, however.

Tension headache not uncommonly develops *after* the diagnosis of hypertension has been made.[29]

True hypertensive headache occurs, though rarely. It may be unilateral or occipital and occurs in the morning. It is most commonly seen in patients with malignant or renovascular hypertension and could be due to the vasoconstrictor effects of angiotensin on cerebral vessels. It is also characteristic of patients with pheochromocytoma.

Epistaxis may be the presenting symptom of any form of hypertension.

Muscle weakness is an occasional symptom in patients with marked hypokalemia secondary to aldosteronoma or diuretic treatment. Also, nocturia and polyuria may occur as a consequence of impaired renal concentrating ability and are suggestive of intrinsic renal disease or aldosteronoma.

Paroxysmal symptoms (the ''five Ps'') suggestive of pheochromocytoma are paroxysms, pallor, pain, palpitations, and perspiration.

The demonstration of normotension interspersed with paroxysms of hypertension is characteristic but not diagnostic of pheochromocytoma. However, it is often difficult to document the paroxysms. Other conditions whose symptoms may also be paroxysmal but lack the associated elevations of blood pressure include panic attacks, hypoglycemia, menopausal hot flashes, migraine and cluster headaches, and carcinoid.

In one series, 30% of untreated hypertensives complained of blurred vision compared with only 15% of normotensives. Such patients do not necessarily have hypertensive retinopathy.[30]

In the same series, 45% of hypertensives complained of depression, compared with only 34% of normotensives.

Finally, claudication suggests the possibility of renovascular hypertension (caused by atheroma) or coarctation.

Diagnostic Studies

Before treatment is started patients with hypertension should be evaluated to determine the type and severity of the hypertension. Patients in different categories or with different types of hypertension may require different strategies or approaches for evaluation.

Patients with Borderline Hypertension. In evaluating patients with borderline hypertension, the following strategy is recommended:

Repeat measurements of blood pressure on successive visits; many patients with borderline pressures will show normal values on repeat testing.

Train patients to take their own blood pressure at home to help identify individuals with "white coat" hypertension.[31]

In patients in whom there is a large disparity between clinic and home blood pressure measurements, 24-hour ambulatory blood pressure recordings may help to determine whether the overall level of blood pressure is within the normal range.[32]

Finally, evaluate other cardiovascular risk factors. A more aggressive workup in borderline patients is warranted if other cardiovascular risk factors such as smoking, high cholesterol, and high blood sugar are present.

Patients Judged to Require Investigation and Possible Treatment. The following additional studies are suggested to assist in evaluating hypertension and elucidating the nature of hypertension in terms of diagnosis and treatment.

Routine Tests (all patients). All patients should be screened for biochemical abnormalities of potassium, calcium, magnesium, BUN/creatinine, cholesterol, glucose, and uric acid levels.

Hypokalemia suggests primary or secondary hyperaldosteronism and may be due to a number of causes, such as diuretic treatment, primary aldosteronism (adrenal tumor), pseudoprimary aldosteronism (adrenal hyperplasia), renovascular hypertension, and licorice intoxication. Calcium levels should be ascertained to detect hypercalcemia, which may suggest hyperparathyroidism. The patient should be screened for hypomagnesemia, which may occur in primary aldosteronism. Also, a BUN/creatinine should be performed to screen for renal disease, which may be the cause or the consequence of hypertension. Cholesterol levels should be checked to detect hypercholesterolemia, which increases risk for any level of blood pressure.

Hyperglycemia increases risk for any level of blood pressure, while hypertension itself may increase the incidence of diabetic complications. Finally, uric acid is often elevated in untreated hypertensive patients and increases further during diuretic therapy. Routine testing should also include urinalysis, which in demonstrating proteinuria or a cellular element may suggest renal disease; and an electrocardiogram, which detects left ventricular hypertrophy or coronary heart disease, both of which are risk factors and may indicate the need for antihypertensive therapy.

Optional Tests. Optional studies should be selected individually on the basis of the physician's clinical judgment and the cost-effectiveness of the procedures for each patient.

Plasma renin activity with 24-hour urine sodium (renin-sodium profile) is helpful for both diagnosis of secondary forms of hypertension and selection of treatment (Table 8–3).[33] A high renin profile suggests renovascular or high renin essential hypertension. A low renin suggests aldosteronoma or low-renin essential hypertension.

Chest x-ray is not usually needed for routine evaluation of patients. However, when indicated, chest radiography may show cardiomegaly suggestive of severe hypertension and poor cardiovascular prognosis. Presence of rib notching may confirm coarctation.

Special Tests for Patients with Suspected Secondary Hypertension. In view of the low incidence of secondary forms of hypertension and the fact that most of these studies are invasive and costly, the following studies are indicated in hypertensive patients only when the index of suspicion for secondary hypertension is high.

Tests for Renovascular Hypertension (Fig. 8–3). The following procedures are indicated to diagnose suspected renovascular hypertension.

Step 1—Obtain a renin-sodium profile. If renin is high, renovascular hypertension is probable. If renin is normal, renovascular hypertension is possible. A low renin excludes renovascular hypertension.

Table 8–3. Renin Profiling in Hypertension

	High Renin	Normal Renin	Low Renin
Percentage of all hypertensive patients	20%	60%	20%
Common in	Malignant hypertension		Blacks, elderly
Secondary hypertension	Renovascular Renin secreting tumor Pheochromocytoma		Adrenocortical disorders Diabetes

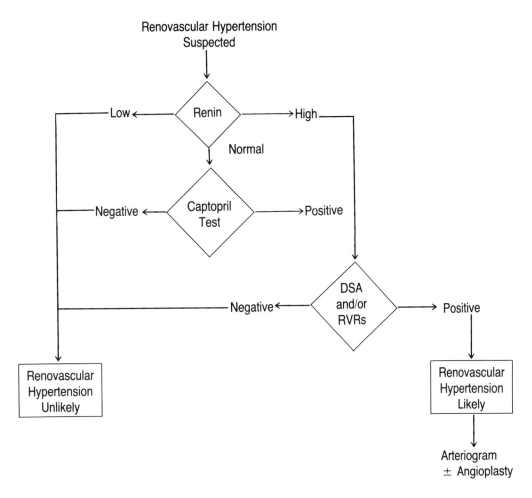

Fig. 8–3. Diagnostic steps in evaluation of renovascular hypertension.

Step 2—Captopril test. A positive captopril test is a highly sensitive and specific test for renovascular hypertension.
Or—Do a renal scan.

Step 3—Obtain renal vein renin measurements, if possible in conjunction with digital subtraction angiography. This will demonstrate the functional significance and anatomy of the renal artery stenoses.

Step 4—Obtain an arteriogram.

The following tests can be used to evaluate renovascular hypertension (Table 8–4).

1. Captopril test. A single oral dose of captopril (25 mg) produces a much larger reactive rise in

plasma renin activity in patients with renovascular hypertension than with essential hypertension or hypertension with renal parenchymal disease. Changes in blood pressure are of less diagnostic value.[34] The diagnostic criteria are a stimulated renin above 12 ng/ml/hour, an increase of renin above 10 ng/ml/hour, and an increase of renin of more than 150%, or more than 400% if baseline renin is less than 3 ng/ml/hour.

2. Renal vein renins[11]: This test, which can be performed as an outpatient procedure, involves taking blood samples from each renal vein and the inferior vena cava (IVC). Unlike renin-sodium profiling, it can be performed while the patient is taking antihypertensive medications, provided that (a) peripheral plasma renin activity is not excessively suppressed (e.g., by beta blockers) and (b) medication does not include angiotensin-converting enzyme inhibitors. The sensitivity of the test may be increased by repeating the measurements 30 minutes after captopril 25 mg po.

The increment of renin between the renal vein

Table 8–4. Sensitivity and Specificity for Screening Tests for Detecting Renovascular Hypertension

Test	Sensitivity	Specificity
Plasma renin activity	75%	70%
IVP	80%	80%
Renal scan	85%	85%
Saralasin test	80%	85%
Captopril test	95%	90%

(V) and renal artery (A)—in practice the IVC level can be substituted for A—is expressed as $(V-A)/A$ and is normally 0.25 on both sides. In renovascular hypertension there is an increased $(V-A)/A$ from the ischemic kidney (usually greater than 0.48) and a decrease from the contralateral kidney (usually near 0, i.e., signifying contralateral suppression of renin secretion). The finding of a markedly asymmetrical renal vein renin pattern, while providing strong evidence for renovascular hypertension, does not indicate whether there is unilateral or bilateral renal artery stenosis; renin secretion lateralizes to the most severely affected side.

An alternative way of expressing renal vein renin data is as the renin ratio between the two renal veins; 1.5 to 1 is usually taken as the cutoff point.

3. Digital subtraction angiography: This procedure can be combined with renal vein renin measurement. Major lesions of the renal artery can usually be visualized, but branch stenoses may be missed.[35] Because of the volume of dye needed, this test should not be performed in patients with elevated serum creatinine.

4. Intravenous pyelogram: This procedure is now obsolete as a screening test for renovascular hypertension because of its relatively low sensitivity and specificity. It is most useful for detecting abnormalities of the collecting system, as in hydronephrosis and reflux nephropathy.

5. Abdominal sonogram: This test is of great value for evaluating renal size in azotemic patients. Bilaterally small kidneys are suggestive of renal parenchymal disease; very unequal size suggests renovascular hypertension; bilaterally enlarged kidneys suggest polycystic disease.

6. Renal scan: Two forms are commonly used: ^{131}I-labeled hippuran, which detects renal blood flow, and ^{99}Tc-DTPA (technetium diethylene triamine pentacetic acid), which detects glomerular filtration. Although the test is comparatively simple to perform, the sensitivity and specificity are relatively low.

7. Saralasin infusion test: In patients whose plasma renin activity is stimulated (e.g., by furosemide given the night before the test), a reduction of supine diastolic blood pressure of more than 5 mm Hg during an infusion of 10 ng/ml/min of saralasin suggests renovascular hypertension.[36]

8. Split-renal function tests: These tests (Howard and Stamey tests) operate on the principle that a reduction of renal perfusion decreases glomerular filtration, urine flow, and urine sodium concen-

tration. Bilateral ureteric catheterization is required. Although these are probably the most accurate of all the tests used to evaluate the effects of renal ischemia, their invasive nature has made them largely obsolete.

TESTS FOR ALDOSTERONE-SECRETING TUMOR (Fig. 8–4).[13,14] The biochemical features of adrenocortical disorders that are associated with hypertension (excluding Cushing's disease, which is not usually confused with the others) are shown in Table 8–5.

The following procedures are indicated to diagnose suspected aldosterone-secreting tumor.

Step 1—Measure serum potassium, urine potassium excretion, serum magnesium, plasma renin activity, and urine/plasma aldosterone after discontinuing antihypertensive medication and while maintaining a normal or high sodium intake. In patients with aldosterone-secreting tumor, a low sodium intake may reverse the hypokalemia. Low serum potassium in the presence of a normal urine potassium is strongly suggestive of primary or secondary aldosteronism.

Step 2—Measure supine (8 A.M.) and upright (12 noon) plasma aldosterone to help differentiate aldosteronoma (in which aldosterone secretion is autonomous, making plasma aldosterone high both times or shows a paradoxical fall when the patient is upright) from pseudoprimary hyperaldosteronism (in which aldosterone secretion is still under physiologic control, and therefore plasma aldosterone is higher when the patient is upright).

Step 3—Perform a CT scan of the adrenals (requiring a high-resolution scanner because tumors are at limits of resolution of conventional scanners). One adrenal enlarged suggests aldosteronoma; both adrenals enlarged suggests pseudoprimary hyperaldosteronism.

Step 4—Perform adrenal vein sampling. The diagnosis of aldosteronoma is confirmed if there is hypersecretion of aldosterone from the side that shows a tumor on the CT scan. Blood samples should be assayed for cortisol as well as aldosterone to confirm correct location of the catheter.

TESTS FOR EVALUATING HYPERALDOSTERONISM (Table 8–5)[13,14]

1. Deoxycorticosterone acetate (Doca) test. This test is used to distinguish the autonomous hyperaldosteronism of aldosteronoma from physiologically suppressible hyperaldosteronism. Plasma and/or urine aldosterone are measured before and after 3 days of Doca (intramuscular q 12 hour for inpatients) or fluorocortisone (0.6 mg po daily for outpatients). Patients with a tumor show no change; those with idiopathic hyperplasia may or may not show suppression.

2. Saline infusion test: This test is also used to test physiologic responsiveness. Infusion of 2 L of normal saline over 2 to 4 hours fails to suppress plasma aldosterone in patients with a tumor.

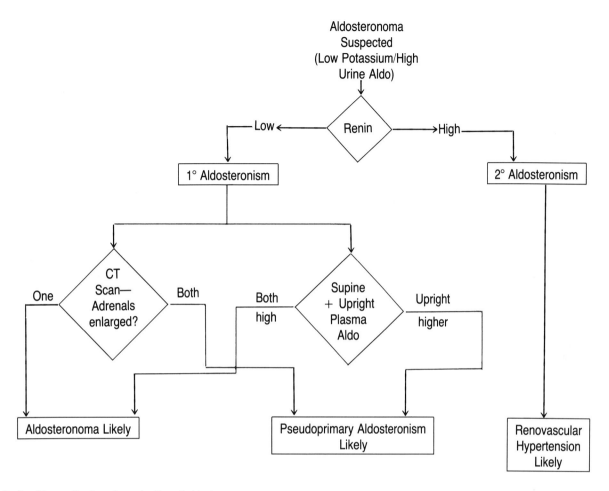

Fig. 8–4. Diagnostic steps in evaluation of aldosteronoma.

3. Iodocholesterol scanning: In patients pretreated with dexamethasone, location of an aldosteronoma can sometimes be achieved if the adrenals are scanned after administration of [131]Iodocholesterol. Small tumors (less than 1 cm in diameter), however, may be missed.

4. Cyproheptadine suppression test: Cyproheptadine, an antiserotoninergic agent, has been reported to suppress plasma aldosterone in patients with idiopathic hyperaldosteronism, but not in patients with an aldosteronoma.[37]

TESTS FOR PHEOCHROMOCYTOMA (Table 8–6). The following procedures are indicated to diagnose suspected pheochromocytoma.

Step 1—Test 24-hour urine for metanephrines, vanillymandelic acid (VMA), or catecholamines.

Step 2—Take plasma catecholamines.

Step 3—Perform a CT scan of abdomen (with a high-resolution scanner).

If the diagnosis is still uncertain and if plasma catecholamines are high:

Table 8–5. Biochemical Features of Adrenocortical Hypertensive Disorders

	Aldosteronoma	Idiopathic Adrenal Hyperplasia	Dexamathasone-Suppressible Hyperplasia	11β-Hydroxylase Deficiency	17α-Hydroxylase Deficiency
Plasma Aldo (supine)	>20 ng/100 ml	<20	Variable	Low	Low
Plasma Aldo (upright)	Falls	Increases	Variable		
PRA	Very low	Low	Low	Low	Very Low
Cortisol	Normal	Normal	Normal	Normal/Low	Low
DOC	Normal/High	Normal	Normal	High	High

Table 8–6. Biochemical Tests for Pheochromocytoma

	Normal Range (mg/day or µg/mg creatinine)	Sensitivity
Urine		
Free catecholamines	<0.1	99
Metanephrines	<1.2	97
VMA	<6.5	90
Plasma	(pg/ml)	
Total catecholamines	900	80

Step 4—Perform a clonidine suppression test. Failure of clonidine to lower elevated plasma catecholamines supports the diagnosis.

If blood pressure is normal between episodes:

Step 5—Perform a glucagon test. IV glucagon may precipitate an attack.

If there is biochemical evidence of pheochromocytoma but the CT scan is nondiagnostic:

Step 6—Arteriography or inferior vena cava catecholamine sampling may localize the position of an extra-adrenal pheochromocytoma.

The following tests are indicated to evaluate pheochromocytoma[16]

1. Plasma catecholamines: These are nearly always above 1000 pg/ml in patients with a pheochromocytoma. Norepinephrine is increased to a greater extent than epinephrine, but both are usually raised. In patients with intermittent elevations of blood pressure, levels may be normal between attacks. The patient should be resting quietly in a supine position when blood is taken. Plasma catecholamines are particularly valuable when taken while the patient is symptomatic.

2. Urine catecholamines and metabolites: Urine may be assayed for free catecholamines or their metabolites (metanephrines or VMA). Patients with small tumors excrete mainly free catecholamines, and those with larger tumors, mainly the metabolites. Metanephrines are probably the best for initial evaluation—false positives are rare and may be due to chlorpromazine. Collections made either over 24 hours or for shorter periods, are expressed as µg per mg of creatinine. Normal values are shown in Table 8–6.

3. Regitine test: Regitine was formerly used to block the effects of circulating catecholamines. This test is nonspecific, potentially dangerous, and obsolete.

4. Glucagon test: In patients with infrequent symptoms and normal basal biochemical tests, this provocative test may occasionally be of value. False positives and false negatives may occur.

5. Clonidine test: In patients with marginally elevated plasma catecholamines, administration of clonidine 0.3 mg po does not lower plasma catecholamines if a pheochromocytoma is present. If plasma catecholamines are elevated from other causes, they should fall to normal levels in 3 hours.

HYPERTENSION IN SPECIAL GROUPS

Children. If hypertension is severe and the patient is young, a secondary cause for hypertension is assumed.[38] Additional clinical features may suggest different causes for hypertension (Table 8–7). Virilization and rapid growth may be seen in patients with 11β-hydroxylase defect. With hypogonadism (in males) and amenorrhea (in females) one should suspect 17α-hydroxylase defect. Children with hypertension and hypokalemia may have dexamethasone-suppressible hyperaldosteronism, adrenal cortical hyperplasia, renin-secreting tumor, or renovascular (fibromuscular) hypertension. The presence of abdominal bruits and weak femoral pulses in children with hypertension may suggest coarctation of the aorta.

As in adults, specialized laboratory studies should be performed (Table 8–8):

1. Renin: A high plasma renin level suggests renovascular hypertension or a renin-secreting tumor. Low renin is seen with hydroxylase defect.

2. Aldosterone: High aldosterone levels are seen with renovascular hypertension, renin-secreting tumor, and hyperaldosteronism. A low level of aldosterone occurs with a hydroxylase defect.

Table 8–7. Diagnostic Clues in Evaluation of Hypertension in Children

Clinical Clues	Disorder
Virilization and rapid growth	11β-hydroxylase defect
Hypogonadism in males and amenorrhea in females	17α-hydroxylase defect
Hypokalemia	Dexamethasone-suppressible hyperaldosteronism Adrenal cortical hyperplasia Renin-secreting tumor or renovascular hypertension
Bruit and weak femoral pulses	Coarctation of the aorta

Table 8–8. Laboratory Tests for Evaluating Hypertension in Children

Disease	Renin	Aldosterone	Urine		Plasma DOC	Plasma Androgens
			DOC	17-oxosteroids		
Renovascular	↑	↑	N	N	N	N
Renin-secreting tumors	↑	↑	N	N	N	N
Hyperaldosteronism	↓	↑	N	N	N	N
Hydroxylase defect						
11β-hydroxylase	↓	↓	↑	↑	↑	↑
17α-hydroxylase	↓	↓	↑	↓	↑	N

3. Urine deoxycorticosterone (DOC) and 17-oxosteroids: If both urine DOC and 17-oxosteroids are elevated, 11β-hydroxylase defect is likely. If DOC is high but 17-oxosteroids are low, 17α-hydroxylase defect is likely. If plasma DOC is high, 11β-hydroxylase or 17α-hydroxylase defects are possible. The presence of high plasma androgens is more likely with 11β-hydroxylase defects.

Pregnant Women. In pregnant women, a diastolic blood pressure above 90 mm Hg in the third trimester is considered abnormal.[39] It is important to distinguish pre-eclampsia from other causes of hypertension. Pre-eclampsia is likely if a primigravid patient with no previous history of hypertension suddenly develops high blood pressure after the twentieth week. A 24-hour urine protein excretion above 300 mg/24 hours favors pre-eclampsia. Serum uric acid elevation also supports the diagnosis of pre-eclampsia and indicates a poor fetal prognosis. Sudden weight gain and edema are more compatible with pre-eclampsia, whereas the absence of these features is more consistent with chronic hypertension. Pre-eclampsia may also be superimposed on chronic hypertension.

Elderly Patients. In elderly patients, isolated systolic hypertension is very common and is thought to occur as a result of decreased arterial compliance.[40] If there is both systolic and diastolic hypertension of recent onset, a renovascular cause should be suspected. In these patients plasma renin activity is likely to be high, in contrast to the majority of elderly patients with essential hypertension, in whom low-renin hypertension is common. In many elderly patients, blood pressure may fall markedly when they stand up and after they eat. It should be remembered that in some patients whose systolic pressure appears to be elevated when measured by auscultatory method, direct intra-arterial readings may show much lower pressures. This has been termed "pseudo-hypertension of the elderly" and is probably another manifestation of decreased arterial compliance.

REFERENCES

1. Pickering, T.G., et al.: Comparisons of blood pressure during normal daily activities, sleep, and exercise in normal and hypertensive subjects. JAMA *247*:992, 1982.
2. Pickering, G.W.: Normotension and hypertension: The mysterious viability of the false. Am J Med *85*:561, 1978.
3. Kannel, W.B., and Gordon, T.: The Framingham Study. An epidemiological investigation of cardiovascular disease. Section 31. DHEW Publication No. (NIH) 70-1083, 1976.
4. Kincaid-Smith, P.: Malignant hypertension. Cardiovasc Rev Reports *1*:42–50, 1980.
5. Naftchi, N.E., Demeny, M., Lowman, E.W., and Tuckman, J.: Hypertensive crises in quadriplegic patients. Changes in cardiac output, blood volume, serum dopamine-β-hydroxylase activity, and arterial prostaglandin PGE₂. Circulation *57*:336–342, 1978.
6. Reis, D.J., and Doba, N.: Hypertension as a localizing sign of mass lesions of brain stem. N Engl J Med *287*:1355–6, 1972.
7. Kuchel, O., et al.: Dopamine surges in hyperadrenergic essential hypertension. Hypertension *4*:845–852, 1982.
8. Rowe, J.W.: Systolic hypertension in the elderly. N Engl J Med *309*:1246–1247, 1983.
9. Tamaki, K., el al.: Evidence that disruption of the blood-brain barrier precedes reduction in cerebral blood flow in hypertensive encephalopathy. Hypertension *6*:(Suppl 1) 75, 1984.
10. The 1984 Report of the Joint National Committee on Detection, Evaluation and Treatment of High Blood Pressure. Arch Intern Med *144*:1045–1047, 1984.
11. Vaughan, E.D., el al.: Clinical evaluation of renovascular hypertension and therapeutic decisions. Urol Clin N Am *11*:393–407, 1984.
12. Kincaid-Smith, P.: Parenchymatous diseases of the kidney and hypertension. *In* Hypertension. Edited by J. Genest, et al. New York, McGraw-Hill, 1983, pp. 989–1006.
13. Weinberger, M.H., et al.: Primary aldosteronism. Diagnosis, localization, and treatment. Ann Intern Med *90*:386–389, 1979.
14. Biglieri, E.G.: Adrenocortical components in hypertension. Cardiovasc Rev Reports *3*:734–738, 1982.
15. Liddle, G.W., Bledose, T., Coppage, W.S.: A familial renal disorder simulating primary aldosteronism but with negligible aldosterone secretion. Trans Assoc Am Physicians *76*:199–213, 1963.
16. Bravo, E.L., and Gifford, R.W.: Current concepts: pheochromocytoma: diagnosis, localization and management. N Engl J Med *311*:1298–1302, 1984.
17. Liberthson, R.R., Pennington, D.G., Jacobs, M.L., and Daggett, W.M.: Coarctation of the aorta: review of 234 patients and clarification of management problems. Am J Cardiol *43*:835–840, 1979.
18. Baruch, D., et al.: Diagnosis and treatment of renin secreting tumors. Hypertension *6*:760–766, 1984.
19. Hamet, P.: Endocrine hypertension: Cushing's syndrome, acromegaly, hyperparathyroidism, thyrotoxicosis and hypothyroid-

ism. *In* Hypertension. Edited by J. Genest, et al. New York, McGraw-Hill, 1983, pp. 964–975.

20. Whitman, H.H., et al.: Variable response to oral angiotensin-converting-enzyme blockade in hypertensive scleroderma patients. Arthritis Rheum *25*:241–248, 1982.
21. Pickering, T.G., Lockshin, M.D., and Eisenmenger, W.J.: Renin-dependent hypertension in polyarteritis nodosa. Br Med J *1*:1758, 1981.
22. Christlieb, A.R.: Diabetes and hypertension. Cardiovasc Rev Reports *1*:609–616, 1980.
23. Larbi, E.B., Cooper, R.S., and Stamler, J.: Alcohol and hypertension. Arch Intern Med *143*:28–29, 1983.
24. Nicholson, J.P., et al.: Cigarette smoking and renovascular hypertension. Lancet *1*:765–766, 1983.
25. Devereux, R.B., and Reichek, N.: Left ventricular hypertrophy. Cardiovasc Rev Reports *1*:55–61, 1980.
26. Dollery, C.T.: Hypertensive retinopathy. *In* Hypertension. Edited by J. Genest, et al. New York, McGraw-Hill, 1983, pp. 723–731.
27. Sims, E.A.: Mechanisms of hypertension in the overweight. Hypertension *4*(Suppl III): III–43–49, 1982.
28. Robinson, J.O.: Symptoms and the discovery of high blood pressure. J Psychosom Res *13*:157–161, 1969.
29. Stewart, I McD G.: Headache and hypertension. Lancet *1*:1261–1266, 1953.
30. Bulpitt, C.J., Dollery, C.T., and Carne, S.: Change in symptoms of hypertensive patients after referral to hospital clinic. Br Heart J *38*:121–128, 1976.
31. Kleinert, H.D., et al.: What is the value of home blood pressure measurement in patients with mild hypertension? Hypertension *6*:574–578, 1984.
32. Pickering, T.G., Harshfield, G.A., Devereux, R.B., and Laragh, J.H.: What is the role of ambulatory blood pressure monitoring in the management of hypertensive patients? Hypertension *7*:171–177, 1985.
33. Laragh, J.H., Sealey, J.E., Niarchos, A.P., Pickering, T.G.: The vasoconstriction-volume spectrum in normotensive and pathogenesis of hypertension. Fed Proc *41*:2415, 1982.
34. Aldigier, J., et al.: Comparison of the hormonal and renal effects of captopril in severe essential and renovascular hypertension. Am J Cardiol *49*:1447–1452, 1982.
35. Zabbo, A., and Novich, A.C.: Digital subtraction angiography for noninvasive imaging of the renal artery. Urol Clin N Am *11*:409–416, 1984.
36. Krakoff, L.R., Ribiero, A.B., Gorkin, J.U., and Felton, K.R.: Saralasin infusion in screening patients for renovascular hypertension. Am J Cardiol *45*:609–613, 1980.
37. Gross, M.D., Grekin, R.J., Gniadek, T.C., and Villaveal, J.Z.: Suppression of aldosterone by cyproheptadine in idiopathic aldosteronism. N Engl J Med *305*:181–184, 1981.
38. New, M.I., and Levine, L.S.: Hypertension in childhood and adolescence. Cardiovasc Rev Reports *3*:115–119, 1982.
39. Lindheimer, M.D.: Some Unresolved Controversies Concerning the Pathophysiology and Management of Preeclampsia. Vol 4. Controversies in Nephrology. Edited by G.E. Schreiner, et al. Bethesda, Georgetown University, 1984, pp 177–194.
40. Gifford, R.W.: Isolated systolic hypertension in the elderly: some controversial issues. JAMA *247*:781–785, 1982.

CHAPTER 9

RENAL PROBLEMS

Alan S. Kliger, M.D. and Jeffrey S. Berns, M.D.

CLINICAL PROBLEMS

The normal human kidneys perform several functions to maintain the normal internal environment. These functions include:

1. excreting urea and other nitrogenous products of metabolism
2. maintaining constant the body's fluid volume
3. maintaining constant the body's osmolar concentration
4. maintaining constant the extracellular concentration of sodium and chloride
5. participating in the balance of many substances located principally in cells and organs, such as potassium, calcium, magnesium, and phosphorus
6. working with the lungs to maintain the acid-base homeostasis
7. producing substances such as renin and prostaglandin to regulate renal blood flow and systemic blood pressure
8. altering substances such as 25-OH vitamin D to the more active 1,25-$(OH)_2$ vitamin D to effect bone and calcium homeostasis
9. elaborating erythropoietin to enable adequate red blood cell production by bone marrow

Renal dysfunction eventually results in abnormalities of one or more of these processes. Thus, patients with end-stage renal failure may demonstrate total body fluid overload, inability to promptly excrete an ingested sodium load, metabolic acidosis, anemia, hypertension, hypocalcemia, and hyperphosphatemia. Interestingly, however, in the progression of renal disease none of these abnormalities may arise until more than 80% of the normal glomerular filtration rate (GFR) has been lost. The kidney, even when damaged by disease, usually retains its ability to maintain the body's internal integrity until far advanced, irreversible disease is present.

For this reason, signs and symptoms of renal disease other than the metabolic abnormalities of end-stage disease must be determined by the physician seeking the earliest manifestations of diseases of the kidney. Some signs of renal dysfunction can be found during routine outpatient visits, while others require laboratory or radiographic investigations. Such studies include:

1. Examination of the urinary sediment. A freshly voided urine specimen can be tested with a dipstick to detect abnormal albumin, heme pigment, pH, glucose, bilirubin, and other substances. An aliquot of urine can then be centrifuged for 3 to 5 minutes and the sediment examined under the microscope. Abnormal casts, cells, or crystals often lead to a diagnosis of renal dysfunction.
2. Measurement of the glomerular filtration rate. The glomerular filtration rate may be estimated by measuring the renal clearance of creatinine. This is accomplished easily by collecting a timed specimen of urine (often a 24-hour collection) and a simultaneous plasma sample for measurement of creatinine. The creatinine clearance is then calculated as

$$Ccr = \frac{Ucr \times V}{Pcr \times t}$$

where
Ccr = creatinine clearance (ml/min)
Ucr = concentration of creatinine in urine (mg/dl)
V = volume of urine collected (ml)
Pcr = concentration of creatinine in plasma (mg/dl)
t = time of urine collection (min)

3. Quantification of urinary protein excretion. The timed urine collection for creatinine clearance can also be used to measure the amount of urinary protein.
4. Studies of the renal anatomy. Kidney disorders are accompanied at times by abnormalities of their gross appearance. Large or small kidneys, asymmetrical kidneys, hydroureter or hydronephrosis, or tumor mass distorting the kidney, ureter, or bladder can be detected by radiographic or ultrasound examination. Such studies might include intravenous pyelography, renal ultrasonography and Doppler study, radioisotope renal scan, digital intravenous angiography, and renal arteriography.
5. Renal biopsy. Percutaneous biopsy of the kidney and study of the tissue with light and electron microscopy and with immunofluorescent microscopy permits an accurate histologic diagnosis. When abnormal glomerular filtration rate, proteinuria, or hematuria are not explained adequately by other noninvasive studies, renal biopsy is often indicated.

In the sections that follow are discussed the cardinal signs of renal dysfunction, including hematuria, proteinuria, pyuria, oliguria, and polyuria. Next, metabolic derangements of fluids, electrolytes, and the acid-base balance are outlined (see also Chapter 10). Thereafter, specific diseases of the kidney are described.

HEMATURIA

DEFINITION

"Hematuria" means blood in the urine. When "gross hematuria" is present, the urine is discolored by blood and may appear tea colored or cola colored. Smaller amounts of hematuria (up to 10 red blood cells per high power field), or "microscopic hematuria," do not discolor the urine to the naked eye but do reveal red blood cells on microscopic examination. Of normal urine samples, 90% have less than one red blood cell per high power field. More than two or three red blood cells per high power field usually signifies an abnormality of the urinary tract.

PATHOPHYSIOLOGIC CONSIDERATIONS AND DIFFERENTIAL DIAGNOSIS

Bleeding into the urinary system may originate anywhere from the glomerular capillary loop to the end of the urethra. It may result from an inflammatory process that alters the integrity of the glomerular or tubular basement membrane, allowing red cells to enter the urinary space; from tumors altering the vascular bed; from stones abrading the epithelium; or from infections or drugs causing inflammatory cystitis.

It is useful clinically to categorize hematuria as coming from the upper tract (from the kidneys) or from the lower tract (from the ureters, bladder, or urethra) (Table 9–1).[1] Bleeding from the glomerulus results from glomerulonephritis, which may be inflammation limited to the kidney (primary renal disease) or one manifestation of a more widespread disease (systemic renal disease). Glomerulonephritis is often accompanied by proteinuria and an active urine sediment with white blood cells, granular casts, and red blood cell casts. Bleeding from the renal interstitium may result from inflammation, anatomic abnormalities, a bleeding disorder, or infarcted, necrotic tissue. Bleeding from the lower urinary tract commonly results from infection, stones, or tumor in the ureters, bladder, prostate gland, or urethra.

Occasionally, microscopic hematuria may be found in normal individuals after heavy exercise, or in patients with congestive heart failure.

DIAGNOSTIC EVALUATION

Patient History

The physician should look for evidence of acute cystitis or prostatitis, including fever, urinary fre-

Table 9–1. Causes of Hematuria

Bleeding from the kidney
  Glomerulonephritis
    Primary renal diseases
      Recurrent "benign" hematuria
      Acute proliferative glomerulonephritis
      Membranoproliferative glomerulonephritis
      Focal glomerulosclerosis
      Lipoid nephrosis
    Systemic diseases
      Vasculitis (systemic lupus erythematosus, Wegener's granulomatosis, periarteritis nodosa, etc.)
      Endovasculitis (acute and subacute bacterial endocarditis, shunt nephritis)
      Goodpasture's syndrome
      Thrombotic microangiopathy (thrombotic thrombocytopenic purpura, hemolytic-uremic syndrome, peripartum renal failure)
      Malignant hypertension
      Diabetic glomerulosclerosis
    Hereditary diseases
      Alport's syndrome
      Fabry's disease
      Nail-patella syndrome
  Renal interstitial diseases
    Arteriovenous malformations
    Polycystic kidney
    Cystic disease of the renal medulla (medullary sponge kidney, medullary cystic disease)
    Papillary necrosis
    Sickle-cell disease or trait
    Renal infiltrate (e.g., lymphoma, renal cell carcinoma)
    Allergic interstitial nephritis
    Renal infarction
    Trauma
Lower urinary tract bleeding
  Bacterial infection of bladder, prostate, urethra
  Tumors of ureter, bladder, prostate, urethra
  Stones
  Congenital anomalies
  Vascular anomalies
  Allergic cystitis, urethritis
  Trauma
  Foreign bodies

quency, and dysuria (pain on urination). Previous renal stones or migrating colicky pain suggests nephrolithiasis. The possibility of pulmonary tuberculosis or exposure to this infection must be explored. A thorough drug history must be taken, since analgesics may cause papillary necrosis, and other medications may lead to hemorrhagic cystitis. Recent trauma may suggest a cause for sudden hematuria, while sudden flank pain and hematuria without trauma may suggest renal infarction. Abnormalities of other organ systems, such as rash, fever, arthritis, cough, or lung disease, may lead to a diagnosis of a systemic disease. A careful family history must be taken, since patients with sickle cell anemia, polycystic kidney disease, medullary cystic disease, Alport's syndrome, or benign familial hematuria will often report hematuria or kidney disease in family members. Children and an occasional adult will report foreign body insertion into the urethra causing hematuria.

Physical Examination

A careful examination of the blood pressure, fundi, skin, joints, heart, lungs, and abdomen may give clues to a systemic disease. The kidneys are palpably enlarged in polycystic kidney disease, and costovertebral angle tenderness can be elicited with pyelonephritis and sometimes with trauma or renal infarction.

Diagnostic Studies

LABORATORY TESTS

A fresh, concentrated urine sample can provide much information. Urinalysis is best performed on the second voided specimen of the morning. A dipstick examination for pH, protein, "blood" (pigment), and glucose is done, and the spun sediment is examined for cells, casts, bacteria, and crystals. The finding of red cell casts suggests glomerular origin of hematuria, while sheets of white cells suggest infection.

A urine culture for bacteria should be performed and a culture for mycobacteria obtained when tuberculosis is suspected.

A 24-hour collection of urine should be obtained for measurement of protein and creatinine excretion, and the creatinine clearance should be calculated.

Initial blood studies should include a complete blood count, platelet count, coagulation studies (prothrombin and partial thromboplastin times), serum urea, and creatinine levels. If glomerulonephritis is suspected, serology studies should be obtained, including complement (C3, C4), antinuclear antibody, and HB$_s$Ag; an erythrocyte sedimentation rate should be measured. Black patients and others with a positive family history should be screened for sickle cell hemoglobin.

Radiographic studies may also be performed. An *abdominal radiograph* should be examined to locate possible stones or calcium deposition in the kidneys (nephrocalcinosis) and to estimate renal size. A renal ultrasound examination can show kidney size, mass abnormalities, and obstruction with hydroureter or hydronephrosis, without the modest risk of nephrotoxicity from intravenous contrast material. In most patients, an intravenous pyelogram is desirable to examine more carefully the anatomy of the kidneys, ureters, and bladder. At times, a computed tomography (CT) scan can show renal or perirenal disease that is not appreciated with standard pyelography and can also show blood clot within the renal artery or vein. When lower tract bleeding remains in the differential diag-

nosis after these studies, cystoscopy should be performed in adults. Isotopic imaging (renal scan) can show the overall perfusion, filtration, and size of the kidneys; this study can show asymmetrical perfusion or renal infarction. A renal arteriogram shows in detail the renal vascular supply and can determine the presence of A–V malformations, the extent of renal tumors or infarcts, or the aneurysms characteristic of periarteritis nodosum. Renal venography, particularly when coupled to intra-arterial epinephrine injection, can demonstrate the presence of renal vein thrombosis.

Renal biopsy is considered when the evaluation suggests glomerular disorder. A tissue diagnosis can provide prognostic and therapeutic information for the patient and physician.

PROTEINURIA

DEFINITION

Daily protein excretion in the urine exceeding 150 mg is abnormal and usually represents an impairment of the renal function. Normally about 50% of urinary protein is derived from the plasma (principally albumin), and the other 50% from renal tubular cells or the lower urinary tract. Protein excretion exceeding 150 mg/day may be the result of increased filtration or enhanced secretion. Glomerular-derived proteinuria may be marked, exceeding several grams per day of albumin excretion. If abnormal proteins are present in the plasma, these may be filtered and appear in the urine. Tubular-derived proteinuria, a mixture of lower molecular weight proteins, usually is less than 1 g/day.

PATHOPHYSIOLOGIC CONSIDERATIONS

Plasma proteins enter the glomerular capillary and encounter the filtration barrier, the glomerular basement membrane. This barrier is both size- and charge-selective, so that large, negatively charged molecules like albumin are filtered to a very small extent. Filtered albumin enters the proximal renal tubule, and cells of this tubular segment resorb much of this protein. Vacuolization and catabolism of these proteins follow. Therefore, only 20 to 50 mg of albumin move from the proximal tubule to the loop of Henle each day. Small amounts of smaller plasma proteins also are filtered. As the filtrate enters the loop of Henle, the distal tubule, and the collecting duct, cells lining these segments excrete a large glycoprotein, Tamm-Horsfall protein, into the tubular fluid. This uromucoid is the protein of urinary casts, and 30 to 60 mg/day are excreted. Finally, trace amounts of nonplasma proteins enter the urine in the lower urinary tract.[3]

Protein excretion increases transiently above these levels following heavy exercise, emotional stress, fever, or prolonged upright posture. Some patients with congestive heart failure also increase their protein excretion. Most patients with proteinuria have an abnormality of the kidney. Diseases of the glomerulus may increase the basement membrane permeability to albumin dramatically, resulting in increased filtration and excretion. Tubular abnormalities may result in increased lower molecular weight protein excretion. Finally, when a monoclonal gammopathy increases production of immunoglobulin protein fragments, increased glomerular filtration results in proteinuria.

DIFFERENTIAL DIAGNOSIS

Quantification and characterization of increased urinary protein helps to establish the underlying cause of the disorder (Table 9–2). When excretion exceeds 3 g/day and the protein is largely albumin, glomerulonephritis is the likely diagnosis. Mixed proteinuria of less than 1 g/day, in which much nonalbumin protein is present, suggests a tubular origin. Increased light-chain or heavy chain protein fragments of immunoglobulin in the urine suggest the diagnosis of monoclonal gammopathy, multiple myeloma, macroglobulinemia, or heavy-chain disease.

Proteinuria may be a variant of normal renal function, may reflect circulatory diseases, or may be caused by primary glomerular or tubular diseases.

DIAGNOSTIC EVALUATION

Diagnostic Studies[2]

The most common screening test for urinary proteins is a paper strip (''dipstick'') impregnated with tetra-bromphenol and a buffer to maintain the pH at 3.0. The color changes as the protein concentration rises. When urinary protein is detected, a quantitative 24-hour urinary protein excretion is measured and its composition determined by urinary protein electrophoresis. In patients with a positive screening test for urinary protein but no hematuria, hypertension, or renal functional impairment, diagnosis of intermittent or postural proteinuria should be considered before proceeding to a full evaluation. The urine should be tested once or twice more. In children or young adults, postural pro-

Table 9–2. Causes of Proteinuria

Variations of normal kidney function
  Intermittent proteinuria
    Exercise
    Fever
    Emotional stress
    Lordotic position
Proteinuria with normal renal function
  Circulatory disease
    Congestive heart failure
    Constrictive pericarditis
    Renal vein thrombosis
  Increased immunoglobulin
    Multiple myeloma
    Macroglobulinemia
    Monoclonal gammopathy
    Heavy-chain disease
    Idiopathic light-chain disease
Proteinuria of renal origin
  Glomerulonephritis
    Systemic diseases affecting the kidney
      Diabetes mellitus
      Goodpasture's syndrome
      Vasculitis (systemic lupus erythematosus, Wegener's granulomatosis, periarteritis nodosa, etc.)
      Endovasculitis (acute and subacute bacterial endocarditis, shunt nephritis)
      Thrombotic microangiopathy (thrombotic thrombocytopenic purpura, hemolytic-uremic syndrome, peripartum renal failure)
      Multiple myeloma
      Amyloidosis
      Toxemia of pregnancy
      Cryoglobulinemia
      Scleroderma
      Lymphoma
    Inherited diseases
      Fabry's disease
      Nail-patella syndrome
      Alport's syndrome
      Polycystic kidney disease
      Sickle cell disease
    Primary renal diseases
      Minimal change disease
      Mesangioproliferative glomerulonephritis
      Idiopathic membranous glomerulonephritis
      Proliferative glomerulonephritis
        Acute poststreptococcal glomerulonephritis
      Membranoproliferative glomerulonephritis
      Focal hyalinosis and glomerulosclerosis
      Chronic nonspecific glomerulonephritis
      Rapidly progressive glomerulonephritis
      Radiation nephritis
      Heavy metal nephrotoxicity (mercury, gold, bismuth)
      Anticonvulsant glomerulonephritis (trichone, others)
      Other drugs and toxins
        Tolbutamide, probenecid, sulfonamides, penicillamine
        Insect stings, snake bites
Interstitial diseases and tubular dysfunction
  Acute and chronic interstitial nephritis
  Fanconi's syndrome
  Nephrotoxins (beryllium, cadmium, lead, lithium)
  Hypertonic injury
    Radiographic contrast materials
    Mannitol

teinuria can be detected by separate urine collections with the patient supine and upright. The urine dipstick test may not detect the presence of immunoglobulin fragments, so urine should also be tested with 5% sulfosalicylic acid. When protein is present, several drops added to an aliquot of urine results in the formation of a precipitate.

The glomerular filtration rate may be estimated by the creatinine clearance. Blood tests to exclude systemic diseases include complete blood count, platelet count, erythrocyte sedimentation rate, serum glucose or glycosylated hemoglobin, serum protein electrophoresis, cryoglobulin, antinuclear antibody, C3, C4, and HB_sAg.

Patient History and Physical Examination

The remainder of the evaluation will depend upon the information derived from the history and physical examination. The anatomy of the kidney may be examined by intravenous pyelography, ultrasonography, or other methods.

NEPHROTIC SYNDROME

DEFINITION

When diseases of the glomerulus cause sufficient proteinuria to reduce the plasma concentration of albumin, a distinct clinical syndrome may result. The nephrotic syndrome is characterized by massive proteinuria, hypoproteinemia, edema, lipidemia, and lipiduria. If prolonged, severe proteinuria may also lead to protein malnutrition, venous thrombosis, arteriosclerosis, and infection. Some patients also have hypocalcemia out of proportion to hypoalbuminuria, and some have aminoaciduria. The rate of protein excretion necessary to produce this clinical syndrome varies from patient to patient but is usually in excess of 3.5 g/24 hours. It is important to note, however, that the presence of ''full-blown'' nephrotic syndrome carries no specific etiologic significance. The presence of proteinuria with or without the nephrotic syndrome requires the same differential diagnosis and evaluation.[4]

PATHOPHYSIOLOGIC CONSIDERATIONS

Increased excretion of plasma proteins, including most prominently albumin, eventually leads to hypoalbuminemia when the renal excretion rate exceeds the increase in production of new albumin. The lowered intravascular osmotic pressure shifts capillary forces toward greater filtration, and interstitial fluid increases, resulting in clinical edema. The edema increases until interstitial tissue pressure equals the net decrease in osmotic pressure. The loss of intravascular fluid into the interstitial space causes intravascular volume depletion and consequent activation of homeostatic mechanisms to maintain the salt and water balance. This may result in an overall increase in sodium and water content in the nephrotic patient.

Elevated levels of plasma lipids, including cholesterol, phospholipids, and triglycerides, are found. The reason for this increase is not understood completely. Increased albumin synthesis is accompanied by increased synthesis of lipoprotein. In addition, profound hypoalbuminemia inhibits peripheral lipolysis. Both processes result in high levels of plasma lipids.

Lipids enter the urine, where, entrapped in casts, they appear as oval fat bodies. Hyperlipemic states not accompanied by renal disease are not characterized by lipiduria. Thus it is likely that glomerular damage in the nephrotic syndrome allows filtration of plasma lipids across the basement membrane. Some lipoproteins are reabsorbed by tubular epithelial cells, and the remainder result in lipiduria.

Low levels of plasma-ionized calcium may be caused by depressed intestinal absorption of calcium in some patients. This may result from disordered vitamin D metabolism associated with the massive proteinuria in this syndrome.

DIFFERENTIAL DIAGNOSIS

The differential diagnosis for the nephrotic syndrome is the same as that for proteinuria (see previous section on proteinuria).

DIAGNOSTIC EVALUATION

In addition to having the diagnostic studies outlined for proteinuria, patients with the nephrotic syndrome should have calcium, cholesterol, and triglycerides measured. Quantitation of low density lipoproteins (LDL) and very low density lipoproteins (VLDL) may be indicated in patients at risk for accelerated arteriosclerosis. The urine should be examined under a polarized light field to search for doubly refractile fat bodies.

PYURIA

DEFINITION

Pyuria, or "pus in the urine," denotes an increased excretion of white blood cells into the urine. When a urine sediment is viewed under a microscope, more than one or two white blood cells per high power field represents abnormal pyuria.

PATHOPHYSIOLOGIC CONSIDERATIONS

Virtually any inflammatory process of the urinary tract may cause shedding of leukocytes and hence pyuria. Infections, neoplasms, stones or foreign bodies in the lower urinary tract, and primary renal diseases all may induce pyuria. The most common causes of pyuria are listed in Table 9–3.

DIFFERENTIAL DIAGNOSIS AND DIAGNOSTIC EVALUATION

The most frequent diagnosis is infection of the lower urinary tract: bacterial cystitis in women, and prostatitis or urethritis in men. Patients frequently are

Table 9–3. Causes of Pyuria

Lower urinary tract: urethra, bladder, prostate, epididymis, ureter
  Infection
    Bacterial
    Fungal
    Viral or "nonspecific" (commonly prostatitis or urethritis)
  Renal stones
  Neoplasm
  Foreign bodies in urethra or bladder
  Allergic cystitis
  Vaginitis and contamination of urine specimen with cells from the vagina
Upper urinary tract: glomerulus, renal interstitium, papillae, calyces
  Infection
    Pyelonephritis
    Renal tuberculosis
    Infected cyst, diverticulum, or other intrarenal abscess
    Perinephric abscess
  Papillary necrosis
  Chronic interstitial nephritis
  Anatomic defects
    Polycystic kidney disease
    Medullary sponge kidney
  Primary renal diseases
  Neoplasm
    Hypernephroma
  Renal stones

symptomatic, with urinary urgency, frequency, pain, or discomfort, and they sometimes have systemic symptoms of fever, lethargy, nausea, and vomiting. Young women often develop cystitis—so-called honeymoon cystitis—shortly after they become sexually active. Likewise, young men may experience symptomatic prostatitis following a sudden increase or decrease of sexual activity. When high fever, rigor, and flank pain are present, acute pyelonephritis is likely.

A careful history helps to focus on the most likely diagnosis. Is there a history of previous urinary infections, stones, vaginal discharge, fever, weight loss, pain? The physical examination should elicit any percussion tenderness over the kidneys or bladder and must include in women a pelvic examination and in men a rectal, prostate, and epididymis examination.

Laboratory evaluation should first include a urinalysis and culture of a "clean-catch" midstream urine sample. Pyuria alone, without hematuria, proteinuria, or urinary casts, usually suggests lower urinary tract infection, although hematuria and some proteinuria also may be present in uncomplicated lower tract infections. Cellular or granular urinary casts suggest an upper tract source of pyuria. "Sterile pyuria" should raise the question of renal tuberculosis.

When nephrolithiasis is suspected, radiographic studies including a plain film of the abdomen, cone views, oblique views, and nephrotomograms may reveal the presence of radiopaque stones. An intravenous pyelogram (IVP) using intravenous radio contrast materials is very useful in detecting stones, cysts, renal tuberculosis, tumors, and other anatomic abnormalities. CT scan with radio contrast is particularly sensitive to small abnormalities.

When hematuria and proteinuria are found with pyuria, an elevation for primary renal diseases must be undertaken (see sections on hematuria and proteinuria).

OLIGURIA

DEFINITION

A reduction of urine volume below that required to excrete the obligatory solute load is a sign of renal failure and is termed oliguria. The solute load that must be excreted in the urine each day is approximately 700 to 1500 mOsm. Since maximum urine concentration is about 1200 mOsm/kg H_2O, a urine volume of at least 400 to 600 ml is required to excrete this load.

Table 9–4. Laboratory Studies to Differentiate Causes of Oliguria

	Normal Response to Hypovolemia	Acute Renal Failure
Urine osmolality (mOsm/kg H_2O)	>500	<350
Urine/plasma creatinine	>40	<20
Urinary Na concentration	<10	<40
Fractional excretion of Na (%)	<1	>3

PATHOPHYSIOLOGIC CONSIDERATIONS

The physiologic changes of acute renal failure are the subject of intensive investigation and have not been delineated clearly. A drastic reduction of glomerular filtration causes oliguria. However, even if the glomerular filtration rate (GFR) is only 4 ml/minute, each day 5.8 L of tubular fluid are formed. If the obligatory proximal and distal tubular reabsorption rates were 85%, more than 800 ml of urine would still be formed daily. Therefore, many investigators believe that patients with oliguric renal failure have tubular obstruction or defects of the renal tubular cells, with abnormally increased passive "backleak" of tubular fluid.

DIFFERENTIAL DIAGNOSIS

Reduced urine volume may be a normal physiologic response to hypovolemia, a rapidly reversible effect of hypotension, or a sign of renal failure. Since the minimal urine volume required to excrete the daily solute load varies widely from one individual to the next and is dependent upon body size, diet, and maximal urine concentrating capacity, the urine volume is actually a poor way to differentiate among these possible diagnoses. Measurement of renal tubular functions, including sodium reabsorption and concentrating ability, can help differentiate the causes of oliguria (Table 9–4).

DIAGNOSTIC EVALUATION

When a patient presents with oliguria, shock or hypotension must be excluded. Next, a clinical assessment of intravascular volume must be made. When such an assessment cannot be made easily, or when primary heart disease, lung disease, or liver disease complicates the picture, direct measurements of cardiac filling pressures should be made. The pulmonary artery and pulmonary capillary wedge pressures can be measured by inserting an intravenous intracardiac Swan-Ganz catheter.

RENAL TUBULAR ACIDOSIS

When the kidney is unable to excrete acids normally, metabolic acidosis may result. The renal tubule has evolved a complex mechanism for bicarbonate reabsorption and hydrogen ion excretion, a system that regulates buffer base concentration in the plasma and mediates the excretion of fixed acid from the body. Defects in various parts of this system may lead to bicarbonate loss or failure to excrete acids (see Chapter 10). This group of diseases is called renal tubular acidosis (RTA) and will be considered according to the underlying renal tubular defect.

DISTAL RTA (TYPE I, CLASSIC RTA)

DEFINITION

A defect in the distal tubule's normal ability to secrete hydrogen ions into the tubular lumen impairs renal acid excretion and may result in hyperchloremic metabolic acidosis with persistently high urine pH (>5.5).

PATHOPHYSIOLOGIC CONSIDERATIONS

Under normal conditions, the distal tubule and collecting duct of the kidney can secrete hydrogen ions against a steep concentration gradient. Whereas plasma pH is 7.4, the urine pH can be lowered to 4.5. This decrease of nearly 3 units means an almost one thousandfold concentration of hydrogen ions in the urine. This ability of the distal tubule and collecting duct to concentrate hydrogen ions allows the kidney to reabsorb the 5 to 20% of filtered bicarbonate that escapes reabsorption in the proximal tubule and also to titrate intraluminal buffers (e.g., phosphates) and ammonium to complete excretion of the body's acid load.

In distal RTA, this system of final bicarbonate reabsorption and hydrogen ion excretion is impaired, resulting in persistent loss of bicarbonate, even during acidosis. In addition, acid excretion via titratable acids and ammonium is decreased. This combination results in slowly progressive hyperchloremic metabolic acidosis leading to profound acidemia, sometimes with plasma bicarbonate concentrations of less than 10 mEq/L or even 5 mEq/L.

Other metabolic consequences ensue. Chronic bicarbonaturia results in volume depletion and in stimulation of the renin-angiotensin-aldosterone axis. The persistence of bicarbonate in the distal nephron and collecting duct, particularly in the presence of aldosterone, increases potassium secretion, and hypokalemia results. Calcium excretion in the urine is increased as well, since an acidosis suppresses distal tubular calcium reabsorption. Nephrocalcinosis and nephrolithiasis may result and may further damage the renal function, with obstruction, interstitial nephritis, and eventually a fall in glomerular filtration.

DIFFERENTIAL DIAGNOSIS

Many abnormalities have been associated with distal RTA (Table 9–5).[6,7] These include renal disease causing nephrocalcinosis or tubulointerstitial diseases, autoimmune disorders, genetic disease, and drug- or toxin-induced nephropathy.

DIAGNOSTIC EVALUATION

In every patient with hyperchloremic metabolic acidosis, the urine pH should be tested in a fresh specimen with a pH meter. When acidemia is present, a urine pH >5.5 confirms the diagnosis of distal RTA. When acidemia is not present, as measured by the plasma bicarbonate and arterial pH, ammonium chloride may be administered to induce acute acidemia, and the urine pH tested again. In patients with distal RTA, sulfate loading does not increase hydrogen ion excretion as it does in normal subjects. The plasma potassium should be measured and is characteristically depressed, although correction of the acidemia reduces potassium secretion and tends to restore plasma potassium toward normal. The kidneys should be examined by ultrasound or radiography, to search for nephrolithiasis and nephrocalcinosis. The renal function should be measured by estimating the glomerular filtration rate with creatinine clearance, and other distal tubular functions such as concentrating ability should be tested. The urine should be cultured. Plasma calcium concentration and 24-hour urinary calcium excretion should be measured. Where appropriate, tests of the immune system, globulin level, and liver function should be performed.

Table 9–5. Conditions Associated with Distal RTA

Renal diseases causing nephrocalcinosis
  Primary hyperparathyroidism
  Vitamin D intoxication
  Idiopathic hypercalciuria
  Hyperthyroidism
  Medullary sponge kidney
  Fabry's disease
Renal tubulointerstitial diseases
  Chronic interstitial nephritis secondary to obstruction
  Chronic pyelonephritis
  Renal transplantation
  Leprosy
  Hyperoxaluria
  Medullary cystic disease
Autoimmune disorders
  Familial hypergammaglobulinemia
  Hyperglobulinemic purpura
  Cryoglobulinemia
  Sjögren's syndrome
  Thyroiditis
  Pulmonary alveolitis
  Primary biliary cirrhosis
  Chronic active hepatitis
  Systemic lupus erythematosus
Genetic diseases
  Ehlers-Danlos syndrome
  Hereditary elliptocytosis
  Sickle cell anemia
  Carbonic anhydrase B deficiency
Other
  Hepatic cirrhosis
  Empty-sella syndrome
  Idiopathic RTA

(Adapted from Sebastian, A., McSherry, E., and Curtis Morris, R.: Metabolic acidosis with special reference to the renal acidoses. *In* The Kidney. Edited by B.M. Brenner and F.C. Rector, Jr. Philadelphia, W.B. Saunders Co., 1976; and Cogan, M.G., Rector, F.C., and Seldin, D.W.: Acid base disorders. *In* The Kidney. 2nd Ed. Edited by B.M. Brenner and F.C. Rector, Jr. Philadelphia, W.B. Saunders Co., 1981.)

PROXIMAL RTA (TYPE 2)

DEFINITION

The proximal tubule of the kidney is responsible for reabsorbing the bulk of filtered bicarbonate. In the normal kidneys 80% of the filtered load, or approximately 3 mEq/minute, is reabsorbed in this tubular segment. A defect in proximal tubular capacity to reabsorb bicarbonate dramatically increases the delivery of bicarbonate to the distal tubule. Even a normally functioning distal nephron cannot reabsorb this amount of bicarbonate, and much of it is dumped into the urine. This proximal renal tubular acidosis results in a hyperchloremic metabolic acidosis and bicarbonate wasting.

PATHOPHYSIOLOGIC CONSIDERATIONS

When plasma bicarbonate concentration and GFR are normal, the amount of bicarbonate reaching the distal nephron is approximately 0.75 mEq/minute, a load that can be reabsorbed by the distal nephron and collecting duct. Proximal RTA reduces from 80% to some lower figure the amount of filtered bicarbonate that is reabsorbed. The resulting doubled or tripled amount of bicarbonate reaching the latter tubular segments exceeds the segments' bicarbonate reabsorption capacity, and a large bicarbonaturia results, reducing the body's bicarbonate stores and causing the plasma bicarbonate level to fall. Once the level falls below 16 to 18 mEq/L, the amount of bicarbonate escaping the impaired reabsorptive mechanism of the proximal tubule falls. For example, if the proximal reabsorptive rate is reduced from 80% to 50% and plasma bicarbonate is 16 mEq/L, then the rate of delivery of bicarbonate out of the proximal tubule is 1.2 mEq/L, a load that the distal tubule and collecting duct can reabsorb completely. Thus, the plasma bicarbonate concentration falls to the level at which the distal tubule segments can reabsorb the remaining tubular bicarbonate. At this point, the bicarbonaturia ceases, the urine pH falls to normal, and the plasma bicarbonate level stabilizes at this new level.

Other metabolic consequences of proximal RTA include volume depletion, hypokalemia, and hypercalciuria. The hypokalemia is caused by the increased bicarbonate reaching the distal potassium secretory sites. Under circumstances of volume depletion and hyperaldosteronism, potassium secretion is enhanced and hypokalemia results. Unlike distal RTA, correction of acidosis increases delivery of bicarbonate to the distal nephron, and hypokalemia may increase significantly. Hypercalciuria does not lead to nephrocalcinosis or nephrolithiasis in proximal RTA, but it may cause osteomalacia, rickets, and abnormal vitamin D metabolism in children.

DIFFERENTIAL DIAGNOSIS

The reabsorptive defect of proximal RTA may be isolated or may be associated with the other abnormalities of tubular transport present in Fanconi's syndrome. The isolated defect can result from deficient or absent carbonic anhydrase, the enzyme that increases bicarbonate reabsorption by facilitating the interconversion of CO_2, HCO_3^-, and H_2CO_3. Drugs such as the carbonic anhydrase inhibitor acetazolamide,

sulfanilamide, and topical mafenide acetate used on burns can induce proximal RTA.

DIAGNOSTIC EVALUATION

The diagnosis of proximal RTA is suspected in patients with hyperchloremic metabolic acidosis, a serum bicarbonate concentration of approximately 12 to 18 mEq/L, and an acid urine. Features of Fanconi's syndrome particularly suggest this diagnosis. To confirm the diagnosis, bicarbonate is infused to progressively raise the plasma concentration, and the urine is examined for appearance of bicarbonate, heralded by an increasing urine pH. In normal individuals, this increase occurs when the plasma bicarbonate is approximately 24 mEq/L, while bicarbonaturia is seen at much lower plasma bicarbonate concentration in patients with proximal RTA.

Adults with proximal RTA must be examined carefully for signs of Fanconi's syndrome—aminoaciduria, glycosuria, and phosphaturia. When it is present, a careful search for dysproteinemic states such as multiple myeloma and monoclonal gammopathy should be sought, as should the other diseases associated with Fanconi's syndrome (see Fanconi's syndrome).

HYPERKALEMIC, HYPERCHLOREMIC RTA (TYPE 4)

DEFINITION

Disturbances in distal nephron function, resulting in impaired secretion of both hydrogen ions and potassium, result in a hyperkalemic, hyperchloremic metabolic acidosis. Because urinary acidification is intact, the urine pH is characteristically low, but titratable acid and ammonium excretion are reduced, and low doses of alkali will return the plasma bicarbonate to normal.

PATHOPHYSIOLOGIC CONSIDERATIONS AND DIFFERENTIAL DIAGNOSIS

Several abnormalities may cause distal tubular dysfunction and decreased secretion of hydrogen ions and potassium. Intrinsic distal tubular disease associated with unresponsiveness to the effects of aldosterone can cause Type 4 RTA. Hypoaldosteronism, either primary or secondary to depressed renin secretion (syndrome of hyporenin hypoaldosteronism [SHH]) also causes Type 4 RTA. Patients with SHH usually have mild or moderate renal insufficiency, often secondary to diabetic renal disease. Chronic interstitial nephritis and hypertensive nephrosclerosis can also cause SHH. Primary hypoaldosteronism causes a hyperkalemic, hyperchloremic metabolic acidosis, and also renal salt wasting, volume contraction, and a secondary increase in renin secretion. Spironolactone can produce the same clinical picture.

Some patients have been reported who have Type 4 RTA, low renin, and low aldosterone, but also have hypertension, normal GFR, and no tubulointerstitial disease. Increased chloride reabsorption, which leads to decreased potassium secretion, may be the primary defect in those patients. The resulting hyperkalemia suppresses ammonia production and thereby limits renal acid excretion.

DIAGNOSTIC EVALUATION

When hyperkalemia is found in conjunction with hyperchloremic metabolic acidosis, renal function and the renin-angiotensin-aldosterone axis should be examined. The GFR should be measured, as well as fasting glucose and glycosolated hemoglobin. Other distal tubular functions such as concentrating capacity, should also be measured (using the overnight dehydration test) to seek evidence for diffuse distal tubular dysfunction. Aldosterone levels can be measured, particularly in volume-restricted patients, since both hyperkalemia and volume depletion are strong stimuli to aldosterone secretion.

LACTIC ACIDOSIS

DEFINITION

An increased plasma concentration of lactic acid causes an anion gap metabolic acidosis. It is a common and often life-threatening complication of an underlying serious illness (see also Chapter 10).

PATHOPHYSIOLOGIC CONSIDERATIONS

Lactic acidosis may result from increased lactate production, decreased utilization, or both. The normal plasma lactate level of 1.0 mEq/L reflects the balance between lactate production (by erythrocytes, skin,

Table 9–6. Causes of Lactic Acidosis

Relative tissue hypoxia
Sudden strenuous exercise or seizures
Shock: decreased tissue perfusion
Decreased oxygen delivery to tissues
Hypoxemia
Carbon monoxide poisoning
Severe anemia
Drugs and toxins
Ethanol
Phenformin
Salicylates
Epinephrine
Norepinephrine
Predisposing systemic illness
Sepsis
Diabetes mellitus
Hepatic failure
Neoplasms
Idiopathic lactic acidosis

brain, and other tissue at rest, and by skeletal muscle during exercise) and lactate utilization (by liver and kidney). While transient lactic acidosis can be seen with increased production alone (such as with severe exercise or seizures), sustained lactic acidosis results from both increased lactate production and impaired lactate utilization.

Conditions leading to anaerobic glycolysis in skeletal muscle increase lactate release. These conditions include sudden strenuous muscle contractions and tissue hypoxia. Drugs such as salicylates that impair oxidative phosphorylation, others such as epinephrine that increase glycogenolysis and glycolysis, and yet others such as phenformin and ethanol induce lactic acidosis. Several generalized systemic diseases predispose to lactic acidosis. Table 9–6, adapted from Harrington and Cohn,[5] outlines common causes of lactic acidosis.

DIAGNOSTIC EVALUATION

Patients with a large anion gap metabolic acidosis in the clinical settings listed in Table 9–6 almost always have lactic acidosis. When the diagnosis is in doubt, the plasma lactate level can be measured.

ACUTE RENAL FAILURE

DEFINITION

Acute renal failure (ARF) is any abrupt decline in renal function caused by a decrease in the glomerular filtration rate, characterized by elevated plasma creatinine and blood urea nitrogen (BUN) concentrations. Acute renal failure should be diagnosed when the plasma creatinine increases 1.0 mg/dl or more above a previously normal or stable value over a short period of time (i.e., a few days). The volume of urine excreted is frequently diminished (in anuria, less than 100 ml daily; in oliguria, 100 to 400 ml daily) but may be normal or even increased (in polyuria). Patients with daily urine volumes greater than 400 to 500 ml are often said to have "nonoliguric" renal failure.[8]

PATHOPHYSIOLOGIC CONSIDERATIONS AND DIFFERENTIAL DIAGNOSIS

Decreased renal blood flow resulting from intravascular volume depletion, hypotension, systemic vasodilatation, or diminished cardiac output may cause renal hypoperfusion ("prerenal azotemia"). Alterations in renal hemodynamics and hormonal factors (aldosterone, antidiuretic hormone, prostaglandins) and changes in renal sodium and water handling lead to the production of small volumes of concentrated, sodium-poor urine. Enhanced reabsorption of urea (as opposed to creatinine, which is not reabsorbed) causes a disproportionate elevation of BUN compared to the serum creatinine. *Postrenal renal failure* is caused by urinary tract obstruction, which may be at the level of the renal pelvis, ureters, bladder, or urethra. Changes in renal blood flow and intratubular pressure and the associated decline in the glomerular filtration rate vary depending on the duration of the obstruction and the rapidity with which it developed and on whether it is unilateral or bilateral. *Intrinsic acute renal failure* is caused by disease of the glomeruli, blood vessels, tubules (acute tubular necrosis [ATN]), or renal interstitium. The mechanisms leading to azotemia in these renal parenchymal diseases are not well understood. In addition to a decreased glomerular filtration rate there may be intratubular obstruction resulting from sloughed cells or cellular debris and passive "backleak" of tubular fluid across the damaged tubule epithelium.

The disorders that cause acute renal failure are often classified as to whether they are most often associated with prerenal azotemia, renal parenchymal azotemia, or postrenal azotemia. Intrinsic renal disease may be further categorized as glomerulonephritis, vasculitis, interstitial nephritis, or acute tubular necrosis (Table 9–7).

DIAGNOSTIC EVALUATION

A thorough patient history and physical examination are of paramount importance in the approach to the patient with acute renal failure and will often suggest the correct diagnosis. Evidence of volume depletion (dry skin and mucosae with poor skin turgor, orthostatic hypotension, tachycardia, weight loss, etc.) or volume overload (pedal and sacral edema, ascites, pulmonary edema) should be sought. A rectal and pelvic examination as well as percussion of the abdomen (or bladder catheterization) for evidence of a distended bladder may indicate possible urinary tract obstruction. Signs such as fever, rash, purpura, Raynaud's phenomenon, and digital ulceration may be clues to intrinsic renal disease as part of a systemic disorder. An assessment of urine volume should be made, although it is not particularly helpful for determining the cause of acute renal failure. Hemodynamic assessment with central venous pressure monitoring or a Swan-Ganz catheter may be useful.[9]

Microscopic and chemical analysis of the urine often provide useful diagnostic information. Hyaline and fine granular cast are not uncommon in the setting of prerenal or postrenal ARF. Reddish brown coarse granular casts and tubule epithelial cells are seen in the urinary sediment of patients with ATN. Red blood cells may be seen in interstitial nephritis or obstructive uropathy; red blood cell casts are generally diagnostic of glomerulonephritis. Eosinophils may occasionally be seen in the urine of patients with allergic interstitial nephritis or atheroembolic disease. It is important to test the urine with a dipstick to detect proteinuria and blood. A positive test for blood without red blood cells in the urine indicates the presence of myoglobin or hemoglobin in urine.

Alterations in the renal handling of water, sodium, and urea produce characteristic changes in the so called "urinary indices," particularly in oliguric prerenal ARF and ATN (Table 9–4).

In addition to BUN, creatinine, and electrolyte determinations, blood tests may include serum calcium and uric acid concentration, antinuclear antibody (ANA), protein electrophoresis, cryoglobulins, and complement (C3, C4), as clinically indicated. Radiologic studies are rarely necessary in the assessment of ARF; however, renal ultrasonography is valuable for the detection of hydronephrosis and urinary tract obstruction. Plain abdominal films, retrograde pyelography, CT scan, and arteriography may be useful in selected circumstances.

Finally, a renal biopsy may be indicated in patients with ARF of undefined cause with prolonged oliguria, or with evidence of glomerulonephritis or a systemic disease with renal involvement.

Table 9–7. Causes of Acute Renal Failure

Prerenal azotemia
  Volume depletion
    Gastrointestinal losses
      Vomiting
      Diarrhea
      Fistulae
      Hemorrhage
    Renal losses
      Diuretics
      Mineralocorticoid deficiency
      Salt-wasting disorders
      Postobstructive diuresis
      Osmotic diuresis, i.e., glycosuria
    Skin losses
      Burns
      Heat stroke
    Hemorrhage
  Decreased cardiac output
  Redistribution of extracellular fluid
    Hypoalbuminemia
      Nephrotic syndrome
      Cirrhosis
      Malnutrition
    Tissue injury
      Peritonitis
      Burns
      Crush injury
  Peripheral vasodilatation
    Sepsis
    Antihypertensive medication
    Arteriovenous fistulae
  Hepatorenal syndrome

Parenchymal azotemia
  Glomerulonephritis
    Poststreptococcal, other postinfection glomerulonephritis
    Bacterial endocarditis, shunt nephritis, visceral abscess
    Membranoproliferative glomerulonephritis
    Systemic lupus erythematosus
    Goodpasture's syndrome
    Rapidly progressive glomerulonephritis
    IgA nephropathy (Berger's disease)
    Mesangioproliferative glomerulonephritis
    Focal glomerulosclerosis
    Nephrotic syndrome
    Nonsteroidal anti-inflammatory drugs
  Vascular diseases
    Polyarteritis nodosa
    Hypersensitivity vasculitis
    Henoch-Schönlein purpura
    Wegener's granulomatosis
    Hemolytic-uremic syndrome, thrombotic thrombocytopenic purpura
    Cryoglobulinemia
    Thromboembolism, atheroembolism
    Renal artery occlusion
    Renal vein occlusion, thrombosis

    Scleroderma
    Malignant hypertension
  Tubules (ATN)
    Volume depletion
    Hypotension
    Sepsis
    Renal cortical necrosis
    Hemoglobinuria
    Myoglobinuria
    Antibiotics
      Aminoglycosides
      Amphotericin B
    Radiographic contrast
    Heavy metals
    Ethylene glycol
    Cis-platinum, methotrexate
    Acute uric acid nephropathy
  Interstitial nephritis
    Antibiotics
      Penicillin
      Sulfonamides
      Cephalosporins
    Nonsteroidal anti-inflammatory drug
    Diuretics
    Other drugs
      Allopurinol
      Cimetidine
    Hypercalcemia
    Oxalate nephropathy
    Multiple myeloma
    Papillary necrosis
    Transplant rejection
    Sarcoidosis
    Infection
    Lymphoma/leukemia
    Idiopathic

Postrenal azotemia
  Renal pelvis/kidney
    Carcinoma
    Calculi
    Papillary necrosis
    Blood clot
    Fungus balls
  Ureter
    Congenital anomalies
    Retroperitoneal fibrosis
    Carcinoma (primary or metastatic), lymphoma
    Operative complication
    Aortic aneurysm
  Bladder/urethra
    Congenital anomalies
    Carcinoma
    Prostatic hyperplasia (BPH)
    Neurogenic bladder
    Urethral stricture

PIGMENT NEPHROPATHY
(Hemoglobinuria, Myoglobinuria, Rhabdomyolysis)

DEFINITION

Acute renal insufficiency may be induced by release of heme pigment into the circulation. Myoglobin (molecular weight 17,800) is released from striated skeletal and cardiac muscle when rhabdomyolysis (muscle destruction) occurs. Hemoglobin is released during intravascular hemolysis. The proteins haptoglobin and hemopexin bind globin and heme, respectively, but once the capacity of these binding proteins is exceeded, free hemoglobin and myoglobin circulate in the plasma. Pigment nephropathy occurs when free hemoglobin and myoglobin produce acute renal failure.

PATHOPHYSIOLOGIC CONSIDERATIONS

Acute myoglobinuria may result from hereditary muscle diseases such as McArdle's disease or from rhabdomyolysis. Traumatic muscle injury follows crush injuries, toxins, or ischemia; nontraumatic muscle injury follows severe exercise, seizures, or prolonged coma induced by alcohol, narcotics, or other drugs. Myoglobin is released following muscle injuries of crush, ischemia, and exercise, while in the hereditary diseases, when abnormal anaerobic glycolysis disturbs the sarcolemmal membranes, myoglobin is liberated into the circulation following exercise. Toxic muscle injury may result from hypokalemia.

Acute hemoglobinuria may result from marked intravascular hemolysis or severe extravascular hemolysis. Transfusion of incompatible erythrocytes may result in massive hemolysis, acute renal failure, and shock. Relatively small volumes of hemoglobin may be released during prolonged running or soldiers' marches (march hemoglobinuria), following exposure to cold (cold hemoglobinuria) in patients with viral infections, or sporadically in patients with erythrocytes particularly sensitive to complement-induced hemolysis (paroxysmal nocturnal hemoglobinuria). These conditions rarely are associated with acute renal failure.

The mechanism of pigment-induced renal injury is not clear. Many patients have hypotension, intravascular volume depletion, and metabolic acidosis, and are simultaneously exposed to other potential nephrotoxins. Thus, the specific role of the free heme pigment as a nephrotoxin is not known. In rabbits, free heme pigment can induce acute renal failure only in the presence of volume depletion and an acid urine. Volume repletion and alkalinization of the urine prevent depression of glomerular filtration. Hemoglobin and the smaller molecular weight myoglobin are filtered in the glomerulus and enter the tubular fluid. In vitro, heme pigment is converted to ferrihemate in an acid medium, and this substance impairs organic anion transport into tubular cells. However, transfusion of hemoglobin-free incompatible erythrocyte stroma may also result in acute renal failure and in the absence of hemoglobinuria. Furthermore, purified hemoglobin can be infused into well-hydrated animals or man, without resulting renal failure.

DIAGNOSTIC EVALUATION AND DIFFERENTIAL DIAGNOSIS

The routine urinalysis dipstick test for blood will be positive if erythrocytes or free heme pigment is present in urine. Microscopic examination will help differentiate hematuria from free pigmenturia. Free hemoglobin or myoglobin may be measured in the urine. Acute pigment nephropathy must be considered in the differential diagnosis of acute renal failure.

The color of both urine and plasma should be examined in patients suspected of pigmenturia. Patients with hemoglobinuria frequently have pink plasma and clear or red urine, since much pigment is found in the plasma. In contrast, patients with myoglobinuria have clear plasma and red or black urine—the smaller myoglobin molecule is rapidly cleared from plasma by glomerular filtration.

Acute hemolysis may be detected by measurement of free hemoglobin in plasma and urine and by measurement of plasma haptoglobin. When available binding protein is low or absent, a diagnosis of acute hemolysis with hemoglobinuria should be considered.

Rhabdomyolysis releases many intracellular electrolytes, enzymes, and other substances into the circulation. Elevated levels of creatine phosphokinase (CPK), creatine, aldolase, potassium, phosphate, and uric acid suggest a diagnosis of acute myoglobinuria. The observation of continued rhabdomyolysis may be followed by serial measurements of CPK, which may rise to very high levels, and by observation of urine color.

HEPATORENAL SYNDROME

DEFINITION

Hepatorenal syndrome is unexplained renal failure that occurs in patients with cirrhosis of the liver in the absence of anatomic, laboratory, or clinical evidence of other known causes of acute renal failure. In this country, alcoholic liver disease with severe hepatic failure, portal hypertension, some degree of hepatic encephalopathy, and marked ascites provides the usual setting for hepatorenal syndrome. Characteristically, the patient will develop progressive and severe oliguria with some degree of azotemia, producing small volumes of concentrated urine with a urinary sodium concentration less than 10 mEq/L. Hypotension, hypothermia, lethargy, and hyponatremia are common.[10,11]

PATHOPHYSIOLOGIC CONSIDERATIONS

The cause of hepatorenal syndrome is unknown. Vigorous diuretic therapy, sepsis, gastrointestinal hemorrhage, or paracentesis may at times be precipitating factors. Intense renal vasoconstriction, particularly involving the renal cortex, causes a decrease in renal blood flow and glomerular filtration rate. A normal physiologic response to a decrease in ''effective'' vascular volume resulting from peripheral vasodilatation, shunting, ascites, pooling of blood in the portal and splanchnic beds, or true volume depletion (from diuretics, bleeding, etc.) has been proposed as a possible mechanism for this renal vasoconstriction. It has also been suggested that alterations in the synthesis or degradation of vasoactive substances such as angiotensin II, prostaglandins, or catecholamines or in vascular sensitivity to some humoral agent may lead to increased renal arterial and arteriolar tone. The precise pathogenetic mechanisms, however, remain obscure.

DIAGNOSTIC EVALUATION AND DIFFERENTIAL DIAGNOSIS

The diagnosis of hepatorenal syndrome should be made only after other potential causes for oliguria and acute renal failure have been excluded. Particularly troublesome is the differentiation between prerenal azotemia and hepatorenal syndrome. Hemodynamic measurements and/or an empiric trial of plasma volume expansion with colloid solutions are often nec-

Table 9–8. Disorders of Combined Hepatic and Renal Insufficiency

Circulatory insufficiency
    Congestive heart failure and cardiac cirrhosis
    Shock liver
    Sepsis
    Cirrhosis with ascites
Infections
    Hepatitis B
    Epstein-Barr virus
    Cytomegalovirus
    Leptospirosis
    Syphilis
    Brucellosis
Systemic diseases
    Systemic lupus erythematosus
    Cryoglubulinemia
    Sarcoidosis
    Vasculitis
    Reye's syndrome
    Acute fatty liver
    Acute yellow atrophy of pregnancy
    Malignancies
Drugs/toxins
    Acetaminophen overdose
    Mushroom (Amanita phalloides) poisoning
    Rifampin
    Tetracyclines
    Phenytoin
    Inhalation anesthetics
    Carbon tetrachloride
    Heavy metals

essary to make an accurate clinical assessment. Hepatic disease may occur in association with acute renal failure in a number of settings (Table 9–8). In addition, obstructive jaundice appears to predispose patients to acute tubular necrosis. Unfortunately, there are no absolute diagnostic criteria for this almost uniformly fatal disorder.

CHRONIC RENAL FAILURE AND UREMIA

DEFINITION

The progressive, irreversible loss of functioning nephrons eventually leads to chronic renal failure, termed uremia when there are symptoms related to the numerous metabolic and clinical manifestations of end-stage renal disease. As the glomerular filtration rate and tubular function decline, serum creatinine and blood urea nitrogen rise. Hypertension, metabolic acidosis (initially hyperchloremic acidosis with a normal anion gap; later predominantly an acidosis with an elevated anion gap), hyponatremia, hyperkalemia, hyperphosphatemia, hypocalcemia, hyperuricemia, and anemia are typically present. Peripheral and pulmonary edema, pleural and pericardial effusions, hemorrhagic tendencies, hypothermia, peripheral neuropathy, pruritus, and anorexia with nausea and vomiting may be present, particularly with advanced renal failure. Metabolic encephalopathy progressing to seizures and coma may develop in the severely uremic patient.[12]

PATHOPHYSIOLOGIC CONSIDERATIONS

Slowly progressive renal failure, as distinct from acute renal failure, is accompanied by adaptive processes that maintain homeostasis until the renal failure is quite advanced. Eventually, when the number of remaining functioning nephrons is insufficient to meet the excretory needs imposed by diet and metabolism, the signs, symptoms, and laboratory derangements of chronic renal failure ensue. The basis for the progressive nature of renal disease may be abnormalities in glomerular hemodynamics that arise as a result of a chronic reduction in functioning nephrons. As a result of the chronic reduction, increased glomerular capillary blood flow and pressure mediate further nephron damage, and a vicious cycle ensues. It is postulated that the clinical manifestations of uremia are due to abnormally high concentrations of such substances as urea, guanidinosuccinic acid, *myo*-inositol, parathyroid hormone, and poorly defined ''middle molecules'' (molecular weight 300 to 5000 daltons), which impair cellular function. No single chemical abnormality appears to account exclusively for all of the manifestations of uremia.[13]

DIAGNOSTIC EVALUATION AND DIFFERENTIAL DIAGNOSIS

The major causes of chronic renal failure are diabetes mellitus, chronic glomerulonephritis, chronic interstitial nephritis, hypertension and atherosclerotic disease, and polycystic kidney disease. Systemic lupus erythematosus and a variety of other inflammatory, metabolic, or inherited diseases may also lead to chronic renal failure. Occasionally, patients will present initially with azotemia, requiring that a distinction between acute and chronic renal failure be made. A complete history, particularly regarding prior hospitalizations (and any accompanying lab studies), other medical or surgical illness, and drug use (both prescription and nonprescription) is essential. Symptoms of nocturia, oliguria, hematuria, edema, anorexia,

pruritus, and general malaise should be sought. Laboratory abnormalities of anemia, hyperphosphatemia, hypocalcemia, and acidosis are often not helpful as they may develop rapidly with ARF. Bilaterally small kidneys and radiographic evidence of renal osteodystrophy suggest the presence of chronic, rather than acute, renal failure.

RENAL OSTEODYSTROPHY

DEFINITION

The general term renal osteodystrophy refers to the various skeletal abnormalities that occur in patients with chronic renal failure. Osteitis fibrosa caused by secondary hyperparathyroidism and osteomalacia are the most common disorders seen in adults. Growth retardation is very common in the child with chronic renal failure. Bone pain, particularly of the axial skeleton, proximal myopathy and muscle cramps, fractures, periarthritis, spontaneous tendon rupture, metastatic calcification, and pruritus are the most common clinical manifestations of renal osteodystrophy. Hypocalcemia, hyperphosphatemia, and elevated serum parathyroid hormone and alkaline phosphatase levels are typical laboratory abnormalities.[14]

PATHOPHYSIOLOGIC CONSIDERATIONS

Osteitis fibrosa is caused by secondary hyperparathyroidism. As renal function progressively declines, the serum parathyroid hormone (PTH) level rises in response to a decreased ionized calcium concentration in the blood. This hypocalcemia appears to be multifactorial in origin. Phosphate retention and hyperphosphatemia may lower serum calcium levels by directly complexing with calcium, by inhibiting bone resorption, or by suppressing renal hydroxylation of 25-(OH) vitamin D_3 to the active hormone 1,25-(OH)$_2$ vitamin D_3. Decreased 1,25-(OH)$_2$ vitamin D_3 synthesis also caused by a decrease in functional renal tissue, and the resulting decreased gastrointestinal tract calcium absorption, appear to play a key role in the development of secondary hyperparathyroidism as well as in the myopathy and childhood growth retardation of renal osteodystrophy. Skeletal resistance to PTH in patients with renal insufficiency also contributes to the hypocalcemia.

Osteomalacia, or defective mineralization of bones,

is in this country less frequently seen than osteitis fibrosa. Recent studies have suggested that aluminum deposition along the mineralization front of bone is primarily responsible for this disorder.[15] Excess aluminum may come from dietary sources or from the water needed for dialysate solutions. Most dialysate water supplies in this country are treated to remove aluminum. Phosphate-binding antacids (aluminum hydroxide) used to treat hyperphosphatemia may serve as the source of excess aluminum in some patients.

DIAGNOSTIC EVALUATION AND DIFFERENTIAL DIAGNOSIS

In addition to the clinical manifestation and laboratory abnormalities noted above, radiographic studies and bone biopsies help to establish the specific diagnosis of renal osteodystrophy. Fine-grain magnified x-rays of the hands appear to be most sensitive. Subperiosteal, endosteal, and terminal phalanx tuft resorption,, bony erosions, mottling of the skull with areas of lucency, and osteosclerosis of the spine (''rugger jersey'' spine) typify osteitis fibrosa. Osteopenia is common. There are no specific radiographic manifestations of osteomalacia. The use of photon-absorption densitometry and CT scanning of bones has been applied to the diagnosis of uremic osteodystrophy. Bone biopsy specimens reveal an increased number of osteoclasts, increased amounts of woven osteoid, and unmineralized osteoid and peritrabecular fibrosis in osteitis fibrosa. Excess demineralized osteoid as shown by double tetracycline labeling characterizes osteomalacia. Special stains may reveal aluminum deposition in the bones of patients with osteomalacia. Mixed lesions, with features of both osteomalacia and osteitis fibrosa, are not uncommon.

MINIMAL CHANGE NEPHROPATHY

DEFINITION

Minimal change nephropathy (also referred to as lipoid nephrosis or ''nil'' disease) is the most common cause of nephrotic syndrome in children. Approximately 75% of all children with nephrotic syndrome will have minimal change nephropathy. Over 90% of cases of steroid-responsive childhood nephrotic syndrome but only about 15 to 20% of adult cases of nephrotic syndrome are due to this disorder. The hallmark of minimal change nephropathy is the finding of normal-appearing glomeruli seen by light microscopy and of effacement or ''fusion'' of epithelial foot processes seen by electron microscopy. Immunofluorescent staining is negative. No electron-dense deposits are seen either at the basement membrane or in the mesangial area, and there is no cellular proliferation.[16]

PATHOPHYSIOLOGIC CONSIDERATIONS

The pathogenesis of minimal change nephropathy is not clearly defined. Neither immune complexes nor complement activation appears to play an important role. Abnormalities of T-lymphocyte function, lymphokine release, or both have been suggested.

DIAGNOSTIC EVALUATION AND DIFFERENTIAL DIAGNOSIS

The diagnostic approach to minimal change nephropathy is the same as the approach to nephrotic syndrome. It is generally assumed that children (less than 6 to 10 years of age) presenting with nephrotic syndrome, particularly if responsive to corticosteroid therapy, have minimal change nephropathy. Therefore, a renal biopsy is rarely performed in children unless the nephrotic syndrome is resistant to steroid treatment or there is reason to suspect other glomerular diseases. Focal gloermulosclerosis and mesangial proliferative glomerulonephritis may also present with nephrotic syndrome. These glomerular lesions tend to be associated with relatively infrequent steroid-responsiveness and a more pronounced tendency to progress to renal insufficiency. A minimal change nephropathy may occasionally be seen in patients with Hodgkin's disease and other lymphomas.

FOCAL GLOMERULOSCLEROSIS (FOCAL SEGMENTAL GLOMERULOSCLEROSIS)

DEFINITION

Focal glomerulosclerosis is a histopathologic entity that causes nephrotic syndrome; isolated asymptomatic microscopic hematuria or proteinuria is less common. Patients may present with renal insufficiency, and progression to end-stage renal failure occurs in approximately 25 to 50% of patients. Focal glomerulosclerosis may be a variant of minimal change disease. The pathologic changes of focal glomerulosclerosis include focal and segmental glomerular hyaline deposits and mesangial thickening, a variable degree of interstitial fibrosis and tubular atrophy, and foot process effacement on electron microscopy. No immune deposits are present.[17]

PATHOPHYSIOLOGIC CONSIDERATIONS

The pathogenesis of focal glomerulosclerosis is not known. As mentioned above, a relationship to minimal change disease has been suggested. Hemodynamic changes characterized by increased intraglomerular plasma flow and perfusion pressure may induce epithelial and endothelial cell injury, resulting in glomerulosclerosis. The occasionally rapid recurrence (within days) of focal glomerulosclerosis following renal transplantation suggests that some humoral factor(s) may also be involved.

DIAGNOSTIC EVALUATION AND DIFFERENTIAL DIAGNOSIS

The diagnostic approach to nephrotic syndrome is presented above. The diagnosis of focal glomerulosclerosis is a histopathologic one made by renal biopsy. Pathologic changes similar to those seen in focal glomerulosclerosis have been found in association with Berger's disease (IgA nephropathy), intravenous drug abuse, sickle cell nephropathy, reflux nephropathy, massive obesity, and Acquired Immune Deficiency syndrome. Focal glomerulosclerosis is occasionally diagnosed in the setting of steroid-resistant or steroid-dependent nephrotic syndrome in children.

MEMBRANOUS NEPHROPATHY

DEFINITION

Membranous nephropathy is the commonest cause of nephrotic syndrome in adults, accounting for 35 to 50% of cases. In addition to severe proteinuria, hypertension and hematuria may occur. Histologically there is a diffuse thickening of glomerular capillary walls without cellular proliferation on light microscopy; silver impregnation reveals perpendicular extensions from the basement membrane that surround sub-

epithelial deposits. Immunofluorescent studies show diffuse granular IgG (and to a lesser extent C3) staining along the capillary loops. Subepithelial electron-dense deposits, epithelial foot process effacement, and basement membrane thickening are seen on electron microscopy. In advanced lesions, these deposits become incorporated into the basement membrane and may become electron lucent.[18]

PATHOPHYSIOLOGIC CONSIDERATIONS

Membranous nephropathy is thought to result from the binding of free circulating antibody to glomerular basement membrane antigens or to antigens that had previously been deposited on the basement membrane. Circulating immune complexes appear to play no role in the immunopathogenesis of this disorder; rather, in situ immune complex formation appears to be responsible for the glomerular injury leading to abnormal proteinuria.

DIAGNOSTIC EVALUATION AND DIFFERENTIAL DIAGNOSIS

The diagnosis of membranous nephropathy can be made only by renal biopsy. A variety of conditions have been associated with membranous nephropathy, including lupus nephritis, drug toxicity (captopril, gold, penicillamine) and infection (hepatitis B, schistosomiasis, malaria, syphilis). In addition, membranous nephropathy may develop in patients with neoplastic disease, particularly solid tumors. In fact, the presence of the nephrotic syndrome may antedate the clinical diagnosis of carcinoma. Patients with membranous nephropathy appear to be particularly prone to the development of renal vein thrombosis. Although not all patients need undergo renal venography or other diagnostic studies, a high index of suspicion should be maintained should the patient develop an acute decline in renal function, flank pain, or symptoms of thromboembolic disease (in particular, pulmonary embolism).

MEMBRANOPROLIFERATIVE GLOMERULONEPHRITIS (MPGN)

DEFINITION

Membranoproliferative glomerulonephritis, also referred to as mesangiocapillary glomerulonephritis, presents clinically most commonly with heavy proteinuria or nephrotic syndrome. Hematuria, hypertension, and impaired renal function are often present. Progression to chronic renal failure occurs in about 50% of patients. Two main pathologic types have been identified. Type I MPGN is characterized by enlarged, lobulated glomeruli with increased mesangial matrix material and mesangial and polymorphonuclear cell proliferation. On electron microscopy, there is extension of the mesangium between the glomerular capillary basement membranes and the endothelium (interposition), which gives rise to the double-contour appearance ("tramtrack") of the capillary loops seen with PAS or silver stains. Electron-dense deposits are seen in the mesangium and along the subendothelial side of the basement membrane.

Type II MPGN is differentiated from type I MPGN by marked basement membrane thickening caused by a ribbon of electron-dense material deposited along the basement membrane (hence the term "dense deposit disease"). Subendothelial deposits are rarely seen. The immunofluorescent staining pattern of type I MPGN shows mesangial and capillary loop deposits of C3 in association with IgG and other complement components; in type II MPGN there is deposition of C3 only.[19]

PATHOPHYSIOLOGIC CONSIDERATIONS

Pathogenetic schemes for MPGN have centered on the abnormalities of the complement system seen in many patients. In type I MPGN, approximately 50% of patients will present with a low serum C3 level; almost all patients will manifest hypocomplementemia at some point in the course of their disease. In addition, the levels of C1q, C4, factor B, and properdin may be depressed, indicating activation of both the classic and alternate pathways of complement. It has been postulated that immune complexes may serve to activate the classic pathway. Platelet aggregation and release of platelet-derived vasoactive substances may be important factors causing glomerular injury in MPGN.

In type II MPGN, C3 levels are almost invariably depressed; hence, the term "hypocomplementemic glomerulonephritis" is often used. C1q and C4 levels are normal, while factor B and properdin levels may be low. A serum IgG autoantibody directed against the C3 convertase of the alternate pathway (C3bBb) activates the alternate pathway by stabilizing C3 convertase. This C3 nephritic factor (C3NeF) is present in the serum of most patients with type II MPGN but occurs much less commonly and in lower concentrations in patients with type I MPGN. Circulating im-

mune complexes may also play a role in the pathogenesis of type II MPGN. Primary abnormalities of glomerular basement membrane synthesis or degradation have been suggested as well.

DIAGNOSTIC EVALUATION AND DIFFERENTIAL DIAGNOSIS

Idiopathic MPGN occurs primarily in children and young adults, although it may occur at any age. A large number of systemic and infectious diseases have also been associated with MPGN, including systemic lupus erythematosus, essential cryoglobulinemia, chronic active hepatitis, sickle cell disease, infective endocarditis, chronic bacteremia caused by visceral abscesses or infected atrioventricular shunts, malaria, schistosomiasis, malignancy, the lipodystrophies, and hereditary complement component deficiencies. Hypocomplementemia serves to distinguish MPGN from the other primary nephropathies.[20]

MESANGIAL PROLIFERATIVE GLOMERULONEPHRITIS

DEFINITION

In addition to membranoproliferative glomerulonephritis, acute glomerulonephritis (poststreptococcal, endocarditis, etc.), and focal or diffuse proliferative glomerulonephritis associated with systemic lupus erythematosus or other systemic diseases, proliferative changes are frequently seen on renal biopsy without other specific clinical or histopathologic features. The presence of a mild increase in mesangial cellularity and matrix material without capillary loop thickening or other specific immunofluorescence on electron microscopy characterizes this glomerulonephritis. The clinical setting may be recurrent gross or microscopic hematuria, proteinuria, or nephrotic syndrome. The prognosis is generally good for these patients.[21,22]

PATHOPHYSIOLOGIC CONSIDERATIONS

The cause of mesangioproliferative glomerulonephritis is unknown. The frequent temporal association with upper respiratory or gastrointestinal illnesses suggests a possible viral cause, perhaps on an immune basis.

DIAGNOSTIC EVALUATION AND DIFFERENTIAL DIAGNOSIS

Systemic lupus erythematosus and other vasculitis syndromes, MPGN, IgA nephropathy (Berger's disease), Henoch-Schönlein purpura, and acute glomerulonephritis associated particularly with streptococcal infections and subacute bacterial endocarditis may present a similar clinical and histopathologic picture. The lack of well-defined electron-dense deposits and specific immunofluorescence on renal biopsy in a patient without clinical or laboratory evidence of these disorders suggests the diagnosis of idiopathic mesangioproliferative glomerulonephritis.

POSTSTREPTOCOCCAL GLOMERULONEPHRITIS (PSGN)

DEFINITION

Group A β-hemolytic streptococcal infection of the pharynx or skin may produce an acute glomerulonephritis following a 1- to 4-week latent period. Symptoms of hematuria (often described as smoky or tea-colored), edema, particularly periorbital edema in children, congestive heart failure, and oliguria or anuria develop in conjunction with hypertension, evidence of circulatory overload with cardiomegaly, pulmonary congestion, and ascites. Azotemia, which may be severe, is common. Proteinuria is frequent and may be in the nephrotic range; red blood cells and red blood cell and granular casts are seen in the urine sediment. An elevation of the antistreptolysin O (ASO) titer is diagnostic in up to 90% of cases; anti-DNAse-B and antihyaluronidase measurements may be useful to diagnose the remainder of cases, particularly following skin infection. Serum C3 levels are depressed; the levels of C1q, C4, and C2 are usually normal.[23,24]

An acute glomerulonephritis with clinical and histopathologic features similar to those of PSGN may also develop in association with a variety of infections, most notably subacute bacterial endocarditis, "shunt-nephritis," and visceral abscesses.

The pathologic hallmark of poststreptococcal glomerulonephritis is a diffuse glomerulonephritis with endothelial and mesangial cell proliferation and polymorphonuclear leukocyte and mononuclear cell infiltration of the glomeruli. Glomerular crescents may be seen. The most characteristic finding is the presence on electron microscopy of subepithelial electron-dense deposits, so-called humps, which may occasionally be large; the basement membrane itself is not thickened, although the overlying epithelial foot processes are often effaced.

PATHOPHYSIOLOGIC CONSIDERATIONS

The mechanism by which group A β-hemolytic streptococcal (or other) infection leads to acute glomerulonephritis appears to be based on an immune complex deposition. The presence of circulating immune complexes (the antigenic identity of which is not clear) and cryoglobulinemia, complement activation, a latent period, and the deposition of immunoglobulin and C3 in the kidney as shown by immune fluorescent techniques support such a hypothesis. The role of streptococcal antigens per se remains to be defined; deposition of streptococcal antigens in the glomerulus may lead to in situ immune complex formation and complement activation with the subsequent development of the observed proliferative, inflammatory response.

DIAGNOSTIC EVALUATION AND DIFFERENTIAL DIAGNOSIS

As noted above, a variety of infections may provoke an acute glomerulonephritis, particularly subacute bacterial endocarditis, visceral abscesses, and "shunt nephritis." Crescentic rapidly progressive glomerulonephritis (RPGN), lupus nephritis, Henoch-Schönlein purpura, and membranoproliferative glomerulonephritis may be clinically indistinguishable from PSGN. The differential diagnosis of hematuria has been presented above. Renal biopsy is often necessary to establish a correct diagnosis of PSGN. An elevated ASO, antihyaluronidase, or anti-DNAse-B titer in conjunction with a low C3 level helps to establish the diagnosis of PSGN. The anti-nuclear antibody is negative, as are blood cultures in C1q, C4, and C2 levels.

RAPIDLY PROGRESSIVE GLOMERULONEPHRITIS (RPGN)

DEFINITION

Rapidly progressive glomerulonephritis is an uncommon clinicopathologic entity characterized by an

Table 9–9. Classification of Rapidly Progressive Glomerulonephritis

No immune deposits (idiopathic RPGN)
Anti-GBM disease
   Goodpasture's syndrome
   Idiopathic anti-GBM nephritis
   Conversion of membranous GN
Granular immune deposits
   Infections
      Streptococcal
      Visceral abscess
      Shunt nephritis
      Bacterial endocarditis
      Hepatitis B (chronic)
   Systemic diseases
      Systemic lupus erythematosus
      Polyarteritis nodosa and other vasculitides
      Essential mixed cryoglobulinemia
      Wegener's granulomatosis
      Henoch-Schönlein purpura
      Neoplasia
   Primary renal disease
      Idiopathic "immune complex" RPGN
      Membranoproliferative GN
      Berger's disease (IgA nephropathy)

acute nephritic syndrome of oliguria, hypertension, proteinuria, hematuria, and renal failure. Uremia is present in approximately 50% of patients at initial presentation. A viral illness prodrome is frequently reported; hemoptysis and transient pulmonary infiltrates may occur. The renal histologic hallmark is the presence of glomerular crescents that usually involve over 50% of glomeruli. Crescents may be cellular or fibrotic and destroy glomerular architecture. Immunofluorescent studies are of paramount importance in the classification of RPGN (see below and Table 9–9).[25,26]

Goodpasture's syndrome is a disease that particularly affects young men (in a ratio to females of 6 to 8:1), presenting with pulmonary disease that may range from asymptomatic pulmonary infiltrates on chest x-ray to life threatening hemoptysis, and renal disease manifest as RPGN. Goodpasture's syndrome is diagnosed by the demonstration of linear deposition of antiglomerular basement membrane (anti-GBM) antibody by immunofluorescent staining of the kidney. Anti-GBM antibody is also found in the sera of patients with Goodpasture's syndrome. In some patients anti-GBM antibody may cause RPGN without associated pulmonary disease (idiopathic anti-GBM disease); these patients tend to be older than those with Goodpasture's syndrome, and the male to female ratio is more equal. The clinical course of patients with anti-GBM disease is indistinguishable from other patients with RPGN.

PATHOPHYSIOLOGIC CONSIDERATIONS

The inciting factors producing anti-GBM disease are largely unknown. It has been postulated that some toxic or infectius pulmonary injury disrupts the alveolar epithelial lining, thus exposing the alveolar basement membrane. An immunologic response produces antibody to these normally sequestered antigens that cross-reacts with renal GBM antigens, leading to the clinical manifestations of Goodpasture's syndrome. Idiopathic anti-GBM disease may result from renal or other nonpulmonary anti-GBM antibody formation, without immune mediated pulmonary damage. RPGN may be divided into three categories based upon immunofluorescent findings.

DIAGNOSTIC EVALUATION AND DIFFERENTIAL DIAGNOSIS

Approximately 40% of patients with RPGN will have granular immune deposits on immunofluorescence or electron microscopy. Circulating immune complexes and/or a systemic vasculitis appear to be the basis of many of these cases. Another 40% of patients with RPGN have so-called idiopathic RPGN, with no glomerular immune deposits. Glomerular crescents appear to contain cells of renal epithelial and monocyte-macrophage origin. The latter may appear in response to altered T-cell mediated immunity. Local activation of the coagulation process resulting in the deposition of fibrin in and around the glomerulus may also be important in initiating crescent formation and inciting monocyte migration into the glomerulus.

Once a diagnosis of crescentic glomerulonephritis has been made by renal biopsy, diagnostic studies directed at determining a precise origin should include blood cultures, antinuclear antibody, antistreptolysin O, hepatitis B serologic studies, serum cryoglobulins, complement levels, and anti-GBM antibody determinations. Poststreptococcal RPGN and RPGN associated with a vasculitis may be particularly difficult to differentiate from idiopathic RPGN. As noted above, immunofluorescent staining of renal biopsy specimens is necessary for the classification of RPGN into diagnostic categories.

BERGER'S DISEASE (IgA NEPHROPATHY)

DEFINITION

IgA nephropathy is a focal and segmental glomerulonephritis that typically presents with recurrent gross hematuria, frequently following upper respiratory or gastrointestinal viral infections. Proteinuria, occasionally in the nephrotic range, and asymptomatic microscopic hematuria are also common. This disease typically occurs in adolescents and young adults, males more commonly than females. Approximately 10 to 20% of patients may develop hypertension and/or chronic renal failure. Renal biopsy specimens show increases in mesangial matrix and mesangial cell proliferation. Glomerular sclerosis, necrosis, and crescent formation may be seen. Electron-dense mesangial deposits are seen on electron microscopy. Immunofluorescent studies reveal a characteristic intense mesangial IgA staining, usually with IgG and C3 staining as well. IgA staining may also be seen in the capillaries of skin biopsy specimens. Approximately 50% of patients have elevated serum IgA levels.[27]

PATHOPHYSIOLOGIC CONSIDERATIONS

The precise pathogenesis of IgA nephropathy has remained unclear. IgA-containing immune complexes, perhaps related to viral or other environmental antigens, may be deposited in capillaries and the renal mesangium. Activation of complement T-cell regulatory abnormalities, and abnormal reticuloendothelial system clearing of secretory IgA have also been proposed. It has been suggested that IgA nephropathy is a forme fruste of Henoch-Schönlein purpura, which also demonstrates glomerular IgA staining in association with a systemic illness with nonthrombocytopenic purpura, arthralgias, and gastrointestinal symptoms in addition to renal disease.

DIAGNOSTIC EVALUATION AND DIFFERENTIAL DIAGNOSIS

The diagnosis of IgA nephropathy can be made only by renal biopsy; demonstration of IgA staining in dermal capillaries provides suggestive evidence. Benign hematuria is excluded by the presence of significant proteinuria. Focal glomerulosclerosis, mesangial proliferative glomerulonephritis, membranoproliferative glomerulonephritis, and poststreptococcal glomerulonephritis can be excluded by renal biopsy. Serum complements, antinuclear antibody, and antistreptolysin O will be normal or negative in Berger's disease. An IgA mesangial glomerulonephritis has also been described in patients with cirrhosis of the liver and portal-systemic shunting.

RENAL DISEASE OF POLYARTERITIS NODOSA (PAN)

DEFINITION

Polyarteritis nodosa is a systemic necrotizing vasculitis of small and medium-sized muscular arteries. Renal manifestations stem from the arteritis, which may occur alone or in conjunction with a necrotizing or proliferative glomerulonephritis. Hypertension is common and may progress to malignant hypertension. Hematuria, proteinuria, symptomatic renal infarction, and progressive ischemic renal failure result from the arteritis. Acute renal failure, which may present as RPGN, hematuria, and proteinuria, occurs in the presence of glomerulonephritis. There are no diagnostic laboratory features of PAN; diagnosis depends on the demonstration of the characteristic vascular lesions in an appropriate clinical setting.[25,28]

PATHOPHYSIOLOGIC CONSIDERATIONS

As noted above, renal manifestations of PAN result from the arteritis and/or glomerulonephritis seen in this disorder. An immune complex injury and a hypersensitivity reaction pathogenesis have been suggested. Some cases occur in association with hepatitis B viral infection.

DIAGNOSTIC EVALUATION

Biopsy of testis, epididymis, skin lesions, muscle, or nerve may demonstrate the vasculitis. Renal biopsy specimens may reveal a focal, necrotizing glomerulonephritis with crescents, which is compatible with but not diagnostic of PAN. The arterial lesions are usually not seen on percutaneous biopsy specimens. Renal (also mesenteric and hepatic) angiography may be used to demonstrate what are rather characteristic arterial stenoses, occlusions, and microaneurysms.

DIFFERENTIAL DIAGNOSIS

The PAN group of systemic vasculitides includes PAN allergic granulomatosis and hypersensitivity angiitis (microscopic PAN). Allergic granulomatosis is characterized by a small-vessel arteritis and venulitis in addition to medium-sized arterial involvement, with eosinophilia, asthma, and pulmonary infiltrates. Microscopic PAN affects small arteries, arterioles, venules, and capillaries; palpable purpura is the most common manifestation. A focal and segmental glomerulonephritis with a variable degree of cellular proliferation and crescent formation occurs as part of this systemic vasculitis.

Systemic lupus erythematosus, Wegener's granulomatosis, cryoglobulinemia, Henoch-Schönlein purpura, hemolytic-uremic syndrome, thrombotic thrombocytopenic purpura, acute glomerulonephritis, and other causes of RPGN should be included in the differential diagnosis.

THE KIDNEY IN WEGENER'S GRANULOMATOSIS

DEFINITION

Wegener's granulomatosis is a disease characterized by necrotizing granulomatous vasculitis of the upper and lower respiratory tracts, glomerulonephritis, and variable degrees of small-vessel systemic vasculitis. Patients usually present with upper respiratory symptoms such as rhinorrhea that progress to purulent sinusitis, oropharyngeal mucosal ulceration, necrosis of the nasal septum and cartilage, and otitis media. Pulmonary disease is manifest as cough, hemoptysis, and dyspnea with pulmonary infiltrates that typically are multiple, bilateral cavitating nodules but can be highly variable. Renal involvement is characterized by hematuria, pyuria, red blood cell casts, and proteinuria (rarely in the nephrotic range). Renal function may be normal initially, but mild to severe azotemia is common; mild renal insufficiency frequently develops into a rapidly progressive glomerulonephritis (RPGN).

Over 90% of patients have clinical involvement of the upper and/or lower respiratory tracts; glomerulonephritis is apparent in 85 to 95% of patients and is often the major life threatening manifestation of the disease. Arthralgias, arthritis, ocular inflammation, constitutional symptoms, neuropathies, and skin lesions are common, as are anemia, leukocytosis, and an elevated erythrocyte sedimentation rate.[29]

The pathologic hallmark of Wegener's granulomatosis is a granulomatous vasculitis that is best seen on lung or skin biopsy. The renal lesion is initially a focal and segmental necrotizing glomerulonephritis, although diffuse proliferative changes may be seen. Glomerular crescents and fibrinoid necrosis of capillary loops are commonly seen; granulomatous changes rarely are seen on renal biopsy specimens.

PATHOPHYSIOLOGIC CONSIDERATIONS

The cause and pathogenetic mechanism of Wegener's granulomatosis are unknown.

DIAGNOSTIC EVALUATION[35]

The diagnosis of Wegener's granulomatosis is based on the presence of a systemic vasculitis involving the respiratory tract, kidneys, and other organ systems.

There are no specific laboratory findings in Wegener's granulomatosis. As mentioned above, anemia is common, and an elevated erythrocyte sedimentation rate is almost universal. Anti-GBM antibody and antinuclear antibody titers are negative. Lung biopsy, particularly by open thoracotomy, most frequently provides diagnostic histopathology. Renal biopsy may be useful in evaluating the extent of glomerular involvement, particularly crescent formation and necrosis.

DIFFERENTIAL DIAGNOSIS

Wegener's granulomatosis may present as a rapidly progressive glomerulonephritis. In addition, a number of "pulmonary-renal syndromes" need to be considered, including Goodpasture's syndrome, systemic lupus erythematosus, polyarteritis nodosa and hypersensitivity vasculitis, idiopathic RPGN with or without immune deposits, right-sided bacterial endocarditis, sarcoidosis, renal vein thrombosis with pulmonary emboli, and scleroderma. Pulmonary infections or congestive heart failure with coexisting renal disease must also be considered.

RENAL DISEASE IN MULTIPLE MYELOMA

DEFINITION

Multiple myeloma is a malignant disorder of plasma cells. Renal manifestations result from the presence of monoclonal immunoglobulins and light chains, hypercalcemia, infection, and amyloidosis. Proteinuria, comprised primarily of monoclonal light chains (Bence Jones proteinuria), is present in approximately 75% of patients. Hypercalcemia produces defective urinary concentrating ability leading to polyuria and potentially to dehydration; this and direct effects of hypercalcemia may precipitate acute renal failure. Fanconi's syndrome (proximal tubule dysfunction) and urinary acidification defects can occur. Acute renal failure develops in about 5 to 10% of patients with multiple myeloma. In addition to hypercalcemia, dehydration is a very common precipitant of ARF. Intravenous radiographic contrast may also occasionally induce ARF in patients with multiple myeloma. Progressive chronic renal insufficiency occurs in approximately 50% of patients and is second to infection as a leading cause of death in multiple myeloma.

The characteristc pathologic lesion of myeloma kidney is a dense intratubular eosinophilic cast comprised of light chains surrounded by multinucleated giant cells. There is often an accompanying interstitial inflammatory response and fibrosis. Tissue deposition of amyloid or nonamyloid light chains may also occur. Light-chain deposition causes tubular basement membrane thickening and occasionally a glomerular lesion characterized by the formation of PAS-positive mesangial nodules.[24,30]

PATHOPHYSIOLOGIC CONSIDERATIONS

The renal manifestations of multiple myeloma are in large part due to the nephrotoxicity of light chains that are filtered at the glomerulus and metabolized by renal tubule cells (mainly proximal tubule cells). Intratubular precipitation of light chains, a direct cellular toxic effect, and hemodynamic changes caused by rouleaux formation and hyperviscosity lead to a decrement in the glomerular filtration rate and to renal failure. Some light-chain proteins (depending on their particular physicochemical nature) are not readily filtered at the glomerulus but instead appear as amyloid or nonamyloid tissue deposits.[31]

DIAGNOSTIC EVALUATION

A bone marrow examination, as well as serum and urine protein electrophoresis and immunoelectrophoresis, should be performed in all patients with suspected multiple myeloma. In addition, serum calcium and uric acid concentration should be determined. It is important to recognize that urinary dipsticks measure only albumin and do not detect light chains, which can, however, be detected by the sulfosalicylic acid test. The classic heat test for the detection of Bence Jones proteinuria (in which a precipitate forms when urine is heated to 45 to 53° C, and then redissolves with continued heating to 100° C; the precipitate forms

again upon cooling) is insensitive. Urinary immunoelectrophoresis should be performed.

DIFFERENTIAL DIAGNOSIS

Hypercalcemia, dehydration, and nephrotoxins (particularly antibiotics) should be excluded in every patient with known multiple myeloma and renal failure. Multiple myeloma occasionally presents as the first clinically apparent manifestation of renal failure and hence must be considered in every patient with unexplained acute or chronic renal insufficiency. Amyloidosis, Waldenström's macroglobulinemia, lymphoma, chronic lymphocytic leukemia, and "benign" monoclonal gammopathy may be associated with urinary light-chain excretion.

RENAL AMYLOIDOSIS

DEFINITION

Amyloid is a β-pleated fibrillar protein derived from immunoglobulin light chains (AL-amyloid) or serum amyloid protein (protein A, AA-amyloid); other proteins may also be incorporated. Primary amyloidosis and amyloidosis associated with multiple myeloma are generally of the AL type, whereas secondary amyloidosis caused by chronic infections or inflammatory disorders is usually of the AA type. In addition to the primary, secondary, and myeloma-associated forms, amyloidosis may also be localized or familial (familial Mediterranean fever, most commonly).[32,33]

Proteinuria is the most common manifestation of renal amyloid deposition; nephrotic syndrome with massive protein excretion is also frequent. Renal insufficiency is present in approximately 50% of cases and may progress to severe renal failure. All patients have albumin in their urine. Monoclonal light chains are excreted by approximately 70% of patients as well.

PATHOPHYSIOLOGIC CONSIDERATIONS

Amyloid proteins are products of plasma cells. The varied manifestations of amyloidosis result from infiltration and replacement of normal tissue with amyloid deposits, which are identified by the characteristic green birefringence with polarized light after Congo red staining. Characteristic short, fine nonbranching fibers with a 55A periodicity are seen on electron microscopy. In addition to excessive amyloid production, impaired monocyte degradation also contributes to tissue deposition.[24]

DIAGNOSTIC EVALUATION

A bone marrow biopsy should be performed on all patients to determine the degree of plasmacytosis. In addition, a serum and urine protein electrophoresis and immunoelectrophoresis should be performed. A tissue diagnosis should first be sought with a rectal biopsy; if negative, biopsy of gingiva or skin or a subcutaneous fat aspiration may be helpful. A renal biopsy will demonstrate amyloid deposition if these other, less invasive procedures are nondiagnostic.

DIFFERENTIAL DIAGNOSIS

Amyloidosis should be considered in any patient with multiple myeloma or a chronic inflammatory or infectious disease who develops proteinuria. Albuminuria in patients with multiple myeloma, as opposed to Bence Jones proteinuria, generally signifies the presence of amyloidosis.

RENAL DISEASE IN CRYOGLOBULINEMIA

DEFINITION

Cryoglobulins are abnormal serum immunoglobulins that precipitate when stored at 4°C for 24 to 72 hours. A classification scheme has been developed based upon immunologic characteristics of the cryoglobulin: Type I consists of monoclonal cryoglobulins, usually IgM or IgG; type II is a mixed cryoglobulin consisting of a monoclonal component (usually IgM) with antibody activity against polyclonal IgG; type III is also a mixed cryoglobulin in which both components are polyclonal. Types II and III comprise circulating immune complexes and are frequently associated with a vasculitis and glomerulonephritis. Patients with type I cryoglobulins may also develop renal disease.[34]

Types I and II cryoglobulinemia are associated with hematologic malignancies and lymphoproliferative disorders, particularly multiple myeloma and Waldenström's macroglobulinemia. Type II also occurs in the setting of chronic lymphocytic leukemia, lympho-

cytic lymphoma, or Sjögren's syndrome. Many cases of type II and III cryoglobulinemia are not associated with another underlying disorder and are termed essential mixed cryoglobulinemia. Collagen vascular diseases, particularly systemic lupus erythematosus, rheumatoid arthritis, and Sjögren's syndrome, and a variety of infections may also be associated with mixed cryoglobulinemia.

Renal disease develops in up to 50% of patients with mixed cryoglobulinemia, initially microscopic hematuria and proteinuria that may rapidly progress to an acute nephritis with edema, hypertension, red cell casts, and acute renal failure or nephrotic syndrome.

PATHOPHYSIOLOGIC CONSIDERATIONS

The mixed cryoglobulins behave as circulating immune complexes and incite a hypocomplementemic systemic small-vessel vasculitis. The C1q and C4 levels are often low, with a normal or only slightly depressed C3. In vivo cold precipitation may also occur, particularly with very high concentrations of cryoglobulins. Renal disease, purpura, Raynaud's phenomenon, cutaneous ulceration, arthralgias, neuropathies, and hepatosplenomegaly result. The renal lesion is a diffuse proliferative glomerulonephritis with endothelial and mesangial cell proliferation and some degree of polymorphonuclear leukocyte infiltration. The glomerular changes may resemble membranoproliferative glomerulonephritis with mesangial interposition and "tram-tracking" of the basement membrane. Small-vessel arteritis is commonly seen. Large periodic acid-Schiff-positive, eosinophilic subendothelial masses may be present. These deposits as well as the glomerular capillary walls usually stain for IgM and IgG, predominantly by immunofluorescence; IgA and complement staining may also be present. Electron microscopy reveals subendothelial and mesangial deposits, with mesangial proliferation and interposition. The large masses seen on light microscopy, which appear to contain fibrillar or annular structures, are deposits of cryoglobulins.

DIFFERENTIAL DIAGNOSIS

The renal manifestation of mixed cryoglobulinemia clinically may appear similar to poststreptococcal and membranoproliferative glomerulonephritis but can be differentiated by the systemic manifestations of mixed cryoglobulinemia and the presence of microscopic subepithelial "lumps" seen in poststreptococcal GN. Lupus nephritis with diffuse proliferative glomerulonephritis may appear in conjunction with mixed cryoglobulinemia. Renal disease caused by cryoglobulins frequently follows a flare-up of the cutaneous lesions. Glomerular crescents of RPGN are rarely seen in cryoglobulinemia. Pertinent laboratory studies (in addition to a properly obtained blood sample for cryoglobulins, observed for at least 72 hours) should include serum complements, erythrocyte sedimentation rate, antinuclear antibody titer, rheumatoid factor, antistreptolysin-O, hepatitis B surface antigen, serum protein and immunoelectrophoresis, and tests of liver function. A bone marrow examination may be indicated as well. Skin biopsy may reveal the presence of a small-vessel vasculitis.[25]

LUPUS NEPHRITIS

DEFINITION

Renal disease in systemic lupus erythematosus (SLE) may take the form of proteinuria, nephrotic syndrome, hematuria, hypertension, an active urinary sediment, acute renal failure, or chronic progressive renal insufficiency. Some manifestation of renal involvement occurs in 50 to 70% of all patients with SLE. The diagnosis of SLE rests on a constellation of clinical and serologic findings. Levels of antibody to native double-stranded DNA and C4 tend to correlate, though imprecisely, with activity of renal disease.[35] A variety of pathologic changes may be seen; such as mesangial matrix increase, mesangial cell proliferation, hyaline thrombi, fibrinoid necrosis, crescent formation, and interstitial infiltrates and scarring. Immune deposits may be seen in the mesangium, subendothelial space, or subepithelial space. Broad classifications, based upon histologic, immunofluorescent, and electron microscopic changes have identified four major types of lupus nephritis: minimal or mesangial nephritis, focal proliferative nephritis, diffuse proliferative nephritis, and membranous nephritis.[24]

PATHOPHYSIOLOGIC CONSIDERATIONS

Immunologic factors appear to be responsible for SLE and its renal manifestations. Deficient T-lymphocyte suppressor function and hyperactive B-cell function result in autoantibody and immune complex formation. Glomerular trapping immune complexes, in situ antibody deposition, and complement activation mediate renal injury. Genetic predisposition appears to

be important in some instances. A viral cause has been suggested but remains unproven.

DIAGNOSTIC EVALUATION

No single clinical or laboratory abnormality confirms the diagnosis of lupus nephritis. Measurement of antinuclear antibody, antinative DNA antibody, and serum complement components can be used to support the diagnosis. The creatinine clearance and 24-hour urinary protein excretion should be determined. The role of a renal biopsy in the management of the patient with lupus nephritis is controversial; prognostic information can be obtained from the renal pathologic changes that are seen, but it is not clear to what extent the therapeutic approach to any given patient is enhanced.

DIFFERENTIAL DIAGNOSIS

Because lupus nephritis generally presents in a patient with established multisystem disease, the diagnosis of lupus nephritis is usually not difficult. Acute glomerulonephritis, RPGN, vasculitides, bacterial endocarditis, mixed cryoglobulinemia, thrombotic thrombocytopenic purpura (TTP), and Goodpasture's syndrome may present with similar manifestations.

RENAL DISEASE IN HENOCH-SCHÖNLEIN PURPURA (HSP)

DEFINITION

Henoch-Schönlein purpura is characterized by a cutaneous leukocytoclastic vasculitis with gastrointestinal, joint, and renal manifestations. Skin lesions typically involve the lower extremities and buttocks and evolve from an urticarial or erythematous rash into purpuric lesions. Transient arthralgias are common. Gastrointestinal manifestations include abdominal colic, vomiting, hemorrhage, and intussusception. Renal involvement may present as gross or microscopic hematuria, proteinuria, or the nephrotic syndrome. Acute renal failure, if present, may range from transient mild azotemia to rapidly progressive glomerulonephritis. Chronic renal failure may subsequently develop. Most cases of HSP occur in children, but adults may also develop this disease.[25]

PATHOPHYSIOLOGIC CONSIDERATIONS

The histopathologic renal lesion of HSP is a focal or diffuse mesangial proliferation, with a variable number of crescents. Fibrinoid necrosis and intracapillary thrombosis may be seen. On electron microscopy there are electron-dense mesangial and subendothelial deposits. Immunofluorescent studies reveal heavy mesangial staining with IgA; C3, IgG, and other immunoglobulins and complement components are also usually present. Skin biopsies may reveal dermal capillary IgA staining, much as has been reported in patients with Berger's disease. The relationship between these disorders, if any, is unclear.[24]

HSP frequently occurs following an antecedent pharyngitis or respiratory illness, and there is a strong history of allergy in approximately 25% of patients. No specific infectious agent has been clearly implicated. IgA-containing immune complex deposition in the glomeruli with subsequent activation of the alternate complement pathway and local coagulation may cause the renal injury.

DIAGNOSTIC EVALUATION

The clinical presentation of HSP in a young child is usually sufficiently characteristic for extensive diagnostic evaluation to be unnecessary. The platelet count and hematocrit are normal, antinuclear antibody and antistreptolysin-O measurements are negative, elevated serum IgA levels are present in approximately 50% of cases, and serum complement levels are usually normal.

DIFFERENTIAL DIAGNOSIS

IgA nephropathy (Berger's disease) is considered by some to be a form of HSP that is limited to renal involvement. Post-streptococcal glomerulonephritis may present renal manifestations similar to HSP. The absence of thrombocytopenia excludes hemolytic-uremic syndrome and thrombotic thrombocytopenic purpura. Systemic lupus erythematosus and other systemic vasculitides must be considered. Other causes of RPGN and proteinuria and hematuria must be considered.

THROMBOTIC THROMBOCYTOPENIC PURPURA (TTP) AND HEMOLYTIC-UREMIC SYNDROME (HUS)

DEFINITION

Thrombotic thrombocytopenic purpura is a clinical syndrome that typically occurs in young adults, especially females, characterized by thrombocytopenic purpura, microangiopathic hemolytic anemia, neurologic abnormalities, fever, and renal involvement. Renal manifestations, which occur in approximately 80% of patients, may include proteinuria, hematuria (gross or microscopic), and some degree of azotemia, which occasionally may be severe. Hemolytic-uremic syndrome typically presents in infants or young children following a prodromal gastrointestinal or respiratory illness with the abrupt onset of acute renal failure, thrombocytopenic purpura, microangiopathic hemolytic anemia, and gastrointestinal bleeding. There may be oliguria or anemia, hematuria, and proteinuria.[36] As may be seen, the distinction between TTP and HUS is not clear; the two disorders probably represent variations of a single clinical spectrum. Occurrence in older patients and more-widespread organ involvement tend to lead to a diagnosis of TTP, whereas, more-pronounced renal manifestations have been associated with HUS.

The renal pathologic findings in both TTP and HUS include thickening of glomerular capillary and arterial walls as a result of endothelial cell swelling, hyaline fibrin thrombi, fibrinoid necrosis of glomerular capillaries and arterioles, and aneurysmal dilatation of arterioles.[24]

PATHOPHYSIOLOGIC CONSIDERATIONS

The manifestations of both HUS and TTP result from the effects of vascular endothelial damage and localized intravascular coagulation. Disseminated intravascular coagulation (DIC) appears not to be pathogenetically important. Abnormalities in prostacyclin (PGI_2) or other plasma factors have been suggested by clinical studies in which plasma exchange or infusion reverses the manifestations of these disorders. The etiologic factors that can incite TTP and HUS are probably multiple. Most cases have no apparent precipitant, but infection with viruses, salmonella, shigella, and streptococci; Escherichia coli toxins; drugs (penicillamine, vaccines); and immunologic factors have been implicated.

DIAGNOSTIC EVALUATION AND DIFFERENTIAL DIAGNOSIS

Systemic lupus erythematosus, malignant hypertension, pre-eclampsia, sepsis with DIC, nonbacterial thrombotic endocarditis, acute glomerulonephritis, and disseminated carcinomatosis may present with features that overlap with those of the highly variable HUS and TTP. Negative blood cultures, Coomb's test and autoimmune serologic studies, the absence of DIC (normal prothrombin and partial thromboplastin times), and normal serum complements characterize TTP and HUS. The abrupt onset of illness in a previously healthy adult or child (except for prodromal symptoms with HUS) suggests the diagnosis of TTP or HUS.[37]

RENAL DISEASE IN SCLERODERMA

DEFINITION

Scleroderma, or progressive systemic sclerosis, frequently involves the kidneys, producing proteinuria, hypertension, and azotemia. The hypertension may be mild to moderate and asymptomatic, or it may be severe and abrupt in onset with the clinical findings of malignant hypertension. Acute renal failure may develop, sometimes in association with malignant hypertension. Pathologic findings consist of small arterial and arteriolar fibrinoid necrosis and intimal proliferation with perivascular fibrosis and thrombi in these vessels and within glomeruli.[38]

PATHOPHYSIOLOGIC CONSIDERATIONS

Immunologic factors, microvascular abnormalities, and abnormalities of collagen synthesis have been suggested as pathogenetic mechanisms, but the precise cause of scleroderma is unknown. The renal disease is due partly to the anatomic vascular changes; vasospasm and renal ischemia, which may be renin mediated, appear to play a role as well.

DIAGNOSTIC EVALUATION AND DIFFERENTIAL DIAGNOSIS

Scleroderma rarely produces clinically apparent renal disease without established cutaneous and vasomotor manifestations or esophagus dysmotility. Some patients, however, may present initially with renal disease, manifest by proteinuria or acute renal failure. Malignant hypertension in the setting of renovascular disease or previously diagnosed essential hypertension may pose a diagnostic problem; renal angiography and/or biopsy may be useful under some circumstances.

DIABETIC NEPHROPATHY

DEFINITION

Diabetic glomerulosclerosis is a common cause of nephrotic syndrome and end-stage renal failure in adults, particularly affecting patients with juvenile-onset insulin-dependent diabetes. Approximately 30 to 50% of patients with juvenile-onset diabetes who have had diabetes mellitus for over 20 to 30 years will ultimately develop renal failure; in contrast, only about 5% of adult-onset diabetic patients ever develop significant renal disease. The earliest manifestation of diabetic nephropathy is actually an increase in the glomerular filtration rate associated with generalized renal hypertrophy. There are no readily detectable clinical manifestations of renal disease for the first 10 to 20 years. Proteinuria then develops as the first manifestation of diabetic glomerulosclerosis; nephrotic syndrome is common. With onset of proteinuria, the GFR begins to decline, and over 50% of these patients will progress to end-stage renal disease and require dialysis or transplantation within 3 to 5 years. In addition to glomerular disease, diabetic patients may develop chronic interstitial fibrosis and tubular atrophy, papillary necrosis, renal arteriosclerosis, and neurogenic bladder dysfunction.[39,40]

The pathologic changes of diabetic glomerulosclerosis (Kimmelstiel-Wilson syndrome) include glomerular basement thickening, a diffuse increase in intercapillary mesangial matrix material, and the pathognomonic nodular sclerosis that occurs in 40 to 50% of patients with diabetic nephropathy.

PATHOPHYSIOLOGIC CONSIDERATIONS

Although there may be some element of genetic susceptibility, a metabolic basis for the renal lesions is probable. Abnormal basement membrane synthesis and degradation and abnormal amino acid and carbohydrate content appear to be responsible for the development of diabetic glomerulosclerosis. There is no evidence as of yet, however, to suggest that good metabolic control with insulin therapy is able to stop the progression of established diabetic nephropathy.

DIAGNOSTIC EVALUATION

The diagnosis and aggressive treatment of hypertension is essential to the management of the diabetic patient with renal disease. Similarly, evidence of urinary tract obstruction and infection should be sought. Quantification of urinary protein losses and measurement of the creatinine clearance should be made; renal function may be followed by serial determination of serum creatinine. Because of the high risk of precipitating acute renal failure, intravenous pyelography and other diagnostic intravenous contrast studies should be avoided in the diabetic patient with even mild renal insufficiency.

DIFFERENTIAL DIAGNOSIS

Unless there has been an abrupt change in renal function in a patient with a previously stable clinical course, the diagnosis of diabetic nephropathy is usually clear-cut. Although diabetic retinopathy is extremely common in patients with diabetic nephropathy, its absence by no means excludes diabetic nephropathy as the cause of a patient's renal disease. Neurogenic bladder dysfunction and papillary necrosis may contribute to a decline in GFR in the diabetic patient.

POLYCYSTIC KIDNEY DISEASE (PCKD)

DEFINITION

Adult-type polycystic kidney disease, a major cause of end-stage renal failure, is an autosomal-dominant inherited disorder presenting with signs and symptoms related to enlarging, cystic kidneys and renal insufficiency. Cysts may be present in a variety of other organs besides the kidneys, particularly the liver. Intracranial aneurysms may be present in 10 to 30% of patients with PCKD. Flank or abdominal pain, hematuria, palpable abdominal masses, proteinuria, uri-

nary tract infection, hypertension, and progressive renal insufficiency are the predominent clinical manifestations. The genetic penetrance is 100%, although clinically evident disease often does not become apparent until beyond the third or fourth decade of life.[41]

PATHOPHYSIOLOGIC CONSIDERATIONS

The cysts of PCKD develop as segmental dilatation of the proximal and distal tubules and retain at least some of the transporting characteristics of renal epithelia. The precise mechanisms responsible for cyst formation are not known. Hyperplasia of tubular epithelial cells (perhaps induced by an environmental toxin in genetically predisposed individuals) causing tubular obstruction and dilatation, an inherited defect of the tubular basement membrane, and disordered epithelial growth and function have been suggested as possible causes. The development of end-stage kidney disease is related in part to replacement of normal renal parenchyma by large cysts; hypertension, infection, and perhaps primary abnormalities in glomerular function may also be involved.[42]

DIAGNOSTIC EVALUATION

The asymptomatic patient with a positive family history of PCKD is best evaluated by ultrasonography, which may show typical bilateral cystic changes 10 to 20 years before clinical manifestations appear. PCKD probably develops only very rarely in an individual who still has a normal ultrasound exam at age 35 to 40. Once a diagnosis of PCKD is made, periodic evaluation for hypertension, urinary tract infection, and developing azotemia is necessary.

DIFFERENTIAL DIAGNOSIS

Polycystic kidney disease should be considered in any patient presenting with hematuria, bilateral abdominal masses, proteinuria, or repeated urinary tract infections, particularly if there is a family history of PCKD. Chronic renal failure is typically a late manifestation. PCKD may be distinguished from other cystic diseases of the kidneys such as simple renal cysts, infantile PCKD, medullary sponge kidney, and medullary cystic disease on the basis of family history, symptoms and signs, and radiologic studies.

ALPORT'S SYNDROME

DEFINITION

While the term "hereditary nephritis" encompasses a variety of familial renal diseases, Alport's syndrome refers to an inherited glomerular disease characterized by the onset in childhood or early adulthood of hematuria, proteinuria, and progressive renal failure in association with sensorineural hearing loss. Ocular abnormalities (lenticonus, macular pigmentation, myopia) and platelet abnormalities may also be present. Recurrent hematuria, either gross or microscopic, is the most frequent presenting abnormality. Proteinuria, which may be in the nephrotic range (greater than 3 g/day), is common. Chronic renal failure progressing to end-stage kidney failure usually develops before the third to fifth decade in affected men but is much less common in women, in whom all manifestations of the disease seem to appear less frequently. The mode of inheritance has not been clearly defined; autosomal dominant and x-linked transmission have been suggested.[43]

PATHOPHYSIOLOGIC CONSIDERATIONS

Irregularity of the glomerular basement membrane, with splitting of the lamina densa and with areas of focal thickening or thinning seen on electron microscopy, is the pathologic hallmark of Alport's syndrome. Alterations in basement membrane antigens and biochemical composition as the result of abnormal persistence of a neonatal glomerular basement membrane may be the primary inherited defect.[44]

DIAGNOSTIC EVALUATION

The diagnosis of Alport's syndrome is made by renal biopsy, which on light microscopy reveals normal glomeruli or mild and focal increases in cellularity and mesangial matrix, and on electron microscopy reveals the characteristic irregular, splintered glomerular basement membrane. The 24-hour protein excretion rate and creatinine clearance should be measured; ocular and audiometric examinations should be performed. Family members may be evaluated by periodic urinalysis for the presence of hematuria or proteinuria.

DIFFERENTIAL DIAGNOSIS

Alport's syndrome must always be considered in the setting of recurrent gross or microscopic hematuria or proteinuria in boys and young men. Berger's disease (IgA nephropathy), mesangial proliferative glomerulonephritis, benign hematuria, and other renal and urologic causes of hematuria should be excluded (see sections on hematuria and proteinuria).

INHERITED RENAL TUBULE DISORDERS

DEFINITION

There are a number of inherited abnormalities in the transport properties of the nephron. Hartnup disease is an autosomal recessive disorder characterized by a pellagra-like rash, cerebellar ataxia, and amino aciduria. Cystinuria, also inherited in an autosomal recessive manner, presents with complication of urinary calculi (obstruction, infection, and renal failure) caused by precipitation of cystine in the renal tubules. Renal glucosuria is the presence of glucose in the urine without hyperglycemia or other evidence of diabetes mellitus. Familial hypophosphatemic rickets is a sex-linked disorder characterized by rickets or osteomalacia with hypophosphatemia and normal serum calcium levels, with low $1,25\text{-}(OH)_2\text{-}D_3$ and with normal serum parathyroid hormone levels. Fanconi's syndrome is described below.[45]

PATHOPHYSIOLOGIC CONSIDERATIONS

Inherited renal tubule disorders result from abnormalities in renal and gastrointestinal tract epithelial transport. Defective neutral amino acid transport results in Hartnup disease. The clinical findings of Hartnup disease are due to intestinal malabsorption rather than the renal transport defect. Cystinuria is caused by a defect in cystine and dibasic amino acid (lysine, arginine, ornithine) transport. Other specific amino acid transport abnormalities have also been identified. Renal glucosuria may be due to either a decreased number of glucose transporting units in the proximal tubule cell membrane or a decreased affinity of the transporter for glucose, resulting in abnormal glucosuria. Familial hypophosphatemic rickets, also called vitamin D-resistant rickets, appears to be due to defective tubular phosphate reabsorption with abnormal vitamin D and parathyroid hormone metabolism and to abnormal gastrointestinal tract absorption of calcium and phosphate.

DIAGNOSTIC EVALUATION AND DIFFERENTIAL DIAGNOSIS

Cystinuria should always be considered in the patient presenting with radiopaque renal calculi, especially with early onset of stone disease (on the average at about 20 years of age, as opposed to 40 to 50 years for onset of other major stone types) and multiple bilateral stones. The cyanide-nitroprusside test is used to screen for cystinuria; excretion of greater than 600 mg of cystine daily is diagnostic. Renal glycosuria may occur as a primary disorder or as part of Fanconi's syndrome. Because blood glucose levels are normal despite persistent asymptomatic glucosuria, the distinction from diabetes mellitus should be apparent. The glucose oxidase method should be used to document the presence of glucosuria, excluding fructosuria, galactosuria, etc. Familial hypophosphatemic rickets (vitamin D-resistant rickets) must be differentiated from vitamin D-dependent rickets and vitamin D deficiency. Symptomatic hypocalcemia, elevated parathyroid hormone levels, and vitamin D responsiveness characterize the latter two disorders; vitamin D deficiency is of course not an inherited disorder.

FANCONI'S SYNDROME

DEFINITION

Fanconi's syndrome is a disorder of renal proximal tubule transport associated with glucosuria, amino aciduria, and phosphaturia. There may also be abnormal urinary losses of uric acid, potassium, bicarbonate, and calcium. Rickets and growth failure or osteomalacia are the usual clinical manifestations.[45]

PATHOPHYSIOLOGIC CONSIDERATIONS AND DIFFERENTIAL DIAGNOSIS

Abnormal cellular metabolism leads to a generalized defect in the proximal tubule reabsorption of glucose, amino acids, and phosphate, causing Fanconi's syndrome.

Fanconi's syndrome may be inherited as a primary

renal tubule disorder but in children is most often associated with cystinosis. Wilson's disease, glycogen storage disease, galactosemia, and fructose intolerance may also lead to inherited Fanconi's syndrome. Multiple myeloma, heavy metal poisoning, and outdated tetracycline administration may cause an acquired Fanconi's syndrome. Fanconi's syndrome must be considered in the patient with a renal tubular acidosis (see section on RTA).

DIAGNOSTIC EVALUATION

A careful family, developmental, and medical history should be obtained. Measurement of urinary and serum amino acids, phosphorus, and glucose are needed. In the adult patient with Fanconi's syndrome, a serum protein electrophoresis should be obtained to exclude multiple myeloma.

NAIL-PATELLA SYNDROME

DEFINITION

Nail-patella syndrome (hereditary arthro-onychodysplasia) is an autosomal dominant trait characterized by hypoplasia or absence of the patellae, by bilateral conical iliac horns, by subluxation of the radial heads, and by atrophic or dystrophic fingernails. Proteinuria, which may range from asymptomatic mild proteinuria to a full-blown nephrotic syndrome, occurs in approximately 40% of patients. Chronic renal failure may occasionally develop.

Light microscopic examination of the kidney is initially normal, but glomerular sclerosis with tubular loss and interstitial fibrosis may develop. Electron microscopy reveals a characteristic thickening of the glomerular basement membrane, which contains irregular lucent areas. With phosphotungstic acid staining, fibrils with the periodicity of collagen may be seen in these lucent areas, as well as in the mesangium, interstitium, and subendothelial space.[46]

PATHOPHYSIOLOGIC CONSIDERATIONS

The precise pathogenetic mechanism for the glomerular lesion of nail-patella syndrome is not known. It has been suggested that abnormal collagen metabolism leads to increased quantities of circulating collagen fragments that are subsequently trapped in glomeruli.

DIAGNOSTIC EVALUATION

As there are no specific tests for nail-patella syndrome, the diagnosis depends upon the constellation of appropriate radiographic, clinical, and renal histopathologic findings.

TOXEMIA OF PREGNANCY

DEFINITION

Toxemia is a disease or group of diseases occurring during gestation or in the early puerperium, characterized by hypertension, proteinuria, and edema.[47] Seizures and coma occur commonly, and their appearance in toxemia is called "eclampsia." "Pre-eclampsia" is the term used to designate toxemia in the absence of seizures. Toxemia is more frequent in women with diabetes mellitus, pregnant with twins, with hydramnios, and with hydatidiform mole. Toxemia is usually a disease of the second half of gestation, occurring only rarely before the twenty-fourth week of gestation. The presence of hypertension or proteinuria during the first trimester suggests underlying renal disease or hypertension present before the pregnancy. The disease often recurs in subsequent pregnancies, and fixed hypertension will develop in 50% of women with repeated toxemia.

PATHOPHYSIOLOGIC CONSIDERATIONS[48]

Hypertension in toxemia, as in other forms of hypertension, is associated with increased peripheral vascular resistance. Arterioles have increased sensitivity to vasopressor substances, such as angiotensin and norepinephrine in patients with toxemia. The intravascular volume is increased during normal pregnancy, as are the renal blood flow and glomerular filtration rate. In toxemia, renal blood flow and GFR normally do not rise and may even fall. Under these conditions, sodium retention develops, and the usual natriuresis of increased blood pressure does not occur, resulting in edema, volume expansion, and hypertension. In the kidney, glomerular capillaries demonstrate endothelial cell swelling, with fibrinogen deposits in a subendothelial location. Neither cell proliferation nor

immunologic damage is seen, and complete resolution of these changes occurs in some patients, though persistent abnormalities are found in others. These renal changes are presumed responsible for the proteinuria, which may range from 0.5 to 30 g/24 hours.

Cerebral hemorrhage is the most common cause of death in toxemia, with precapillary thrombosis and subsequent hemorrhage and infarction. Cerebral vasoconstriction may predispose to these abnormalities.

DIAGNOSTIC EVALUATION AND DIFFERENTIAL DIAGNOSIS

When women develop hypertension and proteinuria during pregnancy, toxemia must be differentiated from pre-existing hypertension or renal disease. Pregestational blood pressure readings or urinalyses must be consulted. Often, because measurement of blood pressure is not recorded regularly until a young woman's pregnancy, other clues such as a family history of diabetes, obesity, or hypertension, might be needed to suggest underlying disease. When hypertension without proteinuria is seen in late pregnancy, the diagnosis is usually essential hypertension. Likewise, proteinuria in the first trimester usually means primary renal disease rather than toxemia. Systemic causes such as diabetes, systemic lupus erythematosus, or vasculitis should be excluded, and primary renal diseases such as glomerulonephritis, chronic or acute interstitial nephritis, or polycystic renal disease must be considered.

Evaluation should include quantitation of the GFR and protein excretion with a 24-hour collection of urine, ultrasound evaluation of the kidneys, and measurements of plasma glucose, creatinine, uric acid, platelet count, complement, and antinuclear antibody (ANA). The plasma uric acid measurements may be particularly helpful. The clearance of uric acid is reduced in toxemia, and plasma uric acid levels rise frequently. The level of uric acid can be used to assess the severity of toxemia; plasma urate rises to approximately 5 mg/dl in mild toxemia, and to over 7.5 mg/dl in severe toxemia.

NEPHROLITHIASIS

DEFINITION

Nephrolithiasis is the formation of kidney stones in the pelvis or calyces of the upper urinary tract. These stones may be composed of various compounds and may take many forms. They may be single or multiple or may grow and merge into a staghorn calculus, a single mass filling the collecting system.[49]

PATHOPHYSIOLOGIC CONSIDERATIONS

Renal stones are crystalline substances, mixed with some water and protein. They can be classified according to crystalline analysis. When these substances are present in urine in concentrations equal to their solubility products, a saturated solution forms. Further addition of the substance forms a supersaturated solution, until a critical concentration is reached, the formation product. Further addition of the substance causes crystalline precipitation. The supersaturated solutions are stabilized by urinary citrate, pyrophosphate, and other substances. It is generally believed that stone formation occurs because the urinary concentration of stone-forming substances is increased by high excretion rates or low urine volume, because concentrations of urinary inhibitors to stone formation such as citrate are reduced, or because a scar or anomaly in the collecting system predisposes to stone nucleation.

DIAGNOSTIC EVALUATION

A complete history should be elicited, with particular attention to all stone events, family history of stone disease, dietary history, or evidence of hyperparathyroidism (GI disease, bone disease, CNS disturbances), joint disease, or inflammatory bowel disease. Stones should be collected by straining the urine and should be submitted for crystallographic analysis. Anatomic evaluation of the urinary tract with an intravenous pyelogram and quantitation of the "stone burden" with cone and oblique views of the kidneys should be performed. Blood is tested for calcium and albumin, phosphorus, uric acid, creatinine, bicarbonate, and chloride. A 24-hour urine is collected for creatinine, calcium, and uric acid, and the volume is noted. The urine pH is recorded, and if pH is >5, the patient is asked to test the urine pH at home several times. The urine is also cultured.

Patients found to have hypercalciuria are then evaluated as below (see Hypercalciuria).

DIFFERENTIAL DIAGNOSIS

Calcium oxalate stones are the most common type of stones, representing 75% of all upper tract stones. About half are pure calcium oxalate, the other half mixed with calcium phosphate. While an exact cause of stone formation may be unclear in any given patient, certain risk factors predispose to calcium oxalate stone formation. These include hypercalciuria (> 4 mg/kg/day calcium excretion in the urine), hyperoxaluria (> 50 mg/day), hyperuricosuria (> 1000 mg/day uric acid excretion in the urine), dehydration with low urine volume, diets high in protein or sodium or high in oxalate in patients with enteric hyperoxaluria, ingestion of vitamins A, D, or C, and a positive family history of nephrolithiasis.

Cystine stones are caused by cystinuria, which is an autosomal recessive inborn error of cystine, ornithine, lysine, and arginine (COLA) transport in the renal and intestinal epithelial cells. In patients homozygous for this disorder, these dibasic amino acids are not reabsorbed from the tubular fluid and appear in high concentration in the urine. Of these, only cystine is insoluble, forming stones in the collecting systems, sometimes even into staghorn calculi.

Uric acid stones result from uric acid, the poorly soluble end product of purine metabolism. One quarter of uric acid is excreted in the gut; the rest is excreted in the urine. Uric acid is filtered at the glomerulus, reabsorbed, and secreted by the renal tubule. Its solubility in urine is dependent on pH; uric acid is relatively insoluble at the usual acid pH and becomes much more soluble as the pH rises. Thus the main risk factors for uric acid stone formation include hyperuricosuria, decreased urine volume, and urine acidity. In patients with gout and hyperuricemia, 20% form uric acid stones. Other groups at risk of uric acid nephrolithiasis include patients receiving uricosuric drugs and patients with inflammatory bowel disease or ileostomy.

Magnesium ammonium phosphate stones, or triple phosphate stones (struvite), are found in patients with chronic urinary tract infections. Infections with urea-splitting organisms raise the urine pH, resulting in supersaturation of magnesium ammonium phosphate and carbonate-apatite. Mineralization of large, gelatinous matrix concretions may lead to large staghorn calculi. Patients at risk of developing these stones include those with anatomic or functional anomalies predisposing to infection, such as ureteral reflux or obstruction, nephrostomy drainage, ileal loop bladder, neurogenic bladder, and medullary sponge kidney; and patients with previously infected stones or those with urologic manipulation.

Calcium phosphate stones are precipitated only in persistently alkaline, sterile urine. Patients at risk include those with distal renal tubular acidosis or patients who chronically ingest absorbable antacids or other alkalies, thus always excreting their alkali load.

HYPERCALCIURIA

DEFINITION

The urinary excretion of calcium depends upon many factors, including dietary calcium, sodium, carbohydrate, and protein; levels of parathyroid hormone and vitamin D metabolites; and the integrity of kidney function. The dietary factors in particular can vary widely in a single patient, and thus a definition of hypercalciuria is difficult without also specifying the patient's diet in the period during which calcium excretion is measured. With ingestion of 1000 mg/day of calcium without excessive protein or sodium, hypercalciuria is defined as calcium excretion rates exceeding 300 mg/day for males and 250 mg/day for females, or exceeding 4 mg/kg/day for either sex.[59]

PATHOPHYSIOLOGIC CONSIDERATIONS

Under normal conditions, the body's calcium economy is maintained when renal calcium excretion is equal to gut calcium absorption. Most calcium is located in bone, which is in dynamic equilibrium with the extracellular fluid. Increases in renal excretion of calcium can result from increased gut absorption of calcium (hyperabsorption), from net movement of calcium out of bones into the extracellular space (bone resorption), and from decreased renal tubular resorption of calcium (renal hypercalciuria).

Table 9–10. Hypercalciuria

Hyperabsorption
  Idiopathic absorptive hypercalciuria
  Primary hyperparathyroidism
  Sarcoidosis
  Vitamin D excess
  Normal pregnancy and lactation
Bone resorption
  Distal renal tubular acidosis
  Immobilization
  Rapidly progressive osteoporosis
  Malignant osteolysis
Renal leak
  Furosemide administration
  Chronic hypoparathyroidism
  Uncontrolled diabetes mellitus
Endocrine abnormalities
  Glucocorticoid excess
  Acromegaly
  Thyrotoxicosis

DIAGNOSTIC EVALUATION

Hypercalciuria should be confirmed by 24-hour urine collection on a diet as described above. The serum calcium, phosphorus, HCO_3, chlorine, and sodium should be measured. The urine pH should be tested. Levels of circulating parathyroid hormone and $1,25\text{-}(OH)_2\text{-}D_3$ can be measured, and values of urinary excretion of total and nephrogenous cyclic AMP may be obtained. In patients with possible absorptive hypercalciuria or primary hyperparathyroidism, the renal excretion of calcium should be measured with the patient on a calcium-restricted diet or in the fasting state. An oral calcium tolerance test may be helpful in these disorders.[49]

Underlying disorders as listed in Table 9–10 should be considered and excluded by history, bone radiographs, glucose tolerance tests, or other appropriate studies.

DIFFERENTIAL DIAGNOSIS

Table 9–10 lists the differential diagnosis of hypercalciuria. Many of these entities are complex, with combined mechanisms causing increased calcium excretion. For example, primary hyperparathyroidism causes hyperabsorption of gut calcium, increased bone resorption, and also lower renal leak. Nonetheless, the major defect is hyperabsorption, and hence hyperparathyroidism is listed under hyperabsorption.

REFERENCES

1. Glassock, R.J.: Clinical aspects of acute, rapidly progressive, and chronic glomerulonephritis. *In* Strauss and Welt's Diseases of the Kidney. Edited by L.E. Earley and C.W. Gottschalk. Little, Brown and Co., Boston, 1979.
2. Bia, M.J., and Kliger, A.S.: The laboratory in renal diseases. *In* Laboratory Medicine in Clinical Practice. Edited by H.N. Mandell. Boston, John Wright PSG Inc., 1983.
3. Kassirer, J.P., and Gennari, F.J.: Laboratory evaluation of renal function. *In* Strauss and Welt's Diseases of the Kidney. Edited by L.E. Earley and C.W. Gottschalk. Boston, Little, Brown and Co., 1979.
4. Earley, L.E., Forland, M.: Nephrotic syndrome. *In* Strauss and Welt's Diseases of the Kidney. Edited by L.E. Earley and C.W. Gottschalk. Boston, Little, Brown and Co., 1979.
5. Cohen, J.J., and Kassirer, J.P. (eds.): Acid/Base. Boston, Little, Brown and Co., 1982.
6. Sebastian, A., McSherry, E., and Curtis Morris, R.: Metabolic acidosis with special reference to the renal acidoses. *In* The Kidney. Edited by B.M. Brenner and F.C. Rector, Jr. Philadelphia, W.B. Saunders Co., 1976.
7. Cogan, M.G., Rector, F.C., and Seldin, D.W.: Acid base disorders. *In* The Kidney. 2nd Ed. Edited by B.M. Brenner and F.C. Rector, Jr. Philadelphia, W.B. Saunders Co., 1981.

8. Brenner, B.M., and Lazarus, J.M. (eds.): Acute Renal Failure. Philadelphia, W.B. Saunders Co., 1983.
9. Bastl, C.P., Rudnick, M.R., and Narins, R.G.: Diagnostic approaches to acute renal failure. In Contemporary Issues in Nephrology. Acute Renal Failure (Vol. 6). Edited by B.M. Brenner and J.H. Stein. New York, Churchill Livingstone, 1980.
10. Levenson, D.J., Skorecki, K.L., and Narins, R.G.: Acute renal failure associated with hepatobiliary disease. In Acute Renal Failure. Edited by B.M. Brenner and J.M. Lazarus. Philadelphia, W.B. Saunders Co., 1983.
11. Vaamonde, C.A., and Papper, S.: The kidney in liver disease. In Strauss and Welt's Diseases of the Kidney. Edited by L.E. Earley and C.W. Gottschalk. Boston, Little, Brown and Co., 1979.
12. Rose, B.D.: Pathophysiology of uremia. In Pathophysiology of Renal Disease. Edited by B.D. Rose. New York, McGraw-Hill, 1981.
13. Knochel, J.P., and Seldin, D.W.: The pathophysiology of uremia. In The Kidney. Edited by B.M. Brenner and F.C. Rector, Jr. Philadelphia, W.B. Saunders, 1981.
14. Coburn, J.W., and Llach, F.: Renal osteodystrophy and maintenance hemodialysis. In Replacement of Renal Function by Dialysis. Edited by W. Drukker, F.M. Parsons, and J.F. Maner. Boston, Martinus-Nijhoff, 1983.
15. Ott, S.M., et al.: The prevalence of bone aluminum deposition in renal osteodystrophy and its relation to the response to calcitriol therapy. N Engl J Med 307:709, 1982.
16. Hoyer, J.R.: Idiopathic nephrotic syndrome with minimal glomerular changes. In Contemporary Issues in Nephrology. Nephrotic Syndrome (Vol. 9). Edited by B.M. Brenner and J.H. Stein. New York, Churchill Livingstone, 1982.
17. Goldszer, R.C., Sweet, J., and Cotran, R.S.: Focal segmental glomerulosclerosis. Annu Rev Med 35:429, 1984.
18. Arnaout, M.A., Rennke, H.G., and Cotran, R.S.: Membranous glomerulonephritis. InContemporary Issues in Nephrology. Nephrotic Syndrome (Vol. 9). Edited by B.M. Brenner and J.G. Stein. New York, Churchill Livingstone, 1982.
19. Kim, Y., and Michael, A.F.: Idiopathic membranoproliferative glomerulonephritis. Annu Rev Med 31:273, 1980.
20. Donadio, J.R., Jr., and Holley, K.E.: Membranoproliferative glomerulonephritis. Semin Nephrol 2:163, 1983.
21. Brown, E.B., et al.: The clinical course of mesangial proliferative glomerulonephritis. Medicine 58:295, 1979.
22. Cohen, A.H., and Border, W.A.: Mesangial proliferative glomerulonephritis. Semin Nephrol 2:228, 1982.
23. Glassock, R.J., Cohen, A.H., Bennett, C.M., and Martinez-Maldonado, M.: Primary glomerular disease. In The Kidney. Edited by B.M. Brenner and F.C. Rector, Jr. Philadelphia, W.B. Saunders Co., 1981.
24. Heptinstall, R.H.: Pathology of the Kidney. 3rd Ed. Boston, Little, Brown and Co., 1983.
25. Couser, W.G., et al.: Acute renal failure associated with renal vascular disease, vasculitis, glomerulonephritis, and nephrotic syndrome. In Acute Renal Failure. Edited by B.M. Brenner and J.M. Lazarus. Philadelphia, W.B. Saunders Co., 1983.
26. Lewis, E.J., and Schwartz, M.M.: Idiopathic crescentic glomerulonephritis. Semin Nephrol 2:193, 1982.
27. Kincaid-Smith, P., and Nicholls, K.: Mesangial IgA nephropathy. Am J Kidney Dis 3:90, 1983.
28. Fauci, A.S. (moderator): The spectrum of vasculitis: Clinical, pathologic, immunologic, and therapeutic considerations. Ann Intern Med 89 (Part 1):660, 1978.
29. Fauci, A.S., Haynes, B.F., Katz, P., and Wolff, S.M.: Wegener's granulomatosis: Prospective clinical and therapeutic experience with 85 patients for 21 years. Ann Intern Med 98:76, 1983.
30. DeFronzo, R.A., Cooke, C.R., Wright, J.R., and Humphrey, R.L.: Renal function in patients with multiple myeloma. Medicine 57:151, 1978.
31. Martinez-Maldonado, M., Benebe, J.E., and Lopez-Novoa, J.M.: Acute renal failure associated with tubulointerstitial disease, including papillary necrosis. In Acute Renal Failure. Edited by B.M. Brenner and M.J. Lazarus. Philadelphia, W.B. Saunders Co., 1983.
32. Kyle, R.A., and Greipp, P.R.: Amyloidosis (AL): Clinical and laboratory features in 229 cases. Mayo Clin Proc 58:665, 1983.
33. Glenner, G.G.: Amyloid deposits and amyloidosis: The β-fibrilloses. N Engl J Med 302:1283, 1980.
34. Brouet J-C., et al.: Biologic and clinical significance of cryoglobulins: A report of 86 cases. Am J Med 57:775, 1974.
35. Glassock, R.J., and Cohen, A.H.: Secondary glomerular diseases. In The Kidney. Edited by B.M. Brenner and F.C. Rector, Jr. Philadelphia, W.B. Saunders Co., 1981.
36. Goldstein, M.H., Churg, J., Strauss, L., and Gribetz, D.: Hemolytic-uremic syndrome. Nephron 23:263, 1979.
37. Ridolfi, R.L., and Bell, W.R.: Thrombotic thrombocytopenic purpura: Report of 25 cases and review of the literature. Medicine 60:413, 1981.
38. Cannon, P.J., et al.: The relationship of hypertension and renal failure in scleroderma (progressive systemic sclerosis) to structural and functional abnormalities of the renal cortical circulation. Medicine 53:1, 1974.
39. Arieff, A.I., and Myers, B.D.: Diabetic nephropathy. In The Kidney. Edited by B.M. Brenner and F.C. Rector, Jr. Philadelphia, W.B. Saunders Co., 1981.
40. Friedman, E.A.: Diabetic nephropathy: strategies in prevention and management. Kidney Int 21:780, 1982.
41. Gardner, K.D., Jr.: Cystic Diseases of the Kidney. New York, Wiley, 1976.
42. Grantham, J.J.: Polycystic kidney disease: a predominance of giant nephrons. Am J Physiol 244:F3, 1983.
43. Gubler, M., et al.: Alports' syndrome: a report of 58 cases and a review of the literature. Am J Med 70:493, 1981.
44. Habib, R., et al.: Alports' syndrome: experience at Hopital Necker. Kidney Int. 21(Suppl 11):S-20, 1982.
45. Defronzo, R.A., Thier, S.O.: Inherited disorders of renal tubule function. In The Kidney. Edited by B.M. Brenner and F.C. Rector, Jr. Philadelphia, W.B. Saunders, Co., 1981.
46. Suki, W.N., and Caskey, C.T.: Hereditary chronic nephropathies. In Strauss and Welt's Diseases of the Kidney. Edited by L.E. Earley and C.W. Gottschalk. Boston, Little, Brown and Co., 1979.
47. Eastman, N.J., and Hellman, L.M. (eds.): Williams' Obstetrics. New York, Meredith Publishing Co., 1966.
48. Ferris, T.F.: The kidney and pregnancy. In Strauss and Welt's Diseases of the Kidney. 3rd Ed. Edited by L.E. Earley and C.W. Gottschalk. Boston, Little, Brown and Co., 1979.
49. Broadus, A.E.: Nephrolithiasis. In Endocrinology and Metabolism. Edited by P. Felig, J.D. Baxter, A.E. Broadus, and L.A. Frohman, New York, McGraw-Hill Book Co., 1981.

GENERAL REFERENCES

Arieff, A.I., and DeFronzo, R.A. (eds.): Fluid, Electrolytes and Acid Base Disorders. New York, Churchill Livingstone, 1985.
Brenner, B.M., and Rector, F.C., Jr. (eds.): The Kidney. Philadelphia, W.B. Saunders Co., 1981.
Brenner, B.M., and Stein, J.H. (eds.): Contemporary Issues in Nephrology. Acid Base and Potassium Homeostasis. (Vol. 2). New York, Churchill Livingstone, 1978.
Earley, L.E., and Gottschalk, C.W. (eds.): Strauss and Welt's Disease of the Kidney. Boston, Little, Brown & Co., 1979.
Felig, P., Baxter, J.D., Broadus, A.E., and Frohman, L.A. (eds.): Endocrinology and Metabolism. New York, McGraw-Hill Book Co., 1981.

CHAPTER 10 # WATER, ELECTROLYTE, AND ACID-BASE PROBLEMS

Charles F. Abboud, M.D., B.Ch. and Alan S. Kliger, M.D.

DISORDERS OF WATER AND SODIUM BALANCE

INTRODUCTION

The maintenance of normal volume and osmolality of body fluids requires that the input of water and solutes equal the output. Since the major solute of the extracellular fluid (ECF) is sodium, the maintenance of normal volume and osmolality depends on the regulation of the balance of water and sodium.

Water Balance. Water is added to the body in three ways: contained in foods (average 800 to 1000 ml/day); consumed as liquid (average 1 to 2 L/day); and generated from food combustion (300 to 400 ml/day). The water input is regulated by the thirst mechanism. Water is lost from the body via four routes: insensible loss through skin and lung (average 800 to 1000 ml/day); in sweat (varying from less than 200 ml to greater than 8 L/day depending on temperature, humidity, and level of physical exertion); in feces (100 to 200 ml/day); and in urine (average 1 to 2 L/day). The water output is regulated primarily by changes in urine volume determined mostly by secretion of antidiuretic hormone (ADH), which is also called arginine vasopressin (AVP).

Control of Water Balance. The input and output of water are regulated by changes in the volume of the liquid ingested, which is controlled by thirst, and in urine volume, which is controlled by AVP. Thirst and AVP secretion are regulated primarily by hypothalamic neurons in response to changes in plasma osmolality and volume; increased plasma osmolality causes shrinkage and stimulation of the hypothalamic osmoreceptors leading to increased AVP secretion and increased thirst. Osmoreceptors are extremely sensitive to changes in plasma osmolality, even to a change of less than 1%.

In extreme circumstances, decreased plasma volume sensed by volume receptors in the atria or pulmonary vessels, carotid sinuses, and aortic arch can also lead to increased thirst and AVP secretion. Volume stimuli can override the effects of osmolality stimulus.

Sodium Balance. Of total body sodium, 35 to 40% is in the skeleton. Of this amount, 65 to 70% is unexchangeable or slowly exchangeable. Sodium is the major cation of the extracellular fluid, with plasma concentration of 135 to 145 mEq/L.

The daily intake of sodium can vary markedly depending on the individual's diet and habits. The average diet contains 100 to 400 mEq of sodium per day. This sodium input does not appear to be physiologically regulated. Sodium is lost from the body by three routes: in sweat, in which sodium loss depends on the volume and the degree of adaptation to a hot environment and can vary from negligible to several hundred mEq/day; in feces, in which sodium loss is normally negligible but can exceed 1000 mEq/day in diarrheal states; and in urine, in which sodium loss averages 100 to 400 mEq/day but can vary from negligible to greater than 600 mEq/day.

Sodium balance is achieved by matching output to input. The output is regulated primarily by changing the amount of sodium excreted in the urine. The three main regulators of renal sodium excretion are glomerular filtration rate (GFR), aldosterone, and atriopeptin.

The changes in GFR play a minor role. Aldosterone causes increased sodium reabsorption by the distal nephron. Aldosterone secretion is stimulated by increased plasma angiotensin II levels, increased serum potassium, decreased serum sodium (minor effect), and increased serum ACTH (minor effect). Atriopeptin is an atrial peptide synthesized in the atrial cardiocyte and secreted in response to atrial stretch by volume expansion. It has diverse effects, aimed at restoring circulatory volume to normal; it causes an increase in the glomerular filtration rate (GFR), pronounced natriuresis and diuresis, inhibition of aldosterone secretion by adrenocortical zona glomerulosa, and suppression of arginine vasopressin (AVP) released by the hypothalamus. Renal sodium excretion can be adjusted to wide ranges of sodium intake. Significant sodium depletion does not occur unless renal sodium conservation is abnormal, for example, from primary renal disease or mineralocorticoid lack, or when extrarenal losses (for example, gastrointestinal losses) are combined with inadequate intake. Similarly, sodium overload implies a defect in renal sodium excretion.

HYPONATREMIA

Definition. Hyponatremia is defined as a decrease in serum sodium concentration below 135 mEq/L. It is usually indicative of hypo-osmolality of the body fluids caused by excess water relative to solute. It is not synonymous with sodium depletion.

Pathophysiologic Considerations (Table 10–1). The commonest cause of hyponatremia is defective urinary dilution. The normal renal response to dilution of body fluids is a water diuresis. For an individual to be able to excrete a water load, several processes must be intact: the secretion of AVP or ADH must be suppressed, sufficient sodium and water must reach the

Table 10–1.   Causes of Hyponatremia

Pseudohyponatremia
  Hyponatremia with normal serum osmolality
    Hyperlipidemia
    Hyperproteinemia
      Multiple myeloma
      Waldenström's macroglobulinemia
  Hyponatremia with serum hyperosmolality
    Hyperglycemia
    Mannitol infusion
    Ingestion of toxins
      Ethylene glycol
      Ethyl alcohol
      Methanol
"True" hyponatremia—hyponatremia with hypo-osmolality
  With volume overload
    Congestive heart failure
    Cirrhosis
    Nephrotic syndrome
    Acute or chronic renal failure
  With volume contraction
    Renal losses
      Diuretics
      Salt-losing states
        Renal tubular acidosis
        Postobstructive states
        Medullary cystic disease
        Osmotic diuresis
        Mineralocorticoid deficiency
    Extrarenal losses
      Gastrointestinal
        Vomiting
        Diarrhea
        External fistulas
        Nasogastric suction
      Third space
        Burns
        Pancreatitis
        Peritonitis
  With clinically euvolemic state
    Decreased solute renal load
      Dietary protein and sodium restriction
      Beer potomonia
    Primary polydipsia

With clinically euvolemic state (cont.)
  Syndrome of inappropriate ADH release (SIADH)
    Hypothalamic
      CNS disease
        Head injury
        Subdural hematoma
        Meningitis
        Encephalitis
        Brain abscess
        Guillain-Barré syndrome
        Acute intermittent porphyria
        Brain tumor
        Idiopathic
    Drugs that increase AVP release
      Chlorpropamide
      Carbamazepine
      Clofibrate
      Nicotine
      Opiates
      Barbiturates
      Vincristine
      Cyclophosphamide
    Drugs that increase AVP effect
      Chlorpropamide
      Indomethacin
      Oxytocin
  Ectopic AVP Secretion
    Neoplasm
      Oat-cell carcinoma of lung
      Thymoma
      Pancreatic carcinoma
      Duodenal carcinoma
    Pulmonary disease
      Pneumonia
      Tuberculosis
      Abscess
      Aspergillosis
    Exogenous
      AVP or analogues
  Metabolic
    Pure glucocorticoid deficiency
    Hypothyroidism
    Acute intermittent porphyria
    Severe potassium depletion
  Reset osmostat
    Sick cell syndrome

diluting segment of the nephron, ascending limb, and distal and collecting tubules, and the nephron segments must function normally in reabsorption of sodium while remaining impermeable to water. Therefore, as is discussed below, a defect in water diuresis will occur with inappropriate secretion of ADH, when sodium reaching the diluting segments is insufficient because of either decreased GFR or enhanced proximal tubular reabsorption, and with defective sodium transport or excessive water permeability even in the absence of ADH, which occurs in intrinsic renal disease.

The secretion of ADH is "appropriate" in terms of homeostatic needs when it occurs in response to serum hyperosmolality or to hypovolemia. When the secretion of ADH occurs in the absence of these stimuli, it is "inappropriate," leading to clinical manifestations designated "syndrome of inappropriate ADH (SIADH)." Basically, there are three possible causes of SIADH. One cause, impairment of hypothalamic function producing a change in the set point of ADH release, arises in the presence of hypothalamic disease, extrahypothalamic CNS disease of various origins, metabolic diseases (such as myxedema or intermittent porphyria), and the use of certain drugs that may enhance ADH secretion and ADH effect on the distal nephron (for example, chlorpropamide, carbamazepine, and vincristine). Another cause of SIADH is the presence of faulty stimuli from volume receptors. This may occur when fluid is sequestered on the venous side of the circulation (right-sided heart failure, ascites, etc.), with mechanical positive pressure breathing, or after commissurotomy for mitral stenosis. The volume receptors will sense an apparent decrease in the blood volume and lead to stimulation of ADH secretion. Finally, secretion of ADH by ectopic extrahypothalamic tissue that is not subservient to homeostatic needs (for example, certain malignant tumors and granulomatous pulmonary diseases) may cause SIADH.

Insufficient sodium delivery to the diluting renal segment because of decreased GFR or increased proximal tubular reabsorption also causes hyponatremia. Under normal conditions, the minimum urinary osmolality that can be achieved is 50 mOsm/kg H_2O. The excretion of a high volume of urine, for example 10 L, requires excretion of 500 mOsm of solute. If the daily urine solute excretion falls, the maximum daily rate of urine formation will be reduced. This decrease in urine solute excretion can be observed in dietary sodium and protein restriction without parallel reduction in water intake, as is seen in beer potomania when large volumes of beer are ingested in association with dietary restrictions of sodium and protein. Decrease in urine solute excretion is also observed in reduction of solute delivery to the diluting segments and collecting ducts with sustained release of ADH, which is seen in volume-contracted states, e.g., untreated Addison's disease, and in disorders characterized by edema formation and reduction of effective circulating volume (intractable congestive heart failure, advanced hepatic cirrhosis with ascites, and nephrotic syndrome).

Rarely, hyponatremia can occur in the absence of a defect in water diuresis. In essential reset hyponatremia, suppression of ADH release occurs at plasma osmolality lower than normal. The effective circulating volume is normal. Affected patients develop brisk water diuresis when the serum sodium is reduced sufficiently, in contrast to patients with SIADH. Sick cell syndrome, which occurs in debilitated or severely ill patients, is believed to be due to redistribution of sodium from ECF to intracellular fluid (ICF) compartments because of impaired activity of membrane-bound Na/K ATPase. Finally, a primary increase in water ingestion, seen in psychogenic polydipsia, is a rare cause of hyponatremia because the kidney's ability to maximally dilute urine is impaired.

Clinical Presentation. Neurologic dysfunction is the principal clinical feature of hyponatremia. The severity of the signs and symptoms depends on the ab-

solute level of serum sodium and on the rapidity of its development. Symptoms include headache, confusion, muscle cramps, weakness, lethargy, apathy, agitation, nausea, vomiting and anorexia, altered levels of consciousness, and seizures. Deep tendon reflexes may be depressed. Hypothermia and Cheyne-Stokes respiration are present.

Acute hyponatremia leads to brain swelling and manifestations of CNS dysfunction when the serum sodium falls to 120 mEq/L or less. Untreated it is nearly always fatal and represents a medical emergency. In chronic hyponatremia, however, loss of brain solutes, principally potassium and chloride, minimizes the brain swelling, and the CNS manifestations are far less common even when serum sodium is 110 mEq/L or less.

Diagnostic Evaluation and Differential Diagnosis (Fig. 10–1). The physician must exclude pseudohyponatremia and hyponatremia caused by osmotic diuresis from the diagnosis.

Hyponatremia may on occasion be associated with hyperlipidemia and hyperproteinemia (pseudohyponatremia) as a consequence of a decrease in the aqueous phase of plasma because of the high lipid or protein content. Sodium concentration per liter of plasma water and plasma osmolality are normal.

The effects of osmotic agents such as mannitol can imitate those of hyponatremia. Significant hyperglycemia causes osmotic equilibration and movement of water from the intracellular to the extracellular fluid compartments with proportionate lowering of serum sodium. An increase of plasma glucose by 180 mg/dl will result in reduction of serum sodium by approximately 5 mEq/L. This is further modified by the sustained sodium and water diuresis from the severe hyperglycemia. A similar mechanism occurs with administration of osmotic agents such as mannitol.

If pseudohyponatremia and hyponatremia due to osmotic diuresis are excluded, then the patient has true hyponatremia.

In determining the cause of hyponatremia, the history and the physical examination may provide important clues to the differential diagnosis of the causes of hyponatremia. The physician should seek clinical evidence of volume expansion (for example, congestive heart failure, cirrhosis, nephrosis, etc.); clinical evidence of volume depletion (for example, the patient's use of diuretics or laxatives, or renal and extrarenal losses); evidence of CNS disease, pulmonary disease, ectopic neoplasm, and endocrine metabolic disease (for example, hypothyroidism, Addison's disease, and acute intermittent porphyria); and evidence of the use of drugs, for example, diuretics, drugs that

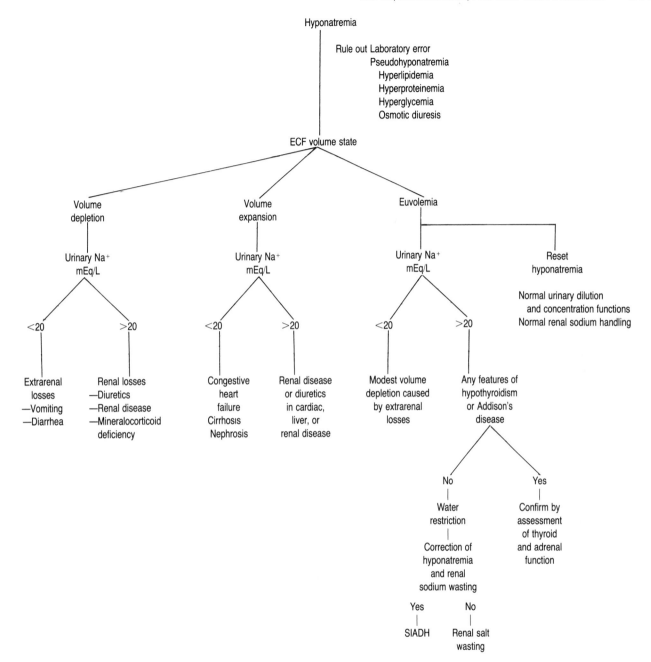

Fig. 10–1. Diagnostic approach to hyponatremia.

increase AVP release (such as chlorpropamide and opiates), ADH and its analogues, and oxytocin.

The first step in the diagnosis of hyponatremia is to rule out sodium depletion and decreased ECF volume. Here the hyponatremia is asymptomatic and the diagnosis is implied by the presence of features of decreased ECF volume. One should look for evidence of weight loss, poor skin turgor, flat neck veins when the patient is supine, a standing drop in the mean arterial blood pressure of greater than 10 mm Hg and a rise in the heart rate greater than 20 beats/minute, relative increases in hematocrit, total proteins, albu-

min, BUN, and uric acid, low measurement of central venous pressure, and high urinary osmolality. If dehydration is confirmed and the cause is not apparent, determine if the sodium loss is renal or extrarenal by measuring urinary sodium concentration.

The physician must rule out edematous states such as congestive heart failure, liver cirrhosis with ascites, or nephrosis. The principal manifestations here are those of the underlying disease; the hyponatremia is asymptomatic unless there is vigorous diuresis or excessive oral or parenteral dilute fluid administration.

Also, dilutional hyponatremia must be ruled out.

The diagnosis is evident from the history: the patient is postoperative, has acute or chronic renal failure, and shows no evidence of dehydration.

SIADH is characterized by ECF volume expansion, hyponatremia, and ECF hypo-osmolality; nonmaximally dilute urine that is usually hypertonic relative to plasma; continued excretion of ingested sodium despite hyponatremia; elevated AVP levels inappropriate for the levels of serum sodium; and reversal of hyponatremia and renal sodium loss by water deprivation.

When all the foregoing criteria are met the diagnosis of SIADH is made easily. An important differential diagnosis relates to patients with modest volume contraction in whom signs of volume depletion may be absent. If the volume depletion is due to extrarenal fluid losses, the urinary sodium is less than 20 mEq/L, and the serum creatinine and uric acid are increased. In contrast, in SIADH, the urinary sodium is greater than 20 mEq/L, and serum creatinine and uric acid are normal or low.

The most difficult differential diagnosis is that between SIADH and hyponatremia related to modest volume contraction from renal salt wasting (due to adrenocortical failure or to intrinsic renal disease). Both disorders have hyponatremia, ECF hypo-osmolarity, and increased urinary sodium. Adrenocortical insufficiency is suspected in the presence of hyperpigmentation, hyperkalemia, or hypoglycemia and is confirmed by specific tests documenting hypocortisolism (see Chapter 11, The Syndrome of Adrenocortical Insufficiency). A useful diagnostic maneuver to differentiate between SIADH and renal salt wasting resulting from intrinsic renal disease is to perform a water restriction test: water is restricted to 600 to 800 ml/day; patients with SIADH exhibit a characteristic response in 2 to 3 days, consisting of weight loss of 2 to 3 kg, correction of hyponatremia, and cessation of salt wasting; however, patients with intrinsic renal disease and renal salt wasting show no correction of hyponatremia or salt wasting.

Essential hyponatremia occurs in association with a variety of chronic illnesses. Affected patients are asymptomatic, do not have evidence of ECF volume depletion (unless caused by the primary disease), and show normal urinary dilution with water loading, normal urinary concentration during water deprivation, and normal sodium excretory responses to sodium loading or restrictions. The differential diagnosis from SIADH is based on the results of water restriction or loading: if the serum sodium is less than 125 mEq/L, fluid is restricted to 800 to 1000 ml/day or less for 2 to 3 days; the characteristic responses in SIADH have been mentioned above. If the serum sodium is greater

Table 10–2. Causes of Hypernatremia

Decreased water intake with normal renal conservation of water
  Disorder of thirst
    Adipsia
    Obtundation or coma
    Essential hypernatremia
Increased water losses with inadequate intake of water
  Extrarenal
    Excessive sweating and insensible losses
    Diarrheal disorders, especially in children
  Renal
    Diabetes insipidus
      Central
      Nephrogenic
    Osmotic diuresis
      Glycosuria
      Mannitol
      Urea
    Chronic renal failure
    Diuretics
    Recovery phase of acute renal failure
Excessive sodium intake with limited access to water
  Bicarbonate: during cardiopulmonary resuscitation or treatment of lactic acidosis
  Hypertonic saline
  Hypertonic dialysate
Miscellaneous
  Cushing's syndrome
  Hyperaldosteronism

than 125 mEq/L, 2 to 3 L of fluid are administered daily by mouth or IV; in SIADH the urine osmolarity is greater than 100 mOsm/kg H_2O (may even exceed plasma osmolality) despite progressive dilution of body fluids, and the urinary sodium excretion will exceed the intake.

Once the diagnosis of SIADH is made, a search for its origin (e.g., neoplasm, diseases of the central nervous system, or pulmonary disease) is in order. A careful history will exclude causative drugs.

HYPERNATREMIA

Definition. Hypernatremia is defined as an elevation of serum sodium concentration above 145 mEq/L.

Pathophysiologic Considerations (Table 10–2). Hypernatremia is indicative of a deficit in body water relative to sodium. It can result from decreased water intake or increased water loss, from water and sodium loss with water loss exceeding the sodium loss, or from sodium overload.

Because of the exquisite sensitivity of the thirst mechanism to changes in ECF osmolality, hypernatremia usually occurs only in patients who are comatose or who are otherwise unable to communicate thirst. It is rare in conscious patients other than infants, in patients with adipsia, and in those with essential hypernatremia. Essential hypernatremia, which may be congenital or acquired, is a rare disorder in which the thirst centers and osmoreceptors are apparently insensitive to osmotic stimuli while they remain normally responsive to volume mediated stimuli.

Increased water losses can occur in extrarenal disorders by the loss of water through the skin (from increased sweating, strenuous activity in high humidity, fever, or extensive burns), through the lungs (during increased respiration), and through the gastrointestinal tract, from diarrhea, especially in infants (see Table 10–1).

Renal water losses occur in diabetes insipidus. Central neurohypophyseal diabetes insipidus is due to partial or complete lack of antidiuretic hormone leading to failure of renal water conservation, passage of large amounts of dilute urine, and ECF hyperosmolality; it responds to hormone replacement with vasopressin. Nephrogenic diabetes insipidus is a polyuric disorder caused by unresponsiveness of the renal tubule to AVP, which leads to passage of large amounts of dilute urine, plasma hyperosmolality, and unresponsiveness to exogenous AVP. It may be hereditary, as an X-linked recessive disorder primarily in males, or may be secondary to systemic diseases such as Sjögren's disease, hypokalemia, or hypercalcemia, or secondary to the use of drugs such as lithium, tetracycline, and methoxyflurane.

Increased renal loss of water and solute with water loss exceeding salt loss occurs in osmotic diuresis during uncontrolled glycosuria, from mannitol administration to reduce increased intracranial pressure, from urea diuresis precipitated by increased tissue breakdown (for example, from burns), from increased protein or amino acid intake, from oral or IV alimentation, or from the use of diuretics.

Excessive sodium intake, particularly if renal function is impaired, can cause hypernatremia. This is seen when bicarbonate is administered (during cardiopulmonary resuscitation or in the management of metabolic acidosis), when hypertonic saline is administered, or when salt is accidentally substituted for sugar in the preparation of infant-feeding formulas.

Minimal persistent hypernatremia may be seen in some patients with Cushing's syndrome and hyperaldosteronism. The adrenal steroid's stimulation of renal tubular absorption of sodium is accompanied by some impairment of thirst, which fails to restore normal body fluid osmolality.

Clinical Presentation. Hypernatremia produces ECF hyperosmolality and dehydration of cells, particularly in the central nervous system (CNS). Symptoms range from somnolence, confusion, and increased neuromuscular irritability with twitching or seizures, to respiratory paralysis and death. The manifestations are variable, depending on the degree of hypertonicity and the rate of its development. In acute hypertonicity, symptoms appear when serum osmolality is greater than 320 mOsm/kg H_2O. Coma and ultimately death ensue with hyperosmolality greater than 360 mOsm/kg H_2O. Chronic hypertonicity produces fewer CNS manifestations because the brain cells accumulate idiogenic osmols that minimize the tendency of brain cell shrinkage.

Manifestations of ECF volume depletion are minimal in hypernatremia (because the loss of water occurs from both intracellular and extracellular fluid compartments) unless the fluid losses are profound.

Diagnostic Evaluation. The diagnosis of hypernatremia is dependent on the determination of serum sodium and serum osmolality (calculated or measured) (Fig. 10–2). The patient history and physical examination will give clues regarding decreased water intake (in patients with adipsia, in comatose patients, or in infants), increased renal losses (osmotic diuresis and nephrogenic or central diabetes insipidus and their causes), increased extrarenal losses (through the skin, lungs, or gastrointestinal tract), and increased sodium load (oral, intravenous, or through dialysis).

The presence of hypotonic urine in the presence of serum hyperosmolality indicates diabetes insipidus. Administration of exogenous AVP will differentiate central diabetes insipidus (DI) (responsive to AVP) from nephrogenic DI (unresponsive to AVP). If the urine is isotonic or hypertonic relative to serum osmolality, the clinical setting and appropriate laboratory studies can exclude decreased water intake, extrarenal water losses, salt loading, osmotic diuretics, primary aldosteronism, and Cushing's syndrome. If these are excluded, the water deprivation test and exogenous AVP administration are needed to rule out partial diabetes insipidus (see Polyuria). In the absence of diabetes insipidus, the possibility of essential hypernatremia should be considered.

POLYURIA

Definition. Polyuria is defined as a urinary output of more than 2.5 L/24 hours.

Pathophysiologic Considerations. Polyuria may be due either to osmotic diuresis caused by an increased solute load with obligatory water loss, or to a primary water diuresis (Table 10–3).

Osmotic diuresis results from the presence of osmotically active solute in the distal tubular fluid. This may be observed in diabetes mellitus, the most common cause, in which glucose is the solute load; in chronic renal failure, in which the total solute load may be normal but the decrease in functioning neph-

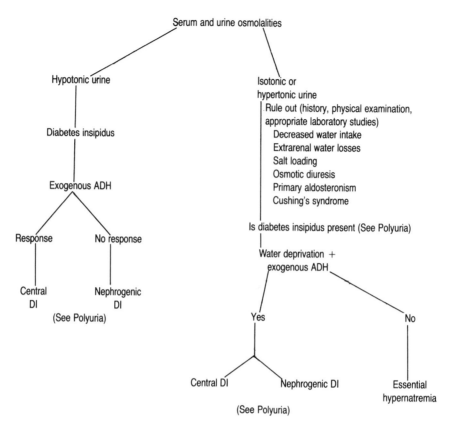

Fig. 10–2. Diagnostic approach to hypernatremia.

rons leads to increase in solute load per nephron, to solute diuresis, and to polyuria of moderate severity; in relief of obstructive uropathy which may have the same mechanism as in chronic renal failure, as well as a possible defect in concentrating ability; during the recovery phase of acute tubular necrosis in which osmotic diuresis is related partly to elimination of water and electrolytes that were retained during the phase of oliguria, and partly to incomplete recovery of tubular function; in massive protein breakdown with increased generation of urea, e.g., large hematoma, burns, etc.; and in diuretic therapy and natriuresis.

Diabetes Insipidus

Diabetes insipidus (DI) may result from failure to secrete the antidiuretic hormone (neurohypophysial DI), from failure of renal responsiveness to AVP (nephrogenic DI), or from primary polydipsia caused by increased water intake and suppression of AVP release.

The causes of central or neurohypophysial diabetes insipidus are outlined in Table 10–3. The basic defect is impairment of secretion of AVP. In the absence of AVP, the distal nephron is rendered impermeable to water, leading to increased renal free-water clearance and hypotonic urine, increased serum osmolality, and increased thirst. If the patient can respond to thirst and

available water is ingested, serum osmolality is normalized.

Primary or idiopathic central DI is the most common cause of spontaneous DI and is due to the loss of AVP neurosecretory cells of indeterminate origin. It affects both sexes, though males more commonly, and it can occur at any age after infancy. No hypothalamic-pituitary organic lesion is identified, and the other hypothalamic-pituitary-endocrine functions are normal. Familial DI is rare and appears to be inherited as autosomal dominant and usually begins in childhood.

Secondary central DI is caused by any lesion that can damage or impair the function of the neurohypophysial system and can be post-traumatic, inflammatory, vascular, neoplastic, or functional. Post-traumatic DI is an increasingly important cause of transient or permanent DI. It can follow head injury, particularly if the injury is associated with basilar skull fracture and avulsion of the pituitary stalk. More commonly, it follows neurosurgical procedures in or around the hypothalamic-pituitary area. Postsurgical DI may show the triphasic response: polyuria occurs in the initial stage as a result of impairment of AVP secretion and may last for hours or days. It is followed by a period of normal urine output and even oliguria, which may last from one to a few days and is due to the

Table 10–3. Causes of Polyuria

Osmotic diuresis
  Diabetes mellitus
  Chronic renal failure
  Relief of obstructive uropathy
  Recovery from acute tubular necrosis
  Diuretic therapy
  Massive protein breakdown, e.g. large hematoma
Water diuresis
  Central or neurohypophyseal diabetes insipidus
    Primary
      Idiopathic
      Hereditary
    Secondary
      Post-traumatic
        Head injury
        Neurosurgery
      Inflammatory
        Sarcoidosis
        Histiocytosis X
        Tuberculosis, syphilis
        Postencephalitic
      Vascular—aneurysm
      Neoplastic
        Primary (e.g. craniopharyngioma, germinoma, and glioma)
        Secondary
          Metastatic
          Leukemia
      Functional
        Drugs
          Narcotic antagonists
          Clonidine
        Anorexia nervosa
  Nephrogenic diabetes insipidus
    Primary
      Hereditary familial: types I and II
      Polycystic disease
      Medullary cystic disease
      Obstructive uropathy
      Pyelonephritis
      Sickle-cell disease or trait
      Amyloidosis
      Light-chain nephropathy
      Radiation nephritis
    Secondary
      Electrolyte disturbances
        Hypercalcemia
        Hypokalemia
      Dietary abnormalities
        Chronic overhydration
        Extreme protein restriction
        Marked salt restriction
      Drugs
        Lithium carbonate
        Demeclocycline
        Amphotericin
        Methoxyflurane
        Colchicine
        Vinblastine
        Nonsteroidal anti-inflammatory agents

release of AVP from the damaged neurohypophysial tissue. This second phase in turn may be followed by the recurrence of polyuria, which may remain permanently and is due to the lack of AVP from irreversible damage to the AVP-producing cells.

Inflammatory diseases of the hypothalamus resulting in secondary central DI are caused by sarcoidosis, histiocytosis X, tuberculosis, and other granulomatous diseases or a sequela of encephalitis. Other causes of DI include vascular diseases, for example, aneurysm; neoplastic diseases, which include primary neoplasm such as craniopharyngioma, glioma, dysgerminoma, or metastatic disease from other malignancies, notably carcinoma of the breast or lung, or from leukemic infiltrates; and functional impairment of AVP secretion, as occurs in anorexia nervosa.

In secondary neurohypophysial DI the causative lesion and other hypothalamic-pituitary-endocrine deficits are usually present. It is important to note that pituitary tumors confined to the sella do not cause DI despite destruction of the posterior pituitary lobe because AVP neurons have many axons that terminate in the median eminence and upper stalk, above the sella, and hence escape destruction by the pituitary tumor. Pituitary tumors can, therefore, cause DI only if they extend above the sella and impinge on the median eminence and upper stalk.

In nephrogenic DI, the basic defect is renal unresponsiveness to AVP, leading to water diuresis, plasma hypertonicity, increased AVP secretion, and increased thirst. Responsiveness to thirst by increased water intake attempts to restore the plasma tonicity to normal. The causes of nephrogenic DI are outlined in Table 10–3. Primary or familial nephrogenic DI is inherited as a sex-linked dominant trait with variable penetrance. Affected patients may have a complete (Type I) or partial (Type II) resistance to AVP and present with manifestations of DI, hypertonic dehydration, growth disturbance, and occasional mental retardation.

Secondary nephrogenic DI is due to recognizable diseases of the renal parenchyma underlying the AVP resistance. These include primary renal disease or renal disease secondary to electrolyte disturbances (hypercalcemia or hypokalemia), or to the use of drugs, notably lithium carbonate or demeclocycline.

Primary polydipsia or compulsive water drinking is more common than true DI. Here, the basic defect is inappropriately high water intake, which leads to plasma hypotonicity and suppression of AVP release. The distal nephron is thus rendered impermeable to water, resulting in water diuresis and restoration of plasma tonicity towards normal. Functional primary polydipsia occurs chiefly in middle-aged individuals, more commonly in females who have a long history of psychiatric disturbance and hysterical conversion symptoms. Organic primary polydipsia is rare and results from a central hypothalamic lesion, e.g., encephalitis or histiocytosis X, which affects the thirst center causing insatiable thirst. The syndrome may also result from intake of drugs that cause dryness of the mouth and increase fluid intake (e.g., phenothiazines and antihistamines).

Clinical Presentation. *Signs.* There may be no abnormal physical findings. Specific findings that may be present relate to dehydration (if there is a problem with compensation by increased water intake in neurohypophysial or nephrogenic DI) or to an underlying disorder, e.g., visual field defect, galactorrhea, hypopituitarism in hypothalamic-pituitary disease, or evidence of uremia or diabetes mellitus.

Symptoms. The clinical manifestations of DI are determined by normality of the thirst mechanisms and availability of water for ingestion. If the thirst mechanism is normal and water is available and ingested, the symptoms are those of polyuria and polydipsia; urine volumes may range from 3 to 20 L/day, nocturia is present, and, in children, nocturnal enuresis may occur. Polydipsia, sometimes with preference for cold water, is present. In neurohypophysial DI, the onset is usually dramatic; in primary polydipsia and nephrogenic DI, it is usually gradual. If the thirst mechanism is impaired or water is not available (for example, with adipsia caused by hypothalamic thirst center damage, loss of consciousness resulting from injury or anesthesia, or enforced restriction of water intake during medical workup), the compensatory increase in water intake does not occur; significant dehydration, volume depletion, and hyperosmolarity occur rapidly, manifest as somnolence, confusion that can progress to stupor, convulsions, collapse, and death from cardiorespiratory arrest.

In compulsive water drinking, the onset of polyuria and polydipsia is usually gradual. There is marked fluctuation in the amount of water ingested and in the urinary output from day to day. There is usually no preference for ice water, nocturia is absent, symptoms may be intermittent or recurrent, and the patient may have symptoms of underlying psychiatric illness. Additional symptoms related to the underlying cause may be present.

Diagnostic Evaluation and Differential Diagnosis (Fig. 10–3). *Patient History and Physical Examination.* The central questions in diagnosing polyuria are whether the polyuria is related to osmotic or to water diuresis, and, if related to primary water diuresis, whether it is due to central or nephrogenic DI or to primary polydipsia, and what the underlying disease process is.

In the history and physical examination, helpful clues may be obtained relating to the onset, duration, course, and severity of the disorder and whether the symptoms are persistent or intermittent; evidence of the presence of diabetes mellitus, chronic renal failure, or other causes of osmotic diuresis; any past or present psychiatric difficulties; any evidence of nephrourologic disease to suggest nephrogenic DI; any other evidence of hypothalamic disease, e.g., visual field defect, increased intracranial pressure, pituitary dysfunction, or galactorrhea; any underlying disease for hypothalamic dysfunction, e.g., head trauma or neurosurgery, systemic disease such as sarcoidosis or histiocytosis, anorexia nervosa, or malignancy; drug history, e.g., drugs that cause nephrogenic DI or diuretics; and family history of central or nephrogenic DI. An assessment of the state of hydration is important.

Polyuria due to osmotic diuresis can be diagnosed from the history, physical examination, standard laboratory tests, and by the finding of the offending solute in the urine.

Diagnostic Studies. URINE OSMOLALITY. This test provides important information regarding the normality of the hypothalamic AVP secretion and the distal nephron responsiveness to the hormone. In the normal individual under circumstances of water lack, urine is maximally concentrated, and the urine osmolality approaches 800 to 1200 mOsm/kg H_2O; under circumstances of water excess the urine is maximally dilute, and the urine osmolarity is between 50 to 90 mOsm/kg H_2O. As an isolated observation, urine osmolality is often not helpful. It needs to be correlated with plasma osmolality or ECF volume state. The urine specific gravity is a crude index of urine concentration. If used, it may be affected significantly by urea, protein, glucose, or radiopaque dye, which contribute very little to osmolality.

SERUM OSMOLALITY. This test is normally maintained within the narrow range of 280 to 295 mOsm/kg H_2O. For accurate determination of serum osmolality, blood must be drawn without the use of tourniquet and studied promptly. Again, as a single observation, serum osmolality is of little value in the evaluation in the problems of water balance. It needs to be correlated with concomitant urine osmolality. If the measurement of serum osmolality is not possible, one can use the clinical calculation:

serum osmolality

$$= 2 \times \text{serum Na} + \frac{\text{glucose mg/dl}}{18} + \frac{\text{BUN mg/dl}}{2.8}$$

This calculation correlates well with the measurement of osmolality.

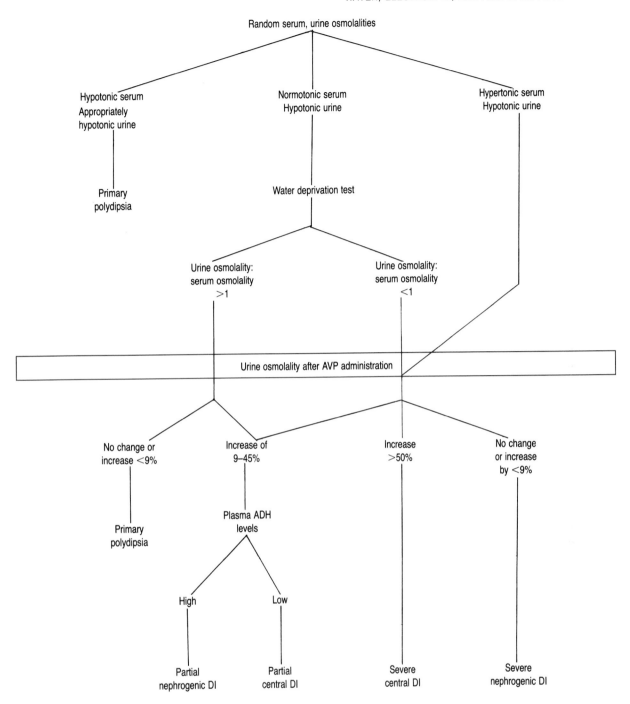

Fig. 10–3. Diagnostic approach to suspected diabetes insipidus (polyuria, dilute urine).

DEHYDRATION TEST. The underlying physiologic principle of this test is that water deprivation normally stimulates secretion of optimal amounts of AVP, producing maximal effects on the renal tubule, water conservation, and increased urinary osmolality, the magnitude of which is limited by mainly the renal medullary osmolality. The objectives of this test are to establish the ability of the hypothalamus to secrete AVP and of the kidneys to respond to the secreted hormone.

The patient is weighed before the test, and the serum and urine osmolalities are obtained. Fluid intake is restricted. Hourly urine volume and urine osmolality are obtained until the urine osmolalities plateau, with change of less than 30 mOsm/kg H_2O in two consecutive hourly samples. Blood is then drawn without the use of tourniquet for plasma osmolality, and an aliquot is set aside for AVP assay if the dehydration tests prove equivocal. Five units of aqueous AVP are then given subcutaneously, and urine and plasma osmolalities are measured 1 hour after the administration of AVP.

In the normal individual with dehydration, AVP secretion is maximum, and urine osmolality increases above serum osmolality and shows no significant change (a change of 9% or less) after the administration of AVP.

In patients with partial neurohypophysial DI, there is submaximal endogenous AVP release, and urine osmolality may be greater than serum osmolality after dehydration but shows a further rise after exogenous AVP administration by 9 to 50% over the maximum dehydration-induced osmolality.

In patients with complete neurohypophysial DI, there is no endogenous AVP release. Urine osmolality is less than serum osmolality and shows a rise in osmolality greater than 50% above the maximum dehydration-induced osmolality after exogenous AVP administration.

In complete nephrogenic DI, there is maximal endogenous AVP release during water deprivation but no renal response, so the urine osmolality is less than the serum osmolality and exogenous AVP administration does not cause a rise in urine osmolality above that induced by dehydration (less than 9%).

In partial nephrogenic DI, endogenous AVP release is maximal during dehydration, the renal response to this endogenous AVP is partial, and exogenous AVP administration may cause a further rise in urine osmolality above that induced by dehydration (greater than 9%). This response may cause difficulty in differential diagnosis with partial central DI (see below).

In compulsive water drinkers, the response to the dehydration test may be normal or subnormal. The subnormal response, which can cause diagnostic difficulties, is due to the fact that the high urinary flow leads to washout of solutes from the renal medulla, loss of renal hyperosmolar gradient, and diminished ability to concentrate urine even in the presence of optimal endogenous AVP secretion. With water restriction over a few days, the renal medullary hypertonicity and normal responsiveness to AVP are restored.

Several points about the dehydration test need to be emphasized. In primary polydipsia the patients are overhydrated, and prolonged water deprivation may be needed to reach plateau in urine osmolality. Also, patients with DI may tolerate dehydration poorly. Careful surveillance is in order with periodic checks of weight and ECF volume state during the test. Finally, patients, particularly those with primary polydipsia, may surreptitiously ingest water during the period of dehydration.

HYPERTONIC SALINE INFUSION. The water deprivation test has largely supplanted the hypertonic saline infusion test in the diagnosis of suspected diabetes insipidus syndrome. The saline infusion test, however, is still useful to assess osmoreceptor function and to determine the threshold of AVP release. The test is based on the fact that infusion of hypertonic saline leads to the increase in serum osmolality. If AVP secretion and renal responsiveness to AVP are normal, antidiuresis occurs. Antidiuresis will not occur in neurohypophysial or nephrogenic DI.

The test is done by giving an oral waterload (20 ml/ kg) by mouth over 10 to 15 minutes. At the same time, a slow infusion of 5% sodium chloride is started at 0.5 ml/minute. When sustained diuresis has been present for six to eight successive collections, 15 minutes each, the rate of infusion of 5% saline is increased to 0.05 ml/kg/minute until a definite fall in three or more subsequent 15-minute urine volumes is noted or until severe headache and thirst intervenes. Plasma osmolality is checked to document the achievement of a hyperosmolar state. Plasma and urine samples are checked for osmolality and free water clearance is carefully calculated. The test is contraindicated in any patient who cannot tolerate acute volume expansion.

AVP LEVELS. A radioimmunoassay for AVP is available in only a few centers at present but should become generally available in the near future. The average concentration of plasma AVP in healthy adults in a normal state of hydration and in the supine position is 1.4 to 2.7 pg/ml. There is an overlap in AVP levels between normal and DI patients. Single measurements are therefore not helpful and need to be correlated with plasma and urine osmolalities. In central DI, serum osmolality is high and plasma AVP levels are inappropriately low; in nephrogenic DI serum osmolality is high and AVP levels are appropriately high. In primary polydipsia, serum osmolality is low and AVP levels are appropriately low.

Differential Diagnosis. The differentiation between central or nephrogrenic DI and primary polydipsia is usually straightforward and based on the following principles. In central DI, a deficiency of AVP secretion leads to water diuresis, polyuria with dilute urine, and hypertonic dehydration. The plasma osmolality and/or serum sodium is elevated. The water balance disorder does not respond to fluid restriction but is corrected by the administration of exogenous vasopressin. In nephrogenic DI, there is renal unresponsiveness to AVP that leads to water diuresis, polyuria with dilute urine, and an elevated plasma osmolality and/or serum sodium. The water balance disorder does not respond to fluid deprivation, and unlike central DI it is not corrected by the administration of exogenous AVP. In primary polydipsia, excessive water intake leads to overhydration, hypotonicity of body fluids, suppression of AVP secretion, water diuresis, and polyuria with dilute urine. In response to water deprivation, AVP secretion is resumed, renal water conservation follows, and the urine concentration rises. Since endogenous AVP secretion and response to water deprivation are optimal, exogenous AVP administration will not lead to further increase in the concentration of urine.

The first step in differentiating central or nephrogenic DI and primary polydipsia is to obtain random serum and urine osmolalities. In a patient with polyuria, the finding of a low urine osmolality and a high serum osmolality rules out the diagnosis of primary polydipsia and leads to consideration of central or nephrogenic DI. Exogenous AVP is administered (as in the water deprivation test). A response to exogenous AVP indicates central DI, while absence of response points to nephrogenic DI. If, in a patient with polyuria, urine and serum osmolalities are found to be low, the diagnosis is compulsive water drinking and primary polydipsia.

If the urine is hypotonic and the serum osmolality is normal (compensated state), the next step is to proceed with the water deprivation test as described above. A diagnosis of complete neurohypophysial DI is made on the basis of a urine osmolality less than serum osmolality, and a rise in urine osmolality following the administration of exogenous AVP greater than 50% above the maximum dehydration-induced osmolality. A diagnosis of partial neurohypophysial DI is made on the basis of a urine osmolality, which may be lesser or greater than the serum osmolality after dehydration but rises following exogenous AVP administration by 9 to 50% over the maximum dehydration-induced osmolality.

When central DI is documented, a search for its cause is initiated, and radiologic studies of the hypothalamic pituitary area (skull x-ray, CT scan), visual field examination, and assessment of pituitary functions are in order. If no cause is delineated, the CT scan is negative, the visual fields are normal, and the other pituitary functions are normal, the diagnosis of idiopathic DI is probable. Follow-up with periodic reassessment is advised since a secondary cause may make its appearance known at some future date. If no cause is delineated, the CT scan is negative, and the visual fields are normal, but there is evidence of other pituitary dysfunction, the diagnosis is probably secondary diabetes insipidus, and the patient is evaluated periodically. The presence of a cause points to sec-

ondary DI and prompts initiation of appropriate management.

In complete nephrogenic DI, urine osmolality at the end of the dehydration test is less than serum osmolality, and exogenous AVP administration (or a rise of less than 9%) does not cause a rise in urine osmolality above that induced by dehydration.

In the usual case of primary polydipsia the response to the water dehydration test is normal: urine osmolality is greater than serum osmolality, and there is no significant change (a change of 9% or less) in urine osmolality after the administration of exogenous AVP.

There are three problems in the differential diagnosis of polyuria. In partial nephrogenic DI, because there is maximal AVP response to water deprivation and a partial renal response, the urine osmolality may exceed serum osmolality at the end of the water deprivation test, and exogenous AVP administration may cause a further rise (greater than 9%) in urine osmolality above that induced by dehydration. The differential diagnosis here is partial central DI. Diagnosis is best made by measurement of plasma AVP at the end of water deprivation. In partial central DI, plasma AVP levels are low relative to plasma osmolality. In contrast, in partial nephrogenic DI, plasma AVP levels are appropriately high relative to the plasma osmolality. If AVP assays are not available, an alternative would be to perform a closely monitored therapeutic trial with standard doses of AVP or its analogues. If no effect is observed in 1 to 2 days, a diagnosis of nephrogenic DI is entertained. If, however, exogenous AVP therapy leads to decreased polyuria and normalization of plasma osmolality, the diagnosis is central DI. If polyuria is decreased without affecting thirst or if water intoxication develops, the diagnosis is primary polydipsia.

In some patients with primary polydipsia, chronic excessive water intake and the resulting water diuresis may "wash out" renal medulla, decreasing its hypertonicity. With water deprivation such patients may not be able to concentrate their urine maximally, and exogenous AVP administration will not improve their concentrating ability. A picture similar to nephrogenic DI is thus obtained. Obtaining plasma AVP values at the end of the water deprivation test is not helpful in the differential diagnosis since in primary polydipsia with renal medullary washout and in nephrogenic DI plasma AVP values are appropriately high for the corresponding plasma osmolality. Differentiation is best made by restricting water for a few days and observing the patient. Water restriction will restore renal medullary tonicity in patients with primary polydipsia, and normal response to water deprivation ensues. It will not have an effect on patients with nephrogenic DI, who will continue to show impaired response to water deprivation.

The presence of cortisol is essential for renal free-water clearance. If ACTH deficiency and cortisol lack accompany central DI, the lack of cortisol may mask the symptoms of polyuria and polydipsia. "Spontaneous amelioration" of symptoms during the course of central DI should prompt consideration of ACTH cortisol deficiency. Administration of cortisol for replacement therapy in such patients unmasks the presence of DI.

DISORDERS OF SERUM POTASSIUM

INTRODUCTION

Potassium plays an important role in the excitability of nerves and muscles, in cell metabolism, and in other physiologic processes. The serum potassium concentration is kept within narrow limits, and a small change can have significant adverse effects, particularly on the transmembrane potential of cardiac and skeletal muscle cells. Hyperkalemia leads to depolarization of cells, which is particularly significant in cardiac muscle and which results in abnormal impulse conduction and potentially life threatening cardiac arrhythmias. Hypokalemia causes hyperpolarization of cells, particularly significant in skeletal muscles, leading to muscle weakness and even paralysis.

Maintenance of plasma potassium can be affected by balance between potassium input and output, and by distribution of potassium between ECF and ICF.

Potassium Input. The average American's diet contains 50 to 100 mEq/day of potassium but can increase to 500 mEq/day if large quantities of potassium containing foods are eaten. In starvation, e.g., anorexia nervosa, less than 10 mEq/day may be ingested. Potassium intake is not physiologically regulated.

Potassium Output. Potassium can be lost from the body by three routes: in sweat, whose potassium concentration is similar to plasma; in feces, which normally contain 5 to 10 mEq/day but that may contain more than 100 mEq/day in diarrheal states; and in urine, averaging 45 to 90 mEq/day but varying from less than 10 to greater than 500 mEq/day.

Potassium-transcellular Distribution. Potassium is pumped into cells by a sodium-potassium ATPase–dependent mechanism and passively diffuses out of cells. A change in plasma potassium can result from changes in its active uptake by the cells (accelerated by insulin and beta adrenergic agonists and decreased by digitalis) from a change in the passive diffusion of potassium from cells (increased by cellular injury and death, hemolysis, and acidosis, and decreased by alkalosis), or from both.

Potassium balance is achieved by changing potassium output to match potassium input. The output is regulated primarily by the kidney. Potassium is reabsorbed and secreted by the proximal and the distal tubules. The potassium in the glomerular filtrate is extensively absorbed. Less than 10% reaches the distal nephron regardless of the intake and output. Potassium balance is regulated primarily in the distal tubule and occurs by changing the rate of potassium secretion. Potassium secretion is increased by an increase in plasma potassium; by increased sodium reabsorption in the distal tubule resulting from aldosteronism or from enhanced sodium delivery to the distal tubule, e.g., by diuretics; by impermeant anions in the tubular fluid delivered to the distal nephron, e.g., sulfate; by an increased rate of tubular fluid flow; and by alkalosis.

HYPOKALEMIA

Definition. Hypokalemia is defined as a serum potassium less than 3.6 mEq/L (normal 3.6 to 4.8 mEq/L).

Pathophysiologic Considerations (Table 10–4). In general, hypokalemia may result from inadequate potassium intake or one of three pathophysiologic events: transcellular shift of potassium from ECF into ICF, excessive extrarenal losses from skin or gastrointestinal tract, and excessive renal losses.

Reduced potassium intake occurs in starvation, alcoholism, anorexia nervosa, and geophagia (ingested clay binds potassium and prevents its absorption from the GI tract) and can cause potassium depletion and hypokalemia. In the face of inadequate intake, maximal renal conservation of potassium requires 7 to 10 days, and during this period the net renal potassium loss may be as much as 150 to 200 mEq.

Extrarenal potassium losses can occur in vomiting, which causes hypokalemia in part because of the loss of gastric juice (which contains 5 to 10 mEq of potassium per liter) but mostly because of increased renal potassium losses (see below). Diarrhea from any cause can result in excessive stool losses of potassium (diarrheal fluid contains 40 to 60 mEq of potassium per liter). This is especially true with colonic villous adenoma and with noninsulin-secreting pancreatic islet cell tumors. Excessive sweating also causes potassium loss; the concentration of potassium in sweat is equal

Table 10–4. Causes of Hypokalemia

Alterations in internal potassium balance
  Alkalosis
  Hypokalemic periodic paralysis
  Barium poisoning
  Treatment of megaloblastic anemia
  Leukemia
  Administration of glucose and insulin
Alterations in external potassium balance
  Decreased potassium intake
    Starvation
    Alcoholism
    Anorexia nervosa
    Geophagia
  Increased gastrointestinal secretion
    Loss of gastric fluid
    Diarrhea
    Noninsulin-secreting tumor of pancreas
    Villous adenoma
    Laxative abuse
  Ureterosigmoidostomy
  Increased renal potassium losses
    Diuretics
    Osmotic diuresis
      Glycosuria
      Mannitol
      Hypertonic sodium compounds
      Recovery from acute tubular necrosis
      Relief of urinary tract obstruction
    Loss of gastric fluid
    Hypermineralocorticoid states
      Aldosteronism
      Cushing's syndrome
      Adrenogenital syndrome
      Licorice
    Intrinsic renal disease
      Renal tubular acidosis
      Potassium-losing nephritis
    Liddle's syndrome
    Bartter's syndrome
    Magnesium deficit
    Certain antibiotics
      Carbenicillin
      Gentamicin
      Amphotericin B
    Leukemia

to or slightly higher than plasma potassium concentration.

In all forms of extrarenal losses, the associated volume depletion leads to secondary hyperaldosteronism and increased renal potassium loss, which contributes to the hypokalemia.

Increased renal potassium losses can result from several influences. All diuretics (except spironolactone, triamterene, and amiloride) can cause hypokalemia. The increased urinary potassium loss is caused by enhanced sodium delivery to the distal tubule, increased tubular flow rate, and volume depletion and secondary hyperaldosteronism.

Osmotic diuresis from significant glycosuria, from therapy with mannitol, hypertonic saline, or bicarbonate solution, or from increased urea (during recovery from acute tubular necrosis or after relief of urinary tract obstruction) can cause increased renal potassium losses.

Loss of gastric fluid from any disorder can produce hypokalemia related to loss of potassium in gastric juice; increased renal potassium loss from metabolic alkalosis, volume depletion and secondary aldosteronism; and transcellular potassium entry from ECF into ICF because of the metabolic alkalosis.

Renal potassium losses can result from disorders associated with increased mineralocorticoid activity of any origin (see Chapter 11, The Syndrome of Primary Aldosteronism) such as primary and secondary aldosteronism, Cushing's syndrome, adrenogenital syndrome (11- and 17-hydroxylase deficiency congenital adrenal hyperplasia), excessive licorice ingestion and Bartter's syndrome.

Another cause, Liddle's syndrome, is a rare disorder of indeterminate origin characterized by a defect in distal sodium to potassium transport.

Intrinsic renal disease, including type I distal RTA, type II proximal RTA, and potassium-losing pyelonephritis can also result in renal potassium loss, as can use of antibiotics such as carbenicillin, amphotericin B, and gentamicin; magnesium depletion; acute myeloid leukemia; and ureterosigmoidostomy.

Transcellular shifts of potassium from ECF to ICF can occur in alkalosis, hypokalemic periodic paralysis, barium poisoning, treatment of megaloblastic anemia, leukemia, and the use of IV glucose and insulin. Hypokalemic periodic paralysis is a rare familial autosomal dominant disorder of uncertain origin characterized by intermittent attacks of weakness that may progress to flaccid paralysis and that may be precipitated by a high carbohydrate diet, IV glucose and insulin, exercise, alcohol, infection, trauma, or stress. It can also be sporadic and can occur in association with thyrotoxicosis.

Clinical Presentation. Patients with mild to moderate degrees of potassium deficiency can be asymptomatic. When symptomatic, their symptoms include weakness, which can be generalized but especially affects proximal muscle groups and, if severe, can lead to paralysis; generalized or localized paresthesias; nocturia, polyuria, and decreased renal concentrating ability (hypokalemic nephropathy and nephrogenic DI); enhanced cardiac toxicity of digitalis; and rhabdomyolysis and myoglobinuria, which can result when large amounts of potassium are lost from skeletal muscle. Signs include proximal muscle weakness, hypoactive DTRs, paralytic ileus, orthostatic hypotension caused by impairment of vascular reflexes, and positive Chvostek's and Trousseau's signs as a result of the associated metabolic alkalosis.

The electrocardiogram reveals decreased amplitude of the T wave and increased amplitude of the U wave. In more severe degrees of hypokalemia, there is depression of ST segment, slight prolongation of the PR interval, and appearance of ectopic beats.

Diagnostic Evaluation.

Patient History and Physical Examination (Fig. 10–4). Hypokalemia should be suspected in the appropriate clinical setting and the presence of a potential cause and suggestive clinical manifestations.

The cause of hypokalemia is usually evident from the history and physical examination. The clinical setting can give clues regarding potassium intake (starvation, anorexia nervosa, and geophagia), gastroin-

testinal potassium loss, vomiting, nasogastric suction, diarrhea, mucus in the stools, fistulas, drugs and toxins (alcohol, diuretics, glucose and insulin, licorice, treatment of megaloblastic anemia, and the antibiotics carbenicillin, gentamicin, and amphotericin), hypertension, evidence of Cushing's or adrenogenital syndrome, leukemia, hypokalemic periodic paralysis, and family history. It is important to remember, however, that patients with potassium deficiency resulting from chronic laxative abuse, psychogenic self-induced vomiting, and surreptitious use of diuretics may not volunteer an accurate history and that patients with villous adenoma may report normal bowel movements. (In such patients, close questioning may provide information regarding increased mucus.)

Diagnostic Studies. If the clinical setting is not re-

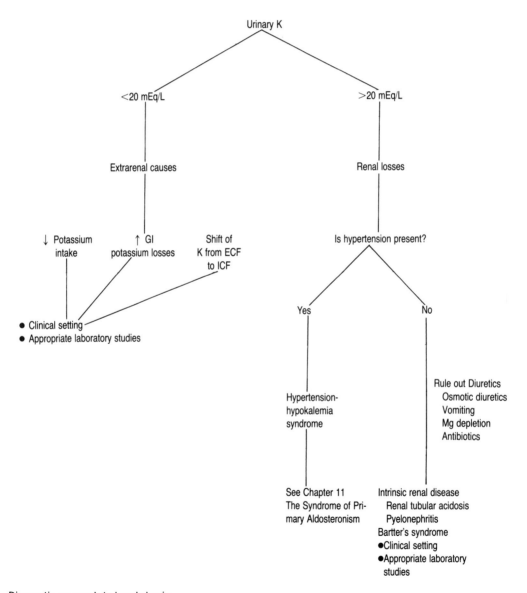

Fig. 10–4. Diagnostic approach to hypokalemia.

vealing, several studies may be of help. It is important to repeat the biochemical determination to rule out laboratory error.

Measurement of urinary potassium excretion is required to assess the presence or absence of inappropriate kaliuresis (i.e., potassium excretion increased relative to the level of serum potassium). Prior to the determination of urinary potassium, the physician should ensure that the patient has been off diuretics and off potassium supplements for at least 3 days, that urinary creatinine is measured concomitantly to ensure completeness of urine collection, that urinary sodium is at least 100 mEq/day to ensure adequate delivery of sodium to distal tubules where potassium is secreted, and that the patient is hypokalemic at the time of collection. In a hypokalemic patient, a urinary potassium excretion less than 30 mEq/L points to extrarenal losses, while a urinary potassium greater than 30 mEq/L points to renal losses. It is important to remember that hypokalemia caused by renal losses may be associated with urine potassium of less than 30 mEq/L in severely depleted patients, in mineralocorticoid excess when sodium intake is low and in diuretic therapy that was stopped at the time of the examination.

Measurement of blood pH may also assist the diagnosis. Most potassium-depleted patients have normal or increased blood pH. Hypokalemia associated with acidosis points to renal tubular acidosis, diarrhea, diabetic ketoacidosis, and treatment with carbonic anhydrase inhibitors.

The presence of hypertension with hypokalemia points to either primary hyperaldosteronism, secondary aldosteronism (except that caused by Bartter's syndrome and volume depletion), Cushing's syndrome, the use of licorice, or Liddle's syndrome. (See Chap 11, The Syndrome of Primary Aldosteronism.)

HYPERKALEMIA

Definition. Hyperkalemia is defined as a serum potassium concentration greater than 5.0 mEq/L (normal 3.6 to 4.8 mEq/L).

Pathophysiologic Considerations (Table 10–5). In general, hyperkalemia results from one of two mechanisms: a shift of potassium from intracellular to extracellular fluid space, or impaired renal excretion of potassium. If renal function is intact, increased intake of potassium is almost never responsible for hyperkalemia.

Hyperkalemia caused by transcellular shifts can result from several factors. In both respiratory and metabolic acidosis, the movement of hydrogen ions into cells for buffering is associated with an outward shift

Table 10–5. Causes of Hyperkalemia

Alterations in internal potassium balance
  Acidemia
  Hypertonicity
  Insulin deficiency
  Hypoaldosteronism
  Drugs
    Digitalis glycosides
    Succinylcholine
    Arginine and lysine hydrochloride
  Tissue breakdown
    Rhabdomyolysis
    Hemolysis
    Burns
    Chemotherapy of leukemia
  Hyperkalemic periodic paralysis
Alterations in external potassium balance
  Increased potassium intake
    Salt substitutes
    Potassium replacement therapy (oral or IV)
    Potassium salts of antibiotics
    Blood transfusions (hemolyzed)
  Decreased potassium renal excretion
    Renal insufficiency
      Acute
      Chronic
    Hypoaldosteronism
      Addison's disease
      Selective
    Tubular unresponsiveness to aldosterone
      Potassium-sparing diuretics
      Systemic lupus erythematosus
      Amyloidosis
      Renal transplants
      Sickle-cell disease
      Congenital defects in potassium secretion
      Chronic interstitial nephritis

of potassium and hyperkalemia; marked hyperkalemia may be present even in the face of decreased total body potassium. Also, any condition associated with rapid tissue breakdown can lead to release of intracellular potassium into the ECF. This may be seen in rhabdomyolysis, burns, massive hemolysis, tumor necrosis, and chemotherapy of neoplastic disorders.

Use of drugs may also cause transcellular shifts and hence hyperkalemia. In digitalis overdose, hyperkalemia may be related to inhibition of the sodium-potassium ATPase–dependent mechanism and inability of cells to maintain intracellular potassium. Succinylcholine and other depolarizing muscle relaxants can cause hyperkalemia, especially in patients with renal failure or neuromuscular disease, by cell membrane depolarization and outward redistribution of potassium. Arginine hydrochloride, which is used as a growth hormone provocative test or in the treatment of metabolic alkalosis, can cause hyperkalemia due to the arginine-potassium exchange mechanism.

In addition, hyperosmolality of any cause leads to

movement of intracellular fluid and potassium into the ECF.

Hyperkalemia in patients with diabetes mellitus may be related to decreased insulin levels, metabolic acidosis, hypertonicity, selective hypoaldosteronism, and chronic renal failure.

Hyperkalemic periodic paralysis is a rare inherited disorder of unknown cause characterized by spontaneous episodes of hyperkalemia, muscle weakness, and paralysis. The episodes begin abruptly and may be precipitated by stress, alcohol, and physical exercise.

Hyperkalemia caused by impaired renal excretion is the most common cause of hyperkalemia and is seen in acute and chronic renal failure; in mineralocorticoid-deficient states as in Addison's disease, selective aldosterone deficiency, enzyme defects of aldosterone synthesis, and end-organ resistance to aldosterone; and in the use of potassium-sparing diuretics spironolactone, triamterene, and amiloride, which cause pharmacologic blockade of distal renal potassium excretion.

An exogenous potassium load does not cause hyperkalemia unless renal function is impaired. It can be seen with oral or IV preparations of potassium, including potassium chloride, potassium iodide, potassium penicillin preparations, and salt substitute, and with administration of old bank blood.

Clinical Presentation. The manifestations of hyperkalemia relate to the heart and skeletal muscle system and are caused by a decrease in the resting electric potential of muscle cells and subsequent prevention of repolarization. Muscle weakness is a dominant manifestation; it initially affects the lower extremities and later progresses to quadriplegia, respiratory paralysis, and death. Cranial nerve and sensory functions are not affected. Alterations in cardiac excitability lead to cardiac arrhythmias and electrocardiographic changes. The earliest electrocardiographic change, which occurs when the serum potassium approaches 6 mEq/L, consists of peaked T waves and a shortened QT interval resulting from an increased rate of repolarization. As serum potassium rises further, a slowing of conduction occurs with widening of the QRS and prolongation of the PR interval. As serum potassium reaches 8.0 to 9.0 mEq/L, failure of conduction occurs with disappearance of the P wave; ventricular fibrillation or asystole may be the terminal event. The electrocardiogram is very important in the assessment of the cardiotoxic effects of hyperkalemia. In the presence of hypocalcemia, hyponatremia, and acidosis, the electrocardiographic changes appear with lower serum potassium levels.

Diagnostic Evaluation and Differential Diagnosis.

Spurious elevations of serum potassium (pseudohyperkalemia) may result from hemolysis and release of intracellular potassium either during venipuncture or in vitro in the blood container, from tight application of a tourniquet and release of potassium from ischemic forearm muscles, and from thrombocytosis and leukocytosis in which potassium is released from in vitro clotting of these cells. Pseudohyperkalemia should be suspected when electrocardiographic abnormalities are absent despite an apparently marked increase in serum potassium. A repeat study with careful venipuncture and collection of a blood sample will obviate pseudohyperkalemia caused by hemolysis or tourniquet application; prompt separation of plasma from the cellular blood components and determination of plasma potassium levels will clarify the problem of pseudohyperkalemia related to thrombocytosis and leukocytosis. In these circumstances, the serum, but not the plasma potassium, is elevated.

In evaluating hyperkalemia, the physician must determine the possible causes (Fig. 10–5). In considering the possibility of transcellular shift, a careful history and physical examination and appropriate laboratory studies will exclude drug history (digitalis overdose, succinylcholine, arginine hydrochloride, hypertonic saline, or mannitol), acidosis (clinical setting, arterial blood gases, blood pH, or serum bicarbonate), tissue breakdown, and hyperkalemic periodic paralysis (characteristic episodes and family history).

Impairment of renal potassium excretion should be inferred by evidence of acute or chronic renal failure (clinical setting and serum creatinine) or a drug history (use of spironolactone, triamterene, and amiloride).

To rule out a mineralocorticoid deficient state, the physician should use determinations of plasma aldosterone, plasma renin activity (PRA), and serum cortisol. In selective aldosterone deficiency, low aldosterone, high PRA, and normal serum cortisol are present. The etiologic diagnosis of selective aldosterone deficiency is based on the clinical setting and appropriate laboratory studies, drug history (heparin), and hormonal studies (congenital adrenal hyperplasia). The diagnosis of hyporeninemic hypoaldosteronism is based on the clinical setting of hyperkalemia, low aldosterone, and low renin activity that is unresponsive to volume contraction.

The physician should evaluate the patient for evidence of end-organ resistance to aldosterone, which is characterized by hyperkalemia, high plasma aldosterone, and high PRA. The etiologic diagnosis depends on the clinical setting (systemic lupus, renal transplant, or sickle-cell disease).

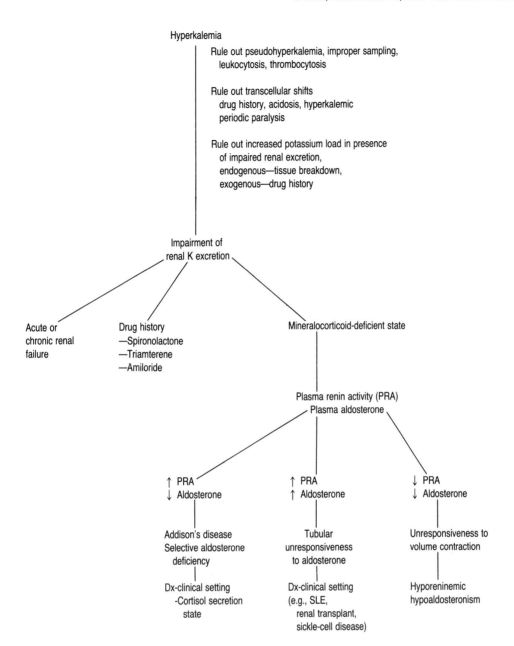

Fig. 10–5. Diagnostic approach to hyperkalemia.

DISORDERS OF SERUM PHOSPHATE

INTRODUCTION

Approximately 85% of total body phosphate is in bone. Of the remainder, greater than 99% is intracellular and consists primarily of organic phosphates (e.g., phospholipids, nucleic acids and nucleotides, and phosphoproteins). Inorganic phosphate, existing primarily as anions of HPO_4^- and $H_2PO_4^-$, is required for synthesis of organic phosphates and is also important as a body buffer. In plasma, two thirds of the total phosphate is in phospholipids and is bound to plasma protein; 90% of the remainder is in inorganic phosphate, of which 50% is ionized and 50% complexed. Plasma phosphate refers to the inorganic component, which in normal adults is 2.7 to 4.5 mg/dl and in children is 4.0 to 7.0 mg/dl.

The factors that affect serum phosphate are the min-

Table 10–6.   Causes of Hypophosphatemia

Decreased input
  TPN with nonphosphate-containing solutions
  Phosphate-binding gels
  Malabsorption
Intracellular phosphate shift
  Glucose infusion
  Insulin infusion
  Alkalosis, respiratory and metabolic
Increased renal losses
  Fanconi's syndrome
    Multiple myeloma
    Cystinosis
    Heavy metal poisoning
    Systemic lupus erythematosus
    Wilson's disease
  Vitamin D-resistant rickets
    Familial
    Sporadic
      Mesenchymal tumors
  Hyperparathyroidism
  Diuretics
  Glycosuria
  ECF volume expansion
  Hypercalcemia
  Hypokalemia
  Idiopathic hypercalciuria
  Ureterosigmoidoscopy

eral homeostatic system (parathyroid hormone [PTH] and vitamin D) shifts between ECF and ICF, and renal tubular and gastrointestinal phosphate transport.

Phosphate, whose intake approximates 1200 mg/day, is nearly ubiquitous in food; a normal diet precludes phosphate deficiency. It is excreted in stools (400 mg) and in urine (800 mg). The renal handling of phosphate is the major regulator of phosphate balance. About 9000 mg of phosphate are filtered daily by the glomeruli, of which 90% is reabsorbed, primarily by the proximal tubule. Factors that affect renal handling of phosphate include PTH, dietary phosphate, and ECF volume. PTH, one of the major regulators of renal handling of phosphate, decreases phosphate renal reabsorption by the proximal tubule. A low-phosphate diet increases the reabsorption of phosphate by a non-PTH mechanism. Extracellular fluid volume expansion leads to increased phosphate excretion (see Chapter 11).

HYPOPHOSPHATEMIA

Definition. Hypophosphatemia refers to a serum phosphate level less than 2.7 mg/dl in adults and 4.0 mg/dl in children. It is a common metabolic abnormality, estimated to occur in 10 to 15% of hospitalized patients.

Pathophysiologic Considerations (Table 10–6). Hypophosphatemia may result from redistribution of phosphate from ECF to ICF and true body deficit induced by gastrointestinal or renal losses.

Redistribution of phosphate from ECF to ICF is the most common cause of hypophosphatemia in a hospital setting. The prime factor is an increase in the utilization of intracellular inorganic phosphate in the metabolic pathway of glycolysis. This increase occurs with glucose infusion, insulin infusion in the therapy of diabetic ketoacidosis, alkalosis (especially of the respiratory type), acute alcoholism, gram-negative septicemia, and salicylate poisoning.

A true body deficit can result from several problems. Decreased tubular reabsorption (increased renal loss) of phosphate is an important cause of hypophosphatemia. It can occur because of an intrinsic defect in tubular transport function or because of the presence of parathyroid hormone and other factors that affect proximal tubular reabsorption. An intrinsic defect in tubular transport can occur as part of a generalized tubular disorder (Fanconi's syndrome) with concomitant glycosuria, aminoaciduria, and bicarbonaturia and occurs in multiple myeloma, cystinosis, Wilson's disease, heavy metal poisoning, and systemic lupus erythematosus. Another possible intrinsic defect in tubular transport is an isolated defect in phosphate reabsorption in vitamin D-resistant rickets, which can occur either as a sex-linked dominant disorder or as a sporadic disorder in adults possibly seen in association with certain mesenchymal tumors (see Chapter 11, Hypocalcemia).

Decreased proximal tubular reabsorption of phosphate also occurs in hyperparathyroidism, the use of certain diuretics, glycosuria, ECF volume expansion, nonparathyroid hypercalcemia, hypokalemia, idiopathic hypercalciuria, ureterosigmoidostomy.

Gastrointestinal losses occur in various states of malabsorption. Diarrheal stools have a very low phosphate content. Hypophosphatemia in malabsorption is usually due to vitamin D deficiency, hypocalcemia, and secondary hyperparathyroidism.

Inadequate dietary intake is a rare cause of hypophosphatemia. The only important cause of decreased phosphate intake is related to the use of large amounts of phosphate-binding gel or in the use of total parenteral nutrition with nonphosphate-containing solutions.

Clinical Presentation. The clinical manifestations of hypophosphatemia result from a decrease in generation of high-energy phosphate bonds, alteration of the cell membrane and mitochondrial integrity, and decrease in 2–3 DPG concentration with subsequent tissue hypoxia.

Mild hypophosphatemia is usually asymptomatic. In acute significant hypophosphatemia, the patient

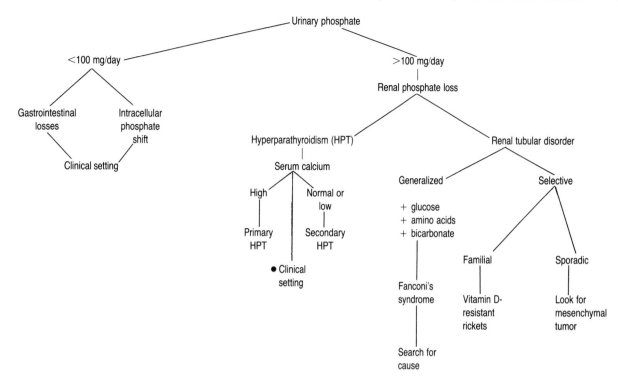

Fig. 10–6. Diagnostic approach to hypophosphatemia.

shows neuromuscular disturbances such as anorexia, nausea, irritability, apprehension, confusion, paresthesias, dysarthria, seizures, and coma. In chronic hypophosphatemia, skeletal manifestations predominate, such as proximal muscle weakness, hypotonia without atrophy, normal deep tendon reflexes, and muscle enzymes. Rhabdomyolysis may occur in severe hypophosphatemia. Hypophosphatemia may also present with osteomalacia or rickets (see Chapter 11, Osteomalacia and Rickets).

Diagnostic Evaluation (Fig. 10–6). Because the normal renal response to hypophosphatemia is a decrease and virtual elimination of phosphate from the urine, measurement of urine phosphate is an important diagnostic tool. If the serum phosphate is less than 2.0 mg/dl and renal handling of phosphate is normal, the urine is usually phosphate free or contains less than 100 mg of phosphate/day. This normal renal response indicates that the hypophosphatemia is related either to gastrointestinal losses or to redistribution from ECF to ICF. The diagnosis depends on the clinical setting.

If, in the presence of hypophosphatemia, the renal phosphate loss is documented (greater than 100 mg/day), the differential diagnosis includes hyperparathyroidism or a primary renal abnormality. Primary hyperparathyroidism is evident by hypercalcemia and an appropriately elevated serum PTH. In secondary hyperparathyroidism, the calcium may be normal or low, and the clinical setting will point to the cause. Renal tubular disorder may be selective or generalized (phosphaturia, glycosuria, aminoaciduria, and bicarbonaturia point to Fanconi's syndrome). In the presence of an isolated renal phosphate handling defect, a family history points to vitamin D-resistant rickets, while no family history should prompt a search for occult mesenchymal tumors.

HYPERPHOSPHATEMIA

Definition. Hyperphosphatemia is defined as a serum phosphate level above 4.5 mg/dl in adults and above 7.0 mg/dl in children. It is a less common metabolic disturbance than hypophosphatemia but can carry considerable risk to the patient because of the possibility of acute hypocalcemia and of extravascular calcification, which may produce cardiac or renal failure.

Pathophysiologic Considerations (Table 10–7). In general, hyperphosphatemia can result from phosphate loading in the presence of impaired renal function, decreased renal phosphate excretion in the presence of maintained phosphate intake, and release of phosphate from intracellular sites.

Phosphate loading can occur via the oral route (phosphate laxatives and enemas, vitamin D intoxication, and accidental or deliberate overdose of phosphate salts) or the IV route (phosphates used in the treatment of hypercalcemia or hypophosphatemia). Increased

Table 10–7. Causes of Hyperphosphatemia

Increased input (exceeding renal excretory capacity)
　Exogenous (phosphate loading)
　　Oral or IV
　Endogenous
　　Release from intracellular sites
　　　Rhabdomyolysis, severe burns, acidosis, therapy of leukemia
　　　　or lymphoma
　　Increased bone resorption
　　　Multiple myeloma
　　　Paget's disease
　　　Metastatic carcinoma
　　　Prolonged immobilization
　　　Hyperparathyroidism
Decreased output
　Decreased renal excretion
　　Renal failure
　　Hypoparathyroidism
　　Pseudohypoparathyroidism
　　Thyrotoxicosis
　　Acromegaly
　　Diphosphonates
　　Tumoral calcinosis
　　Magnesium deficiency

bone resorption leading to hyperphosphatemia occurs in multiple myeloma, Paget's disese, metastatic carcinoma, prolonged immobilization, and secondary hyperparathyroidism caused by renal disease.

Decreased renal phosphate excretion in the presence of maintained phosphate intake can occur with decreased GFR in chronic and acute renal failure and with increased renal tubular phosphate reabsorption as a result of hypoparathyroidism, pseudohypoparathyroidism, magnesium deficiency, thyrotoxicosis, acromegaly, use of diphosphonates, and tumoral calcinosis (a rare, specific renal tubular defect associated with large masses of calcium phosphate precipitation adjacent to various joints).

Release of phosphate from intracellular sites can occur in acute rhabdomyolysis (following trauma, thermal injury, or narcotic overdose), treatment of leukemia or lymphoma with cytotoxic agents or irradiation, severe burns, and metabolic and respiratory acidosis (which block the incorporation of inorganic phosphate into ATP).

Clinical Presentation. Though hyperphosphatemia itself causes no symptoms, symptoms may arise from coexistent hypocalcemia from increased entry of calcium and phosphate into bone and soft tissue and formation of calcium phosphate colloid in the blood. Acute hyperphosphatemia, by whatever mechanism, can cause hypocalcemia and tetany and can lead to vascular and other soft tissue calcification.

Diagnostic Evaluation. The most important diagnostic step is to differentiate among an exogenous phosphate load (by noting a history of administration

of phosphate compounds), an endogenous load (for example, in the clinical setting of rhabdomyolysis, cytotoxic drug treatment, and states associated with increased bone resorption or acidosis), and reduction in renal phosphate excretion. Decreased phosphate clearance can occur in acute or chronic renal failure (high serum creatinine), hypoparathyroidism (hypocalcemia and inappropriately low serum PTH), pseudohypoparathyroidism (with characteristic somatic features, hypocalcemia, and elevated serum PTH), acromegaly or thyrotoxicosis (clinical features and appropriate hormonal studies), and tumoral calcinosis (with a clinical setting of soft tissue calcification).

DISORDERS OF SERUM MAGNESIUM

INTRODUCTION

About 50 to 60% of the total body magnesium is in the bone serving a structural role. Most of the remainder is in the intracellular fluid where it is an essential cofactor for enzymatic reactions and has a role in nerve and muscle function. The normal concentration of magnesium in plasma ranges from 1.5 to 2.5 mEq/L; 30% of plasma magnesium is bound to plasma proteins, 50% is ionized, and 20%, complexed. The levels in plasma are kept within narrow limits, but the controlling factors are largely unknown.

The average diet contains 500 mg of magnesium, which is actively absorbed in the gut by a mechanism enhanced by vitamin D. The ionized and the complex plasma fractions are filtered by the glomeruli; 90 to 99% of the filtered magnesium is reabsorbed, and only 2 to 20 mEq are excreted per day. Magnesium excretion is decreased by parathyroid hormone, and changes in magnesium excretion generally parallel changes in calcium excretion. The renal excretion can be reduced to less than 2 mEq/day but cannot be totally eliminated. Therefore, individuals who ingest a low-magnesium diet (e.g., chronic alcoholics) can experience magnesium depletion. The capacity for renal excretion is large, and magnesium overload does not occur in the presence of normal renal function.

HYPOMAGNESEMIA

Definition. Hypomagnesemia is defined as a decrease in serum magnesium levels below 1.5 mEq/L.

Table 10–8. Causes of Hypomagnesemia

Decreased input
  Diet poor in magnesium
  Intravenous fluid (poor in magnesium) therapy
  Chronic alcoholism
  Gastrointestinal loss
    Vomiting
    Nasogastric suction
    Fistula
    Diarrhea
    Malabsorption
Increased urinary loss
  Diabetic ketoacidosis
  Chronic alcoholism
  Diuresis—osmotic, postobstructive, postrenal transplant
  Diuretics
  Magnesium-losing nephropathy
    Gentamicin
    Cis-platinum
    Amphotericin
  Renal tubular acidosis
  Hyperparathyroidism
  Hypoparathyroidism
  Hyperthyroidism
  Primary aldosteronism
  Bartter's syndrome
Intracellular shift of magnesium
  Hungry bone syndrome

It is a much more frequent metabolic derangement than hypermagnesemia.

Pathophysiologic Considerations (Table 10–8). Hypomagnesemia can result from decreased oral intake; increased losses, renal or gastrointestinal; and temporary magnesium shifts from ECF to ICF.

Decreased intake or absorption occurs in starvation, malnutrition, intravenous fluid therapy, chronic alcoholism, and increased GI losses from vomiting, nasogastric suction, fistula, ileostomy, diarrhea, or steatorrhea.

Increased urinary loss can occur in diabetic ketoacidosis (tissue catabolism and osmotic diuresis), chronic alcoholism, osmotic diuresis (osmotic saline diuresis, after renal transplantation, and after relief of urinary tract obstruction), use of diuretics, and in magnesium-losing nephropathy (from primary renal tubular defect, or from the use of gentamicin, cis-platinum, or amphotericin); increased urinary loss may also occur in endocrinopathies such as primary hyperparathyroidism, hypoparathyroidism, hyperthyroidism, primary aldosteronism, and Bartter's syndrome.

Increased loss into bone can follow parathyroidectomy for primary hyperparathyroidism associated with osteitis fibrosa cystica—the so-called hungry bone syndrome.

Clinical Presentation. The manifestations of hypomagnesemia are similar, if not identical, to those of hypocalcemia. Clinical manifestations may include ap-

athy, irritability, confusion, palpitations, anorexia, nausea, vomiting, tremors, twitches, spasms, myoclonus, spasticity, tonic-clonic convulsions, or frank tetany. Nystagmus and hyperactive reflexes may be present. Cardiac arrhythmias can occur, especially in digitalized patients, because of increased sensitivity of the heart to digitalis. They may range from ectopic beats to ventricular fibrillation and asystole in severe hypomagnesemia.

If chronic and severe, hypomagnesemia leads to suppression of PTH secretion and increased tissue resistance to PTH, and hence to hypocalcemia and its manifestations.

Diagnostic Evaluation. Hypomagnesemia should be suspected in the appropriate clinical setting in patients with suggestive symptoms and in patients presenting with hypocalcemic syndrome. It is confirmed by serum magnesium determination. The etiologic diagnosis is usually obvious on the basis of history and physical examination, which give clues to decreased intake, increased output, and transcellular magnesium shift. Laboratory studies are dictated by the clinical suspicion of its presence.

The diagnosis of hypomagnesemia is confirmed by serum magnesium of less than 1.5 mEq/L. A normal serum magnesium, however, does not rule out magnesium depletion. Serum magnesium levels may remain normal until a total body deficit of magnesium of greater than 20% is produced. In the presence of a normal serum magnesium, magnesium depletion can be diagnosed by performing the magnesium tolerance test. In the presence of an IV magnesium load, a normal person would excrete almost all the dose into the urine, while one with magnesium deficiency will retain varying portions of the dose, depending on the degree of deficiency.

HYPERMAGNESEMIA

Definition. Hypermagnesemia is defined by serum magnesium levels greater than 2.5 mEq/L.

Pathophysiologic Considerations (Table 10–9). Hypermagnesemia results from an imbalance between the intake of magnesium and its excretion or from transcellular shift of magnesium from ICF to ECF compartments.

Increased magnesium input can occur from the use of magnesium-containing laxatives or antacids, from parenteral administration of magnesium as part of treatment of eclampsia, and from accidental or deliberate poisoning. Since the kidney excretes magnesium efficiently, large doses are needed to cause hypermagnesemia in the absence of renal failure.

Decreased magnesium output in urine can occur in

Table 10–9. Causes of Hypermagnesemia

Increased input
  Increased intake
    Magnesium-containing antacids and laxatives
    Parenteral magnesium (treatment of eclampsia)
    Magnesium poisoning
  Increased efflux from cells
    Diabetic ketoacidosis
    Severe burns
    Starvation
    Rhabdomyolysis
Decreased output
  Decreased urinary excretion
    Renal failure
    Familial benign hypocalciuric hypercalcemia
    Hypothyroidism

chronic renal failure, familial benign hypocalciuric hypercalcemia, and hypothyroidism.

Increased efflux of magnesium from ICF to ECF occurs in diabetic ketoacidosis, starvation, severe burns, or rhabdomyolysis.

Clinical Presentation. Hypermagnesemia is rarely encountered in clinical practice except in renal failure when magnesium-containing antacids are used to treat hyperphosphatemia. The clinical features are related to the effects of hypermagnesemia on CNS or neuromuscular function and on the cardiovascular system. Serum magnesium less than 3 mEq/L, as seen in chronic renal failure, is usually asymptomatic. Significant hypermagnesemia can cause anorexia, nausea, vomiting, lethargy, confusion, impairment of neuromuscular ganglionic transmission, respiratory depression, dilated pupils, loss of DTRs, flaccid paralysis, bladder atony, ileus, cardiac conduction defects (heart block), and peripheral vasodilation (hypotension).

Diagnostic Evaluation. The physician should be alert to the potential presence of hypermagnesemia in the setting of renal insufficiency, increased input, and increased efflux from cells. It is documented by measuring serum magnesium.

DISORDERS OF ACID-BASE BALANCE

INTRODUCTION

The normal metabolic processes continuously generate hydrogen ions (H^+). Approximately 24,000 mM of carbonic acid (from complete combustion of carbohydrates and fatty acids to CO_2 and H_2O) and 50 to 100 mM of nonvolatile acids (from sulfur-containing amino acids and organic phosphates) are produced every 24 hours. Many pathophysiologic states are associated with acid and alkali loads and deficits. Despite these perturbations to the body fluids, the H^+ concentration (and pH) have to be maintained within a narrow range (pH of ECF is normally between 7.35 and 7.45) to preserve the action of vital enzyme systems in the body.

There are three main defenses against changes in pH: extracellular and intracellular buffers, the kidneys, and the lungs. Chemical buffering of H^+ concentration by extracellular and intracellular buffer systems is the immediate defense against changes in pH caused by acid or alkali loads or deficits. The bicarbonate buffer system ($HCO_3/PaCO_2$) is the principal extracellular buffer. The major intracellular buffers are proteins, organic phosphates, and bone.

The Henderson-Hasselbalch equation for calculating the pH reads

$$pH = pK + \frac{\log base}{acid}$$

where pK is the dissociation constant. Applied to the bicarbonate buffer system,

$$pH = 6.1 + \frac{\log HCO_3}{\alpha \, PaCO_2}$$

where α is .03 mM/L/mm Hg at 38° C. At a pH of 7.4, the ratio of HCO_3 to $PaCO_2$ is 20 to 1. It is the ratio of HCO_3 to $PaCO_2$, rather than the concentration of each, that determines blood pH. This extracellular buffer is of singular importance, since two separate mechanisms exist for adjusting this ratio: renal regulation of bicarbonate, and respiratory regulation of $PaCO_2$.

The role of the respiratory system in H^+ homeostasis is to alter the partial pressure of CO_2 ($PaCO_2$) in body fluids. The respiratory system serves two important functions: to excrete approximately 24,000 mM of carbon dioxide produced daily by aerobic cellular metabolism (failure of which function results in the accumulation of H_2CO_3 and in acidosis), and to vary the $PaCO_2$ as an adaptive mechanism in response to changes in H^+ concentration induced by nonrespiratory abnormalities. This ventilatory adaptation is mediated by arterial and central chemoreceptors sensitive to H^+ concentration. The respiratory response to changes in blood pH is almost instantaneous. Acidosis stimulates and alkalosis depresses ventilation.

The renal regulatory responses consist of excretion or retention of H^+ ions and excretion or regeneration of lost buffers. In acidosis there is stimulation of renal H^+ secretion, NH_3 production (so that more H^+ can be excreted as NH_4), and bicarbonate reabsorption and generation. In alkalosis there is prompt excretion of bicarbonate. The renal regulation is influenced by a number of factors: CO_2 tension of body fluids, ECF volume, aldosterone, and body potassium stores. Hypercapnia, decreased ECF volume, increased aldosterone, and severe potassium depletion increase H^+ secretion and bicarbonate regeneration, whereas hypocapnia, increased ECF volume, decreased aldosterone, and hyperkalemia decrease hydrogen secretion and increase bicarbonate loss.

Acid-base disturbances can therefore result from a primary alteration in the serum bicarbonate concentration, referred to as "metabolic disorder"; a rise in serum bicarbonate concentration is termed metabolic alkalosis, and a fall, metabolic acidosis. Acid-base disturbances also result from a primary alteration in the arterial Pa_{CO_2}, referred to as "respiratory disorder." A rise or fall in Pa_{CO_2} defines respiratory acidosis or alkalosis, respectively.

Simple disturbances include both the primary alteration and the expected compensation. Mixed disturbances are those in which two or more primary alterations coexist (e.g., respiratory acidosis with superimposed diuretic-induced metabolic alkalosis).

METABOLIC ACIDOSIS

Definition. Metabolic acidosis is characterized by an increase in blood H^+ (decrease in pH) and a primary fall in ECF bicarbonate concentration.

Pathophysiologic Considerations (Table 10–10). Metabolic acidosis may be caused by one of two basic mechanisms: loss of bicarbonate or accumulation of acid other than carbonic acid. It is classified as either metabolic acidosis with normal anion gap or metabolic acidosis with increased anion gap. Sodium is the principal cation in the ECF; serum sodium concentration is greater than the sum of serum chloride and serum bicarbonate concentration. The difference between serum sodium and the sum of serum chloride and bicarbonate is referred to as the unmeasured anions or the anion gap. The normal value is 10 to 12 mEq/L. (The remaining ions include primarily sulfate, phosphate, lactate, ketoacids, albumin, and other proteins, which are generally not reported with routine serum electrolyte measurements.)

Metabolic acidosis with normal anion gap can be caused by several disorders, one of which is impairment of renal absorption of bicarbonate, which occurs in proximal RTA type 2, in patients who are volume expanded (dilutional acidosis), in the use of carbonic anhydrase inhibitors such as acetazolamide, and in primary hyperparathyroidism. Metabolic acidosis with

Table 10–10.   Causes of Metabolic Acidosis

Increased anion gap
  Ketoacidosis
    Diabetes mellitus
    Starvation
    Alcohol induced
  Lactic acidosis
  Chronic renal failure
  Ingestion of
    Methyl alcohol
    Ethylene glycol
    Paraldehyde
    Salicylate
Normal anion gap (hyperchloremic acidosis)
  Loss of bicarbonate
    Gastrointestinal
      Diarrhea
      Pancreatic fistula
    Renal
      Renal acidification defects
        Renal tubular acidosis
        Proximal
        Distal
        Hyperkalemic
      Dilutional acidosis
        Rapid isotonic saline infusion
      Carbonic anhydrase inhibitors
        Acetazolamide
      Ureterosigmoidostomy-ileostomy
  Ingestion of acid or potential acid
    Parenteral hyperalimentation
    Ammonium chloride
    Calcium chloride
    Hydrochloric acid

normal anion gap is also caused by failure of bicarbonate regeneration, which occurs in distal gradient limited RTA type 1, chronic interstitial renal disease with hyporeninemic hypoaldosteronism, and the use of drugs such as triamterene, spironolactone, and amiloride. It can also be caused by extrarenal loss of bicarbonate, which occurs with loss of pancreatic and small-bowel secretion of any cause, in diarrheal states and ileal drainage, and within the colon in exchange for chloride in ureterosigmoidostomy. Finally, it results from administration of acidifying salts, which occurs with ammonium chloride, lysine or arginine hydrochloride, and hyperalimentation without administration of adequate amounts of bicarbonates or bicarbonate-yielding solutes.

Metabolic acidosis with increased anion gap occurs in reduced acid excretion in acute or chronic renal failure leading to retention of sulfates, phosphates, and other organic acid anions and to decreased renal ability to excrete ammonia and conserve bicarbonate. However, the most common cause of acute metabolic acidosis with increased anion gap is accumulation of organic acids, which occurs in lactic acidosis and ketoacidosis.

In lactic acidosis, lactate is generated from the reaction

$$pyruvate + NADH \rightleftharpoons lactate + NAD$$

The reaction is catalyzed by the enzyme lactate dehydrogenase. The concentration of lactate in the cytosol is proportionate to the concentration of pyruvate and to the NADH to NAD ratio. Increased lactate production occurs with an increased concentration of pyruvate or with an increased NADH to NAD ratio. Lactate is normally produced in red cells, skin, and brain and it is metabolized by the liver and kidney. Lactate blood levels are normally from 0.5 to 1.5 mM/L. Increased pyruvate levels result from either an increased rate of formation from glycolysis and amino acids or a decreased rate of utilization to CO_2, fat synthesis, and gluconeogenesis. An increased NADH to NAD ratio results from hypoxemia or from generation of NADH in another reaction.

Lactic acidosis is caused most commonly by tissue hypoxia, seen in shock, severe hypoxemia, severe anemia, carbon monoxide poisoning, and very strenuous exercise. It can also be caused by drugs and toxins such as ethanol, biguanides, fructose, salicylates, methanol, and ethylene glycol. Other causes of lactic acidosis include liver failure; neoplasia, leukemias, and solid tumors; uncontrolled diabetes mellitus; and inborn errors of metabolism.

Ketoacidosis, the other cause of acute metabolic acidosis with increased anion gap (see Chapter 11, Hyperglycemia and Diabetes Mellitus), occurs in alcoholic ketoacidosis, diabetic ketoacidosis, and starvation. It results from the accumulation of beta hydroxybutyric and acetoacetic acids.

Finally, metabolic acidosis with increased anion gap occurs from ingestion of toxins, such as salicylates (acetylsalicylic acid), paraldehyde (unidentified organic acids), methanol (formic acid), and ethylene glycol (glyoxylic-oxalic acid).

Compensation for Metabolic Acidosis. In metabolic acidosis, there is a primary fall in ECF bicarbonate concentration. The acidemia stimulates the respiratory center, leading to an increase in the rate and particularly the depth of respiration (Kussmaul's breathing) and reduction in blood Pa_{CO_2}. The fall in the blood Pa_{CO_2} has been found to equal 1.1 to 1.3 times the fall in bicarbonate (in mEq/L) from the normal.

Clinical Presentation. There are few specific manifestations of metabolic acidosis. In acute metabolic acidosis, hyperventilation (Kussmaul's breathing) is evident and may be intense. Hyperventilation may not be evident in chronic metabolic acidosis. Other nonspecific manifestations include fatigue, confusion, and drowsiness. In severe acidosis, coma may result from

Table 10–11. Causes of Metabolic Alkalosis

Exogenous base administration
  Bicarbonate
    Sodium bicarbonate therapy of acidosis
  Carbonate
    Antacids/milk alkali syndrome
  Acetate
    Hyperalimentation
    Renal dialysis
  Citrate
    Transfusions
Gastrointestinal acid loss
  Gastric
    Vomiting
    Nasogastric suction
    Gastrostomy
  Increased mineralocorticoid activity
    Hyper-reninemic states
      ECF volume contraction
      Renal artery stenosis
      Magnesium deficiency
      Bartter's syndrome
    Primary hypermineralocorticoid state
      Primary hyperaldosteronism
      Cushing's syndrome
      Adrenogenital syndrome
      Licorice ingestion
Increased tubular lumen negativity
  Nonreabsorbable anions
Increase pa_{CO_2}
  Posthypercapnia
? Decreased parathyroid hormone/increased serum calcium
  Hypoparathyroidism
  Hypercalcemic states

increased cerebrospinal fluid H^+ concentration and from CNS depression; there is a decrease in cardiac contractility and in inotropic response to catecholamines, and there is an increase in the risk of cardiac arrhythmias and congestive heart failure; in addition, vasodilation and hypotension are present.

METABOLIC ALKALOSIS

Definition. Metabolic alkalosis is the most common acid base disorder and is characterized by increase in ECF bicarbonate and elevation of pH.

Pathophysiologic Considerations (Table 10–11). Two conditions must be met for metabolic alkalosis to occur: the first is either loss of acid or increase of alkali, which acts to increase bicarbonate concentration; the second is failure of the kidneys to excrete excess bicarbonate because of stimulation of bicarbonate reabsorption by a volume (chloride) deficit as part of the effort to conserve sodium, because of hypermineralocorticoidism, and because of potassium depletion.

Addition of bicarbonate from exogenous substances that either contain or will generate bicarbonate in the body can result in metabolic alkalosis if taken in quantities that exceed bicarbonate excretory capacity of the kidney. These substances include sodium bicarbonate; calcium bicarbonate lactate or gluconate; potassium citrate, acetate, or carbonate; milk alkali; citrated blood; and acetate (dialysis).

Excessive loss of hydrogen ions from the body can result from gastrointestinal acid loss caused by vomiting, nasogastric suction, gastrostomy, or chloridorrhoea, and from renal regeneration and retention of bicarbonate. This regeneration and retention can occur in the use of diuretics such as thiazides and loop diuretics (e.g., furosemide and ethacrynic acid). Diuretics lead to stimulation of H^+ secretion and generation of bicarbonate because of ECF volume contraction, potassium depletion, and secondary aldosteronism. Regeneration and retention of bicarbonate also results from mineralocorticoid excess, whether primary or secondary. Mineralocorticoid excess leads to reabsorption of sodium and secretion of potassium and hydrogen in the distal nephron, resulting in potassium wasting, increased renal acid excretion, and bicarbonate regeneration. Regeneration and retention occurs also in Liddle's syndrome, which is characterized by increased sodium avidity by the distal nephron, hypertension, hypokalemia, and metabolic alkalosis; in Bartter's syndrome, which is characterized by salt wasting leading to increased H^+ secretion and by renal bicarbonate regeneration, secondary hyperaldosteronism, hypokalemia, and metabolic alkalosis; and in administration of large amounts of impermeable anions (e.g., carbenicillin.) Transient metabolic alkalosis can occur following acute improvement in the ventilatory status in patients with chronic hypercapnia (posthypercapnic alkalosis) or delayed conversion of accumulated organic acids, which can occur after insulin therapy for diabetic ketoacidosis, in the recovery phase of lactic acidosis, and following high-efficiency hemodialysis.

Compensation for Metabolic Alkalosis. In metabolic alkalosis, there is increase in ECF bicarbonate. The alkalemia leads to depression of the respiratory center through its effects on arterial and central H^+ receptors. This depression is followed by increase in $Paco_2$, which is linearly related to the increase in bicarbonate in a ratio of 0.6:0.8. Arterial hypoxemia may occur in severe cases.

Clinical Presentation. The adverse effects of metabolic alkalosis include a shift to the left in the oxyhemoglobin dissociation curve (thus interfering with oxygen release at the tissue level), muscular irritability, blunting of the hypoxic respiratory drive, and susceptibility to cardiac arrhythmias.

The clinical manifestations include hypopnea without symptoms; somnolence, obtundation, and coma; rarely, the syndrome of tetany with muscle spasms, positive Trousseau's and Chvostek's signs, and hyperactive TDRs; and muscular weakness, hyporeflexia, and cardiac arrhythmias contributed to, in part, by the associated hypokalemia.

RESPIRATORY ACIDOSIS

Definition. Respiratory acidosis is characterized by increased $Paco_2$ in the lungs and hence in the blood, by increased H^+ concentration, and by acidosis.

Pathophysiologic Considerations (Table 10–12). Respiratory acidosis results from a reduction of the normal effective alveolar ventilation. Essentially, it results from impairment of the ventilatory drive and ventilatory mechanisms. Acute respiratory acidosis results from CNS depression caused by narcotic overdose, anesthesia, CNS disorders, paralysis of respiratory muscles (e.g., from hypokalemia, myasthenia, and aminoglycoside antibiotics), and airway obstruction by foreign body, asthma, trauma, or flail chest. Chronic respiratory acidosis results commonly from chronic obstructive bronchopulmonary diseases, obesity, and the syndromes of reduced thoracic compliance.

Compensation in Respiratory Acidosis. In acute respiratory acidosis almost all the H^+ is buffered within cells. Since extracellular bicarbonate cannot buffer CO_2, the extent to which the H^+ buffering occurs is limited. Increased bicarbonate is generated within the cells and added to the ECF. For each 10 mm Hg rise in $Paco_2$, serum bicarbonate is increased by 1 mEq/L.

Within a few hours renal mechanisms come into play and are optimal in 2 to 5 days. There is increased urinary ammonium (NH_4) excretion, increased urinary net acid excretion, and increased generation of bicarbonate, which is added to the body fluids. For each 10-mm rise above normal in Pco_2, blood bicarbonate increases by 3 to 4 mEq/L.

Clinical Presentation. The clinical manifestations of respiratory acidosis result from the acidosis and the associated hypoxemia resulting from the alveolar hypoventilation. There is increased respiratory effort with dyspnea (which may be blunted in chronic respiratory acidosis) unless the patient is oversedated, comatose, or paralyzed. Somnolence, confusion, and obtundation may follow. Asterixis may be noted. There is dilatation of conjunctival and superficial facial blood vessels, and the optic fundi show dilated and engorged vessels. Frank papilledema may occur.

Table 10–12. Causes of Respiratory Acidosis

Acute	Chronic
Ventilatory disorders	Ventilatory disorders
Severe pulmonary edema	Chronic obstructive bronchopulmonary disease
Severe pneumonia	Far-advanced interstitial fibrosis
Adult respiratory distress syndrome	Kyphoscoliosis-arthritis
Flail chest	Fibrothorax
Pneumothorax	Hydrothorax
Hemothorax	Muscular dystrophy
Airway obstruction	Polymyositis
Severe bronchospasm	
Laryngospasm	
Aspiration	
Obstructive sleep apnea	
Severe hypokalemia	
Myasthenic crisis	
Perfusion disorders	
Massive pulmonary embolism	
Cardiac arrest	
Respiratory drive disorders	Respiratory drive disorders
Central	Central
Anesthesia	Chronic sedative and tranquilizer overdose
Drugs (e.g., sedatives)	Obesity hypoventilation syndrome
Trauma	Myxedema
Stroke	Brain tumors
Central sleep apnea	Brain stem infarcts
	Bulbar poliomyelitis
Spinal cord—peripheral nerves	Spinal cord—peripheral nerves
Cervical cord injury	Poliomyelitis
Guillain-Barré syndrome	Multiple sclerosis
Drugs (e.g., succinylcholine, curare, aminoglycoside)	Amyotrophic lateral sclerosis
Neurotoxins (e.g., botulism, tetanus)	Diaphragmatic paralysis
Acute failure of mechanical ventilation	

RESPIRATORY ALKALOSIS

Definition. Respiratory alkalosis is characterized by a primary decrease in $PaCO_2$ leading to an increase in blood pH and a decrease in serum bicarbonate.

Pathophysiologic Considerations (Table 10–13). Respiratory alkalosis occurs when hyperventilation reduces $PaCO_2$. Acute respiratory alkalosis is most commonly seen as a result of severe anxiety (hyperventilation syndrome), stimulation of the respiratory center by cerebral disease, acute salicylism, fever, septic states, pneumonia, pulmonary embolism, and congestive heart failure. Transient respiratory alkalosis follows the correction of metabolic acidosis, particularly diabetic ketoacidosis, because of a lag in the rise of serum bicarbonate. Alkalosis can be produced iatrogenically by injudicious mechanical ventilatory support. Chronic respiratory alkalosis can occur in acclimatization response to high altitudes, pulmonary fibrosis, advanced hepatic insufficiency, and pregnancy, among other causes.

Compensation in Respiratory Alkalosis. Respiratory alkalosis is characterized by a primary reduction of blood $PaCO_2$ and decreased blood H^+ concentration.

To compensate, there is immediate intracellular buffering of bicarbonate resulting in decreased serum bicarbonate concentration. For each 10 mm Hg decrease in arterial $PaCO_2$ below normal, there is a decrease in serum bicarbonate of about 2 mEq/L.

Renal compensation sets in within hours and is complete in 2 to 5 days. It is characterized by decreased renal H^+ secretion, decreased net acid secretion, and decreased bicarbonate reabsorption leading to decreased serum bicarbonate. For each 10-mm fall in blood $PaCO_2$ serum bicarbonate falls 5 to 6 mEq/L.

Clinical Presentation. Clinical manifestations include increased rate or depth of ventilation (these may be minimal in chronic respiratory alkalosis) and tetanic syndrome, which includes paresthesias, muscle cramps, carpopedal spasms, and, in severe cases, laryngeal spasm and seizures. There may be positive Chvostek's and Trousseau's signs and hyper-reflexia.

DIAGNOSTIC EVALUATION OF ACID-BASE DISTURBANCES

Suspicion regarding the presence of an acid-base disturbance is based on awareness of the clinical set-

Table 10–13.   Causes of Respiratory Alkalosis

Corticol influences
  Anxiety
  Pain
  Fever
  Voluntary
  CNS disorders
    Injury
    Inflammation
    Decreased blood supply
    Tumor
Hypoxemia
  High altitude
  Other low ambient Pa_{O_2} conditions
  Pulmonary shunts
  Pulmonary ventilation perfusion abnormalities
  Pulmonary diffusion defects
Physical
  Irritative lesions of the air passageways (e.g., inflammation, spasm, tumor)
  Stiff lungs (e.g., edema, fibrosis)
Miscellaneous
  Drugs
    Salicylates
    Nicotine
    Xanthines (e.g., aminophylline)
    Catecholamines
  Liver cirrhosis
  Gram-negative septicemia
  Pregnancy
  Heat exposure
  Mechanical ventilation
  Recovery from metabolic acidosis

tings in which these disorders can occur and on the knowledge of pertinent clinical and biochemical abnormalities that can result from these disorders. A careful patient history and physical examination may suggest the specific type of disturbance, e.g., chronic renal failure, COPD, pneumonia, sepsis, diabetes, vomiting, the use of drugs such as diuretics or sedatives, and the use of alcohol.

Diagnostic Studies

Simultaneous arterial pH, blood gases, serum bicarbonate, and serum electrolytes should be ordered.

Serum chloride can be helpful in assessing the acid-base disorder. The level of serum chloride is compared with that of serum sodium. It is important to remember that serum sodium changes only as a result of changes in hydration, whereas serum chloride changes as a result of changes in hydration and in acid-base balance. Therefore, changes in serum chloride that are not reflected by proportionate changes in serum sodium suggest an acid-base disorder. A disproportionate decrease in serum chloride suggests metabolic alkalosis or respiratory acidosis, while a disproportionate increase suggests metabolic acidosis or respiratory alkalosis.

Serum potassium can also be helpful. Potassium transcellular shifts occur in primary acid-base disorders, with metabolic acidosis leading to hyperkalemia and with metabolic alkalosis to hypokalemia. The combination of hypokalemia and increased serum bicarbonate suggests metabolic alkalosis, while hyperkalemia with reduced serum bicarbonate suggests metabolic acidosis. Failure of patients with significant acid-base disorders to show these changes in serum potassium should suggest significant derangement of body potassium homeostasis. The physician should also calculate the anion gap (see above). Increased anion gap results from accumulation of acid anions in the extracellular fluid (e.g., acetoacetate, lactate) and points to metabolic acidosis.

Finally, the expected degree of compensation should be calculated. Mixed acid base disturbances exceed the physiologic limits of compensation.

Metabolic Acidosis. The characteristic laboratory features include reduced serum bicarbonate and decreased pH together with compensatory decrease in Pa_{CO_2}. Hyperkalemia is often present because of the shift of potassium out of cells, perhaps masking significant potassium depletion. The etiologic diagnosis of metabolic acidosis depends on the clinical setting and the calculation of the anion gap.

A normal anion gap in metabolic acidosis signifies hyperchloremic acidosis caused by extrarenal loss of bicarbonate from the body, failure of the kidney to excrete H^+ ions and regenerate bicarbonate, or excessive intake of acidifying salts. The diagnosis is made by taking the patient's history, performing a physical examination, assessing urine acidity, and performing additional appropriate studies. A metabolic acidosis with increased anion gap implies decreased acid excretion from renal failure, increased acid production from lactic acidosis or ketoacidosis (uncontrolled diabetes mellitus, starvation, and alcoholism), or organic acids from an exogenous source. Diagnosis depends on the history, collateral clinical findings, and chemical analysis of the blood BUN, creatinine, ketone bodies, lactate, and toxicology screen.

To determine if a mixed acid-base disorder is present, the compensatory limits should be considered. In pure increased anion gap acidosis, the increase in the anion gap above the normal value should be approximately equal to the decrease in bicarbonate below the normal value. In a mixed acid-base disorder this relationship does not hold; e.g., in patients with diabetic ketoacidosis and protracted vomiting, the increase in the anion gap is greater than the decrease in bicarbonate, reflecting a mixed disturbance of metabolic acidosis and metabolic alkalosis.

If Pa_{CO_2} is higher than expected in metabolic acidosis, a diagnosis of coexisting respiratory acidosis

Table 10–14. Compensatory Responses and Limits in Primary Acid-Base Disorders

Acid-Base Disorder	Primary Response	Compensatory Response
Metabolic acidosis	Loss of HCO_3^- or gain of H^+	Increase in ventilation; chemical buffering
Metabolic alkalosis	Gain of HCO_3^- or loss of H^+	Decrease in ventilation; chemical buffering
Respiratory acidosis	Hypoventilation	HCO_3^- generation cellular buffering
Respiratory alkalosis	Hyperventilation	Cellular buffering, renal HCO_3^- loss

(Adapted from Dubose, T.D., Jr.: Clinical approach to patients with acid-base disorders. Medical Clinics of North Am. Acid-Base Disorders. July '83.)

may be made, e.g., severe pulmonary edema with respiratory acidosis and metabolic acidosis (lactic acidosis from hypoxemia). If Pa_{CO_2} is lower than expected, a coexistent respiratory alkalosis is present, e.g., in salicylate intoxication or in patients with severe liver disease (lactic acidosis with central hyperventilation and respiratory alkalosis).

In pure hyperchloremic acidosis, the increase in chloride above the normal value should be equal to the decrease in serum bicarbonate below normal. If this is not present, a mixed disturbance is suggested.

Metabolic Alkalosis. The diagnosis of metabolic alkalosis is made on the basis of the clinical setting and characteristic laboratory features, which include increased serum bicarbonate, increased pH, and increase in Pa_{CO_2}. The serum potassium is often reduced by the same mechanism that causes the metabolic alkalosis, e.g., diuretics or by a transcellular shift of potassium from ECF to ICF. The etiologic diagnosis of metabolic alkalosis depends on consideration of the clinical setting, e.g., vomiting, use of diuretics, and mineralocorticoid excess, and on appropriate laboratory studies.

The urinary chloride is a useful index in distinguishing metabolic alkalosis caused by volume contraction from that caused by primary mineralocorticoid excess. In volume contracted states, except those caused by Bartter's syndrome and the use of diuretics, the urinary chloride is less than 10 mEq/L. The combination of postural hypotension, hypokalemic metabolic alkalosis, and urinary chloride greater than 20 mEq/L should suggest diuretic abuse or Bartter's syndrome. A urinary chloride greater than 20 mEq/L is most commonly seen in disorders associated with volume expansion, such as hyperaldosteronism, Cushing's syndrome, licorice abuse, Liddle's syndrome, and adrenogenital syndrome. The diagnosis is by the clinical setting and the appropriate hormonal studies.

The physician must determine if there is a mixed acid-base disorder. In metabolic alkalosis, the increase in Pa_{CO_2} amounts to 0.6 to 0.7 mm Hg for each 1.0 mEq/L increase in serum bicarbonate. Arterial blood gases and electrolyte values that do not fit imply a superimposed or mixed acid-base disorder.

If Pa_{CO_2} is greater than expected, the physician should suspect associated respiratory acidosis, e.g., in patients with COPD who are receiving diuretics and whose salt intake is restricted because of cor pulmonale.

If Pa_{CO_2} is less than expected, suspect associated respiratory alkalosis, e.g., in critically ill surgical patients on mechanical ventilators who are receiving nasogastric suction or massive blood transfusions.

For metabolic alkalosis associated with metabolic acidosis, see above under Metabolic Acidosis.

Respiratory Acidosis. The diagnosis depends on the clinical setting and the characteristic laboratory features of increased Pa_{CO_2}, decreased pH, and increased serum bicarbonate. Patients are invariably hypoxemic, and secondary polycythemia occurs in chronic hypercapnic states. Etiologic diagnosis depends on careful history and physical examination.

The physician must determine if there is a mixed acid-base disorder. In uncomplicated respiratory acidosis, the increase in serum bicarbonate is rarely above 32 mEq/L. Values greater than 32 mEq/L suggest concomitant metabolic alkalosis, e.g., in patients with COPD treated with diuretics and salt restriction. A value of serum bicarbonate less than 26 mEq/L suggests concomitant metabolic acidosis, e.g., in chronic lung disease with hypoxemia and lactic acidosis.

Respiratory Alkalosis. The diagnosis rests on the clinical setting, decreased Pa_{CO_2}, increased pH, and decreased serum bicarbonate (rarely below 15 mEq/L). Acute hypocapnia causes a decrease in serum phosphate of as much as 1.5 to 2.5 mg/dl. The etiologic diagnosis of respiratory alkalosis depends on the history and physical examination. The physician must assess the possibility of a mixed acid-base disorder. The compensatory limits in acute respiratory alkalosis consist of a decrease in serum bicarbonate by 2.0 mEq/L for each 10 mm Hg decrease in Pa_{CO_2}, while compensatory limits for chronic respiratory alkalosis consists of a decrease in serum bicarbonate of 5.0 mEq/L for each 10 mm Hg decrease. Values outside these limits suggest combined metabolic disturbance. A greater fall in serum bicarbonate suggests coexistent metabolic acidosis, while a lesser fall suggests coexistent metabolic alkalosis.

GENERAL REFERENCES

DISORDERS OF WATER AND SODIUM BALANCE

Andreoli, T.E.: The polyuric syndromes. In Physiology of Membrane Disorders. Edited by T.E. Andreoli, J.F. Hoffman, and D.D. Fanestil. New York, Plenum Medical Book Co., 1978, 1063–1091.
Beal, T., et al.: Clinical disorders of water metabolism. Kidney Int 10:117, 1976.
Humes, M.D., Narins, R.G., and Brenner, B.M.: Disorders of water balance. Hosp Pract 14:133, 1979.
Lifschitz, M.D., and Stein, J.M.: Hormonal regulation of renal salt excretion. Semin Nephrol 3:196, 1983.
Miller, M., et al.: Recognition of partial defects in antidiuretic hormone secretion. Ann Intern Med 73:721, 1970.
Moses, A.M., Miller, M., Streeten, D.M.P.: Pathophysiologic and pharmacologic alterations in the release and action of ADH. Metabolism 25:697, 1976.
Moses, A.M., Notman, D.: Diabetes insipidus and syndrome of inappropriate antidiuretic hormone secretion (SIADM). Adv Intern Med 27:73, 1982.
Narins, R.G., et al.: Diagnostic strategies in disorders of fluid, electrolyte, and acid base homeostasis. Am J Med 72:496, 1982.

POLYURIA

Miller, M., et al.: Recognition of partial defects in antidiuretic hormone secretion. Ann Intern Med 73:721, 1970.
Moses, A.M., Miller, M., Streeten, D.H.P.: Pathophysiologic and pharmacologic alterations in release and action of ADH. Metabolism 25:697, 1976.
Robertson, G.L.: Thirst and vasopressin function in normal and disordered states of water balance. J Lab Clin Med 101:351, 1983.
Robinson, A.G.: Disorders of antidiuretic hormone secretion. Clin Endocrinol Metab 14:55, 1985.

DISORDERS OF SERUM POTASSIUM

Cohen, J.J.: Disorders of potassium balance. Hosp Pract 16:119, 1979.

DeFronzo, R.A.: Hyperkalemic and hyporeninemic hypoaldosteronism. Kidney Int 17:118, 1980.
Genari, F.J., and Cohen, J.J.: Role of the kidney is potassium homeostasis. Lessons from acid base disturbances. Kidney Int 8:1, 1975.
Kunau, R.T., and Steis, D.H.: Disorders of hypo- and hyperkalemia. Clin Nephrol 7:173, 1977.
Nardone, D.A., McDonald, W.J., and Girard, D.E.: Mechanisms in hypokalemia: clinical correlation. Medicine 57:435, 1978.

DISORDERS OF SERUM PHOSPHATE

Fitzgerald, F.T.: Hypophosphatemia. Adv Intern Med 23:137, 1978.
Janson, C., Birnbaum, G., and Baker, F.J.: Hypophosphatemia. Ann Emerg Med 12:107, 1983.
Knochel, J.P.: Hypophosphatemia. West J Med 134:15, 1981.
Slatopolsky, E., Rutherford, W.E., Rosenbaum, R., et al. Hyperphosphatemia. Clin Nephrol 7:138, 1977.

DISORDERS OF SERUM MAGNESIUM

Cronin, R.E., and Krochel, J.P.: Magnesium deficiency. Adv Intern Med 28:509, 1983.
Dirko, J.H.: The kidney and magnesium regulation. Kidney Int 23:271, 1983.
Wackes, W.E.C.: Magnesium and Man. Cambridge, Mass, Harvard University Press, 1980.

DISORDERS OF ACID BASE BALANCE

Adrogué, H.J., Wilson, H., and Boyd, A.E.: Plasma acid base patterns in diabetic ketoacidosis. N Engl J Med 307:1603, 1982.
Emmett, M., and Narins, R.G.: Clinical use of the anion gap. Medicine 56:38, 1977.
Gabow, P.A., et al.: Diagnostic importance of the increased anion gap. N Engl J Med 1980, 303:854, 1980.
Halperin, M.L., et al.: Metabolic acidosis in the alcoholic: a pathophysiologic approach. Metabolism 32:308, 1983.
Kreisberg, R.A.: Lactate homeostasis and lactic acidosis. Ann Intern Med 92:227, 1980.
Kurtzman, N.A., and Batlle, D.C. (guest eds). Symposium on acid base disorders. Med Clin North Am 67:1983.
Rector, F.C., and Cogan, M.G.: The renal acidoses. Hosp Practice 99:111, 1980.
Seldin, D.W., and Rector, F.C.: The generation and maintenance of metabolic alkalosis. Kidney Int 1:306, 1972.
Schwartz, W.B., and Cohen, J.J.: The nature of the renal response to chronic disorders of acid base equilibrium. Am J Med 66:417, 1978.

CHAPTER 11

ENDOCRINE AND METABOLIC PROBLEMS

Charles F. Abboud, M.D., B.Ch.

THE SYNDROME OF HYPOPITUITARISM

DEFINITION

Hypopituitarism is the syndrome that results from failure of the anterior pituitary gland to produce one, more than one, or all of its hormones.

PATHOPHYSIOLOGIC CONSIDERATIONS
(Table 11–1)

The pituitary gland is composed of two anatomically distinct parts: the anterior lobe, or adenohypophysis, and the posterior lobe, or neurohypophysis. The anterior lobe is an endocrine gland that secretes at least eight identifiable hormones. It is under the control of the hypothalamus through the hypothalamic regulatory hormones, which are secreted by the neuroendocrine cells of the medial basal hypothalamus and are transported to the anterior lobe by the hypothalamic pituitary portal venous system. The anterior pituitary cell types, their hormones, and their hypothalamic regulators are outlined in Table 11–2. The posterior pituitary lobe is not an endocrine gland. It functions as a storehouse for two hypothalamic hormones, vasopressin (ADH or AVP) and oxytocin. These hormones are synthesized in the neurons of the supraoptic and paraventricular hypothalamic nuclei and pass along the axons through the median eminence and pituitary stalk; they are stored in nerve terminals in the posterior lobe until they are discharged into the circulation to meet physiologic needs.

Hypopituitarism can be caused by intrinsic pituitary disease resulting from absence or destruction of hormone-secreting cells of the pituitary; by intrinsic hypothalamic disease that leads to deficiency or loss of the hypothalamic regulatory hormones with resultant lack of stimulation of pituitary hormone secretion; or by extrasellar or parasellar disease that impinges on, infiltrates, or destroys the hypothalamic-pituitary unit.

Intrinsic Pituitary Disease. Pituitary adenomas represent 10 to 15% of all intracranial neoplasms. They arise from the anterior lobe and essentially are all benign. Malignant primary tumors of the anterior lobe and posterior lobe tumors are extremely rare. Most of the adenomas are functioning tumors that hypersecrete anterior pituitary hormones singly or in combinations. More than 50% of these tumors are prolactin-produc-

ing (hyperprolactinemic syndrome), 10 to 15% are GH-producing (gigantism or acromegaly), and 10 to 15% are ACTH-producing (Cushing's disease and Nelson's syndrome). Rarely, gonadotropins, thyrotropin, or alpha glycoprotein subunits are produced by these tumors. Less than 20% of pituitary adenomas are nonfunctioning. Pituitary tumors usually occur as isolated endocrine tumors. Rarely they occur as part of multiple endocrine neoplasia type I or Werner's syndrome, a familial autosomal dominant disease in which patients may have tumors or hyperplasia of the anterior pituitary, parathyroid, or endocrine pancreas.

Craniopharyngioma, a squamous cell tumor that develops from Rathke's pouch remnants, is the most common hypothalamic-pituitary–area tumor in children. Two thirds of these tumors are suprasellar; one third occur within or extend into the sella. Most are cystic; some are solid or mixed. The cysts are filled with yellowish brown fluid resembling motor oil. Craniopharyngiomas have a propensity toward calcification.

Sheehan's syndrome (postpartum pituitary necrosis) is another intrinsic pituitary disease. The pituitary gland is markedly increased in size during pregnancy primarily because of hyperplasia and hypertrophy of lactotroph cells under the influence of rising estrogen secretion. Vasospasm of the hypophyseal vessels occurs in association with severe hemorrhage and hypotension in the immediate postpartum period, leading to ischemic necrosis of the pituitary. The degree of necrosis depends on the severity of the hemorrhage. As many as 30% of women experiencing hemorrhage and vascular collapse during delivery will develop some degree of hypopituitarism. Clinical hypopituitarism does not occur until about 70 to 75% of the anterior pituitary is destroyed. Complete hypopituitarism, which requires destruction of at least 90% of the gland, is less common at present because of great improvements in obstetric care.

Pituitary apoplexy refers to intrapituitary hemorrhage usually associated with functioning or nonfunctioning pituitary tumors. Rarely it occurs in normal glands in diabetic patients with cerebrovascular disease or in patients with sickle-cell disease. Pituitary apoplexy is a medical emergency because of the effects of the rapidly expanding mass and because of acute ACTH-adrenocortical failure. In those patients who recover spontaneously, anterior pituitary failure may occur, though posterior pituitary function is almost always preserved.

The use of radiation therapy in the treatment of malignancies of the head and neck, such as nasopharyngeal carcinoma and brain tumors, can lead to pituitary and hypothalamic damage and is an increas-

Table 11—1. Causes of Hypopituitarism

Primary: pituitary	Functional (continued)
Congenital	Anorexia nervosa
Idiopathic	Systemic disease
Traumatic	Renal, hepatic failure
Neurosurgical (pituitary tumors, breast carcinoma, diabetic retinopathy)	Uncontrolled diabetes mellitus
Radiotherapeutic (to sella or nasopharynx)	Drugs, e.g., vincristine
Inflammatory/infiltrative	Hormones
Infectious, e.g., TB, syphilis, fungal	Glucocorticoids
Sarcoidosis, hemochromatosis	Gonadal steroids
Autoimmune hypophysitis	Thyroid hormones
Vascular	Organic
Ischemic necrosis	Traumatic
Postpartum pituitary necrosis (Sheehan's)	Neurosurgery
Diabetes mellitus	Irradiation
Temporal arteritis	Inflammatory/infiltrative
Sickle-cell disease and trait	Sarcoidosis
Eclampsia	Histiocytosis X
Pituitary apoplexy	Neoplastic
Neoplastic	Primary
Primary	Gliomas
Pituitary tumors	Ectopic pinealoma
Craniopharyngiomas	Craniopharyngioma
Metastatic	Metastatic
Miscellaneous	Lymphoma and leukemia
Primary empty sella	Idiopathic
Idiopathic	Extrasellar disease
Secondary: hypothalamic	Parasellar tumors
Destruction of pituitary stalk	Meningioma
Trauma	Optic nerve glioma
Neurosurgical	Chordoma
Compression by tumor or aneurysm	Cysts, e.g., arachnoid
Hypothalamic or other CNS disease	Nasopharyngeal carcinoma
Functional	Sphenoid sinus mucocele
Stress—psychogenic	Aneurysm of internal carotid
Nutritional	Cavernous sinus thrombosis
Starvation	
Obesity	

ingly recognized cause of hypopituitarism. Spread of infections from contiguous structures, e.g., sphenoid sinus or meninges, or from distant sites, as occurs in septicemia, are rare causes of hypopituitarism. Sarcoidosis, another cause, may involve the hypothalamic-pituitary area and present with diabetes insipidus or hypopituitarism. Lymphocytic hypophysitis, believed to be due to an autoimmune disorder, is rare and may occur as part of a polyendocrine deficiency syndrome in association with Hashimoto's thyroiditis, parathyroid, adrenocortical, or gonadal autoimmune endocrinopathy, pernicious anemia, etc. The incidence of clinical hypopituitarism in primary empty sella syndrome is less than 10%. The cause of the pituitary dysfunction is unknown. No underlying disease is identifiable in idiopathic hypopituitarism, which is as-

Table 11—2. Hormones of the Hypothalamic-Pituitary Unit

Pituitary Cell	Pituitary Hormone	Major Hypothalamic Regulatory Hormone(s)
Somatotroph	Growth hormone (GH)	Growth hormone inhibitory hormone (Somatostatin)
		Growth hormone releasing hormone (GHRH)
Lactotroph	Prolactin (PRL)	Prolactin inhibitory hormone (Dopamine)
Gonadotroph	Follicle stimulating hormone (FSH)	Gonadotropin releasing hormone (GnRH)
	Luteinizing hormone (LH)	
Corticotroph	Corticotropin (ACTH)	Corticotropin releasing hormone (CRH)
	B-Lipotropin (B-LPH)	
	B-Endorphin (B-END)	
Thyrotroph	Thyrotropin (TSH)	Thyrotropin releasing hormone (TRH)

sociated most frequently with unitropic or multitropic pituitary failure. It can be sporadic or familial.

Intrinsic Hypothalamic Stalk Disease. Pathologic processes involving the stalk are most frequently due to trauma (e.g., basilar skull fractures and neurosurgical procedures); mass (e.g,, parasellar tumor or aneurysm that impinges on the stalk and its blood supply); or pituitary stalk section as an alternative procedure to hypophysectomy. Hypothalamic diseases cause hypopituitarism by impairing secretion of the hypothalamic regulatory hormones. They are functional when the impairment of function is not due to a recognizable structural disease, and are organic when there is structural disease caused by congenital, traumatic, inflammatory, infiltrative, vascular, or neoplastic disease process (see Table 11–2). The degree and the extent of the deficiencies depend on the extent of the pathologic process and its location—the closer to the median eminence, the greater the possibility of multiple deficiencies. Functional hypothalamic hypopituitarism may be related to emotional stresses, marked changes in body weight including malnutrition and obesity, anorexia nervosa, systemic diseases such as congestive heart failure and renal failure, drugs such as sex steroids (e.g., oral contraceptives) and primary thyroid and adrenal disorders and diabetes mellitus. Treatment with supraphysiologic doses of glucocorticoids for a prolonged period leads via a negative feedback effect to ACTH deficiency and atrophy of the pituitary corticotrophs and the adrenal cortices.

Kallmann's syndrome refers to a familial isolated hypogonadotropic hypogonadal state that occurs predominantly in males. Secondary to inadequate gonadotropin-releasing hormone (GnRH) secretion, it is frequently associated with hyposmia or anosmia (caused by hypoplasia of the olfactory lobes) and with other developmental defects, including harelip, cleft palate, facial fusion abnormalities, and cryptorchidism. It presents with failure of sexual maturation and anosmia. Careful testing of sense of smell is indicated because affected individuals may be unaware of their olfactory dysfunction.

Extrasellar Diseases. These can cause hypopituitarism by impinging on, displacing, or destroying the hypothalamic-pituitary unit. They include suprasellar cysts, meningiomas, optic nerve gliomas, carotid aneurysm, chordomas, sphenoid sinus mucocele, and nasopharyngeal carcinoma.

CLINICAL PRESENTATION

The clinical manifestations of hypopituitarism result from the hypopituitarism itself and from the cause of hypopituitarism.

Clinical Manifestations Related to Hypopituitarism

Hypopituitarism of any cause can affect one, more than one, or all of the anterior pituitary hormones, and for each hormone the deficiency can be partial or complete. Isolated hormone deficiency is very rare. The usual clinical picture is a composite of several hormonal deficiencies and depends on the patient's age at the time of onset and on the extent and duration of the hormone deficiency. With progressive anterior pituitary failure, e.g., that caused by a slowly expanding mass such as a pituitary tumor, deficiency usually affects first the growth hormone axis, followed in sequence by the gonadotropin, TSH, ACTH, and prolactin axes. It is important to remember, however, that hypopituitarism can afffect the endocrine axis in any sequence or combination, and that prolactin secretion may be increased if the cause of hypopituitarism is a prolactinoma or suprasellar disease. The dominant clinical picture of hypopituitarism in childhood is failure of normal linear growth. In adolescents it is failure or arrest of sexual maturation; in adults it is that of hypogonadism.

Gonadotropin (LH and FSH Deficiency). Hypogonadism is the most common clinical presentation of hypopituitarism in the adult. In premenopausal women, the resulting decrease in ovarian function is manifested by oligomenorrhea, infertility, and hypoestrogenic manifestations that include decreased vaginal secretion, dyspareunia, decreased libido, breast atrophy, and osteoporosis. In the adult male the resulting decrease in testicular function is manifested by decreased libido, potency impairment, decrease in ejaculate volume, infertility, decreased beard and body hair growth, muscle weakness, and fatigue. In prepubertal individuals, gonadotropin lack leads to failure of development of puberty, growth of genitalia, secondary sexual characteristics, and pubertal growth spurt; epiphyseal closure is delayed. Gonadotropin deficiency in postmenopausal women and in children does not cause clinical manifestations.

On examination, the physician may find evidence of decreased vaginal cornification and of uterine and breast atrophy in premenopausal women. In men the testes and the prostate are small and soft, beard and body hair growth may be decreased, and muscle development may be poor. In prepubertal children there is evidence of failure of sexual maturation and eunuchoidism. In prepubertal males the genitalia are infantile, the testes are prepubertal and soft, sexual hair growth is absent, muscle development is poor, and the voice is high pitched. In prepubertal females there is evidence of sexual infantilism. In both sexes the skin is thin and delicate, with fine wrinkling around the mouth and the eyes giving an appearance of premature aging.

Thyrotropin (TSH) Deficiency. Lack of TSH leads to hypothyroidism. The clinical manifestations are similar to those of primary hypothyroidism (see Hypothyroidism) but are less severe. They include physical and mental slowing, lethargy, fatigue, weight gain, dry skin, cold intolerance, and constipation. On examination there is evidence of dryness and pallor of the skin, hypothyroid facies, and absence of palpable thyroid tissue.

Corticotropin (ACTH) Deficiency. ACTH deficiency leads to decreased production of cortisol and adrenal androgens by the adrenal cortex. Aldosterone secretion is preserved since its primary regulator is the renin-angiotensin system. Cortisol deficiency is potentially life threatening, and ACTH lack is the most serious endocrine deficiency in patients with pituitary disease. The symptoms include decreased vigor, decreased appetite, weight loss, fatigue and weakness, depression with occasional psychosis, and diminished tanning after exposure to sunlight. In the face of an acute medical or surgical illness, the patient with ACTH lack may have an acute adrenocortical crisis, which may be lethal (see The Syndrome of Adrenocortical Insufficiency). Fasting hypoglycemia manifestations may occur. On examination, skin and nipple pigmentation is reduced. The patient may have hypotension, but evidence of hypovolemia is usually not present unless in the setting of vomiting or diarrhea.

Decreased adrenal androgens are of no consequence in men. In women, however, they lead to loss of libido and of axillary and pubic hair.

Growth Hormone (GH) Deficiency. Lack of growth hormone in children causes shortness of stature and retardation of linear growth and epiphyseal development. Because of associated delayed gonadal maturation, patients may continue to grow slowly past the usual age of puberty. Hypoglycemia may occur in affected children because GH is a counter-regulatory hormone to insulin. On examination, affected children are found to have shortness of stature with increased truncal fat and a puffy appearance even when euthyroid; their upper to lower segment ratio is less than one, and they may show evidence of delayed gonadal maturation. In adults, GH deficiency is clinically silent.

Prolactin (PRL) Deficiency. The only clinical expression of prolactin deficiency is failure of lactation in the postpartum state. This is classically associated with Sheehan's syndrome (postpartum pituitary necrosis). The incidence of prolactin deficiency in other pituitary disease is not known. The characteristic sign is the absence of milk secretion in the postpartum state.

Clinical Manifestations Related to the Cause of Hypopituitarism

Clinical manifestations related to the cause include evidence of space-occupying lesions in the hypothalamic-pituitary area such as headaches, decreased visual acuity or visual field defect, diabetes insipidus, and other evidence of hypothalamic dysfunction related to suprasellar mass lesions; and diplopia and facial hypesthesia caused by parasellar extension affecting the III, IV, VI, and branches of the V cranial nerves. (See Enlargement of the Sella.) Other manifestations include evidence of pituitary hypersecretion in functioning pituitary tumors or with hyperprolactinemia related to hypothalamic stalk damage. Other features include manifestations of causes of functional hypothalamic disease, and those of multiple endocrine neoplasia type 1 in some patients with pituitary tumors.

Some pertinent points need to be stressed concerning the presentation of hypopituitarism. The manifestations of hypopituitarism are usually of gradual onset. The decline in health may be unnoticed by the patient or family members or may be attributable to nonpituitary causes. Acute presentations of hypopituitarism also may occur, however. Acute disturbance of consciousness varying from faintness, drowsiness, confusion, stupor, or coma may be related to acute adrenocortical insufficiency, severe hypothyroidism, hypoglycemia, or water intoxication from cortisol deficiency, alone or in combination. The acute disturbance in consciousness may be precipitated by acute medical or surgical illness or administration of CNS depressants, to which hypopituitary patients are particularly sensitive. Acute hypopituitarism may develop in the context of pituitary apoplexy.

Two pertinent points relating to ACTH deficiency deserve emphasis. First, because cortisol clearance is decreased in hypothyroidism, ACTH deficiency may not be apparent if hypothyroidism is present concomitantly. If ACTH impairment is only partial, normal serum cortisol levels may be maintained. Therefore, in patients with pituitary disease who have hypothyroidism, it is critical to establish that ACTH secretion is normal prior to initiating thyroid hormone therapy, because treatment with thyroid hormone replacement accelerates cortisol metabolism in such patients and may precipitate adrenocortical crisis. Second, ACTH deficiency may mask the manifestations of diabetes insipidus (DI) because cortisol is required for renal free-water clearance. The manifestations of DI may be unmasked after glucocorticoid replacement.

DIFFERENTIAL DIAGNOSIS

The differential diagnosis of primary target gland failure (thyroid, adrenal, or gonad failure, singly or in combination) is based on the clinical and laboratory features mentioned above. Other associated pituitary function abnormalities, diabetes insipidus, or anatomic evidences of hypothalamic-pituitary disease further point to hypopituitarism.

The major differential diagnosis of isolated gonadotropin deficiency in a prepubertal individual is constitutional delayed adolescence. Absence of puberty by age 16 in females and by age 18 in males raises the question of hypogonadotropic hypogonadism or constitutional delayed adolescence. In both entities, serum sex steroid levels are low and serum LH and FSH levels are inappropriately low. Examination of the sense of smell is important, since hyposmia or anosmia indicate Kallmann's syndrome. In the absence of hyposmia or anosmia there is no clear test to help in the differential diagnosis. Follow-up is important because, whereas patients with constitutional delayed adolescence will mature spontaneously, organic gonadotropin deficiency is permanent.

Anorexia nervosa is a syndrome seen almost exclusively in young females and manifested predominantly by weight loss, amenorrhea, and behavioral disorder. The age of onset is usually less than 25 years. Weight loss can be extreme and accompanied by a distorted and implacable attitude toward eating and weight. These patients deny their illness and fail to recognize their nutritional needs. Some may manifest unusual hording and handling of food. Bulimia (excessive food intake) and vomiting are seen in 50% of these patients. Amenorrhea occurs in all young female patients with anorexia nervosa, and in 25% of them it precedes the weight loss. Other features include bradycardia, hypotension, constipation, impairment in temperature regulation (inability to shiver and inability to maintain body temperature in the face of hypo- or hyperthermia), lanugo hair growth, hypercarotenemia, and in severe cases, dependent edema. Endocrine findings include hypogonadotropism, normal or increased serum GH levels, normal serum thyroxine and TSH levels but reduced serum T_3 and increased reversed T_3 levels, serum cortisol levels that are generally elevated and show normal responsiveness to provocative stimulatory tests, decreased 24-hour urinary 17-ketogenic and 17-ketosteroids, and normal serum prolactin.

Anorexia nervosa is often confused with hypopituitarism because of the presence of hypogonadotropism, low-normal serum thyroxine, low serum T_3, and low 24-hour urinary 17-ketogenic and 17-ketosteroids. It can be distinguished from hypopituitarism by the evidence of severe weight loss, the characteristic psychopathology, the preservation of axillary and pubic hair, and the normal growth hormone, ACTH, and prolactin axis function.

DIAGNOSTIC EVALUATION

Patient History and Physical Examination

In the history and physical examination one needs to consider the patient's age at onset of the disease and the duration and course of the disease; evidence of hypopituitarism, whether monotropic, multitropic, or pantropic; evidence of hyperpituitarism pointing to functioning pituitary tumors; evidence of extrasellar disease including visual field defects, optic pallor, papilledema, other evidence of increased intracranial pressure, and ophthalmoplegia; history of postpartum bleeding and shock followed by failure to lactate and to resume menstrual function, or a history suggestive of pituitary apoplexy, head trauma, or cranial irradiation; causes of functional hypopituitarism, such as drugs (e.g., glucocorticoids or oral contraceptives), weight loss or gain, anorexia nervosa, emotional stresses, systemic illness, and other endocrine disease, e.g., primary thyroid or adrenal disease, diabetes mellitus, or systemic disease (sarcoidosis, histiocytosis, exemia chromatosis, or malignancy); and associated parathyroid and endocrine pancreas problems in multiple endocrine neoplasia type I. The physician should consider, in the prepubertal hypogonadal patient, evaluation of the sense of smell. Hyposmia or anosmia and the presence of other congenital defects in such a patient points to Kallmann's syndrome.

Diagnostic Studies

GENERAL

A moderate anemia is often present, generally resulting from thyroid hormone deficiency and, in males, from impaired erythropoietin production caused by decreased testosterone levels. The anemia is usually normochromic-normocytic. Carbohydrate metabolism is usually not altered in hypopituitarism per se; however, the development of hypopituitarism in patients with insulin-requiring diabetes mellitus requires a significant decrease in insulin dosage because of the absence of the counter-regulatory cortisol and growth hormone; such diabetic patients will have an increased tendency for hypoglycemic reactions.

SPECIFIC (Table 11–3)

Endocrine Tests. The endocrine laboratory findings may include evidence of hypopituitarism, hyperpituitarism due to causative pituitary tumors (see Enlargement of the Sella) and central diabetes insipidus resulting from damage to the hypothalamous stalk by the cause of hypopituitarism (Table 11–4).

Serum Prolactin. This is a very useful determination in suspected hypothalamic-pituitary disease. High val-

Table 11–3. Anterior Pituitary Provocative Tests

Hormone	Provocative Tests	Response	Comments
Growth Hormone (GH)	*Stimulation Tests in Suspected Hypopituitarism* *Insulin Hypoglycemia* After an overnight fast, give regular crystalline insulin, 0.1–0.15 μ/kg, by IV bolus. In patients with hypopituitarism, give 0.05 μ/kg; and if insulin resistance is present (obesity, Cushing's, acromegaly), give 0.15–0.3 μ/kg; determine plasma glucose, serum GH (and serum cortisol, if needed; see below) at 0, 30, 60, 90, and 120 minutes.	A normal response is an increase in serum GH by >5 ng/ml or to a level >10 ng/ml (10–15% of normals may not respond). A normal response indicates an intact hypothalamic-pituitary GH axis. An impaired response cannot differentiate a hypothalamic from a pituitary GH disorder. An impaired response can occur in nonpituitary disorders, e.g., obesity, primary hypothyroidism, thyrotoxicosis, hypogonadism, Cushing's syndrome.	For effective challenge, plasma glucose should drop at least 50% or to a level below 40 mg/dl or to symptomatic hypoglycemic levels. If these criteria are not reached, repeat the insulin dose in 45–60 minutes. Significant hypoglycemia may develop with ischemic cardiovascular and cerebrovascular symptoms, lethargy, stupor, or seizures. A physician should be present throughout the test. 50% glucose should be available and given IV promptly if serious hypoglycemic symptoms develop. The test is contraindicated in the presence of convulsive disorder, in ischemic cardiovascular and cerebrovascular disease, and in elderly patients.
	Propranolol-Glucagon Test After an overnight fast, 40 mg of propranolol are given PO at 7 A.M. and glucagon, 1 mg, is given intramuscularly or subcutaneously at 9 A.M. Serum GH (and serum cortisol, if needed; see below) are obtained at 2 and 3 hours after the administration of glucagon.	The parameters of the normal response are as listed under the insulin test. 10–20% of normals may have an impaired response.	Nausea, vomiting, weakness, pallor, and apprehension may occur. The test is contraindicated in heart block, asthma, congestive heart failure, and diabetes mellitus.
	L-dopa Test After an overnight fast, 500 mg of L-dopa are given by mouth (in a child, 10 mg/kg to a maximum of 500 mg). Serum GH is sampled at 0 minutes and hourly for 3 hours.	The same as under the insulin test.	Transient nausea, vomiting, vertigo, and hypotension may occur. Keep the patient recumbent during the test.
	Arginine Stimulation Test After an overnight fast, L-arginine, 0.5 g/kg to a maximum dose of 30 g, is given IV over 30 minutes. Serum GH is obtained at 0 and every 30 minutes for 2 hours.	The same as under the insulin test. About 30–35% of normals have no response.	No side effects; contraindicated in severe renal or liver failure.
	Sleep Samples for serum GH are obtained 60 and 90 minutes after clinically evident deep sleep.	See under insulin test. Incidence of response in the normal is 20–90%.	Safe test. Useful as screening tests in children.
	Exercise Sample for serum GH at 0 minutes and 20, 40, and 60 minutes after 15–20 minutes of strenuous exertion.	See insulin test.	Useful screening test particularly in children. Avoid the test in the presence of heart disease or other conditions in which strenuous exertion is contraindicated.
	Tests in Suspected Acromegaly and Gigantism *Glucose Suppression Test* A standard oral glucose tolerance test. Blood samples are obtained at 0 minutes, 1, 2, and 3 hours after the administration of glucose.	Normal response is suppression of serum GH to below 3 ng/ml. Patients with acromegaly show lack of suppression, partial suppression, or paradoxic stimulation.	Normal suppression excludes acromegaly or gigantism. Impaired suppression may also be seen in acute illness, chronic renal failure, cirrhosis, anorexia nervosa, and uncontrolled diabetes mellitus.

Table 11–3.   Anterior Pituitary Provocative Tests (*Continued*)

Hormone	Provocative Tests	Response	Comments
	TRH Test Give TRH 500 mg IV bolus, obtain samples for serum GH at 0, 30, and 60 minutes after the TRH.	The normal individual shows no serum GH response. In 70% of acromegalics, there is an increase in serum GH.	Useful if fasting GH and GH responses to an oral GTT are equivocal.
	L-Dopa Test See above.	For normal responses, see above. 60–70% of acromegalic patients show paradoxic suppression of serum GH.	Useful when fasting GH and GH responses to an oral GTT are equivocal.
Prolactin (PRL)	Stimulation Tests TRH After an overnight fast, 500 μg of TRH are given IV bolus. Serum prolactin (and serum TSH, if needed; see below) is obtained at 0, 30, and 60 minutes after TRH. The dose in children is 10 μg/kg or 200 μg/1.7 m².	PRL responses vary according to age, sex, basal level of hormones, etc. Each lab should standardize its normal responses. In general, serum prolactin should at least double. Absence of response indicates impaired lactotroph-prolactin axis.	Mild transient nausea, flushing, urge to urinate, peculiar taste in the mouth. No serious side effects. No known contraindications. Absence of response may be seen in nonpituitary disorder as anorexia nervosa, thyrotoxicosis, malnutrition, and Cushing's syndrome.
	Chlorpromazine Test After an overnight fast, 25 mg of chlorpromazine in the adult (0.4 mg/kg in a child) is given IM. Serum prolactin is sampled at 0 minutes and every 30 minutes for 2 hours.	Same as under TRH test. Absence of response implies impairment in hypothalamic-pituitary prolactin control.	May cause hypotension, dizziness, and idiosyncratic reaction. Contraindicated in chlorpromazine drug allergy. Impaired response may occur in anorexia nervosa, thyrotoxicosis, malnutrition, and Cushing's syndrome.
	Suppression Tests No clinical utility in hypothalamic pituitary disease.		
Gonadotropins LH and FSH	Stimulation Test Gonadotropin Releasing Hormone (GnRH) Can be done at any time of the day. 100 μg of GnRH is given as bolus IV. Blood samples for LH and FSH are obtained at 0 minutes and 30 and 60 minutes after GnRH.	Normal responses vary widely depending on the age, sex, and phase of menstrual cycle in women. Each lab should standardize its normal response.	No side effects and no contraindications. In a single test, absence of response cannot differentiate pituitary from hypothalamic hypogonadism. Normal response does not exclude pituitary disease.
	Clomiphene Stimulation Test Clomiphene is a sex-steroid receptor–competitive inhibitor at the hypothalamic level. In adult males, 100 mg by mouth are given twice a day for 10 days. Serum LH, FSH, and testosterone are drawn before and on the 10th day of drug administration. In adult females, 50–100 mg by mouth is given daily for 5 days, and serum LH and FSH are obtained before the test and on the 5th day. Samples are also obtained on the 10th and 15th days.	In adult males, increase in LH (50–250%), FSH (30–200%), and testosterone (30–200%) on day 10 of drug administration. In adult females, similar increase in LH and FSH on day 5, followed by another surge of LH on day 10 or 15; check also for parameters of ovulation. A normal response implies normal hypothalamic-pituitary gonadotropin axis.	No risks in males. In females, risks of hyperstimulation syndrome and multiple ovulation. No contraindications. Impaired response occurs in hypothalamic as well as in pituitary diseases.
Corticotropin (ACTH)	Stimulation Test Insulin Hypoglycemia Test See under GH.	Plasma cortisol should rise by at least 10 μg/dl or to a maximum of over 20 μg/dl. A normal response indicates normal hypothalamic-pituitary adrenal axis. An impaired response can occur in hypothalamic, pituitary, or adrenal disorder.	See under GH. For effective challenge, plasma glucose should drop to a level adequate to produce symptomatic hypoglycemia with apprehension, tachycardia, sweating, etc. For precautions—as under GH.
	Propranolol Glucagon Test See under GH.	Same as under insulin hypoglycemia test above.	Same as under insulin test under GH.

Table 11–3.   Anterior Pituitary Provocative Tests *(Continued)*

Hormone	Provocative Tests	Response	Comments
	Standard Metapyrone Test Metapyrone is an 11-hydroxylase blocker. It decreases adrenal cortisol production. A normal axis responds by increasing ACTH secretion, steroidogenesis, and levels of 11-deoxycortisol (compound F). Metapyrone is given 500 mg by mouth every 4 hours for 6 doses in the adult (300 mg/m^2 body surface area in divided dosage in children). 24-hour urine for ketogenic or 17-hydroxysteroid, serum cortisol, and serum 11-deoxycortisol on the day before and the day after metapyrone.	In the normal, urinary ketogenic or 17-hydroxysteroids increase 2–4 times above the basal value. Serum 11-deoxycortisol rises to >7.5 µg/dl. A drop in serum cortisol testifies to adequate blockade by metapyrone.	A normal response indicates normal hypothalamic-pituitary adrenal axis. An impaired response can occur in adrenocortical insufficiency due to either hypothalamic-pituitary or adrenal disease. In suspected ACTH-cortisol lack, metapyrone may cause further decrease in cortisol and may precipitate adrenocortical crisis. Test should be done in hospital under close medical supervision. Patients on phenytoin may give false negative results (rapid inactivation of metapyrone). The response may be blunted during recovery from suppression of hypothalamic-pituitary adrenal axis by exogenous steroids.
	Overnight Metapyrone Test Metapyrone is given by mouth at midnight as a single dose, 2.0 g if weight is <70 kg, 2.5 g if weight is 70–90 kg, 3 g if weight is >90 kg. Obtain blood sample for serum cortisol and serum 11-deoxycortisol at 8 AM the day following metapyrone.	Serum 11-deoxycortisol rises to >7.5 µg/dl. Drop in serum cortisol testifies to adequate blockade by metapyrone.	As under standard metapyrone test. The test is safe, has no known contraindication, and may be done under close supervision as an outpatient.
	Suppression Tests Overnight Dexamethasone Standard Low-Dose 2-mg Dexamethasone High-dose 8-mg Dexamethasone (See *Cushing's Syndrome*)		
Thyrotropin (TSH)	*Stimulation Test* *TRH Test* See under Prolactin. Sample TSH at 0, 30, and 60 minutes after TRH administration.	A rise in serum TSH occurs. Normal responses should be standardized by each laboratory. In general, peak values of TSH are at least two-times the basal values.	In hypothyroid patients, absence of response indicates pituitary disease, whereas a delayed response occurs in hypothalamic disease. Impaired responses are seen also in thyrotoxicosis, and in euthyroid patients, elderly patients, and patients with renal failure.
	Suppression Test Of no clinical utility in evaluation of hypothalamic-pituitary disease.		

ues in a hypopituitary patient exclude prolactin deficiency and are usually seen in patients with prolactinomas or organic hypothalamic-stalk disease. Low values of serum prolactin are seen in association with extensive pituitary destruction present in Sheehan's syndrome and large nonprolactin-producing pituitary tumors. In these instances prolactin secretion is not responsive to provocative stimuli, e.g., TRH or chlorpromazine (Table 11–3). Testing for prolactin deficiency is rarely necessary, however, since prolactin deficiency is usually asymptomatic (except in failure of lactation in postpartum pituitary necrosis), and effective therapy is not presently available.

Serum Growth Hormone (GH). In interpreting basal serum GH values, it is important to remember the effects of the episodic and labile GH secretion and the limitation of the radioimmunoassay (RIA) such that the presently available assays cannot distinguish between low-normal and low values seen in hypopituitarism. Therefore, a high-normal or high basal serum GH excludes growth hormone deficiency. Because low basal values may be seen in normal individuals, diagnosing growth hormone deficiency requires provocative tests to document decreased GH reserve in hypopituitarism. Many provocative tests are available (Table 11–3). The two most commonly used tests are the insulin tolerance and L-dopa stimulation tests. A failure to induce a growth hormone response to pro-

Table 11–4. Endocrine Studies in Hypopituitarism

Low serum GH unresponsive to provocative tests
Low serum prolactin unresponsive to provocative tests
Male—low sperm count, low serum testosterone, inappropriately low serum LH and FSH
Female—low serum estradiol, inappropriately low serum LH and FSH
Low serum cortisol, inappropriately low serum ACTH or stepwise response to exogenous ACTH
Low serum T_4 and free T_4 (or free thyroxine index), inappropriately low serum TSH

vocative tests is the most common endocrine abnormality in hypothalamic-pituitary disease.

Documenting GH deficiency with provocative tests for GH reserve is essential in hypopituitary children because of the potential of GH replacement therapy. In the child, lack of GH response to at least two provocative stimuli is needed to establish a diagnosis of growth hormone deficiency. In the adult, these provocative tests are useful (growth hormone deficiency is a very sensitive indicator of hypothalamic-pituitary disease) but not essential, because there is no need for GH replacement in the adult.

There are several important considerations in interpreting GH response to provocative tests. All tests should be performed in the fasting state because postprandial hyperglycemia may suppress GH release; also GH responses to all provocative tests may be impaired in obese patients, in patients on high doses of glucocorticoids, or in these with significant hypothyroidism or hypocortisolism. In the hypopituitary patient with TSH and ACTH deficiencies, GH stimulation tests should be performed after adequate thyroid and cortisol substitution therapy. Because estrogens enhance GH response to the various provocative stimuli, estrogen pretreatment can be used prior to conducting a provocative test.

Serum LH and FSH. In patients with suspected gonadotropin lack, the first step is the evaluation of gonadal function. Normal gonadal function implies normal hypothalamic-pituitary-gonadal axis function. A normal semen analysis in the adult male and a history of regular menstrual function in the adult female exclude hypogonadotropism. Serum testosterone in the adult male and serum estradiol in the adult female during the reproductive phase of life are indices of gonadal function. Low sex steroid levels document hypogonadism. Measurement of basal serum LH and FSH is necessary to differentiate between primary gonadal (hypergonadotropic) and secondary hypothalamic-pituitary (hypogonadotropic) hypogonadism. In primary gonadal failure, the lack of negative feedback by the sex steroids causes elevated serum LH and FSH. In hypogonadism resulting from hypothalamic-pitui-

tary disease, LH and FSH levels are low or low-normal (inappropriately low for concomitant levels of sex steroid).

It is useful to remember that the secretion of gonadotropins is episodic. For accurate evaluation, three basal blood samples should be drawn 30 minutes apart and the pooled sample assayed for serum LH and FSH. Serum LH and FSH levels should always be interpreted in view of the prevailing gonadal function. Low levels of LH and FSH alone cannot be used to diagnose hypopituitarism because they can be present in eugonadal individuals.

Gonadotropin-releasing hormone (GnRH) has been approved by the FDA for the assessment of gonadotropin reserve. Theoretically, patients with hypothalamic lesions should have normal LH and FSH response to GnRH, and patients with pituitary disease should fail to respond. Practically speaking, however, the GnRH test has not been found to be helpful in the differential diagnosis between hypothalamic and pituitary causes of hypogonadism because patients with pituitary hypogonadism may have normal or exaggerated responses to GnRH, while patients with hypothalamic hypogonadism may have blunted responses with initial testing.

The clomiphene test can be used to assess the integrity of the hypothalamic-pituitary gonadal axis (Table 11–3). A normal response indicates a normal axis, while an impaired response can be seen in hypogonadotropism of any cause, without distinguishing between hypothalamic and pituitary causes.

Serum TSH. Measurement of circulating thyroxine (T_4) levels is the most reliable test to exclude hypothyroidism. The tests selected are either total thyroxine and free thyroxine (FT_4) or total T_4 and resin T_3 uptake (RT_3U) and the calculated free thyroxine index (FTI). A normal total and free thyroxine (or free thyroxine index) rules out hypothyroidism, while low values point to hypothyroidism, if the euthyroid sick syndrome is excluded (see Hypothyroidism). Serum T_3 is not a good test for hypothyroidism because it may be normal in hypothyroid patients and low in euthyroid patients when peripheral T_4 to T_3 conversion is reduced.

Serum TSH is critical in the differential diagnosis of hypothyroidism. In primary thyroid failure, serum TSH is high because of lack of negative feedback inhibition. In hypothyroidism caused by hypothalamic-pituitary disease, however, the serum TSH is low-normal or low and always inappropriately low for the levels of circulating T_4.

The TRH test may be helpful in differentiating hypothyroidism caused by pituitary disease from that caused by hypothalamic disease. In pituitary hypothyroidism, serum TSH responsiveness to TRH is usually blunted or absent, while in hypothalamic hypothyroidism the TSH response is usually normal but delayed.

Serum ACTH. In patients with suspected ACTH deficiency, one needs to assess basal ACTH-cortisol production and to demonstrate whether the hypothalamic-pituitary-adrenal axis can respond to stress normally.

In suspected adrenocortical insufficiency, reliance is based on the measurements of plasma cortisol or cortisol's urinary metabolites (17-hydroxycorticoids and 17-ketogenic steroids) and serum ACTH. (The implications of these biochemical measurements are discussed in full in The Syndrome of Adrenocortical Insufficiency.) A plasma cortisol level greater than 20 mμ/dl excludes adrenocortical insufficiency. A normal plasma cortisol value if less than 20 μg does not exclude partial adrenocortical insufficiency. In this circumstance, a provocative test is needed to document adrenocortical insufficiency and to define at which level of the axis the impairment is present (Table 11–3). It is important to remember that a "normal plasma cortisol" in an acutely ill patient (in whom plasma cortisol should be high) points to adrenocortical insufficiency.

A blunted plasma cortisol response to a cosyntropin provocative test indicates unresponsive adrenals and can be due to primary adrenocortical failure or to adrenocortical atrophy resulting from hypothalamic-pituitary failure and ACTH deficiency. The differential diagnosis between these two entities is based on measurement of serum ACTH, which is high in primary adrenocortical failure and inappropriately low in hypothalamic-pituitary ACTH deficiency. If serum ACTH measurements are not available or are unreliable, a long ACTH stimulation can be used. Absence of response to prolonged ACTH stimulation indicates primary adrenocortical failure. In adrenocortical failure secondary to hypothalamic-pituitary disease there is a progressive stepwise response to ACTH stimulation.

A normal plasma cortisol response to cosyntropin indicates responsive adrenal cortex and excludes primary adrenocortical failure. However, it does not exclude recent or partial ACTH deficiency. In such cases an insulin tolerance test or a metapyrone test (Table 11–3) is needed to evaluate hypothalamic-pituitary adrenocortical reserve. A normal response to either test indicates a normal hypothalamic-pituitary-adrenal axis. An impaired response by itself implies a defect in the axis but does not localize its level. However, an impaired response to either test in patients with normal Cosyntropin responsiveness points to second-

ary adrenocortical insufficiency caused by hypothalamic-pituitary disease.

Other Tests. A standard skull x-ray and sellar tomography may reveal symmetrical or asymmetrical sellar enlargement, erosion of the sellar confines, and calcification within or outside the sella. (See Enlargement of the Sella.) A CT scan of the hypothalamic-pituitary area employing the newest generation of CT scanners is the most useful radiologic tool for the study of hypothalamic-pituitary disease. It demonstrates the presence and extent of a space-occupying lesion, shows degenerative changes within the mass including necrosis or bleeding, and evaluates the ventricular system. It can also demonstrate an empty sella. Carotid angiography is necessary only to rule out a carotid aneurysm. A full ophthalmologic study is needed to evaluate the fundus for optic pallor or papilledema, to evaluate the visual fields, to rule out chiasmal syndrome, and to test extraocular muscle function to exclude parasellar space-occupying lesions.

Other laboratory tests that can be used in the assessment of the hypopituitary patient include the delineation of the hyperfunctioning pituitary tumors, and, in those patients with pituitary tumor-induced hypopituitarism, an assessment of parathyroid and endocrine pancreas function to rule out multiple endocrine neoplasia type I.

Diagnostic approach

In diagnosing hypopituitarism, the physician must document the presence of hypopituitarism and delineate its cause.

For trophic hormone deficiencies, the diagnosis rests on the evaluation of the function of the target gland. If target gland failure is present, additional studies are required to distinguish between primary target gland failure and target gland failure secondary to hypothalamic-pituitary disease.

In the hypothyroid patient, a high serum TSH or the presence of a goiter points to primary hypothyroidism. An inappropriately low serum TSH and an atrophic thyroid gland confirm the diagnosis of TSH deficiency.

In suspected hypogonadism, presence of anosmia or hyposmia strongly suggests Kallmann's syndrome. High serum LH and FSH point to primary gonadal failure. In hypogonadism secondary to hypothalamic-pituitary disease, the serum LH and FSH levels are inappropriately low.

If a hypocortisol state is present, a diagnosis of primary adrenocortical failure is supported by the presence of hyperpigmentation, low aldosterone, and low sex steroid levels and is documented by an elevated serum ACTH level or lack of adrenocortical responsiveness to exogenous ACTH stimulation. In adrenocortical failure secondary to hypothalamic-pituitary disease, there is pallor, loss of tanning ability, absence of mineralocorticoid deficiency, inappropriately low serum ACTH levels, and presence of adrenal responsiveness to prolonged exogenous ACTH stimulation.

For the nontropic hormones, GH and PRL, a basal high-normal or high value excludes deficiency; otherwise, a provocative test is needed to assess hormone reserve. Clinically, such provocative tests are needed to document growth hormone deficiency only in hypopituitary children. Failure to respond to provocative tests indicates deficiency, if nonpituitary causes of nonresponsiveness, e.g., obesity, glucocorticoid excess, and thyroid dysfunction can be excluded.

In determining the cause of hypopituitarism, suspected functional causes must be removed or corrected (Fig. 11–1). Normalization of pituitary function lends support to functional hypopituitarism.

If functional causes are excluded or if hypopituitarism persists despite removal or correction of a functional cause, the next step is to evaluate for organic hypothalamic-pituitary disease. This evaluation is based on the clinical setting and appropriate laboratory and radiologic studies. The presence of diabetes insipidus or hypothalamic vegetative dysfunction indicates suprasellar disease; their occurrence in a patient with pituitary tumor points to presence of suprasellar tumor extension.

The diagnosis of pituitary tumors is based on the clinical setting, the finding of sellar enlargement, or documentation of a sellar mass on CT scanning; a definitive diagnosis of pituitary tumor can be made if a pituitary hypersecretory clinical syndrome is present. Nonfunctioning pituitary tumors cannot be differentiated from other sellar masses solely on the basis of sellar x-rays or CT scan findings because other, nonpituitary, space-occupying lesions may have similar radiologic findings; a definitive diagnosis in such cases is based on exploration and pathologic examination of excised tissue.

A craniopharyngioma is the most common space-occupying lesion in the hypothalamic-pituitary area in children. It presents with manifestations of a space-occupying lesion in the hypothalamic-pituitary area, endocrine dysfunction including hypopituitarism, diabetes insipidus, and hyperprolactinemia, and manifestations of hypothalamic syndrome including obesity or emaciation, somnolence or hyperkinetic behavior, adipsia or hypodipsia, and temperature disturbances such as poikilothermia. Suprasellar or intrasellar calcifications on skull films or CT scan strongly point to the diagnosis. Such calcifications are present in only 75% of children and 35% of adults with the disease. The ultimate diagnosis depends on findings at surgical exploration.

The diagnosis of postpartum pituitary necrosis de-

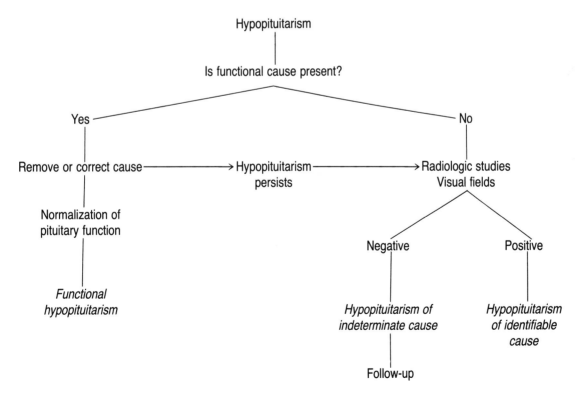

Fig. 11–1. Diagnostic approach to suspected hypopituitarism.

pends on the clinical history of hemorrhage and vascular collapse during delivery, followed by inability to lactate and to re-establish normal menstrual function in the postpartum period. It is important to note that because some cases develop slowly or lead to partial pituitary failure, presence of postpartum lactation cannot be used to exclude the existence of partial pituitary failure. The diagnosis rests on the clinical setting and the exclusion of other causes of hypopituitarism, notably, space-occupying lesions in or around the hypothalamic-pituitary area.

If no cause is found to explain the hypopituitarism, the patient is said to have "hypopituitarism of indeterminate cause." These patients may harbor an organic disease that is too small to be delineated by our presently available radiologic tools. A close long-term follow-up is mandatory, since an organic lesion may make its appearance known sometime during the follow-up.

Diagnostic Pitfalls

Several problems can be encountered in the evaluation of hypopituitarism. One pitfall is failure to determine the extent and the degree of hypopituitarism. It is important to remember that hypopituitarism may affect one or all of its hormones, and for each hormone affected the deficiency can be partial or complete. It is important to evaluate all pituitary functions in patients with suspected hypopituitarism.

Another problem is failure to rule out functional causes. These are important causes of hypopituitarism because they are common and potentially reversible.

Also, the physician might fail to look for organic cause and to follow closely those patients with hypopituitarism in whom such an organic cause is not found. Hypopituitarism may precede the clinical appearance of its cause by a long time.

A final problem is failure to look for other evidences of multiple endocrine neoplasia type I in those in whom the hypopituitarism is caused by a pituitary tumor.

SHORT STATURE

DEFINITION

Short stature is defined as a height of less than the third percentile according to standard age and height graphs and tables for normal population. The definition is arbitrary since 3% or less of the normal population have shortness of stature as it is defined.

Table 11–5. Causes of Short Stature

Intrauterine growth retardation
  Genetic, e.g., osteochondrodystrophies
  Chromosomal, e.g., Turner's syndrome 45 XO, autosomal trisomy
  Infections, e.g., congenital rubella
  Drug induced, e.g., warfarin, aminopterin, hydantoin
  Idiopathic
  Fetal malnutrition
    Multiple fetuses
    Inborn errors of metabolism (glycogen storage disease)
    Placental insufficiency
    Maternal causes (vascular disease, undernutrition, drugs
Disorders of postnatal growth
  Intrinsic shortness of stature
  Chromosomal
    Trisomy 21
    Turner's syndrome 45/XO
    Pseudohypoparathyroidism
    Pseudopseudohypoparathyroidism
  Genetic
    Mucopolysaccharidosis
    Osteochondrodystrophies
    Fragilitas ossium
    Osteogenesis imperfecta
    Rickets
  Nutritional
    Deficient intake
      Socioeconomic, e.g., protein calorie malnutrition
      Psychiatric, e.g., emotional deprivation
    Mechanical disorders, e.g., esophageal or pyloric stenosis
    Malabsorption syndromes
  Chronic systemic disease
    Congenital heart disease with hypoxia
    Chronic renal, respiratory, and hepatic disorders
    Acid-base or electrolyte abnormalities
    Chronic infections
    Anemia
  Endocrine
    Growth hormone deficiency (GH) (congenital or acquired)
    GH resistance—Laron dwarfism
    Mutant GH molecule with decreased bioactivity
    Somatomedin resistance
    Uncontrolled diabetes mellitus
    Hypothyroidism
    Addison's disease
    Cushing's syndrome
    Precocious puberty syndrome
    Pseudohypoparathyroidism
    Rickets
  Neurologic
    Midline craniofacial defects
    Septo-optic dysplasia
    Intracranial hypertension

PATHOPHYSIOLOGIC CONSIDERATIONS

Short stature is the result of a pathologic process that slows or stops linear growth (Table 11–5).

Constitutional delay in growth and adolescence is the most common cause of shortness of stature. It usually affects males. The birth length and weight are normal, the slow growth pattern beginning at about 2 years of age. Height throughout childhood is below average, and the bone age is similarly retarded. Puberty and the attendant growth spurt are delayed, but growth is prolonged because of late epiphyseal fusion. Eventually these patients attain normal height and development. There is often a strong family history for slow maturation and delayed onset of adolescence.

In familial (genetic) shortness of stature the birth weight and height are somewhat reduced, and the height curve advances below and parallel to the third percentile. The height is normal based on midparental stature, and the weight is appropriate for height. Bone age is usually normal or mildly retarded, and puberty is normal. There is a positive history for shortness of stature.

Most babies with low birth weight for their gestational age tend toward the mean in height and weight in childhood. However, some may develop shortness of stature, especially those whose low birth weight resulted from intrauterine infections, e.g., rubella; from placental insufficiency; or from autosomal, chromosomal abnormality.

Hormonal factors have little effect on growth in utero. After birth, thyroid hormone and growth hormone are essential for normal growth. Androgens and possibly estrogens are responsible for the adolescent growth spurt and closure of the epiphysis.

Growth hormone (GH) abnormalities may be congenital or acquired, sporadic or familial. They include GH deficiency, which may occur as an isolated hormone deficiency or as part of the spectrum of pituitary insufficiency; decreased somatomedin generation, as in Laron dwarfism and in African pygmies. GH deficiency usually arises from hypothalamic dysfunction rather than from pituitary disease, and most cases are idiopathic and present as a monotropic GH deficiency. The second most common cause of GH deficiency is tumor in the hypothalamic-pituitary area. Other causes of GH deficiency include congenital hereditary GH deficiency in association with multiple congenital anomalies, and GH deficiency caused by other acquired organic hypothalamic-pituitary diseases including trauma, infection, and irradiation. Emotional psychosocial deprivation is an important cause of decreased linear growth in the early years. The psychosocial deprivation is associated with temporary hypothalamic dysfunction leading to growth hormone deficiency and occasional ACTH deficiency. In congenital GH deficiency, the birth weight and the height are normal, and growth is normal during the first 6 to 12 months. The pattern of slow growth begins at 1 to 2 years of age and shows progressive deviation below the third percentile. In acquired GH deficiency there is initially a period of normal growth followed by growth cessation. Epiphyseal development is progressively delayed, and puberty is delayed if associated gonadotropin deficiency is present.

Hypothyroidism may be congenital or acquired and may be due to primary thyroid failure or failure secondary to hypothalamic-pituitary disease. It leads to deceleration or complete cessation of linear growth and bone maturation. The earlier the onset, the more marked the impairment. Dental development is delayed. Puberty is usually delayed but rarely may be precocious.

In sexual precocity of any cause, skeletal growth and maturation are initially accelerated but ultimate height is reduced because of premature closure of the epiphysis (see Precocious Puberty). Glucocorticoid excess (Cushing's syndrome), whether of exogenous or endogenous origin, is always accompanied by growth retardation because of decreased growth hormone release, decreased growth hormone peripheral action, and the catabolic effects of glucocorticoid excess. Growth arrest seems to be the most sensitive indicator of glucocorticoid excess and may be the only distinct clinical sign of childhood Cushing's syndrome. In poorly controlled diabetes mellitus there is a decrease in height and bone maturation.

Turner's syndrome (45/XO) is the most common cause of shortness of stature related to sex chromosome abnormality. It is characterized by shortness of stature, gonadal dysgenesis, and characteristic physical anomalies. Turner's syndrome can be suspected in infancy by multiple loose skin folds in the posterior neck, pitting edema of dorsum of hands and feet, and increased elbow carrying angle. In early childhood the growth curve is slow and three to four standard deviations from the mean. Sexual development is impaired, and the adolescent growth spurt is absent. Somatic anomalies such as ptosis, webbed neck, low posterior occipital hairline, increased carrying angle, broad chest with widely set apart nipples, numerous nevi, and short third and fourth metacarpals and metatarsals are present. There is increased incidence of hypertension, coarctation of the aorta, renal abnormalities, diabetes mellitus, otitis media, and Hashimoto's thyroiditis. Varying degrees of skeletal and sexual development abnormalities are present in Turner's mosaics.

Chondrodystrophies are a heterogenous group of bone diseases that characteristically disturb length and shape of long bones, trunk, and skull. Disproportionate short stature is the distinguishing characteristic.

Nutritional disorders and chronic systemic disease frequently cause shortness of stature by impairing cellular nutrition and environment. The age of onset and the subsequent growth curves are related to the cause.

Bone age is retarded in proportion to the decreased height.

CLINICAL PRESENTATION

Symptoms are mainly shortness of stature and the attendant emotional disturbance, especially in boys, and symptoms of the cause.

Shortness of stature is the dominant sign. Other signs are usually related to the cause of the disorder. In the physical examination, the physician should carefully document height, weight, skeletal proportions, span, maturation of features, dental development, and, if the patient is adolescent, features of puberty.

1. Use charts relating height to age as an indication of the rate of growth and compare it to normal.
2. Measure skeletal proportions. The lower segment is the distance from the top of the symphysis pubis to the floor. The upper segment is obtained by subtracting the lower segment from the total height. At birth the ratio of upper to lower segment is about 1.7:1. Because the limbs normally grow more rapidly than the trunk, by age 10 to 11 the ratio reaches unity and remains there. Hypothyroid children retain infantile proportions, while those with shortness of stature resulting from pituitary or other diseases (excluding skeletal diseases) have proportions that correspond to the chronological age.
3. Measure the arm span, which largely reflects the length of the arms. In normal adults the span is similar to the height. In eunuchoidism both span and the lower segment are increased.
4. Chart the weight in relation to age using special Tanner's charts. The weight-to-age chart should not be interpreted rigidly because of considerable variation in bony structure and lean body mass. If the impaired growth is related to malnutrition, weight is likely to be reduced to a greater extent than height.
5. Note maturation of the features. Facial appearance is an important guide to skeletal maturity. Hypopituitary dwarfs do not show the lengthening of the nose and the jaw that occurs at normal puberty, and their appearance remains somewhat juvenile.
6. Check for development of primary and secondary dentition.

DIAGNOSTIC EVALUATION AND DIFFERENTIAL DIAGNOSIS (Fig. 11–2)

Patient History and Physical Examination

The history and physical examination are extremely important in narrowing the diagnostic possibilities.

The physician should obtain previous heights and weights for given ages from the family physician, school health records, and annual school photos, and plot a graph to compare these parameters with those of normal peer group. Careful inquiry should be made into the child's health from birth to the time of the examination and the age of achieving the standard milestones of infancy, childhood, and puberty; maternal health during pregnancy, including diseases, drugs used prior to or during pregnancy, and the nature of labor and delivery; information regarding height, weight, and pace of maturation and health of other family members; emotional stresses within the family; any disease of a major organ system and any endocrinopathy; a family history of hereditary inborn errors of metabolism, genetic disorders, social history, or psychosocial deprivation; and medications taken, especially glucocorticoids for asthma or inflammatory bowel disease.

A thorough examination is required to assess, in addition to body measurements, the state of general health and the presence of underlying endocrinopathy, underlying chronic disease, and genetic disorders. The degree of pubertal development in adolescent patients should be ascertained.

Diagnostic Studies

Ultimate height depends not only on the rate of linear growth but also on its duration. The actual height at any given age should always be assessed in relation to the bone maturity or bone age. X-rays of the left wrist and hand and occasionally the knee are obtained. Radiograms should be assigned a precise bone age, although this radiologic tool is limited because of the wide normal variations, and because in some bone dystrophies and dysplasias the overall skeletal maturation may not correlate with rates of linear growth.

Laboratory studies should aim at the exclusion of systemic illness and endocrine disorder. At a minimum these should include hematocrit and blood count, routine urine analysis and serum creatinine, serum electrolytes, fasting plasma glucose, liver function tests, and total and free thyroxine (or free thyroxine index). Additional laboratory studies are ordered based on evidence obtained from the history and physical examination. A buccal smear and chromosomal evaluation should be obtained on all girls presenting with shortness of stature.

The first step in the differential diagnosis is to categorize the disorder of growth by the relationship between height age (HA) and weight age (WA) and to define whether the primary disturbance is that of height or weight. A child with a primary disorder of linear growth has a weight that is appropriate for his height

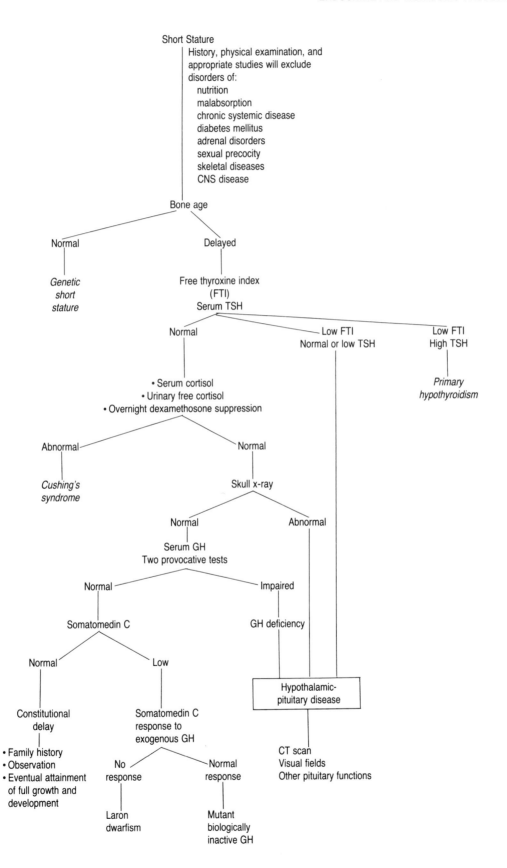

Fig. 11—2. Diagnostic approach to short stature.

(WA = HA). In contrast, a child with a primary nutritional disorder has a height age that is considerably closer to the norm than the weight age (WA < HA). The second step is to assess bone age and to determine whether it is appropriate for the chronologic age. It is important to remember that all correctable diseases that interfere with growth do so by interfering with the progression of bone growth and hence with bone age.

Patients with intrinsic familial genetic shortness of stature usually grow below but parallel to the third percentile. Their bone age is equal to the chronologic age, the child is in good health and well-proportioned, puberty is normal, and family history is positive.

Patients who have a subnormal growth rate (those whose bone age is equal to height age and less than chronologic age) are those with arrested growth resulting from endocrine, metabolic, or severe systemic disease.

In hypothyroidism, serum total and free thyroxine (or free thyroxine index) are low. Serum TSH is increased in primary hypothyroidism but is inappropriately low in hypothyroidism caused by hypothalamic-pituitary disease. X-rays of the different parts of the skeleton may reveal epiphyseal dysgenesis (the epiphyses are misshapen with irregular margins and fragmentation) and may give a clue to the time of onset of hypothyroidism.

Growth retardation may be the only sign of childhood Cushing's syndrome. The height age and bone age are reduced. The diagnosis is by the clinical setting, the finding of increased urinary free cortisol, and failure of suppression of cortisol secretion by the standard low-dose dexamethasone suppression test (see Cushing's Syndrome).

The diagnosis of sexual precocity is not difficult and is based on the clinical setting and appropriate hormonal and radiologic studies.

The diagnosis of growth hormone deficiency is based on the assessment of GH secretory responses to provocative stimuli. Low basal levels may be found in normal children. It is important to remember that 10% of children will not respond to any single definitive provocative test and that the diagnosis of growth hormone deficiency can be made with certainty only if growth hormone response is subnormal to two provocative tests. Serum somatomedin C measures a peptide produced by the liver in response to growth hormone. In childhood the levels increase with age and hence should be interpreted with age adjustment. Low somatomedin levels are seen in growth hormone deficiency but can also be seen in most systemic illnesses, malnutrition, and Laron dwarfism.

In emotional psychosocial deprivation, serum GH levels are low and unresponsive to provocative stimuli.

The emotional disturbance may be obvious in all cases of GH deficiency. A careful assessment of the child's environment and family relationships is important. The impaired growth is reversible with improvement in the child's emotional environment and health.

In Laron dwarfism, serum growth hormone levels are increased but serum somatomedin levels are decreased and do not rise after exogenous GH administration.

In somatomedin resistance, both serum growth hormone and somatomedin levels are normal.

Shortness of stature caused by secretion of abnormal forms of GH is rare. The serum GH levels by RIA are normal or increased but by bioassays are decreased. Somatomedin levels are decreased and can be increased by exogenous GH therapy.

If GH deficiency is documented, a CT scan of the pituitary area to rule out space-occupying lesion, a visual field examination, and an endocrine assessment of the other pituitary hormones are in order.

Turner's syndrome should be suspected in any girl with shortness of stature. The presence of characteristic somatic anomalies and a Barr body–negative buccal smear (except in mosaics) point to the diagnosis, which is confirmed by karyotyping. GH dynamics and serum somatomedin levels are normal.

Systemic disease must be severe to impair growth. If the patient looks well and the physical examination is normal except for the patient's shortness of stature, and if routine urinalysis, serum creatinine, chemistry group, and hematology groups are normal, it is very unlikely that shortness of stature is caused by disease of major organs. However, malabsorption syndromes must always be excluded in any child with shortness of stature without obvious cause. The diagnosis of a chronic systemic disease is made according to the clinical setting and standard laboratory and radiologic studies.

Delayed growth is present when the child has a retarded bone age but continues to grow at a normal pace below the third percentile. This pattern of growth is most commonly due to a constitutional delay in growth and adolescence. The child appears to be in good health, the body proportions are normal, the height age and bone age are similarly retarded, and though puberty and attendant growth spurts are delayed the patient eventually attains normal height and development. There is a strong family history for slow maturation and delayed onset of adolescence.

Skeletal diseases are usually so characteristic as to be easily recognized on clinical examination and confirmed by appropriate radiologic studies.

TALL STATURE

DEFINITION

Tall stature is defined as a height in greater than the 97th percentile according to standard age and height graphs and tables for the normal population. This definition is arbitrary and implies that 3% of the normal population have tall stature.

PATHOPHYSIOLOGIC CONSIDERATIONS AND DIFFERENTIAL DIAGNOSIS

Tall stature occurs either because of inherent growth capability or because of a persistently excessive rate of bone growth (Table 11–6). Intrinsic tallness usually occurs as a constitutional variation of normal in families of above-average stature. The growth rates are normal and are above and parallel to the 97th percentile. The bone age is normal.

Patients with familial early maturation grow at a rapid pace during childhood. Their bone age and height age are advanced in proportion to their chronologic age. They achieve adolescence and adult height at the earliest limits of normal. Their ultimate height is average. There is a positive family history for early development and the parents are of average height.

Children with sexual precocity of various origins have supranormal growth rates early in the course of their disease, and their bone age is advanced and mark-

Table 11–6. Causes of Tall Stature

Physiologic
  Familial, genetic, or constitutional tall stature
  Familial early maturation
Pathologic
  Endocrine
    Gigantism, acromegaly
    Hyperthyroidism
    Precocious sexual maturation (e.g., congenital adrenal virilizing
      hyperplasia)
  Chromosomal
    XXY—Klinefelter's syndrome
    XYY
  Miscellaneous
    Marfan's syndrome
    Homocystinuria
    Marfanoid state in MEN type III
    Cerebral gigantism (Sotos' syndrome)
    Obesity
    Beckwith-Wiedemann's syndrome
    Lipodystrophy

edly out of proportion to height and chronologic age. The degree of disproportion depends on the age of onset and the amount of sex hormone overproduction. Untreated, sexual precocity results in premature epiphyseal fusion and cessation of growth at an early age, ultimately leading to shortness of stature.

In pituitary gigantism, hypersecretion of growth hormone is due to a somatotroph pituitary tumor. The disease is characterized by supranormal growth rates, normal bone age, and in many cases associated acromegalic features. Hyperthyroidism in childhood leads to acceleration of linear growth and bone maturation and may ultimately compromise the adult stature. Obese children are usually taller than lean children of comparable age and have advanced bone age, height age, and dental maturation. They usually have early adolescence and are of average height as adults.

Chromosomal abnormalities leading to tall stature include 47/XYY syndrome and Klinefelter's syndrome (47/XXY and its variants) (see Delayed Puberty in Males). Marfan's syndrome is characterized by tall, slender stature with arachnodactyly, kyphoscoliosis, pectus excavatum or carinatum, hypotonic muscles with hyperextensible joints, lens subluxation (upward), myopia with blue sclera, dilation of the ascending aorta, and potentiality of dissecting aneurysm. Though the cause of the disorder is indeterminate, the disorder may result from a defect in mucopolysaccharide metabolism and is inherited as an autosomal dominant disorder. The intelligence of affected patients is normal.

Homocystinuria is an autosomal recessive disorder characterized by decreased activity of cystathione synthetase leading to accumulation of homocystine and methionine and a deficiency of cystathione and cystine. It resembles Marfan's syndrome except that mental retardation, osteoporosis, increased tendency to fracture, joint contracture, medial degeneration of the aorta, and arterial thrombosis are frequent. A marfanoid habitus may be found in patients with multiple endocrine neoplasia type III, which is a familial autosomal dominant disorder characterized by the presence of medullary thyroid carcinoma, pheochromocytoma, mucosal neuromas, and ganglioneuromatosis.

Lipodystrophy is a disorder of unknown cause characterized by partial or generalized fat loss present from birth. Other characteristics include muscle hypertrophy, abdominal protuberance, penile and clitoral enlargement, acanthosis nigricans, liver and renal disease, hyperglycemia, hyperlipemia, hypermetabolism, and acromegaloid features. Half the patients are mentally retarded. Soft tissue x-rays demonstrate characteristic lack of fat-muscle interface. Congenital overgrowth may be seen with hyperinsulinism, erythroblastosis fetalis, cerebral gigantism (Sotos' syndrome), and Beckwith-Wiedemann's syndrome.

CLINICAL PRESENTATION

An above-average height is often a social disadvantage for girls but rarely so for boys, and consequently females more frequently present for evaluation of tall stature. In addition to the presenting symptom, other symptoms and signs may include those of the primary disease.

DIAGNOSTIC EVALUATION

The history and physical examination are critical in the diagnostic evaluation (Fig. 11–3). Previous heights and weights for given ages are obtained by consulting school health records, the family physician, and annual school photos. A graph of these parameters is plotted and compared with those of a normal peer group. Eval-

uation is warranted if the height falls above the 97th percentile or if there is an inappropriate increase in the rate of growth. A family history is important. The physician should seek evidence of precocious puberty, goiter and hyperthyroidism, acromegalic changes with pituitary mass, visual defects and hypopituitarism, lipodystrophy, Marfan's syndrome, homocystinuria, multiple endocrine neoplasia type III, mental retardation, and obesity.

The initial diagnostic step is the examination of the relationship between chronologic age, height age, bone age, and growth rate.

If the growth rate is normal and the bone age equals the chronologic age, the differential diagnosis includes familial intrinsic tallness, Marfan's syndrome, homocystinuria, and multiple endocrine neoplasia type III. The diagnosis is based on the clinical setting and on appropriate special laboratory or radiologic studies.

Pituitary gigantism is characterized by supranormal growth velocity with normal bone age. The diagnosis

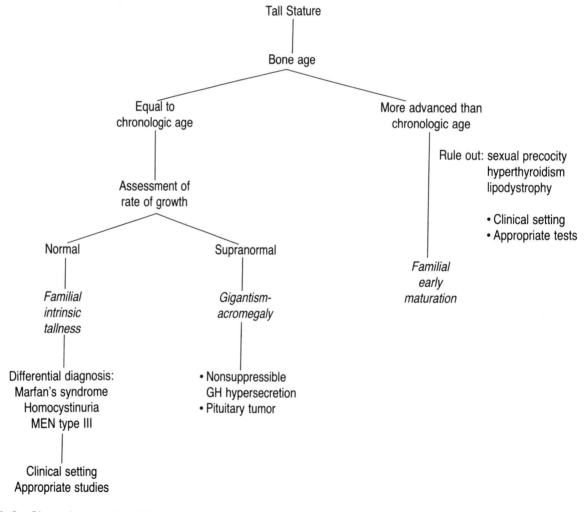

Fig. 11–3. Diagnostic approach to tall stature.

is confirmed by documentation of GH secretion not suppressible by glucose load, elevated serum somatomedin C levels, and the finding of pituitary tumor on radiologic studies of the sella (see Acromegaly and Gigantism).

Disorders characterized by supranormal growth rate but advanced skeletal age (bone age is equal to height age but greater than chronologic age) include familial early maturation or advanced growth related to sexual precocity, hyperthyroidism, or lipodystrophy. The diagnosis is based on the clinical setting and appropriate diagnostic studies.

ENLARGEMENT OF THE SELLA

DEFINITION

Sellar enlargement refers to expansion of the sella turcica by a space-occupying lesion in or adjacent to the pituitary gland.

PATHOPHYSIOLOGIC CONSIDERATIONS

To understand the pathophysiologic considerations, clinical manifestations, and diagnostic evaluation of sellar enlargement, the physician needs to know the anatomic relationship of the pituitary gland and the sella turcica. The pituitary gland is a small ovoid body that weighs about 500 to 1000 mg. It is made up of two anatomically distinct components: the anterior lobe (or adenohypophysis), and the posterior lobe (or neurohypophysis). It lies within the sella turcica, a midline concavity in the sphenoid bone in the middle cranial fossa.

The sella has three bony walls: the anterior wall; the floor; and the posterior wall (the dorsum sella). A fold of dura, the diaphragm sella, forms the superior boundary of the sella, from which the dura extends downward to line the bony walls. The diaphragm sella has a central opening through which passes the pituitary stalk, which connects the median eminence of the hypothalamus and the pituitary gland, and the hypothalamus-hypophyseal portal venous system vessels. In the anatomic relationship of the sella and the pituitary gland, the sphenoid sinuses lie anterior and inferior to the sella; lateral to the sella on each side is the cavernous sinus within the walls of which lie the internal carotid artery and the third, fourth, sixth, and branches of the fifth cranial nerves; and superior to the sella are the subarachnoidal cisterns, the optic chiasm, and the hypothalamus (Fig. 11–4).

Basically, sellar enlargement can be caused by cysts, hyperplasia, or tumors of the pituitary gland; and by space-occupying lesions of the extrasellar structures that encroach on the sella (Table 11–7). The commonest causes of sellar enlargement are pituitary adenomas, empty-sella syndrome, and craniopharyngiomas. The other causes are rare.

Primary pituitary tumors account for more than 50% of the causes of sellar enlargement. The majority are slow-growing, benign adenomas of the anterior pituitary gland. Adenocarcinoma of the anterior pituitary and neurohypophysial tumors are exceedingly rare. Pituitary adenomas are relatively common intracranial neoplasms, found in 20 to 25% of pituitaries in routine autopsy studies. Clinically significant pituitary adenomas represent 10 to 12% of all intracranial neoplasms. They can be classified according to tinctorial, immunohistochemical, or ultrastructural qualities. However, the important classifications from the clinical standpoint relate to the size and function of the tumors. Pituitary microadenomas have a diameter of 10 mm or less and are intrasellar, whereas a macroadenoma has a diameter of more than 10 mm and may or may not extend outside the limits of the sella. A functioning pituitary tumor hypersecretes any of the anterior pituitary hormones singly or in combination; a nonfunctioning tumor does not have clinically recognizable endocrine function.

Prolactin-producing tumors, prolactinomas, are the most common pituitary adenomas. Nonfunctioning pituitary tumors constitute less than 10% of all tumors. Pituitary adenomas are usually sporadic but can be familial and can occur in association with tumors or hyperplasia of the parathyroid glands and endocrine pancreas as a part of multiple endocrine neoplasia (MEN) type I syndrome. The clinical manifestations of pituitary tumors include hypersecretory states produced by functioning pituitary tumors, hypopituitarism that results from compression or infiltration of the normal pituitary tissue by the tumor, and anatomic effects of encroachment on the extrasellar structures by pituitary tumors large enough to grow outside the sellar confines. The manifestations are usually of insidious onset but can present acutely as pituitary apoplexy caused by hemorrhagic infarction of the tumor.

Empty sella syndrome accounts for 20 to 30% of all causes of sellar enlargement and can be either primary or secondary. Primary empty sella occurs spontaneously. The central opening of the diaphragm is normally about 3 mm in diameter. In about 40% of normal individuals, the opening is larger and cerebrospinal fluid from the subarachnoid cisterns can herniate

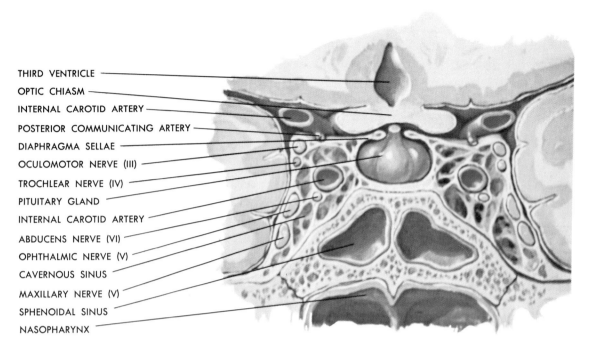

THIRD VENTRICLE
OPTIC CHIASM
INTERNAL CAROTID ARTERY
POSTERIOR COMMUNICATING ARTERY
DIAPHRAGMA SELLAE
OCULOMOTOR NERVE (III)
TROCHLEAR NERVE (IV)
PITUITARY GLAND
INTERNAL CAROTID ARTERY
ABDUCENS NERVE (VI)
OPHTHALMIC NERVE (V)
CAVERNOUS SINUS
MAXILLARY NERVE (V)
SPHENOIDAL SINUS
NASOPHARYNX

Fig. 11—4. Relationship of the pituitary gland to the cavernous sinus. (© Copyright 1959, CIBA Pharmaceutical Company, Division of CIBA-GEIGY Corporation. Reproduced with permission from The CIBA Collection of Medical Illustrations by Frank H. Netter, M.D. All rights reserved.)

into the sella to a variable extent. Primary empty sella syndrome occurs when the CSF fluid is present in such quantities as to cause sellar enlargement and compress and flatten the normal pituitary gland to the floor of the sella. The compressed gland is usually normal but may harbor a coincidental adenoma. Secondary empty sella follows neurosurgical or radiotherapeutic ablative treatment of pituitary tumors; these result in loss of volume of intrasellar contents, allowing herniation of the cerebrospinal fluid into the sella, occasionally carrying the optic chiasm. The clinical manifestations of empty sella syndrome include sellar enlargement; hypopituitarism (from damage to the pituitary gland) or visual field defects (from pressure on or torsion of the optic chiasm), which occur very rarely, if at all, with primary empty sella, but more commonly in association with the secondary type; and coincidental pituitary hypersecretory states if the compressed gland harbors an adenoma.

Craniopharyngioma is the most common cause of sellar enlargement in the young individual. This squamous cell tumor develops from remnants of Rathke's pouch and is usually suprasellar, although about 30% of craniopharyngiomas occur within or extend into the sella. Most of these tumors are cystic, but some are solid or mixed and show great propensity toward calcification. The cystic contents are filled with yellowish brown fluid that resembles motor oil. The clinical manifestations of craniopharyngioma result from compression or infiltration of the surrounding structures and include vegetative and endocrine dysfunction resulting from hypothalamic-pituitary stalk impairment, obstructive hydrocephalus resulting from impingement on the third ventricle, and varying degrees of hypopituitarism, which can result from hypothalamic damage or from damage to the pituitary gland itself.

Primary failure of the pituitary-target glands (thyroid, adrenal cortex, or gonad) leads to loss of the inhibitory target hormone feedback, to hypertrophy and hyperplasia of the appropriate pituitary trophic hormone cells, and to hypersecretion of the trophic hormone. In longstanding primary target gland failure such hypertrophy and hyperplasia can be significant enough to cause sellar mass and enlargement. Rarely, other inflammatory, infiltrative, and neoplastic processes cause sellar expansion (Table 11–7).

CLINICAL PRESENTATION

Sellar enlargement may be clinically silent. When present, clinical manifestations are caused by compression and infiltration of the pituitary gland and its surrounding structures by the underlying disease process (Table 11–8).

Signs

Abnormal signs may include visual impairment of variable type and degree. It is important to consider

Table 11–7. Causes of Sellar Enlargement

Pituitary
  Neoplasms
    Primary
      Adenoma
        Functioning
        Nonfunctioning
      Adenocarcinoma (rare)
      Neurohypophyseal tumors (rare)
    Secondary
      Metastatic
      Multiple myeloma
  Hyperplasia
    Primary hypothyroidism
    Primary hypogonadism
    Primary adrenocortical failure
  Cysts
    Epidermoid
    Dermoid
    Arachnoid
Nonpituitary
  Empty-sella syndrome
    Primary
    Secondary
  Craniopharyngioma
  Optic glioma
  Meningioma
  Hypothalamic
    Neoplasms
      Primary (e.g., glioma, germinoma)
      Metastatic
    Infiltrative (e.g., sarcoidosis or histiocytosis)
  Carotid artery aneurysm
  Chordoma
  Sphenoid sinus
    Mucocele
    Carcinoma
  Increased intracranial pressure (e.g., aqueductal stenosis)

Table 11–8. Clinical Manifestations Associated with Enlarged Sella

Chronic
  Mass lesion effects
    Headaches
    Superior extension
      Chiasmal syndrome: impaired visual acuity and fields
      Hypothalamic syndrome:
        Disturbance in thirst, appetite, satiety, weight, sleep and temperature
        Diabetes insipidus
      Obstructive hydrocephalus
      Frontal lobe dysfunction
    Lateral extension
      Cranial nerve III, IV, V, VI impairment
      Temporal lobe dysfunction
    Inferior extension
      Nasopharyngeal mass
      CSF rhinorrhea
  Hormonal effects
    Hyperpituitarism: excess of one or more hormones
      GH: gigantism, acromegaly
      PRL: hyperprolactinemic syndrome
      ACTH: Cushing's disease, Nelson's syndrome
      TSH: thyrotoxicosis
      LH-FSH: gonadal dysfunction
      Alpha-glycoprotein subunit: no recognizable features
    Hypopituitarism: deficiency of one or more hormones
      GH—child: shortness of stature, hypoglycemia
            adult: asymptomatic
      PRL—adult female: failure of postpartum lactation
      ACTH: hypocortisolism
      TSH: hypothyroidism
      LH-FSH: hypogonadism
  Associations
    Multiple endocrine neoplasia type I
      Pituitary tumor
      Parathyroid tumor or hyperplasia
      Endocrine pancreas tumor or hyperplasia
    Primary target gland failure
      Thyroid
      Adrenal
      Gonad
Acute
  Pituitary apoplexy

the distribution of fibers in the optic chiasm and the chiasm's anatomic location. Fibers from the nasal retinae cross at the optic chiasm into the contralateral optic tract; before crossing, the upper nasal fibers, which accept the lower temporal field, loop into the ipsilateral tract, while those of the lower nasal fibers, which accept the upper temporal field, loop into the contralateral optic nerve before joining the optic tract. The temporal fibers that serve the nasal fields do not cross. The chiasm usually lies centrally on top of the diaphragm sella, although it may be located somewhat anteriorly (prefixed) or posteriorly (postfixed) to the usual central location. Impingement on the chiasmal area may, therefore, lead to bitemporal hemianopia (loss first of upper and then of lower temporal quadrants) from pressure on the chiasm, to homonymous hemanopia from pressure on the optic tract, or to scotomas from pressure on the optic nerve. The visual losses may be asymmetrical and frequently may be restricted to one eye. Optic atrophy and blindness may be the ultimate result.

Other abnormal signs may include decreased visual acuity from damage to the macular fibers in the chiasm; papilledema in the presence of obstructive hydrocephalus; extraocular palsy from IIIrd, IVth, or VIth cranial nerve damage; facial hypoesthesia from damage to the Vth cranial nerve; evidence of hypothalamic vegetative dysfunction (e.g., inanition or obesity, poikilothermia, or behavioral abnormalities); signs of pituitary hypofunction (e.g., hypogonadism, shortness of stature, hypothyroidism, or hypocortisolinism); signs of hyperfunctioning pituitary tumors such as galactorrhea, evidence of acromegaly or giantism, Cushing's disease, or Nelson's syndrome; and nasopharyngeal mass from inferior extension of the expanding pituitary tumor.

Symptoms

Many patients are asymptomatic, the sellar enlargement being detected in routine skull x-rays obtained in the evaluation of head injury, headaches, sinus, or neck problems. Once symptomatic, the patient may complain of headaches that are usually nonspecific and may be frontal, retro-orbital, occipital, or generalized. The patient may have chiasmal symptoms, which include decreased visual acuity and visual field impairment; symptoms of impairment of the vegetative hypothalamic functions, which include disorders of temperature regulation, sleep, appetite satiety, thirst, and behavior; diabetes insipidus from damage to the neurohypophysial neurons and axons in the anterior hypothalamus, median eminence, and upper stalk; symptoms of pituitary hormone hypersecretion, e.g., amenorrhea-galactorrhea, acromegaly, Cushing's disease, and symptoms from functioning pituitary tumors; manifestations of hypopituitarism from damage to the adenohypophysis; ptosis, diplopia, or facial pain from invasion of the cavernous sinus and contents; psychomotor seizures, memory disturbances, and anosmia from extension of pathologic process into temporal or frontal lobes; and CSF rhinorrhea from leakage of CSF through the sellar bony confines through the sphenoid sinus and into the nasopharynx. The onset of symptoms is usually insidious and progression is slow, except in pituitary apoplexy, in which the patient may present with acute onset of severe headaches, visual loss, diplopia, photophobia, ptosis, nausea, vomiting, and altered consciousness.

DIFFERENTIAL DIAGNOSIS

In most cases, the diagnosis is obvious from the results of the clinical, radiologic, ophthalmologic, and endocrine evaluations. Rarely, surgical exploration and excisional biopsy may be needed for definitive diagnosis.

The presence of a pituitary hypersecretory state (acromegaly, Cushing's disease, Nelson's Syndrome, TSH-induced thyrotoxicosis) points to a functioning pituitary tumor as the cause of the sellar enlargement. Hyperprolactinemia, however, can be caused not only by a prolactinoma but also by any other hypothalamic-pituitary–area mass lesion (caused by interference with dopamine, the hypothalamic-prolactin–inhibitory factor). A value of serum prolactin greater than 200 mg/ml (normal, 0 to 20 mg/ml) is diagnostic of a prolactinoma. Lower values can be seen with prolactinoma

or other mass lesions, for example, craniopharyngioma.

Hypopituitarism in a patient with sellar enlargement could be caused by a pituitary tumor or by any other hypothalamic-pituitary mass (caused by compression and infiltration of the hypothalamic-pituitary unit).

Sellar enlargement in a patient who has normal pituitary functions and has no evidence of extrasellar mass effects strongly suggests primary empty sella. The diagnosis is confirmed by a CT scan with or without the use of metrizamide. If CT scanning is not available, a pneumoencephalographic study is required for diagnosis of the empty sella.

Increasing sellar enlargement, visual dysfunction, or pituitary function impairment occurring after treatment of pituitary tumor raise suspicion of a recurrent pituitary tumor or of a secondary empty sella. Diagnosis is by CT scan with or without metrizamide or if CT scan is not available, pneumoencephalography. Occasionally, surgical exploration is necessary for the differentiation.

Sellar mass in a patient who has primary target gland failure (primary hypothyroidism, primary adrenocortical failure, or primary hypogonadism) raises the question of secondary hyperplasia of the anterior pituitary from absence of negative feedback or of another coincidental sellar mass. If treatment with target gland hormone replacement leads to regression of the sellar mass, the diagnosis is secondary pituitary hyperplasia. If regression of the sellar mass does not occur, the presence of a coincidental sellar space-occupying lesion is pursued in the investigative manner outlined above.

Craniopharyngioma is suspected in the presence of a sellar enlargement in the young individual with impairment of growth or sexual development or with obstructive hydrocephalus. Suprasellar and sellar floccular calcification and characteristic CT findings point to craniopharyngioma.

Optic glioma is suspected in young children with visual disturbances, enlargement of the optic foramina, or chiasmal syndrome. Nodular calcification may be present in one third of the patients.

Suprasellar meningioma usually occurs in middle-aged females. The sella is usually normal, with thickening and hyperostosis of the neighboring bone.

In chordoma the mass lesion is parasellar or suprasellar and occasionally calcified; there is evidence of destruction of the sphenoid and clivus, and the sella may be ballooned or eroded on one side.

In carotid aneurysm there is often parasellar calcification in the wall of the aneurysm, and angiography is the definitive diagnostic test.

The diagnosis of metastasis as the cause of sellar

mass is based on evidence of a primary malignant disease. Occasionally, when the primary tumor is occult, the presentation may resemble that of a pituitary tumor, and the diagnosis is only made after excisional biopsy.

The diagnosis of sarcoidosis or histiocytosis X is usually supported by other evidence of the systemic disease and occasionally is made only after excisional biopsy.

DIAGNOSTIC EVALUATION

The diagnostic evaluation of a patient with sellar enlargement should define the nature of the space-occupying lesion and assess its effects on the extrasellar anatomic structures and on the function of the hypothalamic-pituitary unit.

Patient History and Physical Examination

The history and physical examination should include a detailed assessment of the anatomic and functional manifestations of the space-occupying hypothalamic-pituitary–area lesion, assessment of the lesion's onset, duration, and course, examination for a primary tumor elsewhere (in the breast or lung), examination for systemic disease (e.g., sarcoidosis or histiocytosis X), and assessment of a personal or family history of other manifestations of multiple endocrine neoplasia type I.

Diagnostic Studies (Table 11–9)

The objectives of the investigation are to assess the presence and degree of sellar expansion, of pituitary dysfunction, and of extrasellar effects, and to assess the nature and extent of the expanding mass.

RADIOLOGIC STUDIES

Standard skull films and sellar tomograms are evaluated for the size of the sella, changes in its contour, thinning and erosion of its confines, and sellar and extrasellar calcification. Additionally, the presence of myelographic dye (from previous myelography) within the sella is diagnostic of an empty sella. Enlargement of the sinuses and prominence of external occipital protruberance may point to acromegaly. These radiologic studies are limited because of the great variation in the size of the normal sella and by the fact that decalcification and thinning of the sellar confines can be found in normal individuals who do not harbor a sellar space-occupying lesion.

CT scan of the pituitary area employing the newest generation of CT scanners and using coronal and axial views of the sella is the most helpful radiologic tool available at present. The resolving power is improved by the intravenous administration of iodide-containing

Table 11–9. Diagnostic Approach to the Enlarged Sella

Are there extrasellar effects
  History and physical examination including neurologic evaluation
  Complete ophthalmologic evaluation
    Visual acuity
    Fundi
    Extraocular muscles
    Visual fields (perimetry)
Is there endocrine dysfunction
  Pituitary
    Hyperpituitarism or hypopituitarism
      Basal hormone ± provocative test
      Target gland hormone(s) + trophic pituitary hormone
    Hypothalamic
      Diabetes insipidus or SIADH: serum/urine osmolality and additional studies as needed
    Pituitary target gland failure
      Target gland hormone and trophic pituitary hormone
    MEN I, if needed
      Parathyroid: serum calcium ± iPTH
      Pancreas: fasting plasma glucose ± serum insulin, serum gastrin, etc.
What is the cause
  Clinical setting
  CT scan with contrast ± metrizamide
  Carotid angiography
  Neurosurgical exploration

contrast media. CT scanning can identify a sellar mass as small as 3 to 4 mm in diameter, and extrasellar extension, if present. The sellar mass may be hypo- or hyperdense, may increase the volume of the sella contents, and may cause the pituitary stalk to deviate, as well as causing thinning and erosion of the sellar floor. CT scanning can also identify an extrasellar mass, its nature and extent, and its effect on the ventricular pathways. For any mass, a CT scan can identify whether it is solid, cystic, or mixed, and if solid, whether it is complicated by necrosis or hemorrhage. Calcification within the mass is identifiable even before becoming apparent on standard skull films. In addition, CT scanning can identify an empty sella and aneurysm and vascular tumors (for example, meningioma). CT scanning after the introduction of metrizamide into the subarachnoid space can be used for better delineation of a suprasellar space-occupying lesion and the empty sella.

Other radiologic studies include carotid angiography for diagnosing aneurysm and defining a tumor with characteristic vascularity, e.g., meningioma. Pneumoencephalography has been superseded by the non-invasive CT scanning in the diagnosis of empty sella. Nuclear magnetic resonance is not widely available at present, and experience is limited in sellar radiology.

OPHTHALMOLOGIC EVALUATION

Full ophthalmologic examination should be an integral part of the evaluation of patients with an enlarged sella and should include formal visual field charting (Goldman perimeter) using small colored targets and assessment of visual acuity, of the optic disk for papilledema or atrophy, and of extraocular muscle function.

ENDOCRINE EVALUATION

Complete evaluation of anterior and posterior pituitary functions is important to rule out anterior pituitary hypofunction (see The Syndrome of Hypopituitarism), anterior pituitary hyperfunction (see Hyperprolactinemia and Galactorrhea, Acromegaly and Gigantism, and Cushing's Syndrome).

ACROMEGALY AND GIGANTISM

DEFINITION

Acromegaly and gigantism refer to the syndromes that result from chronic growth hormone (GH) hypersecretion in the adult (acromegaly) or in children and adolescents (gigantism). These are rare diseases, with reported incidence of approximately 400 new cases per year in the US.

PATHOPHYSIOLOGIC CONSIDERATIONS
(Table 11–10)

The most common cause of the syndrome is primary pituitary disease caused by a GH-producing anterior pituitary tumor. Approximately 10 to 15% of all pituitary tumors secrete GH and cause the syndrome. These tumors vary in size and extent and may be less than 1 cm in diameter (microadenoma) and intrasellar, or greater than 1 cm in diameter (macroadenoma) and associated with extrasellar extension. The vast majority of these tumors are benign but may be locally invasive. The tumors may hypersecrete other pituitary hormones in addition to GH. They usually occur sporadically but rarely may occur as part of familial MEN

Table 11–10. Causes of Acromegaly-Gigantism

Primary: pituitary GH-producing tumor
GH only
GH and other pituitary hormones
Secondary: GH-RH-producing tumor
carcinoid: bronchial, foregut, pancreas
Ectopic GH-producing tumors, e.g., lung, liver

type I in association with parathyroid and endocrine pancreatic tumor or hyperplasia.

Rarely the syndrome may be caused by excessive GH secretion and somatotrope hyperplasia or adenomatous hyperplasia, secondary to excessive stimulation by a growth hormone-releasing hormone (GH-RH)–secreting tumor. Such tumors include carcinoid tumors of the bronchus, foregut, or pancreas; and neuronal tumors in the hypothalamus (hamartoma) or in the pituitary (gangliocytoma or choristoma). In these cases, removal of the GH-RH–secreting tumor leads to normalization of GH secretion and regression of the somatotrope hyperplasia.

Ectopic production of GH by nonpituitary tumors is very rare and has been described in breast, ovarian, or bronchial cancers. In such cases, the GH hypersecretion is modest and usually is not associated with clinical acromegaly.

CLINICAL PRESENTATION

The clinical features of acromegaly-gigantism are related to the functional and anatomic effects of the pituitary tumor. These effects include GH hypersecretion with or without hypersecretion of other pituitary hormones, anatomic sellar and extrasellar effects from tumor growth, and syndrome of hypopituitarism. In addition, in some patients the clinical features may include those of associated endocrine hyperfunction in multiple MEN type I (primary hyperparathyroidism and tumors of the endocrine pancreas). The disease affects both sexes equally, and the manifestations of acromegaly often begin in the third or fourth decade of life.

Signs

Acromegalic features are often brought to the patient's attention by relatives, friends, or the attending physician. Examination of the patient's photographs over the years usually gives a good indication of the time of onset and progression of the disease.

Cutaneous changes include thickening with increased porosity, oiliness, increased perspiration (a sensitive clinical indicator of disease activity), hyperpigmentation, coarsening of body hair, pedunculated epithelial tags (fibroma molluscum), and, occasionally, acanthosis nigricans. The calvarium is thickened, and the facial features are coarse, with prominent supraorbital ridges and skin folds. Increased length and thickness of the mandible leads to prognathism, underbite, spacing of the teeth, and malocclusion. The tongue is enlarged and furrowed and may show indentations from the teeth, and the salivary glands, especially the submandibular glands, are prominent.

The chest is barrel shaped, and kyphosis may be present. The voice is deep, husky, and resonant. The soft tissues of the hands and feet have a rubbery, spongy texture, and the fingers are spade-like. Hypertension is present in about 25 to 50% of patients and is usually mild and responsive to drug therapy. Cardiac examination may reveal findings of systolic click murmur syndrome, arrhythmias, cardiomegaly, and, rarely, congestive heart failure. Features of carpal tunnel syndrome, peripheral neuropathy, proximal myopathy, and degenerative joint disease may be present. Exophthalmos is present in a few patients but may be masked by prominence of the supraorbital ridges. Acromegalic patients have increased incidence of glaucoma. A diffuse or nodular goiter is present in many patients. Occasionally the patient may exhibit manifestations of thyroid dysfunction. (Hyperthyroidism may be due to TSH hypersecretion by the pituitary tumor or associated Graves' disease or toxic nodular goiter; hypothyroidism may occur as a part of hypopituitarism.)

Other findings that may be seen in some patients include findings related to pituitary tumor extrasellar growth, e.g., visual field defects, decreased visual acuity, hypothalamic impairment caused by superior extension of the tumor, and extraocular muscle palsy and facial hypesthesia caused by lateral extension of the tumor. In addition may be seen associations of multiple endocrine neoplasia type I, e.g., lipomas and evidence of primary hyperparathyroidism or tumors of the endocrine pancreas.

Gigantism develops when growth hormone hypersecretion occurs in childhood before epiphyseal fusion. Because of the frequent association of gigantism with hypogonadism, epiphyseal closure is delayed and the period available for growth is prolonged, allowing patients to reach enormous physical proportions. Myopathy, severe peripheral motor and sensory neuropathy, and hypopituitarism may be prominent late in the course of the disease.

Symptoms

Typically, the onset of acromegaly-gigantism is insidious, and the course covers many months to years. Usually the earliest symptoms are coarsening of the facial features and soft-tissue swelling of hands and feet, leading to an increase in hat, ring, glove, and shoe size. The patient may complain of thickening of skin, increased porosity, hyperpigmentation, oily skin and acne, coarsening of body hair, mild hirsutism, increased perspiration, offensive body odor, and fatigue. Additional symptoms of tissue effects of GH hypersecretion may include acroparesthesias, nerve entrapment syndromes (e.g., carpal tunnel syndrome), peripheral neuropathy, and proximal muscle weakness;

Raynaud's phenomena; joint complaints with features of degenerative joint disease, especially of the spine, hips, or knees, or with painful swelling of finger joints and wrist that may simulate rheumatoid arthritis; symptoms of hypertension or cardiac arrhythmias, and congestive heart failure often resistant to standard therapy; daytime somnolence, excessive snoring, and sleep apnea that may be central, obstructive, or mixed; and symptoms of clinical diabetes mellitus, which can occur in about 10% of patients. Other symptoms may be related to associated pituitary hormone hypersecretion, e.g., amenorrhea-galactorrhea in females and decreased libido and potency in males from hyperprolactinemia, or TSH-induced thyrotoxicosis; symptoms of hypopituitarism caused by anterior pituitary impairment by the tumor mass; the effects of extrasellar extension of the tumor, which may include headaches, visual difficulties, diplopia, or facial pain; and symptoms related to the features of multiple endocrine neoplasia type I.

DIFFERENTIAL DIAGNOSIS

Pachydermoperiostosis (Touraine-Solente-Golé syndrome) is a familial condition characterized by coarsening of the acral features, thickening of the skin, and hypertrophic osteoarthropathy, including clubbing of the fingers. Patients with this syndrome bear clinical resemblance to patients with acromegaly; however, they have normal growth hormone levels and secretory dynamics and do not have evidence of pituitary abnormality. Other differential diagnoses include patients on long-term therapy with phenytoin who may have an acromegaloid appearance, and patients with lipodystrophy or cerebral gigantism whose conditions may be confused with gigantism caused by growth hormone–producing pituitary tumor. In all these conditions the serum GH levels and GH-secretory dynamics are normal.

DIAGNOSTIC EVALUATION

The diagnostic approach is concerned with documenting the presence of acromegaly-gigantism and identifying its cause (Fig. 11–5).

Patient History and Physical Examination

The history and physical examination give important clues relating to onset, duration, and course of the disease; severity of its clinical manifestations; its neurologic, articular, cardiovascular, endocrine, and other complications; complications of extrasellar extension and hypopituitarism; association with MEN type I; and

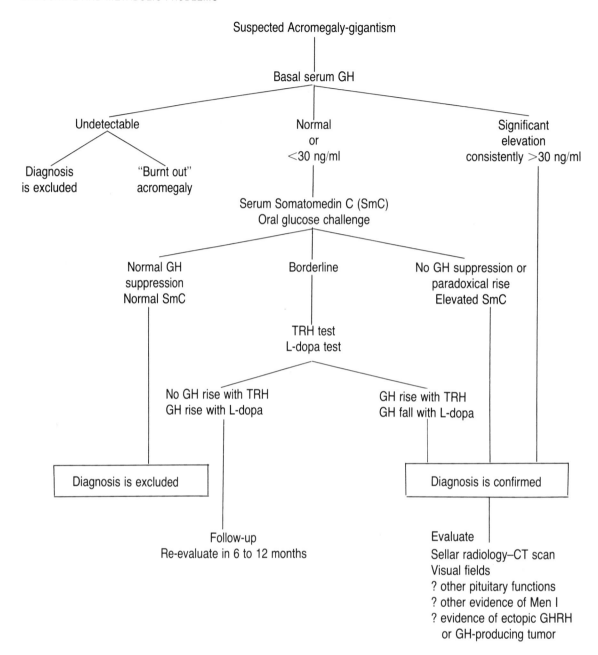

Fig. 11–5. Diagnostic approach to suspected acromegaly-gigantism.

the presence of ectopic GH- or GH-RH–producing tumors.

There is usually no problem in the diagnosis of flagrant cases. The challenge is to make the diagnosis early, because, untreated, chronic disease can cause irreversible physical changes, increase patients' morbidity (by the effects of tumor, GH hypersecretion, and other endocrine dysfunctions), and increase mortality (from hypertension, diabetes, and cardiovascular effects). The syndrome should be considered in the differential diagnosis of increased perspiration, oiliness of the skin, hyperpigmentation, menstrual irreg-

ularities, galactorrhea, hypertension, diabetes, premature and significant degenerative joint disease, carpal tunnel and other entrapment neuropathies, peripheral neuropathy, sellar enlargement, and chiasmal syndrome, and in the setting of MEN type I.

The diagnosis depends on documenting evidence of growth hormone hypersecretion. A high or normal basal serum GH level that fails to be suppressed normally during an oral glucose tolerance test is the definitive diagnostic test. In borderline cases, diagnostic support may be obtained from the finding of an elevated serum somatomedin C level or paradoxic serum

GH response to TRH or L-dopa. The physician must also document the presence and the extent of pituitary tumor by radiologic studies.

Diagnostic Studies

Once the diagnosis of acromegaly or gigantism is made, full ophthalmologic evaluation should be performed to rule out extrasellar extension of the tumor. Also, other pituitary functions should be assessed to exclude other pituitary hormone hypersecretion or the complication of hypopituitarism (see The Syndrome of Hypopituitarism). An assessment should be made of the presence of other endocrine abnormalities, including associated thyrotoxicosis or multiple endocrine neoplasia type I. Finally, consideration of the unlikely possibility of a GH- or a GH-RH–producing tumor should be considered.

LABORATORY TESTS

General. Growth hormone hypersecretion may cause hyperphosphatemia, abnormal glucose tolerance or frank diabetes mellitus, hypercalciuria, occasional mild hypercalcemia, hypertriglyceridemia, increased 24-hour urinary 17-ketogenic steroids and 17-ketosteroids, increased skeletal muscle CPK, and increased plasma and red blood cell volumes.

Specific (see Table 11–3).

Basal Serum GH. This is measured by RIA. The normal values are less than 5 ng/ml in males and less than 10 ng/ml in females.

Most acromegalic patients have elevated basal serum GH levels. An elevated basal serum GH is not diagnostic of acromegaly, because mild to moderate elevations of serum GH can be seen also in nonacromegalic patients as a result of stress, fasting, anorexia nervosa, malnutrition, and the use of estrogen. A basal value of serum GH greater than 50 ng/ml, however, is diagnostic of acromegaly. Because 10% of patients with acromegaly have basal serum GH falling within the normal range, a normal basal GH level does not exclude acromegaly. An undetectable basal serum GH level is never seen in active acromegaly, however, and therefore excludes the diagnosis.

Serum Somatomedin C. GH exerts its growth-promoting effects on the peripheral tissues indirectly via somatomedins, which are polypeptides produced primarily by the liver and fibroblasts. Somatomedins measurements by RIA are presently available. The normal values depend on the type of assay used. Such values are not influenced by daily serum GH level fluctuations and are better indicators of GH bioactivity than are serum GH levels measured by RIA.

A highly specific radioimmunoassay for Somatomedin C (Sm C) is now generally available and has proved to be of considerable utility in the diagnosis and treatment of growth hormone related disorders. Sm C values vary considerably with age; they are low during the first few years of life, rise gradually to a peak between 13 and 15 years of age, and thereafter gradually diminish. Sm C levels are increased in virtually all patients with active acromegaly or gigantism. It should be noted that Sm C levels may be elevated into the ''acromegalic'' range in normal adolescence during the pubertal growth spurt and in normal pregnancy; interpretation of Sm C values under these physiologic conditions should, therefore, be made cautiously.

Plasma Growth Hormone Releasing Hormone (GHRH). This assay is presently available only in certain pituitary research centers. It may help in the identification of those rare patients in whom the acromegaly is due to ectopic GHRH production.

Provocative Tests. In the oral glucose tolerance test, 100 g of glucose are given by mouth, and blood samples for plasma glucose and serum GH are obtained at 0 minutes and at 1 and 2 hours after glucose administration. In the normal, serum GH is suppressed during the test to a value less than 3 ng/ml. Failure of such suppression is the sine qua non for the diagnosis of acromegaly and gigantism. No serum GH suppression is evident in 60% of patients with the syndrome; 25% show some partial suppression but not into the normal range, and 15% show paradoxic serum GH elevation.

In the TRH test, 500 μg of TRH are given as an IV bolus, and blood samples for serum GH are obtained at 0 minutes and 30 to 60 minutes after TRH administration. In the normal, there is no GH response to TRH. About 70% of acromegalic patients show GH secretory response to TRH.

In the L-dopa test, 500 mg of L-dopa are given by mouth, and blood samples for serum GH are obtained at 0 minutes and hourly for 3 hours after L-dopa administration. In the normal, serum GH is increased in response to L-dopa. Many acromegalic patients display paradoxic suppression of serum GH.

Abnormal GH secretory responses to these provocative tests are also seen in uremia, cirrhosis, depression, and anorexia nervosa. These entities do not pose any problems in differential diagnosis, however.

RADIOLOGIC STUDIES

Skull x-rays reveal sellar enlargement in greater than 90% of patients in association with enlargement of the frontal sinuses and increased prominence of the external occipital protuberance. Sellar tomography may be helpful in those with normal sella on standard skull films to show demineralization or erosion of the sellar confines and asymmetrical sellar enlargement. The best radiologic tool is CT scan of the pituitary area, which shows the pituitary tumor and its extent and delineates extrasellar extension. Metrizamide study, pneumoencephalography, and carotid angiography are not usually needed.

Other useful radiographic findings to support the diagnosis include thickening of the soft tissue of the heel pad to greater than 22 mm, tufting of the ends of the distal phalanges, and widening of the joint spaces because of thickened articular cartilage. A chest x-ray may show cardiomegaly and evidence of an ectopic GH– or GH-RH–producing tumor. Magnetic resonance imaging of the sella is not widely available at present and experience with it is limited. It may prove helpful in sellar radiology in the future.

HYPERPROLACTINEMIA AND GALACTORRHEA

DEFINITION

Hyperprolactinemia is defined as a serum prolactin level above the normal range. Galactorrhea refers to secretion of milk by the breasts that is not related to pregnancy or breast-feeding. Since prolactin is a necessary requirement for initiation and maintenance of milk production, galactorrhea is a manifestation of derangement in prolactin physiology.

PATHOPHYSIOLOGIC CONSIDERATIONS
(Table 11–11)

Prolactin is a peptide hormone secreted by the lactotroph cell of the anterior pituitary gland. Its secretion is regulated by hypothalamic inhibition primarily by dopamine. Hyperprolactinemia can be either physiologic or pathologic.

Physiologic hyperprolactinemia can occur in pregnancy and lactation. Prolactin levels start to rise between the first and second months of pregnancy and continue to rise, reaching peak levels of several hundred ng/ml at term. The increased production is due to hypertrophy and hyperplasia of the lactotroph cell caused by rising estrogen levels during pregnancy. After delivery, in those women who do not breast-feed, prolactin levels drop rapidly, returning to normal in 1 to 2 weeks. In those who do breast-feed, serum prolactin levels are high for the first few weeks, with

Table 11–11. Causes of Hyperprolactinemia

Physiologic
  Newborn
  Pregnancy and lactation
  Stress
Pathologic
  Pituitary disease
    Prolactinoma
    Acromegaly
    Cushing's disease
    Primary empty-sella syndrome
  Hypothalamic disease
    Traumatic, e.g., stalk section, irradiation
    Inflammatory, e.g., sarcoidosis
    Infiltrative, e.g., histiocytosis X
    Neoplastic
      Primary, e.g., glioma, ectopic pinealoma
      Parasellar, e.g., craniopharyngioma
      Secondary—metastatic
  Functional
    Drugs
      DA receptor antagonists
        Phenothiazines, butyrophenones
        Thioxanthenes, metoclopramide, sulpiride, pimozide
        Monoamine inhibitors or depletors (alphamethyldopa, reserpine)
      Estrogens
      TRH
      Narcotics—morphine, codeine, heroin
      Catechol-reuptake interfering drugs
        Amphetamines
        Tricyclic antidepressants
      Cimetidine (iv)
      Calcium-channel blockers
    Primary hypothyroidism
    Renal and hepatic failure
    Chest wall disease
    Thoracic spinal lesion
  Ectopic
    Bronchogenic carcinoma
    Hypernephroma
  "Idiopathic" of indeterminate origin

sharp surges in prolactin secretion during suckling. Despite continued lactation, basal levels and post-suckling surges decrease, and prolactin levels return to normal in a few months.

Physiologic hyperprolactinemia can also be produced by stressful events, including surgery, anesthesia, exercise, hypoglycemia, and pelvic examination.

Pathologic hyperprolactinemia can result from hypersecretion of prolactin by the pituitary lactotroph because of primary pituitary disease or secondary to hypothalamic abnormality; very rarely it can also result from excessive production of prolactin by extrapituitary ectopic tumor, e.g., bronchogenic carcinoma and hypernephroma.

Prolactinomas, prolactin-producing pituitary tumors, comprise 60 to 70% of all pituitary tumors and are the most common organic cause of hyperprolactinemia. They are variable in size (tumors less than 1 cm in diameter are called microadenomas, and those more than 1 cm are called macroadenomas) and in extent (they may be confined to the sella or have extrasellar extension). The tumors are preponderately benign. The course of microadenoma is unknown; at least a few will increase in size and become macroadenomas. The sex distribution of prolactinomas is approximately equal, although microadenomas are found much more commonly in young females, presumably because of earlier recognition of the endocrine consequences of hyperprolactinemia.

Hyperprolactinemia may occur with other pituitary tumors. Functioning pituitary tumors may produce more than one pituitary hormone, and hyperprolactinemia has been noted in patients with acromegaly and Cushing's disease. Alternatively, a nonfunctioning tumor may be associated with hyperprolactinemia if it has a suprasellar extension impinging on the pituitary stalk or hypothalamus and interfering with hypothalamic inhibition of the prolactin reaction.

Organic hypothalamic and pituitary stalk disorders can be associated with hyperprolactinemia because of interruption of hypothalamic dopamine inhibitory regulation. Craniopharyngiomas are the most common nonpituitary tumors causing hyperprolactinemia. Other hypothalamic tumors (primary or metastatic), space-occupying lesions impinging on the hypothalamic stalk area (e.g., meningioma), infiltrative disorders such as sarcoidosis or histiocytosis X, hypothalamic irradiation, and pituitary stalk section can also lead to hyperprolactinemia. In such disorders hyperprolactinemia may be the only demonstrable hormonal abnormality, although these disorders frequently lead to hypopituitarism, diabetes insipidus, and vegetative hypothalamic dysfunction, which may include disturbances in sleep, temperature, appetite, and thirst.

Mild hyperprolactinemia is found in about 15% of all patients with primary empty sella. Other significant pituitary dysfunction is almost never found, and only rarely do visual field defects caused by traction on the optic nerves and chiasm occur. The physician should search for coexistent microadenoma in patients with hyperprolactinemia and primary empty sella.

Drugs are the most common cause of hyperprolactinemia. Among the offending drugs are those that deplete the hypothalamus of dopamine (e.g., alpha methyldopa) or antagonize the action of dopamine at the pituitary level (DA receptor–blocking agents, such as phenothiazines). Estrogens cause lactotroph hyperplasia and an increase in synthesis and release of prolactin. Drug-induced hyperprolactinemia usually resolves in a few days to a few weeks following the discontinuation of the offending drug.

Hyperprolactinemia is estimated to occur in about 20 to 30% of patients with primary hypothyroidism, while primary hypothyroidism probably is present in about 5% of all hyperprolactinemic patients. The cause of the hyperprolactinemia is uncertain but probably is related to changes in hypothalamic dopamine turnover and is corrected by thyroid hormone replacement. In addition, in primary hypothyroidism there is loss of negative feedback by thyroid hormones, a rise in TSH secretion, and TSH cell hypertrophy and hyperplasia. This increase in TSH cell mass may give rise to a pituitary mass and sellar expansion. Therefore, primary hypothyroidism can be associated with hyperprolactinemic syndrome and a sellar mass that can be misdiagnosed as a prolactinoma.

Chest wall lesions including those produced by trauma, thoracoplasty, pneumonectomy, radical mastectomy, herpes zoster, and other lesions involving the fourth to the sixth intercostal nerves can cause mild hyperprolactinemia by activation of the afferent sensory mechanisms.

Hyperprolactinemia occurs in 20 to 40% of patients with renal failure and in nearly all patients requiring hemodialysis. The cause is indeterminate. The elevated prolactin levels are not changed by recent hemodialysis but are corrected by renal transplant. Liver failure, especially with hepatic encephalopathy, can also cause hyperprolactinemia primarily by a decrease in the clearance of prolactin.

Ectopic production of prolactin by nonpituitary tumors is rare and has been reported to occur in bronchial carcinoma, hypernephroma, and testicular tumors of germ-cell origin.

CLINICAL PRESENTATION

The clinical manifestations of hyperprolactinemia include those related to hyperprolactinemia itself and those due to its cause. Hyperprolactinemia results in inhibition of gonadal function primarily by suppression of gonadotropin-releasing hormone (GnRH) release and hypogonadotropism, and to some extent by the direct inhibitory effect of hyperprolactinemia on gonadal tissues. Hyperprolactinemia also results in a galactogenic effect on the breast tissues, and in increased androgen production by the adrenal cortex, with ACTH playing a permissive role. The clinical manifestations related to hyperprolactinemia are the same regardless of the cause.

Signs

In adult females, signs include the presence of galactorrhea, spontaneous or expressible; evidence of hypoestrogenism; and hyperandrogenicity. In adult males one may find evidence of hypogonadism, small, soft testes, and a small, soft prostate. Gynecomastia and galactorrhea are rare. In prepubertal children there may be features of failure of sexual development.

In both sexes and at all ages additional clinical manifestations include visual acuity and field abnormalities, optic atrophy and papilledema, and cranial nerve III, IV, and VI dysfunction related to parasellar space-occupying lesions; evidence of hypopituitarism; evidence of other pituitary hormone hypersecretion (functioning pituitary tumors); goiter or features of thyroid dysfunction; chest wall lesions; and evidence of ectopic tumor, systemic disease, or renal and liver failure.

Symptoms

In adult females in the reproductive phase of life, hyperprolactinemia presents with ovulatory and menstrual dysfunction (in 60 to 90% of patients). Such dysfunction includes inadequate luteal phase, oligo- or anovulation, infertility, oligo- or amenorrhea, and symptoms of hypoestrogenism, including decreased vaginal secretion, dyspareunia, hot flashes, and osteopenia in long-standing cases. Hyperprolactinemia also presents with decreased libido; hirsutism and acne; and, in 30 to 60% of patients, galactorrhea, which can be variable in quantity, spontaneous or expressible, milky turbid or clear, and unilateral or bilateral. Menstrual abnormalities and galactorrhea may be present concurrently but either may precede or follow the other.

In adult males, decreased libido and potency impairment are the most common symptoms. In some males oligospermia or azospermia and infertility may be the presenting features. Gynecomastia and galactorrhea are rare in hyperprolactinemic males.

In both sexes, few patients with hyperprolactinemia are entirely asymptomatic. In prepubertal patients, hyperprolactinemia may present with delayed pubertal and sexual maturation.

Some additional comments related to the clinical presentations are in order.

Although galactorrhea in the nulliparous female is always abnormal, expressible galactorrhea can be demonstrated in as many as 25% of women who have been pregnant and who have breast-fed in the past and therefore may not be clinically important in most of these patients. It assumes clinical importance if it is present in more than a tiny drop, if 12 months or more have elapsed since the last pregnancy, or if it is associated with menstrual dysfunction. Spontaneous galactorrhea in any woman is always clinically important.

The breast secretions in galactorrhea are usually milky white but may be turbid or clear. In suspected cases the secretion should be placed on a slide and stained with Sudan IV; the presence of fat globules indicates galactorrhea. A brownish breast discharge is usually related to fibrocystic breast disease. If the expressed fluid is dark or bloody, breast neoplasm should be suspected.

Galactorrhea may be present only transiently and intermittently, or it may not even be apparent to the patient. A careful breast examination including an attempt at expression of breast secretions is required in all patients with suspected hypothalamic-pituitary disease. A complex endocrine milieu (estrogen, progesterone, thyroxine, cortisol, insulin, and growth hormone), in addition to prolactin, is necessary for the initiation of lactation.

Absence of galactorrhea in some patients with documented hyperprolactinemia is probably due to associated deficiency of gonadal hormones, which are required to initiate lactation. Also, although enhanced prolactin secretion is necessary for the initiation of milk production, galactorrhea can be maintained in the presence of minimally or intermittently elevated prolactin levels. Therefore, hyperprolactinemia is not always demonstrated in patients with galactorrhea.

Clinical experience indicates that approximately one third of patients with secondary amenorrhea, one third of patients with post-pill amenorrhea, and greater than two thirds of patients with amenorrhea and galactorrhea have demonstrable hyperprolactinemia. Presence of galactorrhea in a patient with normal menstrual function is usually not indicative of hyperprolactinemia. When hyperprolactinemic amenorrheic patients are evaluated, it is found that 40 to 50% of them present after discontinuation of oral contraceptives, 5 to 15% have onset in the postpartum period, and 20 to 40% have spontaneous onset of symptoms. Of patients with polycystic ovarian syndrome, 5% have hyperprolactinemia, and some of these patients may harbor a prolactinoma.

In men, recognition of hyperprolactinemia is frequently delayed because decreased libido and potency impairment may be dismissed by both the patient and his physician as resulting from psychiatric factors. In those who harbor a pituitary tumor, marked hyperprolactinemia and a macroprolactinoma are usual at the time of presentation. Early diagnosis of prolactinoma in men rests on a high index of suspicion.

DIAGNOSTIC EVALUATION

Patient History and Physical Examination

Diagnostic evaluation starts with a careful history and physical examination. Careful inquiry is made relating to pregnancy, use of drugs, gonadal function, libido and fertility, headache, visual abnormalities and other pituitary dysfunctions, cranial trauma or irradiation, chest wall lesion, thyroid disease, renal or liver failure, and other systemic disease. In the physical examination in women, the physician should evaluate the secondary sex characteristics for the hypoestrogenic state or hirsutism, evaluate the breast for galactorrhea, and evaluate the pelvis for the possibility of pregnancy or polycystic ovaries. In the male attention is paid to the size and consistency of the testes and prostate, and the patient is examined for gynecomastia or galactorrhea. In both sexes, it is important to assess the visual fields, other pituitary functions, thyroid function, and the presence of a goiter.

Diagnostic Studies

LABORATORY TESTS

Serum Prolactin (PRL). Measurement of serum PRL by specific and sensitive radioimmunoassays is widely available. Normal levels are 0 to 20 ng/ml in males and 0 to 23 ng/ml in females. In the normal individual, secretion of prolactin is episodic and labile. Diurnal variation occurs, with maximum levels reached during sleep and in the early hours of the morning. Stress can cause a moderate increase in serum prolactin. When sampling for the hormone, errors in timing should be avoided. Sampling is best done in the morning between 9 A.M. and 12 noon with the patient at rest and before breast and pelvic examination. If serum prolactin is found to be normal or mildly elevated in a patient suspected of having hyperprolactinemia, a repeat determination obtaining samples on successive days (or multiple samples every 30 to 60 minutes for three or four times with prolactin assayed in the pooled sample) should be made. In hyperprolactinemic states, serum prolactin values can vary from slight elevation to a level greater than 10,000 ng/ml. The levels fluctuate during the day. In those with mild hyperprolactinemia, levels in the normal range can be found intermittently. In the future, a sensitive bioassay of serum prolactin utilizing Nb2 lymphoma, a cell bioassay system, may become available and prove to be a useful adjunct in the assessment of hyperprolactinemic states.

Provocative Tests. Many stimulation tests (e.g., TRH, chlorpromazine) and suppression tests (e.g., L-dopa, L-dopa-carbidopa) are available. They demonstrate differences in prolactin secretion between normal individuals and those with pathologic hyperprolactinemia. Unfortunately, none of these tests has proved to be reliable in the differential diagnosis of tumorous and nontumorous hyperprolactinemia.

The test that has been used most extensively is the TRH test (Table 11–3). The normal response is a rise in serum prolactin that occurs early, peaks at 30 minutes, and starts its return to baseline by 60 minutes. Each lab should standardize its normal response. The majority of patients with prolactinomas do not show a response to TRH. Such lack of response, however, may be seen in hypothalamic causes of hyperprolactinemia. Patients with hyperprolactinemia caused by drugs or primary hyperthyroidism usually show hyperresponsiveness to TRH. This test is essentially free of hazards, though some patients may complain of transient urinary urgency, headache, nausea, and dizziness.

Additional Endocrine Studies. Additional endocrine studies include assessment of gonadal function, which in the male involves semen analysis, serum testosterone, LH, and FSH, and in the female, serum estrogen, LH and FSH, and tests to assess ovulatory function, including basal body temperature, serum progesterone, or endometrial biopsy (see Infertility). Other endocrine studies include tests of thyroid function to rule out primary hypothyroidism, such as serum total and free thyroxine (or free thyroxine index) and serum TSH and tests to rule out the presence of hypopituitarism, if organic hypothalamic-pituitary disease is suspected (see The Syndrome of Hypopituitarism). If a pituitary tumor is the cause of hyperprolactinemia, a search for other evidence of multiple endocrine neoplasia type I is in order (serum calcium, fasting plasma glucose, and other tests, as indicated).

RADIOLOGIC STUDIES

The primary goal of radiologic studies is to assess the hypothalamic-pituitary area for the presence of a space-occupying lesion. Standard skull films may show evidence of sellar enlargement or of suprasellar calcification of craniopharyngioma. In patients with normal skull films, polytomography or coned views of the sella may be of help to delineate subtle changes in sellar contour or symmetry. These studies have significant false negative and false positive results. More than 50% of patients with microprolactinomas have a normal sella. On radiologic examination, subtle sellar demineralization or erosive changes may be present in patients with normal pituitary glands. Sellar enlargement is not pathognomonic of pituitary tumor because it may occur in patients with parasellar mass lesions and in primary empty sella syndrome.

The most reliable radiologic diagnostic tool is the CT scan of the hypothalamic-pituitary area (with contrast utilizing the newest generations of CT scan and obtaining both axial and coronal sellar cuts). CT scanning can delineate microadenomas as small as 3 to 4 mm in diameter, can define tumor size and extent (sellar with or without extrasellar extension), and can identify hypothalamic and parasellar space-occupying lesions and primary empty sella. Pituitary microadenomas are recognized as hypo- or hyperdense sellar abnormalities associated with upward bulging of the diaphragm and deviation of the pituitary stalk.

Negative radiologic studies do not exclude the diagnosis of prolactinoma because very small prolactinomas may be missed. Positive radiologic studies support the diagnosis of prolactinoma, but the physician needs to consider the other space-occupying lesions that can give similar radiologic findings, e.g., craniopharyngioma. Rarely, angiography (to exclude aneurysm) and metrizamide scan (to delineate small suprasellar mass lesions or an empty sella) may be needed. Magnetic resonance imaging of the sella is not widely available at present and experience with it is limited. It may prove very helpful in sellar radiology in the future.

Diagnostic Approach

In the diagnostic evaluation of hyperprolactinemia and galactorrhea (Fig. 11–6), the physician must rule out pregnancy and take a careful drug history. If the patient is taking a drug that can cause hyperprolactinemia, a decision has to be made whether the drug can be discontinued. If the drug is discontinued, serum prolactin is rechecked in a few weeks. If the repeat serum prolactin is normal, a diagnosis of drug-related hyperprolactinemia is made. If the drug cannot be discontinued, or if the hyperprolactinemia persists despite discontinuation of the drug, the workup is continued to rule out organic disease.

A careful history and physical examination and appropriate laboratory and radiologic studies are usually sufficient to rule out a chest wall lesion, renal or hepatic failure, systemic disease, or metastatic disease.

The next step is to rule out primary hypothyroidism. Thyroid function tests should be carried out in all hyperprolactinemic patients because many patients with primary hypothyroidism are asymptomatic and findings may be subtle. Serum total and free thyroxine (or free thyroxine index) and serum TSH are obtained. If the thyroid function tests indicate primary hypothyroidism, thyroid hormone replacement therapy is instituted. If the hyperprolactinemic state and its manifestations resolve, a diagnosis of primary hypothyroidism-induced hyperprolactinemia is made. If no resolution occurs, a search for other causes of hyperprolactinemia is continued.

The next step is to rule out a pituitary tumor or other hypothalamic-pituitary mass lesions. The diagnosis of pituitary tumor is based on consideration of the levels of the serum prolactin and on the findings on radiologic examination, especially a CT scan of the pituitary area. Most patients with serum prolactin of greater than 100 ng/ml and almost all patients with prolactin levels greater than 250 ng/ml harbor a pituitary tumor. A substantial portion of patients with serum prolactin between 25 and 100 ng/ml have pituitary tumors; therefore, marginally elevated values do not rule out a tumor. Radiologic studies, especially CT scan of the hypothalamic-pituitary area, are crucial for the diagnosis of pituitary tumor in these cases. A mass lesion supports the diagnosis of tumor, but definitive proof may come only with surgery. Pituitary function tests are of limited value in differentiating prolactinomas from other causes of hyperprolactinemia. The TRH can be helpful in borderline cases. Absence of response to TRH suggests the presence of a prolactinoma. In all patients, careful, complete ophthalmologic evaluation including visual field assessment by perimetry is required.

Pituitary function tests should be performed in all patients with suspected hypothalamic-pituitary disease to rule out the presence of other pituitary hypersecretory states or of complicating hypopituitarism (see The Syndrome of Hypopituitarism, Enlargement of the Sella).

In those patients with pituitary tumors it is important to determine whether there are manifestations of other endocrine tumors in the multiple endocrine neoplasia type I syndrome. Serum calcium, fasting plasma glucose, serum gastrin, and other tests are performed as deemed appropriate.

If after a thorough evaluation no discernible cause is found, the hyperprolactinemia is considered to be of indeterminate origin. A follow-up is critical in these patients because some of them may harbor microadenomas or other hypothalamic-pituitary space-occupying lesions below the limits of radiologic detection and on follow-up may show evidence of a mass. The serum prolactin should be checked every 3 to 6 months and a CT scan repeated in 1 to 2 years or earlier if deemed necessary by the development of new symptoms.

HYPOTHYROIDISM

DEFINITION

Hypothyroidism refers to the constellation of signs and symptoms that result from the exposure of the tissues to decreased levels of thyroid hormones.

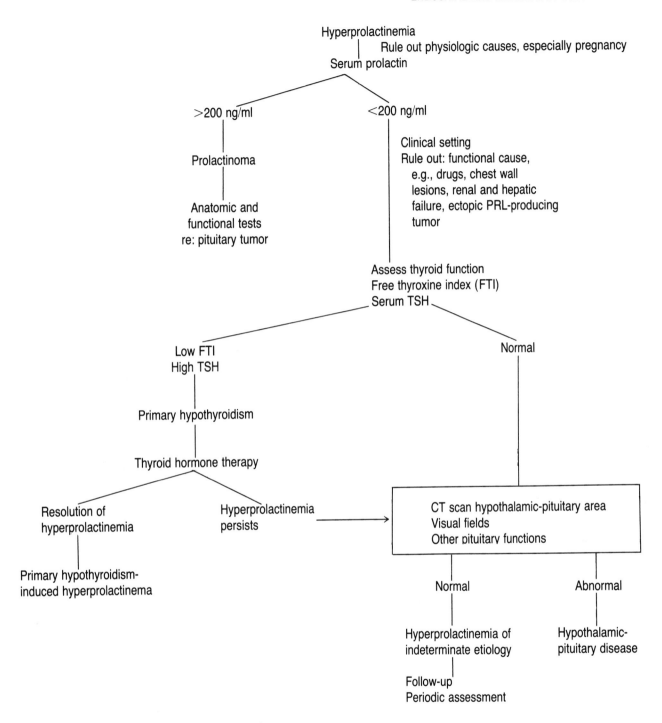

Fig. 11–6. Diagnostic approach to hyperprolactinemia.

PATHOPHYSIOLOGIC CONSIDERATIONS

The hypothalamic-pituitary-thyroid axis is responsible for the maintenance of a euthyroid state, wherein the production of the thyroid hormones thyroxine (T_4) and triiodothyronine (T_3) by the thyroid gland is adequate to meet physiologic body needs. This axis operates as a classic closed negative feedback system (Fig. 11–7).

Hypothyroidism results from deficiency of thyroid hormones, which may be due either to primary or thyroprivic hypothyroidism caused by intrinsic thyroid disease (95%) or to trophoprivic hypothyroidism caused by lack of stimulation by TSH (5%). Lack of TSH can result from intrinsic pituitary disease (secondary hypothyroidism) or from inadequate TSH secretion because of hypothalamic disease (tertiary hy-

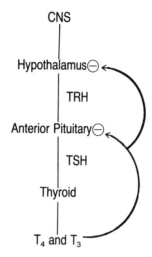

CNS

Hypothalamus⊖

TRH

Anterior Pituitary⊖

TSH

Thyroid

T₄ and T₃

TRH = Thyrotropin-releasing hormone
TSH = Thyrotropin or thyroid-stimulating hormone
T₄ = Thyroxine
T₃ = Triiodothyronine

Fig. 11–7. The hypothalamic-pituitary-thyroid axis.

Table 11–12. Causes of Hypothyroidism

Primary thyroid failure (thyroprivic) (95%)
  Structural
    Congenital developmental defect
      Agenesis
      Maldevelopment
      Maldescent
    Primary atrophic
      Spontaneous
      Postablative
        Postsurgical
        Postradioiodide therapy
        Postneck irradiation
    Hashimoto's thyroiditis
    Hypothyroid phase of subacute or painless thyroiditis
    Riedel's thyroiditis
    Infiltrative diseases, e.g., sarcoidosis
    Neoplastic
      Anaplastic carcinoma, lymphoma
  Functional
    Iodide deficiency
    Goitrogens
      Drugs
        Thionamides
        Iodides
        Lithium
        Phenylbutazone
        Paraminosalicylic acid
        Resorcinol
        Thioureas
        Perchlorate
    Dietary; e.g., Cruciferae family
  Hereditary dyshormonogenesis
Hypothalamic pituitary disease (trophoprivic) (5%)
  Functional
    Transient: after withdrawal of thyroid hormone therapy in a
      euthyroid individual
  Organic
    Trauma, e.g., neurosurgical
    Developmental defects
    Irradiation
    Vascular accidents
      Postpartum necrosis
      Pituitary apoplexy
    Tumor
      Primary
        Pituitary adenomas
        Hypothalamic tumors
        Craniopharyngioma
      Metastatic
Tissue resistance to thyroid hormone (very rare)

pothyroidism). The causes of hypothyroidism are outlined in Table 11–12.

Hashimoto's thyroiditis (chronic lymphocytic thyroiditis, struma lymphomatosa) is the most common cause of primary hypothyroidism in iodine-sufficient parts of the world. It commonly presents in the fifth or the sixth decades although it can occur at any age, and occurs in females 15 times more frequently than in males. Hashimoto's thyroiditis is believed to be an organ-specific autoimmune disease characterized by lymphocytic infiltration, germinal center formation, follicular destruction, fibrosis, and scarring. The pathologic changes lead to goiter and impairment of thyroid function to a variable degree. About 25% of patients are hypothyroid at presentation; the remainder are euthyroid, with normal or raised serum TSH levels. Some of those who are euthyroid with raised TSH levels develop overt hypothyroidism at some time in the future. Rarely, there is a phase of hyperthyroidism in the evolution of the disease. Antibodies to various thyroid antigens, among them thyroglobulin and thyroid microsomes, are found in the serum of most patients.

Spontaneous primary atrophic hypothyroidism is believed to be due to an autoimmune disease characterized by lymphoid infiltration and prominent destruction, fibrosis, and atrophy of the thyroid gland. There is considerable evidence indicating that spontaneous primary atrophy of the thyroid and Hashimoto's thyroiditis are closely related; possibly primary atrophic hypothyroidism is the end stage of previously unrec-

ognized Hashimoto's thyroiditis. Patients affected by either Hashimoto's thyroiditis or primary atrophic hypothyroidism have a positive family history and an increased frequency of other autoimmune diseases, including Addison's disease, diabetes mellitus, hypoparathyroidism, premature gonadal failure, pernicious anemia, Sjögren's syndrome, chronic active hepatitis, systemic lupus erythematosus, and rheumatoid arthritis.

Postablative hypothyroidism accounts for one third of cases of acquired hypothyroidism. It develops after surgical or radioactive iodine treatment of hyperthyroidism and may be transient or permanent, clinical or subclinical.

Transient postsurgical hypothyroidism occurring during the first 6 months after surgery is present in about 25% of patients. It may resolve spontaneously but is usually permanent if it persists beyond 6 months. Of patients developing hypothyroidism, 15% do so within the first year. Half of those who will remain euthyroid have raised TSH levels and will presumably be at an increased risk of developing hypothyroidism in the future. Long-term follow-up is justified.

Postradioactive iodine treatment hypothyroidism is more common than hypothyroidism following surgery. It is estimated that 25% of patients will have hypothyroidism at the end of the first year after therapy, and that every year an additional 2 to 4% will develop hypothyroidism. The cumulative incidence in some centers is 80% after 15 years. The early development of hypothyroidism after radioactive iodine treatment is to some extent dose related, whereas the late development probably depends on such factors as autoimmune destruction and inability of the surviving irradiated cells to replicate. The likelihood of thyroid failure is increased by multiple therapeutic doses of radioactive iodine.

Iodine given to normal individuals in sufficient doses will transiently inhibit thyroid hormone synthesis and release (Wolff-Chaikoff effect). In some patients, an intrinsic thyroid defect permits a persistent inhibition. In such cases, the suppression of thyroid hormone synthesis and release causes a compensatory increase in TSH secretion, resulting in a goiter. Hypothyroidism results if the inhibition is severe and the compensatory increase in TSH fails to restore hormone synthesis and release to normal. Patients with Graves' disease particularly after radioactive iodine treatment, patients with Hashimoto's thyroiditis, and the normal fetus are particularly sensitive to exogenous iodine. This may be administered in an inorganic form (most commonly in patients with chronic respiratory diseases who are prescribed expectorants containing potassium iodide) or in an organic form (radiocontrast iodide containing agents and drugs such as amiodarone). Pregnant women should not be exposed to iodides because iodides can cross the placenta and cause iodide-induced goiter and hypothyroidism in the fetus. Lithium carbonate used for the treatment of manic-depressive psychosis is a common cause of drug-induced goiter, since lithium cation, like iodide, inhibits the release of thyroid hormones from the gland. Other goitrogens, e.g., thionamides, phenylbutazone, and para-aminosalicylic acid, can cause a goiter and hypothyroidism.

Subacute thyroiditis and painless lymphocytic thyroiditis are causes of transient hypothyroidism. Initially in their evolution, the inflammatory follicular destruction leads to the release into the circulation of hormone-rich stored colloid, resulting in the transient thyrotoxic state. As the inflammation resolves, a transient phase of hypothyroidism follows and may last a few weeks until the follicles have fully recovered their hormone secretory function.

Infiltrative disorders of the thyroid are a rare cause of hypothyroidism. The gland may be involved by such infiltrative processes as Riedel's thyroiditis, sarcoidosis, hemochromatosis, amyloidosis, lymphoma, or metastatic malignancy.

Hypothyroidism caused by iodide deficiency is a major cause of goiter and hypothyroidism worldwide. Certain areas such as the Indies, the Himalayas, and central Africa have dietary iodine deficiency, leading to failure of thyroid hormone synthesis, a compensatory increase in TSH, and endemic goiter. The goiter usually appears in adolescence and is diffuse; in later life, it may become nodular. The majority of the patients are euthyroid, but hypothyroidism may occur in severe cases. Iodine deficiency, goiter, and hypothyroidism are eliminated by iodine prophylaxis.

Dyshormogenesis is a rare disorder caused by a genetically determined defect in hormone synthesis inherited as an autosomal recessive trait. Several forms have been described, the most common of which is Pendred's syndrome, which results from a deficiency of the intrathyroidal peroxidase system necessary for oxidation of iodide to iodine and is associated with nerve deafness. If the enzyme deficiency is severe, congenital hypothyroidism or hypothyroidism occurring in early childhood results. If the deficiency of enzyme is minor, the presentation is usually in childhood or adolescence as a diffuse or occasionally a nodular goiter; the compensatory increase in TSH can maintain euthyroidism.

In trophoprivic hypothyroidism, the thyroid gland is intrinsically normal but is deprived of stimulation by pituitary TSH. This entity is due most commonly to the presence of pituitary tumor, to postpartum pituitary necrosis, or to extrasellar disease. Hypothalamic hypothyroidism is less common and results from inadequate secretion of TRH. Trophoprivic hypothyroidism is usually associated with other hypothalamic-pituitary endocrine dysfunction and with evidence of causative lesion.

In peripheral resistance to thyroid hormone, the intrinsic thyroid gland activity is normal, but the target tissues throughout the body fail to respond to normal circulating thyroid hormone. The levels of T_4 and T_3 are increased, and because of their impaired effectiveness, TSH levels are increased, resulting in a goiter. Most patients are clinically euthyroid or marginally hypothyroid.

CLINICAL PRESENTATION

Signs

In flagrant hypothyroidism, the patient is slow in demeanor and has a husky, low-pitched voice with slow speech. The eyelids, hands, and feet are puffy, the nails and hair are dry and brittle, and there may be patchy alopecia. The skin is pale or carotinemic, dry, and rough. Absence of the lateral third of the eyebrow is a common but nonspecific sign.

Cardiovascular signs include bradycardia, hypertension, silent precordium, distant heart sounds, cardiac enlargement, and, rarely, evidence of cardiac failure. In severe cases, there may be signs of pericardial or pleural effusions, ascites, or synovial effusion. The deep tendon reflexes show characteristically delayed relaxation, most obvious at the ankle. Signs of carpal tunnel or, rarely, of cerebellar disease may be present. In primary hypothyroidism, the patient may have a goiter of variable size that may be diffuse, firm, rubbery, and bosselated (in Hashimoto's thyroiditis), soft to firm (in goitrogen-induced hypothyroidism), or hard and fixed and obstructive (in Riedel's thyroiditis). The goiter may be nodular. Signs of autoimmune associations including vitiligo or other evidence of autoimmune endocrine disease may be present. In trophoprivic hypothyroidism, no palpable thyroid tissue is present in the neck, and there may be other evidence of hypopituitarism and of the cause of the secondary or tertiary hypothyroidism.

Symptoms

In the adult with hypothyroidism, common complaints include physical, emotional, and mental slowing with decreased energy level, drive, and stamina, easy fatigability, somnolence, decreased concentration and memory (perhaps raising the question of dementia), and symptoms of agitation, depression, and, rarely, paranoia and frank psychosis. In addition, the patient may complain of cold intolerance and thickened, dry skin, puffiness of the face, hands, and feet, and brittle hair and nails; muscle aches, stiffness, and arthralgias; weight gain despite normal or decreased appetite, and constipation; hoarseness of the voice, slowness of speech, and progressive deafness; symptoms of carpal tunnel syndrome, peripheral neuropathy, and, rarely, cerebellar ataxia; dyspnea on exer-

tion and angina; and decreased libido and potency in males, menorrhagia in premenopausal women, and, occasionally, amenorrhea and galactorrhea. In addition, the patient may complain of symptoms referable to the cause of the hypothyroidism, goiter, hypothalamic-pituitary disease, and associations of autoimmune thyroid disease. The patient may be asymptomatic, especially early in the course or in transient hypothyroidism, e.g., following subacute or painless thyroiditis.

DIFFERENTIAL DIAGNOSIS

The differential diagnosis includes nephrotic syndrome, in which facial puffiness, pallor, anemia, high cholesterol, low serum T_4 (caused by TBG loss in the urine), and low serum T_3 (caused by euthyroid sick syndrome) may raise suspicion of hypothyroidism. In the nephrotic syndrome, however, the free thyroxine, free thyroxine index, and serum TSH are normal.

Muscle stiffness, myalgias, and arthralgias may raise the question of primary muscle or joint disorder.

Primary hypothyroidism may be associated with hyperprolactinemia, amenorrhea, galactorrhea, and a sellar mass caused by TSH cell hyperplasia. The differential diagnosis here is that of prolactinoma. Primary hypothyroidism should always be considered in the differential diagnosis of the hyperprolactinemic state. Serum thyroxine and TSH are critical measurements in this situation.

Hypothyroidism should enter into the differential diagnosis of menorrhagia, dementia, cerebellar ataxia, hyperlipidemia, cardiomegaly, pericardial effusion, pleural effusion, anemia, habitual constipation, syndrome of inappropriate ADH and hyponatremia, and isosexual precocious puberty.

DIAGNOSTIC EVALUATION

The objectives of the diagnostic approach are to confirm the presence of hypothyroidism and to identify its cause.

Patient History and Physical Examination

In the history, attention is paid to the age of onset of symptoms, their duration, and course; previous thyroid disease and goiter, previous thyroid surgery, radioiodine treatment, or irradiation of the neck, exposure to goitrogenic drugs; geographic location and dietary goitrogens, autoimmune endocrinopathies or systemic disease; hypothalamic-pituitary disease; a recent pregnancy or delivery; and family history of autoimmune thyroid or other endocrine disease or of congenital dyshormonogenesis.

In the physical examination, attention is paid to the presence of goiter and its characteristics and the presence of other evidence of hypothalamic-pituitary disease or other autoimmune or systemic disease. Absence of palpable thyroid tissue in a hypothyroid patient points to primary atrophic thyroid failure, postradioiodine or postsurgical hypothyroidism, or hypothalamic-pituitary hypothyroidism. A diffuse goiter in a hypothyroid patient could be related to Hashimoto's thyroiditis, goitrogen-induced hypothyroidism, iodine deficiency, or congenital dyshormonogenesis.

Diagnostic Studies

GENERAL

Routine laboratory studies may show anemia, which is usually normocytic and normochromic and caused by thyroid hormone deficiency but which may be microcytic and hypochromic (blood loss resulting from menorrhagia and from decreased iron absorption from associated achlorhydria), or which may be macrocytic and hyperchromic (associated pernicious anemia or folate deficiency).

The sedimentation rate is usually elevated. Serum sodium may be low (inappropriate ADH), and the serum calcium may be transiently elevated. Increased serum enzyme levels including SGOT, LDH, and CPK of skeletal muscle origin may be found in up to 80% of hypothyroid patients. Serum uric acid and creatinine may be mildly elevated. Serum cholesterol and triglycerides may be elevated with lipoprotein phenotype of type II-A or type IV.

Endocrine studies in patients with primary hypothyroidism may show evidence of associated autoimmune endocrinopathy and, in patients with trophoprivic hypothyroidism, evidence of other pituitary hormone dysfunction. Patients with primary hypothyroidism may show impaired growth hormone response to an insulin hypoglycemia test, impaired pituitary ovarian function, hyperprolactinemia, decreased 24-hour urinary 17-hydroxycorticosteroids, 17-ketogenic steroids, and 17-ketosteroids with normal serum cortisol, and findings of inappropriate ADH, all of which resolve with thyroid hormone replacement therapy.

A chest x-ray may show enlargement of the cardiac silhouette resulting from pericardial effusion and may also show evidence of a pleural effusion. If the heart is small on chest x-ray in a hypothyroid patient, trophoprivic hypothyroidism should be suspected.

The electrocardiogram shows sinus bradycardia, low voltage, and nonspecific ST-T wave changes. Echocardiogram reveals the presence and the degree of pericardial effusion.

SPECIFIC (Table 11-13)

Circulating Thyroid Hormones. The most important test in documenting hypothyroidism is a determination of the serum thyroxine (T_4) level. Since serum thyroxine measures both the bound and the free thyroxine fractions, and since it is the free, biologically active fraction that determines the thyroid function state, a measurement of the free thyroxine (FT_4) or an assessment of the thyroxine-binding proteins is essential in the interpretation of the total serum T_4 value. The most commonly used index of thyroxine-binding proteins is the resin T_3 uptake (RT_3U) (which should not be confused with serum T_3). The total T_4 and the RT_3U may be combined to give the free thyroxine index (FTI), which correlates well with the free T_4 concentration.

Serum total thyroxine is reduced in hypothyroidism and in euthyroid patients with decreased thyroxine-binding globulin (from the effect of androgen, glucocorticoid, phenytoin, salicylates, nephrosis, liver disease, genetic influences, etc.). The free thyroxine and the free thyroxine index are reduced in hypothyroidism but normal in euthyroid patients with decreased thyroxine-binding globulin. In hypothyroidism, therefore, the levels of serum total thyroxine and free thyroxine (or the free thyroxine index) are decreased. Decreased values can also be found in patients with nonthyroidal illness (see below).

Serum triiodothyronine (serum T_3) is not helpful in the diagnosis of hypothyroidism. It can be low in euthyroid patients with nonthyroidal illness and can be normal in 20 to 25% of patients with overt hypothyroidism.

Serum Thyrotropin (TSH). In primary hypothyroidism, the decrease in circulating thyroid hormone levels leads to decreased negative feedback on the hypothalamic-pituitary unit and to an appropriate increase in serum TSH levels. In trophoprivic hypothyroidism, which is due to pituitary (secondary) or hypothalamic (tertiary) hypothyroidism, the serum TSH is inappropriately low for the reduced level of serum thyroid hormones. An increased serum TSH in a hypothyroid patient is diagnostic of primary hypothyroidism. In fact, serum TSH is the most sensitive index presently available for the diagnosis of primary hypothyroidism. A normal serum TSH excludes the diagnosis of primary hypothyroidism.

TRH Test. This test assesses the function of the TSH secretory mechanism. It is simple and free of significant side effects. Each laboratory should standardize its normal ranges. In primary hypothyroidism, basal serum TSH is elevated, and the TSH response to TRH is exaggerated and prolonged. Since the elevated basal TSH already points to the diagnosis of

Table 11–13. Common Laboratory Tests in Thyroid Dysfunction

Tests	Determinants	Hypothyroidism	Hyperthyroidism
Total Thyroxine (TT₄) Normal, 5.0–12.5 μg/dl	Thyroid function; thyroxine-binding globulin TBG; TT₄ measures both bound (99.95%) and free (0.05%) T₄.	Decreased in primary, secondary, and tertiary hypothyroidism. Can be decreased in euthyroid patients with: a. Low serum-binding proteins (androgen and anabolic steroid therapy, marked hypoproteinemia, genetic TBG absence or deficiency, glucocorticoid excess, chronic liver disease, acromegaly). b. Inhibitors of serum T₄ binding (salicylates, clofibrate). c. T₃ therapy. d. Euthyroid sick syndrome.	Increased in 80–90% of hyperthyroid patients. May be normal in: a. T₃ toxicosis. b. In hyperthyroidism associated with decreased serum-binding protein, inhibition of serum protein binding, and in the euthyroid sick. May be increased in euthyroid patients with: a. Increased TBG (estrogens, pregnancy, acute hepatitis, acute intermittent porphyria, perfenazine, genetic). b. Increased albumin or prealbumin. c. Peripheral resistance to thyroid hormones. d. D T₄ therapy. e. Euthyroid sick syndrome.
Free Serum Thyroxine (FT₄) Normal, 0.7–1.8 ng/dl	Thyroid function.	Decreased. May be decreased in euthyroid patients with euthyroid sick syndrome.	Increased. May be increased in euthyroid patients with: a. Euthyroid sick syndrome. b. Peripheral tissue resistance to thyroid hormone.
Free Thyroxine Index (FTI) Normal, 5.0–10.0 (Laboratory dependent)	Total thyroxine and an indirect measure of TBG binding (T₃ resin uptake, R T₃ U). It is equivalent to the free serum thyroxine.	Decreased. May be decreased also in euthyroid sick patients.	Increased in 80–90% of hyperthyroid patients. May be increased in euthyroid patients with: a. Euthyroid sick syndrome. b. Peripheral resistance to thyroid hormone. c. Genetic albumin- and prealbumin-binding protein abnormality. d. Anti-T₄ antibodies. e. D T₄ toxicosis.
Serum Tri-iodothyrine (T₃) Normal, 90–230 ng/dl	Thyroid function, thyroid-binding globulin levels, peripheral T₄ to T₃ conversion. Measures both bound (99.5%) and free (0.5%) T₃.	Decreased. May also be decreased in euthyroid patients with decreased T₄ to T₃ conversion. a. Neonatal and elderly patients. b. Acute or chronic illness (euthyroid sick). c. No carbohydrate intake and caloric deprivation (malnutrition, anorexia nervosa, uncontrolled DM). d. Drugs (propylthiouracil, propranolol, glucocorticoids, certain iodinated contrast agents, and amiodarone).	Increased in all patients with thyrotoxicosis except those who have associated euthyroid sick syndrome. May also be increased in euthyroid patients with: a. Increased TBG (see above under Total Thyroxine). b. Peripheral resistance to thyroid hormone.
Serum Thyrotropin (TSH) Normal, 0.5–6.0 U/ml	Hypothalamic-pituitary-thyroid axis function.	Increased in primary hypothyroidism; normal or low in secondary and tertiary hypothyroidism. Serum TSH may be low or undetectable in 10–20% of euthyroid patients.	Serum TSH is low or undetectable in all types of thyrotoxicosis except those due to pituitary TSH hypersecretion (tumor or hyperplasia).
TRH Test Each laboratory should standardize its normal responses.	Pituitary TSH responsiveness.	Exaggerated response in primary hypothyroidism; blunted response in secondary pituitary-hypothyroidism; delayed response in tertiary hypothalamic-hypothyroidism. Response may be blunted in euthyroid patients, especially elderly patients and in those with euthyroid sick syndrome. Blunted or absent response is also seen in those with Cushing's syndrome and thyrotoxicosis.	Blunted response in all cases of thyrotoxicosis except those due to TSH pituitary hyperplasia. Blunted response may be seen in euthyroid patients, especially elderly and euthyroid sick patients, and those with Cushing's syndrome.

primary hypothyroidism, there is usually no need for the TRH test in a primary hypothyroid patient. In those patients with borderline TSH values, an exaggerated response to TRH points to primary hypothyroidism.

The TRH test can be used to distinguish between secondary pituitary hypothyroidism and tertiary hypothalamic hypothyroidism. In patients with secondary hypothyroidism, the TSH response to TRH is usually blunted, whereas in tertiary hypothyroidism, the response is usually normal but delayed.

Antithyroid Antibodies. When present in high titers, antithyroid antibodies point to autoimmune thyroiditis (Hashimoto's thyroiditis or primary atrophic thyroid failure) as the cause of the hypothyroidism. The presence of significant titers of antithyroid antibodies does not, however, give information about the thyroid functional state.

Diagnostic Approach

The diagnostic approach to hypothyroidism is outlined in Figure 11–8. The first step is to obtain a serum total thyroxine and free thyroxine (or a free thyroxine index). Normal values exclude the diagnosis of hypothyroidism. Low values point to hypothyroidism and should prompt a TSH determination. A high TSH in the presence of hypothyroidism points to primary hypothyroidism; if the serum TSH is inappropriately low, a diagnosis of hypothalamic-pituitary hypothyroidism is made. The TRH test can be used to distinguish between pituitary hypothyroidism (no response) and hypothalamic hypothyroidism (normal but delayed response).

In determining the cause of hypothyroidism, a diagnosis of primary hypothyroidism should prompt several considerations. The physician should evaluate the patient for iatrogenic or natural goitrogens. If discontinuation of exposure to goitrogen leads to recovery of a euthyroid state, a diagnosis of goitrogen-induced hypothyroidism is made. Also, the patient should be examined for the presence of diffuse bosselated goiter, which in the hypothyroid patient points to Hashimoto's thyroiditis. Significant titers of antithyroid antibodies support the diagnosis. A careful evaluation for other autoimmune endocrinopathies is in order. Screening of immediate relatives for thyroid or autoimmune endocrinopathy is optimal. The physician must evaluate the causes of transient hypothyroidism. In these situations, the necessity for continued thyroid hormone therapy, if given, should be reviewed at some future date.

If the diagnosis of trophoprivic hypothyroidism is made, a search for other manifestations of pituitary dysfunction and extrasellar effects and radiologic evaluation of the sella are in order.

If the thyroid hormones are found to be low in an acutely ill patient, the differential diagnosis is mainly between euthyroid sick syndrome and hypothyroidism. Serum T_3 has no utility in this situation since it can be normal in hypothyroidism and can be low in both entities. The most helpful step in the diagnosis is serum TSH determination; an elevated serum TSH is diagnostic of primary hypothyroidism. A normal or low TSH indicates either the euthyroid sick syndrome or trophoprivic hypothyroidism. A serum prolactin and cortisol can be obtained. If the serum prolactin is normal and cortisol is greater than 20 mg/dl (indicating a normal stressed ACTH adrenal axis), secondary hypothyroidism is unlikely. In this instance, the patient

may, if necessary, be treated with thyroid hormone, and the thyroid state can be rechecked after the resolution of the acute illness. If the prolactin levels are high or serum cortisol is less than 20 mg/dl in the acutely ill patient, the possibility of hypothalamic-pituitary disease should be evaluated.

Special Considerations

Transient Hypothyroidism. This can occur after thyroid surgery or radioactive iodine treatment or in the recovery phase of subacute or silent thyroiditis. It can be found in the neonate of mothers with autoimmune thyroid disease, presumably because of transplacental transfer of blocking antibodies to the TSH receptor, or it can occur in the neonate owing to maternal exposure to iodides or goitrogens. Transient hypothyroidism can also occur in the period following the discontinuation of prolonged thyroid hormone therapy in euthyroid patients. Also, it can be found in postpartum hypothyroidism, which develops in a small group of women with chronic thyroiditis who usually have significant titers of antithyroid antibodies. The mechanism of postpartum hypothyroidism is unknown; although the hypothyroidism is usually transient, permanent hypothyroidism may occur.

Subclinical Hypothyroidism or Impaired Thyroid Reserve. This entity describes clinically euthyroid patients who have serum T_4 levels in the low-normal range but have raised serum TSH levels. It is encountered most commonly after radioiodine or surgical treatment of hyperthyroidism or in patients with autoimmune thyroiditis. It may remain stable for many years or may progress to frank hypothyroidism.

Cretinism. Neonatal hypothyroidism affects 1 in 5000 births. Untreated, affected individuals will develop cretinism and severe mental retardation. Prompt recognition and therapy are imperative. Every newborn should undergo screening by measurement of T_4 and TSH in either cord or infant blood. The following manifestations should prompt suspicion of neonatal hypothyroidism: postmaturity and increased birth weight; evidence of delayed skeletal maturation (large posterior fontanelle, low nasal bridge); history of respiratory distress syndrome, especially in infants with birth weight greater than 2.5 kg; hypothermia; persistence of physiologic jaundice beyond 3 days; large tongue and hoarse cry; edema of the feet, eyelids, or labia; constipation; somnolence; or feeding problems.

In infancy, hypothyroidism leads to delay in reaching normal developmental milestones and to appearance of features of cretinism at about 6 to 12 months. These include short stature, coarse features with a broad, flat nose, widely set eyes, protruding tongue,

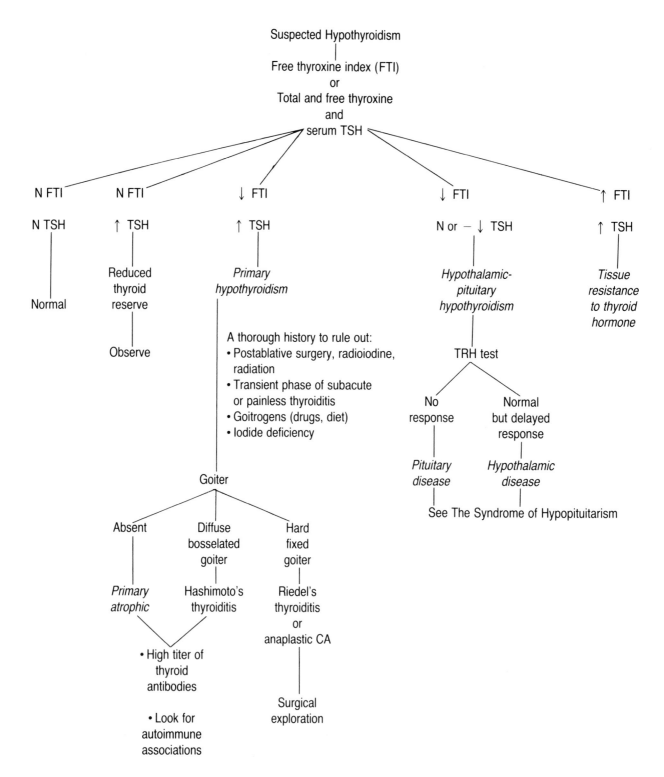

Fig. 11–8. Diagnostic approach to suspected hypothyroidism.

sparse hair, dry skin, protuberant abdomen with umbilical hernia, lethargy and hypotonia, and retarded mental development. Radiologic studies show retarded bone age, epiphyseal dysgenesis, and delayed dental development.

Juvenile Hypothyroidism. Juvenile hypothyroidism has presentations that include many of the features of adult hypothyroidism. Additional prominent features include slowing in linear growth rate leading to short stature with infantile body proportions (increased upper to lower segment ratio); deterioration in school performance; commonly, retardation of sexual maturation and delayed puberty, and, rarely sexual precocity; marked delay in bone age; epiphyseal dysgenesis; and sellar enlargement caused by increased pituitary mass from the hyperplastic TSH cells.

Myxedema Coma. This is a rare entity and usually affects elderly patients with severe long-standing hypothyroidism. It is characterized by gradual onset of lethargy, progressing to stupor or coma, alveolar hypoventilation, hypoxia and hypercapnia, and dilutional hyponatremia. Predisposing factors include cold exposure, trauma, infections (especially pneumonia), or administration of CNS depressants. The patient usually appears myxedematous. The body temperature is low, and the true degree of hypothermia may not be appreciated unless a low-reading rectal thermometer is used. Shivering is characteristically absent. Other findings include bradycardia, hypotension poorly responsive to vasopressors, shock, and seizures. The CSF pressure and protein concentration are high. The mortality rate is extremely high. Prompt recognition and treatment are mandatory because, even with the best treatment, mortality is greater than 50%.

Withdrawal of Thyroid Hormone Therapy. The physician frequently withdraws thyroid hormone therapy to evaluate the need for continuation of thyroid hormone therapy in a patient already receiving thyroid hormone but with no reliable previous diagnosis of hypothyroidism. The preferred method of assessment is to discontinue the thyroid hormone and measure total T_4 and free T_4 (or the free thyroxine index) and serum TSH in 6 to 8 weeks, a period adequate to allow recovery of a suppressed but normal hypothalamic-pituitary-thyroid axis.

Euthyroid Sick Syndrome. Acute medical and surgical illness can cause certain alterations in thyroid physiology. These changes may simulate the biochemical features of hypothyroidism and include reduced serum T_3 resulting from decreased conversion of T_4 to T_3 by the extrathyroidal tissues, notably the liver and kidney, with shift to conversion to reverse T_3 (rT_3). This results in a low serum T_3, raised serum rT_3, and normal T_4. Another feature is reduced serum T_3 and

serum T_4 resulting from a decreased level of thyroid-binding globulin because of decreased hepatic synthesis or decreased binding capacity of TBG. Another change may be a low TSH and a blunted TSH response to TRH caused by inhibition of secretion of TSH.

THYROTOXICOSIS

DEFINITION

Thyrotoxicosis refers to the constellation of signs and symptoms that result from the exposure of the tissues to increased levels of thyroid hormones.

PATHOPHYSIOLOGIC CONSIDERATIONS

The causes of the thyrotoxic state are listed in Table 11–14. The excess thyroid hormones can be derived from an endogenous or exogenous source. Endogenous hyperthyroidism can result from primary glandular thyroid disease (nodular goiter, subacute thyroiditis, painless thyroiditis, or thyroid malignancy), from stimulation of the thyroid gland by identifiable stimulators (Graves' disease, pituitary TSH hypersecretion, trophoblastic HCG hypersecretion), or from ex-

Table 11–14. Causes of Thyrotoxicosis

Endogenous
  Primary thyroid disease
    Toxic nodular goiter
      Spontaneous
        Single nodule
        Multinodular
      Iodine induced
    Thyroiditis
      Subacute
      Painless lymphocytic
    Functioning thyroid malignancy
  Excess thyroid stimulators
    Thyroid-stimulating immunoglobulins
      Graves' disease
    TSH
      Hypothalamic pituitary disease
        Idiopathic
        Tumor
    HCG (TSH-like effect)
      Trophoblastic disease
  Ectopic
    Struma ovarii
Exogenous
  Iatrogenic
  Factitious

trathyroidal sources (struma ovarii). Exogenous hyperthyroidism is usually caused by iatrogenic administration of supraphysiologic doses of thyroid hormones; rarely, it may be due to the factitial or surreptitious ingestion of thyroid hormones. Graves' disease and toxic nodular goiter account for more than 90% of all cases of thyrotoxicosis.

Graves' disease, the most common cause of hyperthyroidism, is believed to be an expression of an autoimmune thyroid disorder with familial predisposition. Its characteristic manifestations include diffuse goiter, thyrotoxicosis, ophthalmopathy, and, rarely, pretibial myxedema and acropachy. These manifestations need not appear together and in a given individual tend to run largely independent courses. The thyroid gland is enlarged and hypervascular, shows abundant small follicles with hyperplastic follicular cells, and has variable degrees of lymphocytic infiltration. The orbital contents, except for the globe, are infiltrated with inflammatory lymphocytes, plasma cells, and mast cells; the extraocular muscles are predominantly involved, initially with enlargement, later with degeneration, and ultimately with fibrosis of the muscle fibers. The dermopathy is characterized by lymphocytic and mucopolysaccharide infiltration, and by consequent thickening of the dermis. Acropachy results from subperiosteal bone formation in the distal part of the extremities. The hyperthyroidism in Graves' disease probably results from the presence of circulating stimulatory immunoglobulins directed against the TSH receptor on the thyroid cell. The pathogenesis of the other manifestations is unknown at present. Other nonstimulatory antibodies directed against other thyroid components such as thyroglobulin and microsomes are present in a significant proportion of patients, often in high titers. There is an increased incidence of other autoimmune disorders such as Addison's disease, and other autoimmune endocrinopathies, myasthenia gravis, and systemic lupus erythematosus.

Toxic nodular goiter is the second most common cause of hyperthyroidism. Within the thyroid gland are one or more autonomous nodules that hypersecrete thyroid hormones and cause TSH suppression and involution of the remaining normal thyroid tissue. If the autonomous tissue is in one area of the thyroid, a single toxic nodule results; if it is in more than one area, it leads to toxic multinodular goiter. The origin of toxic nodular goiter is at present unknown.

Subacute thyroiditis (see Painful Goiter), a presumed viral infection, causes an acute inflammation of the thyroid with polymorphonuclear infiltration and occasional giant-cell formation, rupture of the thyroid follicles, and discharge of stored thyroid hormones into the circulation, causing thyrotoxicosis. The disease

and the resulting thyrotoxicosis last a few weeks. A transient phase of hypothyroidism may follow until the regeneration of the follicles is complete, at which time euthyroidism is restored. The disease is self-limiting but may have a number of relapses and remissions.

Painless lymphocytic thyroiditis (transient silent thyroiditis) is an increasingly recognized entity of indeterminate origin. The thyroid gland shows follicular destruction and lymphocytic infiltration. As in subacute thyroiditis, hyperthyroidism results from follicular rupture and access of large amounts of stored hormone to the circulation. This is followed by transient hypothyroidism before euthyroidism is restored with follicular regeneration. The disease is transient and self-limiting and tends to undergo remissions and relapses.

Widely metastatic functioning follicular carcinoma of the thyroid is very rarely associated with hyperthyroidism.

Chronic ingestion, in supraphysiologic doses, of either or both the thyroid hormones, T_4 and T_3, can cause a thyrotoxic state, exogenous hyperthyroidism. Such ingestion may be inadvertent (iatrogenic) or surreptitious (factitial). Here the pituitary TSH secretion is suppressed, leading to involution and atrophy of the thyroid gland.

Very rarely, diffuse thyroid enlargement and hyperthyroidism can result from inappropriate excessive secretion of TSH by the anterior pituitary gland. The cause of this TSH hypersecretion may be a TSH-producing pituitary tumor or hyperplasia of indeterminate cause.

Exposure of some individuals to excess iodine (from bread and dairy product iodide supplementation, iodine-containing radiographic contrast media, and certain cardiac drugs, e.g., amiodarone and benziodarone) may lead to the development of iodide-induced thyrotoxicosis. Such individuals may or may not have an underlying thyroid disorder, e.g., nodular goiter or Graves' diathesis. The mechanism underlying development of iodide-induced thyrotoxicosis has not been established.

Hyperfunctioning ectopic thyroid tissue, either in dermoid tumors or teratomas of the ovary (struma ovarii) or in a lingual thyroid, is a very rare cause of thyrotoxicosis. HCG, a glycoprotein with an alpha subunit identical to that of TSH and with a distinctive beta subunit, possesses weak thyroid-stimulating activity. Trophoblastic disease such as choriocarcinoma, molar pregnancy, or embryonal carcinoma of the testes can produce excessive quantities of HCG and hyperstimulation of the thyroid, resulting in thyrotoxicosis.

CLINICAL PRESENTATION

The clinical manifestations of thyrotoxicosis are a composite of manifestations of the effects on tissue of excess thyroid hormones, which therefore are nonspecific and common to all causes of the syndrome, and manifestations specifically related to the cause of the syndrome and its associations.

Clinical Manifestations Related to All Types of Thyrotoxicosis

Thyrotoxicosis leads to an increased metabolic rate, excessive catabolism, and an increase in tissue sensitivity to catecholaminergic stimulation.

SIGNS

The patient is typically hyperkinetic and restless. The skin is warm, moist, and soft and the scalp hair is fine. There is a fine tremor of hands and fingers. Onycholysis (nail separation from nail bed–Plummer's nails) and palmar erythema may be seen. Sinus tachycardia is present even at rest and during sleep, and the pulse pressure is wide. The precordium is hyperactive and the heart sounds are loud and ringing. A functional systolic murmur and occasionally a scratchy systolic sound along the left sternal border (Lerman-Means scratch) may be heard. Cardiac arrhythmias are common and invariably supraventricular; atrial fibrillation and, less commonly, paroxysmal atrial tachycardia can develop, particularly in the older patient. High output failure may occur rarely and characteristically is resistant to standard treatment with digitalis and diuretics. It is important to remember that the cardiovascular manifestations may be the sole presentation of thyrotoxicosis. It is estimated that 10% of patients with otherwise unexplained atrial fibrillation have thyrotoxicosis as the cause of the arrhythmia. Muscle weakness and wasting may be obvious, especially in the proximal girdle muscles. Thyrotoxicosis of any cause, through enhanced sympathetic activity, leads to increased activity of Müller's muscle, resulting in decreased blinking, staring, lid retraction (the rim of sclera is exposed above the limbus), and lid lag (when the patient moves eyes from upward to downward gaze).

SYMPTOMS

Common presenting symptoms include easy fatigability, weight loss despite an increase in appetite, heat intolerance, increased sweating, palpitations, nervousness, emotional lability, a decrease in concentration ability and in performance, disturbed sleeping patterns, and inability to "unwind." Muscle weakness can be prominent, with difficulty in such activities as household chores involving the use of the humero-scapular muscles, climbing stairs, arising from the sitting position, and, rarely, hoarseness and difficulty in swallowing. Cutaneous manifestations particularly noted by affected women include a change in skin texture with increased smoothness and softness, and a change in texture of scalp hair, which becomes fine and resistant to hair styling. Occasionally a patient may complain of severe pruritus. Palpitations and dyspnea on exertion are prominent, and some patients may complain of symptoms of tachyarrhythmias. Appetite may become voracious. In most patients the increased caloric intake does not meet the excessive caloric expenditure, resulting in weight loss, but in a few patients intake may exceed the expenditure, leading to weight gain. Many patients complain of hyperdefecation with frequent passage of small amounts of well-formed stool. An increased tendency to symptomatic osteoporosis occurs particularly in middle-aged and elderly women. Because of changes in sex steroid-binding globulin and an increase in the ratio of free estrogen to testosterone, male patients may complain of decreased libido and potency and of gynecomastia, while female patients frequently may have menstrual irregularities with oligomenorrhea.

Clinical Manifestations Related to the Cause of Thyrotoxicosis

Graves's disease can occur in any age and either sex but characteristically affects female adults in the third and fourth decades. The patient may complain of a goiter or a feeling of tightness in the neck. Symptoms related to the characteristic infiltrative ophthalmopathy include redness of the eyes, swelling of the lids, a feeling of "sand" or irritation in the eyes, photophobia, and excessive tearing. In advanced cases, proptosis, diplopia, and inability to close the lids may develop, leading to corneal ulceration, infection, and decreased vision. One may find scleral injection, chemosis (edema of the subconjunctival space), proptosis, and impaired extraocular muscle function, especially limitation of upward gaze caused by tethering fibrosis of the inferior rectus and inferior oblique muscles. In advanced cases, corneal ulceration may result from proptosis and inability to close the eyelids. Optic nerve dysfunction leading to papilledema, optic atrophy, visual field abnormalities, and blindness may occur.

Symptoms of the other mesenchymal manifestations include skin rash, particularly over the anterior tibial areas, and bony tenderness in the distal extremities. The goiter in Graves' disease varies in size; it is usually two to three times the normal size but may be within the normal range in few patients. It is diffuse, smooth, soft to firm in consistency, mobile, and nontender. A bruit may be heard over the gland.

Pretibial myxedema and acropachy develop in about 5% of patients with Graves' disease. When they occur it is usually in those patients who have infiltrative ophthalmopathy. Pretibial myxedema usually affects the skin of the pretibial area. The affected skin is raised, erythematous, and indurated, and it has a peau d'orange appearance, first in plaques and later perhaps becoming confluent. Acropachy is associated with clubbing and bony swelling and tenderness over the distal extremities. Other associations of Graves' disease include lymphadenopathy and splenomegaly, and periodic hypokalemic paralysis, particularly in patients of Japanese origin. Some manifestations may be related to autoimmune phenomena that may occur in association with Graves' disease, including vitiligo, pernicious anemia, Addison's disease, diabetes mellitus, and myasthenia gravis.

Patients with toxic multinodular goiter are usually middle-aged and usually female, with a long history of multinodular goiter. The thyroid gland is enlarged, usually to a significant but variable degree. The gland is firm, irregular, nodular, mobile, and nontender. Cardiovascular and myopathic symptoms of thyrotoxicosis predominate in this age group. Tachycardia frequently with atrial fibrillation, congestive heart failure resistant to standard therapy, and weakness and wasting of muscle, frequently with loss of appetite rather than with hyperphagia, can dominate the picture (apathetic thyrotoxicosis). The nervous manifestations common in the young thyrotoxic patient with Graves' disease are less common with toxic nodular goiter. Because the goiter may be large, obstructive symptoms may be present with dysphagia and dysphonia. Hoarseness of the voice should suggest malignancy.

Toxic adenoma primarily affects females in their fourth to fifth decade. The patient usually gives a history of a long-standing, slowly progressive thyroid nodule. On examination of the thyroid, a single nodule greater than 3 cm in diameter that is firm, smooth, mobile, and nontender is found. The rest of the gland is characteristically not palpable.

In subacute thyroiditis the patient's primary complaints are related to the inflamed thyroid and consist of pain in the thyroid area often radiating to the jaw and ears, increased by swallowing and neck movement, and associated with exquisite tenderness of the enlarged thyroid. Systemic upset with malaise and fever is common. The gland is enlarged focally or diffusely and is exquisitely tender.

In painless thyroiditis the gland is normal in size or modestly enlarged, firm, painless, mobile, and nontender.

In patients with surreptitious thyroid hormone ingestion, no thyroid tissue is palpable in the neck.

Patients with a TSH-producing tumor may complain of visual abnormalities related to extrasellar extension of the pituitary tumor and manifestations of hypopituitarism related to deficiency of other pituitary hormones. The thyroid gland is diffusely and modestly enlarged, mobile, and nontender. Visual field defects and signs of hypopituitarism may be seen.

Patients with struma ovarii may complain of abdominal pain and swelling (ascites) and are found to have a pelvic mass. The thyroid gland is small.

Patients with trophoblastic disease have primary manifestations of the cause and a small goiter.

In metastatic follicular thyroid cancer there is usually a history of thyroid surgery related to the disease and evident metastatic disease in neck, lungs, and bones.

DIFFERENTIAL DIAGNOSIS

An anxiety state and neurasthenia have many features that resemble thyrotoxicosis, including fatigue, irritability, and palpitations in young female patients. Unlike in thyrotoxicosis, the hands are cool and clammy, the sleeping pulse rate is normal, there is usually no goiter, and thyroid function tests are always normal.

Diabetes mellitus may resemble thyrotoxicosis because of weight loss despite a good appetite, weakness and wasting, and occasional diarrhea. The diabetic patient may also have associated goiter caused by Hashimoto's thyroiditis. In addition, the thyrotoxic patient may have impaired carbohydrate tolerance. The diabetic patient has other diabetic stigmata, and the thyroid function tests are normal (or low if Hashimoto's thyroiditis is present).

Pheochromocytoma resembles thyrotoxicosis because of hypermetabolism and increased adrenergic activity. In pheochromocytoma, hypertension is present, and the patient does not have a goiter (unless medullary carcinoma of the thyroid in MEN II or III is associated). The thyroid function tests are normal and catecholamines and their metabolites are increased in plasma or urine.

Chronic obstructive pulmonary disease and cirrhosis of the liver have many features that raise the question of thyrotoxicosis. In both these entities, thyroid function tests are normal.

Thyrotoxicosis should enter into the differential diagnosis of tachyarrhythmias, congestive heart failure of indeterminate origin (particularly if resistant to standard therapy), myopathy, weight loss, chronic diarrhea, and osteoporosis, even though the typical features of presentation of thyrotoxicosis may be absent. Total and free serum thyroxine (or the free thyroxine index) should be obtained in all these patients.

Acute medical and surgical illness can cause certain alterations in thyroid physiology and circulating thyroid hormone levels. The physician needs to consider these changes when interpreting thyroid function tests in the presence of such an illness. These changes include high serum T_4 and low serum T_3 caused by decreased conversion of T_4 to T_3 by the peripheral tissues and continued secretion of TSH, and low TSH and blunted TSH response to TRH caused by inhibition of secretion of TSH. One can see that thyroid function tests in a euthyroid sick individual can raise the question of hyperthyroidism. Serum T_3 should be measured; if it is increased, one can safely make the diagnosis of hyperthyroidism. If the serum T_3 is normal, one cannot exclude the diagnosis of hyperthyroidism, and a TRH test should be done. If the TSH response is normal, the diagnosis of hyperthyroidism is excluded. A blunted TSH response to TRH is not helpful in the differential diagnosis. In this instance, it would be advisable to treat the patient temporarily as a hyperthyroid patient (with antithyroid drug and beta adrenergic blockers) and to reassess the thyroid function state after the resolution of the acute illness.

DIAGNOSTIC EVALUATION

The diagnostic approach has as its two goals to ascertain the presence of thyrotoxicosis and to determine its cause. The approaches are outlined in Figure 11–9.

Patient History and Physical Examination

In the history and physical examination, attention is paid to onset, duration, and course of the signs and symptoms; drug history, with particular attention to exposure to iodides (which may cause hyperthyroidism or may interfere with the interpretation of the I_{131} uptake), to thyroid hormones (for therapeutic purposes, or accessible from family, workplace, etc.), and to beta blockers (which may mask the signs and symptoms of thyrotoxicosis). Attention is paid also to systemic symptoms, fever, malaise, or local symptoms (pain and tenderness may point to subacute thyroiditis); recent miscarriage or abortion (trophoblastic disease) or known pelvic mass (struma ovarii); family history (familial autoimmune thyroid or other endocrine disease); remissions and relapses (Graves' disease, subacute thyroiditis, silent thyroiditis); long history of goiter (nodular goiter); manifestations of ophthalmopathy or dermopathy (Graves' diathesis); or pituitary tumor (TSH-producing pituitary tumor).

On examination, attention is paid to the presence or absence of goiter and, if present, to the characteristics of goiter—whether it is diffuse, nodular, painful, or tender. A search should be made for findings of ophthalmopathy or dermopathy and for a pelvic mass.

Diagnostic Studies

LABORATORY TESTS

General. Routine laboratory studies may reveal a mild degree of anemia, granulocytopenia, and lymphocytosis. The serum calcium may be mildly elevated. Liver function abnormalities may be present (mild elevation in SGOT, alkaline phosphatase, and bilirubin). The electrocardiogram shows sinus tachycardia. Urinary 17-hydroxysteroids may be increased (increased hepatic cortisol degradation) but the plasma cortisol remains normal.

Specific (Table 11–13).

Circulating Thyroid Hormone Levels. The thyroid gland produces two hormones, thyroxine (T_4) and triiodothyronine (T_3). In 80% of thyrotoxic patients both of these hormones are produced in excess. In about 20% of patients, however, the thyrotoxic gland produces T_3 preferentially. Because of their availability, serum T_4 measurements by radioimmunoassay are the most commonly used tests in the diagnosis of thyrotoxicosis.

It is important to remember that the thyroid hormones are present in the circulation in two forms: a form bound to binding proteins (thyroxin-binding globulin, albumin, and prealbumin) representing 99.95% of T_4 and 99.5% of T_3, and the free, biologically active form representing 0.05% of T_4 and 0.5% of T_3. While circulating T_4 is derived exclusively from the thyroid gland, serum T_3 is derived from two sources: 20% from thyroid secretion and 80% from deiodination of T_4 to T_3 by peripheral tissue deiodinase. Taking these facts into consideration, one can deduce that the levels of circulating T_4 and T_3 depend on a number of variables, the two major ones being glandular hormone production and the quantity and binding capacity of the circulating binding proteins. Peripheral tissue activity and hormone clearance are important variables in euthyroid sick syndrome.

The two major causes of an elevated total T_4 (TT_4) are hyperthyroidism and states associated with increased binding globulin. The differentiation is made by assessing the binding protein levels or capacity by direct measurement (radioimmunoassay) or indirect measurement (the T_3 RU) or by measurement of the free, biologically active fraction of the hormone (FT_4). The most common tests used to document hyperthyroidism are the serum total thyroxine and the T_3 resin

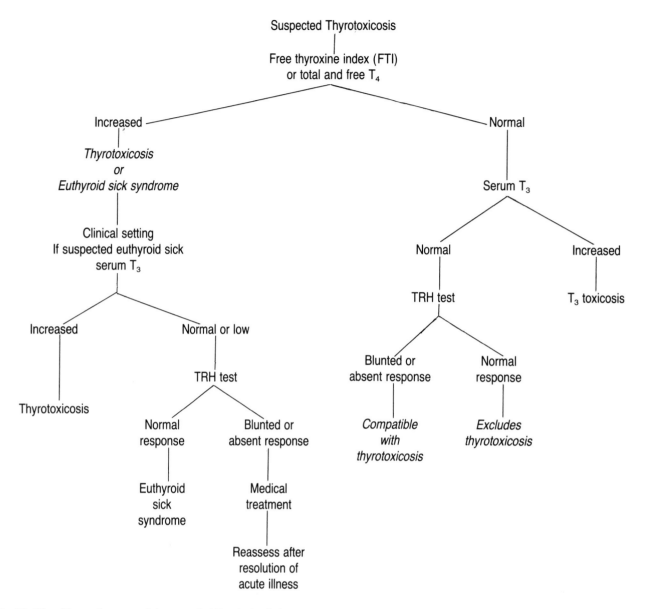

Fig. 11–9A. Diagnostic approach to suspected thyrotoxicosis I.

uptake. For the sake of convenience, the serum TT_4 and the RT_3U have been combined by arithmetic multiplication to give the so-called free thyroxine index (FTI). In most clinical situations, the FTI closely parallels the level of the free, biologically active T_4 and is therefore considered by many authorities to be the best single test of thyroid function. An increased total and free serum thyroxine or an increased free thyroxine index are virtually diagnostic of hyperthyroidism.

Serum triiodothyronine (T_3) should be measured in a patient suspected of having thyrotoxicosis but with normal TT_4 and FT_4 (or FTI). Elevated serum T_3 in this setting, in the absence of increased TBG binding capacity, is diagnostic of T_3 toxicosis.

Tests of Thyroid Autonomy. If the levels of free

thyroxine index and serum T_3 are borderline, a TRH test or a T_3 suppression test may be performed. A blunted TSH response to TRH or failure of T_3 suppression in a patient suspected of having thyrotoxicosis documents autonomy of the thyroid gland and provides strong support for the diagnosis of thyrotoxicosis.

In a normal individual, TSH secretion usually rises in response to the administration of TRH. In the usual case of thyrotoxicosis, increased thyroid hormone levels lead to suppression of pituitary TSH secretion and blunting of TSH responsiveness to exogenous TRH. Elderly euthyroid patients and euthyroid patients with autonomous hormone secretion, e.g., simple nodular goiter, will also have blunted TSH responsiveness to TRH. A normal TSH response to TRH excludes the

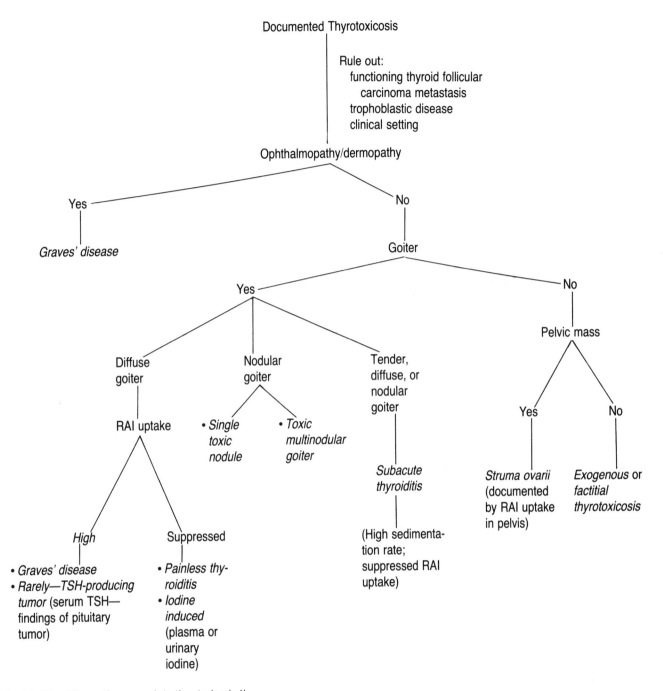

Fig. 11–9B.   Diagnostic approach to thyrotoxicosis II.

diagnosis of hyperthyroidism, whereas blunted response is compatible with, but alone is not diagnostic of, thyrotoxicosis. The test has no significant side effects.

An alternative test to assess autonomy of the gland is the T_3 or T_4 suppression test. Every 8 hours for 7 days 25 μg of T_3 is given by mouth (or, alternatively, T_4 is given as a single dose of 3 mg by mouth). A radioactive iodine uptake is done before and on the seventh day of T_3 administration. A normal suppres-

sion response is a decrease of the radioactive iodine uptake by 50% or more. Absence of such normal suppression indicates autonomy and can be seen in hyperthyroidism and in euthyroid patients with autonomous thyroid tissue, e.g., nodular goiter and euthyroid Graves' disease. This test has the disadvantages of involving administration of potent hormones (which can increase thyrotoxicosis and be hazardous in those patients with cardiovascular disease) and requiring two radioactive iodine uptake tests (contraindicated in pregnancy and in childhood). It has been supplanted by the TRH test.

Radioiodine (I$_{131}$) Uptake. This is an index of thyroid activity. A tracer dose is given and accumulation of I$_{131}$ in the thyroid gland is measured at 2, 4, 6, or 24 hours. The uptake is influenced by dietary iodine intake and the iodide pool. Each lab must establish a local normal range.

For clinical purposes the I$_{131}$ uptake is routinely measured at 24 hours. It is elevated in patients with Graves' disease, in most patients with nodular goiter, and in those with TSH-producing pituitary tumor. It may be normal in some toxic nodular goiter patients and in those with trophoblastic disease. The I$_{131}$ uptake is suppressed in thyrotoxicosis associated with thyroiditis, thyrotoxicosis-facticia, iodide-induced thyrotoxicosis, struma ovarii, and functioning metastases from thyroid carcinoma.

The utility of the I$_{131}$ in the diagnosis of thyrotoxic state is in identifying those forms of thyrotoxicosis associated with suppressed uptake and, in equivocal cases, as a part of the T$_3$ suppression test.

Radioisotopic Scanning. This is useful in the thyrotoxic patient to delineate a "hot nodule" in toxic nodular goiter, ectopic sites such as stroma ovarii, and metastatic follicular carcinoma causing thyrotoxicosis. A scan should not be done in patients with diffuse thyroid enlargement because it provides little information beyond that obtained by careful palpation of the thyroid gland.

Special Tests. Pituitary secretion of TSH will be suppressed in all cases of hyperthyroidism (except those caused by inappropriate TSH secretion). The commercial assays of serum TSH presently available are insufficiently sensitive to distinguish between the low but normal and the subnormal serum TSH levels in thyrotoxic patients. In the future, advent of highly sensitive assays for serum TSH determination may replace serum T$_4$ and T$_3$ as primary screening tests for thyrotoxicosis.

Plasma iodide measurement is useful in distinguishing between the various diagnostic alternatives in patients with thyrotoxicosis and low I$_{131}$ uptake. The normal value for plasma iodide is below 1 μg/dl. Values greater than 5 μg/dl indicate iodide contamination of the body iodide pool.

Antibodies against the TSH receptors include thyroid-stimulating immunoglobulins (TSI) and thyrotropin-displacing activity (TDA) and are found in 85 to 90% of patients with Graves' disease. They can be used to confirm the presence of Graves' diathesis. A positive test is not necessarily indicative of the presence of hyperthyroidism. These tests are not widely available yet.

A small amount of thyroglobulin (TG) is normally secreted from the thyroid and can easily be detected with current radioimmunoassay techniques. Serum thyroglobulin can be valuable in differentiating thyrotoxicosis facticia (when the serum TG levels are suppressed) from other causes of thyrotoxicosis in which there is very low radioactive iodine uptake (where serum TG is normal).

Diagnostic Approach

The first step is to obtain a serum TT$_4$ and FT$_4$ or an FTI. The causes of elevated values of these parameters are outlined in Table 11–13. Elevated values are diagnostic of thyrotoxicosis if one excludes the euthyroid sick syndrome and the rare entities of familial disalbuminemic hyperthyroxinemia or the presence of anti-T$_4$ antibodies. Normal values in a patient suspected of thyrotoxicosis should prompt measurement of serum T$_3$. An elevated serum T$_3$ in the absence of causes of increased TBG points to T$_3$ toxicosis. A normal serum T$_3$, however, does not exclude the diagnosis. Serum T$_3$ may be normal in thyrotoxic patients because of decreased deiodination of T$_4$ to T$_3$ (in patients with concomitant severe illness, liver disease, or malnutrition, in those on steroids or propranolol, or in iodide-induced thyrotoxicosis). When the complicating illness subsides, serum T$_3$ levels become elevated again.

In patients with equivocal thyroid hormone measurements, the TRH test should be done. A normal TSH response to TRH excludes the diagnosis of thyrotoxicosis, whereas a blunted or absent response provides strong support for the diagnosis. The advent of highly sensitive serum TSH assays may replace the TRH test in the diagnosis of hyperthyroidism in the future.

Once thyrotoxicosis is confirmed, the next step is to identify its cause. Major reliance is placed on the history and the physical examination, particularly as they relate to the nature and the characteristics of any goiter and the presence or absence of evidence of Graves' mesenchymal manifestations (infiltrative ophthalmopathy or dermopathy).

The diagnosis of Graves' disease is confirmed if a thyrotoxic patient has infiltrative ophthalmopathy or dermopathy. If these mesenchymal manifestations are not present, the characteristics of the goiter become crucial in identifying the origin of the thyrotoxic state.

If the thyrotoxic patient has a diffuse goiter, the possibilities are Graves' disease, painless lymphocytic thyroiditis, and the rare TSH-producing pituitary tumor. A suppressed I$_{131}$ uptake in a patient with diffuse, nontender goiter is compatible with painless thyroiditis if exposure to excess iodide is excluded (in this case the plasma and the urinary iodides are increased). An increased I_{131} uptake is almost always diagnostic of Graves' disease. In the rare TSH-producing pituitary tumor, serum TSH is increased (in contradistinction to all other causes of thyrotoxicosis, in which the serum TSH is suppressed) and the patient has radiologic evidence of pituitary tumor.

If the gland has a single palpable nodule greater than 3 cm in diameter or if the gland is large and multinodular, the diagnosis of toxic nodular goiter is made.

If the patient has a painful tender goiter, often with systemic upset such as fever and malaise, the diagnosis of subacute thyroiditis is very likely. It is confirmed by a high sedimentation rate and suppressed I_{131} uptake.

If the thyrotoxic patient has no identifiable goiter, the diagnosis of factitial thyrotoxicosis or struma ovarii needs to be considered. A pelvic mass favors struma ovarii; a suppressed I_{131} uptake in the neck but uptake and localization in the pelvis is diagnostic. If the uptake is suppressed and no ectopic sites of uptake are delineated, the diagnosis of factitial thyrotoxicosis should be seriously considered. Serum thyroglobulin (TG) is suppressed in thyrotoxicosis factitia.

The diagnosis of functioning metastatic thyroid malignancy and HCG-producing trophoblastic disease can be made without difficulty on the basis of the clinical setting.

The diagnosis of iodide-induced thyrotoxicosis is supported by a history of iodide exposure, a suppressed I_{131} uptake, and high plasma or urinary iodides and it is confirmed if the disorder resolves when the exogenous iodide is withdrawn.

Special Considerations

Thyrotoxic Crisis or Storm. The clinical picture in a thyrotoxic crisis is a dramatic increase in all the symptoms and signs of thyrotoxicosis. Crisis occurs rarely in untreated or inadequately treated patients and is precipitated by surgical emergency or complicating acute medical illness, usually sepsis. It may also occur postoperatively in thyrotoxic patients who are poorly prepared for surgery. It is characterized by fever to 41°C (106° F), tachycardia, extreme restlessness and irritability, vomiting, diarrhea, hypotension, delirium, and coma. It can be associated with acute adrenocortical insufficiency. The differential diagnosis includes postoperative hemorrhage, sepsis, or transfusion or drug reaction. When it is suspected, blood should be drawn for circulating thyroid hormone measurements, and treatment for thyrotoxic crisis should be instituted promptly because the entity has a very high mortality rate.

Postpartum Thyrotoxicosis. One third of the patients with this increasingly recognized entity have typical Graves' disease, another third have transient thyrotoxicosis with increased radioactive iodine uptake, and another third have transient thyrotoxicosis with suppressed radioactive iodine uptake. The thyrotoxicosis may be self-limited to a few weeks or a few months and may be followed by a period of hypothyroidism before gland function returns to normal. The whole process may recur after another pregnancy.

EUTHYROID DIFFUSE AND NODULAR GOITER

DEFINITION

Goiter refers to enlargement of the thyroid gland. From the clinical standpoint, it can be given an "anatomic classification" based on the structure of the thyroid and a "functional classification" based on the state of thyroid function, divided into hypothyroid, euthyroid, or hyperthyroid goiters. This chapter will deal with the clinical manifestations and diagnosis of euthyroid diffuse or nodular goiter.

PATHOPHYSIOLOGIC CONSIDERATIONS

Euthyroid goiter can result from several pathogenetic mechanisms.

Partial interference with thyroid hormone biosynthesis and release, from whatever cause, leads in sequence to an initial decrease in thyroid hormone's circulating levels, a decrease in negative feedback, an increase in pituitary TSH secretion, enlargement of the thyroid and compensatory stimulation of thyroid hormone biosynthesis, and restoration of euthyroidism. The goiter is initially diffuse but in long-standing cases tends to become nodular.

Inflammation of the thyroid or stimulation of thyroid activity by a non-TSH mediated stimulus, e.g., thyroid-stimulating antibodies, can also cause euthyroid goiter, as occurs in Graves' disease and Hashimoto's thyroiditis. The functional state of the thyroid reflects the net effect of the variable impairment of function by the thyroid inflammatory process and the stimulation of hormonogenesis by the non-TSH mediators. Such a patient may, therefore, be euthyroid or may show varying degrees of hyper- or hypothyroidism.

Euthyroid goiter can also result from diffuse infiltration of the thyroid gland by a chronic inflammatory or degenerative process (e.g., Riedel's thyroiditis, sar-

Table 11–15. Causes of Diffuse Goiter

Simple goiter
Hashimoto's thyroiditis
Euthyroid Graves' disease
Congenital dyshormonogenesis
Goitrogens
   Drugs
      Antithyroid
      Iodides
      Lithium
      Sulfonamides
      Sulfonylureas
      Methylxanthines
      Aminoglutethimide
      Ethionamide
   Diet
      Brassica family
      Soybeans
      Iodides (seaweed)
      Contaminated water
Iodide deficiency
Riedel's thyroiditis
Infiltrative disease (e.g., sarcoidosis, amyloidosis)
Lymphoma

coidosis, or amyloidosis) or by a neoplastic process (primary or metastatic). The causes of euthyroid diffuse goiter are outlined in Table 11–15, and those of euthyroid nodular goiter in Table 11–16.

Simple goiter is the most common cause of diffuse or multinodular euthyroid goiter that does not result from an inflammatory or neoplastic process. Its prevalence shows marked geographic variation. The cause is unknown, although it is likely that genetic factors, minor degrees of iodine deficiency, a thyroid enzymatic defect, or exposure to goitrogens are important in its development. Initially the gland is diffusely enlarged and may pass through cycles of activation and regression resulting from changing needs for thyroid hormone or from variation in the activity of the biosynthetic process. For reasons unknown, the phases of activity and inactivity ultimately affect the gland nonhomogeneously, leading to the production of nodules. Simple goiter is always more common in females (in a ratio of females to males of from between 5 and

Table 11–16. Causes of Nodular Goiter

Single nodule (see Single Thyroid Nodule)
Multinodular
   Simple
      ?Iodide deficiency
      Goitrogens
      Congenital dyshormonogenesis
   Hashimoto's thyroiditis
   Lymphoma
   Carcinoma
      Primary
      Metastatic

10 to 1). Diffuse goiter is commonly seen during adolescence or pregnancy, whereas simple multinodular goiter rarely presents before middle age.

Chronic Hashimoto's thyroiditis is a common chronic progressive autoimmune inflammatory disease of the thyroid. It usually affects the gland diffusely and uncommonly may cause focal involvement. It can affect any age and sex but is most frequently seen in middle-aged females. A family history of autoimmune thyroid disease is common. The dominant clinical manifestation is a diffuse asymptomatic goiter of gradual onset. The patient may be euthyroid or hypothyroid, depending on the degree of inflammation and scarring and on response to compensatory TSH secretion. Occasionally the disease can present with hyperthyroidism. (See Thyrotoxicosis.)

Graves' disease (see Thyrotoxicosis) may present infrequently with diffuse euthyroid goiter with or without the other Graves'-specific mesenchymal infiltrative manifestations of ophthalmopathy or dermopathy.

Thyroidal dyshormonogenesis refers to defects in the enzymatic biosynthetic process of thyroid hormone formation, which can be inherited as an autosomal recessive trait and can cause varying degrees of impairment of thyroid hormone synthesis. If the defect is partial, the compensatory increase in TSH secretion causes a goiter, and euthyroidism is maintained. If the impairment is more severe, goiter and the hypothyroid state result.

Iodine is the essential substrate for thyroid hormone synthesis; though iodine deficiency has been corrected in developed countries by supplementation of dietary sources with iodine, it still exists in many areas throughout the world (for example, South America, the Himalayas, and central Africa). The goiter is initially diffuse but may become nodular. In most instances the euthyroid state is maintained, but in a few affected individuals hypothyroidism may ensue.

Goitrogens are a group of exogenous substances that have the capacity to inhibit thyroid hormone biosynthesis. This inhibition leads to compensatory TSH hypersecretion and development of a goiter. In most individuals, a euthyroid state is maintained. In a few patients, however, particularly those with decreased thyroid reserve caused by chronic thyroiditis, iodine deficiency, or surgically or radioiodine-treated Graves' disease, hypothyroidism may result. Table 11–15 lists the iatrogenic and naturally occurring goitrogens.

Riedel's thyroiditis is a rare disorder of unknown cause characterized by sclerosing fibrous infiltration of the thyroid gland and extrathyroidal tissues. It leads to an extremely firm to hard goiter and ultimately to hypothyroidism. The spread of the process outside the thyroid can affect the surrounding muscles of the neck and the trachea, leading to obstructive manifestations of dyspnea, stridor, dysphagia, and hoarseness of the voice. There may be association with retroperitoneal fibrosis and sclerosing cholangitis. Riedel's thyroiditis may be difficult to differentiate from carcinoma of the thyroid, and exploration and biopsy may be needed for diagnosis and management of the obstruction.

Lymphoma and primary or metastatic carcinoma are rare cause of diffuse or multinodular goiters. (See Single Thyroid Nodule.)

CLINICAL PRESENTATION

Signs

In diffuse goiter the thyroid enlargement is variable, usually two to three times the normal size, and the goiter is usually soft to firm, nontender, and mobile during deglutition. In nodular goiter the enlargement is asymmetrical, and the nodules of variable size and consistency. Occasionally such a gland feels irregular and lobulated but lacks distinct nodules. Rarely a nodule may feel hard because of calcification that occurs after hemorrhage into a nodule. The physician should be alerted to the probability of malignancy by a dominant nodule (especially if it is rapidly growing), fixation of the goiter to surrounding structures, hoarseness of the voice, or presence of cervical lymphadenopathy. In chronic Hashimoto's thyroiditis, the goiter usually involves the gland diffusely in a lobulated or bosselated manner, is rubbery in consistency, and may have a prominent pyramidal lobe. Less often, Hashimoto's thyroiditis may present with focal enlargement of the thyroid gland or a rapid diffuse enlargement that may be painful and tender. The trachea, particularly in nodular goiter, may be displaced to one side. Encroachment on the superior mediastinum may occur with large goiters associated with retrosternal extension. In such individuals, elevation of the arms above the head results in suffusion of the face, dizziness, and occasional syncope (Pemberton's sign). In patients with euthyroid Graves' disease, other Graves' mesenchymal manifestations of ophthalmopathy or dermopathy may be apparent.

Symptoms

Patients with euthyroid goiter are usually asymptomatic, and the goiter, often of many years' duration, is first noted by relatives or friends or by the attending physician during a general examination. If the goiter is moderate to large in size, the patient may complain of a tight sensation in the neck, of social embarrassment, or of obstructive manifestations of dysphagia or stridor. Hoarseness of the voice generally indicates

malignancy of the thyroid or an infiltrative disease, such as Riedel's thyroiditis. Rarely, hemorrhage into a cyst or a nodule of a multinodular goiter may cause painful tender swelling of a few days' duration.

DIAGNOSTIC EVALUATION

Patient History and Physical Examination

Workup of a patient with euthyroid diffuse or nodular goiter should begin with a careful history and physical examination. Important is information regarding the mode of onset and rate of change in size of the goiter; the presence of pain, tenderness, or obstructive or infiltrative manifestations; the clinical assessment of thyroid function; the presence of Graves' ophthalmopathy or dermopathy; a drug history; and family history.

Diagnostic Studies

The objective of laboratory testing is to assess the goiter anatomically and functionally.

An anatomic assessment of the nature, size, and extent of the goiter includes a chest x-ray to look for evidence of retrosternal extension, tracheal deviation or compression, and calcification within the goiter. In addition, a barium swallow with esophageal roentgenography may be of additional help in some cases. A thyroid scintiscan may show a patchy or diffuse uptake and aids in the characterization of a dominant nodule in a multinodular goiter (see Single Thyroid Nodule). If a retrosternal extension is suspected, scintiscan is preferably done with I_{131} because the gamma rays from technetium and I_{123} may not be strong enough to penetrate the sternum. Finally, fine needle aspiration cytology or open biopsy may be needed for diagnosis, particularly if a neoplastic process is suspected.

Functional assessment, based on the evaluation of the thyroid function state, is best done by measuring total and free serum thyroxine, or by performing a total thyroxine and resin T_3 uptake and calculating the free thyroxine index. If hypothyroidism is suspected, a serum TSH should be obtained. On the other hand, if hyperthyroidism is suspected, a serum T_3 may be helpful to rule out T_3 hyperthyroidism if the levels of thyroxine are borderline or normal. Tests of thyroid regulation, a TRH test, or a T_3 suppression test help in demonstrating autonomy. In multinodular goiter there may be a tendency for hyperthyroidism of the apathetic type to develop later in life (see Thyrotoxicosis). A radioactive iodine uptake is usually not helpful in the evaluation of diffuse or nodular euthyroid goiters though it is certainly of importance in the differential diagnosis of a hyperthyroid goiter. Antithyroid antibodies are helpful in the diagnosis of Hashimoto's thyroiditis and Graves' disease. In these autoimmune thyroid diseases, antibodies present in the serum bind to various antigens of thyroid tissue. The most important of these antibodies is the thyroid antimicrosomal antibody. Titers in excess of 1/100 are significant and are found in 95% of patients with Hashimoto's thyroiditis, 55% of patients with Graves' disease, and about 10% of adults with no apparent thyroid disease. Antithyroglobulin antibodies are also present in the serum of about 60 to 70% of patients with Hashimoto's thyroiditis. TSI and TDA are antibodies directed against the thyroid TSH receptor. They are present in the serum of patients with Graves' disease, and their presence provides support for the diagnosis of Graves' diathesis.

Diagnostic Approach

The approach to the diagnosis of diffuse and multinodular goiter is outlined in Figures 11–10 and 11–11.

The first step in the diagnostic process is the assessment of thyroid function. If the patient with a diffuse or nodular goiter has thyroid hypofunction or hyperfunction, the evaluation proceeds along the same steps as for hypothyroidism or thyrotoxicosis. (See Figs. 11–7 and 11–9.)

If the patient has a euthyroid diffuse goiter, attention is paid to a history of exposure to goitrogens and to the onset and course of the goiter.

If there is a history of exposure to a goitrogen, a tentative diagnosis of goitrogen-induced goiter is made. Resolution of the goiter on discontinuation of the exposure to the goitrogen confirms the diagnosis.

If there is no history of exposure to a goitrogen and the goiter is of gradual onset and slow progression, the differential diagnosis includes euthyroid Graves' disease, Hashimoto's thyroiditis, and simple goiter. The diagnosis of euthyroid Graves' goiter depends upon the presence of ophthalmopathy or dermopathy, thyroid autonomy as documented by a TRH test or a T_3 suppression test, or thyroid-stimulating immunoglobulins in the patient's serum. The diagnosis of Hashimoto's thyroiditis is entertained in the presence of a characteristic bosselated goiter, other autoimmune disease entities, and strongly positive thyroid antibody titers. Rarely, tissue diagnosis is needed for confirmation. The diagnosis of simple diffuse goiter is supported by occurrence in adolescence or pregnancy; by absence of mesenchymal manifestations of Graves' disease, thyroid autonomy, thyroid antibodies, and thyroid stimulators; and by spontaneous resolution of the goiter in a few months to a few years.

If the diffuse goiter is of rapid onset and progression,

diagnostic considerations include Hashimoto's thyroiditis and lymphoma. Thyroid antibodies in high titers are typical of Hashimoto's thyroiditis. If these antibodies are absent or are present only in a low titers, a radioactive iodine uptake should be obtained. A normal or increased radioactive iodine uptake favors Hashimoto's thyroiditis. The diagnosis of lymphoma of the thyroid rests on biopsy of thyroid tissue.

Riedel's thyroiditis always raises the suspicion of malignancy because of its hard consistency and signs of infiltration of the extrathyroidal structures. Evidence of mediastinal or retroperitoneal fibrosis favors a diagnosis of Riedel's thyroiditis. The definitive diagnosis rests on surgical exploration and biopsy. The diagnosis of amyloidosis or sarcoidosis is suspected in the presence of other evidence of the systemic disease. Biopsy may be necessary for confirmation.

If the goiter is multinodular and has a dominant nodule, the diagnostic approach is similar to that of a single thyroid nodule. (See Single Thyroid Nodule.)

If the multinodular goiter is associated with features suggestive of malignancy (for example, hard consistency, fixation, hoarseness of the voice, or the presence of cervical nodes), tissue examination is mandatory. Otherwise, the differential diagnosis of a multinodular goiter rests between simple multinodular goiter and Hashimoto's thyroiditis. The presence of associated autoimmune endocrinopathies or systemic diseases and thyroid antibodies in high titers are characteristic of Hashimoto's thyroiditis. Biopsy is not needed for this differential diagnosis because the two disorders are benign, and the exact diagnosis is not essential for management.

SINGLE THYROID NODULE

DEFINITION

Single thyroid nodule refers to a single discrete mass identified in the thyroid gland. It is variable in size, location within the gland, consistency, function, and its clinical implications. Thyroid nodules occur in 2 to 4% of the adult population and are twice as common in females than males.

PATHOPHYSIOLOGIC CONSIDERATIONS

Clinically, thyroid nodules can be classified as single (solitary) or multinodular. It should be noted that

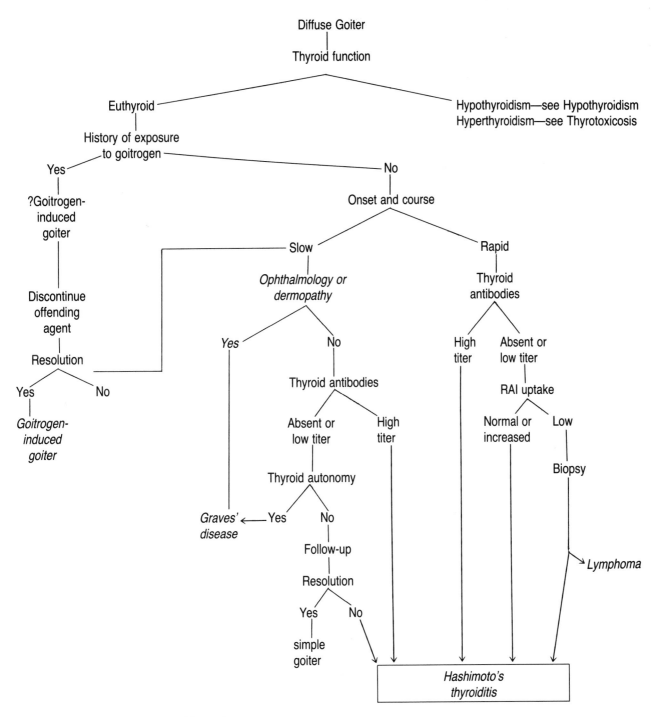

Fig. 11–10. Diagnostic approach to diffuse goiter.

a thyroid gland with a clinically discrete solitary nodule is often found to be multinodular upon radioisotopic scanning, ultrasonography, or surgery. The clinical classification is very helpful, however, because a gland with a solitary nodule is more likely to harbor a malignancy than multinodular glands are. The causes of single thyroid nodule are outlined in Table 11–17.

Adenomas account for the majority of benign sol-

itary nodules. They are usually microfollicular but can be colloidal, macrofollicular, fetal, embryonal, or Hürthle cell in type. Follicular adenomas can function and produce T_4, T_3 or both, occasionally leading to a thyrotoxic state.

Cysts can develop within a thyroid adenoma by central degeneration or by hemorrhage into an adenoma with subsequent liquefaction of the hematoma.

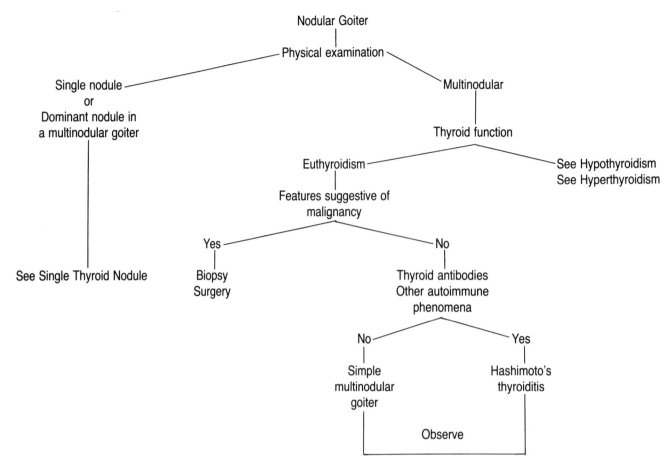

Fig. 11–11. Diagnostic approach to nodular goiter.

Focal thyroiditis, multinodular goiter with a single dominant nodule, remnant hyperplasia following radioiodine or surgical management of certain thyroid disorders, and infiltrative diseases of the thyroid (for example, amyloid) can present as solitary nodules.

Neoplastic diseases of the thyroid can be primary, i.e., originating in the gland itself, or metastatic, i.e., arising from malignancies of extrathyroidal tissues. The primary thyroid malignancies are classified according to the cell of origin into follicular types, which can be differentiated (papillary and follicular carcinoma) or undifferentiated (anaplastic carcinoma); a parafollicular C cell type (medullary carcinoma); or a lymphocyte cell type (lymphoma). Because of a rich blood supply the thyroid is a common site of metastases from malignancies of the kidney, pancreas, esophagus, rectum, lung, melanoma, etc. Clinical metastatic thyroid disease is, however, rare.

Papillary carcinoma is the most common type, accounting for more than 60% of all thyroid cancers. It can occur at any age but characteristically affects young patients. Females are affected two to three times more often than males. The disease usually runs an

indolent course. Pathologically it is composed of closely packed cells arranged in layers covering fibrovascular stalk with little attempt to form follicles, it is not encapsulated, and it may be multifocal. Typically it spreads by lymphatics to the regional cervical lymph nodes and by local invasion. Hematogenous dissemination is rare. Papillary cancers do not have the ability to synthesize thyroid hormones and do not lead to thyroid dysfunction. The affected patient may present with a solitary thyroid nodule, with cervical lymphadenopathy without a clinically apparent thyroid mass, with recent onset of enlargement of one area of long-standing nodular goiter, especially in elderly patients, and, rarely, with fine stippled calcifications in the thyroid area on neck x-rays caused by calcium-containing psammoma bodies.

Follicular carcinoma accounts for about 25% of thyroid cancer and usually affects individuals in middle age, more frequently females. It is usually single, encapsulated, and composed of follicles of varying size and differentiation. It spreads especially to bones and lung, characteristically by the hematogenous route. Malignant follicular tissue retains some ability to form

Table 11–17. Causes of Single Thyroid Nodule

Benign
  Adenoma
    Follicular
    Colloid
    Macrofollicular
    Fetal
    Embryonal
    Hürthle cell
  Cysts
  Focal thyroiditis
  Dominant nodule in a multinodular goiter
  Remnant hyperplasia, postsurgical or postradioiodide therapy
  Infiltrative (e.g., amyloid)
Malignant
  Primary
    Thyroid follicle
      Differentiated
        Papillary
        Follicular
      Undifferentiated
        Anaplastic
    Parafollicular–C cell
      Medullary carcinoma
  Secondary
    Metastatic (e.g., kidney, pancreas)
  Lymphoma

thyroid hormones. A patient who has follicular thyroid carcinoma may present with a solitary thyroid nodule, with effects of metastatic disease (e.g., bone pain or fracture) or, rarely, with thyrotoxicosis caused by excessive thyroid hormone formation by widespread follicular metastatic disease.

Anaplastic carcinoma accounts for less than 10% of thyroid cancers and characteristically affects middle-aged and elderly patients, females more than males. It is a rapidly growing, invasive, undifferentiated cancer that spreads by local invasion, by lymphatics, and through the circulation, and it is fatal within 1 year of diagnosis. It can present with a rapidly enlarging, sometimes painful, tender thyroid mass, with local invasive manifestations including hoarseness of the voice (caused by recurrent laryngeal palsy), stridor (tracheal compression), dysphagia (esophageal compression), or ulceration of the overlying skin, and with metastatic manifestations, e.g., cervical lymphadenopathy.

Medullary carcinoma of the thyroid is a distinctive thyroid malignancy that arises from the parafollicular C cells and accounts for about 5% of all thyroid malignancies. It usually occurs in a sporadic form (80%) or as an autosomal dominant familial form (20%). Pathologically, it is characterized by the presence of neoplastic parafollicular cells with amyloid deposits. It spreads by local invasion or by lymphatic or hematogenous routes. The parafollicular cells have a dis-

tinctive endocrine function: they all produce excess calcitonin, and some may produce excess ACTH, prostaglandin, serotonin, and other amines. Medullary carcinoma of the thyroid may be associated with hyperplasia or neoplasia of the adrenal medulla and parathyroid glands in an autosomal dominant familial syndrome known as Sipple's syndrome or multiple endocrine neoplasia. This is subdivided into two subtypes: type II, in which the patient has a normal phenotype, and type IIB (or type III), in which the patient has a marfanoid habitus, mucosal neuromas, and ganglioneuromatosis of the gastrointestinal tract. Medullary carcinoma can present with nodular goiter, metastatic disease, ectopic humoral syndromes (e.g., carcinoid, Cushing's syndrome, or watery diarrhea), and other manifestations of multiple endocrine neoplasia type II or III. It can be detected through family screening of a patient within a kindred of MEN II and III.

Lymphoma of the thyroid may occur as a primary extranodal form of malignant lymphoma. It accounts for less than 1% of all thyroid malignancies and usually affects middle-aged or elderly women. The usual presentation is of a rapidly enlarging and usually painless firm thyroid mass.

CLINICAL PRESENTATION

Signs

The principal signs are those related to the nodule itself and include size, consistency, surface characteristics, mobility or fixation, and absence or presence of tenderness. Careful palpation of the rest of the thyroid gland may reveal other nodules. The neck is examined for tracheal deviation and cervical lymph node enlargement. Note is taken of the absence or presence of hoarseness, stridor, or dysphagia. Signs of metastasis may be noted on the general exam. In some patients, signs of association of medullary carcinoma, including mucosal neuromas and marfanoid habitus may be seen. The blood pressure should be specifically checked to ascertain or rule out associated pheochromocytoma. A vocal cord check may reveal paresis or fixation of a vocal cord.

Symptoms

The patient may be asymptomatic, the nodule having been noted by the spouse, friends, or relatives, or discovered incidentally by the physician during a general examination. Infrequently the patient seeks medical attention because of a history of radiation exposure or as a part of family screening for multiple endocrine neoplasia type II or III. When symptomatic, the patient may complain of pain or tenderness in the thyroid area (caused by hemorrhage into the nodule or anaplastic carcinoma), hoarseness, stridor or dysphagia (caused by infiltration of the surrounding tissues by malignancy), or cervical lymphadenopathy, bone pain or fracture, abdominal pain, etc. (related to metastasis). Infrequently the presentations are with symptoms referable to hyperthyroidism (toxic nodule or metastatic follicular carcinoma), hypothyroidism (destruction of the gland by inflammatory or neoplastic process), ectopic humoral syndromes associated with medullary carcinoma (carcinoid, ectopic ACTH syndrome, etc.), or associations of medullary cancer (pheochromocytoma or hyperparathyroidism).

DIFFERENTIAL DIAGNOSIS

Nonthyroid neck masses usually do not pose difficulty in the differential diagnosis because, unlike thyroid masses, they do not move with deglutination. It is important to remember, however, that the thyroid mass may lose this feature if fixed to the surrounding structures by the underlying disease.

Parathyroid adenomas, carcinomas, and cysts are very rare and are frequently associated with hypercalcemia. Most palpable thyroid-area nodules in primary hyperparathyroidism are nodules of the thyroid itself. Thyroglossal cyst is a remnant of the embryologic descent of the thyroid from its point of origin in the base of the tongue to the thyroid area. It usually appears at puberty and presents as a midline swelling in the anterior neck slightly to one side of the midline that moves upward on protrusion of the tongue. If superficial it may transilluminate.

A branchial cyst originates in the remains of the branchial cleft and presents as a fluctuant cystic swelling in the lateral part of the neck. It may arise at any age but usually occurs in patients younger than age 40. Agenesis of the thyroid lobe implies failure of development of one lobe of the thyroid and is associated with hyperplasia of the contralateral lobe, which may suggest a unilateral thyroid nodule. Radioisotopic scanning shows the thyroid lobe to be the only functioning tissue and may simulate a hot nodule. Exogenous TSH administration is helpful in the differential diagnosis; such administration prevents further thyroid tissue from becoming evident in agenesis of the thyroid lobe. By contrast, however, if one is dealing with an autonomous thyroid hot nodule, the remnant of the normal thyroid tissue is suppressed, and exogenous TSH will make it become apparent.

DIAGNOSTIC EVALUATION

It is usually difficult to distinguish with absolute certainty between malignant and benign thyroid nod-

Table 11–18.   Factors in Single Thyroid Nodule that Increase Suspicion of Malignancy

Young age of patient
Male patient
Characteristics of nodule
   Recent growth
   Firm to hard consistency
   Fixation
   Hoarseness, stridor, dysphagia
   Cervical nodes
   ?Metastasis
Family history of thyroid cancer
   Medullary cancer
   Papillary cancer
Previous irradiation to neck
Appearance while the patient is on thyroid hormone therapy
No regression on thyroid hormone therapy
Cold on scan
Solid or mixed cystic-solid on ultrasonography
Suspicious cytology on fine needle aspiration

ules on clinical grounds alone. The physician's primary goal is to decide whether the thyroid nodule is more likely benign or malignant. If the nodule is suspected of being benign, a course of observation (with or without thyroid hormone suppression) is undertaken. If the nodule is suspected of being malignant, the patient is referred for surgical excision. The diagnostic evaluation hence includes an assessment of the known clinical risk factors and the use of laboratory, radiologic, and cytopathologic studies.

Patient History and Physical Examination

The clinical risk factors that point to increased risk of malignancy are listed in Table 11–18. Most important to consider are the patient's age, sex, and family history, the nodule's growth pattern, a history of irradiation in the patient, and the physical characteristics of the nodule.

Most nonmalignant nodules occur in patients above age 40; 50% of papillary cancers occur in those below age 40. Therefore, the younger the patient, the more likely the risk of cancer. The risk of malignancy in a single nodule in a child or adolescent is about 50%, whereas that in an adult is about 10 to 20%.

For benign thyroid disease, the female to male ratio is about 8 to 1, whereas for malignant disease the ratio is about 2 to 1. The ratio of malignant tumors to benign tumors is much higher in males.

Medullary carcinoma is familial in about 20% of cases as MEN type II and III. Papillary and follicular carcinoma may also occur as a part of familial multiple hamartoma syndrome (Cowden's disease).

A nodule of recent onset, one exhibiting progressive enlargement over a few weeks to a few months, or one that has appeared in a patient on thyroid hormone therapy has increased risk for malignancy.

External irradiation of the head, neck, or upper thorax for the treatment of a variety of benign conditions was commonly employed a few decades ago. Such conditions included enlargement of the tonsils or adenoids, thymus or cervical nodes, hemangiomas, keloids and acne, tinea capitis, and proptosis. Such irradiation, especially in childhood, has resulted in increased incidence of head and neck tumors (including thyroid, parathyroid, salivary, and neurogenic tumors) with a latency period that may be as long as 40 years or more. The risk of development of thyroid cancer is dependent on the dose of external irradiation. In a patient with a palpable thyroid nodule with a history of such irradiation, the risk of thyroid cancer may be between 20 and 50%.

A single nodule in an otherwise normal gland is more likely to represent a neoplasm, benign or malignant, with a risk of malignancy of about 20%. Multiple nodules in an enlarged gland usually represent benign, multinodular goiter (one exception to this is the multinodular glands in a previously irradiated gland). A nodule that is firm to hard in consistency or fixed to the surrounding structures is more likely to be malignant. Association with cervical lymphadenopathy or with fixation of vocal cord from recurrent nerve paralysis is virtually diagnostic of malignancy.

Diagnostic Studies

Thyroid function tests should be performed. Total and free thyroxine (or total thyroxine and resin T_3 uptake and calculation of the free thyroxine index), serum T_3, and serum TSH may be needed to assess thyroid function and to exclude hyper- or hypothyroidism. Thyroid antibody titers may be needed to support the diagnosis of autoimmune thyroid disease. If thyrotoxicosis is found in a patient who harbors a single thyroid nodule, the nodule is most likely to be a benign functioning adenoma, but it is important to remember that a malignant nodule may coexist with Graves' disease. The presence of hypothyroidism or significant titers of thyroid antibodies in a patient with single thyroid nodule increases the likelihood of focal thyroiditis as the cause of the nodule, but malignancy may coexist with chronic thyroiditis.

Other blood tests should be employed selectively. A basal serum calcitonin as well as determination of calcitonin levels following calcium and pentagastrin stimulation may be required if medullary carcinoma of the thyroid or multiple endocrine neoplasia type II or III is suspected. These provocative tests involve the administration of calcium 5 mg/kg/over 4 hours intravenously with serum calcitonin measurements at 0, 30, 60, 90, 120, and 240 minutes, or the administration of pentagastrin 0.5 mg/kg IV and sampling for serum

calcitonin at 0, 1, 2, 3, 6, and 9 minutes. Serum thyroglobulin may be elevated, not only in malignancy of the thyroid but also in a number of benign thyroid nodules, and therefore is not useful in the differential diagnosis between benign and malignant nodules.

Radioisotopic scanning plays an important role in the diagnostic evaluation of thyroid nodules. Functioning thyroid tissue can concentrate iodide or technetium, and studies using radioisotopes of iodine or technetium can identify active thyroid tissue within and outside the thyroid gland. In the normal patient, diffuse activity is present throughout the gland. When the nodule has increased uptake compared to the remainder of the gland, it will appear "hot" relative to the less active or suppressed surrounding tissue. In most instances, a hot nodule is due to an autonomously functioning benign adenoma; the incidence of malignancy in such a hot nodule is extremely low. When the nodule is inactive, it will not concentrate the radioisotope and thus will appear "cold" relative to the surrounding normal active thyroid tissue. The incidence of malignancy in cold nodules is about 20%. A "warm" nodule has an activity that falls between cold and hot nodules. The incidence of malignancy in warm nodules is about 10%.

It is important to note that the majority of malignant tumors are cold on scanning, but that the majority of cold nodules are benign. Because small cold nodules can be obscured by overlying functional tissue, the gland has to be scanned in the lateral and oblique angles in addition to the standard AP projections. Rarely, thyroid cancers can transport iodide but not organify it and can appear hot on technetium scan but cold on radioactive iodine scan.

The chief values of radioisotopic scanning in a patient with a single thyroid nodule are to identify the patient who has a hot nodule and to identify the typical patchy appearance of multinodular goiter. In both these circumstances, the incidence of malignancy is quite low. Scanning may be useful in the initial screening of patients with a history of neck irradiation, even in the absence of a palpable abnormality.

High resolution ultrasonography in the evaluation of a single thyroid nodule is of distinctive value in that it allows differentiation of cystic, solid, or mixed-solid cystic nodules, and in that it can demonstrate other nodules in the thyroid in addition to the palpable lesion. A cyst less than 4 cm in diameter is rarely malignant. Ultrasonography cannot differentiate benign from malignant lesions if the cyst is greater than 4 cm or if the nodule is solid or mixed. If more than one nodule is found in the thyroid, it is safe to assume a benign multinodular goiter.

In fine-needle aspiration cytology, thyroid tissue is

obtained for cytologic examination using a fine needle (size 23) introduced into the thyroid nodule through the overlying skin. The cytologic findings correlate very well with the histology of the resected nodule. This simple, safe office procedure, which does not require anesthesia, has emerged as the most accurate test currently available in the differential diagnosis between benign and malignant thyroid nodules and as the most accurate method for selecting patients for surgery. The critical factor is the availability of cytopathologic expertise. The frequency of false positive and false negative tests is about 5%. Fine needle aspiration cytology's limitations are its vulnerability to sampling error and the cytopathologist's inability to distinguish between well differentiated follicular carcinoma and follicular adenoma. It is important to remember that fine needle aspiration does not exclude malignancy if such is suspected on clinical grounds.

The rationale underlying thyroid hormone suppressive therapy is that benign nodules are TSH responsive while malignant nodules are not. If TSH is suppressed, a benign nodule would decrease in size while a malignant nodule would remain the same size or enlarge further. LT_4 is given in the dose of 0.15 to 0.2 mg/day to suppress TSH secretion, and the nodule is re-evaluated after 3 to 6 months of such therapy. The test is limited by variation in the examiner's measurements, which can be circumvented by ultrasonographic measurement of the nodule size, and by the facts that benign lesions may remain stable or enlarge, and thyroid cancer may occasionally show temporary regression on therapy.

Diagnostic Approach

The diagnostic approach to a patient with a single thyroid nodule is outlined in Figure 11–12. The first step is radioisotopic scanning. If the nodule is found to be hot, the likelihood of malignancy is very low, and the major concern is to rule out thyrotoxicosis.

If the nodule is cold or warm, evaluation of the clinical risk factors is important. If such evaluation points toward a high risk of malignancy, no further studies are done and surgery is recommended. If clinical evaluation of the risk factors shows that the risk of malignancy is relatively low, fine needle aspiration cytology should be performed, if available. If the cytology is benign, the patient is started on T_4 suppression and re-evaluated in 3 to 6 months. If the nodule shrinks, T_4 can be continued indefinitely. If the nodule fails to shrink or grows in the period of observation, surgery is recommended. If the cytology is reported to be suspicious or malignant, surgery should be recommended.

If fine-needle aspiration cytology is not available,

an ultrasonographic examination can be done. A cyst less than 4 cm in diameter is very rarely malignant, whereas one greater than 4 cm in diameter is suspicious. The cyst is aspirated and cytologic examination of the fluid is undertaken. If the aspirated fluid is clear or straw colored and the cytology is benign, the patient is put on thyroid hormone suppressive therapy. If there is no recurrence, thyroid hormone is continued indefinitely. If the aspirated fluid contains old or new blood and the cytology is suspicious, or if the cyst recurs on thyroid hormone suppression, the risk of malignancy is increased and surgery is recommended. If the nodule is a solid or mixed cystic-solid on ultrasonography, suppressive T_4 therapy is started. If the nodule shrinks, T_4 is continued indefinitely. If no shrinkage occurs, surgery is recommended.

If the above diagnostic approach is followed, the incidence of malignant lesions at the time of surgery will be in the range of 30 to 40%.

PAINFUL GOITER

DEFINITION

Painful goiter refers to focal or diffuse painful thyroid gland enlargement.

PATHOPHYSIOLOGIC CONSIDERATIONS

The causes of a painful goiter are listed in Table 11–19. Subacute de Quervain's thyroiditis (or acute nonsuppurative thyroiditis, granulomatous thyroiditis) is an uncommon inflammatory thyroiditis believed to be induced by a virus (e.g., mumps, Coxsackie, or adenovirus). The gland may be diffusely or focally involved with intense infiltration and disruption of the follicles by polymorphonuclear leukocytes associated with giant-cell reaction. It is followed in a few weeks to a few months by resolution of the inflammatory process and regeneration of the thyroid follicular structure.

Acute suppurative thyroiditis is a rare disorder that results from bacterial infection of the thyroid gland (Staphylococcus aureus, Streptococcus hemolyticus, Pneumococcus, etc.). The infection reaches the gland by direct spread from neighboring structures or through the blood circulation from distant sites. It is characterized by focal and diffuse inflammation and evidence

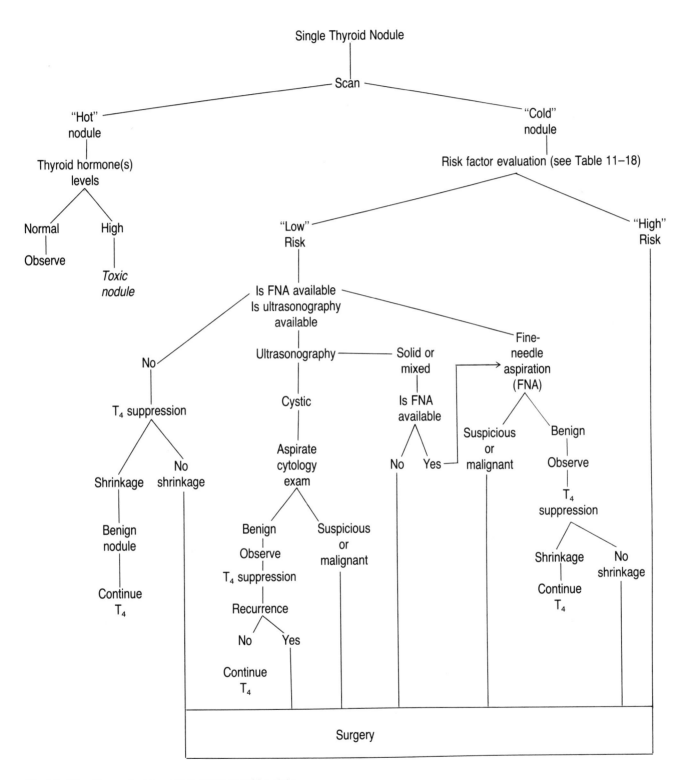

Fig. 11–12. Diagnostic approach to single thyroid nodule.

Table 11–19. Causes of Painful Thyroid Area Mass

Thyroidal
    Inflammatory
        Subacute thyroiditis
        Acute suppurative thyroiditis
        Hashimoto's thyroiditis (rare)
    Degenerative
        Hemorrhage into cyst or adenoma
    Neoplastic
        Anaplastic carcinoma
        Lymphoma
Extrathyroidal
    Infected thyroglossal duct cyst

of suppuration, necrosis, or hemorrhage. Cervical lymphadenopathy may occur.

Hemorrhage into a thyroid adenoma or cyst, Hashimoto's thyroiditis, lymphoma, anaplastic carcinoma, and infected thyroglossal cysts are other causes of a painful, tender thyroid-area mass.

CLINICAL PRESENTATION

Signs

Physical examination may show fever, a thyroid mass that may be focal (subacute or suppurative thyroiditis, hemorrhage into a nodule, or anaplastic carcinoma) or diffuse (subacute thyroiditis, Hashimoto's thyroiditis, or lymphoma), tenderness that may be exquisite, cervical lymphadenopathy (suppurative thyroiditis or anaplastic carcinoma), or an anterior neck mass moving up with protrusion of the tongue (infected thyroglossal cyst).

Symptoms

A symptom common to all the causes of painful goiter is pain of varying degree in the thyroid area, radiating to the angle of the jaw and the ears and aggravated by swallowing, moving the neck, and coughing. It is associated with tenderness, perhaps exquisite, in the thyroid area. Other features depend on the origin. Systemic symptoms may be present, such as fever of varying degree (subacute or suppurative thyroiditis), associated with chills or rigors (suppurative thyroiditis), malaise, a feeling of ill health, a history of recent upper respiratory tract infection (subacute thyroiditis), a source of bacteremia (acute suppurative thyroiditis), and symptoms of hyperthyroidism (subacute thyroiditis).

DIFFERENTIAL DIAGNOSIS

In subacute thyroiditis, the patient is usually female, 20 to 50 years old, who presents with pain and tenderness in the thyroid area. The patient frequently has systemic symptoms consisting of fever of variable degree, malaise, a feeling of ill health, and a history of recent upper respiratory viral infection. Upon examination, there is exquisite tenderness of the thyroid, which may be focally or diffusely enlarged. The overlying skin is normal, and no lymphadenopathy is detected. Features of mild hyperthyroidism caused by the release of preformed colloid into the circulation from the damaged follicles may be exhibited by 75% of patients for a few weeks. It is followed in less than 50% of patients by a period of hypothyroidism lasting for a few weeks before full regeneration and recovery of follicular function and euthyroid state. Permanent hypothyroidism develops in less than 5% of patients.

Subacute thyroiditis is characterized in many patients by exacerbations and remissions, but the total duration of the illness usually is 2 to 6 months. The symptoms and the signs respond dramatically to salicylates or steroids. The white count is usually normal but may be elevated. Thyroid antibodies may appear transiently in low titers. The two hallmark laboratory abnormalities are significant elevation of the sedimentation rate (which may exceed 100 mm in the first hour) and suppression of the radioactive iodine uptake, primarily caused by the inability of the damaged follicular cell to trap iodine. Because of the suppressed radioactive iodine uptake, thyroid scanning is not possible.

In acute pyogenic thyroiditis, the patient presents characteristically with extremely painful and tender thyroid swelling, usually focal and confined to a single lobe; with high fever and possibly rigors and chill, with dysphagia and dysphonia or stridor; and in the setting of an adjacent or distant acute bacterial infection. On examination the patient is febrile and looks toxic. There is erythema and heat over the thyroid area, very tender focal or diffuse goiter, and a demonstrable source of infection. Laboratory studies show neutrophilic leukocytosis and an elevated sedimentation rate. Euthyroidism is the rule. The radioactive iodine uptake is normal, and scanning shows a cold area corresponding to the involved area of the thyroid. Needle aspiration and cultures reveal suppuration and a pathogenetic organism.

Hemorrhage into a thyroid adenoma or cyst manifests itself with rapid onset of painful tender focal thyroid enlargement. Systemic symptoms are conspicuously absent. The lymph nodes are not palpable, and thyroid function is normal. The white count and sedimentation rate and the radioactive iodine uptake are normal. A scan reveals a cold area corresponding to the affected nodule. Resolution is rapid and occurs in few days.

Hashimoto's thyroiditis usually presents as a painless, diffuse goiter in a euthyroid or hypothyroid patient. Occasionally it may present acutely with rapid onset of a painful, tender goiter. Systemic symptoms are usually absent. The gland is found to be diffusely enlarged, firm, and bosselated. No lympadenopathy is detected. Thyroid function is normal or decreased. The white count is usually normal. The sedimentation rate may be increased, and thyroid antibodies are present in most patients and in very high titers. (See Hypothyroidism.)

Lymphoma of the thyroid predominantly affects females over age 60 and presents with rapid, diffuse, firm enlargement of the thyroid, which occasionally is painful and tender. Systemic symptoms are usually absent. The majority of patients remain euthyroid, although rarely primary hypothyroidism may be present. The sedimentation rate is increased. The radioactive iodine uptake may be normal but usually is reduced, and scanning is often not possible because of reduced uptake. Diagnosis is based on pathologic examination of tissue obtained by open biopsy.

Anaplastic carcinoma usually presents with a rapidly enlarging thyroid mass that is occasionally painful and tender and commonly associated with compressive manifestations of stridor, dysphagia, or hoarseness. Examination shows a hard, fixed thyroid mass with cervical lymphadenopathy. The patient remains euthyroid, the radioactive iodine uptake is normal, and the mass is cold on scan.

Infected thyroglossal cyst may present with a painful and tender mass that lies in the anterior neck slightly to one side of the midline. The overlying skin is usually inflamed, and the mass may move up with protrusion of the tongue. The white count and the sedimentation rate may be mildly elevated. Thyroid function is normal. The radioactive iodine uptake and scan are normal. Fine needle aspiration of the mass may show the infected cyst content.

DIAGNOSTIC EVALUATION

The diagnostic approach rests primarily on the clinical picture, the use of standard laboratory tests, and the presence or absence of thyroid dysfunction.

Patient History and Physical Examination

In the history and physical examination, consideration is given to rapidity of onset, duration, and course of the disease; systemic features; prior viral upper respiratory tract disease or local cervical or distant bacterial infection; the characteristics of the painful thyroid-area mass (whether it is focal or diffuse, or mobile or fixed; if it moves with deglutition or protrusion of

the tongue; and if it is accompanied by cervical lymphadenopathy); and an assessment of thyroid function.

Diagnostic Studies

Laboratory tests that may be helpful in the differential diagnosis include white count and differential, sedimentation rate, thyroid hormone levels to assess thyroid function, thyroid antibodies (when autoimmune thyroid disease is suspected), and a radioactive iodine uptake (and scan when possible). Only rarely are fine needle aspiration and open biopsy needed for the differential diagnosis.

EXOPHTHALMOS

DEFINITION

Exophthalmos refers to abnormal prominence of one or both eyes, usually caused by disease of the orbit or its contents.

PATHOPHYSIOLOGIC CONSIDERATIONS

Exophthalmos usually results from an orbital mass, an inflammatory process, or a vascular abnormality that displaces the eye globe forward. It may be unilateral or bilateral (Table 11–20).

Graves' ophthalmology is an inflammatory process in which the orbital tissues, exclusive of the globe, are edematous and infiltrated with lymphocytes, mast cells, plasma cells, and mucopolysaccharides. Predominantly affected, the orbital muscles are swollen, with degeneration of the muscle fibers and ultimate fibrosis. The cause is uncertain and may be related to an immunologic reaction involving antigen antibody complex binding to intraorbital tissues and a local cell-mediated immune reaction. The clinical manifestations of congestion, proptosis, and ophthalmoplegia are a result of increased intraorbital pressure, increased volume of orbital contents, and extraocular muscle dysfunction; they are usually bilateral but may be unilateral and can affect patients of any age but usually females in their fourth and fifth decades.

Orbital pseudotumor is a localized, inflammatory infiltration of the orbital tissues of unknown cause. It usually affects one eye at the onset but may become bilateral, and it has a variable but self limiting course that may be characterized by remissions and relapses. The clinical manifestations are those of orbital inflam-

Table 11-20.   Causes of Exophthalmos (Proptosis)

Inflammatory
   Graves' disease
   Pseudotumor
   Orbital cellulitis
   Sarcoidosis
   Vasculitis, e.g., Wegener's granulomatosis
Traumatic
Vascular
   Shunts
Cysts
   Dermoid
   Epidermoid
Neoplasm
   Primary
      Hemangioma
      Lymphangioma
      Optic nerve glioma
      Neurofibroma
      Rhabdomyosarcoma
      Lacrimal gland tumor
   Metastatic
      Neuroblastoma
      Lung, breast
   Hematologic
      Lymphoma
      Leukemia
Miscellaneous
   Uremia
   Cirrhosis
   COPD
   Superior vena cava obstruction
   Cushing's syndrome
   Familial

mation, exophthalmos, and, in some cases, systemic manifestations. It can affect patients of any age but usually those in their sixth or seventh decade. In a variant of pseudotumor, the Tolosa-Hunt syndrome, the inflammation is localized near the supraorbital fissure, optic canal, or cavernous sinus. Its cause is unknown.

Orbital cellulitis, the most common cause of exophthalmos in early childhood, may occur following trauma, from hematogenous spread, or, more commonly, from spread of infection from adjacent sinuses, especially the ethmoid sinuses. It is characterized by orbital congestion, inflammation, and proptosis. Systemic symptoms may be present. Early diagnosis and treatment is important to prevent visual impairment. A variety of systemic inflammatory diseases may involve the orbit, including sarcoidosis, amyloidosis, connective tissue disease, and vasculitis, and can produce proptosis, extraocular muscle enlargement, and involvement of the lids. Involvement of other organ systems may be apparent.

Vascular shunts, which may follow trauma, are usually unilateral but can be bilateral, and can present with congestion, proptosis, and ophthalmoplegia. Or-

bital cysts, which include epidermoid and dermoid cysts, can present with a unilateral mass effect and proptosis. In addition, these cysts may rupture, causing an orbital inflammation.

Primary and metastatic neoplasms can also be causes of exophthalmos. Among the primary neoplasms are hemangioma, lymphangioma, optic nerve glioma, meningioma, rhabdomyosarcoma, and tumors of the lacrimal gland. Among metastatic lesions occurring in adults are metastasis of breasts and lungs; neuroblastoma and Ewing's sarcoma occur in children.

Lymphoma can present with unilateral or bilateral exophthalmos. It may also involve the paraorbital tissues including the lacrimal system, upper lids, and forehead. There may be evidence of systemic disease. Intraorbital foreign bodies may produce orbital inflammation and proptosis.

CLINICAL PRESENTATION

Graves' disease is associated with two groups of clinical ophthalmologic findings: those related to the thyrotoxicosis per se and therefore common to all types of hyperthyroidism; and those that result from the characteristic infiltrative process specific for Graves' disease.

The thyrotoxic eye signs result from sympathetic overactivity and spasm of Müller's muscle and usually abate when the thyrotoxic state is reversed. These signs include retraction of the eyelids, resulting in widening of the palpebral fissure, and exposure of a rim of sclera above the superior margin of the limbus. Lid retraction gives the patient a wide-eyed, staring look and is associated with infrequent blinking. It may be asymmetrical. Other signs are lid lag when the patient looks down and globe lag when the patient looks up. In addition, the movements of the lids are jerky and a tremor of the lightly closed lids is usually present.

Graves' infiltrative ophthalmopathy is present clinically in about 50% of patients with Graves' disease, although ultrasonographic and CT studies have shown characteristic orbital changes in virtually all patients. It follows a course independent of thyrotoxicosis and can be present in those with present or past thyrotoxicosis and even in those with euthyroid Graves' disease. Symptoms of Graves' infiltrative ophthalmopathy include a sense of irritation and foreign body in the eyes, increased tearing and photophobia, redness of the eye, sense of pressure behind the eye, exophthalmos, swelling and often incomplete closure of the lids and periorbital edema, and double vision, blurring of vision, and, ultimately, decreased vision. Physical examination signs may reveal edematous and reddened lids, injected and edematous conjunctivae (chemosis),

Table 11–21. The "No Specs" Classification of Thyroid Ophthalmopathy

Class	Description
0	No physical symptoms and signs
1	Only signs; no symptoms. Signs are limited to lid retraction, stare, and lid lag
2	Soft tissue involvement
3	Proptosis
4	Extraocular muscle involvement
5	Corneal involvement
6	Sight loss (optic nerve involvement)

and exophthalmos, usually bilateral although often slightly asymmetrical.

True unilateral exophthalmos is rare; when it occurs, it usually does so in the absence of Graves' hyperthyroidism, and eventually the other eye is affected. It is usually accompanied by periorbital edema, which masks the degree of exophthalmos. Extraocular muscle impairment may be apparent and can affect any extraocular muscle; the most common finding is limitation of the upward gaze which is related to fibrous thickening of the inferior rectus and oblique muscles.

Ophthalmoplegia usually occurs with other ophthalmologic Graves' findings but can occur alone. The lacrimal glands may be enlarged. Ophthalmologic examination should include assessment of the fundus, visual acuity, visual fields, and intraocular tension. A simple classification of thyroid ophthalmopathy proposed by the American Thyroid Association, the "NO SPECS" classification, is shown in Table 11–21.

In addition to the ophthalmic findings, the patient may manifest a diffuse goiter of variable size, findings of thyrotoxicosis, or Graves' dermopathy (see Thyrotoxicosis).

Patients with pseudotumor oculi may have similar eye complaints; however, orbital pain is a prominent symptom. The signs of inflammation and proptosis in pseudotumor are usually unilateral but rarely may be bilateral. In association with orbital cellulitis, there may be fever, pain, soft-tissue edema, and restriction of eye movement. The other clinical findings depend on the cause: e.g., neurofibromatosis, or cafè-au-lait spots in patients with optic glioma; systemic evidence of vasculitis in Wegener's granulomatosis; and sarcoidosis, lymphoma, and evidence of primary tumor (breast, lung, melanoma, etc.).

DIFFERENTIAL DIAGNOSIS

If the exophthalmos is bilateral, the main differential diagnosis is among Graves' disease, other inflammatory states, pseudotumors, Wegener's granulomatosis, and lymphoma. If the exophthalmos is unilateral, the main differential diagnosis is between Graves' disease and orbital mass.

The diagnosis of Graves' ophthalmopathy is based on the presence of specific patterns of eye findings characteristic of Graves' ophthalmopathy, abnormalities of thyroid function and regulation, and the characteristic swelling of the extraocular muscles on ultrasonography or CT scan examination. The presence of thyroid-stimulating and thyroid-binding immunoglobulins supports the diagnosis. (See Thyrotoxicosis.)

In orbital pseudotumors, the dominant symptoms are those of orbital pain, restricted eye movements, and proptosis. If orbital pseudotumors are severe, vision may be decreased. Systemic symptoms may be present, including fever, malaise, and anorexia. Examination shows the presence of signs of orbital inflammation, exophthalmos, and maybe ophthalmoplegia. There is no eyelid retraction. The abrupt onset of symptoms associated with orbital pain, the absence of any abnormality of thyroid function or regulation, and response to treatment with steroids point to the diagnosis of pseudotumor. Biopsy of intraorbital tissue is sometimes necessary to exclude systemic disease or neoplasia.

In orbital cellulitis, there is evidence of orbital congestion, pain, proptosis, and ophthalmoplegia. Systemic symptoms may be present. There may be a history of trauma or of adjacent sinusitis. Bone tenderness on examination of the sinuses may be present. There may be leukocytosis and an increased sedimentation rate. Orbital x-rays show opacification of the involved sinuses without bone destruction.

In Wegener's granulomatosis, there is evidence of bilateral orbital disease, nasolacrimal duct obstruction, epistaxis, and saddlenose deformity. There may be systemic findings including hemoptysis, hematuria, arthralgias, and arthritis. The diagnosis is confirmed by biopsy of the nasal mucosa.

Diagnosis of sarcoidosis and amyloidosis is based on the presence of systemic features, on appropriate laboratory and radiologic studies, and on biopsy.

The diagnosis of vascular shunts is based on a careful evaluation of the history for trauma and on ultrasonography or a CT evaluation, which may show dilatation of the orbital vessels. The definitive diagnosis is by angiography.

The diagnosis of orbital cysts is made by the characteristic appearance on orbital scans.

Careful palpation, ultrasonography or CT scan examination, and biopsy may be indicated for the diagnosis of neoplasms.

Systemic involvement and evidence of involvement of paraorbital structures including the lacrimal system, upper eyelids, and forehead may point to lymphoma.

Biopsy is needed for confirmation and histologic classification.

Conventional orbital x-rays and orbital CT usually allow identification of foreign bodies.

DIAGNOSTIC EVALUATION

The diagnostic evaluation is based on documenting the presence of exophthalmos and defining its cause. In adults, the distance from the lateral orbital rim to the corneal apex, as checked by an exophthalmometer, ranges between 12 mm and 20 mm and is usually 16 mm. Exophthalmos is present if the exophthalmometer reading is greater than 20 mm in one eye. An asymmetry between the two eyes of more than 3 mm, even if the two readings fall within the normal range, is suggestive of unilateral exophthalmos.

The physician must rule out pseudoexophthalmos, which is simulation of an abnormal prominence of the eye or a true asymmetry that is not due to a mass or inflammatory process or a vascular abnormality. Pseudoexophthalmos may be due to asymmetrical orbital size on a congenital, post-traumatic, postsurgical, or postirradiation basis; to asymmetrical palpebral fissure caused by lid retraction, facial nerve palsy, lid scar, ectropion or entropion, or contralateral ptosis; to an enlarged globe related to myopia trauma or glaucoma; to contralateral enophthalmos from Horner's syndrome, orbital fracture, or small globe; and to extraocular muscle abnormality related to postsurgical muscle recession, paralysis, or paresis.

Patient History

A detailed history is important in determining the cause of exophthalmos. The physician should inquire about the onset and progression of symptoms; an abrupt onset and rapid progression indicate orbital pseudotumor, or cellulitis, whereas a gradually progressive course with exacerbations and partial remissions is characteristic of endocrine Graves' ophthalmopathy. In addition, constitutional symptoms are important. A history of fever, malaise, and weight loss points to systemic diseases and raises the question of lymphoma or vasculitis. The physician should also ask about a history of orbital trauma or recurrent sinus infections. Past or present history of goiter or thyrotoxicosis, and a positive family history of thyroid disease increase the likelihood of endocrine ophthalmopathy.

Physical Examination

Physical examination should include a complete examination of the eye for congestive signs, exophthalmos, and extraocular muscle dysfunction; in addition, a detailed examination of the media and fundi, of vis-

ual acuity, of the visual fields, and of intraocular pressure are in order. The orbits and the paraorbital tissues should be examined for masses or tenderness and the thyroid should be examined for goiter. A general examination for evidence of thyrotoxicosis, systemic diseases such as sarcoidosis, Wegener's granulomatosis or lymphoma, and evidence of a primary neoplasm in the breast or lung should be performed. Finally, the extremities should be examined for pretibial myxedema and acropachy.

Diagnostic Studies

Laboratory tests that aid in the differential diagnosis include complete blood count and sedimentation rate, and thyroid function tests, including total and free serum thyroxine or free thyroxine index, serum T_3, radioactive iodine uptake, and, if necessary, tests of thyroid autonomy including a TRH test or a T_3 suppression test. Also, serum levels of thyroid-stimulating and thyroid-binding immunoglobulins and antithyroid antibodies should be obtained, and orbital roentgenography, including ultrasonography and CT scanning, should be performed.

HYPOCALCEMIA

DEFINITION

Hypocalcemia is defined as a decreased total serum calcium. Calcium exists in plasma in three forms: an ionized, biologically active fraction (50%); a protein-bound fraction, bound chiefly to albumin (40%); and a small fraction complexed to citrate and other plasma anions (10%). A low total serum calcium can result from a decrease in the ionized fraction (true hypocalcemia) or from a decrease in the bound calcium caused by a decrease in serum albumin (the ionized calcium remaining normal) (pseudohypocalcemia). Hypocalcemia may be asymptomatic and detected by routine standard biochemical testing or may be symptomatic and potentially life threatening.

PATHOPHYSIOLOGIC CONSIDERATIONS

Normal serum calcium is maintained within a relatively narrow physiologic range (8.9 to 10.1 mg/dl). The homeostatic influences that participate in the maintenance of normal serum calcium include parathyroid hormone (PTH) and vitamin D. PTH stimulates release

Table 11–22. Causes of Hypocalcemia

Disorders of decreased parathyroid hormone synthesis and action
  Hypoparathyroidism
    Postsurgical
    Idiopathic (spontaneous)
      Familial
      Sporadic
    Congenital
      diGeorge's syndrome
    Infiltrative
      Amyloidosis
      Hemochromatosis
    Postirradiation (I^{131})
  Pseudohypoparathyroidism
    Type I
    Type II
  Magnesium deficiency
  Renal failure
Disorders of vitamin D availability, metabolism, or action
  Vitamin D deficiency
    Nutritional
    Malabsorption syndromes
    Hepatic and biliary cirrhosis
    Anticonvulsant drugs
  Vitamin D–dependent rickets
  Vitamin D–resistant rickets
    Familial
    Sporadic
  Renal failure
Removal of calcium from serum
  Phosphate excess
    Renal failure
    Iatrogenic
    Rapid cell or tumor lysis
  Increased bone avidity for calcium
    Postparathyroidectomy for primary HPT
    Malignancy
      Osteoblastic metastases
      Rapid healing of osteolytic lesions by chemotherapy
Miscellaneous
  Acute pancreatitis
  Neonatal hypocalcemia
  Drugs
    Mithramycin
    EDTA
    Fluoride intoxication
  Citrated blood
  Excess calcitonin
    Medullary carcinoma of thyroid (very rare)

of calcium from bone, reabsorption of calcium by the renal tubule, and biosynthesis of the active metabolite of vitamin D, $1,25(OH)_2D$, by stimulation of renal 1-hydroxylase enzyme activity. Vitamin D, principally $1,25(OH)_2D$, stimulates the absorption of calcium from the intestine and facilitates the action of PTH on bone. Hypocalcemia results from impairment in these homeostatic mechanisms resulting from deficiency or impaired activity of PTH or vitamin D. Table 11–22 outlines the various causes according to the underlying disorder in calcium metabolism. Several of the causes

disturb more than one basic mechanism of calcium homeostasis. The most frequent causes of hypocalcemia are chronic renal disease, hypoparathyroidism, and magnesium deficiency.

Disorders of Parathyroid Hormone. Disorders of parathyroid hormone are of two types: impaired secretion, or hypoparathyroidism, and impaired end-organ response, or pseudohypoparathyroidism.

Postoperative hypoparathyroidism, the most common cause of hypoparathyroidism, is due to excision or damage of the parathyroid glands or impairment of their blood supply during surgery for thyroid disorders or primary hyperparathyroidism, or from radical neck dissection for malignancy. Patients undergoing second or third thyroid-area explorations are particularly prone to develop the disease. It usually develops several days after the operation, but months or years can pass before the diagnosis is made. It can be transient or permanent, partial or complete, clinically latent or overt.

Spontaneous hypoparathyroidism is rare and occurs in either familial or sporadic form. Familial hypoparathyroidism is of two types: a sex-linked recessive disorder predominantly affecting males that manifests in the first year of life and that is mild and not associated with other abnormalities, and an autosomal recessive or dominant trait with variable penetrance that is more severe, usually appears before age 30, and is presumably autoimmune in origin. This latter type is frequently associated with mucocutaneous candidiasis, Addison's disease, primary gonadal failure, primary hypothyroidism, pernicious anemia, and diabetes mellitus. Patients with sporadic, spontaneous hypoparathyroidism may have similar clinical expressions but a negative family history.

Congenital hypoparathyroidism is caused by absence of the parathyroid glands because of failure of development of the third and fourth bronchial clefts; the thymus also fails to develop, with consequent severe immunologic deficiency leading to early death because of infection and hypocalcemia. Rarely, parathyroid failure may result from postirradiation damage from radioactive iodine treatment for hyperthyroidism, or from infiltration of the glands, e.g., by hemochromatosis, amyloidosis, or metastatic disease.

Pseudohypoparathyroidism is a rare sex-linked dominant familial disorder characterized by peripheral tissue unresponsiveness to PTH, hyperplasia of the parathyroid glands and elevated levels of circulating PTH, and distinctive somatic defects that may include short stature, a round face, obesity, shortened third and fourth metacarpals and metatarsals, subcutaneous calcification, exostoses, and variable degree of subnormal intelligence. Pseudohypoparathyroidism is of two

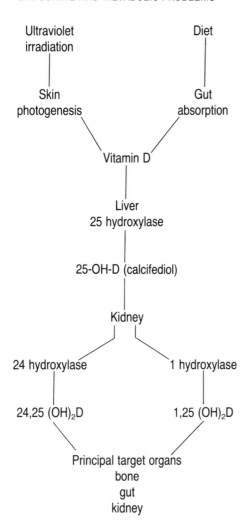

Fig. 11–13.   Vitamin D metabolism.

types: Type I is characterized by failure of PTH to activate renal adenylate cyclase; type II is characterized by defective intracellular action of cyclic AMP. Pseudopseudohypoparathyroidism is characterized by somatic features typical of pseudohypoparathyroidism but shows no evidence of tissue resistance to PTH; it occurs in the same families as pseudohypoparathyroidism and is transmitted as a sex-linked dominant trait.

Hypomagnesemia, occurring in such conditions as malnutrition, malabsorption, and chronic alcoholism, is becoming an increasingly recognized cause of hypocalcemia. Hypomagnesemia causes a state of functional hypoparathyroidism because of decreased PTH secretion and decreased peripheral responsiveness to PTH. It is clinically important because it is a common cause of hypocalcemia and because its recognition leads to avoidance of unnecessary and expensive diagnostic evaluation.

Vitamin D Disorders (Fig. 11–13). Among vitamin D disorders causing hypocalcemia is altered availability of vitamin D caused by decreased intake or decreased gastrointestinal absorption, in the presence of little or no exposure to ultraviolet irradiation from the sun. In the U.S., nutritional vitamin D deficiency is unusual (because of fortification with vitamin D of foods such as milk and bread) except in elderly institutionalized patients. Gastrointestinal disease with malabsorption of vitamin D is the most frequent cause of vitamin D deficiency.

Reduced 25-OH-D can result from decreased availability of D_3, as mentioned; from increased metabolism of 25-OH-D to inactive metabolites (therapy with phenobarbital, phenytoin, and aminoglutethimide may induce microsomal enzymes, causing rapid breakdown of 25-OH-D); from loss through abnormalities of enterohepatic circulation, in particular biliary cirrhosis; and from excessive urinary loss, as occurs in the nephrotic syndrome (25-OH-D is bound in plasma to specific vitamin D-binding proteins).

Chronic renal insufficiency is the most common cause of hypocalcemia caused by altered metabolism of vitamin D resulting from decreased availability or action of 1,25-OH_2D. Hypocalcemia results from failure of conversion of 25-OH-D to 1,25-$(OH)_2D$, hyperphosphatemia, and subnormal PTH response at the bone level. Vitamin D-dependent rickets caused by defective 1-hydroxylation of 25-OH-D and vitamin D-resistant rickets caused by target organ resistance to 1,25-$(OH)_2D$ are rare causes of hypocalcemia.

Removal of Calcium from Serum. Hyperphosphatemia is a common pathophysiologic mechanism for hypocalcemia. It may be due to acute and chronic renal disease, increased intake of phosphate either orally or intravenously (severe hyperphosphatemia is rare with increased intake of phosphate unless there is impaired renal function), and rapid cell lysis, as occurs with rhabdomyolysis or in the treatment of certain lymphoproliferative disorders. The mechanism of hypocalcemia is not well understood but may be related to decreased 1-hydroxylase renal activity and to an increase in the solubility product of calcium and phosphate leading to deposition of calcium in the soft tissues and bone. Hypocalcemia may also develop as a consequence of rapid deposition of calcium into bone, which can be seen in osteoblastic metastasis, particularly with tumors of the prostate, breast, and lung; in patients with rapid healing of osteolytic malignant lesions after successful chemotherapy; and following removal of a parathyroid adenoma, particularly in hyperparathyroid patients with significant bone disease.

Miscellaneous Causes of Hypocalcemia. Hypocalcemia can occur in pancreatitis, in which it may be related to local precipitation of calcium salts of fatty acids in the pancreatic area, to decreased PTH secretion, and to increased PTH resistance. Neonatal hypocalcemia may be due to vitamin D deficiency, parathyroid hypofunction in infants of hyperparathyroid mothers, magnesium deficiency, and hyperphosphatemia from a high content of phosphate in cows' milk. Citrate administration may also cause hypocalcemia because citrate in transfused blood may bind ionized calcium; hypocalcemia is occasionally seen after multiple transfusions with citrated blood. Other causes of hypocalcemia include drug therapy with mithramycin (which inhibits bone resorption), and acute fluoride intoxication, which can cause a marked hypocalcemia because of formation of insoluble precipitate with calcium in bone.

CLINICAL PRESENTATION

The clinical manifestations of the hypocalcemic syndrome result from the hypocalcemia and its cause. The manifestations attributed to hypocalcemia depend on the degree of hypocalcemia and the rapidity of its development. They are due primarily to disturbances in neuromuscular function, which consist of increased excitability of sensory and motor nerves.

Other signs and symptoms that may be present in the hypocalcemic patient are those of the cause of the hypocalcemic syndrome.

Signs

Two classic physical findings may be seen in hypocalcemic states: Chvostek's sign and Trousseau's sign. Chvostek's sign consists of contraction of facial muscles (mouth, nostril, orbicularis oculi) in response to tapping over the facial nerve in front of the ear. This sign, however, is present in 10 to 15% of normal people. Trousseau's sign is the induction of a carpopedal spasm by inflating a sphygmomanometer to a level above the systolic pressure for 3 minutes. This sign is a more reliable sign of hypocalcemia because it may occur in only 1% of normal subjects. Because both signs may be absent in patients with hypocalcemia, their absence does not exclude the diagnosis. Other signs of hypocalcemia include dry, puffy skin, scanty body and scalp hair, hypoplasia of the teeth that develops during periods of hypocalcemia, deformed nails, bilateral subcapsular cataracts, and, rarely, papilledema associated with benign intracranial hypertension, cardiac arrhythmias, and congestive heart failure.

Chronic hypocalcemia may be clinically silent until the calcium balance is stressed, for example, with the use of a calciuric diuretic such as furosemide, or in situations of increased calcium demand, such as pregnancy.

Symptoms

Hypocalcemic patients may be asymptomatic or may complain of numbness and tingling of the hands, feet, tongue, and perioral region. There may be muscle spasms that may involve any muscle group but characteristically the carpopedal group. In carpopedal spasm, the elbows, wrists, and metacarpophalangeal joints are flexed, the interphalangeal joints are extended, and the thumb is adducted and lies across the palm. If severe, hypocalcemia can result in generalized convulsions and laryngeal stridor, which can lead to life threatening respiratory embarrassment. Rarely, chronic hypocalcemia may present with symptoms of psychic disturbances, including depression, irritability, and memory loss; Parkinsonism or choreoathetosis; nausea, vomiting, and abdominal pain; congestive heart failure, which is usually resistant to standard treatment and reversible only with calcium replacement; benign intracranial hypertension; skin, hair, and fingernail abnormalities and delayed dental development; and intestinal malabsorption.

DIFFERENTIAL DIAGNOSIS

Hypocalcemia should enter into the differential diagnosis of tetany. Other causes of tetany include hypomagnesemia, hyperventilation, metabolic alkalosis, and pheochromocytoma. The serum calcium is normal in all these disorders except hypomagnesemia.

Hypocalcemia should also enter into the differential diagnosis of seizure disorder, Parkinsonism, choreoathetosis, benign intracranial hypertension, dementia, psychoneurosis or psychosis, congestive heart failure resistant to standard therapy, and intestinal malabsorption. The diagnosis of hypocalcemia is based on the awareness of the clinical settings in which it can occur and on laboratory documentation of true hypocalcemia.

DIAGNOSTIC EVALUATION

Patient History and Physical Examination

The diagnostic approach is outlined in Figure 11–14. Hypocalcemia may be detected by routine screening in an asymptomatic patient or may be looked for in a patient who has suggestive symptoms and signs or a disorder known to be associated with hypocalcemia. Hypocalcemia is present if the total serum calcium is less than 8.9 mg/dl.

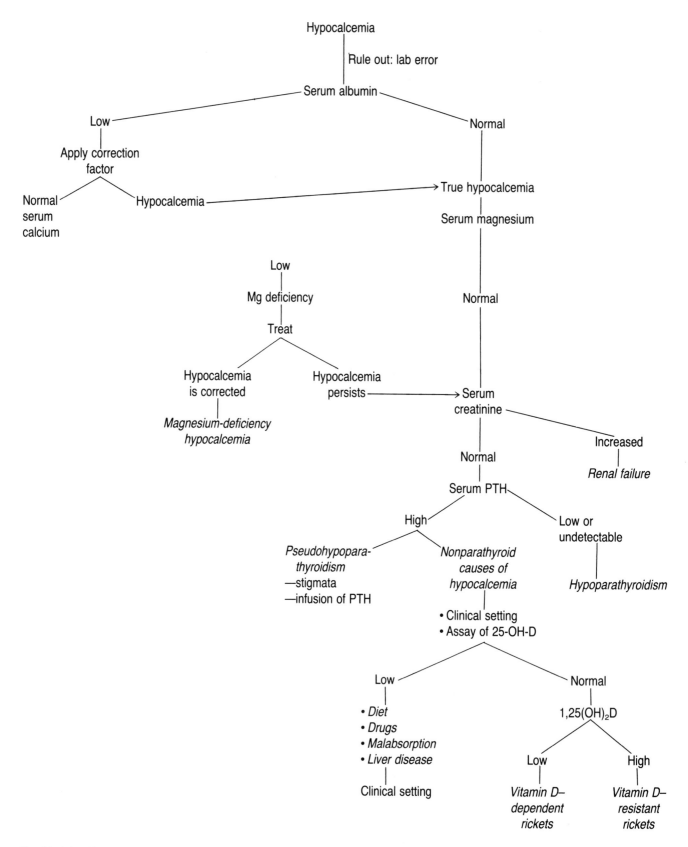

Fig. 11—14.   Diagnostic approach to hypocalcemia.

Table 11–23.   Common Laboratory Tests in Calcium Disorders

Test	Determinants	Hypocalcemic Syndrome	Hypercalcemic Syndrome
Serum Calcium Normal, 8.9–10.1 mg/dl	Serum calcium exists in three forms—ionized (50%), complexed (10%), and protein bound chiefly to albumin (40%). The determinants for the ionized biologically active fraction are parathyroid hormone, vitamin D, bone turnover, and renal excretion. For the protein-bound fraction, the determinants are serum albumin and, to a lesser extent, globulin levels. Serum calcium always has to be evaluated concomitantly with serum albumin concentration. A change of 1.0 g/dl in serum albumin will change total calcium by approximately 0.8 mg/dl in the same direction.	Decreased. May be normal in hypocalcemic patients with increased serum protein levels and may be decreased in eucalcemic patients with decreased serum proteins.	Increased. May be normal in hypercalcemic patients with low serum proteins and may be high in eucalcemic patients with hyperproteinemia.
Serum Ionized Calcium Normal, 4.75–5.20 mg/dl at pH 7.40	Parathyroid hormone, vitamin D, and bone turnover. It is not affected by changes in plasma proteins.	Decreased.	Increased.
Serum Phosphate Normal, 2.5–4.5 mg/dl in adults and 4.0–7.0 mg/dl in children	Renal function: parathyroid hormone, vitamin D, bone turnover, and diurnal variation.	Increased in hypocalcemia due to hypoparathyroidism, pseudohypoparathyroidism, and renal insufficiency; but may be normal in these disorders if there is dietary restriction or administration of aluminum hydroxide gel. It is decreased in hypocalcemia associated with secondary hyperparathyroidism except that of renal failure. May be increased in eucalcemic patient with (a) increased phosphate load especially in the presence of renal impairment and (b) renal failure.	May be normal, decreased, or increased. Low serum phosphate is common in primary HPT except in the presence of renal failure but may also be low in other hypercalcemic states. Serum phosphate may be increased in renal failure. If increased in the absence of renal failure, it points to nonparathyroid cause; e.g., thyrotoxicosis, acromegaly, and sarcoidosis.
Urinary Calcium Normal in adult males, <250 mg/day; in adult females, <200 mg/day	Parathyroid hormone, vitamin D, bone turnover, renal function, and sodium excretion.	No clinical utility.	Low values <150 mg/24 hours favor familial benign hypocalciuric hypercalcemia or the use of thiazides. Values are normal or modestly elevated in primary HPT. More profound hypercalciuria occurs in nonparathyroid cause of hypercalcemia.
Serum Parathyroid Hormone (PTH) ≤70 μLEq/ml	Parathyroid function. Serum PTH is measured by IRA. Keep in mind the heterogeneity of circulating PTH and the variable specificity of anti-PTH antibodies. 10–25% of normal may have undetectable levels because of assay sensitivity.	Decreased or absent in hypocalcemia due to hypoparathyroidism and magnesium deficiency. Increased in pseudohypoparathyroidism and in hypocalcemic syndromes associated with secondary HPT due to vitamin D deficiency or resistance, and renal insufficiency.	Suppressed levels indicate nonparathyroid cause. Serum PTH is elevated in >90% of patients with primary HPT to a degree appropriate to the level of hypercalcemia. 10% of patients with primary HPT have normal serum PTH levels (although normal, levels are inappropriately high for the level of serum calcium). Serum PTH may be modestly elevated in ectopic PTH humoral syndrome but without correlation to the degree of hypercalcemia.
Urinary Cyclic AMP (cAMP)	Filtered cAMP and renal-generated (nephrogenous) cAMP.	No clinical utility.	Decreased values point to a nonparathyroid cause. Increased in hyperparathyroidism but values overlap with the normal (less so with a nephrogenous cAMP). May be increased in hypercalcemia of malignancy.

Table 11–24. Laboratory Findings in Hypocalcemic States

Disorders	Serum Calcium	Serum Phosphate	Serum Magnesium	Serum Creatinine	Serum PTH	25-OH-D	125-(OH)₂-D
Hypoparathyroidism	↓	↑	N	N	↓	N	↓
Pseudohypopara-thyroidism	↓	↑	N	N	↑	N	↓
Chronic renal failure	↓	↑	↑	↑	↑	N	↓
Hypomagnesemia	↓	N	↓	N	↓	N	↓
Vitamin D deficiency	↓	↓	N	N	↑	↓	↓
Hungry bone syndrome	↓	↓	↓	N	↑	N	↑

↓ = decreased
↑ = increased
N = normal

Diagnostic Studies

LABORATORY TESTS (Tables 11–23, 11–24)

Serum Calcium. As mentioned, calcium in the plasma exists in three forms: ionized (50%), protein-bound (40%), and complexed to citrate and other plasma anions (10%). It is the decrease in the ionized fraction that results in the symptoms and signs of hypocalcemia. Measurement of the total serum calcium is the most readily available and least expensive means of documenting hypocalcemia. The normal range for serum calcium is 8.9 to 10.1 mg/dl. Serum calcium, however, must always be evaluated concomitantly with serum albumin concentration. One gram of albumin per deciliter of plasma will bind about 0.8 mg/dl of calcium. When serum albumin concentration deviates from normal, appropriate correction of serum calcium must be made to assess whether hypocalcemia is present; 0.8 mg/dl of calcium should be added to the measured serum calcium levels for each 1 g/dl decrease in serum albumin from the normal of 4.0 g/dl. Since stored plasma may yield an artifactual decrease in circulating calcium concentration, it is important to use fresh serum for calcium measurement.

Serum Ionized Calcium. Direct determination of the ionized calcium can be made using a special calcium ion-selective electrode, the measurement being made after serum has been corrected to a pH of 7.4. The range of normal for ionized calcium is 4.75 to 5.20 ng/dl. Although measurement of ionized calcium is ideal for definition of hypocalcemia, it is rarely necessary because the same information can be obtained from consideration of total calcium and serum albumin.

Serum Phosphate. The normal range for serum phosphate in the adult in a fasting morning sample is 2.5 to 4.5 mg/dl. Serum phosphate is markedly influenced by diet (increased protein or increased phosphate intake will increase serum phosphate; increased carbohydrate intake or decreased phosphate intake will decrease serum phosphate). Diurnal variations in serum phosphate are partly related to the diurnal change in cortisol. Hypocalcemia caused by hypoparathyroidism and renal insufficiency is associated with hyperphosphatemia. The diagnosis of hypoparathyroidism is virtually certain if hypocalcemia and hyperphosphatemia are found in the absence of renal failure. However, hyperphosphatemia may not be found in some patients with hypoparathyroidism who are relatively phosphate depleted because of dietary restriction or administration of aluminum hydroxide gel. Hypocalcemia caused by secondary hyperparathyroidism of any cause is associated with a low serum phosphate, except in renal failure.

Serum Parathyroid Hormone (iPTH). Determination of serum levels of PTH by radioimmunoassay is important in the differential diagnosis of the hypocalcemic syndrome. It is probably the best currently available test of parathyroid function. Each lab should standardize its normal range. Most normal individuals have measurable quantities of PTH in the serum, but 10 to 20% have undetectable levels because of assay insensitivity. Therefore, it is of utmost importance in assessing iPTH concentration that it be assessed concomitantly with the serum calcium concentration. Undetectable PTH in the presence of hypocalcemia confirms the diagnosis of hypoparathyroidism, if hypomagnesemia is excluded. Increased values of iPTH in the range appropriate to the degree of hypocalcemia exclude the presence of hypoparathyroidism and suggest pseudohypoparathyroidism, vitamin D deficiency, or renal failure.

Other Tests. Other tests needed in the evaluation of the hypocalcemic patient include serum magnesium. The normal range for serum magnesium is 1.8 to 2.7 mEq/L. In magnesium depletion the serum magnesium is usually low but may be normal (in this instance urinary magnesium is less than 1 mEq/day). Also, serum creatinine or BUN is needed as an index of glomerular function. Radioimmunoassays for 25-OH-

D and 1,25(OH)₂D are now commercially available; the normal range for 25-OH-D is 26.5 ± 5.3 ng/ml, and for 1,25(OH)₂D is 34.1 ± 9.8 pg/ml. Vitamin D assays are useful in the diagnosis of various disorders of vitamin D metabolism, which include decreased availability (low levels), decreased hepatic 25-hydroxylation (low levels), decreased renal 1-hydroxylation (low 1,25(OH)₂D but normal 25-OH-D), and decreased tissue responsiveness (normal or high 1,25(OH)₂D and 25-OH-D).

PTH administration for measurement of responsiveness to PTH is helpful in the diagnosis of pseudohypoparathyroidism: 600 to 800 units/day of PTH subcutaneously or intramuscularly for 3 days will show impaired calcemic or phosphaturic response in these patients.

The electrocardiogram usually shows prolongation of the QT interval. Occasionally it may also show cardiac arrhythmias.

RADIOLOGIC STUDIES

X-rays of the hand may show the short metacarpals in pseudohypoparathyroidism or evidence of subperiosteal bone resorption in secondary hyperparathyroidism. Skull x-rays may show basal ganglia calcification.

The radiologic appearance of bone is usually normal, but occasionally osteosclerosis may be apparent. Basal ganglia calcification may be seen on skull films. Subcutaneous calcification may be seen in patients with pseudohypoparathyroidism.

Diagnostic Approach

The first step is to rule out pseudohypocalcemia related to hypoproteinemia. This can be achieved by adjusting total serum calcium for changes in serum proteins. If hypoalbuminemia is present, the correction factor is applied by adding 0.8 mg/dl of calcium to the measured serum calcium for each 1 g/dl decrease in serum albumin from the normal of 4.0 g/dl. Pseudohypocalcemia can also be ruled out by determining the ionized serum calcium. If the serum total calcium is still low after the application of the correction factor in hypoproteinemic states or if the ionized calcium is low, true hypocalcium is present.

Clinical clues that may be helpful in suggesting the cause of hypocalcemia include history of neck surgery, socioeconomic nutritional problems, malabsorption, liver or renal disease, rickets or osteomalacia, malignant tumors with metastasis, rapid cell or tumor lysis, acute pancreatitis, skeletal features of pseudohypoparathyroidism, associated autoimmune endocrinopathy, or a family history of hypoparathyroidism or other autoimmune endocrinopathies, or of pseudohypoparathyroidism or pseudopseudohypoparathyroidism. A

drug history is important, particularly as it relates to the use of anticonvulsant therapy, oral or intravenous phosphate, fluoride, mithramycin, or multiple transfusion of citrated blood.

The definitive etiologic diagnosis rests on consideration of the clinical setting and on the measurement of serum phosphate, creatinine, magnesium, and parathyroid hormone.

An elevated serum phosphate with normal serum creatinine and serum magnesium points to parathyroid hormone deficiency or tissue resistance. Hypoparathyroidism is present if the serum PTH in this setting is low or low-normal in the presence of hypocalcemia. Postsurgical hypoparathyroidism is obvious from the history and physical examination. Otherwise, one should consider autoimmune hypoparathyroidism and look for other associated autoimmune endocrinopathies.

The diagnosis of pseudohypoparathyroidism is based on the typical somatotype, family history, normal or increased serum PTH, and impaired calcemic or phosphaturic response to the administration of exogenous parathyroid hormone.

The diagnosis of hypomagnesemia is based on the awareness of the clinical setting, presence of hypomagnesemia or a urinary magnesium less than 1 mEq/24 hours, and resolution of the hypocalcemia with replenishment of the magnesium stores. If with such replenishment resolution of the hypocalcemia does not occur, a search for other mechanisms for hypocalcemia should be in order.

An elevated serum creatinine, and normal or high serum phosphate point to renal failure.

A low serum phosphate and normal serum creatinine should prompt consideration of a vitamin D disorder unrelated to renal insufficiency. A low serum 25-OH-D points to nutritional disorder, use of drugs, or liver disease. The diagnosis is made by the clinical setting and appropriate laboratory or radiologic studies. If the serum 25-OH-D is normal, the levels of 1,25(OH)₂D should be checked. In this setting, a low serum 1,25(OH)₂D points to vitamin D-dependent rickets, whereas normal or high serum 1,25(OH)₂D points to vitamin D-resistant rickets.

Two points deserve to be stressed. First, hypocalcemia after parathyroidectomy may be related to hypoparathyroidism (from injury to the residual parathyroid tissue, or from chronic suppression of normal parathyroid tissue from prolonged preoperative hypercalcemia or associated magnesium depletion) or to the hungry bone syndrome (deposition of calcium, phosphate, and magnesium into bone when the stimulus to bone resorption has been removed by parathyroidectomy). Serum phosphate provides a reliable guide to the differential diagnosis. It is increased in hypoparathyroidism and decreased in the hungry bone syndrome. If the serum phosphate determination is inconclusive, determination of serum PTH is in order; it is decreased in hypoparathyroidism and increased in the hungry bone syndrome.

Second, serum calcium should be checked yearly in those who have had anterior neck surgery and those who are suspected of having multiple autoimmune endocrinopathies.

HYPERCALCEMIC SYNDROME

DEFINITION

The hypercalcemic syndrome refers to the symptoms and signs that result from persistent elevation of serum calcium. It is encountered in clinical practice frequently, with an estimated incidence of 2%. Hypercalcemic syndrome varies in severity; it can be asymptomatic, noted accidentally by routine laboratory screening tests, or it can be a life threatening illness.

PATHOPHYSIOLOGIC CONSIDERATIONS

Basically, hypercalcemia may develop from increased bone resorption, increased intestinal absorption, or decreased urinary excretion. In many disorders more than one mechanism is involved. The causes are outlined in Table 11–25.

Hyperparathyroidism (HPT). Primary hyperparathyroidism denotes autonomous secretion of parathyroid hormone by a primary parathyroid glandular disorder. This disorder is usually a single or multiple parathyroid adenoma (80% and 3%, respectively), hyperplasia of all the parathyroid glands (15%), or adenocarcinoma (2%). The adenoma is usually of the chief-cell variety. It can be ectopic in 6 to 10% of cases, lying in the thyroid or thymus, behind the esophagus, or in the pericardium. Hyperplasia, usually of the chief-cell type, may be symmetrical or asymmetrical.

Primary hyperparathyroidism may occur as an isolated disease or may be familial (as familial primary hyperparathyroidism or as a part of multiple endocrine neoplasia type I or type II). In multiple endocrine neoplasia type I, primary hyperparathyroidism is associated with endocrine pancreatic tumors and pitui-

Table 11–25. Causes of Hypercalcemia

Pseudohypercalcemia
  Hyperproteinemic states
    Macroglobulinemia (e.g., sarcoidosis)
    Lymphoma
    Multiple myeloma
  Laboratory error
Hyperparathyroidism (HPT)
  Primary
  Tertiary (rare)
  Ectopic
Neoplasia
  With bone metastasis
  Hematologic
    Leukemia
    Multiple myeloma
  Humoral
    Ectopic PTH
    Prostaglandins
    Osteoclast activating factors
      Lung carcinoma (epidermoid, large cell)
      Hypernephroma
      Epidermoid tumors of head, neck, esophagus
      Hepatobiliary and gastrointestinal tumors
Drugs
  Thiazides
  Vitamin D
  Vitamin A
  Alkali antacids
  Lithium carbonate
Nonparathyroid endocrine disorders
  Hyperthyroidism
  Hypothyroidism
  Pheochromocytoma
  Adrenal insufficiency
  Acromegaly
  Vipoma
Granulomatous disorders
  Sarcoidosis
  Mycobacterial
  Fungal
Immobilization
Familial benign hypocalciuric hypercalcemia (FBHH)
Renal disorders
  Diuretic phase of acute renal failure
  Postrenal transplantation
Idiopathic hypercalcemia of infancy

tary adenomas; in type II, it is associated with medullary carcinoma of the thyroid and pheochromocytoma. The presence of parathyroid hyperplasia should raise the possibility of multiple endocrine neoplasia or of familial primary hyperparathyroidism.

Tertiary hyperparathyroidism results from neoplastic adenomatous change that can occur in hyperplastic glands in the setting of secondary hyperparathyroidism.

Rarely, hyperparathyroidism can be ectopic due to the secretion of parathyroid hormone or parathyroid hormone-like substances by nonparathyroid neoplasms, usually of the bronchus, kidney, intestine, ovary, testes, liver, etc.

Primary hyperparathyroidism is the most common cause of hyperparathyroidism and has been diagnosed with increasing frequency since the advent of routine multichannel analyzers. It is estimated to be present in 0.12% of the U.S. population. Inappropriate hypersecretion of parathyroid hormone causes hypercalcemia directly by increasing bone resorption and decreasing urinary calcium excretion and indirectly by stimulating renal 1-hydroxylase enzyme, leading to increased circulating $1,25(OH)_2D$ and increased intestinal calcium absorption. A modest hypercalciuria is usually present. In addition, increased PTH leads to enhanced renal phosphate excretion and hypophosphatemia, and enhanced urinary cyclic AMP generation and excretion.

Malignant Disease. This is the most common cause of hypercalcemia detected in the hospital setting (70%). It is most commonly associated with metastasis to bone, in which the hypercalcemia is explained primarily by osteolytic action of tumor cells on bone, although humoral local factors may be responsible. The extent of clinical metastatic disease need not correlate with the degree of hypercalcemia. Metastatic carcinoma of the breast is a frequent cause; hypercalcemia may appear following the initiation of estrogen, androgen, or progestational therapy.

Hypercalcemia can also develop in the absence of apparent skeletal metastasis. This is often termed pseudohyperparathyroidism. Possible causes include tumoral production of PTH or PTH-like peptides (uncommon), stimulation of generation of prostaglandins, especially of E series, by the tumor, and generation of osteoclast-activating factor (OAF) peptide. Lung carcinoma (epidermoid and large cell), renal cell tumors, epidermoid tumors of the head, neck, and esophagus, and hepatobiliary and gastrointestinal tumors are the most common neoplasms causing hypercalcemia without apparent bone involvement. In pseudohyperparathyroidism, the parathyroid glands are normal, and surgical excision of the causative tumor leads to normalization of serum calcium, whereas a recurrence of the tumor will lead to a recurrence of the hypercalcemia.

Hypercalcemia can occur in 20 to 30% of patients with multiple myeloma, presumably caused by osteoclast-activating factor elaborated by the myeloma cells. Hypercalcemia can occur in acute lymphocytic leukemia and, rarely, in Hodgkin's disease, lymphosarcoma, and reticulum cell sarcoma.

Familial Benign Hypocalciuric Hypercalcemia. This is a newly recognized syndrome characterized by mild hypercalcemia, a low urinary calcium of less than 150 mg/day, and a benign course free of significant complications. It is familial, inherited as autosomal dominant, and almost always manifests in affected individuals by age 10. The parathyroid glands are usually hyperplastic and the serum PTH is normal or slightly increased, but for any given serum calcium level, the serum PTH is lower than that in primary hyperparathyroidism. It responds poorly even to subtotal parathyroidectomy. The cause is unknown but possibly is related to increased sensitivity of the renal tubule to the calcium-conserving effect of PTH. It is usually recognized when there is failure to find parathyroid adenoma during an operation for presumed primary HPT or as a result of family screening after the syndrome has been detected in one member.

Drugs. Overdosage with vitamin D or one of its metabolites or analogues can cause hypercalcemia from increased calcium intestinal absorption and increased bone resorption (hypervitaminosis D). This is a rare cause of hypercalcemia and usually follows the ingestion of doses equivalent to an excess of 100,000 units of vitamin D for many months to years and is seen in patients receiving vitamin D therapy for hypoparathyroidism or for a uremic bone disease. It can also occur in individuals prone to self-medication with large doses of vitamins and minerals. It is characteristically reversed by glucocorticoid therapy.

Hypervitaminosis A is another rare cause of hypercalcemia caused by increased bone resorption from increased secretion of PTH. It is seen in young children and elderly females who have been given doses a hundred times the normal physiologic requirements (3000 IU in children and 5000 IU in adults), and in hunters who have ingested large quantities of polar bear liver. A painful periostitis, especially of the ulnae, clavicles, and metatarsals, occurs in affected patients and has a characteristic radiologic finding.

Thiazides are a frequent cause of mild hypercalcemia. The exact cause is uncertain and may be related to diuretic-induced hemoconcentration, reduced urinary excretion of calcium, or potentiation of PTH's effect on bone. Diuretics may cause a transient small rise in serum calcium in patients who have no detectable disorder of calcium metabolism. Persistent mild hypercalcemia, however, is noted most commonly in patients with an underlying disorder characterized by rapid bone turnover, for example, primary HPT and multiple myeloma.

In the milk-alkali syndrome (Burnett's syndrome), chronic ingestion of calcium (dietary or pharmaceutical) and absorbable alkali can cause hypercalcemia, mild systemic alkalosis, and azotemia. The syndrome is now rare because nonabsorbable antacids have replaced the absorbable types in the treatment of peptic ulcer disease and reflux esophagitis. Affected patients can exhibit metastatic calcification, e.g., band keratopathy, and the hypercalcemia can respond to withdrawal of the offending agent.

Lithium carbonate used in doses typical for manic-depressive illness can cause mild hypercalcemia, presumably related to an altered set-point in the control of PTH secretion.

Other Causes. Sarcoidosis and other granulomatous diseases including tuberculosis and histoplasmosis may cause hypercalciuria and hypercalcemia by excessive sensitivity to vitamin D and enhanced synthesis of $1,25(OH)_2D$ by the enzyme 1-hydroxylase present in granulomatous tissue. Thus, hypercalcemia is encountered more commonly in the summer months, is increased by ultraviolet irradiation, and is dramatically reversed by the administration of glucocorticoids, which decrease the generation of $1,25(OH)_2D$. Rarely, hypercalcemia is related to granulomatous invasion of the bone with increased bone resorption or to hyperglobulinemia with increased calcium binding in plasma. Hypercalcemia occurs in about 10 to 20% of patients with sarcoidosis, predominantly in patients with chronic or generalized disease.

Hypercalcemia may develop during the diuretic phase of acute renal failure, particularly that caused by rhabdomyolysis. These patients are commonly hypocalcemic during the oliguric phase (hyperphosphatemia, deposition of calcium in damaged tissues, and low $1,25(OH)_2D$ resulting in secondary hyperparathyroidism). Hypercalcemia develops in the diuretic phase, is transient, lasting from 1 to 3 weeks, and is related to the secondary hyperparathyroidism and immobilization. Hypercalcemia may also develop in postrenal transplant patients. In the pretransplantation period, hypocalcemia is common, related to decreased $1,25(OH)_2D$ levels, hyperphosphatemia, and vitamin D and PTH resistance with ensuing secondary hyperparathyroidism. After renal transplant, these biochemical abnormalities are corrected and transient hypercalcemia may occur.

Hypercalcemia may also occur in nonparathyroid endocrine disorders. Mild hypercalcemia occurs in about 25% of patients with thyrotoxicosis. In this clinical setting, increased bone resorption from the thyrotoxicosis results in hypercalcemia, hypercalciuria, and suppressed PTH. It resolves with the treatment of the thyrotoxicosis. Rarely, hypercalcemia may be seen in hypothyroidism due to a mechanism yet unknown, and it responds to thyroid hormone therapy. Pheochromocytoma can be associated with hypercalcemia caused by increased catecholamines and increased PTH secretion (this resolves after the removal of the pheochromocytoma); Primary HPT can coexist with pheochromocytoma in multiple endocrine neoplasia type II and, rarely, type III. Hypercalcemia can be observed in adrenal insufficiency, especially in acute adrenal failure. The mechanism is not well understood but may be related to extracellular fluid depletion and hemoconcentration, enhanced renal tubular reabsorption of calcium, and relative hypervitaminosis D. It is corrected by glucocorticoid replacement. Hypercalcemia occurs rarely in acromegaly and is related to increased bone turnover with resorption greater than formation. Significant hypercalciuria is common in acromegalic patients. Acromegaly may be associated with primary HPT in multiple endocrine neoplasia type I.

Immobilization will not cause hypercalcemia unless the patient has rapid bone turnover, especially in young patients and adult patients with Paget's disease, primary HPT, thyrotoxicosis, etc. With total immobilization and prolonged bed rest, the rate of bone resorption exceeds that of formation; hypercalciuria and hypercalcemia may result.

Idiopathic hypercalcemia of infancy is a rare disorder characterized by an inborn error of calcium metabolism, hypercalcemia, and hypercalciuria, peculiar elfin facies, retardation of skeletal and mental development, renal impairment, multiple congenital cardiovascular abnormalities, and diagnostic bone changes (sclerotic changes in frontal and basal regions of the skull, and dense rings of bone near epiphysial margins of long bones).

CLINICAL PRESENTATION

Clinical manifestations reflect both the degree and the duration of hypercalcemia. Acute hypercalcemia developing over several days and weeks is manifested by anorexia, nausea and vomiting, azotemia, and marked neurologic manifestations ranging from lethargy to coma. Chronic hypercalcemia, however, may be asymptomatic or may present with specific features related to several organ systems.

Renal manifestations include polyuria, polydipsia, vasopressin-resistant diabetes insipidus caused by a defect in renal concentration ability, and dehydration; renal colic and obstructive uropathy caused by renal stones, usually calcium oxalate or phosphate; nephrocalcinosis; and chronic renal failure.

Neurologic effects are also present. Calcium has a depressive effect on the central nervous system. It may impair nerve conduction and neuromuscular function and lead to fatigue, weakness (especially proximal muscle weakness), and even paresis, to impairment of mental status (lethargy, confusion, stupor, or even coma and abnormal electroencephalographic findings), and to mild personality disturbances, depression, or even organic psychosis.

Gastrointestinal manifestations include anorexia, nausea, vomiting, constipation, and increased incidence of peptic ulcer and pancreatitis. Hypercalcemia may be associated with cardiovascular problems of hypertension, bradycardia, arrhythmias, and potentiation of digitalis toxicity. Metastatic calcification may occur, with increased deposition of calcium salts in soft tissues, lungs, kidneys, blood vessels, joints, eye, and skin, leading to such complaints as red eyes, pruritus, and joint pain. On examination, one may find evidence of dehydration (nausea, vomiting, and vasopressin-resistant diabetes insipidus), hypotonia, hyporeflexia, bradycardia, and hypertension. Band keratopathy is present in about a third of patients with chronic hypercalcemia; it may be apparent as diffuse, hazy-gray corneal opacities running concentrically within limbus on nasal or temporal sides, or both, and characteristically is separated from the limbus by a clear margin; most often it is demonstrable only by slit lamp examination. In addition, the physician may see evidence of proximal weakness, ectopic conjunctival calcification, and, rarely, a palpable mass in the neck (an incidental thyroid mass, medullary carcinoma of the thyroid, or, rarely, parathyroid carcinoma). A short QT interval and arrhythmias may be apparent on the electrocardiogram. In addition, patients may have the clinical manifestations of the underlying disorder.

DIAGNOSTIC EVALUATION

Diagnostic Studies (see Table 11–23)

The major goals of the laboratory tests are to demonstrate and confirm hypercalcemia and to delineate its cause. The most important of these tests are the serum calcium, the serum immunoreactive parathyroid hormone (iPTH) (or, if such radioimmunoassay is not available, various parameters to measure the biologic effects of PTH), and other tests as needed by the clinical setting.

LABORATORY TESTS

Serum Calcium. The total serum calcium concentration must always be evaluated concurrently with the serum albumin concentration, and if the serum albumin deviates from the normal, appropriate correction of the serum calcium must be made. A serum calcium consistently above 10.1 mg/dl, in the presence of normal serum albumin concentration, denotes hypercalcemia. In hypercalcemia, the level of serum calcium may be variable and some help in the differential diagnosis. A level greater than 13 to 14 mg/dl should

raise the suspicion of malignancy; thiazide diuretics cause mild hypercalcemia with levels equal to or less than 10.5 mg/dl. A level greater than 10.5 mg/dl in a patient on thiazide diuretics should prompt a search for another cause of hypercalcemia.

Serum Ionized Calcium. Ionized calcium is not affected by changes in serum protein concentration. Although this measurement is ideal for assessing true hypercalcemia, it is not needed in the usual cases; the same information can be obtained from consideration of the total serum calcium and serum albumin concentrations.

Serum Phosphate. The normal range in the adult is 2.5 to 4.5 mg/dl. Since serum phosphate may change with diurnal variation and with the level of dietary intake, a fasting morning sample on an adequate phosphate diet is required. Hypophosphatemia is a common finding in primary HPT but is nonspecific because it may occur in hypercalcemia of any cause. Hyperphosphatemia occurs in the presence of renal failure; its occurrence in the absence of renal failure favors a nonparathyroid cause for the hypercalcemia (e.g., thyrotoxicosis or acromegaly).

Twenty-Four–Hour Urinary Calcium. The normal range for urinary calcium in male adults on a normal or low-calcium diet is less than 250 mg/day, and in adult females less than 200 mg/day. Because calcium excretion parallels sodium excretion and is altered by factors such as sodium intake and the use of diuretic, it is imperative to obtain simultaneous urinary sodium measurements. Urinary calcium should be measured in all hypercalcemic patients. In hypercalcemic patients with normal renal function, there is an increased filtered load of calcium; only in hyperparathyroidism is there increased tubular reabsorption of the filtered calcium. Therefore, the finding of normal to mildly elevated urinary calcium (less than 400 mg/24 hours) in a hypercalcemic patient with normal renal function favors primary HPT. In nonparathyroid causes, more profound hypercalciuria is usually found. A low urinary calcium, less than 150 mg/24 hours, raises the possibility of benign familial hypocalciuric hypercalcemia or the use of thiazide diuretics.

Serum Parathyroid Hormone (iPTH). Serum PTH measured by radioimmunoassay is probably the best test of parathyroid function currently available. It has simplified the diagnosis of primary HPT and obviated the need for multiple indirect tests of parathyroid function. It is important to keep in mind the heterogeneity of circulating PTH. The antibodies available in different labs can measure intact PTH, as well as its amino or its carboxy terminals, accounting partly for the variation in the normal ranges from one laboratory to another. Most assays use the antiserum directed against the carboxy terminal that measures intact hormone and the carboxy terminal fragment as well. This assay will give a good separation of patients with primary HPT from normal subjects.

Of patients with primary HPT, 90% have elevated serum PTH, while 10% have PTH within the normal limits. It is of utmost importance that serum PTH be assessed concomitantly with serum calcium. A suppressed PTH value in the hypercalcemic patient indicates nonparathyroid hypercalcemia; a ''normal'' PTH in the presence of hypercalcemia indicates inappropriate PTH secretion because normal parathyroid secretion should be suppressed in the presence of hypercalcemia. Therefore, a ''normal'' or a high PTH in the face of hypercalcemia indicates inappropriate PTH secretion caused most commonly by primary hyperparathyroidism, or, rarely, by ectopic hyperparathyroidism.

Serum PTH should also be assessed concomitantly with serum creatinine; the half-life of the carboxy terminal, which is cleared by the kidney, is long, and any decrease in the glomerular filtration rate will cause accumulation of this parathyroid fragment.

Urinary Cyclic AMP (UcAMP). Urinary cyclic AMP includes filtered cAMP (plasma cAMP) and cAMP generated through the effect of PTH on the renal tubule (nephrogenous fraction, NcAMP). NcAMP can be used as an indirect assay of PTH action. Since the plasma level and the filtered cAMP tend to remain fairly constant, the use of UcAMP is of almost equal value and easier. These laboratory parameters are advantageous in that they involve an incubation period of hours rather than days and hence are particularly useful when urgent decisions regarding a hypercalcemic patient have to be made. The values are elevated in 90% of patients with primary HPT. Unfortunately, because high values may also be obtained in patients with hypercalcemia of malignancy, normal or increased values do not help in the differential diagnosis of primary HPT and hypercalcemia of malignancy, though low values rule out a diagnosis of primary HPT and suggest a nonparathyroid cause of hypercalcemia.

Steroid Suppression Test. This can be used in equivocal cases. The underlying principle is that steroids do not suppress hypercalcemia of primary HPT but do so in some cases of nonparathyroid hypercalcemia. Cortisone acetate is given in the dose of 120 mg/day (or, alternatively, prednisone, 30 mg/day) is given for 5 to 10 days. The purpose of the test is to demonstrate whether a suppression of serum calcium greater than 1 mg has or has not occurred. Suppression characteristically occurs in patients with vitamin D intoxication, multiple myeloma, breast carcinoma, and lymphoproliferative disorders. However, some patients with pri-

mary HPT, especially those with radiologic bone disease, may show suppression.

Miscellaneous Tests. Another test is the serum chloride/phosphate ratio. In primary HPT, there is a tendency towards hyperchloremia and hypophosphatemia. A serum chloride greater than 103 mEq/L and a chloride/phosphate ratio greater than 33 is seen in most patients with primary HPT. In nonparathyroid hypercalcemia, the ratio is less than 30 but overlap may occur.

Assessment of acid-base balance should also be done. In primary HPT there is a mild degree of proximal renal tubular acidosis. In nonparathyroid hypercalcemia, PTH is suppressed and metabolic alkalosis ensues. However, presence of renal impairment complicates the interpretation.

Serum alkaline phosphatase should be measured. Most patients with primary HPT have normal alkaline phosphatase; bone alkaline phosphatase may be increased in hyperparathyroid bone disease, Paget's disease and thyrotoxicosis, and hepatic alkaline phosphatase may be increased in metastasis, granulomas, and hepatobiliary malignancy.

The presence of anemia and a high sedimentation rate suggest nonparathyroid cause of hypercalcemia, particularly malignancy, but have been recorded in primary HPT.

Polyclonal hypergammaglobulinemia suggests multiple myeloma or sarcoidosis but has also been observed in primary HPT.

Tests of renal handling of phosphate including tubular reabsorption of phosphate (TRP) and maximum tubular reabsorption of phosphate (TmP/GFR) have been of limited use since the advent of serum PTH determinations. PTH increases phosphate excretion; TRP and TmP/GFR are reduced in most patients with primary HPT. TRP is also affected by renal function, dietary intake, and circadian rhythm and is of limited use because of overlap between values in the normal and primary HPT. TmP/GFR gives better discrimination.

RADIOLOGIC STUDIES

Bone changes of osteitis fibrosa cystica are pathognomonic of hyperparathyroidism. X-rays of the hands, skull, and clavicle may show the characteristic findings. Subperiosteal resorption is best demonstrated on magnified fine-grain industrial radiographs of the hand and, particularly, on the radial surface of the middle phalanx, especially the index finger. Generalized osteopenia with bone cysts, brown tumors, and erosion of the distal phalangeal tufts or distal ends of the clavicle may be apparent. Extensive areas of demineralization alternating with areas of increased bone density in the skull give a picture of "salt and pepper."

An excretory urogram may show evidence of urolithiasis, nephrocalcinosis, or causative hypernephroma.

Other radiologic studies are indicated depending on the clinical setting. A chest x-ray may show evidence of sarcoidosis or other granulomatous disease or underlying lung tumor. Bone survey and bone scan may show evidence of metastatic disease or multiple myeloma.

Diagnostic Approach

The diagnostic approach is outlined in Figure 11–15. To determine if true hypercalcemia is present, the physician needs to rule out inappropriate sampling (postprandial or after prolonged use of phlebotomy tourniquet, because volume depletion may cause minimal increase in serum calcium); it is important to make certain of the use of cork stoppers, acid-washed glassware, and calcium-free disposable syringes. It is also important to rule out pseudohypercalcemia caused by hyperproteinemia. A simultaneous serum albumin concentration should be checked. If the serum albumin is high, a correction formula is applied by the subtraction of 0.8 mg calcium to the measured calcium level for every 1.0 g increase in serum albumin. It is also important to rule out a lab error and to confirm the presence of hypercalcemia by more than one serum calcium determination.

To determine the cause of hypercalcemia, helpful clues can be obtained from the clinical evaluation, such as clinical evidence of chronicity (by obtaining previous serum calcium determinations, if possible, or a history of renal colic, documented renal stones or nephrocalcinosis, or subperiosteal bone resorption). Hypercalcemia of a few years' duration makes diagnosis of primary HPT extremely likely, whereas a hypercalcemia of recent detection without evidence of chronicity should prompt a thorough search for other causes of hypercalcemia.

A drug history is important, especially as it relates to thiazides, vitamins A and D, absorbable antacids, oral calcium agents, and milk. Also important is a history of exposure to TB or other granulomatous disease; a history of immobilization, other endocrinopathy, systemic symptoms suggestive of malignancy, sarcoidosis, etc: a family history of primary hyperparathyroidism or multiple endocrine neoplasia type I or II; evidence of primary neoplasm in the bronchus, kidney, breast, prostate, gonads, liver, gastrointestinal tract, pancreas, etc., clinical evidence of sarcoidosis, erythema nodosum, uveitis, lymphadenopathy, or Paget's disease; band keratopathy, which points to hy-

percalcemia of long duration and favors primary HPT; and a thyroid-area mass, which is usually a coincidental thyroid nodule but may be due to medullary carcinoma of the thyroid or parathyroid carcinoma.

If the hypercalcemia is drug associated, the drug is discontinued and the patient observed. Normalization of serum calcium points to drug-induced hypercalcemia; persistence of hypercalcemia dictates further evaluation.

It is important to remember that because thiazides rarely cause hypercalcemia with serum calcium greater than 10.5 mg/dl, other causes of hypercalcemia should be considered in a patient taking thiazides. Also, the urinary calcium is usually low in thiazide-induced hypercalcemia. If hypercalciuria is present, one should look for other causes. Hypercalcemia caused by thiazide administration resolves in 3 weeks after the discontinuation of thiazide. If hypercalcemia is due to vitamin D intoxication, it may persist for months after the discontinuation of the drug.

Serum PTH is the next critical assessment in hypercalcemic patients. If the parathyroid glands are normal, plasma levels of calcium greater than 10.1 mg/dl should suppress the parathyroid glands and lead to undetectable levels of serum PTH. Autonomous production of PTH can lead to a normal serum PTH in the face of hypercalcemia or a frankly elevated serum PTH. A normal or elevated serum PTH in the face of hypercalcemia can be seen in primary hyperparathyroidism or in ectopic pseudohyperparathyroidism.

The diagnosis of primary HPT is suggested by mild to moderate hypercalcemia of long duration with chronic complications (such as nephrolithiasis, periosteal bone resorption, pancreatitis, peptic ulcer, and band keratopathy), and it is associated with hypophosphatemia, a high chloride/low serum bicarbonate, and urine calcium of less than 400 mg/24 hours. In this setting, the finding of a normal or elevated serum PTH, which shows a positive correlation with a degree of hypercalcemia, is diagnostic of primary hyperparathyroidism.

An elevated serum PTH may be found in some patients with hypercalcemia of malignancy. An absolute discrimination between primary HPT and hypercalcemia of malignancy cannot be made on the basis of any single test. Hypercalcemia of malignancy should be suspected in the presence of moderate to severe hypercalcemia greater than 13 to 14 mg/dl, a short, rapidly progressive course, weight loss, absence of evidence of chronicity (such as urinary calculi, nephrocalcinosis, subperiosteal resorption, and band keratopathy), normal or mildly decreased serum phosphate, serum chloride less than 102 mEq/L, and normal or elevated serum bicarbonate. Serum PTH in such

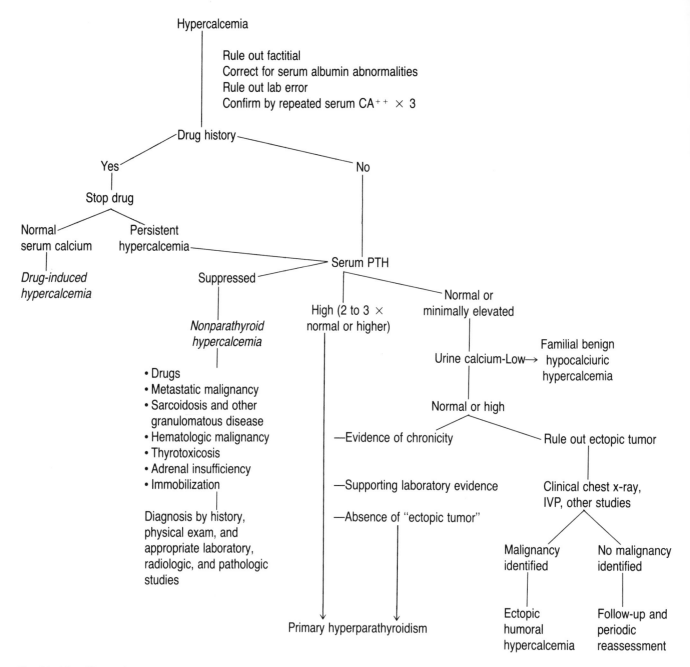

Fig. 11–15. Diagnostic approach to hypercalcemic disorders.

patients is normal or mildly elevated, is rarely greater than twice the upper limit of normal, and shows no correlation with the serum calcium level. In addition, most of these patients have clinically overt lesions (evident on clinical evaluation, chest x-ray, and excretory urogram) and do not constitute a diagnostic problem.

Once the provisional diagnosis of primary HPT is made, an assessment of the severity of the disease is in order as a prelude to determining therapy. The severity of the disease is assessed using the level of serum

calcium, an excretory urogram to look for evidence of nephrocalcinosis or renal stones, and an abdominal x-ray to look for pancreatic calcification. In addition, associated metabolic bone disease is assessed using parameters of alkaline phosphatase, hand x-rays on industrial films looking for evidence of subperiosteal bone resorption, and bone densitometry studies.

Several tests have been devised for the preoperative localization of parathyroid lesions. These include parathyroid ultrasonography or CT scanning, isotope scanning, arteriography or venography, and venous sampling. Because of the high cost to benefit of these procedures, they are not recommended for routine use prior to initial neck exploration. Localization, however, is indicated prior to any parathyroid reexploration.

In all patients presumed to have primary hyperparathyroidism, a 24-hour urine calcium should be checked. A low urinary calcium in a patient who is not on thiazide therapy points to familial benign hypocalciuric hypocalcemia. The diagnosis is supported by the mild to moderate elevation in the serum calcium, the absence of complications, and the positive family history.

A suppressed, undetectable serum PTH in a hypercalcemic patient indicates a nonparathyroid cause of the hypercalcemia, including the use of drugs, metastatic malignancy, sarcoidosis and other granulomatous disease, hematologic malignancy, other endocrinopathy, and immobilization. The diagnosis is made on the basis of the clinical setting and appropriate laboratory, radiologic, and pathologic studies.

In evaluating such a patient, a drug history is critical. The diagnosis of metastatic malignancy is based on the clinical setting, bone x-rays or scans, and tissue diagnosis. A diagnosis of hematologic malignancies is based on the clinical setting, bone x-rays and scans, protein studies in the serum or the urine, marrow aspiration, and steroid suppressibility.

In sarcoidosis, hypercalcemia is usually associated with severe disseminated disease. Findings of pulmonary involvement may be apparent on the chest x-ray or in abnormal pulmonary function tests (exercise-induced hypoxia and abnormal carbon monoxide diffusion); serum angiotensin-converting enzyme levels are elevated. The hypercalcemia is steroid suppressible, and noncaseating granulomas can be demonstrated by liver or lymph node biopsy (the latter usually by scalene node).

Thyrotoxicosis is usually evident on clinical evaluation but may be occult in elderly patients. Diagnosis is made by elevated thyroid hormone levels (see Thyrotoxicosis). Treatment of thyrotoxicosis leads to normalization of the serum calcium.

The diagnosis of adrenal insufficiency is supported by finding low cortisol levels unresponsive to provocative tests (see The Syndrome of Adrenocortical Insufficiency). Glucocorticoid therapy leads to normalization of the hypercalcemia.

Idiopathic hypercalcemia of infancy is diagnosed on the basis of the age distribution, clinical setting, and distinctive clinical features.

Immobilization as a cause of hypercalcemia is evident in the clinical setting.

It is important to remember that primary hyperparathyroidism may be associated with any of the nonparathyroid causes of hypercalcemia.

If, as happens rarely, diagnostic uncertainty persists despite intensive evaluation, two options are available. Observation is a reasonable option if no life threatening problems are present. The serum calcium is checked every few weeks, and the patient is asked to return promptly if clinical deterioration occurs. A repeat evaluation is performed in 3 to 6 months. In most cases, the repeat evaluation will yield the diagnosis or strengthen the suspicion enough so that other steps can be taken.

If a life threatening hypercalcemic problem is present, the main thrust of the evaluation should be to assess whether the patient has a surgically correctable parathyroid disorder. Hand x-rays on industrial films to look for subperiosteal resorption as an indicator of parathyroid hormone excess, ultrasonography or CT of the neck, or CT of the chest to localize parathyroid adenoma are in order. In some centers, venous catheterization with sampling for PTH at different sites can be done; a gradient between a given site and peripheral venous blood shows the source of parathyroid hormone overproduction. In nonparathyroid hypercalcemia, no such gradient is found.

URIC ACID DISORDERS

Uric acid is the major product of purine metabolism and is formed by the oxidation of purine bases derived from endogenous and exogenous nucleoproteins. Its formation occurs predominantly in the liver and intestinal mucosa.

The uric acid biosynthetic pathway is shown in Figure 11–16. The purine nucleotides adenylic acid (AMP), inosinic acid (IMP), and guanylic acid (GMP) are the end products of purine biosynthesis and are utilized for the synthesis of the nucleic acids, cyclic AMP, cyclic GMP, ATP, and certain cofactors. They can be synthesized in one of two ways: either directly, from purine bases guanine, hypoxanthine, and adenine, or de novo, beginning with nonpurine precursors and progressing to the formation of IMP, which is the common intermediate purine nucleotide. The nucleotides are degraded via the steps outlined in Figure 11–16 with the end product being uric acid. The regulation of this synthetic pathway is complex. It appears that the intracellular concentration of phosphoribosylpyrophosphate (PRPP) is the major determinant of synthesis of uric acid.

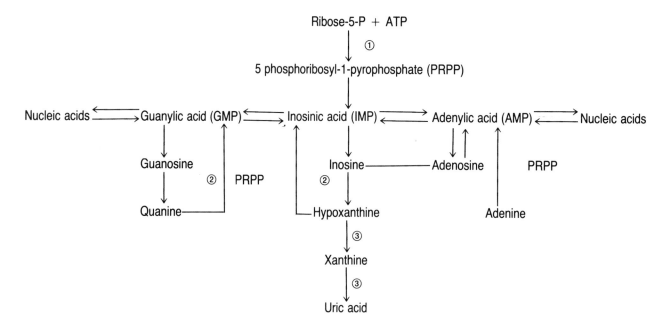

① PRPP synthetase
② Hypoxanthine guanine phosphoribosyltransferase (HG-PRT)
③ Xanthine oxidase

Fig. 11–16. Outline of purine metabolism.

The average adult excretes 400 to 800 mg of uric acid per day; two thirds are excreted by the kidney and one third by the gastrointestinal tract. The renal handling of urate is complex. It is freely filtered by the glomeruli, with 98 to 100% of the filtered urate reabsorbed by the proximal tubule (presecretory reabsorption). Secretion occurs in subsequent segments of the proximal tubule with partial reabsorption by the distal proximal tubule (postsecretory absorption). Excreted urate arises almost entirely from tubular secretion.

HYPERURICEMIA

Definition. Hyperuricemia refers to serum uric acid levels above the upper limit of the normal range defined as the mean serum urate +/− 2 SD in a healthy population matched by age and sex. The upper limit of normal in males is 7.0 mg/dl, and in females, 6.0 mg/dl. Age and sex affect urate levels. In children, the average serum uric acid level is 3.6 mg/dl. Serum uric acid increases at puberty, more so in boys than girls. In males, the levels plateau at age 20 and remain stable thereafter. In females, the levels remain stable between the age of 20 and 40 and increase after the menopause.

Pathophysiologic Considerations. Hyperuricemia can result from increased synthesis of uric acid from endogenous purines, decreased renal excretion of urate, or a combination of both defects. Abnormalities of gastrointestinal absorption or excretion have not been implicated as cause of hyperuricemia. Hyperuricemia can be primary when it is the central manifestation of the disease, or secondary when it is due to another disease or results from the use of drugs (Table 11–26).

Overproduction of Uric Acid. This may result from an acceleration of the rate of purine synthesis de novo or from an increased turnover of purines. Overproduction of uric acid accounts for less than 15% of all cases of primary hyperuricemia.

Hypoxanthine-guanine phosphoribosyltransferase (HG-PRT) catalyzes the conversion of hypoxanthine to IMP and guanine to GMP. Its partial deficiency leads to decreased consumption and accumulation of PRPP and increased synthesis of purines and uric acid. It is inherited in an X-linked manner, males being affected through carrier females. It is characterized by onset of gouty arthritis at a young age (15 to 30 years), high incidence (75%) of uric acid stones, and occasional occurrence of mild neurogenic dysfunction characterized by dysarthria, hyperreflexia, incoordination, or mental retardation.

Lesch-Nyhan syndrome is due to a more severe deficiency of HG-PRT. It is a rare X-linked disorder occurring in 1 out of every 100,000 births, and is

Table 11–26. Classification of Hyperuricemia and Gout

Primary
  Idiopathic (>99%)
    Normal urinary excretion (80–90%)
    Increased urinary excretion (10–20%)
  Associated with specific defects (<1%)
    Partial deficiency of HG-PRT
    Increased activity of PRPP synthetase
Secondary
  Associated with increased de novo synthesis
    "Complete" deficiency of HG-PRT: Lesch-Nyhan syndrome
    Glycogen storage type I disease (von Gierke's) disease
  Associated with increased nucleic acid turnover
    Myeloproliferative or lymphoproliferative disorders
    Multiple myeloma
    Secondary polycythemia
    Pernicious anemia
    Certain hemoglobinopathies
    Infectious mononucleosis
    Sarcoidosis
    Chemotherapy and radiation of malignant neoplasms
    Psoriasis
    Sickle-cell disease
  Associated with decreased renal clearance of uric acid
    Reduced renal functional mass
      Renal failure
      Polycystic kidney
      Lead nephropathy
    Inhibition of secretion and/or increased reabsorption
      Drugs, toxins
        Diuretics
        Low-dose salicylate, probenecid, sulfinpyrazone
        Pyrazinamide
        Nicotinic acid
        Ethambutol
        Ethanol
      Endogenous metabolic products
        Starvation
        Diabetic ketoacidosis
        Lactic acidosis
        Maple syrup urine disease
      Hyperparathyroidism
      Hypoparathyroidism
      Pseudohypoparathyroidism
      Hypothyroidism

characterized by profound overproduction of uric acid, hyperuricemia, a neurologic disorder with components of self-mutilation, choreoathetosis, spasticity, mental retardation, and retardation of growth.

Several families have been reported to have increased activity of PRPP synthetase leading to increased intracellular PRPP and increased purine and uric acid synthesis. Affected patients develop gout in the second or third decade of life and have a high incidence of uric acid stones.

Secondary hyperuricemia caused by increased production is seen in patients with glucose-6-phosphate deficiency (glycogen storage type 1 disease) and increased turnover of nucleic acids, resulting from mye-loproliferative and lymphoproliferative diseases, multiple myeloma, secondary polycythemia, pernicious anemia, certain hemoglobinopathies, infectious mononucleosis, psoriasis, and some cancers.

Reduced Urate Excretion. As mentioned, excretion of urate is dependent on glomerular filtration, tubular reabsorption, and tubular secretion; accordingly, decreased excretion may be due to decreased filtration, increased absorption, or decreased secretion. In primary hyperuricemia, which results from reduced excretion, all these factors may be operative. Secondary hyperuricemia, resulting from reduced urate excretion, is seen with decreased glomerular filtration rate (renal failure); decreased urate secretion (polycystic kidneys, lead nephropathy); the use of diuretics, low-dose aspirin, pyrazinamide, nicotinic acid, ethambutol, and ethanol; adrenal insufficiency and nephrogenic DI; diabetic ketoacidosis, starvation, alcoholic ketoacidosis, lactic acidosis, and maple syrup urine disease (competitive inhibition of uric acid secretion by excess organic acids); and hyperparathyroidism, hypoparathyroidism, pseudohypoparathyroidism, and hypothyroidism caused by an unknown mechanism.

Clinical Presentation. Hyperuricemia may be asymptomatic or can present as an integral part of gout. Gout is characterized by several abnormalities that may occur singly or in combination: hyperuricemia; precipitation of monosodium urate as deposits (tophi) throughout the body with a special predilection for joints, periarticular cartilage, bone or bursae, and subcutaneous tissue (a notable exception is the central nervous system); recurrent clinical attacks of arthritis; and nephropathy and, frequently, nephrolithiasis. Gout can be primary or secondary. Primary gout is due to an inborn error of metabolism involving uric acid synthesis and excretion. Its mode of inheritance is unknown. Fewer than one third of the patients have a family history of clinical gout, but many of their close relatives are found to have hyperuricemia. Primary gout affects males predominantly (greater than 90%), with peak incidence in the fifth decade. It is very rare prior to age 20. Secondary gout occurs in association with hyperuricemia from numerous other causes. In secondary hyperuricemia, gout is a very uncommon complication.

Other clinical features that may be associated with hyperuricemia include neurologic abnormalities of choreoathetosis, spastic cerebral palsy, aggressive behavior, and compulsive self-mutilation in Lesch-Nyhan syndrome, and those features of other underlying disorders affecting uric acid production and renal excretion.

Diagnostic Evaluation. The objectives of the diagnostic approach to hyperuricemia are to define its cause, assess the presence and the extent of damage of the tissues and organs, and identify associated abnormalities.

If the patient gives a history of nephrolithiasis, an excretory urogram is in order. If a stone is recovered, it should be analyzed. The most important single test in hyperuricemic patients is the determination of 24-hour urinary excretion of uric acid, which is collected after 3 days of moderate purine restriction. A urinary urate greater than 600 to 800 mg/day points to overproduction of uric acid. In such patients, it is necessary to exclude secondary causes of uric acid overproduction (Table 11–26) and to measure erythrocyte HG-PRT and PRPP synthetase levels.

The differential diagnosis of the causes of hyperuricemia depends primarily on the clinical setting.

HYPOURICEMIA

Hypouricemia is defined as a level of serum uric acid less than 3.0 mg/dl in males and less than 2.0 mg/dl in females.

Hypouricemia may be caused by decreased production of uric acid in xanthinuria, phosphoribosylpyrophosphate deficiency, and severe liver disease, and with the use of allopurinol. It may also be caused by increased renal excretion, which may be congenital (Fanconi's syndrome, Wilson's disease, Hartnup's disease) or acquired (from toxins). It can also be seen in the syndrome of inappropriate ADH and with the use of drugs such as salicylates (in large doses), methyldopa, clofibrate, phenylbutazone, sulfinpyrazone, and phenothiazines (Table 11–27).

Table 11–27. Causes of Hypouricemia

Decreased production
  Use of allopurinol
  Xanthinuria
  Phosphoribosylpyrophosphate deficiency
  Severe liver disease
Increased renal excretion
  Congenital
    Fanconi's syndrome
    Wilson's disease
    Hartnup's disease
  Acquired
    Toxins
Miscellaneous
  SIADH
  Drugs
    Salicylates (large doses)
    Methyldopa
    Clofibrate
    Phenylbutazone
    Sulfinpyrazone
    Phenothiazines

HYPERGLYCEMIA AND DIABETES MELLITUS

DEFINITION

Diabetes mellitus is a metabolic disorder in which the basic defect is absolute or relative lack of insulin. It is manifest in its complete form by hyperglycemia, accelerated atherosclerosis, microvascular disease (retina and kidney), and neuropathy. It affects about 5% of the population in the U.S.

PATHOPHYSIOLOGIC CONSIDERATIONS AND CLASSIFICATION

A classification developed by the National Diabetes Data Group (NDDG) from the National Institute of Health, Bethesda, MD, distinguishes a number of classes according to the degree and pathogenesis of the metabolic abnormality.

Type I, insulin dependent, ketosis-prone diabetes mellitus (juvenile onset diabetes mellitus) is characterized by severe absolute insulin deficiency, the patient's dependence on exogenous insulin therapy (except maybe in the initial stages), and high predisposition to ketosis. It affects 10 to 20% of the diabetic population, usually appearing in patients less than 20 years of age with a peak at 12 years of age, but it can occur at any age. Both genetic and environmental factors are involved in its pathogenesis; there is concordance in twins in about 25 to 50% of cases, frequent association with certain histocompatibility antigen HLA types, and association with abnormal immune responses, including islet-cell antibodies. Certain cases result from viral infection (e.g., enteroviruses and mumps). Some patients may show a remission of up to several months after initial insulin therapy has restored the metabolic balance. This ''honeymoon'' or ''brush effect'' is transient and is followed by recurrence of insulin deficiency and symptomatic diabetes mellitus.

Type II, noninsulin dependent, ketosis-resistant diabetes mellitus is characterized by partial insulin deficiency, resistance to the development of ketosis, and, in most patients, insulin resistance at target tissues. It affects 80 to 90% of the diabetic population and can occur at any age but usually appears in the older obese patient. Genetic susceptibility is strong, and twin concordance is 100%. Environmental factors such as obesity play a definite role in the development of the disease.

Diabetes associated with certain conditions, gestational diabetes mellitus, and impaired glucose tolerance are described below.

DIAGNOSTIC EVALUATION

Patient History and Physical Examination

Type I diabetes mellitus usually has a dramatic onset related to abrupt severe insulin deficiency. It usually presents with polyuria, polydipsia, polyphagia with associated weight loss, severe dehydration, ketoacidosis, and, eventually, coma. Nocturnal enuresis may signal the onset in very young children. On examination the physician may find varying levels of impairment of consciousness, depending on the degree of hyperosmolarity; features of dehydration, including dry tongue and skin, loss of skin turgor, tachycardia, a weak, thready pulse, and hypotension; and weight loss. In some individuals may be found an enlarged liver, eruptive xanthomas, and lipemia retinalis, a result of the associated hyperlipidemia (triglyceride levels greater than 2000 mg/dl).

Type II diabetes mellitus usually has an insidious onset. Usually the patient is initially asymptomatic, and the diagnosis is suggested by the presence of glycosuria or is made by the finding of fasting hyperglycemia. Patients may complain of blurring of vision and myopia; generalized pruritus; and episodes of recurrent infections, carbuncles, furuncles, urinary tract infections, monilial vaginitis in females, and balanitis in males. Occasionally the patient may present with evidence of chronic diabetic complications (neuropathy, nephropathy, or retinopathy) without symptoms relating to the glucose intolerance. Patients may develop polyuria, polydipsia, and polyphagia under certain conditions when the insulin output is stressed, e.g., in pregnancy, with infection, and with the use of certain drugs. Occasionally the patient can present with hyperosmolar nonketotic coma. Some patients may present with transient postprandial hypoglycemia. The diagnosis should be suspected in women who have delivered large babies (greater than 9 pounds) or who have had a history of hydramnios, pre-eclampsia, and unexplained fetal losses.

Chronic Complications

Arteriosclerosis, which appears earlier and is more extensive in the diabetic patient than in the general population, can present clinically as peripheral vascular disease (with intermittent claudication, gangrene, and impotence), coronary artery disease (with angina and myocardial infarction), and cerebrovascular disease (e.g., stroke). Coronary heart disease accounts for 70% of deaths in the diabetic population. It tends to involve the proximal and distal vessels in both the right and the left coronary systems. Atypical manifestations may occur. Angina may present with epigastric distress, heartburn, and neck or jaw pain. Myocardial infarction may be silent (in 15% of cases) because of autonomic neuropathy; it should be suspected in those patients with sudden onset of left ventricular failure. Diabetes mellitus may also be associated with cardiomyopathy and heart failure (in 17% of cases) in the absence of other identifiable causes and with a normal coronary arterial system by angiography. Peripheral vascular disease has a higher frequency of distal involvement, particularly in the lower extremities. The usual presentation is intermittent claudication that may progress to pain at rest. It is important to remember that arteriography should be avoided if the patient has diminished renal function because acute tubular necrosis may develop; it should be reserved for patients who are candidates for vascular surgery.

Microvascular Complications

The characteristic diabetic microvascular lesion is basement membrane thickening and accumulation of periodic acid Schiff-positive material. Retinopathy will eventually develop in 90% of diabetic patients. Present in at least 50% of patients who have had diabetes for approximately 15 years and in more than 90% who have had diabetes for 30 years, it is a leading cause of blindness in the U.S.

Simple background nonproliferative retinopathy can manifest early with increased capillary permeability (detected by fluorescein angiography), occlusion and dilation of capillaries (microaneurysms), and dilated veins. Intraretinal hemorrhages—"dot" in the deep retinal layers and "blot" in the superficial layers—may occur. The patient may develop exudates, "cotton wool" from microinfarcts and "hard" from leakage of protein and lipids from the damaged capillaries. The retinal ischemia can lead to retinal and macular edema, which is the most common cause of decreased vision in simple retinopathy. In most patients, simple retinopathy tends to remain stable. In 10 years, 10 to 15% of patients progress to proliferative retinopathy.

Proliferative retinopathy results from new vessel formation, which occurs in response to the underlying retinal ischemia. New vessels may develop over any portion of the retina but mostly around the optic disc and will penetrate into the vitreous, resulting in two complications, preretinal and vitreous hemorrhage, and retinal detachment from the growth of fibrous tissue into the vitreous and the fibrous tissue's subsequent contraction. This type of retinopathy can present with sudden loss of vision in one eye and is the leading cause of blindness in the 20- to 64-year-old age group in the U.S.

Other ophthalmologic problems in the diabetic patient include temporary changes in the lens shape and marked fluctuation of the visual acuity resulting from hyperglycemia; increased frequency of cataract (perhaps due to the polyol pathway) and glaucoma (posthemorrhagic and fibrous scarring of the outflow tract of the canal of Schlemm); neoproliferation of the vessels of the iris; and, occasionally, isolated primary pupillary abnormalities such as anisocoria and Argyll Robertson pupil (decreased reactivity to light but normal reactivity accommodation). Ophthalmologic evaluation is critical in all diabetic patients at least annually. Proliferative retinopathy may also be caused by sickle cell anemia, retinal vein obstruction, and retrolental fibroplasia.

Nephropathy

In early diabetes mellitus the kidneys are enlarged and the glomerular filtration rate is increased. After a number of years, characteristic lesions appear: glomerulosclerosis (nodular, Kimmelstiel-Wilson syndrome, diffuse, or exudative), arteriosclerosis of glomerular arteries and renal arteries and their major branches, and peritubular deposits of glycogen, fat, and mucopolysaccharides. Nephropathy may be manifested by proteinuria of variable degrees (full-blown nephrotic syndrome is rare); change in the renal threshold for glucose; hypertension and uremia; and increasing insulin sensitivity, necessitating a decrease in insulin dosage. A very high percentage of patients with diabetic nephropathy have simultaneous diabetic retinopathy. Other renal problems that can complicate the diabetic state include urinary tract infection (atonic bladder or prostate hypertrophy); hypertensive renal disease, which may be present in up to 50% of those with diabetes mellitus; and renal papillary necrosis and renal infarction.

Neuropathy

The nerves in a diabetic patient may show segmental demyelination, axonal degeneration, and basal lamina thickening. Unlike the other chronic consequences of diabetes mellitus, neuropathy may occur early in the disease, but the frequency and severity increase in proportion to the duration and the severity of the hyperglycemia. Neuropathy is clinically evident in about 30% of individuals with diabetes of more than 10 years' duration.

Peripheral polyneuropathy is the most commonly encountered type. It is usually bilateral and symmetrical and affects the lower extremities more commonly than the upper. It presents with numbness, paresthesias or hyperesthesia, or deep-seated moderate to severe pain that is worse at night. Onset may be insidious or acute, often occurring during the loss of diabetic control secondary to infection or other stresses. Peripheral polyneuropathy also presents with abnormalities of proprioceptive fibers, leading to gait abnormalities and development of Charcot's joints (painless progressive destruction of articular cartilage and joint architecture and function; x-rays commonly reveal loss of arch and multiple fractures of the tarsal bones). There may also be development of neurotrophic ulcers, particularly on the plantar aspect of the feet, that may be complicated by osteomyelitis. Examination will show absence of deep tendon reflexes and decreased vibration sense.

Mononeuropathy can affect any single nerve trunk and characteristically can present with sudden wristdrop, footdrop, or painful diplopia resulting from III, IV, or VI cranial nerve dysfunction (in the cranial nerve dysfunctions presentation, pain precedes the development of paralysis by 5 to 10 days. When the third nerve is involved there is a characteristic sparing of the pupillary fibers in more than 80% of cases. Aneurysms or intracranial mass lesions generally involve both the pupillary fibers and the fibers to the extraocular muscles). There is a high degree of spontaneous reversibility, usually over several weeks.

Radiculopathy is a sensory syndrome that can present with pain in the distribution of one or more spinal nerves, usually in the chest wall, abdomen, and lower extremities. It is also usually self-limited.

Autonomic neuropathy can involve virtually every organ system, the gastrointestinal tract being the prime target. Although constipation is the most common manifestation of this autonomic neuropathy, it tends to be overshadowed by the common, distressing diabetic diarrhea, which consists of intermittent explosive diarrhea not preceded by cramps and seemingly worse at night. Radiologic studies may demonstrate characteristic patterns of disordered small-bowel motility. Steatorrhea suggests the possibility of coexisting celiac disease or other causes of malabsorption.

Diabetic gastroparesis may present with early satiety and nausea or vomiting. Radiologic and electrophysiologic studies may reveal impaired peristalsis and delayed gastric emptying. This complication is important because, as a result of the inconsistency of food absorption, there may be unpredictable swings in plasma glucose and in levels of diabetic control. Esophageal dysfunction and dysphagia may also occur.

Genitourinary involvement includes urinary bladder dysfunction, which occurs in more than 50% of patients with diabetes of greater than 20 years' duration, and can present as hesitancy, delayed and incomplete emptying, and residual urine. A voiding cystometrogram may reveal decreased propulsive efforts and increased residual urine. Urinary bladder dysfunction may be complicated by bacteriuria initially and later by overt urinary tract infection. It leads to loss of utility of the double-voided urine as an index of diabetes control.

Potency impairment occurs in more than 50% of men with long-standing diabetes and may be the initial presentation of the diabetic syndrome. Another cause of potency impairment in diabetic patients is penile vascular insufficiency caused by aortoiliac occlusive disease (Leriche's syndrome). The diabetic male patient may also have retrograde ejaculation.

Features of cardiovascular autonomic neuropathy may include manifestations of orthostatic hypotension, cardiac arrest, and sudden death. Irregularity of sweating and partial and total anhidrosis may be observed and a patchy distribution of sweating may be particularly evident in the face. An unusual variant of autonomic instability may be manifested in some diabetic patients by gustatory sweating after eating.

Diabetic neuromuscular disease presents with symmetrical painless atrophy and weakness of the intrinsic muscles of the hand that may be associated with sensory impairment and occurs more commonly in elderly patients and in males.

Diabetic amyotrophy refers to a progressive weakness and wasting involving the pelvic girdle and anterior thigh compartments, most commonly the quadriceps femoris. It is usually accompanied by severe pain and may be distributed asymmetrically. It is found characteristically in elderly men and generally resolves in 2 to 4 months from the time of diagnosis. A similar but less painful variant occurs in the upper extremities.

In diabetic neuropathy the electromyogram may show a reduction in motor and sensory nerve conduction velocity, evidence of denervation and fasciculation, and characteristic distribution of nerve dysfunction. Cerebrospinal fluid examination may show a slight increase in protein content.

Diabetic foot ulcers result from the effects of neuropathy and vascular disease. Abnormal pressure distribution results in callus formation, ill-fitting shoes lead to blisters, and foreign bodies lead to abrasions and punctures. These ulcers are painless and are frequently complicated by infection and osteomyelitis.

Infections

Although infections may not occur more frequently in a diabetic patient than in a nondiabetic patient, they tend to be more severe because of the presence of hyperglycemia (which impairs leukocyte function) and because of associated macro- and microvascular disease, which decreases the regional blood flow. In diabetic patients there is an increased frequency of cutaneous infections (Staph infections, furuncles, pyoderma, and carbuncles), urinary tract infections (cystitis, pyelonephritis, papillary necrosis), lung infections (pneumonia), extremity infections (gram-negative and anaerobic infections), and genital tract infections (vulvovaginitis and balanitis). Three unusual conditions appear to have specific relationships to the diabetic syndrome: malignant external otitis, rhinocerebral mucormycosis, and emphysematous cholecystitis.

Dermatologic Complications

A variety of cutaneous lesions may occur in the diabetic patient. Necrobiosis lipoidica diabeticorum consists of plaque-like lesions with central yellowish areas surrounded by a brownish border, usually occurring over the anterior surfaces of the legs. Ulceration may occur. Diabetic dermopathy consists of small-rounded plaques with a raised border occurring over the anterior tibial surfaces that may ulcerate centrally and crust at the edges. As these lesions heal, there is a depressed scar and diffuse brown discoloration. Bullosis diabeticorum is rare and consists of bullous lesions that may be superficial with clear serum or may be mildly hemorrhagic. Joint contractures may occur in patients with type I diabetes mellitus and in patients who appear to have accelerated development of diabetic complications.

Acute Metabolic Complications

Diabetic ketoacidosis (DKA) occurs in insulin-dependent diabetic patients of any age but predominantly as a complication of type I diabetes. It is initiated by acute insulin deficiency and an increase in the contrainsulin hormones glucagon, epinephrine, cortisol, and growth hormone. Diabetic ketoacidosis involves enhancement of glycogenolysis and gluconeogenesis and impairment in the peripheral utilization of glucose. These lead to severe hyperglycemia, osmotic diuresis, dehydration, and volume depletion. In addition, they cause increased free–fatty acid release from fat depots, uptake and oxidation, and ketone body formation by the liver, leading to ketoacidosis, which may ultimately produce cardiovascular failure and death.

Diabetic ketoacidosis usually evolves over several days but can appear as a fulminant disorder in a few hours. The onset is with anorexia, nausea and vomiting, polyuria and polydipsia, and, occasionally, abdominal pain (with or without pancreatitis). Untreated, ketoacidosis progresses to altered consciousness and coma. Infections, acute medical or surgical illness (e.g., myocardial infarction or acute pancreatitis), omission or reduction of prescribed insulin, emotional stress, and pregnancy are frequent precipitating factors. On occasion, no obvious precipitating factor may be delineated.

Physical findings include evidence of volume depletion with tachycardia and hypotension; hyperpnea with Kussmaul's breathing, which appears when the pH falls below 7.3 and may disappear with progressive acidosis from the patient's exhaustion; and acetone breath. Body temperature may be normal or decreased in uncomplicated ketoacidosis; fever suggests the presence of infection. The reflexes are usually normal and the Babinski response is flexor.

Laboratory evaluation shows the presence of significant glycosuria, hyperglycemia, hyperosmolarity, dehydration, hypovolemia, electrolyte depletion, ketonuria, ketonemia, and metabolic acidosis. Leukocytosis may be a feature of diabetic ketoacidosis and may not indicate an infection. Serum sodium tends to be low (due to a shift of water from intracellular to extracellular fluid space because of hyperosmolarity and artifactual decrease from the severe hyperlipidemia). Serum potassium may be normal or increased despite a significant total body potassium deficit (effects of catabolic state, intracellular potassium loss caused by acidosis, and prerenal failure). Similarly, serum phosphate may be high initially despite depletion of body stores. Severe hyperlipidemia (type IV or V) may occur because of hepatic overproduction of very low density lipoprotein (VLDL) and impaired lipoprotein lipase activity. Prerenal azotemia is present, reflecting volume depletion; serum amylase may be elevated in uncomplicated ketoacidosis, but frank pancreatitis may occur.

Hyperosmolar, nonketotic coma (HNKC) is less common than DKA and usually occurs in the setting of type II diabetes. It is characterized by marked hyperglycemia and absence of ketoacidosis. The cause of the absence of ketoacidosis is not known but may be related to the presence of insulin in quantities adequate to prevent full activation of the ketogenic process. HNKC commonly occurs in the elderly patient who lives alone or in a nursing home and develops a stroke or an infection that worsens the hyperglycemia and prevents adequate water intake. It may follow procedures such as peritoneal dialysis or hemodialysis, tube feedings of high-protein formulas, high carbohydrate infusion loads, use of osmotic agents such as mannitol, and use of steroids, immunosuppressive

drugs, and diuretics. It can also occur in patients with type I diabetes given insulin sufficient to prevent ketosis but insufficient to control the hyperglycemia.

HNKC is characterized clinically by effects of extreme hyperglycemia, hyperosmolarity, and volume depletion. It is usually preceded by a more prolonged period of polyuria, polydipsia, and increasing and progressive dehydration that may range from 5 to 21 days and culminates in frank coma, acute renal shutdown, thrombosis, vascular collapse, and lactic acidosis. Central nervous system manifestations may dominate the clinical picture with clouded sensorium evolving to coma, seizures, and transient hemiplegia. Occasionally, HNKC may be complicated by acute pancreatitis and bleeding from disseminated intravascular coagulation. HNKC may be confused with primary cerebrovascular disease. A high index of suspicion for infection should be maintained because these infections are common, particularly pneumonia and gram-negative sepsis.

Laboratory findings show significant hyperglycemia, with plasma glucose ranging from 600 to 2400 mg/dl, generally around 1000 mg/dl. Serum osmolarity is extremely high, with values greater than 325 mOsm kg/H_2O common, but because of the hyperglycemia the absolute serum sodium values are often not elevated. Significant hypokalemia and prerenal azotemia may be present. A mild metabolic acidosis may be found with plasma bicarbonate levels around 20 mEq/L and arterial pH levels as low as 7.2 because of starvation ketosis, renal insufficiency, and lactic acidosis. The mortality rate is very high, greater than 50%, thrombotic events being the principal causes of death.

Diagnostic Studies

In the diagnostic approach to diabetes, the physician must determine if the patient has diabetes mellitus and if there is a secondary cause for the diabetic syndrome. A series of tests may help establish whether diabetes mellitus is present.

Fasting Plasma Glucose. This is obtained in the morning 10 to 16 hours after the last meal and before ingestion of noncaloric stimulants and smoking. The normal fasting plasma glucose is less than 115 mg/dl. In nonpregnant adults, values of 140 mg/dl or greater on two or more separate occasions confirm the diagnosis of diabetes. It is important to remember that glucose values obtained from whole blood are 15% lower than plasma glucose values. Plasma or serum glucose measurements are more frequently used clinically because they are independent of hematocrit, more closely approach glucose levels in interstitial tissue, and lend themselves to automated analytic procedures.

Oral Glucose Tolerance Test (OGTT). The main function of this test is to establish or refute the diagnosis of diabetes mellitus in the following circumstances: when the fasting plasma glucose values are borderline (between 115 and 139 mg/dl); when the patient presents with symptoms related to diabetes mellitus or its known chronic complications and the fasting plasma glucose is normal or borderline; and when a diagnosis of diabetes mellitus in pregnancy must be made.

The test is done in the morning with the patient at rest. A blood sample is drawn for fasting plasma glucose. An oral glucose load of 1.75 g/kg of the patient's ideal weight (but not exceeding 75 g) in less than 400 ml of water is ingested over a 5-minute period, and blood samples for plasma glucose are collected every 30 minutes for 2 hours. Standardization of the GTT is essential for its interpretation; it should be performed in the morning after 10 to 12 hours of fasting in an otherwise healthy and unstressed individual. The patient should be prepared for the test by eating an unrestricted diet containing at least 150 g of carbohydrates per day and engaging in normal levels of exercise for at least 3 days prior to the day of the test. The physician must be aware of the various drugs that affect glucose homeostasis (psychoactive drugs such as amitriptyline, haloperidol, imipramine, and lithium carbonate; hormones such as corticosteroids, catecholamines, and oral contraceptives; alcohol in large amounts; caffeine, clonidine; and diphenylhydantoin).

A diagnosis of diabetes mellitus is made if, on two separate occasions, the fasting plasma glucose is less than 140 mg/dl and the 2-hour value and one additional value between ½ and 1½ hours are 200 mg/dl or greater. A 2-hour plasma glucose value of less than 140 mg/dl effectively rules out the diagnosis of diabetes. The diagnostic criteria should be adjusted according to the patient's age; as compared with younger individuals, in patients beyond age 50, a progressive rise in glucose values is observed, with an increase of 10 mg/dl/decade.

A diagnosis of impaired glucose tolerance is made if the fasting plasma glucose is less than 140 mg/dl, the 2-hour value is 140 to 200 mg/dl, and the intervening values are 200 mg/dl or greater. Over time patients with impaired glucose tolerance may decompensate to frank diabetes, may revert to normal glucose tolerance, or may remain unchanged. They should be re-evaluated periodically or if clinical indications develop. Because many of these patients may never develop diabetes, they should not be labeled as diabetic or prediabetic and should not have to suffer the so-cioeconomic sanctions that frequently accompany such a diagnosis.

Patients with previous abnormality of glucose tolerance have a previous history of documented hyperglycemia that has subsequently returned to normal. They include those with gestational diabetes and those who developed hyperglycemia during the acute phase of myocardial infarction, during serious trauma or sepsis, or during ingestion of diabetogenic drugs.

Patients with potential abnormality of glucose tolerance have normal glucose tolerance but are at an increased risk of developing diabetes compared to the general population. They include the monozygotic twins or other first-degree relatives of diabetic patients, obese individuals, and mothers who have delivered babies of greater than 9 pounds.

Intravenous Glucose Tolerance Test. Intravenous glucose tolerance tests should be reserved for patients who have significant gastroenterologic problems such as malabsorption and impaired absorption caused by hyper- or hypothyroidism and for patients who have had a gastrectomy. The preparation for the test is similar to OGTT. Glucose is given in 0.5 g/kg dose and is infused as a 25 or 50% solution within 3 to 4 minutes. Blood sampling is done at 3, 5, and 10 minutes and at 10-minute intervals for 1 hour. The results are expressed as K values, which represent the coefficient of glucose disappearance in percentage per minute. The glucose values in mg/dl are plotted against time, and from the graph is determined the time interval during which the plasma glucose values have fallen from a certain level to half that level (t½). The K value is then calculated as follows:

$$K = \frac{0.693}{t\frac{1}{2}} \times 100\%/min$$

A K value of less than 0.9 is indicative of diabetes mellitus, values between 0.9 and 1.2 are borderline, and those 1.3 or greater are normal.

Special Diagnostic Considerations

Glycosuria. The presence of glucose in the urine is highly suggestive but not diagnostic of diabetes mellitus and should prompt further evaluation. Glucose can occur in the urine despite normoglycemia in disorders associated with abnormalities of renal glucose handling; these include Fanconi's syndrome, chronic renal failure, and the benign familial disorder of the renal tubule, "renal glycosuria," which occurs predominantly in males and is manifested only by a defect in renal glucose reabsorption. The use of the copper reduction reaction (e.g., Clinitest) can be positive if reducing substances other than glucose are present, e.g., fructose, galactose, pentose (present with inborn errors of metabolism), and lactose (in pregnancy). The presence of these substances does not pose any problems if urine is tested with glucose-specific strips. The only pitfall of using glucose-specific paper strips is that false negative results may be obtained if the patient has alcaptonuria or if present in the urine are strong reducing agents that interfere with oxidation of chromogen, e.g., ascorbic acid, salicylic acid, levodopa, 5-OH-indoleacetic acid, and beta-hydroxybutyric acid.

Random Plasma Glucose. In adults a random plasma glucose greater than 200 mg/dl can be indicative of diabetes mellitus, but diagnosis should be made only if fasting plasma glucose is greater than 140 mg or a diagnostic oral GTT is found.

Two-Hour Postprandial Glucose Level. A 2-hour postprandial glucose level is of questionable value as a screening test. The quantity of carbohydrate ingested, other constituents of the meal, and the patient's prior nutritional state may combine to produce false negative or false positive results. Screening is better performed by measuring a 2-hour sample after proper preparation and a defined glucose load is administered. A 2-hour plasma glucose value of less than 140 mg/dl effectively rules out the diagnosis of diabetes. A higher value should prompt an oral glucose tolerance test.

Pregnancy. Clinical experience has shown that early detection and optimal management of diabetes during pregnancy can prevent congenital malformation and reduce neonatal morbidity and mortality. Screening for glucose intolerance is advisable in all pregnancies, especially when the patient is obese, has had five or more children, or has family history of diabetes in first-degree relatives, history of spontaneous abortions, stillbirth, or fetal malformation, previous delivery of offspring weighing greater than 9 pounds, or history of previous neonatal hypoglycemia.

In the oral glucose tolerance test during pregnancy, 100 g of glucose are given orally. The diagnostic criteria are those of O'Sullivan and Maher. Two or more of the following plasma glucose values must be met or exceeded: fasting—105 mg/dl; 1 hour—190 mg/dl; 2 hours—165 mg/dl; 3 hours—145 mg/dl. By these criteria, 2 to 3% of all pregnancies in the U.S. are attended by gestational diabetes. The status of the carbohydrate intolerance should be reclassified in the postpartum period. Reclassification can fall into three categories: diabetes mellitus, impaired glucose tolerance, and normal with previous abnormality of glucose tolerance. In these latter patients continued monitoring is indicated because of the high likelihood of subsequent development of carbohydrate intolerance or even type II diabetes.

Diabetes in Childhood. The vast majority of diabetic children have type I diabetes and present with classic symptoms. The diagnosis can be made if the random plasma glucose is greater than 200 mg/dl. If the patient is asymptomatic, an oral glucose tolerance test with the same preparation and a glucose load of 1.75 g/kg of ideal body weight to a maximum of 75 g is given. A diagnosis of diabetes is made if the fasting plasma glucose is equal to or greater than 140 mg/dl and the 2-hour value and one intervening plasma glucose value are equal to or greater than 200 mg/dl. If the test is done using capillary blood, the criteria for diagnosis are the fasting blood sugar equal to or greater than 120 mg/dl, and the 2-hour value and one intervening value equal to or greater than 200 mg/dl. A diagnosis of impaired glucose tolerance is made if the fasting plasma glucose is less than 140 mg/dl but the 2-hour postprandial plasma glucose is greater than 140 mg/dl (the corresponding values for capillary blood are: fasting—less than 120 mg/dl; 2-hour postprandial—greater than 120 mg/dl).

Diagnosis of the Acute Metabolic Complications

The criteria for the diagnosis of diabetic ketoacidosis are significant hyperglycemia, hyperketonemia, and metabolic acidosis. The diagnosis of DKA is usually not difficult but may require differentiation from other common causes of metabolic acidosis with an increased anion gap, e.g., lactic acidosis, uremia, alcoholic ketoacidosis, and certain poisoning.

The first step in the diagnosis of DKA is to test the urine for glucose and ketones. If the urine is negative for ketones, another cause for acidosis is likely; if it is positive, differentiation between DKA and starvation ketosis can best be accomplished by checking the plasma for ketones or using a semiquantitative nitroprusside test (ketosticks or acetest tablets). If plasma ketones are present, serial dilutions of the plasma are checked. A strong test with undiluted plasma can result from starvation ketosis whereas a strong reaction beyond one-to-one dilution is presumptive evidence of DKA. A sample of blood is obtained for glucose, urea creatinine, sodium, potassium chloride, and bicarbonate, and arterial blood gases are obtained for $PaCO_2$ and pH. One can use Dextrostix or Chemstrip to rapidly determine the presence of hyperglycemia while awaiting the more accurate plasma glucose determinations from the lab. A positive nitroprusside test with an elevated anion gap in excess of 15 confirms hyperketonemia (the anion gap can be calculated by subtracting the sum of serum chloride and serum bicarbonate from the serum sodium).

It is important to remember that the nitroprusside

tests react with acetoacetate and to a slight extent with acetone but do not react with beta-hydroxybutyric acid, the ketone with the greatest concentration in blood and urine. Diagnostic difficulties may therefore be encountered, though rarely. Since the changes in the total ketoacid load may not be reflected by changes in acetoacetate concentration (e.g., concomitant lactic acidosis, alcoholic ketoacidosis, or hypoxia may decrease acetoacetate and increase beta-hydroxybutyrate concentration) severe DKA may be present irrespective of the results of the nitroprusside testing of ketone reactivity in serum or plasma.

It is vital to look for precipitating causes, which may be multiple, especially in elderly patients. Infection is the most important cause identified in 40% of all cases and should be actively sought; however, in a small percentage of patients no cause can be identified.

Ketoacidosis also occurs in nondiabetic alcoholic patients who had a chronic heavy drinking bout until 1 to 3 days before presentation and present with persistent anorexia, abdominal pain, nausea, vomiting, consequent food abstention, and ketosis. Because alcohol metabolism leads to the production of hydrogen and transformation of NAD to NADH, increased production of beta-hydroxybutyric acid (which is not measured by the standard nitroprusside test) may occur. In addition, there is increased lactate formation and decreased gluconeogenesis. In such alcoholic patients, diagnosis is made by the presence of metabolic acidosis with elevated anion gap and plasma glucose levels that are variable and may be hypoglycemic to mildly hyperglycemic. Alcoholic diabetics may present with a complex mixture of alcoholic and diabetic acidosis.

The diagnosis of hyperosmolar nonketotic coma is based on the clinical setting, the significant hyperglycemia with plasma glucose values generally around 1000 mg/dl but ranging from 600 to 2400 mg/dl, significant dehydration, absence of Kussmaul's breathing and acetone on the breath, and absence of evidence of ketoacidosis. A mild metabolic acidosis may be present due to starvation ketosis, renal insufficiency, or lactic acidosis.

Hypoglycemia in the diabetic patient should be suspected in a patient on insulin or oral antidiabetic therapy with a history of a missed meal or unusual vigorous exercise. The onset is sudden but may be gradual with long-acting insulins or oral agents. A preceding febrile illness or other stress is absent. The patient is very weak, the skin moist and pale, the temperature normal or low, the respirations normal and shallow with no acetone breath, the pulse full and bounding, and the blood pressure normal, and there is no evidence of

volume depletion. Rapid confirmation is by Dextrostix or Chemstrip with blood glucose less than 60 mg/dl; serum ketones are usually absent but may be present in trace quantities. Improvement is rapid following carbohydrate administration or glucagon injections.

In lactic acidosis with increased anion gap not accounted for by drug ingestion, uremia, and ketoacidosis, the patient is generally acutely ill, stuporous or obtunded, and tachypneic or hypotensive. Definitive diagnosis is by a blood lactate level greater than 5 mM/L. A determined attempt should be made to assess the predisposing cause.

Secondary Diabetes

The physician must determine if there is a secondary cause for the diabetic syndrome.

Diabetes mellitus may develop secondarily to destructive lesions or surgical removal of the pancreas, or to hypersecretion of hormones with actions that are antagonistic to insulin or that interfere with insulin secretion.

Pancreatic diabetes may be caused by surgical removal of more than two thirds of the pancreas or to chronic relapsing pancreatitis. Pancreatic diabetes differs from spontaneous insulin dependent diabetes by requiring in most cases no more than 20 to 40 units of insulin per day, by a greater tendency to insulin-induced hypoglycemia, by a lessened tendency to ketosis, and by usual association with exocrine pancreatic insufficiency. Hemochromatosis is often associated with "bronze diabetes;" diabetes can be explained by increased insulin resistance resulting from cirrhosis, insulin deficiency caused by the effects of iron deposits in the pancreas, or associated genetic predisposition to diabetes. Pancreatic carcinoma should be considered in the new onset of diabetes in elderly patients, particularly if associated with abdominal pain, weight loss, depression, etc.

Features common to virtually all forms of endocrinopathy-associated diabetes mellitus include reversibility of the hyperglycemia with the cure of the underlying endocrine disorder, and absence in most patients of ketosis because of the ongoing availability of endogenous insulin. In acromegaly the prevalence of glucose intolerance is as high as 60%, fasting hyperglycemia is observed in only 15 to 30% of patients, and less than 10% of patients require insulin. Insulin antagonism may be mediated by a reduction in insulin binding to its receptor.

In Cushing's syndrome, whether of an exogenous or endogenous cause, there is insulin antagonism and increased neoglucogenesis. Fasting hyperglycemia is present in 20 to 25% of patients. The diagnosis of Cushing's syndrome should be considered in any diabetic patient with Cushingoid features, osteoporosis, hypertension, or psychosis.

In pheochromocytoma, excess catecholamines interfere with insulin secretion or its action. The degree of hyperglycemia is usually mild. Glucagon and somatostatin secreting tumors of the pancreas (glucagonoma and somatostatinoma) are rare causes of the diabetic syndrome. In glucagonoma there is weight loss, diarrhea, an erythematous, bullous skin eruption (necrolytic migratory erythema), anemia, hypokalemia, pancreatic tumor, and increased plasma glucagon levels. In somatostatinoma there is weight loss, abdominal discomfort, diarrhea, steatorrhea, hypochlorhydria, increased incidence of cholelithiasis, pancreatic tumor, and high plasma somatostatin levels.

Isolated growth hormone deficiency is associated fairly commonly with glucose intolerance. Diabetes mellitus may coexist with multiple autoimmune endocrine deficiency syndrome (Addison's disease, Hashimoto's thyroiditis, Graves' disease, hypoparathyroidism, primary gonadal failure, pernicious anemia, etc.).

Stress hyperglycemia occurs in association with acute illness, e.g., sepsis, myocardial infarction, burns, stroke, and severe trauma, and results from increased catecholamines and glucagon and decreased insulin release. It may unmask previous mild carbohydrate intolerance. Patients may not have evidence of diabetes before or after the episode. The tests of glucose intolerance should not be performed until several weeks or months after recovery and restoration of adequate nutrition and physical activity. Uremia and liver cirrhosis, particularly when accompanied by portal hypertension, may very commonly be associated with glucose intolerance caused by insulin resistance and hyperglucagonemia.

A large number of congenital or hereditary disorders are associated with increased incidence of diabetes. These include Prader-Willi syndrome, Refsum's syndrome, Friedreich's ataxia, optic atrophy and nerve deafness, and Turner's syndrome. The cause of the increased association is not known.

In all these circumstances associated with secondary diabetes mellitus, the diagnosis is based on the suspicion, clinical setting, and appropriate laboratory studies, hormonal studies, or both.

Lipoatrophic diabetes mellitus is a rare syndrome of uncertain origin characterized by partial or complete absence of fat with apparent muscle hypertrophy, insulin-resistant diabetes mellitus, absence of ketosis, presence of hypermetabolism in association with normal thyroid function, and hepatomegaly that often progresses to cirrhosis. Associated factors include accelerated growth, acromegaloid features, acanthosis nigricans, and clitoromegaly.

HYPOGLYCEMIC SYNDROME

DEFINITION

Hypoglycemic syndrome refers to the symptoms and signs that result from a low blood sugar.

PATHOPHYSIOLOGIC CONSIDERATIONS

Normal plasma glucose is maintained within fairly constant and narrowly defined limits by a balance between the input of glucose into, and its output from, the blood circulation. Immediately after food intake, glucose and amino acids are absorbed into the blood circulation; their rising plasma levels, together with gut hormone responses to the meal, stimulate insulin secretion by the pancreatic beta cells. The rise in insulin levels has several effects. It causes stimulation of glucose transport into muscle and adipose tissue cells, where it is utilized for energy purposes or stored after conversion to glycogen or triglyceride. It also causes stimulation of glucose uptake by the liver and promotion of glycogen storage. In addition, the rise in insulin levels results in inhibition of hepatic glycogenolysis, i.e., the synthesis of glucose from amino acids, lactate, and glycerol.

Postprandially, as the blood glucose levels fall, insulin secretion ceases promptly and release of glucocorticoids and growth hormone increases. This response normally prevents a fall of plasma glucose to hypoglycemic levels. If hypoglycemia occurs despite these hormonal changes, other hormonal responses are triggered. Catecholamines and glucagon act rapidly to inhibit insulin secretion and glucose uptake by the peripheral tissues and to stimulate glucose hepatic production and fatty acid mobilization.

Early in fasting, the plasma glucose levels are maintained by increased production of glucose, almost exclusively by the liver. Glycogen breakdown predominates in the first 24 hours of fasting. During a more prolonged fast, peripheral glucose utilization is decreased and hepatic gluconeogenesis becomes the sole source of plasma glucose. Gluconeogenesis is regulated by hormonal control of the activity of hepatic enzymes, as well as by the release of substrates from the muscles (amino acids) and adipose tissue (glyc-

Table 11–28. Causes of Hypoglycemia

Postprandial or exogenous hypoglycemia
  Reactive, functional, or idiopathic
  "Diabetic"
  Alimentary
Fasting or endogenous hypoglycemia
  Hepatic
    Extensive surgical resection
    Acute fulminant hepatic necrosis
      Viral
      Toxic
    Cirrhosis
    Hereditary enzyme deficiencies
      Glycogen storage diseases
      Galactosemia
      Hereditary fructose intolerance
  Endocrine
    Insulin excess
      Insulinoma
      Insulin and oral hypoglycemic agents
        Therapeutic error
        Factitial
      Autoimmune
    Hypopituitarism
    Cortisol deficiency
  Alcohol
  Severe medical illness
    Chronic renal failure
    Severe malnutrition
    Infection and sepsis
  Extrapancreatic islet tumors
    Mesenchymal tumors
    Hepatoma
    Adrenocortical carcinoma
    GI, bronchial, or pancreatic carcinoma
  Drugs and poisons
    Beta blockers
    Salicylates
    Mushroom poisoning
    Ackee fruit
    Hepatotoxins

erol). The most significant hormonal response to fasting is a marked reduction in circulating insulin levels and an increase in glucagon, cortisol, and growth hormone.

Hypoglycemia is generally caused by a reduced glucose release by the liver and sometimes, in addition, by increased peripheral glucose utilization. It can be due to insulin excess, deficiency of counter-insulin regulatory hormones, and impaired hepatic glycogenolysis and neoglucogenesis caused by primary or secondary hepatic disorders. Based on their relation to food intake, two major patterns of hypoglycemia can be defined: postprandial hypoglycemia, which is provoked by food ingestion and does not occur in the fasting state; and fasting hypoglycemia, which usually follows a period of fasting but can also occur in the postprandial period. The causes are outlined in Table 11–28.

Postprandial or exogenous hypoglycemia is due to asynchronous or excessive insulin secretion relative to prandial plasma glucose levels. It is characterized by symptomatic hypoglycemia occurring 1 to 5 hours following food ingestion. Contrary to popular notion, this entity is uncommon. It can occur as a rare hereditary abnormality seen in children in which hypoglycemia may follow the ingestion of fructose, galactose, or leucine. Reactive, functional, or idiopathic hyperglycemia is the most common type of postprandial hypoglycemia. The symptoms usually appear 3 to 5 hours after a meal, and the manifestations are those of prominent adrenergic response. Neuroglycopenic symptoms usually do not occur. The pathogenesis of reactive, functional, or idiopathic hyperglycemia is still unclear. IV glucose does not produce the symptoms. Glucose tolerance is not impaired, and the serum insulin responses are heterogeneous and can be appropriate or normal, but with delayed responsiveness, or excessive.

Postprandial hypoglycemia does not occur in patients with frank diabetes mellitus. However, in some patients who have impaired glucose tolerance with normal fasting plasma glucose, symptomatic hypoglycemia or "diabetic" hypoglycemia, may develop 4 to 6 hours following glucose ingestion and is attributed to excessive and delayed insulin response to a glucose load.

"Alimentary" hypoglycemia most often follows gastrectomy, jejunostomy, or vagotomy and pyloroplasty. Symptomatic hypoglycemia in alimentary hypoglycemia occurs earlier (1 to 2 hours after a glucose meal) than in other forms of postprandial hypoglycemia. The mechanism is believed to be due to rapid entry of large amounts of glucose into the small bowel, causing a precipitous rise in plasma glucose level and dramatic secretion of insulin. Alimentary hypoglycemia may also occur in patients with thyrotoxicosis or rapid gastric emptying of unknown cause.

Fasting or endogenous hypoglycemia results from several causes. Among the hepatic causes are primary liver disorders. Symptomatic hypoglycemia occurs infrequently in liver disease such as severe cirrhosis or acute fulminant hepatic necrosis of viral or toxic origin, or after extensive surgical resection. Inborn defects of hepatic enzymes required for normal carbohydrate metabolism are rare and include glycogen storage diseases, galactosemia, and hereditary fructose intolerance.

There are several hormonal causes of fasting or endogenous hypoglycemia. Insulinomas are rare islet-cell pancreatic tumors that can occur in all ages but most frequently in patients in the fourth to the seventh decades with slight preponderance in females. Of the affected patients, 80% have a single benign tumor;

10% of the insulinomas are multiple; another 10% are malignant. Of insulinomas, 10% occur in the setting of multiple endocrine neoplasia type I.

Autoimmune hypoglycemia is a rare entity that can occur in patients who have antibodies to insulin (without prior exposure to insulin) or in patients with autoantibodies to insulin receptors of indeterminate cause.

Drug-related hormonal causes are the most common cause of hypoglycemia. Insulin administration in a known diabetic can result in hypoglycemia. The causes of insulin-induced hypoglycemia include excessive insulin dose because of erroneous prescription or inability to measure the correct dose; failure to reduce insulin dose, for example, during weight reduction; associated hypopituitarism or adrenocortical insufficiency, renal or hepatic failure; at the termination of pregnancy in an insulin-requiring woman; or after recovery from stressful situations.

Surreptitious administration of insulin may also cause hypoglycemia, as may excessive dosage in oral antidiabetic therapy related to decreased degradation or excretion, e.g., in kidney failure; potentiation by other drugs, e.g., barbiturates, coumadin, phenylbutazone, salicylates, sulfonamides, thiazide, or MAO inhibitors; or surreptitious administration.

Another hormonal cause, glucocorticoid deficiency, whether related to primary adrenal disease or secondary to hypothalamic-pituitary disease, can cause fasting or late postprandial hypoglycemia because of impairment of hepatic neoglucogenesis. This deficiency can be completely corrected by adequate steroid replacement.

Also, growth hormone deficiency in children can cause clinical hypoglycemia because of enhanced peripheral glucose utilization related to unopposed insulin effects.

In addition to hormonal causes, hypoglycemia associated with severe medical illness can occur in chronic renal failure because of decreased gluconeogenesis by the liver and kidney, decreased availability of amino acid precursors, congestive heart failure, and, rarely, hyperinsulinism; in severely malnourished children or adults; and in infection and sepsis caused by a direct effect of toxin on the liver, decreased liver perfusion, or hyperinsulinism.

Another cause is extrapancreatic islet tumors. Hyperglycemia can occur in patients with tumors of any histologic type but most frequently in those who have mesenchymal tumors, massive fibroma or sarcoma (for example, retroperitoneal or intrathoracic), hepatomas, adrenocortical carcinomas, and gastrointestinal, bronchial, and exocrine pancreatic carcinoma. The cause of the hypoglycemia is not known; it may be related to the presence of nonsuppressible insulin-like activity, or to a substance produced by the tumor that inhibits gluconeogenesis.

Hypoglycemia can be caused by other drugs and poisons. It can be induced by beta adrenergic blockers, salicylates, and other drugs, most commonly in children, that interfere with glucose metabolism in the liver. Ingestion of certain poisonous plants, for example mushrooms, and ackee fruit, and hepatotoxins can cause fatal hypoglycemia.

Alcohol-induced hypoglycemia is probably the most frequent cause of fasting hypoglycemia. It occurs most commonly in chronically malnourished alcoholics who had stopped food and alcohol intake 10 to 20 hours earlier. It can also follow a short drinking spree in healthy adults or children. Hypoglycemia results mainly from inhibition of gluconeogenesis by the products of ethanol metabolism; NADH accumulates in the liver and prevents entry of substrates into the gluconeogenic pathway.

CLINICAL PRESENTATION

Clinical manifestations are related to hypoglycemia and to its cause. The degree of hypoglycemia required to produce symptoms and the clinical manifestations reported by different patients vary widely. However, a similar pattern of symptoms generally recurs in any one individual.

Hypoglycemic symptoms may be hyperepinephrinemic, resulting from sympathetic activation, or neuroglycopenic, resulting from impairment of CNS function. Hyperepinephrinemic symptoms usually occur when the plasma glucose levels fall rapidly. They include sweating, palpitation, tremor, nervousness, hunger, faintness, weakness, or acral and perioral numbness. These features may be blunted or absent in patients treated with beta adrenergic blocking agents, e.g., propranolol. Neuroglycopenic symptoms usually predominate when the plasma glucose levels decline slowly and reach lower levels (40 mg/dl or below). They include headache, diplopia, confusion, inappropriate affect, motor incoordination, and, when hypoglycemia is severe, seizures, coma, and ultimately death. The physical signs include those of adrenergic response, hypothermia, conjugate deviation of the eyes, extensor rigidity of the limbs, trismus, and Babinski's extensor sign.

Hypoglycemic manifestations can mimic a wide variety of neurologic and psychiatric abnormalities, and affected patients are often admitted to neurologic or psychiatric wards. In patients with cerebrovascular disease, hypoglycemic manifestations may occur at higher plasma glucose levels, and the localized neurologic findings may correlate with the underperfused regions of the brain. The manifestations of hypoglycemia are generally reversible, but permanent brain damage can result from a prolonged severe episode.

DIFFERENTIAL DIAGNOSIS

Symptomatic hypoglycemia should be differentiated from anxiety state and psychoneurosis, pheochromocytoma, thyrotoxicosis, and carcinoid syndrome. The most common pitfall is to incorrectly ascribe symptoms of psychoneurosis to functional hypoglycemia. Adherence to the need for demonstration of Whipple's triad before diagnosis of symptomatic hypoglycemia is critical. The diagnosis of the other disorders rests on definitive laboratory studies and absence of hypoglycemia.

DIAGNOSTIC EVALUATION (Fig. 11–17)

Evaluation of a patient for possible hypoglycemia has two diagnostic objectives: to demonstrate that the clinical manifestations are due to hypoglycemia, and to identify the underlying cause.

Patient History and Physical Examination

In determining if the patient has hypoglycemia, a detailed history and examination are often helpful in the diagnostic evaluation.

The important features in the history include the age of onset, duration, and course; whether the hypoglycemic manifestations occur postprandially or during fasting; a history of drugs, e.g., oral antidiabetic agents, insulin, beta adrenergic blockers, etc.; alcohol consumption; occupation (medical, nursing, or paramedical personnel with easy access to insulin or oral agents); clinical evidence of endocrinopathy, e.g., hypopituitarism or hypoadrenalism, liver disease, chronic renal failure, or systemic disease; family history of diabetes (easy access to insulin or oral agents) or multiple endocrine neoplasia type I (pituitary, parathyroid, or endocrine pancreas tumors); and the presence of stigmata of liver or renal disease, endocrine disease, or an abdominal mass (e.g., retroperitoneal, mesenchymal tumors, adrenocortical carcinoma, or hepatoma).

Diagnostic Studies

The most important step in the diagnostic approach to hypoglycemia is to document Whipple's triad, i.e., to show that typical symptoms and chemical hypoglycemia occur during a spontaneous attack or a provocative test, and that the symptoms are relieved promptly by the ingestion or infusion of glucose. The actual level of plasma glucose that defines hy-

poglycemia is controversial. A reasonable diagnostic criterion is a glucose level less than 50 mg/dl in a male and less than 40 mg/dl in female that is associated with clinical symptoms.

It is important to rule out artifactual hypoglycemia. Whole-blood glucose values may be spuriously low in polycythemia vera and in leukemia, but measurement of plasma glucose in these conditions should provide an accurate result. The possibility of a lab error should be excluded by repeat determination.

Fasting Hypoglycemia. In evaluating fasting hypoglycemia, measurement of plasma glucose (to document hypoglycemia) and serum insulin (to categorize its cause) are the two critical laboratory determinations. They can be obtained during a spontaneous attack, after an overnight fast, or after a provoked attack (during a 72-hour fast).

If the patient is observed during a spontaneous attack, a blood sample is drawn for plasma glucose, serum insulin, and other tests as deemed appropriate by the clinical setting. Glucose is then administered promptly. (If the patient has hypoglycemia, glucose will shorten the attack; the prompt relief of the symptoms is an important criterion for the diagnosis of hypoglycemia by Whipple's triad. If, on the other hand, the patient is not hypoglycemic, no harm will have been done by the glucose administration.)

The 72-hour fast should be done in a hospital setting under medical and nursing supervision to ensure prompt treatment of hypoglycemia manifestations when these occur and to monitor the patient to avoid surreptitious food or drug ingestion. A heparin-lock or an IV catheter and saline infusion is set up so that an avenue for glucose administration is available should serious hypoglycemic manifestations develop. At the bedside should be available laboratory test tubes for glucose, insulin, and other laboratory parameters that are deemed necessary, 50% glucose vials, and symptomatic supportive measures to be utilized should the patient develop convulsions. Activity is encouraged and noncaloric beverages are allowed. Sampling for glucose and insulin is done every 2 to 8 hours depending on the history of the patient's tolerance to fasting. When hypoglycemic symptoms develop, a blood sample is obtained for glucose and insulin, and glucose is administered promptly to terminate the test. If symptoms do not develop by the end of this 72-hour fast, the patient should exercise for 2 hours; exercise raises the plasma glucose in normal individuals but decreases the glucose levels in patients with organic hypoglycemia.

Hyperinsulinism. When fasting glucose levels are less than 50 mg/dl, normal insulin production by the beta pancreatic cells is suppressed and serum insulin

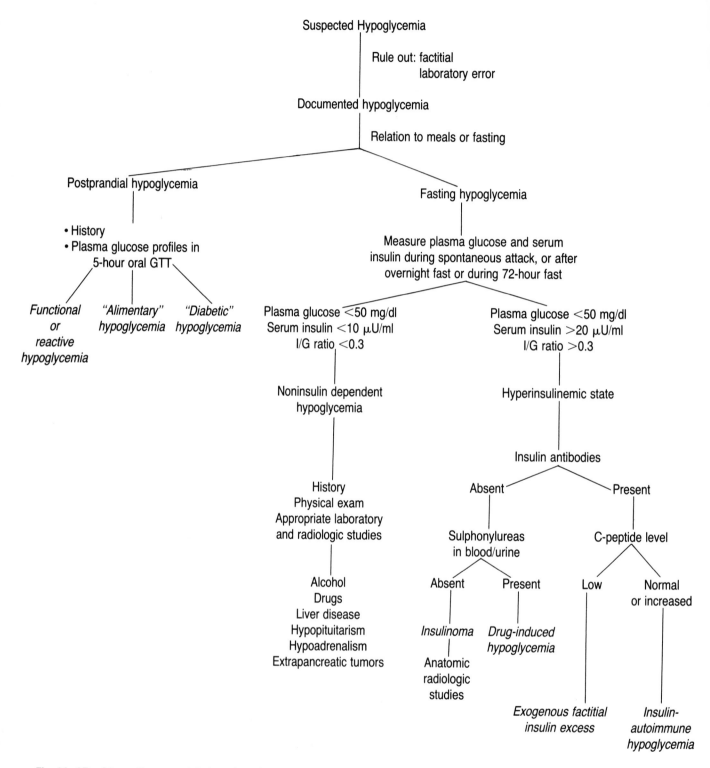

Fig. 11—17.   Diagnostic approach to hypoglycemia.

levels fall to less than 10 μU/ml; when plasma glucose values are less than 40 mg/dl, insulin values should be less than 5 μU/ml. During continued fasting in normal individuals, plasma glucose and serum insulin levels decline together. As a result, the ratio of insulin to plasma glucose remains constant and less than 0.3. Hyperinsulinism is identified by plasma insulin levels greater than 20 μU/ml in association with plasma glucose of less than 50 mg/dl in men and less than 40 mg/dl in women. In the majority of patients with hyperinsulinism, the ratio of insulin to plasma glucose is greater than 0.3.

If hyperinsulinism is present, the diagnostic considerations are insulinoma or the surreptitious administration of insulin or oral antidiabetic agents.

Surreptitious administration of insulin or oral agents occurs most commonly in family members of insulin-dependent diabetics or in hospital personnel who have ready access to insulin and syringes or oral agents. All patients should be examined carefully for injection marks, and if surreptitious administration of insulin is suspected, the hospital room should be searched for hidden insulin and syringes. Detection of insulin antibodies in the plasma of a nondiabetic patient supports the diagnosis (remember that insulin autoantibodies also occur in some individuals who have not received exogenous insulin). The diagnosis is confirmed by the measurement of serum or urinary levels of C peptide, which normally is secreted in equimolar concentration with insulin. It is not present in measurable quantities in exogenous hyperinsulinism. In patients with hyperinsulinism, a high C peptide level implies endogenous insulin secretion, whereas a low C peptide level suggests an exogenous source. The diagnosis of surreptitious ingestion of oral antidiabetic agents as a cause of the hypoglycemic syndrome is confirmed by the measurement of plasma drug levels or urinary metabolites.

The exclusion of surreptitious administration of drugs points to insulinoma as the cause of the hyperinsulinemic state. The diagnosis can be further supported by high serum proinsulin levels. Proinsulin is the single-chain precursor of insulin. In the normal patient, proinsulin constitutes less than 22% of the total immunoreactive insulin. Insulinoma is generally associated with secretion into the circulation of increased amounts of proinsulin. In over 85% of patients with insulinoma, the percentage of proinsulin exceeds 25%, and the more undifferentiated the tumor, the higher the percentage of proinsulin.

The use of an exogenous insulin suppression test can be useful to distinguish physiologically controlled pancreatic beta cell islet from autonomous nonsuppressible insulin production in insulinoma. Suppression is assessed by measuring serum C peptide following the administration of insulin to produce hypoglycemia.

Provocative agents such as tolbutamide, glucagon, leucine, or calcium elicit more insulin secretion from insulinomas than from normal beta cells. These provocative tests can be helpful in selected patients.

Once the diagnosis of insulinoma is entertained, attempts at anatomic delineation of the tumor are in order. Ultrasonography or a CT scan of the pancreas can delineate tumors larger than 2 cm. An angiogram is needed to detect smaller tumors. Serum levels of HCG or its alpha or beta subunits are found to be elevated in two thirds of patients with malignant insulinomas but not in those with benign disease.

If hyperinsulinism is absent in patients with documented hypoglycemia, the differential diagnosis should include hypopituitarism, hypoadrenalism, liver disease, drug-induced hypoglycemia, and extrapancreatic tumor. If the clinical evidence suggests hypopituitarism or hypoadrenalism, cortisol and growth hormone levels after provocative tests are in order. (See The Syndrome of Hypopituitarism.) Severe liver disease or ingestion of alcohol, drugs or toxins can generally be distinguished by the history, physical examination, and liver function tests. In inborn hepatic enzyme defects, symptoms usually begin in infancy, and the diagnosis depends on the clinical setting and appropriate enzyme assays. The diagnosis of primary liver disease is usually obvious, but the physician should remember that if hypoglycemia is noted in the course of cirrhosis, the presence of hepatoma needs to be excluded.

The presence of an extrapancreatic tumor causing hypoglycemia is likely if the clinical findings and specific laboratory tests do not support one of the above conditions, especially if significant wasting or an abdominal mass is present.

It is important to remember that alcohol-induced hypoglycemia is the most frequent cause of fasting hypoglycemia. Its manifestations are often mistakeningly attributed to drunkenness. Plasma glucose should be determined in all symptomatic patients with a history of significant alcohol intake. Diabetic patients on insulin or oral agents are especially susceptible to ethanol-induced hypoglycemia. It is also important to bear in mind that blood alcohol levels may not be elevated when the patient is seen with hypoglycemia.

Postprandial Hypoglycemia. It is important to remember that postprandial hypoglycemia is uncommon, that patients are inclined to attribute a great variety of symptoms to hypoglycemia, that lack of energy, chronic anxiety, lethargy, mental dullness, and similar complaints rarely result from hypoglycemia, and that the physician's responsibility is to demonstrate that these symptoms have been incorrectly attributed to hypoglycemia.

The patient is instructed in the use of glucose oxidase strip reagents (e.g., Chemstrip BG) and asked to measure the plasma glucose at the time of the symptoms. If the levels are greater than 80 mg/dl, the diagnosis of hypoglycemia is ruled out. If the levels are less than 80 mg/dl, a glucose tolerance is indicated. A 5-hour GTT is the procedure of choice to provoke postprandial hypoglycemia. The test must follow a standard protocol (see Hyperglycemia and Diabetes Mellitus) to avoid false positive and false negative results. The patient should avoid drugs known to influence glucose tolerance and ingest at least 50 grams of complex carbohydrates for 3 days before the test. A standard dose of glucose, 1.75 g/kg of ideal weight (but not to exceed 75 g), is given as 50% solution, and blood samples are obtained every 30 minutes throughout the test. The patient is instructed to inform the attendant of any symptoms. The time and the nature of the symptoms should be noted.

No single value is uniformly accepted as evidence of chemical hypoglycemia because plasma glucose may fall to less than 50 mg/dl during a GTT in normal individuals. Values of plasma glucose greater than 65 mg/dl rule out the diagnosis, and a plasma glucose less than 40 mg/dl in association with appropriate symptoms confirms the diagnosis. Since the rapidity of the fall of plasma glucose also contributes to the development of symptoms, the hypoglycemic index can be used as an additional diagnostic criterion in patients who are symptomatic and in whom the plasma glucose falls between 50 and 60 mg/dl. This index takes into account both the rate of decline and the nadir of plasma glucose. The hypoglycemic index is

$$\frac{PGN\ 90\ -\ PGN}{PGN}$$

where PGN is the plasma glucose nadir, and PGN 90 is the plasma glucose 90 minutes before the nadir. A value greater than 1 strongly suggests the diagnosis, whereas a value less than 1 rules it out.

Differentiation between reactive, "diabetic," and "alimentary" postprandial hypoglycemia is based on historical information and on the evaluation of the profile of plasma glucose responses during a glucose tolerance test.

HYPERLIPIDEMIA

DEFINITION

Hyperlipidemia refers to an elevation of serum cholesterol, triglyceride concentrations, or both beyond the normal range.

PATHOPHYSIOLOGIC CONSIDERATIONS

A knowledge of lipoprotein structure, synthesis, and disposal is essential for understanding the causes, clinical manifestations, and diagnosis of hyperlipidemia.

Cholesterol and triglycerides, the major plasma lipids, do not circulate freely in solution in plasma, but are transported in combination with proteins as plasma lipoproteins. These lipoproteins are composed of a central core of apolar lipids (triglyceride and cholesterol esters) surrounded by a surface coat of protein and more hydrophylic lipids (cholesterol and phospholipids, especially lecithin). The protein component, known as apoprotein, not only imparts solubility to the core lipids but also serves to signal for lipoprotein uptake by cellular receptors and to activate enzymes that metabolize the lipid moieties of the lipoprotein. The lipoproteins are subdivided into distinct subtypes based on the chemical composition, size, density, and electrophoretic mobility (Table 11–29).

Chylomicrons (CM) are the largest and least dense lipoproteins. They are composed primarily of triglycerides (85 to 90%), and their major proteins are apoB and apoC. CM are synthesized exclusively in the intestinal mucosa and are the major carriers of exogenous dietary triglycerides from the intestine, via the thoracic duct, to the venous system. Normally they are not present in the postabsorptive state.

Very low density lipoproteins (VLDL), or prebeta-lipoproteins, are composed of triglycerides (55 to 65%) and cholesterol (10 to 20%), combined with several apoproteins (apoproteins B, C, and E). Only 5 to 10% of plasma cholesterol is normally found in VLDL. VLDL are the major carriers of endogenous triglycerides and are synthesized predominantly by the liver and to a lesser extent by the intestinal mucosa; the triglyceride component is formed from fatty acids derived from carbohydrate and CM remnants in the postprandial state and from adipose stores in the fasting state.

The triglycerides in CM and VLDL are hydrolyzed

Table 11–29. Classification and Clinical Manifestations of Hyperlipidemia

Disorder	Abnormal Lipoprotein	Physiologic Abnormality	Electrophoretic Motility	Appearance of Plasma After Overnight Refrig	Cholesterol	Triglycerides	Lipoproteins	Clinical Manifestations	Coronary Heart Disease Risk	Secondary Causes
Type I	Chylomicrons (CM)	Lipoprotein lipase deficiency	Origin	Creamy layer over clear infranatant	N or moderately ↑	↑↑	Chylomicrons	Onset in infancy or childhood: recurrent abdominal pain, pancreatitis, eruptive xanthomas, lipemia retinalis, hepatosplenomegaly	Not increased	Pancreatitis Diabetes mellitus Dysglobulinemia Lupus erythematosus
Type IIa	LDL	Impaired LDL catabolism	Beta	Clear	↑	N	LDL	Tendinous and tuberous xanthomas, xanthelesma, corneal arcus, premature coronary disease; familial type can be diagnosed at birth	Very high	Hypothyroidism Nephrotic syndrome Obstructive liver disease Multiple myeloma Porphyria
Type IIb	LDL and VLDL	Impaired LDL and VLDL catabolism	Beta and prebeta	Clear or cloudy	↑	↑	LDL and VLDL	Same as Type IIa	Same as Type IIa	Same as Type IIa
Type III	B-VLDL	Abnormal remnant catabolism	Beta	Clear or cloudy	↑	↑	B-VLDL	Palmar and tuboeruptive xanthomas; coronary and peripheral vascular disease; diabetes is common	Very high	Diabetes mellitus Obesity Liver disease Hypothyroidism Dysglobulinemia
Type IV	VLDL	Increased endogenous triglyceride input	Prebeta	Clear or cloudy	N or slightly increased	↑	VLDL	Tuberous xanthomas; usually not manifest until early adulthood; diabetes is common	Uncertain	Diabetes mellitus Obesity Alcoholism Pancreatitis Oral contraceptives Steroids Pregnancy Nephrotic syndrome
Type V	VLDL and chylomicrons	Mixed abnormality (I and IV)	Prebeta and CM	Creamy layer over cloudy infranatant	Moderate ↑	↑↑↑	VLDL and CM	Recurrent bouts of abdominal pain; eruptive xanthomas; acute pancreatitis; manifest in adult life; diabetes mellitus	Not increased	Pancreatitis Diabetes mellitus Nephrotic syndrome Alcoholic liver disease Obesity Multiple myeloma

by lipoprotein lipase (LPL), an enzyme present in the capillaries of muscles and adipose tissue. The released free fatty acids and glycerol are used as an energy source or stored in adipose tissue. After the removal of the triglyceride, CM and VLDL are picked up by high density lipoprotein (HDL) and are acted upon by lecithin cholesterol acyl transferase (LCAT). By progressive triglyceride removal and removal of some apoproteins, chylomicrons are transformed into remnant lipoprotein and the VLDL is converted to low density lipoproteins (LDL). VLDL is the main source of plasma LDL.

The major lipid constituents of remnant lipoproteins (also known as intermediate density lipoproteins [IDL] or beta VLDL) are esterified cholesterol and phospholipids, and the major apoprotein is apoB. These are transitional lipoproteins and in the normal individual are present transiently in the circulation in low concentration. They are taken up by the liver for degradation.

Cholesterol, about two thirds of which is as esters, comprises about half of the low density lipoproteins (LDL), or betalipoproteins. Apo B is the sole lipoprotein of LDL. From 50 to 75% of plasma cholesterol is normally found in LDL. LDL is formed from the metabolism of VLDL and is removed from plasma by binding to specific cellular receptors.

High density lipoproteins are the smallest lipoproteins and are composed mainly of proteins (45 to 50%). They are synthesized by the liver and function as a shuttle for cholesterol between cells and the liver. The fraction of total plasma cholesterol in HDL is approximately 25%. The HDL are secreted from both the liver and the intestine as "nascent" lipoprotein that is disc shaped and has a high ratio of phospholipids to cholesterol. HDL accumulates cholesterol from the peripheral tissues and thereby is converted to a more dense particle, called HDL_3. During metabolism of CM and VLDL by HDL and LCAT, HDL_3 is converted to a larger, less dense form of HDL, termed HDL_2.

Hyperlipidemia is always associated with an increased concentration of one or more of these lipoproteins. The type of hyperlipidemia is determined by the type of lipoprotein present in excess. Hyperlipidemia must result from either increased synthesis or diminished removal of plasma lipoproteins and their constituent lipids. Synthesis may be altered by factors that influence availability or production of lipids, formation of protein, coupling of lipid to protein, or secretion of complete lipoproteins. The removal may be altered by abnormalities in enzymatic metabolism of lipids and in the interreaction between apoproteins with specific tissue receptors. Hyperlipidemia may be primary, in which no identifiable cause may be found and which may be familial, or secondary, in which an underlying disorder is apparent. Primary and secondary hyperlipidemias have similar clinical manifestations.

Although there has been some progress in the understanding of the pathogenesis of several genetic forms of hyperlipidemia, the precise pathogenesis of most hyperlipidemias is as yet unknown.

The classification, causes, clinical manifestations, and diagnosis of hyperlipidemias are outlined in Table 11–29.

Type I hyperlipoproteinemia (or hyperchylomicronemia) is a relatively rare disorder due either to congenital deficiency of LPL activity or to a congenital absence of lipase-activating apoprotein CII. It is characterized by inability to remove or clear CM from the blood. Serum cholesterol is normal, and the serum triglyceride is greatly increased. Type I hyperlipoproteinemia is manifested in children or young adults by recurrent pancreatitis, eruptive xanthomas, lipemia retinalis, and hepatosplenomegaly. Secondary causes include pancreatitis, systemic lupus erythematosus, dysgammaglobulinemia, and type I diabetes mellitus.

Type IIa hyperlipidemia (or hyperbetalipoproteinemia) is a genetic disorder of lipid metabolism that is characterized by increased serum cholesterol in association with xanthelasma, tendon and tuberous xanthomas, arcus juvenilis, accelerated atherosclerosis, and early death from myocardial infarction. It is caused by absent or defective LDL cell receptors resulting in delayed LDL clearance, increased levels of plasma LDL, and accumulation of LDL over joints, and pressure points and in blood vessels. The serum cholesterol is increased, and the serum triglyceride is normal. Secondary causes include dietary excesses of cholesterol, hypothyroidism, nephrotic syndrome, obstructive liver disease (lipoprotein X), multiple myeloma, and porphyria.

In type IIb hyperlipidemia, or familial combined hyperlipidemia, there is increased LDL and VLDL. Serum cholesterol and triglycerides are increased.

Type III hyperlipidemia (broad beta disease, or dysbetalipoproteinemia) is characterized by deficiency of apoE III, and accumulation in the serum of a beta-migrating VLDL rich in triglycerides and cholesterol. It is associated with tuboeruptive and pathognomonic planar (palmar) xanthomas and a marked predisposition to severe premature coronary and peripheral artery disease. It appears to result from a defect in the conversion of the triglyceride-rich VLDL to LDL. Serum

triglyceride and cholesterol are increased. It is usually familial but may be seen secondary to diabetes mellitus, obesity, liver disease, hypothyroidism, and dysproteinemias.

Type IV endogenous hypertriglyceridemia (or hyperprebetalipoproteinemia) is a common disorder characterized by a variable elevation of serum triglycerides combined predominantly in VLDL and a possible predisposition to atherosclerosis. It may be associated with mildly abnormal glucose tolerance, obesity, and hyperuricemia. The serum triglycerides are increased, and the serum cholesterol is either normal or increased. It is often familial but may be secondary to diabetes mellitus, obesity, alcoholism, pancreatitis, pregnancy, nephrotic syndrome, and the use of oral contraceptives or glucocorticoid.

Type V hyperlipidemia (mixed hypertriglyceridemia, or hyperprebeta- and hyperchylomicronemia) is an uncommon disorder associated with defective clearance of exogenous and endogenous triglyceride present in VLDL and CM and with the risk of pancreatitis. Serum cholesterol is increased, and the serum triglycerides are greatly increased. It can present with eruptive xanthomas, lipemia retinalis, hepatosplenomegaly, and pancreatitis. It is sometimes familial but may be secondary to pancreatitis, diabetes mellitus, nephrotic syndrome, alcoholic liver disease, obesity, and multiple myeloma.

CLINICAL PRESENTATION

The clinical manifestations of hyperlipidemias relate to ischemic cardiovascular disease and include angina, myocardial infarction, intermittent claudication, and transient or permanent neurologic deficit of cerebrovascular disease. In addition are cutaneous manifestations, skin rash (eruptive xanthoma), nodules (xanthelasma), and cutaneous and subcutaneous xanthomas; premature arcus senilis; and abdominal pain due to acute recurrent pancreatitis.

Type III is characterized by planar xanthomas in the palmar creases. Tuberous xanthomas can occur in types II, III, and IV. When triglycerides reach especially high levels and CM is present, the patient may develop hepatosplenomegaly, eruptive xanthomas (pinkish yellow papular cutaneous deposits over pressure points and extensor surfaces), lipemia retinalis, and, often, severe abdominal pain caused by pancreatitis. Xanthelasmas are the most common indicators of type II hyperlipidemia, although about 60% of patients with xanthelasmas have normal serum lipids. Patients with type II may also have premature arcus senilis and tendinous xanthomas. Tendon xanthomas in the Achilles tendon and digital extensor tendons are almost always diagnostic of familial hypercholesterolemia; however, they may also occur in two other rare hereditary conditions (beta-sitosterolemia and cerebrotendinous xanthomatosis).

Prospective epidemiologic studies have shown that hypercholesterolemia is a major risk for coronary vascular heart disease because of the atherogenic potency of LDL. Beta VLDL is also highly atherogenic. In general, although plasma triglycerides are not an independent risk for premature coronary artery disease, hypertriglyceridemia is usually associated with reduced levels of HDL that may predispose to coronary disease. Peripheral vascular disease is especially common in type III.

In contrast, HDL, particularly HDL_2, is a protective lipoprotein. It may exert its protective effect by transporting cholesterol from arterial wall to the liver for excretion, or by partially blocking the uptake of LDL cholesterol by endothelial and smooth muscle cells of arteries.

DIAGNOSTIC EVALUATION (Fig. 11–18)

The physician must first determine if the patient has hyperlipidemia. If measurement of lipid and lipoprotein levels is to be useful, one must be aware of several considerations. Because the serum levels of cholesterol and triglyceride are distributed continuously in the population, arbitrary levels must be established to define significant hyperlipidemia. Also, the concentration of lipids increases with age. In addition, chylomicrons may be present in the blood up to 14 hours after a meal; hence, a fasting specimen, taken 12 to 16 hours after the last meal, should be used for measurements of lipids, and the normal ranges must be age- and sex-adjusted. Table 11–30 lists the upper limits of normal for these parameters, which represent the 95th percentile for individuals of the same age and sex. These arbitrary values should not imply that levels of circulating lipids that are prevalent in most of the population are without risk. (Epidemiologic studies have shown that there is a progressive increase in the risk of coronary heart disease as the level of serum cholesterol increases above 180 mg/dl.) In general, levels of serum cholesterol greater than 270 mg/dl and serum triglycerides greater than 190 mg/dl merit investigation.

Another factor to be considered is that lipoprotein concentrations are under dynamic metabolic control

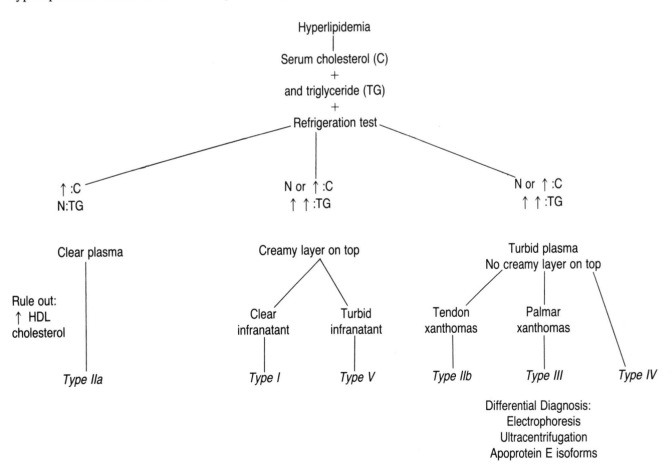

Fig. 11–18. Diagnostic approach to hyperlipidemia.

Table 11–30. Plasma Lipid and Lipoprotein Cholesterol Levels

Sex	Age/years	Plasma Cholesterol mg/dl 95th percentile	Plasma Triglycerides mg/dl 95th percentile	LDL Cholesterol mg/dl 95th percentile	HDL Cholesterol mg/dl 95th percentile
Males	0–14	203	59	132	37
	15–24	218	201	147	30
	25–34	254	266	185	28
	35–44	270	321	189	27
	45–54	277	324	202	28
	55–64	276	289	210	28
	65±	274	267	210	30
Females	0–14	205	131	140	36
	15–24	216	131	135	35
	25–34	216	151	151	37
	35–44	252	191	174	33
	45–54	285	233	215	33
	55–64	300	262	234	36
	65+	303	243	223	33

(From U.S. Department of Health and Human Services. Public Health Service, National Institutes of Health, Lipid Metabolism Branch, NHLBI: The Lipid Research Clinics Population Studies Data Book, Bethesda, NIH Publication No 80–1527, 1980, Vol 1.)

and are readily affected by diet, illness, drugs, and weight change. Patients should maintain the usual diet and alcohol intake, maintain stable weight, and be off all drugs known to influence lipid levels, e.g., steroids or estrogen, for 1 month before samples for lipid analysis are taken. Myocardial infarction or severe stress may increase serum triglycerides and decrease serum cholesterol significantly; thus, 4 to 8 weeks should intervene before lipid studies are conducted on these patients.

Also, if the serum cholesterol and triglycerides are found to be elevated, at least three lipid determinations at weekly intervals are needed to confirm the diagnosis and establish the pretreatment baseline.

A strong argument can be made for screening all individuals for plasma lipids because of the seriousness of the consequences of coronary and peripheral vascular disease, and because of the availability of effective therapy for most hyperlipidemic patients. Since prevention of atherosclerosis is the goal, evaluating plasma lipids is especially important in young subjects. At the very least, plasma lipids should be measured in patients with other coronary risk factors such as hypertension, diabetes mellitus, cigarette smoking, and family history of premature cardiovascular disease or hyperlipidemia; with diseases associated with secondary hyperlipidemia; and with clinical indicators of hyperlipidemia, i.e., those patients with xanthelasma, xanthomas, lipemia retinalis, arcus juvenilis, hepatosplenomegaly, pancreatitis, premature coronary heart disease, peripheral vascular disease, hyperuricemia, and lipemic serum.

Certain diagnostic studies should be performed to determine the presence and type of hyperlipidemia.

Blood is obtained for cholesterol (C), triglyceride (TG), and HDL cholesterol determinations. A 2 ml-aliquot of the blood sample is refrigerated overnight and checked for a creamy layer and turbidity before and after overnight refrigeration. Another aliquot is saved for additional studies should serum triglycerides be elevated.

Measurement of HDL cholesterol is a necessary component of a screening evaluation because measurement of total cholesterol, which includes LDL cholesterol (50 to 75%), HDL cholesterol (25%), and VLDL (5%), may be misleading: If normal, it does not exclude an increased LDL or a decreased HDL, and if increased, it does not mean increased LDL. HDL cholesterol measurement is necessary particularly in subjects with a modest increase in cholesterol (240 to 300 mg/dl). One abnormality associated with increased risk of coronary artery disease is hypoalphalipoproteinemia, or deficiency of HDL. Many of these patients have normal serum cholesterol and triglyceride levels and no clinical stigmata to attract attention.

A reliable estimate of LDL cholesterol is obtained from the following formula:

$$\text{LDL chol} = \text{total chol} - \left(\text{HDL chol} + \frac{\text{plasma TG}}{5} \right)$$

This formula is applicable if the plasma triglycerides are less than 400 mg/dl and the patient does not have type III hyperlipidemia.

In a patient with an elevated serum cholesterol and normal serum triglycerides, if the serum cholesterol is only modestly elevated (up to 290 mg/dl), HDL cholesterol levels should be considered since hyperalphalipoproteinemia may account for the observed hypercholesterolemia. LDL cholesterol should be estimated: a calculated level of LDL cholesterol greater than 200 mg/dl is clinically significant.

Since HDL cholesterol never contributes more than 120 mg/dl of plasma cholesterol, a serum cholesterol greater than 290 mg/dl always represents significant hyperlipidemia, either obstructive liver disease (lipoprotein X) or increased LDL. If obstructive liver disease is absent, the patient's abnormality can be assumed to be due to increased LDL.

Cholesterol levels greater than 350 mg/dl are more suggestive of heterozygous familial hypercholesterolemia. Very high cholesterol levels may be found in the homozygous form of familial hypercholesterolemia. Here, there is no difficulty in the diagnosis because of the patient's youth at onset and positive family history. Very high cholesterol levels may also be found in the adult with combined hyperlipidemia or hypothyroidism.

In the patient with predominant increase in serum triglycerides (plus or minus a moderate increase in serum cholesterol), the differential diagnosis is between increased VLDL, CM, or both. The increase in cholesterol is due to the fact that both VLDL and CM contain cholesterol, and their contribution to the total cholesterol is about 8 to 15% of the triglyceride content. The serum is checked for turbidity and refrigerated overnight. (Serum begins to appear hazy when the level of triglyceride reaches 200 mg/dl.) Plasma turbidity indicates hypertriglyceridemia. CM are the largest and lightest lipoproteins, and on refrigeration overnight they float to the surface and form a creamy layer. Therefore, a creamy layer on top with a clear infranatant points to type I hyperlipidemia, while a creamy layer on top with turbid infranatant points to type V hyperlipidemia.

It is important to check the turbidity before and after refrigeration. A marked increase in turbidity with chilling suggests familial dysbetalipoproteinemia (because of increased tendency of the abnormal lipoprotein to aggregate in the cold).

Elevation of both serum cholesterol and serum triglycerides can be the result of either of two abnormalities: combined hyperlipidemia (or type IIb) in which there is an increase in both LDL and VLDL, or type III hyperlipidemia. The differentiation requires application of additional diagnostic studies. In high-quality agarose gel electrophoresis, patients with type IIb hyperlipidemia show increased prebeta and beta bands that are well resolved from each other; patients with type III hyperlipidemia show a broad beta pattern that obscures the resolution of beta and prebeta lipoprotein bands; prior ultracentrifugation will separate the lipoproteins. Type III hyperlipidemia is confirmed by isoelectric focusing techniques that demonstrate absence or severe deficiency of apoprotein E isoforms.

Appropriate studies are conducted to exclude secondary causes of hyperlipidemia (see Table 11–29). Secondary hyperlipidemia may present as any type of hyperlipidemia, although type IV is the most common presentation.

Since all types of hyperlipidemia may be determined genetically, first-degree family members, especially children, should be screened for abnormal plasma lipids so that treatment can be initiated before irreversible vascular changes occur. Familial hypercholesterolemia can be detected in children at birth, while familial type IV hyperlipidemia is often not manifest until late teens or early twenties.

OBESITY

DEFINITION

Obesity is defined as an excess of adipose tissue. It is an important clinical entity because of its prevalence and its association with certain pathophysiologic complications that can increase morbidity and mortality. Its prevalence increases with age, peaks at about age 50, and decreases in the older age group. It is estimated that 40% of middle-aged females and 20% of middle-aged males in the U.S. are obese. The incidence of complications of obesity increases progressively, parallel to the degree of deviation above average weight.

Several indices have been used to define obesity and its degree. The simplest index of obesity is the body weight. It is important to remember that body weight and the quantity of body fat are distributed continuously in the population and there is no clear dividing line between obese and nonobese individuals. Also, body weight is not always an accurate reflection of total quantity or relative proportion of adipose tissue in the body. In addition, weight adjusted to body size gives a better indication of obesity than body weight alone. For clinical purposes, the percentage of ideal body weight (based on the readily available Metropolitan Life Insurance Company tables) usually gives a close approximation of the presence and the degree of obesity. Obesity can be defined as body weight greater than 20% above mean average body weight. (See also Chapter 19.)

A variety of anthropometric measurements have been found to correlate closely with percentage of body fat. The two most useful of such measurements are weight/height^2 index, in which obesity is defined as an index greater than 27 kg/m^2 in males, and greater than 25 kg/m^2 in females; and triceps skin fold thickness as measured by skin calipers, in which obesity is defined as skin fold thickness greater than 23 mm in males and greater than 30 mm in females.

Indices based on body density, x-ray, distribution of fat-soluble gases, total body water, and total body K-40, which have been used in research, are not necessary for clinical purposes.

PATHOPHYSIOLOGIC CONSIDERATIONS
(Table 11–31)

A gain in adipose tissue is caused by an imbalance between caloric intake and expenditure. The pathogenesis almost always involves a primary increase in caloric intake. However, a reduction in caloric expenditure because of decreased physical activity or decreased thermogenesis may contribute in some circumstances.

Table 11–31. Causes of Obesity

Idiopathic
  Lifelong (familial)
  Adult (sporadic)
Secondary
  Endocrine
    Hypothalamic
      Tumor
        Craniopharyngioma
        Glioma
      Cyst
      Inflammatory and infiltrative
        Sarcoidosis
        Histiocytosis X
        Encephalitis, e.g., tuberculosis
        Leukemia
      Benign intracranial hypertension
      Trauma, e.g., neurosurgical procedures
    Primary empty sella
    Cushing's syndrome
    Insulinoma
    Hypothyroidism
    Hypogonadism
    Polycystic ovary syndrome
    GH deficiency
    Pseudohypoparathyroidism
  Congenital
    Prader-Willi Syndrome
    Laurence-Moon-Biedl Syndrome
  Drugs
    Oral contraceptives
    Cyproheptadine
    Phenothiazines
    Glucocorticoids

Idiopathic obesity affects 99% of obese patients. Its exact cause is uncertain, but possible factors in its pathogenesis include excess lipid deposition related to increased food intake associated with emotional or cultural influences or with unidentified hypothalamic lesions, or related to hyperlipogenesis caused by adipose tissue hypercellularity or increased lipoprotein lipase activity. Idiopathic obesity may also result from decreased lipid utilization caused by defective lipid oxidation, defective thermogenesis, inactivity, or aging, or it may result from decreased lipid mobilization caused by defective lipolysis, decreased lipolytic hormones, or abnormalities of autonomic innervation.

Idiopathic obesity is classified into two major types. Adult onset or sporadic obesity, the most common type, is characterized by adipose tissue hypertrophy rather than hyperplasia; onset of obesity in adult life, patients being of average weight or thin until age 20 to 40 and obesity occurring perhaps after marriage, multiple pregnancies, or cessation of smoking or athletic activities; predominantly "central" distribution of fat, the so-called middle-aged spread; and lack of family history of obesity.

Lifelong obesity is characterized by adipose tissue hyperplasia and hypertrophy; onset of obesity in childhood, patients usually being of normal body weight at birth; occurrence of a large spurt of weight gain at puberty, and in affected females with each successive pregnancy; attainment of gross obesity with weight greater than 175% of ideal body weight; peripheral and central fat distribution; and positive family history.

Secondary obesity accounts for the obesity of a very small minority of patients (less than 1%). It can be caused by hypothalamic lesions of various origins that impair the ventral medial hypothalamic nucleus. It is characterized by marked and almost uncontrollable hyperphagia, average weight gain of 20 to 50 kg (as much as 30 kg may be gained in the first 6 months of onset), and weight ultimately stabilizing below 150 kg. Insulin levels and lipogenesis are increased.

Secondary obesity is frequently seen in certain endocrine disorders, such as Cushing's syndrome of exogenous or endogenous origin, insulinoma, hypothyroidism, hypogonadism, polycystic ovary syndrome, and GH deficiency in childhood (see below).

In secondary obesity, partial lipodystrophy is a rare variant of congenital lipodystrophy in which the subcutaneous fat is totally absent from a portion of the body and in other portions is hypertrophied.

Multiple lipomatosis is a familial disorder in which the triglycerides in subcutaneous deposits are unavailable for mobilization, even during starvation.

Secondary obesity is associated with certain congenital syndromes that manifest in childhood. The

Prader-Willi syndrome is characterized by short stature, delayed osseous maturation, cryptorchidism, mental retardation, and muscle hypotonia; other abnormalities that may occur include strabismus, small hands and feet, and enamel hypoplasia. The Laurence-Moon-Biedl syndrome is characterized by retinitis pigmentosa, polydactyly and syndactyly, mental retardation, hypogonadism, nerve deafness, and variable renal and cardiac abnormalities. Other syndromes associated with obesity include adiposogenital syndrome, Alstrom's syndrome, and pseudohypoparathyroidism.

CLINICAL PRESENTATION

The clinical presentations are related to the obesity per se and its sequelae. Obesity is the most important factor in the emergence of type II diabetes mellitus. In the U.S., greater than 80% of patients with type II diabetes are obese. Obesity decreases insulin receptors and postreceptor activity, leading to insulin resistance and hyperinsulinism, and ultimately to high-output failure of the pancreatic islets.

Obesity is associated with five major risk factors for atherosclerotic cardiovascular diseases: hypertension (increased blood volume, increased salt intake, increased stroke volume, and increased cardiac output to perfuse the excess adipose tissue), diabetes mellitus, hypercholesterolemia (caused by increased cholesterol production), hypertriglyceridemia (due in part to associated hyperinsulinism), and decreased HDL levels. Obese individuals have more atherosclerotic manifestations and are more prone to sudden death than nonobese individuals.

Obesity leads to characteristic respiratory abnormalities. Patients with moderate obesity may have increased work of respiration because of the thick respiratory wall and decreased compliance of the thorax; decreased vital capacity; decreased expiratory reserve; and ventilatory perfusion disturbances. In cases of massive obesity, alveolar hypoventilation occurs, leading to carbon dioxide retention and hypoxia, the so-called obesity hypoventilation or pickwickian syndrome. This syndrome is characterized by daytime somnolence, occasional sleep apnea, fatigue, dyspnea, personality changes, secondary polycythemia, pulmonary hypertension, and eventually cor pulmonale with cardiorespiratory failure.

Gastrointestinal symptoms are frequent in obese individuals. They consist of nonspecific bloating and dyspepsia, increased incidence of diaphragmatic hernia and reflux esophagitis, fatty liver and associated abnormalities of liver function tests, and increased incidence of cholesterol gallstones in obese females.

There is an increased incidence of arthritis in obese individuals, usually of the degenerative joint disease type primarily affecting the spine and the weight-bearing joints. In addition, hyperuricemia and increased incidence of gouty arthritis occur; gouty arthritis can be precipitated during the treatment of obesity with carbohydrate-restricted fad diets, as a result of competition of ketone bodies (produced by starvation ketosis) and uric acid for renal excretion.

There is increased incidence of fungal skin infections and intertrigo of the axillae and groin and under the breasts from the flabby skin and moist cutaneous folds.

In obese women, there is increased incidence of menstrual abnormalities; increased incidence of toxemia and hypertension of pregnancy; and increased obstetric risk because of longer labor, larger babies, and more frequent need of C-sections. In older women, incidence of uterine fibroids and risk of endometrial cancer are increased.

Obese patients are at an increased risk when undergoing surgery because of increased risk in using anesthetics, technical surgical difficulties, and increased postoperative complications of atelectasis, wound infections, and cardiovascular and venous thrombotic abnormalities.

In obesity, there is increased incidence of varicose veins, venous stasis, and edema.

DIAGNOSTIC EVALUATION

The objectives of the diagnostic approach are to look for secondary causes and to assess the presence and extent of complications of obesity.

In determining if a secondary cause is present, the history and physical examination are critical. If the history and physical examination are negative for a secondary cause, there is usually no need for additional tests beyond what is appropriate for sound medical practice. If the history and the physical examination are suspicious for a secondary cause, however, appropriate laboratory and radiologic studies are indicated.

The possibility of a hypothalamic lesion as a cause for obesity is supported by the finding of anatomic and functional evidence of hypothalamic-pituitary disease (see The Syndrome of Hypopituitarism). Confirmation is by radiologic studies, primarily CT scan of the hypothalamic-pituitary area, and other radiologic tools in special circumstances, e.g., angiogram to rule out aneurysm. It is important to remember that obesity per se may lead to impairment of growth hormone and prolactin responses to provocative stimuli.

Cushing's syndrome may also be associated with

obesity (see Cushing's Syndrome). In simple obesity, distribution of fat is usually generalized (but may be central), the skin has normal thickness, the striae are pale, muscle strength and bulk are normal, and there is usually no plethora or osteoporosis. Although the 17-ketogenic and 17-ketosteroids are increased, and the overnight dexamethasone suppression test may be abnormal, in simple obesity, plasma cortisol and urinary free cortisol are normal and there is normal responsiveness to the standard low-dose dexamethasone (2-mg) suppression test.

In insulinoma, a modest weight gain of only 6 to 12 kg occurs, a result of the hypoglycemia, increased appetite, and the lipogenic effect of increased insulin. In patients with insulinoma, there is usually a history of episodic hyperepinephrinemic or neurologic symptoms. The diagnosis rests on the demonstration of hypoglycemia, inappropriately increased serum insulin levels, and, during spontaneous or induced episodes, the relief of symptoms with ingestion of glucose. It is important to remember that basal insulin levels are increased in most patients with obesity of any cause (because of insulin resistance), and that some of the insulin provocative tests, e.g., tolbutamide, may not be helpful in the differential diagnosis of insulinoma from obesity because hyper-responsiveness in insulin secretion may also be observed in simple obesity.

In hypothyroidism, weight gain, which is usually modest, can be attributed to the hypothyroidism itself, partly a result of fat but mostly because of retention of fluid and mucin. The physician should be alert to the possible presence of hypothyroidism if the patient has cold intolerance (ordinarily, obese patients have heat intolerance), inappropriate somnolence, dry and yellowish skin, constipation, delayed relaxation phase of deep tendon reflexes, goiter, or a family history. The diagnosis is documented by the finding of low serum T_4 levels (total and free serum thyroxine or free thyroxine index). Serum TSH is critical in the differential diagnosis between primary and secondary hypothyroidism.

Hypogonadism also can be associated with modest weight gain, seen in perimenopausal women and in patients with primary hypogonadism. The diagnosis is based on the clinical and biochemical findings of decreased sex steroid levels. Serum LH and FSH are critical for the differentiation between primary and secondary hypogonadism (see Amenorrhea and Hypogonadism in the Adult Male). Obesity is frequently associated with polycystic ovarian syndrome. Hirsutism, acne, menstrual irregularity, infertility, increased androgen levels that are suppressible with exogenous estrogen, and an increased ratio of LH to FSH are characteristic (see Hirsutism and Virilization).

Obesity may also be encountered in growth hormone deficiency in childhood. The clinical picture, decreased serum growth hormone responses to provocative stimuli, decreased serum somatomedin C levels, and the demonstration of the hypothalamic-pituitary disease point to GH deficiency.

PORPHYRIAS

DEFINITION

The porphyrias are disorders of porphyrin metabolism, characterized chemically by overproduction of porphyrins or porphyrin precursors, and characterized clinically by photosensitivity, episodes of neurologic dysfunction, or a combination of both. They can be hereditary or acquired.

PATHOPHYSIOLOGIC CONSIDERATIONS

Heme is the most important end product of porphyrin metabolism. A constituent of hemoglobin, cytochromes, and peroxidase systems, it has a unique ability to bind and release oxygen. Heme is present in all aerobic cells, particularly bone marrow and liver. Its biosynthetic pathway is illustrated in Figure 11–19 and consists of several steps. First, glycine and succinyl-CoA condense to form delta-aminolevulinic acid (ALA). This reaction is catalyzed by ALA synthetase and is the rate-limiting step in heme synthesis. It is reversibly inhibited in a feedback manner by the final product, heme. Second, two molecules of ALA condense to form the monopyrrole porphobilinogen (PBG), catalyzed by ALA dehydratase. Third, four molecules of monopyrrole PBG combine to form the tetrapyrrole uroporphyrinogen (URO), the first porphyrin in the metabolic pathway. This step is catalyzed by an enzyme complex containing urosynthetase and urocosynthetase. This enzyme complex directs the synthesis of uroporphyrinogen III (URO III), which is the precursor of heme. The synthetase alone directs the synthesis of uroporphyrinogen I (URO I), which cannot be converted to heme and represents a metabolic "dead end." Normally very little porphyrinogen of the I series is formed. Fourth, URO III is decarboxylated to coproporphyrinogen III (COPRO III), which is further decarboxylated to protoporphyrinogen IX (PROTO IX). Fifth, PROTO IX is rapidly oxidized

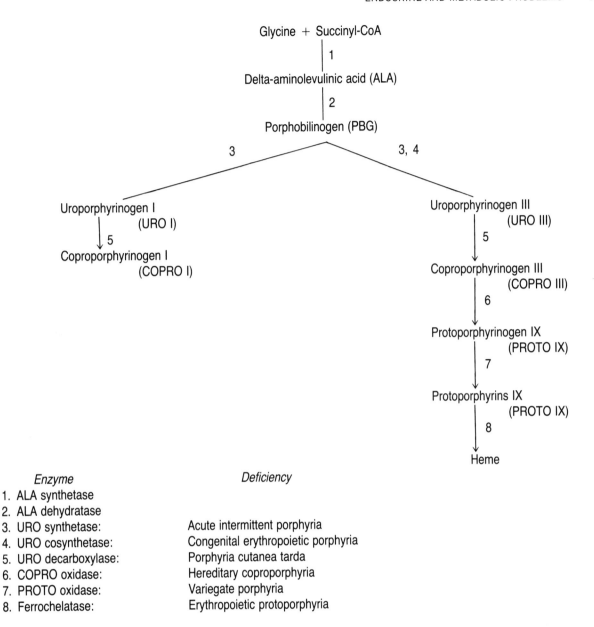

Glycine + Succinyl-CoA
|
1
|
Delta-aminolevulinic acid (ALA)
|
2
|
Porphobilinogen (PBG)

3   3, 4

Uroporphyrinogen I   Uroporphyrinogen III
        (URO I)   (URO III)
| |
5   5
| |
Coproporphyrinogen I   Coproporphyrinogen III
        (COPRO I)   (COPRO III)
                                                         |
                                                         6
                                                         |
                                                   Protoporphyrinogen IX
                                                            (PROTO IX)
                                                         |
                                                         7
                                                         |
                                                   Protoporphyrins IX
                                                            (PROTO IX)
                                                         |
                                                         8
                                                         |
                                                        Heme

Enzyme   *Deficiency*
1. ALA synthetase
2. ALA dehydratase
3. URO synthetase: Acute intermittent porphyria
4. URO cosynthetase: Congenital erythropoietic porphyria
5. URO decarboxylase: Porphyria cutanea tarda
6. COPRO oxidase: Hereditary coproporphyria
7. PROTO oxidase: Variegate porphyria
8. Ferrochelatase: Erythropoietic protoporphyria

Fig. 11–19. Outline of porphyrin metabolism and the porphyrias.

to protoporphyrin IX, which is chelated with iron by ferrochelatase to form heme.

The reduced porphyrinogen intermediates in heme synthesis are colorless and nonfluorescent. Outside the cells, they are rapidly oxidized to form porphyrins, which are red to purple, fluorescent, and photosensitizing.

The porphyrins differ markedly in solubility characteristics. ALA, PBG, and those with many carboxylic acid side chains, e.g., uroporphyrin, are water soluble and excreted mainly in the urine; those with few carboxylic acid side chains, e.g., protoporphyri-

nogen, are lipid soluble and excreted mainly via the bile into feces; those with an intermediate number of side chains, e.g., coproporphyrin, are excreted by both routes.

The porphyrias are caused by enzymatic dysfunction in the heme pathway leading to increased concentration of heme precursors proximal to the defective enzyme in the blood, urine, and feces. The overproduction of porphyrins is associated predominantly with cutaneous photosensitivity; the dermatologic effects are proportional to the approximate concentration of porphyrins in the subcutaneous tissues and depend on the excitation of porphyrins by visible light. Increased circulating ALA and PBG are linked to a variety of neurologic problems.

CLINICAL PRESENTATION

The clinical manifestations and laboratory findings of the porphyrias are outlined in Table 11–32. Porphyria cutanea tarda is probably the most common form of porphyria, followed by protoporphyria. Acute intermittent porphyria is the most commonly recognized form of acute porphyria, except in South Africans of Dutch extraction, in whom variegate porphyria is relatively common. Other types of porphyrias are rare.

Acute Intermittent Porphyria. This autosomal dominant disorder is due to a deficiency of uroporphyrinogen synthetase resulting in increased excretion of ALA and PBG in the urine. It is characterized clinically by acute neurologic attacks. Cutaneous symptoms are not a feature of this type of porphyria. It is more frequently seen in females, the typical patient usually a woman in her twenties.

The acute neurologic dysfunction can affect any part of the nervous system, and the clinical features include abdominal pain, vomiting, and constipation caused by neurogenic motility disturbance of the bowel. There may be a mild leukocytosis, but fever is unusual. This presentation raises the suspicion of a surgical abdomen, prompting, in some patients, repeated laparotomy. Autonomic manifestations include labile hypertension, sinus tachycardia, postural hypotension, sweating, and vascular spasm. In addition, sensory and motor peripheral neuropathy, usually motor, may be caused by peripheral nervous system involvement. There may be organic brain syndrome, seizures, and cerebellar, basal ganglia, hypothalamic, and bulbar manifestations due to CNS involvement. The patient may also have hyponatremia due to SIADH.

The neurologic attack is usually precipitated by drugs, starvation, female sex hormones, or bacterial or viral infection, but can occur without provocation. Among the drugs that have been incriminated in the precipitation of attacks are those, notably barbiturates, that deplete the hepatic regulatory heme pool by inducing cytochrome P_{450}. Other drugs that are incriminated include chlordiazepoxide, chloral hydrate, meprobamate, sulfonamide, griseofulvin, tolbutamide, the anticonvulsants phenytoin and methsuximide, estrogen, progestins, danazol, aminopyrine, methyldopa, chloramphenicol, chloroquine, imipramine, pentazocine, and ergot preparations.

Routine laboratory tests are usually normal, but the serum sodium may be decreased (SIADH), and serum thyroxine may be increased (increased thyroxine-binding globulin) while the free thyroxine is normal; the cholesterol and the LDL levels are often increased. The most useful laboratory tests in the rapid diagnosis of symptomatic acute porphyria is one of the qualitative tests for PBG in the urine, which is almost always strongly positive. If it is negative, a urine sample should be sent for quantitative ALA and PBG determinations. Increased ALA and PBG are present in almost all patients during a neurologic attack. A urine porphyrin screen does not measure PBG and therefore could be misleading in the evaluation of patients with acute abdominal pain. Between attacks, the levels of ALA and PBG may be normal; the diagnosis depends on the family history, quantitative urine and fecal porphyrin excretion, and assay of specific enzymes in the heme pathways.

Hereditary coproporphyria and variegate porphyria

Table 11–32.　Classification and Clinical Manifestations of Porphyrias

Type	Inheritance	Enzyme Deficiency	Clinical Manifestations		Biochemical Findings		
			Abdominal pain/ neurologic	Cutaneous	RBC	Urine	Stools
Acute intermittent porphyria (AIP)	Autosomal dominant	Uroporphyrinogen synthetase	Present	Absent		↑ALA ↑PBG	
Congenital erythropoietic porphyria (CEP)	Autosomal recessive	Uroporphyrinogen co-synthetase	Absent	Present	↑↑URO I ↑↑COPRO I	↑↑URO I ↑↑COPRO I	↑URO ↑COPRO I
Porphyria cutanea tarda (PCT)	Autosomal dominant	Uroporphyrinogen decarboxylase	Absent	Present		↑↑URO I ↑↑URO III ↑COPRO	±↑URO, COPRO ↑↑ISO COPRO
Hereditary coproporphyria (HC)	Autosomal dominant	Coproporphyrinogen oxidase	Present	Present		↑↑URO ↑↑COPRO ↑↑ALA ↑↑PBG	↑↑COPRO
Variegate porphyria (VP)	Autosomal dominant	Protoporphyrinogen oxidase	Present	Present		↑↑COPRO ↑URO ↑ALA ↑PBG	↑↑PROTO
Erythropoietic or erythrohepatic protoporphyria	Autosomal dominant	Ferrochelatase	Absent	Present	↑↑PROTO	normal	↑↑PROTO

can also present with acute neurologic attacks. In these porphyrias, photosensitivity skin lesions are present. The specific diagnosis rests on quantitative determination of urinary and fecal heme precursors (see below).

In lead poisoning, ALA levels may be increased, but PBG levels are normal.

Congenital Erythropoietic Porphyria. This is a very rare autosomal recessive disorder caused by deficiency of uroporphyrinogen I cosynthetase. Symptoms usually begin before age 5, and the presentation is characterized by severe cutaneous lesions on the exposed parts of the body consisting of vesicles or bullae leading to ulceration, infection, scarring, severe deformities, and hypertrichosis; and hemolytic anemia, splenomegaly, and hypersplenism. Acute attacks of abdominal pain with neurologic manifestations do not occur. The urine is noted to be red early in childhood. The teeth are discolored (erythrodontia) and exhibit red fluorescence when exposed to Wood's light.

Laboratory evaluation shows evidence of hemolytic anemia. Fluorescence of normoblasts in marrow and erythrocytes in blood is present. There is a significant increase in URO I and COPRO I, producing the port wine urine. Fecal COPRO I and plasma and erythrocyte URO I and COPRO I are increased. The urinary porphyrin precursors ALA and PBG are normal.

Porphyria Cutanea Tarda. This disorder, which is due to deficiency of uroporphyrinogen decarboxylase, can be inherited as an autosomal dominant disorder. More commonly, it is acquired. It is the most commonly diagnosed porphyria in the U.S., characterized by cutaneous lesions on the exposed parts, with erythema, vesicles, bullae, crusts and scabs, scarring, hirsutism, pigmentation, or depigmentation. Abdominal pain and neurologic attacks do not occur.

The typical patient is a middle-aged male with a history of alcohol abuse, chronic liver disease, or both but the disease is increasingly reported in women taking oral contraceptives and in patients undergoing chronic hemodialysis. A positive family history is usually lacking. Diabetes mellitus, lupus erythematosus, and hemochromatosis occur with increased frequency in affected patients. Severel cases associated with hepatomas have been reported.

Routine laboratory studies may show fasting hyperglycemia, glycosuria, and abnormal liver function tests. The urine is usually red-orange or brown. The key screening test is for urinary porphyrins. Urinary URO is strikingly increased, and the urinary COPRO is mildly increased. Although there may be some increase in ALA, there is no increase in PBG. There is an increase in fecal isocoproporphyrin and no increase in fecal protoporphyrin.

Hereditary Coproporphyria. This rare autosomal dominant disorder is due to coproporphyrinogen oxidase deficiency. It leads to excess excretion of ALA, PBG, URO, and COPRO in urine and excess COPRO in feces. It presents with acute neurologic attacks, as in acute intermittent porphyria (AIP) but, in contrast to AIP, it can cause photosensitivity, which usually does not extend beyond the acute attack.

During an acute neurologic attack, fecal COPRO and urinary ALA and PBG are increased. In asymptomatic patients, fecal COPRO is increased, and the urine may be normal or may show increased COPRO. Hereditary coproporphyria is differentiated from acute intermittent porphyria by the high fecal COPRO.

Variegate Porphyria. This autosomal dominant disorder quite common in South Africans of Dutch descent but very rare in other people, is due to protoporphyrinogen oxidase deficiency. Its presentation is identical to acute intermittent porphyria, but like porphyria cutanea tarda it can also produce cutaneous disease on the exposed portions of the body.

Fecal protoporphyrin is increased during the attacks and in asymptomatic periods. Urinary ALA and PBG are increased during the attack. There is increased urinary URO and COPRO. In addition, a peptide conjugate of porphyrin is characteristically present in the urine and stools of patients (porphyrin X).

In contradistinction to acute intermittent porphyria, variegate porphyria characteristically has cutaneous lesions and increased fecal protoporphyrins.

Erythrohepatic or Erythropoietic Protoporphyria. This is an autosomal dominant disorder caused by ferrochelatase deficiency. It is characterized by cutaneous acute photosensitivity reactions that almost always begin before age 13 and consist of burning, swelling, itching, and redness of the skin (solar urticaria). Itching and burning may occur without the other symptoms. Cutaneous burning can occur indoors and outdoors (window glass can transmit wave lengths responsible for photosensitivity). Bullae, purpura, scarring, hirsutism, and pigmentation are rare. In contrast to congenital erythropoietic porphyria, erythrodontia and fluorescence of the teeth are absent. There is increased incidence of gallstones with increased protoporphyrin in the stones. Rarely, deposition of protoporphyrins in the liver leads to progressive liver disease.

Routine laboratory studies usually show hypochromic microcytic anemia with normal serum iron levels. The urinary porphyrins and porphyrin precursors are normal. The key to the diagnosis is increased protoporphyrin IX in red blood cells, feces, or both. There is fluorescence of normoblasts in the bone marrow and circulating red blood cells. Protoporphyrins can be detected in the liver. The most definitive diagnosis is made by finding decreased ferrochelatase in the tissues.

Differentiation from other acute photosensitivity reactions is by the finding of increased red blood cell (RBC) protoporphyrin levels. However, increased RBC protoporphyrin levels can also be found in iron deficiency, lead intoxication, and hemolysis; in these disorders, however, there is no photosensitivity and plasma protoporphyrin levels are normal. The liver disease associated with erythropoietic protoporphyria shows characteristic fluorescence (Maltese cross) on polarization microscopy.

DIAGNOSTIC EVALUATION

Porphyrias should be considered in patients presenting with dark urine or suggestive cutaneous or neurologic disorders, and in those with a positive family history for the disease. The clinical features and diagnostic laboratory tests are outlined in Table 11–32.

The porphyrias are differentiated on the basis of the specific enzymatic defect in each type and the unique pattern of excretion of heme precursors (ALA, PBG, or porphyrins) associated with each defect. The pattern is best determined with quantitative tests. Qualitative tests such as the Watson-Schwartz test for PBG are best reserved for when quantitative determinations are unavailable or in urgent circumstances. The porphyrins are usually measured spectrophotometrically and fluorometrically after differential extractions. Isomers of porphyrins are usually separated by thin-layer or high-performance liquid chromatographic procedures. ALA and PBG are quantitated by chromatographic methods.

A large variety of pathologic conditions besides porphyrias may cause an abnormality in porphyrin and heme metabolism. Photosensitivity is not a feature of any of these disorders. Those features related to hepatic disease (alcoholic liver disease, cirrhosis of any cause, cholestasis, hereditary tyrosinemia) are characterized principally by a relatively mild increase in urinary COPRO excretion. Those related to hematologic disorders (hemolytic and sideroblastic anemias, iron deficiency, Hodgkin's disease, leukemia) principally show increased erythrocyte protoporphyrin. Lead toxicity results in increased ALA and COPRO but normal or slightly increased PBG. To avoid the major pitfall of concluding that such patients suffer from porphyria, the physician should quantitate fecal, urinary, and erythrocytic porphyrins, and urinary ALA and PBG. None of the patterns in these diseases resembles those associated with porphyrias.

CARCINOID SYNDROME

DEFINITION

Carcinoid syndrome refers to the constellation of symptoms and signs that are related to the anatomic and functional effects of carcinoid tumors. Its primary manifestations are caused by tumoral release into the circulation of serotonin and other biologically active substances.

PATHOPHYSIOLOGIC CONSIDERATIONS

Although carcinoid tumors can occur anywhere in the gut from the gastroesophageal junction to the anus, the syndrome is caused most frequently (80%) by ileocecal tumors with hepatic metastasis; other causes include colon tumors (about 5%) or bronchial tumors (about 5%) and nonbronchial foregut structures and teratomas of the gonads (about 10%). Except for bronchial and gonadal tumors, which have systemic venous drainage, carcinoid tumors that give rise to the syndrome are almost always metastasized to the liver (the humoral substances are deactivated by one passage through the liver; hence the syndrome does not appear until hepatic metastasis releases these active compounds into the circulation).

Other malignancies such as oat-cell carcinoma, nonbeta islet–cell tumors, and medullary carcinoma of the thyroid can secrete biologic amines and give rise to the syndrome.

The foregut carcinoids also can secrete polypeptide hormones and can present with other characteristic endocrine syndromes. The polypeptide hormones that can be secreted by these foregut carcinoids include ACTH, growth hormone–releasing hormone, calcitonin, glucagon, insulin, gastrin, and VIP. There is an increased incidence of carcinoid tumors in patients with multiple endocrine neoplasia type 1.

Among the biologic substances secreted by carcinoid tumors are serotonin (responsible for gastrointestinal hypermotility, bronchoconstriction, vasodilatation, and endocardial fibrosis), kallikrein, which forms kinins from kininogen in the plasma (kallikrein causes vasodilatation and bronchoconstriction and mediates the flush), and histamine, primarily from gastric carcinoid (which causes flushing, hypotension, tremulousness, tachycardia, and increased incidence of peptic ulceration).

CLINICAL PRESENTATION

The clinical manifestations are related to the anatomic and functional effects of the causative tumor and its associations.

Vasomotor paroxysms of flushing are the most common functional manifestation of the syndrome, occurring in 75 to 90% of patients. The typical flush is erythematous, may be red to violet, and involves the "blush area" of the head and neck. It may be precipitated by excitement, exertion, eating, or the use of ethanol, beta adrenergic agonists, or pentagastrin, and it usually lasts 2 to 15 minutes. Tachycardia may be present; the blood pressure is usually normal, although hypotension may be present in some patients. Hypertension is distinctively rare. Borborygmus, abdominal cramping, explosive diarrhea, bronchoconstriction, and wheezing may occur. If prolonged, the paroxysm may be associated with excessive lacrimation and periorbital edema. In chronic cases, telangiectasia, primarily of the face and neck may occur as a result of prolonged vasodilatation.

Among other functional manifestations are chronic diarrhea and malabsorption (60 to 75%). Cardiac manifestations (40 to 50%) are related to the deposition of fibrous tissue on the endothelia of valvular cusps and cardiac chambers, primarily on the right side of the heart. This deposition leads to distortion of the cusps, chordae tendinae, and papillary muscles, and it presents as valvular disease with regurgitation or stenosis, most commonly affecting the tricuspid and pulmonary valves. The cardiac output may be increased because of the release of vasodilators and excessive flow in the metastatic lesions.

Bronchoconstriction and wheezing (15 to 20%) occur as functional manifestations, more severely during the episodic flush.

Gastric carcinoids are associated with unique flushing that is bright red and patchy with sharp borders that tend to coalesce. The flush is especially likely to be precipitated by food. These carcinoids secrete 5-hydroxytryptophan and histamine, the latter causing a high incidence of peptic ulcer. Diarrhea and heart lesions are not prominent with gastric carcinoids. In bronchial carcinoids, flushing is usually prolonged and severe and is associated with periorbital edema, increased lacrimation, salivation, hypotension, tachycardia, anxiety, nausea and vomiting, explosive diarrhea, and bronchoconstriction. These flushes can be prevented by the administration of corticosteroids.

Other endocrine syndromes resulting from the elaboration of polypeptides by carcinoid tumors include Cushing's syndrome, acromegaly, insulinoma, glucagonoma, and watery diarrhea. These may occur in isolation or in association with multiple endocrine neoplasia type 1.

Because of increased shunting of tryptophan to serotonin synthesis, there is decreased synthesis of nicotinic acid, which may lead to pellagra.

Anatomic manifestations are related to the anatomic effects of the tumor mass or metastasis. These include intestinal obstruction or bleeding; tumoral or metastatic necrosis with abdominal pain, tenderness, fever, and leukocytosis; mucosal erosions by bronchial carcinoids and hemoptysis, or obstruction and atelectasis. Metastasis to the liver causes right upper quadrant abdominal pain and tenderness; bony metastases are often osteoblastic.

DIFFERENTIAL DIAGNOSIS

Oat-cell carcinoma of the lung, nonbeta islet-cell tumors of the pancreas, and medullary carcinoma of the thyroid may secrete serotonin and be confused with the typical carcinoid syndrome. Diagnosis is by the clinical setting, appropriate radiologic and laboratory studies, and tissue biopsy. In medullary carcinoma of the thyroid usually there is a goiter, basal calcitonin levels are increased, and the calcitonin response to calcium infusion or pentagastrin is exaggerated. In patients with vipoma, there is evidence of a pancreatic tumor and increased serum VIP levels.

Among other causes of flushing is systemic mastocytosis. This rare neoplastic syndrome is characterized by mast cell proliferation that can be cutaneous or systemic and can involve any tissues in the body except the central nervous system (skin, bone, GI, liver, spleen, lymph nodes, bone marrow). Rarely, it can lead to malignant transformation and mast cell leukemia. Degranulation of mast cells releases the mediators histamine, heparin, and prostaglandin D_2.

Clinical manifestations of systemic mastocytosis include urticaria pigmentosa, which can be isolated or can occur as a part of the systemic illness. It consists of plaque-like or nodular reddish brown lesions that if stroked lead to pruritus and surrounding erythema (Darier's sign). If generalized, urticaria pigmentosa can lead to pruritus and flushing. Systemic mastocytosis also can produce acute episodes that result from extensive urticaria pigmentosa or systemic disease. These episodes are related to increased circulating histamine, PGD_2 and other biologic compounds and are characterized by vasodilation, headache, dizziness, tachycardia, hypotension, syncope, and shock. They can be precipitated by stroking a cutaneous lesion or by ingesting alcohol, morphine, or codeine.

Other manifestations of systemic mastocytosis include gastrointestinal manifestations of anorexia, nau-

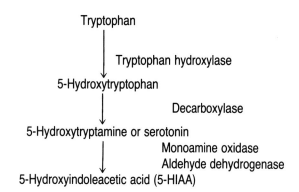

Fig. 11–20. The serotonin pathway.

sea, vomiting, diarrhea, peptic ulceration, malabsorption, and hepatosplenomegaly; osseous manifestations of bone pain with or without fracture, osteoporosis, and osteosclerosis; rhinitis and wheezing; and anemia, leukopenia, thrombocytopenia, and bleeding tendency.

The diagnosis of systemic mastocytosis depends on the pathognomonic cutaneous lesions and Darier's sign, characteristic osseous lesions consisting of adjacent areas of osteoporosis and mottled osteosclerosis; increased urinary histamine and PGD_2 metabolite; and biopsy of the involved organ. Urinary 5-HIAA is usually normal. It is important to remember that some gastric carcinoids may secrete histamine.

In addition to systemic mastocytosis, other causes of flushing include drugs such as nicotinic acid, alcohol, and chlorpropamide. Also, flushing may be caused by pheochromocytoma (see Pheochromocytoma). Either pallor or flushing may be observed during a pheochromocytoma spell. In addition, there are hypertension, increased urinary catecholamines and their metabolites, increased plasma catecholamines, and findings of an adrenal or other catecholaminergic tumor.

Finally, flushing can be postmenopausal flush, easily diagnosed by the age of the patient, absence of other symptoms, and flushing's responsiveness to estrogen therapy.

DIAGNOSTIC EVALUATION

The diagnosis of carcinoid syndrome depends on consideration of the syndrome in the appropriate clinical setting, and documentation of the characteristic biochemical and anatomic alterations related to the causative tumor.

Increased urinary 5-hydroxyindoleacetic acid (5-HIAA) (normal is up to 9 mg/24 hours) is the biochemical hallmark of the syndrome (Fig. 11–20). A value of greater than 25 mg/day is diagnostic, although smaller increases may also be seen in nontropical sprue

and acute intestinal obstruction. It is important to remember that 5-HIAA can be increased by the ingestion of foods containing serotonin (walnuts, bananas, avocados, and pineapple) and that its measurement can be influenced by a number of agents or drugs (e.g., guaiacolate may give false increases; phenothiazines and methenamine mandelate can interfere with the assay). Ideally, all drugs should be discontinued several days prior to the urine collection.

Additional biochemical studies can be helpful in certain circumstances. These include the finding of increased blood or platelet serotonin levels (measurement is not generally available); increased blood 5-hydroxytryptophan levels in foregut tumors; and increased blood and urinary histamine and its metabolites in gastric carcinoids. In the provocative epinephrine test, 5 µg of epinephrine (0.5 ml of 1:1000 solution diluted 100 times) is given IV, causing facial flushing and some dyspnea in a few minutes in patients with carcinoid syndrome. This is a dangerous provocative test that may lead to severe hemodynamic changes and is best avoided.

Delineation of the cause and the sequelae of the syndrome depends on clinical and ancillary laboratory and radiologic studies. The primary goals are to rule out a curable primary carcinoid (of gonadal or bronchial origin); to assess metastatic disease by liver scan, bone radiology, or bone scan; to evaluate hepatic and cardiac function; and to evaluate for possible malabsorption in patients who have significant diarrhea.

THE OSTEOPOROTIC SYNDROMES

DEFINITION

Osteoporosis is defined as a decrease in bone mass that compromises the mechanical support function of the skeleton. The remaining bone is morphologically normal. (See also Chapter 12.)

PATHOPHYSIOLOGIC CONSIDERATIONS
(Table 11–33)

Primary Osteoporosis. In most people, bone mass continues to increase until the fourth decade of life; thereafter, bone loss occurs at the relatively constant rate of approximately 1.5%/year. Though bone turnover may be normal, increased, or decreased, the rate

Table 11–33. Causes of Osteoporosis

Primary (idiopathic)
  Postmenopausal
  Senile
  Juvenile
Secondary
  Endocrine
    Cushing's syndrome
    Thyrotoxicosis
    Hyperparathyroidism
    Hypogonadism
    Diabetes mellitus
  Malignancy
    Multiple myeloma
    Leukemia
    Lymphoma
    Systemic mastocytosis
  Immobilization
    Generalized
    Localized
  Genetic abnormalities in bone collagen synthesis
    Homocystinuria
    Ehlers-Danlos syndrome
    Osteogenesis imperfecta
  Drugs
    Corticosteroids
    Heparin therapy
    Methotrexate
  Nutritional
    Protein malnutrition
    Ascorbic acid deficiency
    Alcoholism
  Gastrointestinal
    Malabsorption
    Gastric surgery

of bone resorption exceeds that of bone formation. Primary osteoporosis is much more common in women than in men and in whites than in blacks. The rate of bone loss in women is accelerated with the decline in ovarian function and loss of estrogen at menopause. Bone loss begins later in life and proceeds at a slower rate in men. This age-related bone loss is universal, but certain individuals appear to be more susceptible than others. Failure to develop sufficient bone mass during adult life, defective intestinal calcium absorption, increased sensitivity to endogenous parathyroid hormone, and genetic, environmental, and dietary factors may be involved. In postmenopausal osteoporosis the skeletal loss occurs most prominently in trabecular bone, and fractures of the vertebrae and wrist are common. In senile osteoporosis, which appears after the eighth decade and affects both sexes equally, the skeletal loss affects both cortical and trabecular bone and characteristically involves the neck and intertrochanteric areas of the femur.

Secondary Osteoporosis. Secondary osteoporosis may be produced by a number of disorders. Cushing's syndrome, whether caused by endogenous cortisol hy-

persecretion or prolonged glucocorticoid therapy, is frequently associated with osteoporosis, which may occasionally be the presenting feature of this syndrome. The osteoporosis results from increased bone resorption and decreased bone formation caused by acceleration of catabolism of $1,25(OH)_2D$, decreased calcium absorption from the gut (antivitamin D effect), secondary stimulation of PTH secretion, and inhibition of osteoblastic activity. Spontaneous symptomless fractures may occur in the vertebrae, ribs, and pubic and ischiatic rami and often heal partially with exuberant callus.

Gonadal hormones play an important role in the maintenance of skeletal mass, and osteoporosis can occur in both primary and secondary hypogonadism. Patients with Klinefelter's and Turner's syndromes are particularly susceptible because the adult skeleton is decreased to begin with, and therefore, age-related bone losses are more significant.

Thyrotoxicosis leads to an increased rate of bone turnover favoring resorption. Osteoporosis may occur in patients with long-standing, unrecognized thyrotoxicosis, especially in elderly patients. It is important to rule out hyperthyroidism as a contributing factor in all patients with osteoporosis.

In primary HPT, excess parathyroid hormone leads to increased bone resorption. Osteoporosis in primary hyperparathyroidism is more common than the specific bone effects of subperiosteal resorption, osteitis fibrosa cystica, and brown tumors.

The osteoporosis in acromegaly is unlikely to be related to growth hormone excess but appears to be more related to concomitant hypopituitarism and gonadal insufficiency.

The role of nutritional deficiency in osteoporosis is not certain. Vitamin C is important for normal collagen synthesis, and its deficiency (scurvy) can be associated with osteoporosis. Osteoporosis can also occur in patients with malnutrition and intestinal malabsorption and is probably related to deficiencies of vitamins, minerals, and protein.

Bone marrow infiltrative diseases, such as leukemia and myeloma, are associated with osteoclast-activating factors in the bone marrow that increase bone resorption on the endostial, trabecular bone surfaces. In systemic mast cell disease, localized as well as generalized osteoporosis can occur as a result of local synthesis of heparin and prostaglandins that can increase bone resorption.

Disuse osteoporosis can also occur. Mechanical stress plays an important role in the maintenance of normal bone mass. Immobilization leads to increased bone resorption, decreased bone formation, and rapid loss of bone mineral leading to bone thinning that may be generalized or focal. Localized osteoporosis can occur in a limb after trauma (post-traumatic or Sudeck's osteodystrophy). Bone turnover is high, favoring more resorption and leading to spotty demineralization and cortical striations. In addition, patients have autonomic dysfunction and increased sweating.

Regional migratory osteoporosis is a localized osteoporosis characterized by high bone turnover that involves the lower extremities. Successive regions exhibit progressive bone loss accompanied by signs of inflammation of the overlying tissue that may simulate inflammatory joint disease. The cause is unknown, and spontaneous recovery usually occurs in 6 to 12 months.

Drug-related osteoporosis can occur in long-term administration of heparin and administration of immunosuppressive agents, e.g., methotrexate.

Chronic excessive ingestion of ethanol, often associated with alcoholic cirrhosis, is frequently associated with osteoporosis because of the direct effect of alcohol on bone and associated malnutrition and liver disease.

Juvenile and idiopathic osteoporosis are observed in adolescence and early adult life; the cause is unknown. The osteoporosis may progress over months or years and in many patients is self-limiting with spontaneous recovery.

Osteoporosis can occur in association with heritable disorders of connective tissue, such as Ehlers-Danlos syndrome, Marfan's syndrome, homocystinuria, and osteogenesis imperfecta (see Miscellaneous Metabolic Bone Diseases).

CLINICAL PRESENTATION

Most patients with uncomplicated osteoporosis are relatively asymptomatic until they develop a complicating fracture, which often occurs after minimal trauma. Because trabecular bone bears the brunt of the disease, fractures typically involve the vertebrae, distal radius, and neck of the femur. In crush vertebral fracture, there is an acute onset of severe localized pain in the back, over the affected vertebrae and with minimal lateral radiation; it is aggravated by movement and weight-bearing and is somewhat relieved by recumbency, lasting 4 to 8 weeks until the fracture is healed. During the acute phase, there is spot tenderness over the back and paraspinal muscle spasm; neurologic signs are rare, and their presence should suggest an alternative diagnosis, e.g., metastatic malignancy or multiple myeloma. The characteristic physical findings of hip fracture are shortening and external rotation of the lower extremity, along with severe pain and loss of motion.

The patient may then be free of symptoms until another fracture occurs. It is important to remember that spine fractures may occur gradually and with very little pain. After repeated compression fractures and anterior wedging of the vertebrae, loss of height, dorsal kyphosis (Dowager's hump), and drooping of the rib cage onto the pelvic brim with pleating of the truncal skin may occur. Chronic and continuous back pain, made worse by standing or sudden movement, may develop secondary to muscle and ligamentous strains.

Other features that may be present are those that relate to the secondary cause of the osteoporosis.

DIFFERENTIAL DIAGNOSIS

Osteomalacia (see Osteomalacia and Rickets) is suggested by the presence of hypocalcemia, hypophosphatemia, increased serum alkaline phosphatase, and compatible underlying disease. In the osteomalacic spine, all the vertebrae are affected simultaneously and in a similar way, unlike in osteoporosis, in which a wide variety of radiologic changes simultaneously affect different vertebrae. Pseudofractures are pathognomonic of osteomalacia. The diagnosis of osteomalacia is confirmed by characteristic bone biopsy findings. It is important to remember that osteoporosis and osteomalacia may coexist.

Metastatic bone disease should be strongly suspected if vertebral collapse occurs above T9 vertebra, if there is a history and findings of a primary tumor known to metastasize to bone, if the process affects the posterior arches of the vertebrae, or if there is elevation of serum or urinary calcium. Scanning procedures with bone-seeking isotopes may be helpful in the differential diagnosis. In the absence of a recent fracture, "hot" spots suggest the presence of tumor or early Paget's disease. Definitive diagnosis is by biopsy.

In occasional patients, Paget's disease of the lytic type may be confused with osteoporosis. In Paget's disease the bone diameter is enlarged and the alkaline phosphatase is increased.

Some late forms of osteogenesis imperfecta may be confused with involutional osteoporosis (see Miscellaneous Metabolic Bone Diseases). Other features of osteogenesis imperfecta and a history are supportive. Definitive diagnosis is by bone biopsy.

DIAGNOSTIC EVALUATION (Fig. 11–21)

The physician must determine if the patient has osteoporosis and must determine its cause.

Suspicion of the presence of osteoporosis depends on awareness of suggestive symptoms and signs and of the clinical setting in which the disorder may occur.

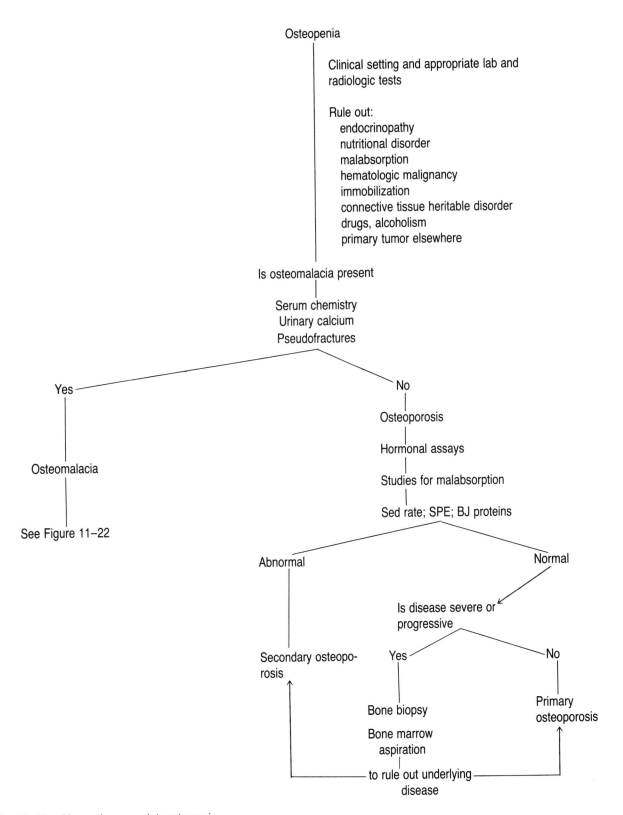

Fig. 11–21. Diagnostic approach to osteopenia.

The diagnosis rests on documenting evidence of bone thinning, which is usually generalized but affects the axial skeleton especially.

X-ray examination of the affected bones is a relatively insensitive diagnostic tool because greater than 30% loss of mineral content has to occur before radiologic changes are apparent. The earliest sign of osteopenia is loss of the horizontal vertebral trabeculi with relative prominence of the residual vertical trabeculi and end plates. Later, the vertical trabeculi are resolved and the vertebrae look like empty boxes. More advanced radiologic changes include ballooning of the intervertebral disc, shortening of the height in the center of the bone, "codfish spine," anterior wedging in the lower thoracic and upper lumbar vertebrae, and vertebral collapse. Trabecular loss may be seen in the femoral head (Singh index). The relation of the cortical width to the total width of the second metacarpal bone in hand x-rays can be useful in the diagnosis; normally, the cortical width is at least 45% of the total width; this percentage is increased in osteoporosis.

Photon beam absorptiometry is considerably more sensitive than skeletal x-rays in detecting bone loss. The distal end of the radius is chosen as representative of trabecular bone, and the mineral content is determined by penetration of the photons through bone. The amount of radiation passing through the tissue is inversely proportional to the density. This method is not useful in establishing the diagnosis because there is overlap in values between osteoporotic patients and controls, but it is useful for follow-up in monitoring the change in bone mass. Dual photon absorptiometry can assess the vertebrae and femoral neck with considerably less overlap between osteoporotic and normal patients than the single photon can.

Laboratory tests are remarkable for their normalcy in osteoporosis that is unassociated with systemic illness. Serum calcium, phosphate, alkaline phosphatase, parathyroid hormone levels, urinary calcium, and hydroxyproline are normal. Serum alkaline phosphatase, however, may be slightly elevated after a recent fracture. Serum protein electrophoresis is normal.

Accurate measurements of height and arm span are important in assessing the development and progress of osteoporosis. Normally, the patient's height equals the arm span. It becomes progressively less than the arm span with recurrent vertebral collapse.

A detailed history and physical examination can provide important clues in the attempt to rule out secondary causes of osteoporosis. The physician should inquire about history of immobilization; exposure to glucocorticoids, heparin, and cytotoxic agents; dietary history, nutritional state, and social habits; and features of chronic disease, endocrinopathy, malabsorption state, or malignancy.

The following tests are recommended: serum calcium, and, if necessary, serum parathyroid hormone to rule out hyperparathyroidism; serum cortisol, 24-hour urinary free cortisol, and a standard low-dose dexamethasone suppression test, if needed, to rule out Cushing's syndrome; serum total and free thyroxine (or free thyroxine index) and serum T_3 to rule out thyrotoxicosis; serum testosterone in men to rule out hypogonadism; sedimentation rate, serum protein electrophoresis, tests for Bence Jones protein in the urine, and bone marrow aspiration, if needed, to search for myeloma; bone marrow aspiration to rule out infiltrative disease of bone marrow such as lymphoma, leukemia, and carcinomatosis; appropriate tests to rule out liver disease, intestinal malabsorption, and renal disease; bone biopsy in osteopenia in all men, in black women, and in all premenopausal white females when the cause is not discernible.

OSTEOMALACIA AND RICKETS

DEFINITION

Osteomalacia in the adult refers to failure of mineralization of bone osteoid, resulting in an excess of unmineralized osteoid and deficiency of mature mineralized bone. In children, rickets is associated, in addition, with failure of maturation of the growth plate at the epiphysis and with gross skeletal deformities.

PATHOPHYSIOLOGIC CONSIDERATIONS

Failure to mineralize osteoid can result from decreased supply of minerals to bone-forming surfaces because of decreased tissue levels of calcium, phosphate, or both; unfavorable milieu for calcification at the mineralization front; and defective biosynthesis of osteoid from abnormal functioning of bone-forming cells or from defective collagen production. The causes are outlined in Table 11–34. The most common causes of osteomalacia in the Western world are malabsorption of vitamin D, disorder of vitamin D metabolism, hypophosphatemic osteomalacia, dietary deficiency of vitamin D in elderly patients, and the use of anticonvulsant drugs.

Disorders of Vitamin D Metabolism. Normal vitamin D metabolism is outlined in Figure 11–13. De-

Table 11–34.　Causes of Osteomalacia

Disorders of vitamin D metabolism
　Vitamin D deficiency
　　Nutritional
　　Malabsorption syndromes
　Defects of 25-OH-D generation
　　Anticonvulsants
　　Severe hepatic disease
　Defects of 1,25 $(OH)_2$ D generation
　　Renal failure
　　Hyperphosphatemia
　Hereditary disorders
　　Vitamin D–resistant rickets (VDRR)
　　　Type I
　　　Type II
Phosphate Deficiency
　Phosphate-binding antacids
　Renal phosphate loss
　　Proximal tubular defects
　　　Isolated
　　　Generalized (Fanconi)
　　Renal tubular acidosis
　　Vitamin D–resistant rickets
　Nonfamilial adulthood hypophosphatemia
　Neoplasms
Abnormal bone cell, matrix, crystal
　Familial hypophosphatasia
　Fibrogenesis imperfecta ossium
　Axial osteomalacia
　Fluoride toxicity
　Aluminum toxicity
　Diphosphonates

ficiency or disordered metabolism of vitamin D leads to decreased calcium absorption from the gut, to a tendency toward hypocalcemia, and to secondary hyperparathyroidism. Increased circulating PTH causes mobilization of calcium and phosphate from bone and causes increased calcium reabsorption and phosphate excretion by the renal tubule. Osteomalacia is due to the limited supply of minerals to osteoid and to the direct effect of vitamin D lack on the calcification front.

Vitamin D deficiency can occur in nutritional deficiency, especially in elderly individuals who eat sparingly and who have poor exposure to the sun. It can also be found in people living in underprivileged areas of the world and in food faddists. Also, malabsorption is one of the most common causes of osteomalacia caused by disordered vitamin D metabolism. It may be due to postgastrectomy syndrome, sprue syndrome with or without gluten enteropathy, small-bowel resection or bypass, pancreatic insufficiency, laxative abuse, or prolonged use of cholestyramine. In malabsorption, there is not only decreased vitamin D absorption, but also interruption of the enterohepatic circulation of 25-OH-D with depletion of body stores of vitamin D.

Defects of 25-OH-D metabolism can occur in severe hepatic disease, e.g., primary biliary cirrhosis, which is associated with decreased levels of 25-OH-D caused by decreased generation and disruption of the enterohepatic circulation; and in long-term anticonvulsant therapy with phenytoin or phenobarbital leading to decreased 25-OH-D levels because of accelerated catabolism of cholecalciferol and 25-OH-D, and to the suppressive effect on the action of 1,25$(OH)_2$D at the gut or bone levels.

Deficiency of 1,25$(OH)_2$D occurs in renal failure from defective 1-hydroxylation resulting from the decreased renal cell mass and from hyperphosphatemia. In these patients there are also decreased tissue effects of 1,25$(OH)_2$D and a tendency toward hypocalcemia and secondary hyperparathyroidism. The majority of patients with chronic renal failure have renal osteodystrophy with the metabolic bone disease, often caused by a mixture of osteomalacia, osteitis fibrosa cystica, and osteosclerosis.

Hereditary disorders of vitamin D metabolism and vitamin D-resistant rickets are uncommon, inherited in autosomal recessive fashion, and present in childhood as rickets. In type I there is failure of 1-hydroxylation of vitamin D; the levels of 25-OH-D are normal, whereas those of 1,25$(OH)_2$D are decreased. In type II there is a decrease or absence of target sensitivity to 1,25$(OH)_2$D, and the levels of 25-OH-D are normal whereas those of 1,25$(OH)_2$D may be increased.

Disorders of Phosphate Metabolism. Phosphate deficiency reduces the calcium and phosphate concentration at the mineralization front and interferes with the metabolism of osteoblasts, impairing matrix formation and leading to osteomalacia. It can occur in inborn or acquired proximal renal tubular defects leading to phosphaturia and hypophosphatemia. Phosphaturia may exist as a single defect, or it may be associated with more complex impairment of renal tubular transport of glucose and amino acids, and with defects of urinary acidification and concentration (Fanconi's syndrome).

Phosphate deficiency also occurs in distal renal tubular dysfunction; X-linked hereditary hypophosphatemia or vitamin D–resistant rickets in which a renal phosphate transport defect is manifest; phosphate depletion caused by decreased dietary intake or intestinal phosphate binding by antacids (aluminum hydroxide); nonfamilial adulthood hypophosphatemia; and neoplasms, including giant-cell tumors, mesenchymal tumors, and angiomatous tumors involving bone and soft tissue that are usually benign but can be malignant; the hypophosphatemia may be related to the production by the tumor of a substance that inhibits 1-hydroxylation of 25-OH-D or that is a potent phosphaturic agent.

Familial Hypophosphatasia. This rare syndrome is characterized by deficiency of alkaline phosphatase in serum, bone, liver, and kidney. Alkaline phosphatase may be required to break down organic phosphate compounds, for example, pyrophosphate, that inhibit mineralization. In the infantile form, which is autosomal recessive, manifestations appear in the first 6 months of life and are characterized by severe rickets and growth failure; it is frequently fatal by 1 to 2 years. In the childhood form, which may be autosomal recessive or dominant, symptoms appear after the first 6 months and are usually less severe. In the adult form, which is autosomal dominant and the least severe type, the presentation is with osteomalacia. In all forms of the disease, the serum alkaline phosphatase is low, the bone isoenzyme is low, and there is marked increase of phosphorylethanolamine and of pyrophosphate in serum and urine.

Fibrogenesis imperfecta ossium is a rare skeletal disorder, characterized by a defect in normal polarization of collagen fibers and defective mineralization of collagen. Primarily it affects middle-aged males and presents with osteomalacia. Its cause is uncertain. In axial osteomalacia, there is a generalized lack of mineralization and accumulation of osteoid in the axial but not in the appendicular skeleton. Its cause is unknown.

Inhibitors of Mineralization. Diphosphonates are synthetic analogues of pyrophosphate that resist hydrolysis and therefore have a more prolonged effect. These compounds coat the bone surfaces, inhibiting mineral deposition and resorption of bone. They are used therapeutically to inhibit bone resorption in the treatment of Paget's disease and to inhibit bone formation in ectopic ossification. Large doses over prolonged periods of time may impair mineralization and lead to osteomalacia. Long-term administration of fluoride leads to accelerated synthesis of matrix and impaired mineralization. Aluminum toxicity in patients with renal osteodystrophy on dialysis, and in those receiving total parenteral nutrition, can inhibit mineralization and induce osteomalacia.

CLINICAL PRESENTATION

Patients with mild osteomalacia are usually asymptomatic or have nonspecific symptoms. Those who have moderate to severe disease have diffuse bone pain and tenderness, muscle weakness, and waddling gait. The clinical manifestations in adults often go unrecognized or are overshadowed by those of the primary disorders. Patients with osteomalacia have few signs, if any, except proximal weakness and waddling gait and deformities that develop as a result of fractures.

In infants and children, rickets is characterized by delayed development, bone pain, and deformities. Young infants with rickets are restless, sleep poorly, and have craniotabes (decreased mineralization of the skull). Older infants show delay in sitting and crawling, bossing of the skull, costochondral beading (rachitic rosary), and delayed fontanelle closure. Later there is enlargement of the epiphysial cartilage at the lower ends of the radius, ulna, tibia, and fibula, delay in walking, and deformities such as bow legs and kyphoscoliosis. In older children and adolescents there is pain on walking and deformities such as bow legs and knock knees.

DIAGNOSTIC EVALUATION

The diagnosis of osteomalacia is suggested by the clinical features of bone pain, tenderness, fractures, deformities, proximal weakness, and waddling gait, and by the occurrence of these features in a clinical setting known to be associated with the presence of osteomalacia or rickets.

Screening tests should include serum calcium, phosphate, and magnesium, serum PTH, alkaline phosphatase, urinary calcium, and, if needed, serum 25-OH-D. Serum calcium is normal or decreased, and serum phosphate is decreased (except in renal insufficiency); serum alkaline phosphatase is increased; and the serum iPTH is variable. Decrease in urinary calcium (caused by secondary hyperparathyroidism) is one of the earliest biochemical abnormalities. Serum 25-OH-D levels are low in vitamin D deficiency. Serum 1,25(OH)$_2$D are low in abnormalities of 1-hydroxylation of vitamin D and are high in target insensitivity to vitamin D.

X-ray studies show osteopenia with a nonspecific decrease in radiodensity and a generalized loss of cortical bone that may be associated with a coarsened trabecular pattern. Looser's zones (milkman's fractures, pseudofractures) are almost pathognomonic of osteomalacia. They represent areas of linear decalcification perpendicular to the periosteal surface and along the course of large blood vessels. They are usually bilateral and symmetrical, occurring in the scapulae, pelvis, and proximal long bones, and they represent stress fractures in which normal healing is impaired because of the mineralization defects. Radiologic findings of associated secondary hyperparathyroidism may be present with subperiosteal resorption, osteitis fibrosa cystica, and cysts. In affected infants and children, radiologic features of rickets include widening and irregularity of the epiphysis, cupping of the metaphysis, bowing of bones, and fractures.

Radionuclide bone scans are especially helpful in detecting the presence of pseudofractures even when skeletal x-rays appear normal.

Definitive diagnosis of osteomalacia rests on a study of bone biopsy; double tetracycline labeling procedure should be done, before the biopsy of the iliac crest is performed to allow quantitation of mineralized bone formed per unit time. The biopsy shows widened osteoid seams, increased bone surfaces covered by osteoid, decreased rate of osteoid mineralization, and low appositional rates.

Clues to the etiologic diagnosis from the history and physical examination include inadequate intake of vitamin D; malabsorption; hepatic or renal disease; use of drugs such as anticonvulsants, phosphate-binding antacids, diphosphonates, fluoride, and aluminum-containing dialysate; presence of mesenchymal neoplasms causing hypophosphatemia; and family history of rickets (vitamin D-dependent or -resistant rickets, renal tubular defects, and hypophosphatasia).

If the cause is not evident after a careful history and physical examination and the biochemical tests mentioned above, additional tests are in order. These may include serum potassium, serum albumin, serum bicarbonate, and blood pH; pH of early morning urine to detect defects in urinary acidification; indices of renal glomerular and tubular functions including serum creatinine and urinary excretion of creatinine, phosphate, glucose, calcium, and potassium; indices of the nutritional state such as red blood cell indices, serum iron and iron-binding capacity, folate, and serum B_{12} screening for malabsorption including 72-hour stool fat excretion, d-xylose excretion, and, if needed, gastrointestinal radiologic studies and bowel biopsy; and liver function tests.

The etiologic diagnostic approach to osteomalacia and rickets is represented in Figure 11–22. A useful classification depends on the assessment of serum calcium, serum phosphate, and serum iPTH. In the presence of a normal serum calcium and serum PTH, a low serum phosphate points to phosphate depletion, while a normal serum phosphate points to either hypophosphatasia or osteomalacia related to abnormal bone cell, matrix, or crystal. (A low serum alkaline phosphatase points to hypophosphatasia, while a normal one points to abnormality in bone cell bone matrix, or bone crystal.)

In the presence of normal or low serum calcium and a high PTH, a high serum phosphate points to hyperphosphatemic osteomalacia caused primarily by renal insufficiency, while a low serum phosphate points ultimately to deficiency of 25-OH-D, deficiency of 1,25(OH)$_2$D, or target insensitivity to 1,25(OH)$_2$D. A low serum 25-OH-D points to vitamin D deficiency and impaired generation or catabolism of 25-OH-D by the liver. Normal serum 25-OH-D and low 1,25(OH)$_2$D points to 1,25(OH)$_2$D deficiency as the cause of the osteopenic syndrome. A normal 25-OH-D and elevated 1,25(OH)$_2$D points to target insensitivity to 1,25(OH)$_2$D.

MISCELLANEOUS METABOLIC BONE DISEASES

PAGET'S DISEASE

Definition and Pathophysiologic Considerations

This is a relatively common disorder characterized by disorganized bone remodeling resulting in structurally weakened bone, skeletal pain, and deformities. It affects about 3% of the population over 45 years old, chiefly middle-aged individuals, and is distributed equally among males and females. It is rare in individuals less than 40 years of age.

The cause is uncertain; genetic or viral influences may play a role in the pathogenesis. The affected bone is enlarged and in the early stages shows excessive bone resorption leading to decreased bone density and lytic lesions. This lytic phase is followed by excessive bone formation and increased density with creation of a distorted trabecular pattern, the so-called mosaic pattern. Rarely, the disease presents in an osteosclerotic fashion. Paget's lesions may be monostotic or polyostotic and affect the axial more often than the appendicular skeleton, with sites of predilection being the sacrum, spine, femur, tibia, skull, and pelvis.

Clinical Presentation

The presentation is variable and covers a spectrum from an asymptomatic disease to a severely crippling bone disease. The major manifestations are pain, due either to direct bone involvement or to complicating degenerative joint disease adjacent to the involved bone; deformity such as bowing of femur or tibia; fractures, e.g., transverse fractures in the femur or tibia; compressive neurologic manifestations caused by bony enlargement, e.g., optic atrophy, sensorineural hearing loss, and vertigo in petrous pyramid involvement; spinal cord, cauda equina, and nerve root compression in vertebral involvement; basilar impres-

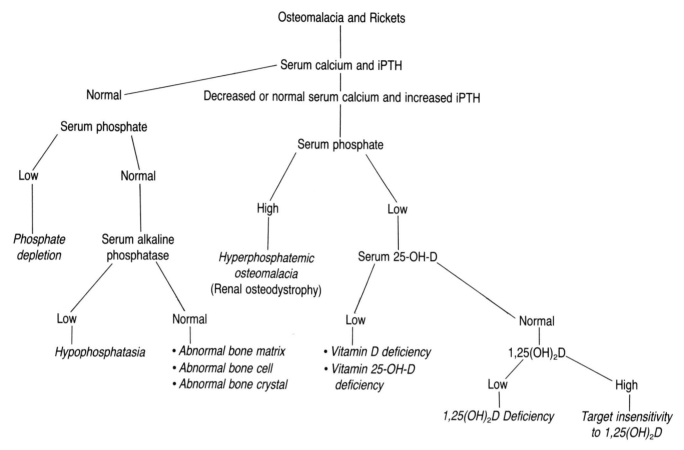

Fig. 11–22. Diagnostic approach to osteomalacia and rickets.

sion and brain stem compression in involvement of the skull; high output cardiac failure in extensive disease caused by increased blood flow through the hypervascular affected bone (usually only in association with some primary cardiac disorder); and malignant transformation of the affected bone, especially the femur and humerus, to osteogenic sarcoma or fibrosarcoma (suspected with a history of increased pain, rapid soft tissue swelling, and rapid increase in alkaline phosphatase). The characteristic signs include deformity and bowing of long bones, enlargement of the skull, erythema and warmth of the overlying skin because of increased blood flow, dorsal kyphosis, and the presence of angioid streaks on fundus examination in 15% of patients with polyostotic disease.

Differential Diagnosis

The major differential diagnosis is osteoblastic metastasis, especially in the pelvis, from prostate carcinoma. An increase in the external dimension of the bone favors Paget's disease. In contrast to pelvic metastasis, in Paget's disease one finds evidence of thickening of pelvic brim and the iliopectineal line (brim sign), and enlargement of the pubic and ischeal bone.

Diagnostic Evaluation

The diagnosis of Paget's disease rests on awareness of a suggestive history and physical findings and the characteristic laboratory and radiologic features. Elevated serum alkaline phosphatase, which reflects increased osteoblastic activity, is the major biochemical abnormality; it correlates well with the extent of active skeletal involvement but may be normal in monostotic disease or late in the disease. Elevated serum acid phosphatase and increased urinary hydroxyproline reflect increased bone resorption. Serum calcium and serum phosphate are usually normal (although hypercalcemia may be present with immobilization after a pathologic fracture or with coexistent primary HPT). The urinary calcium is frequently increased and may play a role in the increased incidence of nephrolithiasis. Serum uric acid is increased because of increased bone cell turnover.

The radiologic features reflect the disorder of bone remodeling. Lytic lesions may appear in the skull (osteoporosis circumscripta), in the long bones (at either end and usually progressing with a sharply defined V shape), or in the vertebrae (picture-frame appearance with central lytic lesion with sclerotic margins); mixed lesions appear in the skull with a honeycomb appearance or as "cotton-wool" lesions, in the long bones as irregular trabeculation and thickened cortex, and in the pelvis as thickening of the iliopectineal line, the so-called brim sign, and enlargement of ischial and pubic bones. Sclerotic lesions may be the dominant lesions, e.g., in the vertebrae or patella. Single or multiple fissure fractures may occur on the convex surface of the involved femur and tibia and may superficially resemble a pseudofracture. CT scanning may be particularly helpful in patients with back pain to define the pagetic, arthritic, and neurologic complications. A bone survey and radioisotopic scanning using bone-seeking radioactive agents, e.g., technetium diphosphonate, outline the extent of the disease. Radioactive scans are more sensitive than the skeletal x-rays in detecting the early stages of Paget's disease; active lesions appear "hot" while inactive lesions are "burnt out."

OSTEOGENESIS IMPERFECTA

This is an inherited generalized disorder of collagen structure of uncertain origin that results in thin bones and increased tendency to fractures. Depending on the age of onset of fractures, this bone disorder presents in two forms: osteogenesis imperfecta congenita, which is present at birth and in which a positive family history is rare, and osteogenesis imperfecta tarda, which appears later in childhood or adulthood and is autosomal dominant in inheritance, and for which a positive family history is common.

Characteristic clinical features include abnormally thin sclera with choroid pigment visible, the so-called blue sclera; hyperextensible joints; paper-thin skin; fractures and deformities; abnormal dental development; and deafness caused by otosclerosis. The serum calcium and serum phosphate are usually normal; increased serum alkaline phosphatase and urinary hydroxyproline may be present. The differential diagnosis is from juvenile osteoporosis: a family history may be helpful in making the correct diagnosis, and bone biopsy is confirmatory.

FIBROUS DYSPLASIA

This rare disease is characterized by fibrous tissue replacement of bone. It can affect any part of the skeleton, in single or multiple sites, especially the femur, proximal tibia, and skull. Onset is usually during childhood and rarely, in young adulthood. It affects both sexes equally. Bone deformities and pathologic fractures occur frequently. Pigmented skin lesions,

café au lait spots, that have irregular borders and end in the midline, are frequently observed. Endocrine and metabolic abnormalities may be associated, usually with the polyostotic type. These abnormalities include isosexual precocity in females, hyperthyroidism, acromegaly and gigantism, glucose intolerance, adrenal hyperplasia, acquired hypophosphatemia, and osteomalacia. The Albright-McCune-Steinberg syndrome consists of polyostotic fibrous dysplasia, pigmented skin lesions, and sexual precocity in girls.

THE SYNDROME OF ADRENOCORTICAL INSUFFICIENCY

DEFINITION

Adrenocortical insufficiency exists when hormonal secretion of the adrenal cortex is inadequate to meet physiologic needs.

Table 11–35. Causes of Adrenocortical Failure

Primary adrenocortical failure
  Glandular disease
    Idiopathic autoimmune
    Granulomatous infection
      Tuberculosis
      Histoplasmosis
      Coccidioidomycosis
      Toxoplasmosis
    Metastatic disease
    Systemic bacterial infections
      Meningococcal
      Staphylococcal
    Infiltrative disorders
      Sarcoidosis
      Amyloidosis
      Hemochromatosis
    Trauma
    Iatrogenic: drugs
      Anticoagulants
      Adrenolytic agents
      Blockers of steroidogenesis
    Adrenoleukodystrophy
  Intrinsic functional derangement
    Congenital adrenal hyperplasia
    Congenital adrenal hypoplasia
    Resistance to ACTH
Secondary adrenocortical failure (see The Syndrome of Hypopituitarism)
  Organic hypothalamic-pituitary disease
  Functional: prior treatment with glucocorticoid
  Peripheral resistance to glucocorticoid effects

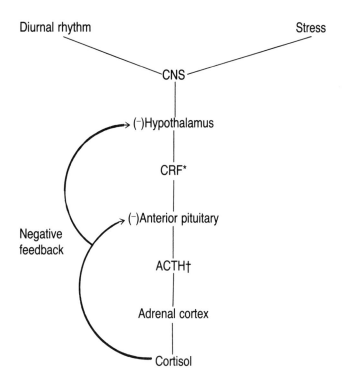

*CRF = Corticotropin-releasing hormone
†ACTH = Corticotropin

Fig. 11–23. The hypothalamic-pituitary-adrenal axis.

PATHOPHYSIOLOGIC CONSIDERATIONS
(Table 11–35)

The adrenal cortex synthesizes and secretes the glu-cocorticoid cortisol primarily by the zona fasciculata, the mineralocorticoid aldosterone by the zona glo-merulosa, and sex steroids, primarily weak androgens, by the zona reticularis.

The secretion of cortisol is regulated by the hypo-thalamic pituitary unit via corticotropin (ACTH). This control includes negative feedback by cortisol, and diurnal rhythm and stress mechanisms integrated by the central nervous system (Fig. 11–23). Aldosterone secretion is regulated primarily by the renin-angioten-sin system through angiotensin II. Other regulators include serum potassium and, to a small extent, ACTH (see Fig. 11–27).

Endocrine failure of the adrenal cortex may be se-lective or global, partial or complete. It may be caused by primary adrenocortical failure, e.g., destruction by autoimmune inflammation or infection, or by second-ary adrenocortical failure caused by absence of normal physiologic stimulation of the adrenal cortex. Second-ary adrenocortical failure includes ACTH lack caused by hypothalamic-pituitary disorders and renin-angio-tensin lack caused by renal disorder. Rarely, endocrine failure of the adrenal cortex is due to peripheral re-sistance to the normally produced steroid.

Primary adrenocortical insufficiency (Addison's dis-ease) is a rare disease. Idiopathic autoimmune inflam-mation is the most frequent cause of spontaneously occurring adrenal insufficiency and in the U.S. ac-counts for greater than 80% of all cases. It may occur as part of a more generalized autoimmune disorder directed against endocrine and related organs. Hash-imoto's thyroiditis is a very frequent association; in addition, associations may include Graves' disease, hypoparathyroidism, primary gonadal failure, diabetes mellitus, pernicious anemia, and chronic active hep-atitis. The association with Hashimoto's thyroiditis is referred to as Schmidt's syndrome.

Less commonly, adrenal destruction may be due to granulomatous diseases including tuberculosis, fungal diseases, and toxoplasmosis, to metastatic disease, to adrenal hemorrhage occurring in the course of menin-gococcemia (Waterhouse-Friderichsen syndrome), or to other disseminated infections, or it may be related to trauma or the use of anticoagulants. Adrenal hem-orrhage is, at this time, probably the second most common cause of adrenal insufficiency in this country. Other rare causes of adrenocortical destruction include infiltrative diseases such as sarcoidosis, amyloidosis, hemochromatosis, and iatrogenic causes that include birth trauma, bilateral adrenalectomy, and the use of adrenolytic drugs, for example, mitotane (O-p′-DDD) and drugs such as aminoglutethimide and metapyrone that block steroid biosynthesis.

Adrenoleukodystrophy is a rare entity that is inher-ited as a sex-linked recessive trait and is characterized by a degenerative process that affects the adrenal cor-tex and the brain and that manifests as variable degrees of adrenal insufficiency, quadriplegia, blindness, de-mentia, and death in childhood.

Congenital adrenal hyperplasia refers to a group of inborn errors of steroid biosynthesis caused by enzy-matic defects that are inherited as autosomal recessive traits. Cortisol secretion is decreased, leading to in-creased ACTH production, steroid precursor build-up, and shunting to unaffected steroidogenic pathways. Insensitivity of glucocorticoid-secreting cells to ACTH is an extremely rare cause of primary adrenocortical insufficiency.

Secondary adrenocortical insufficiency may be due to organic or functional hypothalamic-pituitary dis-orders (see The Syndrome of Hypopituitarism). In or-ganic hypothalamic-pituitary disorders, ACTH lack may occur as an isolated deficiency or as a part of a more generalized anterior pituitary failure. The most common cause of secondary adrenocortical insuffi-ciency is functional ACTH deficiency related to the withdrawal of prolonged supraphysiologic glucocorticoid therapy or the removal of the unilateral cortisol-secreting adrenal tumor. Functional secondary adrenocortical insufficiency may require 6 to 12 months for recovery.

Tissue insensitivity to glucocorticoids is a very rare cause of adrenocortical insufficiency.

Aldosterone deficiency may occur as a part of a general primary adrenocortical failure or as an isolated defect. The major cause of isolated aldosterone deficiency is hyporeninemic hypoaldosteronism. In this condition, decreased renin secretion leads to decreased angiotensin II generation and decreased aldosterone production. It occurs mainly in older patients, especially in those with a mild to moderate degree of renal impairment and with diabetes mellitus. Congenital enzymatic defects in aldosterone biosynthesis are a rare cause of hypoaldosteronism and may be due to congenital deficiencies in the late enzymatic steps of aldosterone biosynthesis or more commonly to the usual causes of congenital adrenal hyperplasia. Transient aldosterone deficiency occurs following removal of an aldosterone-producing tumor. Pseudohypoaldosteronism is a rare congenital insensitivity of the distal tubule to aldosterone. Very rarely, aldosterone deficiency may occur as a result of marked potassium depletion or heparin administration.

CLINICAL PRESENTATION

Clinical features are determined by the nature of hormone deficiencies (cortisol, aldosterone, or sex steroids), the type of hormones that may be secreted in excess (ACTH in primary adrenocortical failure, or increased androgens in congenital adrenal hyperplasia), the rapidity of onset and the course of the disease, and the cause of the adrenocortical insufficiency and its associations.

Signs

The patient usually looks acutely or chronically ill, may be apathetic, lethargic, or confused, and shows evidence of weight loss. Pigmentation is usually the sign that evokes clinical suspicion of Addison's disease. It is present over the entire body, including covered areas, especially the creases of the hands and the axillae, but it is more prominent in the exposed areas, and over extensor surfaces (e.g., elbows, knees, and knuckles) and is particularly likely to affect areas of recurrent minor trauma. The pigmentation affects mucous membranes, especially the buccal mucous membrane along the line where the upper and lower teeth come together, and can also affect rectal and vaginal mucosa. The scars, which are incurred at the time

adrenoinsufficiency is present, are pigmented, and small black freckles may appear, especially over the forehead, face, and neck. Areas of vitiligo may be seen in patients with autoimmune adrenal failure. Hypotension with orthostatism is frequent, as are other signs of dehydration. Muscle weakness is prominent, and the deep tendon reflexes are depressed or absent. The signs of coexistent autoimmune endocrinopathy or pituitary disease may be present. Rarely, calcification of auricular cartilages may be found.

Symptoms

In the usual case, symptoms develop insidiously over several weeks to years, and the course varies in duration and severity, depending on the extent of the destructive process. Common symptoms include decreased strength and stamina, easy fatigability, diffuse musculoskeletal aches, anorexia with altered taste perception and salt craving, nausea, vomiting or occasional diarrhea, and weight loss.

Mental changes are common and include irritability, restlessness, drowsiness, depression, and occasional psychosis. Hyperpigmentation described as "a summer tan that never fades" and the appearance of black freckles are frequent complaints in primary adrenocortical insufficiency. Other frequently encountered complaints include postural dizziness and faintness, changes in hair texture, decreased body hair and menstrual irregularities in females, decreased libido, impotency in males, symptoms of fasting hypoglycemia, and hyponatremia, especially in children. In addition, there may be manifestations of other associated autoimmune endocrinopathy, manifestations of pituitary dysfunction, or manifestations of the cause of the disease. It is important to remember that affected patients may experience minimal symptoms unless exposed to a stressful event; these patients tolerate stress, infections, or surgery very poorly and may develop marked prostration, nausea, vomiting, volume depletion, and dehydration that may progress rapidly into life threatening adrenocortical crisis.

DIFFERENTIAL DIAGNOSIS

Adrenocortical failure is a rare disorder, but frequently must be considered in the differential diagnosis of more common disorders such as anorexia nervosa, general debility associated with chronic infections and malabsorption, pigmentary disorders such as hemochromatosis and uremia, and fasting hypoglycemia. The most common pitfalls are to not consider adrenocortical failure or to attribute its manifestations to other causes. Prudence dictates that the physician keep a high index of suspicion of this potentially life threatening disease and proceed with a screening cosyntropin test when indicated.

DIAGNOSTIC EVALUATION

The goals of the diagnostic approach are to document the presence of adrenocortical insufficiency, to document whether it is due to primary adrenocortical or secondary hypothalamic-pituitary disease, and to delineate its cause.

Patient History and Physical Examination

In the clinical approach, attention should be paid to the onset, duration, and course of symptoms and to the patient's response to stress. History of tuberculosis, other granulomatous disease, infiltrative disease, primary extra-adrenal tumor with suspected metastatic disease, and autoimmune endocrinopathy is important. Drug history, including prior glucocorticoid or ACTH therapy and the use of mitotane, aminoglutethimide, metopyrone, or anticoagulants, prior Cushing's disease with transsphenoidal surgery, and history of hypothalamic-pituitary disease are important factors for consideration. A family history is important as it relates to congenital adrenal hyperplasia or autoimmune polyendocrinopathy.

Diagnostic Studies

GENERAL

General routine laboratory studies may show a normochromic, normocytic anemia with neutropenia, eosinophilia, and a relative lymphocytosis. The anemia can be masked by the dehydration and hemoconcentration. The presence of macrocytic anemia should raise the suspicion of associated pernicious anemia. Chest x-ray may reveal a small heart. Adrenal calcification from granulomatous disease may be apparent on plain abdominal x-ray. The electrocardiogram may show low-voltage, nonspecific ST-T wave changes related to electrolyte abnormalities.

SPECIFIC (Table 11–36)

Plasma Cortisol. Cortisol circulates in the plasma in two forms; 98% is bound to cortisol-binding globulin, and 2% is free. Plasma cortisol measures both the bound and the free. The levels of plasma cortisol can be affected by circadian rhythm, episodic secretion, stress, and factors that affect cortisol-binding globulin. In adrenocortical insufficiency, plasma cortisol values are usually low. Low values, however, are of limited value in diagnoses unless they occur in the setting of an acute illness or are consistently very low on repeated testing. Normal values of plasma cortisol

do not exclude the diagnosis of partial adrenocortical failure. An elevated plasma cortisol value, a value greater than 20 mg/dl, is strong presumptive evidence against the diagnosis. In most circumstances, however, it is necessary to demonstrate that plasma cortisol is not responsive to stimulation with appropriate stimuli (see below).

Urinary Cortisol Metabolites. Urinary 17-hydroxycorticosteroids (17-OHCS) and 17-ketogenic steroids (17-KGS) measure steroid metabolites, predominantly those of cortisol and 11-deoxycortisol. A 24-hour urine collection for these cortisol metabolites provides an integrated assessment of cortisol production and excretion. These assays are subject to interference by commonly used drugs, however, and are altered in many extra-adrenal disease states; therefore, they are not recommended in the assessment of adrenocortical insufficiency. These cortisol metabolites may be increased in congenital adrenal hyperplasia despite the presence of cortisol lack because of increased production of cortisol precursors that can be measured by these assays.

Urinary Free Cortisol (UFC). This represents less than 1% of the total adrenal cortisol secretion, which is filtered by the glomeruli and excreted in an unaltered and unconjugated form. The current clinical assays are insensitive in the lower range and are not useful in the assessment of adrenocortical insufficiency.

Serum ACTH. ACTH is usually secreted episodically, and normal persons may have undetectable values. Low basal values, therefore, do not differentiate the normal individual from one with secondary adrenocortical failure. Once the diagnosis of adrenocortical failure is made, however, basal serum ACTH is very helpful in the differential diagnosis between primary and secondary adrenocortical failure. In primary adrenocortical failure, low cortisol levels lead to a compensatory increase in ACTH production, and the serum ACTH levels are generally greater than 250 pg/ml. In secondary adrenocortical failure related to hypothalamic-pituitary disease, there is ACTH deficiency, and serum ACTH is usually less than 50 pg/ml and inappropriately low for the corresponding plasma cortisol level.

Stimulation Tests. These tests assess the reserve capacity of the hypothalamic-pituitary-adrenal axis and its ability to respond appropriately to stressful situations. Various stimulation tests that act at different sites of the axis can be used to assess its different functions.

ACTH Stimulation Test. Exogenous ACTH administration allows the direct assessment of adrenocortical glucocorticoid reserve. In the normal individual the hypothalamic-pituitary-adrenal axis is intact and the adrenal cortex is primed by endogenous ACTH secre-

Table 11–36. Laboratory Tests in Disorders of Cortisol Secretion

Test	Measurement	Cushing's Syndrome	Adrenocortical Failure
Serum Cortisol Normal: A.M. 7–25 mg/dl P.M. 2–14 mg/dl	Radioimmunoassay (competitive protein-binding assays and fluorometric assays are also available) Serum cortisol measures total plasma cortisol (bound, 98%, and biologically active/free, 2%) Pitfalls include normal variation due to circadian rhythm, episodic secretion, and stress; cross-reactivity with other steroids; and interference with drugs that fluoresce in the fluorometric assay.	Elevated in 70–80% of patients. There is usually loss of diurnal variation. False negatives: 20–30% Can be elevated in non-Cushing's states: acute illness, trauma or surgery, starvation, anorexia nervosa, depression, alcoholism, state of increased cortisol-binding globulin (estrogen, pregnancy, hyperthyroidism, familial, and certain hematologic disorders).	Usually low, but can be normal in partial failure. "Normal" values during acute illness (inappropriately low for the stress). Low values can also be seen in eucortisol individuals with decreased cortisol-binding globulin (congenital, hypothyroidism, liver disease, nephrotic syndrome, and multiple myeloma).
Serum ACTH Normal: Equal or less than 120 pg/dl	Radioimmunoassay Pitfalls 1. Proper collection in heparinized plastic tubes on ice, centrifuged in cold within 1 hour of collection; plasma must be frozen until assayed. 2. Normal variation with circadian rhythm, episodic secretion, and responsiveness to stress.	Levels can be normal, suppressed, or increased. In hypercortisolism, suppressed levels of ACTH are diagnostic of adrenal tumor; normal to moderately elevated levels point to Cushing's disease (40 to 200 pg/ml). Markedly elevated levels point to ectopic ACTH syndrome (100 to greater than 1000 pg/ml); overlap exists between levels in Cushing's disease and those in ectopic ACTH.	Levels can be suppressed, normal, or high. Low serum ACTH levels can be found in the normal (due to assay sensitivity) or in ACTH deficiency. In the presence of subnormal responsiveness to exogenous ACTH (cosyntropin test), levels of serum ACTH greater than 250 pg/ml are diagnostic of primary adrenocortical failure; while levels less than 50 pg/ml are diagnostic of secondary adrenocortical failure.
Urinary 17-hydroxysteroids (17-OHCS) or 17-ketogenic steroids (17-KGS) Normal for 17-OHCS 3 to 10 mg/24 hours or 2.0–6.5 mg/g creatinine Normal for 17-KGS is 4–14 ng/24 hours for males and 2.0–12.0 mg/24 hours for females	17-OHCS are measured by Porter-Silber reaction, and 17-KGS, by oxidation and Zimmerman reaction. Used as index of 24-hour cortisol production. Pitfalls 1. Measure cortisol, steroidogenic precursors, and their metabolites. 2. Need complete 24-hour urinary collection (check urinary creatinine). 3. Susceptible to drug interference, e.g., spironolactone, phenothiazines, etc. 4. Depend on liver function (production) and renal function (excretion).	Elevated in 70% of cases with false negative of 30%. Can also be increased in non-Cushingoid states: obesity, thyrotoxicosis, congenital adrenal hyperplasia of 11- and 21-hydroxylase types, inaccurate collection (greater than 24 hours), and drug interference.	Usually low, but can be normal or high in hypocortisol states caused by congenital adrenal hyperplasia (because of increased cortisol precursors and their metabolites). Can also be low in nonadrenocortical insufficient patients due to incomplete collection, starvation, renal failure, liver disease, pregnancy, hypothyroidism, and drugs that induce hepatic microsomal enzymes, e.g., phenytoin, phenobarbital, primidone, and OPDDD.
Urinary Free Cortisol Normal 0 to 110 μg/24 hours	Radioimmunoassay Measures cortisol filtered and excreted unchanged in the urine—represents 1% of total cortisol daily production. Pitfalls 1. Completeness of the urine collection (check urinary creatinine). 2. Cross-reaction with other steroids. 3. Renal function.	Elevated in greater than 97% of cases with false negatives less than 3%. Can also be increased in noncushingoid states: acute illness, trauma, surgery, alcoholism, and depression.	Low or undetectable, but can be "normal" in partial adrenocortical failure. Assay sensitivity cannot differentiate between low-normal and low values, therefore, has low utility in the diagnosis of adrenocortical failure.

Table 11–36.   Laboratory Tests in Disorders of Cortisol Secretion (Continued)

Test	Measurement	Cushing's Syndrome	Adrenocortical Failure
Overnight Dexamethasone Suppression Test	1.0 mg of dexamethasone is given PO at 11 P.M. Plasma cortisol is measured at 8 A.M. on the following morning. The normal response is plasma cortisol level of less than 5 μg/dl.	A reliable screening test. Patients with Cushing's syndrome have values greater than 10 μg/dl. False negatives are less than 2% but false positives can occur in 1% of outpatient controls, 13% of obese patients, and 25% of hospitalized, chronically sick patients, and in acute illness, anxiety, depression, alcoholism, estrogen, pregnancy, and drugs that accelerate dexamethasone metabolism (e.g., phenytoin and barbiturates).	
Standard Low-dose Dexamethasone Suppression Test	Baseline plasma cortisol and 24-hour urinary cortisol and 17-hydroxysteroids or 17-ketogenic steroids are obtained. Dexamethasone is given PO 0.5 mg every 6 hours for 2 days. Plasma cortisol and 24-hour urinary steroids are measured on day two. The normal response is a plasma cortisol less than 5 μg/dl, 17-OHCS decreased to less than 4 mg/24 hours, and urinary free cortisol decreased to less than 25 μg/24 hours.	This is the standard test for the diagnosis of Cushing's syndrome. Failure of suppression is seen in greater than 95% of patients with a false negative of 5% due to either delayed dexamethasone clearance or periodic hormonogenesis. False positives in control subjects—3% may also be seen with acute and chronic illness, depression, alcoholism, and drugs that interfere with dexamethasone metabolism, e.g., anticonvulsants. It cannot differentiate between the different causes of Cushing's syndrome.	
High-dose Dexamethasone Suppression Test	Baseline plasma cortisol and 24-hour urinary 17-OHCS or 17-KGS and urinary free cortisol. Dexamethasone is given PO 2.0 mg every 6 hours for 48 hours. Plasma cortisol and 24-hour urine collection for steroids are obtained during the second day.	Useful in differentiating Cushing's disease from other causes of Cushing's syndrome. Cortisol production can be suppressed by high-dose dexamethasone in Cushing's disease but not in other causes of the syndrome. Suppression is to below 50% of the baseline levels. *Pitfalls* 1. Failure to suppress in 15 to 30% of patients with Cushing's disease 2. Suppression may occur in some patients with ectopic ACTH tumors, especially bronchial carcinoid.	
Rapid ACTH Stimulation Test (Cosyntropin)	Can be performed on an outpatient basis any time of the day. Synthetic ACTH (cosyntropin) is given in the dose of 250 μg IM or IV. Samples for plasma cortisol (± aldosterone) are obtained before and at 30 and 60 minutes following the injection. The normal response is a plasma cortisol increment greater than 7 μg/dl with peak cortisol levels greater than 18 μg/dl; plasma aldosterone increment greater than 4 ng/dl.		Subnormal cortisol responses establish the diagnosis of adrenocortical failure but cannot differentiate between primary and secondary failure. A normal cortisol response excludes primary adrenocortical failure but can be seen in partial secondary (ACTH) deficient failure. In an adrenocortical deficient patient, subnormal aldosterone responsiveness points to primary adrenocortical failure, whereas a normal aldosterone response points to secondary adrenocortical failure.

Table 11–36. Laboratory Tests in Disorders of Cortisol Secretion *(Continued)*

Test	Measurement	Cushing's Syndrome	Adrenocortical Failure
3-Day ACTH Stimulation Tests	A baseline 24-hour urine for 17-OHCS or 17-KGS, plasma cortisol is obtained. Synthetic ACTH 250 μg or bovine ACTH 40 units are administered IV in 500-ml saline over 8 hours for 3 consecutive days (alternatively, long-acting ACTH gel, 40 units intramuscularly b.i.d. for 3 days). A 24-hour urine for steroids and plasma cortisol is obtained daily. In suspected adrenocortical failure, patients can be simultaneously treated with dexamethasone 0.5 b.i.d.		Useful in the differential diagnosis of primary versus secondary adrenocortical failure. In primary failure, 17-OHCS and plasma cortisol fail to rise even with repeated stimulation. In secondary adrenocortical failure, ACTH stimulates the atrophic adrenals, and a step-wise increase in 17-OHCS values and plasma cortisol to three times the basal level is obtained on the third day.
Standard Metapyrone Test	See Table 11–3	Enhanced responses in Cushing's disease; impaired responses in patients with adrenal tumor or ectopic ACTH. Enhanced responses, however, may be seen in some patients with ectopic ACTH-producing bronchial carcinoids. Generally the test is safe, but it may cause adrenocortical insufficiency during the test in patients with adrenal tumors.	A normal response excludes adrenocortical failure. A subnormal response indicates primary or secondary adrenocortical failure but does not differentiate between them. Since the test can exacerbate adrenocortical insufficiency, it should be done during hospitalization and under careful supervision.
Overnight Metapyrone Test	For procedure see Table 11–3	See under Standard Metapyrone Test	See under Standard Metapyrone Test. Generally safe, can be conducted as an outpatient test.
Insulin Tolerance Test	See Table 11–3	Cortisol responsiveness is suppressed in all patients with Cushing's syndrome. In contrast, patients with depression maintain normal cortisol responsiveness (see text).	A normal response indicates intact hypothalamic pituitary adrenal axis and excludes adrenocortical insufficiency. An impaired response indicates adrenocortical failure but does not identify whether it is primary or secondary failure.

tion and, therefore, is responsive to exogenous ACTH. In adrenocortical failure, the adrenal cortex is damaged by disease (primary adrenocortical failure) or is atrophic because of lack of endogenous ACTH (secondary adrenocortical failure) and, therefore, cannot respond to exogenous ACTH. There are many protocols for the administration of ACTH.

THE SHORT ACTH TEST (COSYNTROPIN OR CORTROSYN). Synthetic ACTH (1 to 24–ACTH) has full biologic potency. When the adrenal function is intact, a rise in plasma cortisol occurs by at least 7 μg/dl or to a level of at least 18 μg/dl. Failure of such response establishes the diagnosis of adrenocortical insufficiency but does not differentiate between its primary and secondary causes. A normal response excludes primary adrenocortical failure but does not exclude partial secondary adrenocortical failure of recent duration.

The cosyntropin test can also be used to measure plasma aldosterone response, and this modification can be used in the differential diagnosis between primary and secondary adrenocortical insufficiency. In primary adrenocortical insufficiency, all zones of the adrenal cortex are destroyed and the cortisol and aldosterone responses to cosyntropin are impaired. In secondary adrenocortical insufficiency, however, the renin-angiotensin-aldosterone system is intact: the cortisol responses to cosyntropin are impaired but the aldosterone responses are normal and rise by greater than 4 ng/dl.

PROLONGED ACTH TEST. Prolonged ACTH stimulation can be done in various ways (Table 11–36). In normal individuals, the response is maximal on the first day of ACTH administration. In patients with primary adrenocortical failure, the adrenal cortex is destroyed and will not increase its steroid output no matter how much and for how long ACTH is given. In patients with secondary adrenocortical failure, there is ACTH deficiency and the adrenal cortex is atrophic. On the first day of ACTH administration there may be little or no response, but by continued daily administration there is a stepwise increase in responsiveness. By the third to the fifth day there is at least doubling of steroid output with serum cortisol of 15 to 40 μg/dl by day 3 and 30 to 60 μg/dl by day 5, and 17-hydroxy steroids of 15 to 40 mg/24 hours on day 3, and 30 to 40 mg/24 hours on day 5.

The major use of the prolonged ACTH test is in the differential diagnosis of primary versus secondary adrenocortical failure. It should be done only after the diagnosis of adrenocortical failure has been made. These tests are rarely used now because of the availability of serum ACTH and aldosterone measurements. The exogenous ACTH tests have rarely been associated with anaphylactic reactions to ACTH.

Metapyrone Test. In the normal, metapyrone blocks 11-hydroxylase in the adrenocortical steroidogenic pathway and decreases cortisol production. There is a compensatory increase in ACTH, increased steroidogenesis, and increased production of the cortisol precursor, 11-deoxycortisol (compound S). This precursor can be measured in plasma and in urine by radioimmunoassay, or its metabolites can be measured as 17-hydroxycorticoids or 17-ketogenic steroids. An increased production of compound S in response to a metapyrone block depends on the presence of a normal hypothalamic-pituitary-adrenal axis. Impaired activity at any level of the axis results in subnormal response.

The overnight metapyrone test is simple, sensitive, and safe and is not usually associated with precipitation of adrenocortical crisis. In the normal, the plasma compound S in the basal state is 0.3 to 1.0 μg/dl; after administration of metapyrone it should exceed 7 μg/dl. If the compound S response is inadequate, the finding of a plasma cortisol level in the same sample in excess of 10 μg/dl indicates inadequate block by metapyrone caused by vomiting or malabsorption of the ingested drug, accelerated metabolism, or failure of the patient to take the medication in the required dosage at the proper time. Cortisol less than 10 μg/dl indicates that an adequate block has been achieved, and failure of compound S to rise indicates hypothalamic-pituitary-adrenal impairment.

The standard metapyrone test (Table 11–36) is indicated if facilities for measurements of the serum 11-deoxycortisol are not available. Patients with normal hypothalamic-pituitary-adrenal responsiveness will show at least doubling of 17-hydroxycorticoids in the urine on the day after the metapyrone. This method of metapyrone administration may induce adrenocortical crisis in patients with adrenocortical insufficiency and must be done in a hospital setting under medical supervision.

Because the reduction of plasma cortisol by metapyrone is critical for ACTH stimulation, administration of glucocorticoid to "cover the patient" will suppress the ACTH response and negate the validity of the test.

Insulin in Hypoglycemia Test. The stress of hypoglycemia leads to stimulation of the hypothalamic-pituitary-adrenal axis and to a rise in plasma cortisol.

A normal response to an insulin hypoglycemic challenge is a plasma cortisol rise of at least 10 μg/dl or to a level over 20 μg/dl. This is the most sensitive of all currently available tests for assessing hypothalamic-pituitary-adrenal function. An impaired response indicates impairment of the hypothalamic-pituitary-adrenal axis but cannot distinguish the level of the impairment.

Diagnostic Approach

The first step in the diagnostic process is the performance of a cosyntropin test. An impaired response indicates adrenocortical failure but does not distinguish between primary or secondary causes of this failure. This differentiation is made by serum ACTH, which will be found to be high in primary adrenocortical failure and inappropriately low in secondary adrenocortical failure. If the serum ACTH assays are not available, a prolonged ACTH stimulation test is done. Absence of response to prolonged ACTH stimulation documents primary adrenocortical failure. A stepwise increase and ultimately normalized response point to a secondary adrenocortical failure.

A normal response to cosyntropin stimulation tests excludes primary adrenocortical failure but does not exclude partial or recent secondary adrenocortical failure. The physician then proceeds with either a metapyrone or an insulin-provocative test as described above. A normal response to metapyrone or to insulin hypoglycemia challenge indicates a normal hypothalamic-pituitary-adrenal axis and excludes adrenocortical failure. An impaired response in a patient who has responded to cosyntropin indicates secondary adrenocortical failure.

If the patient has primary adrenocortical failure, the history, physical examination, and standard radiologic and laboratory tests will point to its cause. If an autoimmune adrenocortical failure is suspected, evaluation of the other endocrine glands for associated autoimmune endocrinopathy is in order. First- and second-degree relatives optimally should be screened for endocrine deficiency syndromes. In secondary adrenocortical failure, the other pituitary functions need to be assessed, and a CT scan of the pituitary area and visual field examination are in order.

The diagnostic approach to adrenocortical failure is outlined in Figure 11–24.

SPECIAL CONSIDERATIONS

Secondary adrenocortical insufficiency differs from primary adrenocortical failure in that ACTH and related peptides are deficient, leading to lightening of pigmentation (rather than hyperpigmentation) and inability to tan. The renin-angiotensin-aldosterone system is usually intact. Although aldosterone responsiveness may be somewhat blunted in chronic hypopituitarism, absolute mineralocorticoid lack does not occur. Patients with secondary adrenocortical failure do not usually show significant signs of volume depletion, significant hypotension and dehydration do not

occur, and the heart is not small on chest x-ray. Because of cortisol lack these patients may exhibit postural hypotension and hyponatremia. Other aspects of hypothalamic-pituitary disease are present with other pituitary dysfunction, and there may be evidence of a space-occupying lesion in or around the pituitary area.

Selected ACTH suppression from exogenous glucocorticoid therapy represents the most frequently encountered form of adrenocortical insufficiency. Pharmacologic doses of glucocorticoid over several weeks to months may suppress the hypothalamic-pituitary axis for up to 1 year after the discontinuation of therapy. This suppression depends on a number of variables, including the type of glucocorticoid given and its potency, duration of action, and route of administration. Clinically, the diagnosis is suggested by the history of glucocorticoid administration and by the paradoxic combination of Cushingoid manifestations and features of adrenocortical insufficiency. The other pituitary hormones are intact.

Adrenal crisis is a life threatening emergency that can result from an inadequate supply of glucocorticoid

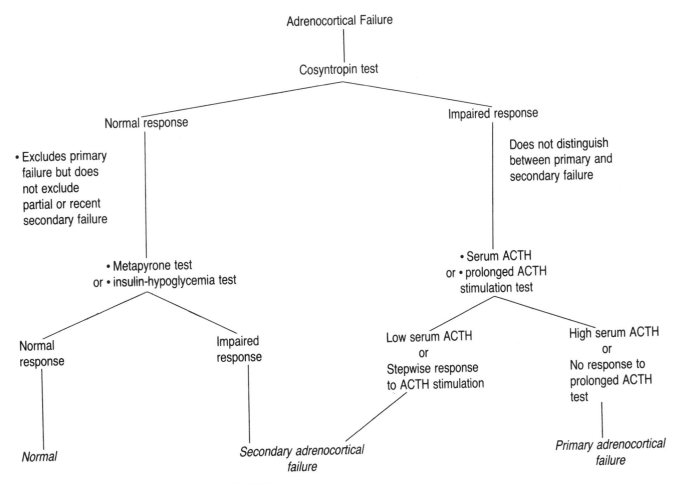

Fig. 11–24. Diagnstic approach to adrenocortical failure.

plus or minus mineralocorticoid. Typically it occurs during infections (viral or bacterial) and may be precipitated by surgery or other stresses. It can occur in any setting of adrenocortical failure, but the most common presentation is in the patient who is on glucocorticoid therapy for physiologic replacement or pharmacologic treatment and in whom glucocorticoid is either omitted or not increased appropriately to meet body needs during intercurrent illness. The clinical features are those of decreased steroid effects and those of the precipitating cause, e.g., pneumonia. The predominant feature is hypotension, and sudden unexpected shock may be the initial presentation. Early on, the patient will exhibit tachycardia, orthostatism, profound dehydration from vomiting and diarrhea, abdominal pain, muscle weakness and fatigue, and fever. With progressive disease, the patient may have impaired consciousness, cardiac arrhythmia, and rapidly progressive disease ending in death. Hyperkalemia, hyponatremia, increased blood urea nitrogen and creatinine, hypoglycemia, and hypercalcemia should all raise the suspicion of adrenocortical insufficiency. A small cardiac silhouette on the chest x-ray and tall, big T waves may be seen on the electrocardiogram.

The most important step in the diagnosis is to suspect the disease in the appropriate setting. Investigation and therapy should be undertaken simultaneously. A blood sample is obtained for serum cortisol and serum ACTH, and normal saline and 5% dextrose in water are started with 1 L given intravenously in 1 hour, 1 L in 2 hours, and 2 to 4 L in the subsequent 21 hours. A synthetic glucocorticoid that will not influence plasma cortisol or urinary metabolites is given. Dexamethasone is preferred, in the dose of 4 mg IV and then 4 mg IM every 6 to 8 hours. A cosyntropin stimulation test followed by prolonged ACTH test is then performed. An important step in the diagnosis is to search for and correct precipitating factors, e.g., infection. It is important to remember that plasma cortisol may turn out to be low or in the low-normal range, i.e., less than 12 μg/dl. This value is inappropriately low in the setting of an acute illness and points to adrenocortical insufficiency, since in acute stressful illness in the normal patient, plasma cortisol is nearly always greater than 25 μg/dl.

CUSHING'S SYNDROME

DEFINITION

Cushing's syndrome refers to the clinical picture that results from prolonged exposure of the tissues to excess glucocorticoids.

Table 11–37. Causes of Cushing's Syndrome

Exogenous (most common)
  Glucocorticoid therapy
  ACTH therapy (rare)
Endogenous
  Bilateral adrenal hyperplasia
    ACTH dependent
      Pituitary-corticotrophic tumor or hyperplasia (70%)
        Primary
        Secondary to excess CRH
      Ectopic ACTH-producing tumor (20%)
    Non-ACTH dependent
      Bilateral nodular adrenal hyperplasia (rare)
  Adrenal tumors (10%)
    Adenoma
    Carcinoma

PATHOPHYSIOLOGIC CONSIDERATIONS

Cortisol is the principal glucocorticoid produced by the adrenal cortex. Its secretion is stimulated by corticotropin (ACTH) from the anterior pituitary, which in turn is stimulated by secretion of corticotropin-releasing hormone (CRH) by the endocrine hypothalamus. Normal production of cortisol is controlled by negative feedback of cortisol on the hypothalamic-pituitary axis, diurnal rhythm with peak ACTH and cortisol secretion in early morning and nadir in the late evening, and stress, which stimulates the axis and results in increased cortisol production. When present, stress overrides the negative feedback and diurnal rhythm influences (Fig. 11–23).

Table 11–37 outlines the various causes of Cushing's syndrome. These include exogenous administration of cortisol or a glucocorticoid analogue or, rarely, of ACTH; and endogenous cortisol overproduction. Overproduction results from autonomous adrenal tumor (adenoma or carcinoma) or nodular hyperplasia; from excess ACTH production caused by hypothalamic-pituitary disease (most commonly a pituitary tumor) and ectopic tumor; and, rarely, from overproduction of corticotropin-releasing hormone (CRH) from hypothalamic disease or an ectopic neoplastic process.

Cushing's disease (70%) is caused by pituitary ACTH secretion resulting from a pituitary tumor or hyperplasia. The majority of the patients have a pituitary microadenoma. Pituitary ACTH hypersecretion leads to bilateral adrenal hyperplasia and enlargement. Adrenal tumors, which account for 10% of causes of Cushing's syndrome, may be adrenal adenoma, which is usually a unilateral small benign tumor, or adrenal carcinoma, which is a unilateral but considerably larger malignant tumor often with signs of local spread or distant metastasis to the liver or lungs. In any cortisol-producing adrenal tumor, the remaining normal cortisol-secreting tissue in the same gland and the contralateral gland is atrophic because of suppression of the hypothalamic-pituitary axis by the hypercortisol state.

Bilateral nodular adrenal hyperplasia is rare, of unknown cause, and is characterized by bilaterally hyperplastic glands with multiple nodules. Ectopic ACTH-producing tumor (20%) results from ACTH production by a bronchial carcinoid (50%), bronchial adenocarcinoma (8 to 10%), thymic tumor (10%), pancreatic tumor (10%), and other tumors (20%). The excess ACTH leads to bilateral adrenal hyperplasia, cortisol overproduction, and suppression of the hypothalamic-pituitary-ACTH axis.

CLINICAL PRESENTATION

The clinical features in Cushing's syndrome are due to the effects of an excess of glucocorticoid hormone; excess of other hormones produced by the pathophysiologic process, e.g., adrenal androgen, mineralocorticoids, or ACTH; and the causative tumor.

Signs

Obesity is seen in the great majority of patients. It is classically central and manifested by a moon face, thick neck with supraclavicular fat pads and buffalo hump, and trunkal obesity with relative sparing of the extremities. Generalized obesity is seen with equal frequency. A minority of patients are not obese but still have central distribution of fat and typical facial appearance. An examination of previous photos and a look at the records of height and weight in childhood are important to document onset and progression of the disease. The skin is thin and plethoric and has characteristic striae that are typically red to purple, depressed below the skin surface, wide, and most commonly abdominal but also present along the breasts, axillae, hips, buttocks, and thighs.

Mucocutaneous fungal infections can be seen. Hyperpigmentation almost always points to an extra-adrenal tumor and occurs especially in ectopic ACTH syndrome. Mild hyperandrogenicity with hirsutism and acne are common in females, but other evidences of virilization are unusual except in adrenocortical carcinoma. Muscle weakness, especially of the proximal muscles, is common. Hypertension is noted in 75 to 85% of patients. Peripheral edema is not frequent and points to ectopic ACTH syndrome. Gynecomastia is unusual and points to an estrogen-secreting adrenocortical carcinoma. A decrease in height and kyphosis may be noted as sequelae of osteoporosis. Patients who have iatrogenic Cushing's syndrome tend to have characteristic additional physical findings that include sub-capsular cataracts, glaucoma, papilledema, benign intracranial hypertension, and avascular necrosis of bone not seen in patients with endogenous Cushing's syndrome.

One can also see signs of the underlying cause, e.g., an abdominal mass in adrenocortical carcinoma, or visual defect and evidence of hypopituitarism in patients with Cushing's disease.

Symptoms

Weight gain and obesity are the most common presenting symptoms (in greater than 90% of patients). The patient may also complain of easy bruising and poor healing of minor abrasions or surgical incisions. Mucocutaneous fungal infections are frequent, including tinea versicolor, candidiasis, and onychophytosis. Of affected females, 65 to 70% complain of mild to moderate hirsutism, acne, or seborrhea. Gonadal dysfunction is very common and manifests itself as amenorrhea and infertility in the majority of affected young females and as decreased libido and potency in affected males.

Of the patients, 75% also have psychiatric problems, which in the majority of patients are mild and consist of increased irritability, emotional lability, depression, disordered sleep, insomnia, and decreased memory. A minority of patients have severe depression, paranoia, psychosis, and suicidal tendency.

More than one half of the patients complain of muscle weakness, especially proximal, manifested by difficulty in climbing stairs or arising from a deep chair. Back pain related to osteoporosis or pathologic fractures is the initial complaint in about 40% of patients. Infrequently the presenting symptoms may be those of renal colic or diabetes or its sequelae. Growth failure is the most common presenting feature in affected children, the shortness of stature being due to decreased growth hormone secretion, decreased somatomedin C generation, and the catabolic effect of increased cortisol. Associated symptoms related to the cause can include abdominal pain, manifestations of hypopituitarism and a sellar mass, or manifestations of the ectopic ACTH-producing tumor. Hyperpigmentation related to increased ACTH production may be noticed.

DIFFERENTIAL DIAGNOSES AND PITFALLS

In simple obesity, the distribution of fat is usually generalized but may be centripetal, and the muscular mass is preserved. Although 17-OHCS or 17-KGS may be mildly elevated and 10 to 15% of patients may have an abnormal overnight dexamethasone suppression test, the plasma cortisol (PC) and urinary free cortisol (UFC) values are normal, and the standard low-dose dexamethasone suppression test shows normal suppressibility.

Some alcoholic patients have clinical and biochemical features of Cushing's syndrome (the so-called alcohol-induced pseudo-Cushing's syndrome). They have increased cortisol production, increased 24-hour urinary free cortisol, and are non-low-dose dexamethasone suppressible. These abnormalities always revert to normal following abstention from alcohol. Alcohol-induced pseudo-Cushing's should be considered in every patient with suspected Cushing's syndrome. If a history of alcohol abuse is present, the alcohol is discontinued, and the steroid tests are repeated in a few weeks to a few months.

Frequently depressed patients are found to have biochemical parameters of hypercortisolism. The cortisol production is increased, the plasma cortisol and 24-hour urinary free cortisol levels are increased, and the patients are not dexamethasone suppressible. However, these patients do not have typical cushingoid manifestations and they maintain normal cortisol responses to an insulin provocative test. (Patients with true Cushing's syndrome have blunted cortisol response to hypoglycemia.) The hypercortisol state reverts to normal upon the patients' recovery from depression.

Patients with acute or chronic illness, especially in a hospital setting, can have increased cortisol secretion and can be nondexamethasone suppressible. Steroid evaluation should be repeated when the illness is resolved.

Estrogens, oral contraceptives, pregnancy, and other causes of increased cortisol-binding globulin may be associated with increased PC, and the overnight dexamethasone suppression may be abnormal. UFC and response to a standard low-dose dexamethasone suppression test, however, are normal.

Few patients with Cushing's syndrome may have normal dexamethasone suppressibility caused by delayed dexamethasone clearance resulting in higher plasma dexamethasone levels (in these patients the urinary free cortisol is increased and helps in the differential diagnosis); or, by periodic or episodic hormonogenesis in patients who may have a pituitary tumor, an ectopic ACTH-producing tumor, or an adrenal tumor. In this state, the cortisol hypersecretion may be cyclic or periodic, lasting for a few weeks to a few months. Between the cycles of activity, cortisol secretion may be normal, and patients may have normal dexamethasone suppression. A repeated evaluation in weeks to months is required to establish the diagnosis.

Of patients with Cushing's disease, 30% may not be high-dose (8-mg) dexamethasone suppressible and may need larger doses of dexamethasone, from 16 to 64 mg/day, to show suppressibility. However, these patients are metapyrone responsive.

Patients with Cushing's syndrome should be differentiated from patients with diabetes mellitus, hypertension and hypokalemia, hyperandrogenicity (for example, polycystic ovarian syndrome), myopathy, nephrolithiasis, or osteoporosis. In all these states, the steroid data are normal.

DIAGNOSTIC EVALUATION (Fig. 11–25)

The diagnosis of Cushing's syndrome should be entertained in obese individuals who have thinning of the skin, muscle weakness, osteoporosis, hypertension, diabetes mellitus, hyperpigmentation, and hyperandrogenicity, and in those patients who have a pituitary tumor, a tumor known to be associated with Cushing's syndrome, or an adrenal tumor.

Patient History and Physical Examination

The history and physical findings are important to give information concerning the onset, duration, course, and degree of hypercortisolism. Additional features important in the general assessment include the presence of hypertension, diabetes, and osteoporosis and evidence of pituitary, ectopic, or adrenal tumors. Hyperpigmentation points to increased ACTH, whereas significant hyperandrogenicity points to an adrenal carcinoma. The history should delineate the presence or absence of depression, alcohol abuse, and the use of drugs such as glucocorticoids or ACTH.

Diagnostic Studies

GENERAL

Routine laboratory studies usually show the hemoglobin and hematocrit to be high-normal. Neutrophilic leukocytosis with decreased lymphocytes and eosinophils may be seen. Hypokalemia and metabolic alkalosis point to ectopic ACTH syndrome or adrenocortical carcinoma. The serum calcium is usually normal, but the urinary calcium may be elevated in up to 50% of patients with Cushing's syndrome. Fasting hyperglycemia is seen in less than 20% of patients, but impaired glucose tolerance is more common. Hypertriglyceridemia may be present. In long-standing cases, decreased renal function may be related to the effects of hypertension, diabetes, renal stones, nephrocalcinosis, and urinary tract infections. Radiologic studies may show osteoporosis. Chest x-ray may reveal cardiomegaly, mediastinal widening resulting from fat accumulation, and rib and vertebral fractures from the osteoporosis. An abdominal x-ray or an intravenous

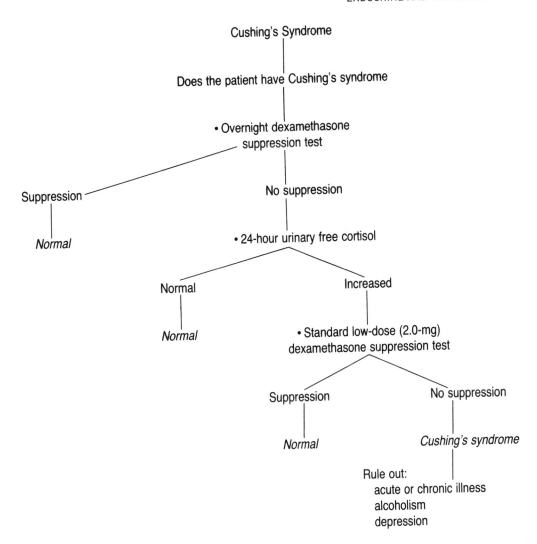

Cushing's Syndrome

Does the patient have Cushing's syndrome

• Overnight dexamethasone
  suppression test

Suppression

Normal

No suppression

• 24-hour urinary free cortisol

Normal

Normal

Increased

• Standard low-dose (2.0-mg)
  dexamethasone suppression test

Suppression

Normal

No suppression

Cushing's syndrome

Rule out:
  acute or chronic illness
  alcoholism
  depression

Fig. 11–25. Approach to the diagnosis of Cushing's syndrome.

pyelographic study may reveal kidney stones or a suprarenal mass (adenoma or carcinoma). An electrocardiogram may show hypertensive changes.

SPECIFIC (Table 11–36)

Plasma Cortisol (PC). In assessing PC, it is important to remember that its secretion is normally episodic, labile, and responsive to stress and shows a diurnal rhythm; and that cortisol circulates in plasma, primarily (98%) bound to cortisol-binding globulin and as free cortisol (2%). In Cushing's syndrome, PC values are usually high and show loss of normal diurnal variation. However, 10 to 20% of patients with Cushing's syndrome have morning PC levels within the normal range. High PC values may be found in non-Cushing's patients because of increased cortisol-binding globulin from the use of estrogen, in pregnancy, on a congenital basis, or in certain hematopoietic disorders. High PC values may also be found in response to stress; stress can also disrupt the normal diurnal rhythm. Because of these considerations, single measurements of PC are usually of little help in the diagnosis of Cushing's syndrome, but a low-normal PC should cast some doubt about the diagnosis.

Urinary Steroid Metabolites. These include 17-hydroxycorticoids (17-OHCS), 17-ketogenic steroids (17-KGS), and 17-ketosteroids (17-KS). Cortisol is degraded and conjugated in the liver, and the soluble metabolites are excreted by the kidneys and can be measured in a 24-hour urine collection. The main advantage of cortisol metabolites measurements is that they provide indices of integrated adrenal activity and are not subject to short-term fluctuations in PC levels. Cortisol metabolites measurements do have significant drawbacks; an accurate 24-hour urine collection is dependent on the patient's cooperation and on nursing diligence; and the production of these cortisol metabolites can be modified by extra-adrenal factors, including body weight (excretion is parallel to body mass—it is increased in obesity and decreased in weight loss), thyroid state (excretion is increased in hyperthyroidism and decreased in hypothyroidism), and drugs, which can interfere with these metabolite measurements. It is important to measure the creatinine content of all 24-hour urine to assess the adequacy of the 24-hour urine collection.

Despite these shortcomings, these measurements are a valuable asset in the study of adrenocortical function. They are usually increased in patients with Cushing's syndrome but can be normal in 10 to 15% of patients and can be increased in noncushingoid states, especially obesity. The 17-KS can be helpful in the differential diagnosis of Cushing's syndrome because they are normal or decreased in patients with adrenal adenomas, modestly elevated in ACTH-dependent Cushing's syndrome, and markedly increased (> 50 mg/4 hours) in the majority of patients with adrenocortical carcinoma.

Urinary Free Cortisol (UFC). Urinary free cortisol represents the free cortisol that is filtered by the glomeruli and excreted in the urine in an unconjugated and unaltered form (only about 1% of the adrenal cortisol's daily production). UFC is currently the most important test in the diagnosis of a hypercortisol state. It is increased in greater than 98% of patients with the syndrome. False negatives are extremely rare, but false positives (2 to 3%) can be seen after acute physical and emotional stress, in acute illness, and in pregnancy.

Overnight Dexamethasone Suppression Test. Dexamethasone is a potent glucocorticoid that suppresses ACTH secretion through the negative feedback effect on the hypothalamic-pituitary axis. It is given in very small quantities, which are not measured by routine lab tests used for the measurements of cortisol and its metabolites.

In the overnight suppression test, dexamethasone obliterates the normal early morning surge of ACTH, and PC the following morning is generally < 5 µg/dl. Patients who have Cushing's syndrome will not show a suppressed cortisol secretion, and PC the following morning is >10 µg/dl. This test has no contraindications or side effects.

False positive results can occur in thyrotoxicosis, and with the use of microsomal-inducing drugs that cause rapid dexamethasone clearance; the most common false positive results occur in 30% of sick or stressed patients, patients with simple obesity (10 to 15%) and patients on oral contraceptives. The test has a very low incidence of false negatives.

The overnight dexamethasone suppression test is the simplest, most reliable outpatient screening test for

Cushing's syndrome. A normal suppressive response essentially rules out the diagnosis. If no suppression occurs, the patient is further evaluated with a 24-hour urinary free cortisol or the performance of a standard low-dose dexamethasone suppression test.

Standard Low-Dose Dexamethasone Suppression Test. Normal individuals will suppress their ACTH adrenal axis in response to this low dose of dexamethasone. This suppression is reflected in a PC of <5 µg/dl, 17-KGS <5 mg, 17-OHCS <4 mg, and UFC <20 µg/24 hours. Failure of suppression establishes the diagnosis of Cushing's syndrome. This test serves as the standard, most discriminating test for the identification of Cushing's syndrome. It is abnormal in 99% of these patients. False positive responses occur in acute illness, alcoholism, and depression; false negative responses occur with rapid dexamethasone clearance caused by drugs and with periodic hormonogenesis (see below). It is important to remember that this test defines the presence of Cushing's syndrome but does not distinguish among its various causes. It is a safe test and is essentially free of side effects.

High-Dose Dexamethasone Suppression Test. The high-dose dexamethasone suppression test is valuable in identifying the cause of Cushing's syndrome. Suppression of cortisol parameters points to Cushing's disease, while failure of suppression should prompt consideration of an adrenal tumor or the ectopic ACTH syndrome. Suppressibility is identified by the suppression of 17-OHCS, 17-KGS, or UFC by greater than 50% of the baseline, and of PC to less than 10 µg/dl.

Metapyrone Test. Metapyrone inhibits 11-hydroxylase, the enzyme that catalyzes the final step in cortisol biosynthesis and that consists of hydroxylation of 11-deoxycortisol (compound S) to cortisol (compound F). Thus, metapyrone in the normal individual would lead to decreased cortisol, a compensatory increase in ACTH, an increase in steroid biosynthesis, and an increased secretion of compound S. The level of compound S can be measured indirectly as 17-KGS or 17-OHCS in a 24-hour urine collection or directly by radioimmunoassay in plasma or urine.

In normal individuals, stimulation of the hypothalamic-pituitary-adrenal axis is reflected by an increase in serum 11-deoxycortisol to >7.5 µg/dl and an increase in 17-KGS or 17-OHCS to two to four times the basal value.

The metapyrone test is important in the differential diagnosis of Cushing's syndrome. Patients with Cushing's disease whose feedback control of ACTH secretion is preserved show metapyrone hyperresponsiveness. Patients with Cushing's syndrome related to an adrenal tumor or an ectopic ACTH syndrome have a suppressed hypothalamic-pituitary axis and are therefore nonresponsive to metapyrone. A few ectopic ACTH-producing tumors, especially bronchial carcinoids, may show metapyrone responsiveness, however. Therefore, although nonresponsiveness to metapyrone rules out Cushing's disease, responsiveness to metapyrone can be seen in patients with Cushing's disease and some patients with ectopic ACTH-producing tumor.

It is important to remember that metapyrone can cause a significant decrease in cortisol production and in patients with adrenal tumors can lead to development of adrenocortical crisis. Although the overnight metapyrone test is safe, extended metapyrone tests should be done only in the hospital setting under close medical supervision.

Serum ACTH. Measurement of ACTH by radioimmunoassay is now available through commercial laboratories. It is one of the most difficult radioimmunoassays to perform reliably, because ACTH is unstable in plasma and adheres to glass. The specimen should be collected in an anticoagulated plastic or silicone coated tube placed on ice, centrifuged in the cold without delay, and frozen until the assay can be performed. Serum ACTH is also secreted episodically with diurnal variation; several blood samples can be collected every 30 minutes three to four times and pooled. Serum ACTH plays an important role in the differential diagnosis of Cushing's syndrome. In most patients with Cushing's disease, serum ACTH is normal (though inappropriately high for the prevailing cortisol levels) or modestly elevated. In patients with ectopic ACTH syndrome, the serum ACTH is moderately to significantly elevated. Patients with adrenal tumors have suppressed ACTH levels.

The Corticotropin-Releasing Hormone (CRH) Stimulation Test. This test, which is still investigational but should become generally available in the near future, is often useful in the differential diagnosis of Cushing's syndrome. In the test, CRH is administered in a dose of 1 to 3 µg/kg of body weight in the normal individual. In response to CRH, ACTH secretion peaks in 10 to 15 minutes (cortisol secretion peaks in 30 to 60 minutes) and may be sustained for several hours; peak ACTH levels are approximately three times the basal levels. In patients with Cushing's disease, the ACTH levels rise in response to CRH; in patients with ectopic ACTH syndrome, the high basal ACTH levels do not rise further; in patients with adrenal tumors, the suppressed basal ACTH levels do not rise. The CRH test should be performed with the patient in a supine position because flushing and occasionally hypotension have been observed after administration of the drug.

Radiologic Studies. A chest x-ray may be helpful in revealing an ectopic source of ACTH such as oat-cell carcinoma, bronchial carcinoid, or thymoma. A CT scan of the adrenals is a critical test in the evaluation of patients with Cushing's syndrome. The CT scan can visualize the adrenals in almost all patients and can identify an adrenal tumor, its location, its size, and the potential presence of metastasis. In patients with Cushing's disease, the adrenals are usually normal in size, whereas in those with ectopic ACTH tumors, the adrenals are usually enlarged. The adrenals are found to be enlarged and nodular in patients with nodular adrenal hyperplasia. CT scanning can be extended to include the rest of the abdomen and the chest in an attempt to identify an ectopic ACTH-producing tumor site. Nuclear magnetic resonance imaging of the sella is not widely available at present and experience with it is limited. It may prove very helpful in sellar radiology in the future.

In patients with suspected Cushing's disease, radiologic study of the sella is in order. A standard skull film may be normal in as many as 50% of patients with pituitary tumors causing Cushing's disease. Abnormal sellar tomography is present in only 60 to 70% of affected patients and is unreliable because of the many false-positive results. A CT scan of the pituitary area employing the new generation of CT scanners can identify a pituitary tumor in about 70 to 80% of patients with Cushing's disease. In such patients, a visual field examination to detect chiasmal syndrome and studies of other pituitary functions are in order.

Selective venous sampling with assays of ACTH from the periphery, from inferior petrosal sinuses that drain the pituitary area, and from ectopic sites can be helpful in the differential diagnosis of Cushing's disease from ectopic ACTH syndrome when other clinical and biochemical tests are equivocal.

Diagnostic Approach

An overnight 1-mg dexamethasone suppression test is performed, and a 24-hour urine is collected for urinary free cortisol assay. If the overnight dexamethasone suppression and UFC are normal, Cushing's syndrome is excluded. If these two tests are definitely abnormal, the diagnosis of Cushing's syndrome is established provided that disease states causing false positive responses are excluded (see below). If the two tests show equivocal or borderline results, the standard 2-day low-dose (2-mg) dexamethasone suppression test is performed. A normal response to this suppression test excludes Cushing's syndrome (with very rare exceptions).

Once the diagnosis of Cushing's syndrome is made, the next step is to define the specific cause of the hypercortisol state and determine whether the causative disease is an adrenal tumor, ectopic ACTH syndrome, or Cushing's disease (Fig. 11–26). In the usual case, differentiation is based on biochemical and anatomic data. The biochemical approach includes the determination of serum ACTH levels and the performance of two provocative tests: the high-dose (8-mg) dexamethasone suppression and the metapyrone stimulation tests. The anatomic approach consists of radiologic studies, especially CT scanning, to identify the site of the pituitary, ectopic, or adrenal tumor.

Patients with Cushing's disease usually present with a classic clinical picture of gradual onset and slow progression. Predominantly they are females between ages 20 and 40. Hyperpigmentation and hyperkalemic metabolic alkalosis are rare. These patients usually have a mild to moderate increase in cortisol secretion associated with a very modest increase in androgen production by the adrenal gland and have normal to modestly elevated plasma ACTH levels (ranging from 40 to 200 pg/ml). Approximately 50% of these patients have ACTH levels consistently within the normal range. In addition, patients with Cushing's disease have an impaired but responsive hypothalamic-pituitary-ACTH axis. Thus, their cortisol secretion is metapyrone responsive and high-dose dexamethasone suppressible. A pituitary tumor is demonstrable radiologically in about 80% of these patients.

The majority of patients with ectopic ACTH-producing tumor are males between ages 50 and 70, and the ectopic tumor is apparent (oat-cell carcinoma, carcinoma of the lung, thymoma, pancreatic tumor, medullary carcinoma of the thyroid, or pheochromocytoma, among other tumors). The disease is of rapid onset and progression. These patients have a severe

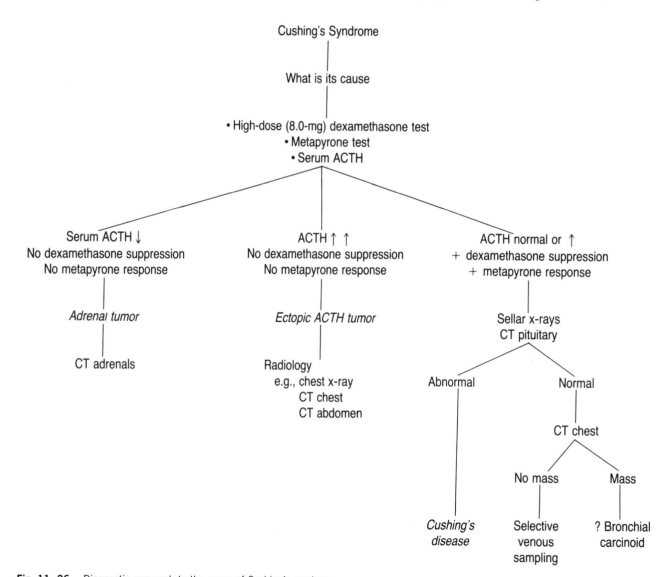

Fig. 11–26. Diagnostic approach to the cause of Cushing's syndrome.

degree of cortisol excess manifested by weakness, debility, hypertension, diabetes mellitus, hypokalemic alkalosis, hyperpigmentation, a high incidence of edema, and weight loss rather than weight gain. The florid cushingoid features are not present. In addition to increased cortisol production, they have increased mineralocorticoid and increased androgen production. Patients with this syndrome frequently have markedly elevated plasma ACTH levels, with 65% of patients having levels above 200 pg/ml. Some of them, however, have levels that overlap with the range seen in Cushing's disease. In the usual ectopic ACTH syndrome, the ectopic tumor is autonomous, and the hypothalamic-pituitary-ACTH axis is suppressed. Therefore, the cortisol secretion is nonmetapyrone responsive and nondexamethasone suppressible.

A minority of patients with ectopic ACTH syndrome, particularly those with benign tumors like bronchial carcinoid, show clinical and biochemical features indistinguishable from those of Cushing's disease. The primary tumor may not be clinically apparent. Differential diagnosis between this entity and Cushing's disease rests on the delineation of the causative tumor by CT scanning or by selective venous sampling procedures.

Patients with adrenal adenomas are usually female and have features of glucocorticoid excess only. The onset is gradual, the cortisol excess is mild to moderate, and the androgen production is low-normal or low. Patients with adrenocortical carcinoma show a rapid onset and progression; the increase in cortisol production is associated with increased mineralocorticoid and androgen production. 17-ketosteroids are markedly elevated, and the patient may have abdominal pain, a palpable mass in the abdomen, or evidence of metastatic disease. In patients with Cushing's syndrome caused by adrenal tumors, plasma ACTH levels are undetectable (less than 20 pg/ml); the hypothalamic-pituitary axis is suppressed, and thus these patients are not metapyrone responsive or high-dose dexamethasone suppressible.

THE SYNDROME OF PRIMARY ALDOSTERONISM

DEFINITION

Primary aldosteronism is a syndrome characterized by autonomous excessive aldosterone secretion by the adrenal cortex that causes sodium retention, potassium wasting, hypertension, and suppression of plasma renin activity. Although it is present in less than 2% of patients with hypertension, it should be considered in the evaluation of hypertensive patients because appropriate treatment is available that can cure or ameliorate the hypertension and associated metabolic abnormalities in most patients.

PATHOPHYSIOLOGIC CONSIDERATIONS

Knowledge of the physiology of aldosterone secretion is basic to the understanding of hyperaldosteronism, its clinical manifestations, and its diagnosis (Fig. 11–27). Aldosterone is the principal mineralocorticoid produced by the zona glomerulosa of the adrenal cortex. Its most important target organ is the distal nephron, in which aldosterone promotes reabsorption of sodium and secretion of potassium and hydrogen ions. The magnitude of this renal effect depends on the salt intake; increased sodium intake leads to increased sodium delivery to the distal nephron, sodium reabsorption, and potassium and hydrogen secretion. Conversely, a decreased sodium intake results in decreased potassium and hydrogen renal losses. Other known extrarenal targets for aldosterone in which aldosterone promotes sodium retention and potassium loss include the sweat and salivary glands, the ileum, and the colon, but these extrarenal actions are ordinarily of minor physiologic importance.

Aldosterone secretion is regulated primarily by the renin-angiotensin system and also by serum potassium and serum ACTH. Renin is a proteolytic enzyme produced in the juxtaglomerular cells of the renal afferent arterioles. Decreased blood volume, decreased blood flow in the afferent renal arterioles, or decreased sodium delivery to the distal tubule and sympathetic stimulation lead to an increase in renin secretion. Renin causes the transformation of angiotensinogen (an α_2 globulin produced by the liver) to angiotensin I, a 10-aminoacid polypeptide, which in turn is converted to angiotensin II, an 8-aminoacid peptide, by the angiotensin-converting enzyme located mainly in the lung. Angiotensin II is rapidly degraded to angiotensin III, a 7-aminoacid compound. Angiotensin II, and to a lesser extent angiotensin III, stimulates the secretion of aldosterone by the zona glomerulosa. The secreted aldosterone causes sodium and water retention by the renal tubule, an increase in blood volume, and therefore a decrease in renin secretion.

A second important factor controlling aldosterone secretion is the potassium ion. Increased serum potassium increases aldosterone secretion; decreased serum potassium has the opposite effect. The potas-

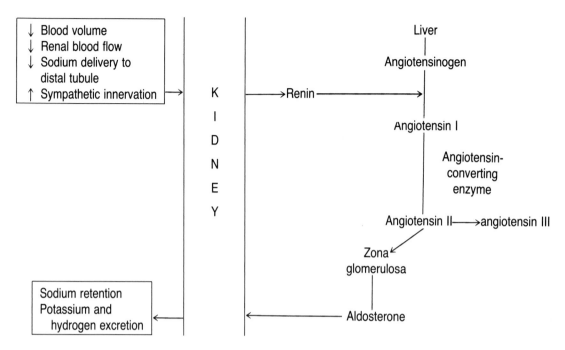

Fig. 11–27. The renin-angiotensin-aldosterone axis.

sium level appears to directly affect the zona glomerulosa. ACTH has a minimal effect on aldosterone secretion; it stimulates aldosterone production acutely, but the effect is not sustained.

Table 11–38 outlines the causes of aldosteronism. In primary aldosteronism, autonomous overproduction of aldosterone by the adrenal cortex is caused by a unilateral adenoma (in 70% of cases), by bilateral hyperplasia of the zona glomerulosa cells with micro- or macronodular changes (in 30% of cases), and, rarely, by carcinoma of the adrenal cortex.

Secondary aldosteronism is due to either increased renin or increased angiotensinogen production. Among the causes of increased renin production without hypertension are a decreased renal perfusion resulting from volume depletion, congestive heart failure, ascites, or nephrosis; excessive potassium intake; and Bartter's syndrome. Among the causes of increased renin production with hypertension are renal artery stenosis; malignant hypertension; primary reninism caused by a renin-producing tumor, which may be renal or ectopic (e.g., pulmonary); and hypertension treated with diuretics. Causes of increased angiotensinogen production include pregnancy and the use of estrogen or oral contraceptives.

Primary aldosteronism leads to increased sodium retention, ECF volume expansion, and suppressed plasma renin activity; and to increased potassium and hydrogen renal excretion, potassium deficiency, hypokalemia, and metabolic alkalosis.

Table 11–38. Causes of Aldosteronism

Primary aldosteronism
  Adenoma (approximately 70%)
  Hyperplasia (approximately 30%)
  Carcinoma
  Glucocorticoid remediable (rare)
Secondary aldosteronism
  With hypertension
    Increased renin
      Renal artery stenosis
      Malignant hypertension
      Primary reninism
        Renal renin tumor, e.g., Wilms'
        Ectopic renin tumor, e.g., pulmonary paraganglioma
    Hypertension and diuretics
    Increased angiotensinogen
      Estrogen: oral contraceptives
  Without hypertension
    Increased renin
      Decreased renal perfusion
        Volume depletion
        Congestive heart failure
        Nephrosis
        Cirrhosis-ascites
      Pregnancy
      Excessive potassium intake
      Bartter's syndrome

CLINICAL PRESENTATION

Primary aldosteronism occurs in approximately 1 to 2% of unselected hypertensive patients. It is twice as common in females and most frequent in the third and fourth decades of life.

Signs

Hypertension is a universal finding. It is usually mild to moderate. Malignant hypertension is very rare. Hypertensive sequelae may occur in long-standing cases. A postural fall in blood pressure without reflex tachycardia can be observed in severely potassium-depleted patients. A positive Trousseau's or Chvostek's sign may be present because of metabolic alkalosis. Clinical edema is rare.

Symptoms

The patient may be entirely asymptomatic. When present, symptoms are related to hypokalemia and consist of fatigue, muscle weakness, and, rarely, paralysis; polyuria, nocturia, and polydipsia usually related to hypokalemic nephrogenic diabetes insipidus or to frank diabetes mellitus caused by impaired insulin secretion; postural dizziness from impaired vascular postural reflexes; and paresthesias and tetany from metabolic alkalosis. Headache is a frequent incidental complaint.

DIFFERENTIAL DIAGNOSIS AND PITFALLS

Several entities should be remembered in the differential diagnosis. Essential hypertension treated with diuretics is probably the most common cause of hypertension and hypokalemia. In addition to causing hypokalemia, diuretics can decrease the extracellular fluid volume and therefore increase renin and aldosterone production. To establish the diagnosis of primary aldosteronism, it is usually necessary to discontinue diuretics for several weeks and proceed with evaluation if hypokelamia persists. (In these weeks, if antihypertensive treatment is required, one can use prazosin or guanadrel because they do not interfere with renin release or aldosterone secretion.) Alternatively, the finding of suppressed renin in the presence of hyperaldosteronism in a patient on diuretic therapy is diagnostic of primary aldosteronism.

Cushing's syndrome may caue hypertension and hypokalemia because of the mineralocorticoid effects of excess cortisol ± corticosterone or DOC. These patients have additional features of cortisol excess, and the diagnosis can usually be made on clinical grounds and from laboratory tests documenting increased cortisol production (see Cushing's Syndrome).

Hypertensive states associated with secondary aldosteronism, including renal artery stenosis, malignant hypertension, renin-secreting tumors, and use of estrogen, must be considered in the differential diagnosis. In these situation, PRA is increased in contrast to its suppression in patients with primary aldosteronism.

Another cause of hypertension associated with suppressed renin is chronic excessive licorice ingestion as occurs in licorice addicts, excessive consumption of soft drinks flavored with licorice, and the long-term use of carbenoxolone, a drug used in the treatment of peptic ulcer. Licorice contains glycyrrhizic acid, which has a direct mineralocorticoid effect on the distal tubule and causes sodium reabsorption and potassium loss. Also, some forms of congenital adrenal hyperplasia, specifically 17-hydroxylase and 11-hydroxylase deficiency states, must be considered in the differential diagnosis. These are associated with mineralocorticoid overproduction of aldosterone precursors and abnormalities of sexual development. Among other causes of hypertension associated with suppressed renin are 11-deoxycorticosterone-producing adrenal tumors and Liddle's syndrome. (This syndrome is presumably a primary renal tubular disorder characterized by excessive reabsorption of sodium and loss of potassium by the distal tubule without any identifiable cause.) In all these states, the history, clinical features, and appropriate laboratory studies, including a suppressed renin and suppressed aldosterone, aid in the differential diagnosis.

Low-renin essential hypertension. In approximately 20% of patients with essential hypertension, PRA is suppressed and unresponsive to acute stimulation with diuresis and upright posture. The cause is indeterminate, but these patients do not have hypokalemia and their plasma or urinary aldosterone levels are normal (although they may be inappropriately high for the simultaneous renin and angiotensin II levels).

Bartter's syndrome is characterized by renal salt loss, ECF volume depletion, normotension, increased renin, increased aldosterone, hypokalemia, and metabolic alkalosis. It usually occurs in early life and is seen in dwarfed and occasionally in mentally retarded patients. Its cause is not clear, but it is presumably due to excessive renal prostaglandin biosynthesis. It is differentiated from primary aldosteronism by its clinical features, normotension, and high PRA.

DIAGNOSTIC EVALUATION (Fig. 11–28)

Patient History and Physical Examination

Primary aldosteronism should be suspected in hypertensive patients who have unprovoked hypokalemia or who exhibit profound hypokalemia soon after the institution of diuretic therapy, and in those with muscle weakness, postural hypotension, diabetes mellitus, or nephrogenic diabetes insipidus.

The history and physical findings should assess the hypertension and its sequelae, clinical manifestations

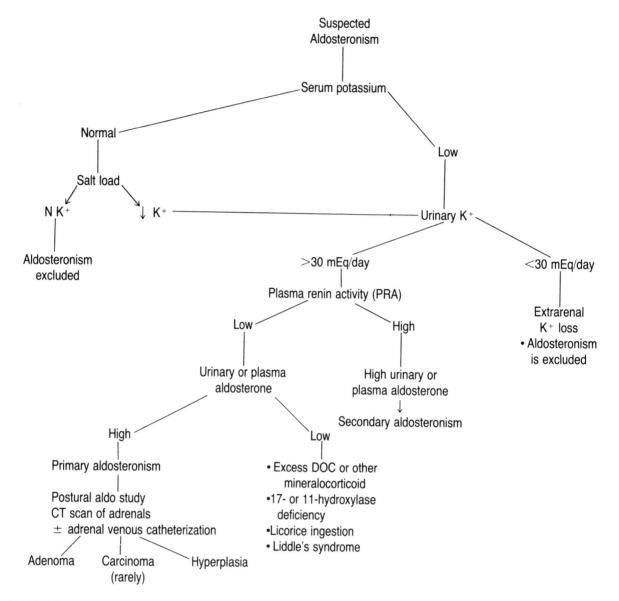

Fig. 11—28. Diagnostic approach to aldosteronism.

of hypokalemia, including muscle weakness, signs of neuromuscular excitability, and orthostatic hypotension. Family history is important in glucocorticoid-remediable hyperaldosteronism.

The diagnosis is based on the presence of hypokalemia (spontaneous or induced by salt loading), inappropriate kaliuresis, elevated plasma aldosterone (PA) or urinary aldosterone (UA) in a sodium replete patient, and suppressed plasma renin activity (PRA) under conditions of maximal stimulation.

The physician must determine the cause of primary aldosteronism. The diagnostic tests to determine if it is adenoma or hyperplasia include PA postural responses; radiologic studies, primarily CT scanning of

the adrenals (supplemented, if necessary, by iodocholesterol scanning and selective adrenal venous sampling); and, if available, plasma levels of 18-hydroxycorticosterone.

Adrenocortical carcinoma is a rare cause of primary aldosteronism. It should be suspected in the presence of evidence of increased secretion of other steroids including cortisol and sex steroids and if a large tumor is identified. Glucocorticoid-remediable hyperaldosteronism is also an uncommon entity characterized by adrenocortical hyperplasia that is familial and primarily affects young males. Its hallmark is that the administration of glucocorticoid in the form of 0.5 to 2 mg dexamethasone daily for 4 weeks will reverse all the clinical and biochemical abnormalities of primary hyperaldosteronism. The serum cortisol and ACTH are within the normal limits.

Diagnostic Studies

GENERAL

Routine laboratory studies may show impaired ability to concentrate the urine, hypernatremia (caused by sodium retention and by water loss from nephrogenic diabetes insipidus), metabolic alkalosis, and hypomagnesemia. Impaired glucose tolerance occurs in about 50% and fasting hyperglycemia in less than 25% of patients. An electrocardiogram may show left ventricular hypertrophy. Prominent T waves and cardiac arrhythmias from hypokalemia are uncommon.

SPECIFIC (Table 11–39)

Serum Potassium. Unprovoked hypokalemia is the hallmark of primary aldosteronism; as many as 50% of spontaneously hypokalemic hypertensive patients will be found to have the disease. Hypokalemia may be mild and intermittent, especially in patients with bilateral hyperplasia. Occasionally the serum potassium may be normal, because low salt intake may lead to decreased delivery of sodium to the aldosterone-responsive distal tubule and to decreased sodium-potassium exchange. In such cases, salt loading will reveal the hypokalemia; this can be accomplished by a diet containing 250 mEq of sodium daily for 5 days. (A 24-hour urine collection for sodium should be undertaken to document the daily intake.) Occasionally the diagnosis of primary aldosteronism is suggested by the occurrence of unusually profound hypokalemia in a patient recently started on diuretic therapy.

Inappropriate Kaliuresis. In a hypokalemic patient, a urinary potassium determination helps in the differentiation between renal and extrarenal potassium losses. A urinary potassium of >30 mEq in the face of hypokalemia points toward renal potassium loss. In primary aldosteronism, the hypokalemia is associated with inappropriate excessive kaliuresis.

Plasma Renin Activity (PRA). Assessment of renin production is critical in the differential diagnosis of states of mineralocorticoid excess. Currently used methods do not assess plasma renin directly, but measure plasma renin activity by quantifying the amount of angiotensin I generated in the patient's plasma over a period of time. The normal values of PRA depend on salt intake and the postural state. PRA is undetectable in primary aldosteronism even under conditions of maximum stimulation.

A suppressed PRA is not specific for primary aldosteronism since it may be found in 20 to 25% of patients with essential hypertension; however, it is a critical test in the differential diagnosis of primary from secondary aldosteronism because the latter is always associated with increased renin production.

The procedure for the evaluation of PRA should be standardized in each laboratory. Numerous procedures are available. In one procedure, a low-salt diet is given for 2 days followed by furosemide, 40 mg by mouth at 6 P.M., repeated at midnight and again at 7 A.M. The patient is then kept in an upright position for 4 hours. Alternatively, 40 mg of furosemide is given intravenously followed by an upright posture for 4 hours. In another procedure, a low-salt diet (10 to 20 mEq sodium per day) is given for 5 days, and on day 6, PRA is determined after 4 hours in an upright position; a urinary sodium is checked to document the state of sodium balance.

It is important to remember that therapy with the aldosterone antagonist spironolactone in patients with primary aldosteronism may lead to the recovery of renin production and an increase in PRA. Therefore, spironolactone should be stopped for 1 to 2 months before the study of PRA.

Aldosterone Measurements. Aldosterone can be measured in the plasma or urine. The plasma measurements ordinarily involve extraction and chromatography of the steroid followed by radioimmunoassay. Urinary measurements are usually done by radioimmunoassay of the 18-glucuronide metabolite of aldosterone. Alternatively, urinary tetrahydroaldosterone can be measured.

Plasma aldosterone (PA) is measured after overnight recumbency. Urinary aldosterone is measured in a 24-hour urine collection. In general, measurement of PA is less reliable than urinary assays in the diagnosis of mild states of aldosterone hypersecretion. PA, however, is of greater utility in the differentiation of causes of primary aldosteronism, because patients who have aldosterone-producing adenoma almost always have a PA >20 ng/dl, whereas those with idiopathic hyperplasia often have PA within the normal limits.

Increased aldosterone production may occur in sodium-depleted normal individuals as well as in patients with primary or secondary hyperaldosteronism. It is therefore necessary to demonstrate that, in patients with primary hyperaldosteronism, the aldosterone secretion is inappropriate for the level of sodium intake and that it is nonsuppressible.

It is important to ensure that the patient is sodium replete and well hydrated during a 24-hour urinary aldosterone collection. The 24-hour urinary sodium should be in excess of 100 mEq. Under these conditions, aldosterone secretion is suppressed in normal subjects but is inappropriately high in patients with

Table 11—39.   Laboratory Tests in Hypermineralocorticoid States

Test	Determinants	Hyperaldosteronism	Comments
Serum Potassium (K+) 3.6—4.8 mEq/L	External balance (potassium intake vs output) and potassium shifts between intracellular and extracellular fluid compartments.	Hypokalemia is the biochemical hallmark of the disease. It occurs in both primary and secondary hyperaldosteronism. Serum K may be normal in patients who are salt restricted (perform salt-loading test).	Serum K may be low in other hypertensive patients who are on diuretics, in hypertensive states due to other mineralocorticoid excess (Cushing's syndrome, increased DOC, licorice, etc.). Hypokalemia may be present in nonmineralcorticoid excess states.
Urinary Potassium Normal, 30—90 mEq/24 hours	Potassium load; renal, glomerular, and tubular function; sodium excretion.	Increased: >30 mEq/L in both primary and secondary hyperaldosteronism. May be normal in salt-depleted patients.	May be increased in hypertension due to other mineralcorticoid excess (Cushing's syndrome, 21-hydroxylase, 11-hydroxylase deficiency, licorice) and in hypertensive patients on diuretics. May be low in hypertensive patients with hypokalemia due to extrarenal potassium loss.
Plasma Renin Activity (PRA) Normal in a sodium-repleted upright patient is ≤ 0.6—4.3 ng/ml/hour. Normal in salt-depleted patients in the upright position is 2.9—24.0 ng/ml/hour.	ECF volume; GFR; sodium in the distal tubule; adrenergic innervation. *Procedure:* 1. Low-salt diet for 2 days; furosemide, 40 mg PO at 6 P.M., midnight, and 7 A.M.; upright posture for 4 hours. 2. 40 mg furosemide IV followed by upright posture for 4 hours. 3. Low-salt diet (10—20 mEq/day) for 5 days and then upright posture on day 6 for 4 hours.	This is a critical test in the differential diagnosis of *primary vs secondary aldosteronism).* PRA is undetectable in primary aldosteronism and is high in hypertensive patients with secondary aldosteronism.	Caution during the provocative testing since severe life threatening volume depletion and hypokalemia may occur with administration of furosemide. PRA may be undetectable also in patients with Cushing's syndrome and other mineralocorticoid excess (licorice, 17- and 11-hydroxylase deficiency) and in Liddle's syndrome. It also can be undetectable in 20—25% of patients with essential hypertension. PRA can be high in normotensive patients with secondary aldosteronism (congestive heart failure, liver cirrhosis, nephrosis, Bartter's syndrome).
Serum Aldosterone Normal, 1—21 ng/dl RIA *Urinary Aldosterone* Normal 2—16 µg/24 hours	Renin-angiotensin-aldosterone axis function. Plasma aldo should be measured after an overnight recumbency; urinary aldo should be measured after adequate sodium repletion (120 mEq/24 hours for at least 4 days).	High; can be normal in aldosteronism if serum potassium is significantly low (correct hypokalemia before measuring aldo levels). High levels cannot differentiate primary from secondary aldosteronism.	Low levels in nonaldosterone hypermineralocorticoid states (Cushing's syndrome, 17- and 11-hydroxylase deficiency, DOC-producing tumor, licorice).
Aldosterone Suppression Test	Renin-angiotensin-aldosterone axis function. Replenish body K before test. Keep a close check on serum K because sodium loading may aggravate hypokalemia. *Procedure* 1. IV saline, 2 L over 4 hours; plasma aldo before and after; normal response is decrease in aldo levels to <8 ng/dl. 2. Sodium intake >150 mEq + Florinef, 0.2 mg every 12 hours for 3 days or DOC, 10 mg IM every 12 hours for 3 days; normal response is urinary aldo <20 µg/24 hours; urinary sodium should be >150 mEq/day.	In primary aldosteronism, there is no suppression. Plasma or urinary aldosterone is suppressed in all other hypertensive patients including those with secondary aldosteronism.	
Plasma Aldosterone after 8 hours of recumbency and again after 4 hours of upright posture.	Aldosterone-producing adenomas are uniquely responsive to ACTH and nonresponsive to angiotensin II; while primary aldosteronism due to hyperplasia is responsive to angiotensin II but not to ACTH.	In hyperplasia, plasma aldosterone rises with upright posture; in patient with adenoma, aldosterone levels fail to rise or may fall.	Best biochemical test to differentiate between primary aldosteronism caused by tumor from that caused by hyperplasia.

aldosteronism, where the aldosterone excretion can be found to be above 17 µg/24 hours.

A short-term IV saline suppression test is suitable for outpatient screening. Two liters of normal saline are given IV over 4 hours, and PA is measured before and after the IV infusion. In normal individuals and in all other hypertensive patients including those with secondary aldosteronism, PA is reduced to less than 8 ng/dl by the end of the infusion. In patients with primary aldosteronism, there is failure of such suppression. Alternatively, the patient is given a sodium intake >150 mEq/day and fludrocortisone acetate (Florinef) 0.2 mg every 12 hours for 3 days (or Doca, 10 mg IM every 12 hours for 3 days). This maneuver will suppress aldosterone production in normal patients and in those with secondary aldosteronism. Patients with primary aldosteronism will have nonsuppressible aldosterone production.

Because significant hypokalemia may decrease aldosterone production, it is important to replenish body potassium stores before aldosterone measurements.

OTHERS

Surgery is the therapeutic option of choice in patients with aldosterone-producing adenoma because it cures or ameliorates the hypertension in the majority of patients and restores normal electrolyte balance in all of them. In patients who have bilateral adrenal hyperplasia, however, although surgery can correct the electrolyte abnormalities, it controls or ameliorates the hypertension in less than a third of the patients. Hence, if surgery is being considered, it is important to try to determine whether a patient with primary hyperaldosteronism has an adenoma or hyperplasia. If surgery is not contemplated, there is little reason to proceed with this differential diagnosis.

The levels of PA provide an initial indication of the underlying disorder. In patients with aldosterone-producing adenoma, plasma aldosterone levels are significantly elevated, and >30 ng/dl.

ACTH plays a minor role in the control of normal aldosterone secretion. Aldosterone adenomas, however, are uniquely responsive to ACTH and nonresponsive to angiotensin II, whereas aldosterone production in bilateral hyperplasia is responsive to antiotensin II and nonresponsive to ACTH. PA is obtained at 8 A.M. after at least 8 hours of recumbent posture, and again after the patient has been upright for 4 hours. In patients with an adenoma, plasma aldosterone fails to rise and may actually decrease because of the diurnal decrease in ACTH. In adrenal hyperplasia, the plasma aldosterone rises with upright posture.

An aldosterone adenoma secretes not only aldosterone but also aldosterone precursors. Measurements of 18-hydroxycorticosterone as well as deoxycorticosterone or corticosterone may be of help in the differential diagnosis. A recent study indicates that patients with aldosterone adenomas have elevated 18-hydroxycorticosterone, while in those with adrenal hyperplasia, the 18-hydroxycorticosterone levels were normal. Unfortunately, these measurements are not generally available.

The localizing technique of choice, a CT scan of the adrenal area, should be performed in all patients. Both adrenal glands can be visualized in greater than 95% of patients. A CT scan can localize adenomas larger than 1 cm in diameter in over 80% of patients with aldosterone-producing adenomas. It is readily available and noninvasive and exposes the patient to less radiation than iodocholesterol scanning.

Adrenal scintiscan with iodocholesterol can also be useful in localization. Radiocholesterol is taken up by both cortisol and aldosterone-producing cells. Dexamethasone is used to suppress the normal adrenal tissue and highlight the adenoma. (0.5 mg of dexamethasone is given every 6 hours for 48 hours before administration of the radiocholesterol and is maintained until the scanning has been performed.) Saturated solution of potassium iodide (SSKI) is used to suppress the uptake by the thyroid. In patients who have an adenoma, there is an early uptake on the side of the adenoma; in those with hyperplasia, there will be diffuse, bilateral uptake of radioactivity.

Radiocholesterol scanning is successful in 80% of patients, but it is time consuming and may take 7 to 18 days. The use of MP-59, a new iodocholesterol scanning agent, reduces the interval between injection and scanning to about 24 hours. The disadvantages of radioisotopic scanning include high irradiation dose, inconvenience, and more extensive patient preparation. The CT scan and MP-59 scanning should be regarded as complementary, not exclusive tests.

Selective adrenal venous sampling for aldosterone for confirmation of the diagnosis and for localization is available in specialized centers. It may be considered if CT scan or radioscanning fails to localize the adenoma. Concomitant cortisol measurements to verify the source of the sample and to allow determination of aldosterone-cortisol ratios will further help with localization. ACTH administration minimizes the episodic changes in serum cortisol and maximizes aldosterone secretion from the adenoma. The test has been falsely localizing in a few patients with adrenal hyperplasia. Selective adrenal venography can be performed at the same time and can reliably localize an adenoma of greater than 1.0 cm, but it can be complicated by adrenal vein rupture with extravasation of the dye and adrenal infarction. Recent studies indicate that the converting enzyme–inhibitor captopril can be used in the differential diagnosis; this inhibitor causes a drop in plasma aldosterone in patients with adrenal hyperplasia but not in those with adenoma.

PHEOCHROMOCYTOMA

DEFINITION

Pheochromocytomas are catecholamine-secreting tumors of neuroectodermal origin that arise from chromaffin cells. They are a rare cause of hypertension, affecting 0.1 to 0.7% of the hypertensive population, but are important because they are potentially curable, frequently fatal if undiagnosed, associated with other potentially fatal but curable disorders, and often familial.

PATHOPHYSIOLOGIC CONSIDERATIONS

Catecholamine-secreting tumors are found at all ages in both sexes, most commonly in patients in their fourth to fifth decades of life. About 90% of these tumors arise from the adrenal medulla. Pheochromocytomas have been called the "10% tumors" in that 10% are bilateral; 10% are multiple; 10% are extra-adrenal and can be found anywhere along the para-ganglionic system, mostly in the abdomen, para-aortic area in the organ of Zuckerkandl, and rarely in the bladder, thorax, neck, or brain; 10% are malignant; 10% occur in children; and 10% are familial.

Familial pheochromocytomas can occur alone or in association with phakomatosis or neuroectodermal tissue diseases (von Recklinghausen's disease, von Hippel-Lindau disease, and tuberous sclerosis); and with multiple endocrine neoplasia (MEN) types II and III, which are autosomal dominant disorders with incomplete penetrance. The most common components of MEN type II are medulllary carcinoma of the thyroid, pheochromocytoma, and primary hyperparathyroidism. The common components of MEN type III are medullary carcinoma of the thyroid and pheochromocytomas; primary hyperparathyroidism is rare. Patients with MEN type III have a marfanoid habitus, mucosal neuromas, thickened corneal nerves, and alimentary ganglioneuromatosis. In familial pheochromocytomas, the tumors can be preceded by adrenal medullary hyperplasia, are bilateral in 50% of cases, and may be latent, with a majority of the patients being normotensive and often asymptomatic. All family members of affected individuals should be screened for pheochromocytoma.

CLINICAL PRESENTATION

The clinical manifestations are related to the effects of the released catecholamines, other hormones produced by the tumor, the anatomic mass of the tumor, and the associations in familial pheochromocytomas.

Signs

Hypertension is the most important clinical sign, being present in greater than 90% of patients. Of these patients, 60% have sustained hypertension with some lability, and about 40% of patients also have distinct crisis or paroxysms. Usually the systolic and the diastolic blood pressures are increased. The hypertension can be severe and resistant to conventional antihypertensive drug treatment. Occasionally, malignant hypertension supervenes. In about 40% of patients, the hypertension is paroxysmal. Patients may also show postural hypotension or may be hypotensive if epinephrine is the predominant secreted catecholamine.

The patient is usually thin, shows manifestations of hypermetabolism and diaphoresis, and has cool, moist hands and feet. Of patients, 15% have a palpable tumor in the abdomen and, rarely, in the neck. Deep palpation of the abdomen may produce a typical paroxysm in about 20 to 50% of patients. Physical examination may disclose associated neurofibromas, café au lait spots, telangiectasia, goiter, marfanoid habitus, or mucosal neuromas.

Symptoms

The classic spells of pheochromocytoma are experienced by more than 50% of the patients. The spell usually begins with nervousness, tremulousness, a feeling of impending doom, awareness of pounding in the chest and forceful heartbeat, severe headaches, profuse sweating, pallor of the skin, and, rarely, flushing. If severe and prolonged, the spell may be associated with nausea or vomiting, visual disturbances, chest or abdominal pain, angina or myocardial infarction, paresthesias, seizures, or cerebrovascular accident. Characteristically, the symptoms and their order of occurrence remain quite similar from one episode to another. About 75% of patients have one or more attacks per week, and 25% have one or more attacks daily. The attack is usually short-lived and in 50% of cases lasts less than 15 minutes. It may occur spontaneously or may be precipitated by a variety of factors including stress, eating, drinking, smoking, straining at stool, micturition, bending, abdominal examination, invasive diagnostic procedures, generally anesthesia, intubation, and medications, e.g., opiates and antidepressants. Following the attack, there is a feeling of fatigue and exhaustion that may last for hours.

Other symptoms that may be experienced by patients with pheochromocytoma include heat intolerance, excessive sweating, weight loss despite normal or increased appetite, severe constipation, symptoms of postural hypotension, changes in sleep pattern, psychoneurosis, occasionally frank psychosis, symptoms of diabetes mellitus, and less commonly, tachy- or bradyarrhythmias, angina, and congestive heart failure. Occasionally the picture may be dominated by acute abdominal pain caused by either hemorrhage in the tumor or associated cholelithiasis. Some patients may present in shock following trauma, surgery, or parturition. Severe peripheral vasoconstrictive manifestations such as Raynaud's phenomenon, purpura, or cutaneous infarcts may be present. Other symptoms such as watery diarrhea (vasoactive intestinal polypeptide [VIP]), Cushing's syndrome (ectopic ACTH produced by the pheochromocytoma or medullary carcinoma of the thyroid), and hypercalcemic manifestations (ectopic humoral hyperparathyroidism or primary hyperparathyroidism associated with multiple endocrine neoplasia) may be due to associated endocrinopathy.

DIFFERENTIAL DIAGNOSIS AND PITFALLS

Pheochromocytoma enters into the differential diagnosis of hypertension, hypoglycemic spells, psychiatric disorders, flushing, endocrinopathies associated with hypermetabolism and weight loss, e.g., thyrotoxicosis or diabetes mellitus, overwhelming infection and shock, and states of severe constipation such as functional bowel disorders or Hirschsprung's disease. The differential diagnosis is based on the history, physical examination, and appropriate laboratory and radiologic studies.

The physician should exclude false positive elevations of catecholamines and their metabolites. If a diagnostic error is to be avoided in the biochemical assessment of patients with suspected pheochromocytoma, the physician should pay particular attention to the details of sample collection, handling, and storage, to potential sources of biologic variation in catecholamine production, and to the effect of drugs.

The most common pitfall is to not consider pheochromocytoma when it is clinically indicated. It should be considered in any hypertensive patient even in the absence of characteristic features such as spells, in patients suspected of having medullary carcinoma of the thyroid or other features of MEN type II or III, in patients with "nonfunctioning" adrenal masses on CT scan of the abdomen, and in patients with other causes of secondary hypertension. Pheochromocytoma may simulate renovascular hypertension because it may be associated with increased renin (volume depletion and direct effect of catecholamines), and extra-adrenal pheochromocytoma may compress the renal artery.

The physician should remember that pheochromocytoma may be simulated rarely by the surreptitious intake of catecholamines by mentally disturbed patients. Such disorder should be suspected if the urinary catecholamines are disproportionately higher than catecholamine metabolites.

Every member of the kindred of a patient with MEN type II and III should be screened periodically for pheochromocytoma; pheochromocytoma should be particularly excluded before thyroid or parathyroid surgery in these patients.

DIAGNOSTIC EVALUATION (Fig. 11–29)

The diagnostic approach depends on clinical suspicion, biochemical confirmation, and anatomic localization.

Patient History and Physical Examination

Patients who should be screened for pheochromocytoma include young hypertensive patients; patients of any age with unexplained severe hypertension; hypertensive patients with persistent or paroxysmal symptoms, weight loss, hypermetabolism, seizures, orthostatic hypotension, hyperglycemia, or hypertensive crisis or unexplained shock during anesthesia, surgery, or delivery; patients with family history of pheochromocytoma or MEN type II or III even in the absence of symptoms or high blood pressure, neurofibromatosis, and other neurocutaneous syndromes; and patients with paradoxical pressure response to guanethidine or ganglion blocking agents.

A careful history and physical examination are essential to assess hypertension and its sequelae, orthostatic hypotension, evidence of peripheral vasoconstriction, hypermetabolism, weight loss, diabetes mellitus, arrhythmias, congestive heart failure, associated endocrinopathy, the presence of abdominal or extra-abdominal mass, and the manifestations of associated disease. The family history is important (history of pheochromocytoma and its sequelae, multiple endocrine neoplasia type II or III, and neuroectodermal diseases).

Diagnostic Studies

In patients suspected of having pheochromocytoma, a 24-hour urine sample for total metanephrines (TMN) vanillylmandelic acid (VMA), urinary total and fractionated catecholamines (UTC), and creatinine is collected, and a blood sample for plasma catecholamines (PC) is obtained. Repeated measurements are needed for verification. Normal values of catecholamines or their metabolites in a hypertensive patient exclude the diagnosis of pheochromocytoma. In patients with abnormal elevation in catecholamine production, a diagnosis of pheochromocytoma is made only after the exclusion of other conditions associated with hypertension and sympathetic discharge (coronary ischemia, paraplegia, diabetic crisis, lead poisoning, acute porphyria, abrupt withdrawal of clonidine, cluster headaches, other causes of hypertension [e.g., renal artery stenosis], diencephalic autonomic epilepsy, use of monoamine oxidase [MAO] inhibitors, posterior fossa

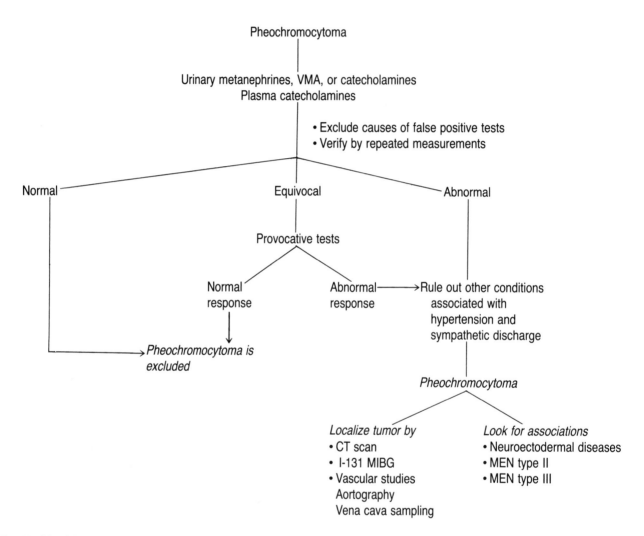

Fig. 11—29. Diagnostic approach to pheochromocytoma.

intracranial tumors, or subarachnoid hemorrhage). Once a diagnosis of pheochromocytoma is made, attempt at tumor localization is pursued, and, in addition, a search for associations of pheochromocytoma including neuroectodermal diseases and multiple endocrine neoplasia is made. If the catecholamine studies are equivocal, they can be repeated. Provocative tests may rarely be indicated.

GENERAL

Routine laboratory studies may show modest elevations in hemoglobin and hematocrit caused by decreased plasma volume or by release of erythropoietin by the tumor; fasting hyperglycemia or impaired glucose tolerance; hypercalcemia that can be due to ectopic humoral syndrome from the tumor or to associated primary hyperparathyroidism; and electrocardiographic changes of left ventricular hypertrophy or evidence of myocarditis. An anteroposterior and oblique film of the chest may be helpful in detecting tumors of the sympathetic chain in the chest.

SPECIFIC (Table 11–40)

Urinary Catecholamines and Metabolites (Fig. 11–30). A complete 24-hour urine collection is assayed for urinary total metanephrines (TMN), vanillylmandelic acid (VMA), and urinary total and fractionated catecholamines (UTC). Traditionally, TMN and VMA have been measured by spectrophotometric assays and UTC by fluorometric assays. Recently, however, measurements of TMN and VMA by high-performance liquid chromatography (HPLC) and of UTC by highly specific radioenzymatic methods have become available. It is essential that these tests be performed by a reliable laboratory.

Urinary catecholamines and metabolites are increased in almost all patients with pheochromocytoma: TMN are increased in greater than 95% of patients, UTC in 90% of patients, and VMA in 85% of patients. If only one of these parameters is to be measured, TMN measurement is preferred by most authorities. It is extremely rare for a patient with pheochromocytoma to have normal results for the three tests.

The pattern of urinary catecholamines and metabolites in patients with pheochromocytoma is variable. In those with large tumors, there is slow synthesis and turnover of catecholamines, and most catecholamines are degraded within the tumor itself, resulting in a low rate of excretion of UTC and a relatively high excretion rate of VMA and TMN. In small tumors, however, there is rapid synthesis and release of catecholamines and preferential excretion of UTC in the urine.

When the 24-hour urine values are equivocal, a spot or timed urine sample should be obtained immediately after a crisis for analyses. Because any severe stress elevates 24-hour urinary catecholamines and their metabolites, measurements should not be obtained during any severe intercurrent illness.

The less differentiated the pheochromocytoma, the more likely it is to produce catecholamine precursors. In those patients suspected of harboring a malignant pheochromocytoma, assays of dopamine and its metabolite, homovanillic acid, are in order.

Plasma Catecholamines (PC). Total and fractionated catecholamines, norepinephrine (NE), epinephrine (E), and dopamine (DA) can be measured by sensitive, specific, simple, and rapid radioenzymatic assays. Proper sampling and handling is essential for reliability. After the patient has fasted overnight, a needle is inserted in a forearm vein, and after the patient has been at rest in a supine position for at least 30 minutes, a blood sample is drawn for plasma catecholamines. A tourniquet is not used. The blood is collected in iced heparinized tubes, and separated in a refrigerated centrifuge at 4° C within an hour, and the plasma is stored at −70° C until it is processed.

In over 90% of patients with pheochromocytoma, PC are elevated in the basal state and rise further during a symptomatic episode. PC levels >2000 pg/ml support the diagnosis of pheochromocytoma, and values between 1000 and 2000 pg/ml are borderline. Normal levels, when the patient is hypertensive, are strong evidence against the diagnosis of pheochromocytoma; it is important to remember that some pheochromocytomas may secrete catecholamines only intermittently. These patients may have normal PC levels at one time or another. PC levels may be increased also in patients who do not have pheochromocytoma (Table 11–40).

Clonidine Suppression Test. Oral clonidine suppresses plasma catecholamines in hypertensive patients without pheochromocytoma but not in patients who harbor the disease. After an overnight fast and with the patient supine after 30 minutes of rest, blood pressure and heart rate are measured serially, and blood is drawn for plasma catecholamines. 0.3 mg of clonidine is given by mouth; the blood pressure and pulse rate are determined every 30 minutes for 3 hours, and blood samples are drawn at 2 and 3 hours following the ingestion of the medication. (After the test is completed, the patient may have symptomatic orthostatic hypotension and should be attended. In addition, the patient is instructed not to drive a car for at least 8 hours after the test.) A normal response is a fall of plasma NE to normal values (≤400 pg/ml) or a fall of at least 40% from basal values. False negatives may occur. The utility of this test in the diagnosis of pheochromocytoma awaits further experience.

Table 11—40.   Common Laboratory Tests in Pheochromocytoma

Test	Procedure	Pheochromocytoma	Comments
Urinary Catecholamines and Metabolites Total catecholamines (TC) <103 µg/24 hours; total metanephrines (TMN) <1.3 mg/24 hours. Vanillylmandelic acid (VMA) N < 9.0 mg/24 hours in the adult. Homovanillic acid N < 8.0 mg/24 hours in the adult.	Needs complete 24-hour urine collection. Check adequacy of urine collection by urinary creatinine. Measurement should be done by a reliable technician. Urinary catecholamines are measured by RIA. TMN and VMA measured by colorimetric or HPLC assays.	Increased in the majority of patients. (TMN >95%; VMA, 85%; TC >90%). Extremely rare to have normal result for the 3 tests in pheochromocytoma. An elevated value should be documented by repeat determination.	If equivocal, repeat determination or check timed sample after acute spell of pheochromocytoma. Increased HVA points to malignant tumors. High values may be seen in nonpheochromocytoma patients; e.g., severe stress, intercurrent illness, acute intermittent porphyria, etc. Urinary TMN may be *increased* by catecholamines, drugs that contain or release catecholamines, L-dopa, ephedrine, methylxanthines, amphetamine, vasodilators, clonidine withdrawal, MAO inhibitors, alcohol, and chlorpromazine. It may be *decreased* by methylglucamine (contrast agent). Urinary catecholamines may be *increased* by catecholamines, drugs that contain or release catecholamines (see above) and methyldopa. Urinary VMA may be increased by catecholamines, drugs that contain or release catecholamines (see above), nalidixic acid, and lithium. It is *decreased* by MAO inhibitors; clofibrate, Methanamine, alcohol, disulfiram, and chlorpromazine. If colorimetric test is done, patient should avoid coffee, tea, chocolate, vanilla, glyceryl guaiacolate, and aminosalicylic acid.
Plasma Catecholamines, Total and Fractionated Normal norepinephrine (NE) = 70–750 pg/ml. Epinephrine (E) <110 pg/ml. Dopamine (DA) <30 pg/ml.	Measured by RIA. Proper sampling and handling are essential. After overnight fast, insert needle in the forearm, rest the patient in supine position for at least 30 minutes, then sample. Do not use tourniquet. Collect blood in iced tube. Separate and refrigerate within 1 hour. Store plasma at −70°C until processing.	Increased in >90% of patients. Total catecholamines >2000 pg/ml support diagnosis. Values 1000–2000 pg/ml are borderline. Normal levels in a hypertensive patient is against the diagnosis of pheo; but normal levels may be seen in pheochromocytoma normotensive patients between spells.	May be increased in nonpheochromocytoma patients with: upright posture, volume depletion, drugs (theophylline derivatives, vasodilators, clonidine withdrawal, desipramine, and drugs containing catecholamines), other concomitant diseases (angina, COPD, congestive heart failure, TIA, depression, hypothyroidism), and laboratory error.
Clonidine Suppression Test	After overnight fast, patient in supine position for 30 minutes, draw blood for plasma catecholamines. Give 0.3 mg clonidine by mouth and sample blood at 2 and 3 hours following medication. Determine pulse and blood pressure before and repetitively during the test. Drowsiness and symptomatic hypotension may occur.	Clonidine suppresses plasma catecholamines in nonpheochromocytoma hypertensive patients (plasma catecholamines may fall to normal or by at least >40% of basal value). Plasma catecholamines are nonsuppressible by clonidine in pheochromocytoma.	False negatives may occur. Utility in diagnosis of pheochromocytoma awaits further experience.

Table 11–40.   Common Laboratory Tests in Pheochromocytoma *(Continued)*

Test	Procedure	Pheochromocytoma	Comments
Intravenous Phentol-amine	Bed rest; record blood pressures until stable; give a test dose of phentolamine, 0.5 mg IV; if no significant hypotension, give 4.5 mg of the drug IV. Check blood pressure every 30 seconds for 5 minutes and then every minute for 10 minutes or until return to baseline. Have norepinephrine available for IV use in case severe hypotension occurs.	In pheochromocytoma, there is a fall of 25/35 mm Hg in blood pressure, which is maximal in 2–3 minutes and lasts 10 minutes.	Should only be done in a hypertensive patient. Test is rarely indicated since it is potentially dangerous. It may be useful as a diagnostic test in patients with life threatening hypertension. False positive responses may occur in uremia and in patients on sedatives and vasodilator drugs. Blood pressure response supports but is not diagnostic of pheochromocytoma.
Histamine or Glucagon or Tyramine Stimulation Test	An IV line in place; administer saline IV as placebo; follow blood pressure until stable; perform cold pressor test; allow blood pressure to return to baseline; give *histamine* (6.25 μg IV, and, if no response, an additional 19.75 μg IV bolus) *or glucagon* (1 mg IV) or tyramine (1 mg IV); check blood pressure every 30 seconds for 5 minutes and then every 60 seconds for an additional 5 minutes; draw blood for catecholamines at 0, 3, 5, and 10 minutes after the administration of the drug. Nitroprusside, phentolamine, and propranolol should be available in case there is an untoward hypertensive response.	In pheochromocytoma, there is a rise in blood pressure within 1–3 minutes after the administration of the drug. It should be in the order of 60/40 mm Hg and should exceed the cold pressor response by 20/10 mm.	These tests are done in patients who are asymptomatic and normotensive at the time of the evaluation. They are indicated rarely because they are potentially dangerous. Blood pressure response supports but is not diagnostic of pheochromocytoma. Biochemical confirmation should be obtained. There are many false negative (for all 3 stimuli) and false positive (for histamine and tyramine) responses.

Pharmacologic Tests. These potentially hazardous tests are rarely indicated at the present time and are reserved for the unusual patient who is suspected of having pheochromocytoma and in whom basal plasma and urinary catecholamine studies are nondiagnostic. These tests are of two kinds: suppressive tests in patients with persistent hypertension, and stimulation tests in patients who are asymptomatic and normotensive at the time of evaluation.

Suppressive Phentolamine Test. The patient is put at bed rest, and blood pressures are recorded until a stable measurement is obtained. A test dose of phentolamine, 0.5 mg, is given intravenously, and if it does not produce significant hypotension, another dose of 4.5 mg is given. The blood pressure is checked every minute for 10 minutes or until the blood pressure returns to basal value. A positive response consists of a blood pressure fall of 35 mm systolic and 25 mm diastolic, which should be maximal in 2 to 3 minutes and last 10 minutes after the administration of the drug. False positive tests are not uncommon and are seen in uremia and in patients receiving sedative, vasodilator, or antihypertensive therapy. Patients with pheochromocytoma may display inordinate sensitivity to the drug. The attendant should have norepinephrine for intravenous use available should severe hypotension occur. The test may be useful as a diagnostic test in patients with life threatening hypertension prior to the initiation of antihypertensive therapy.

Provocative Tests. The patient's blood pressure response to a provocative agent is compared to the response to nonspecific blood pressure effects of the cold

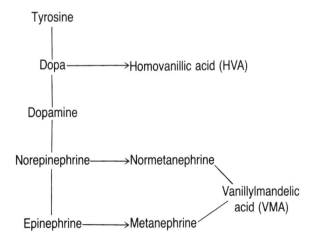

Fig. 11–30. Catecholamine synthesis and degradation.

pressor test. An IV line is secured, and blood pressure is recorded until stable. A cold pressor test is done by placing both hands in ice water for 3 minutes and noting the blood pressure responses. The blood pressure is allowed to return to basal and a provocative agent is then given. This may be histamine base, 6.25 μg, given intravenously and, if there is no response, given 19.75 mg bolus. Histamine initially causes headaches, flushing, and hypotension. Alternatively, glucagon, 1 mg IV, or tyramine, 1 mg IV, can be given. Blood pressure is measured every 30 seconds in the first 5 minutes and then every minute for another 5 minutes. A positive response is a rise in blood pressure within 2 minutes that should be in the order of 60 mm systolic, 40 mm diastolic, and should exceed the cold pressure response by at least 20 mm systolic and 20 mm diastolic. Nitroprusside, phentolamine, and propranolol should be available in case there is an excessive hypertensive response. Histamine and tyramine have many false positive and false negative responses. Glucagon also has many false negative but very few false positive responses. The blood pressure responses to these provocative agents are never diagnostic of pheochromocytoma; biochemical confirmation must be obtained by drawing blood for plasma catecholamines at 0, 3, 5, and 10 minutes after the administration of the drug.

Catecholamines in Platelets. Catecholamine concentrations in platelets are elevated in pheochromocytoma and remain elevated between attacks when the patient may be normotensive. Values are increased also in moderately severe hypertension of any cause but usually are normalized with antihypertensive treatment; in pheochromocytoma, they remain elevated even if the patient is rendered normotensive. This test is not commercially available at present.

Tumor Localization. Accurate preoperative localization of pheochromocytoma is essential. Since 90% of the tumors arise in the adrenal glands and up to 99% of them are intra-abdominal, localization procedures should initially be focused on the abdomen.

X-ray of the abdomen may detect calcification in the adrenal areas in a few patients, but it is rarely helpful. An IVP with nephrotomography will detect tumors larger than 3 cm in diameter.

The major advance in the localization of pheochromocytoma has been the use of the new generation of CT scanners, and CT scanning has emerged as the localization method of choice. It detects the majority of tumors greater than 1 cm in diameter and gives information regarding the location and extent. It may be extended to include the remainder of the abdomen, pelvis, and thorax to locate extra-adrenal tumors. Only the smallest tumors, less than 1 cm in diameter, and

those shielded by clips and other metal objects from previous surgery have escaped detection. The diagnostic accuracy of CT scanning is 90 to 95%. It carries no risk to the patient. Glucagon should not be used during routine CT evaluation for pheochromocytoma because it may induce a dangerous and unexpected rise in blood pressure. Ultrasound examination carries no advantage over CT scanning.

An exciting new development in localization is scintigraphic imaging of pheochromocytoma using ^{131}I metaiodobenzylguanidine (^{131}I-MIBG), which is concentrated in adrenergic neutrotransmitter vesicles. Only abnormal sites of adrenergic tissue such as pheochromocytoma, metastases, or paragangliomas show uptake. The normal adrenals fail to visualize. Rare false negative scans have been reported. Unfortunately, this new technique is not yet commercially available.

Aortography detects almost all pheochromocytomas because most tumors are highly vascular. If all else fails, vena cava catheterization with multiple site sampling for plasma catecholamines may be particularly useful when the tumors are small, multiple, or metastatic. These vascular procedures are invasive and hazardous and can precipitate hypertensive crisis. Pretreatment with alpha blocking agents is mandatory, and a facility should be readily available to treat blood pressure changes or arrhythmias that may occur during these procedures.

Enzymatic conversion of norepinephrine to epinephrine is unique to the adrenal medulla. Tumors of the adrenal medulla and organ of Zuckerkandl produce epinephrine and norepinephrine, while most extra-adrenal tumors produce norepinephrine alone. Although increased plasma or urinary epinephrine strongly suggests adrenal or organ of Zuckerkandl pheochromocytoma, it cannot be used as a definitive localization test because of reports of epinephrine production by other extra-adrenal pheochromocytoma.

AMENORRHEA

DEFINITION

Amenorrhea is the absence of menstruation. It may be physiologic or pathologic. Physiologic amenorrhea occurs in the premenarcheal state, during pregnancy, in early lactation, and after the menopause. Pathologic amenorrhea occurs at any other time and requires evaluation. Conventionally, amenorrhea is classified as primary when there is lack of menarche in a phenotypic female at least 17 years old, and as secondary when there is cessation of menstruation for at least 6 consecutive months in a woman with previously established menstrual function.

PATHOPHYSIOLOGIC CONSIDERATIONS

To understand the etiologic and pathophysiologic considerations of amenorrhea, one needs to keep in mind that a normal menstrual function requires an intact hypothalamus capable of providing an integrating center for the initiation and maintenance of normal menstrual function. The hypothalamus produces gonadotropin-releasing hormone (GnRH) to regulate the production of the two gonadotropins by the anterior pituitary gland. In addition, normal menstrual function requires normal anterior pituitary gonadotropin function, which provides the two gonadotropins, luteinizing hormone (LH) and follicle-stimulating hormone (FSH), to initiate and coordinate the events of the ovarian cycle. Normal ovarian function capable of producing the normal ovarian cycle of follicle development, ovulation, and corpus luteum function is also necessary. As a result of ovarian function, optimal quantity and sequence of steroid hormones are produced to stimulate the endometrium. Also necessary for normal menstrual function are an intact endometrium capable of responding to the ovarian hormones, and an intact genital outflow tract (uterine cavity, cervix, vaginal canal, and vaginal orifice) capable of discharging the shed endometrium. The hypothalamic-pituitary-gonadal axis is shown in Figure 11–31.

Amenorrhea can therefore result from an impairment of function of any components of the endocrine hypothalamic-pituitary-ovarian axis, and from an anatomic abnormality of the genital tract. The causes of amenorrhea are outlined in Table 11–41.

Outflow tract disorders are an uncommon cause of primary amenorrhea and include developmental and acquired entities. The fallopian tubes, uterus, and upper two thirds of the vagina develop from the müllerian ducts, and the lower third of the vagina develops from the urogenital sinus. Developmental anomalies include an imperforate hymen, isolated absence of the uterus, vaginal aplasia, and congenital vaginal atresia. Outflow tract disorders are the least common cause of secondary amenorrhea. They include severe endometritis (postabortive or post partum or caused by tuberculosis or by fungal or other granulomatous disease); overzealous dilatation and curettage (D & C) with destruction of the endometrial basal layer, formation of adhesions, and obliteration of the uterine cavity (Asherman's syndrome); and irreversible endometrial atro-

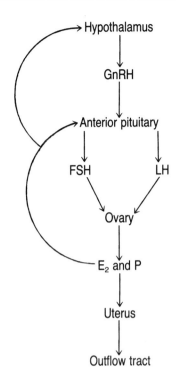

GnRH = Gonadotropin-releasing hormone
FSH = Follicle-stimulating hormone
LH = Luteinizing hormone
E_2 = Estradiol
P = Progesterone

Fig. 11–31. The hypothalamic-pituitary-gonadal axis in the female.

phy caused by prolonged use of progestational agents for contraceptive purposes or in the treatment of endometriosis.

Ovarian defects account for the majority of causes of primary amenorrhea and also include developmental and acquired disorders. Normal ovarian development depends on the absence of the Y chromosome, the presence of two X chromosomes, and normal responsive gonadal tissue. If the Y chromosome is absent and the patient has less than the full complement of XX constitution, e.g., 45/XO, or deletion of short or long arms of one X, normal gonadal development does not occur and fibrous streaks result. The presence of a Y chromosome or its representative H-Y antigen in a genetic female results in mixed gonadal dysgenesis in which the gonad contains variable elements of testicular tissue. Such gonads are predisposed to malignant transformation.

Turner's 45/XO gonadal dysgenesis is the most common cause of primary amenorrhea. It is estimated to affect 1 in 3000 of newborn females. It is characterized by 45/XO karyotype, fibrous gonadal streaks,

Table 11–41. Causes of Amenorrhea

Disorder	Primary Amenorrhea	Secondary Amenorrhea
Outflow tract		
Vagina		
Aplasia	+	
Atresia		
Congenital	+	
Acquired		+
Imperforate hymen	+	
Uterus		
Congenital absence	+	
Endometritis	+	+
Asherman's syndrome		+
Gonadal disorders		
Gonadal dysgenesis		
Classical 45/XO	+	
45/XO variants and mosaics	+	+
46/XX	+	
46/XY	+	
Congenital absence	+	
Testicular feminization	+	
17-hydroxylase deficiency	+	
Autoimmune oophoritis	+	+
Resistant ovary syndrome	+	+
Polycystic ovary syndrome	+	+
Ovarian tumors	+	+
Hypothalamic-pituitary disorders		
Functional		
Stress, diet, exercise	+	+
Postpill		+
Drugs	+	+
Delayed puberty	+	
Systemic disease	+	+
Thyroid disorder	+	+
Adrenal disorders		
Congenital adrenal hyperplasia	+	+
Cushing's syndrome	+	+
Adrenal tumors	+	+
Organic		
Kallmann's syndrome	+	
Isolated gonadotropin deficiency	+	
Craniopharyngioma	+	+
Pituitary tumors	+	+
Other inflammatory degenerative, vascular, neoplastic syndromes	+	+

internal and external female genitalia, short stature, skeletal and developmental anomalies, and, in the adolescent patient, primary ovarian failure and sexual infantilism.

In Turner's mosaics, patients have more than one sex chromosomal line, the most common combination being 45/XO, 46/XX. The degree of ovarian dysgenesis varies depending on the ratio of XO to XX germ cells; it may present with primary or secondary amenorrhea. Affected patients are not invariably short and may have few or many of the physical stigmata of

Turner's syndrome, depending on which tissues get the XO chromosomal line.

46/XX gonadal dysgenesis is characterized by a normal female karyotype, gonadal fibrous streaks, phenotypic female, internal and external female genitalia, and, in the adolescent female, primary ovarian failure with failure of sexual maturation and primary amenorrhea. The patient has eunuchoidal features and does not have the Turner's physical stigmata.

46/XY gonadal dysgenesis is characterized by fibrous streaks with a variable amount of testicular tissue, a female phenotype, and, in the adolescent female, failure of normal sexual maturation and primary amenorrhea; often there is postpubertal virilization as a result of androgen secretion by the dysgenetic gonad. Such gonads are at an increased risk of neoplastic transformation and hence gonadectomy is advisable as soon as the diagnosis is made.

True hermaphrodism is defined by the presence of both ovarian and testicular tissues in either the same or opposite gonads. The karyotype can be 46/XX or 46/XY although some patients have mosaicism. The external genitalia are often ambiguous but can be distinctly female or male. The uterus is present in virtually all patients. At puberty, significant breast development occurs in the majority and menstruation will occur in more than half of the patients. Some patients will present with primary amenorrhea.

Testicular feminization is a hereditary disorder transmitted as X-linked recessive affecting genetic males and characterized by peripheral tissue unresponsiveness to androgen (testosterone and dihydrotestosterone) resulting from an abnormality in cystoplasmic androgen receptors. The vagina is often shallow, ending in a blind pouch, and the testis may be inguinal, leading to suspicion of inguinal hernia, or may be intra-abdominal. These male pseudohermaphrodites are raised as females. In adolescence, with the gonadotropin pubertal surge and increased estrogen production by the testes, normal breast and female secondary sexual maturation occurs except for the absence of sexual hair (which is androgen dependent) and for primary amenorrhea. Gonadectomy is required after completion of pubertal development to forestall the development of neoplastic changes.

Ovarian disorders are common causes of secondary amenorrhea. The most common cause is the polycystic ovary syndrome (see Hirsutism and Virilization). Ovarian destructive processes are an uncommon cause of secondary amenorrhea and premature menopause. These processes include autoimmune oophoritis as part of polyendocrine autoimmune disease that also affects the thyroid, parathyroid, pancreas, and adrenal cortex and has a familial predisposition; various forms of mosaic gonadal dysgenesis that lead to premature exhaustion of the complement of ovarian follicles; abdominal irradiation, and chemotherapy with such agents as cyclophosphamide and vincristine; and ovarian tumors that cause secondary amenorrhea by hormonal abnormalities (hypersecretion of estrogen, androgen, or HCG) or, if bilateral, by destruction of the ovarian tissue.

Hypothalamic-pituitary disease can cause gonadotropin deficiency and amenorrhea by destruction of the pituitary gonadotropin or hypothalamic GnRH cell population by organic diseases of various origins, or by functional suppression of these cells, commonly by a hyperprolactinemic state, nutritional disorder, and anorexia nervosa. (See The Syndrome of Hypopituitarism and Hyperprolactinemia and Galactorrhea.)

Hypothalamic defects are the least frequent cause of primary amenorrhea. Isolated absence of GnRH occurs in females but much less so than in males. In some patients it is associated with anosmia or hyposmia caused by hypoplasia or aplasia of the olfactory lobe (Kallmann's syndrome). This syndrome is familial and may be associated with midline craniofacial defects and other skeletal abnormalities. Constitutional delay in puberty can occur in females but less frequently than in males. It may be genetic, and a parent or a sibling may have experienced a similar delay. The patient has evidence of delayed growth throughout childhood and delayed bone age but will ultimately progress through the normal stages of puberty. Organic hypothalamic-pituitary disease resulting from various causes outlined in Table 11–41 is an uncommon cause of primary amenorrhea. In young adults, craniopharyngioma is the most common space-occupying lesion; prolactinomas do occur but are rare in this age group.

Hypothalamic-pituitary disorders are the most common pathologic cause of secondary amenorrhea and may be either functional or organic. Functional hypogonadotropism results from hypothalamic amenorrhea caused by a defect in cyclic center, inhibition of midcycle GnRH and LH surge, and failure of ovulation. This disorder is seen in the mild forms of anorexia nervosa, in nutritional deficiency, from moderate physical exercise such as running, and from various forms of emotional stress, e.g., in young women in college, in a teenager at camp, during bereavement, etc. Functional hypogonadism also results from more severe suppression of the GnRH gonadotropin axis, and hypogonadotropism from more severe emotional trauma, from more strenuous exercise, after the use of oral contraceptives, from the use of progestational agents, from systemic disease, from thyroid disorders, from uncontrolled diabetes mellitus, from the hyperandrogenic state caused by adrenal or ovarian disorders, and from estrogen-producing tumors. Postpill amenorrhea is common, accounting for approximately 30% of cases of secondary amenorrhea; it occurs in approximately 2% of birth control pill users who may or may not have had prepill menstrual irregularity.

At present, amenorrhea is thought to result from hypothalamic dysfunction. Of patients with postpill amenorrhea, 30% are found to have hyperprolactinemia, and some of these may have underlying pituitary adenoma. In general, spontaneous recovery occurs in a few months unless a pituitary adenoma is present. Psychotropic drugs, especially the phenothiazine family, can cause hypogonadotropism by a direct effect at the hypothalamic level or secondary to hyperprolactinemia from the antidopaminergic effect of these drugs.

Primary hypothyroidism can lead to amenorrhea via three mechanisms: anovulation, which in mild cases may lead to breakthrough bleeding and menorrhagia and in severe cases to amenorrhea; hyperprolactinemia, which can occur in 20 to 30% of patients with primary hypothyroidism and can cause functional suppression of the hypothalamic-pituitary-gonadotropin axis; and autoimmune primary ovarian failure and consequent amenorrhea, which can be associated with autoimmune thyroid diseases. Adrenal disorders can lead to amenorrhea through a hyperandrogenic state (congenital adrenal hyperplasia, Cushing's syndrome, adrenal tumors), through chronic adrenocortical insufficiency by its effects on general health and nutrition; or by its association with autoimmune primary ovarian failure.

Organic hypogonadotropism can be the only manifestation of hypothalamic-pituitary organic disease, or it can occur in association with other pituitary function abnormalities. (See the Syndrome of Hypopituitarism.) Hyperprolactinemia is a common cause of secondary amenorrhea, accounting for 25 to 40% of all cases. Postpartum pituitary necrosis (Sheehan's syndrome), previously a common cause, has declined in incidence with the improvement of obstetric care.

CLINICAL PRESENTATION

Signs

The important signs in primary amenorrhea relate to the secondary sexual characteristics, whether normal, those of sexual infantilism, or those manifesting androgen excess. The physician will also note presence or absence of shortness of stature, physical stigmata of Turner's syndrome, and hyposmia or anosmia. In any amenorrheic patient, evidence of systemic disease, visual field abnormalities, manifestations of hyper- or hypopituitary states, goiter, or galactorrhea are noted. A pelvic exam may show abnormalities of the external genitalia, outflow tract disorders, or pelvic masses.

Symptoms

In primary amenorrhea, "delay" in menarche is what usually prompts the patient or parents to seek medical help. Associated symptoms in patients with primary amenorrhea, which depend on the cause, include those of failure of sexual maturation, shortness of stature, and cyclic abdominal pain caused by cryptomenorrhea. In addition to secondary amenorrhea, adult patients may complain of symptoms of hypoestrogenism such as decreased libido, decreased vaginal lubrication, dyspareunia, hot flashes, and osteopenic manifestations. In both primary and secondary amenorrhea, the patient may also complain of symptoms of androgen excess, of galactorrhea, of symptoms of other pituitary dysfunction, or of thyroid, adrenal, or systemic disease.

DIAGNOSTIC EVALUATION (Table 11–42)

Primary Amenorrhea (Fig. 11–32). In determining if the patient has primary amenorrhea, the first issue the physician must face is whether the complaint of amenorrhea warrants study. Two points need to be kept in mind: first, the mere fact that the parents or patient have sought medical consultation indicates that the issue requires attention for medical, family, or social considerations; second, the process of puberty is a dynamic physiologic process consisting of a series of events encompassing a 3- to 5-year interval. It includes development of secondary sex characteristics, menarche, and pubertal growth spurt, and it varies in onset, duration, and sequence. The onset of puberty with breast and pubic hair development occurs between the ages of 9 and 12 with a mean of 11.2. In the U.S., menarche occurs between ages 10 and 16 years with mean of 12.6 years. Therefore, as a general rule, a girl should be evaluated for primary amenorrhea by age 14, if there is no other evidence of pubertal development, or by age 16, if other pubertal changes have occurred.

The diagnostic approach to primary amenorrhea includes several steps. In clinical evaluation the history can provide clues relating to data on the patient's somatic growth pattern and pubertal development, to development of secondary sex characteristics, to cyclic or abdominal pains in cryptomenorrhea, to the influence of diet, exercise, and stress, to symptoms of hypothalamic-pituitary disease or of systemic illness, and to family history regarding the age of menarche in siblings, the mother, or the grandmother, and history of familial endocrine disease, e.g., congenital adrenal hyperplasia or autoimmune disease.

The physical examination provides clues regarding height. Shortness of stature with primary amenorrhea may be related to Turner's syndrome, constitutional delay of both growth and pubertal development, hypopituitarism, or primary hypothyroidism. The growth charts should be checked. A eunuchoid habitus, in which the arm span is greater than the height and the lower-to-upper segment is greater than one may be seen with any cause of delayed puberty when the growth hormone secretion is normal. The physical exam also provides clues regarding breast development and galactorrhea; secondary sex characteristics; the presence or absence of vaginal or uterine pelvic masses; signs of androgen excess; and somatic anomalies of Turner's syndrome, the presence of hyposmia or anosmia, visual abnormality, pituitary or thyroid dysfunction, or systemic disease.

In the sexually developed patient, pregnancy, though unusual in a girl presenting for evaluation of primary amenorrhea, should always be considered and excluded.

The presence of normal secondary sex characteristics implies adequate estrogen production and, therefore, a normal hypothalamic-pituitary-gonadal axis. It should prompt the physician to consider outflow tract disorders, uterine anomalies, and testicular feminization. Cryptomenorrhea, in which menstruation occurs but does not appear externally because of obstruction, is suggested by the history of monthly lower abdominal pain. On examination, one may find an imperforate hymen (a bluish, bulging hymenal membrane), a pelvic abdominal mass (hematocolpos, which is a distended vagina, or hematometra, which is a distended uterus). Corrective surgery resolves the amenorrhea.

The absence of signs of cryptomenorrhea and outflow tract obstruction points to developmental absence of the uterus. These patients have 46/XX chromosomal constitution, and diagnosis is made by specialized radiographic procedures, e.g., pelvic ultrasonography.

In testicular feminization, the secondary sex characteristics are normal except for the absence of sexual hair because of androgen unresponsiveness. The vagina is a short, blind pouch, and the uterus is absent. Buccal smear is negative, and the karyotype is 46/XY. The testes may be palpable in the inguinal canal. Establishment of this diagnosis implies a need for gonadectomy as soon as the pubertal changes are completed because of the fear of gonadal neoplastic changes.

The diagnosis of endometrial diseases resulting from such causes as endometritis is supported by the history, absence of menstrual response to estrogen-progester-

Table 11–42. Laboratory Tests in Adult Female Hypogonadism

Tests	Determinant(s)	Hypogonadism	Comments
Serum Estradiol Normal, 3–40 ng/dl	Hypothalamic-pituitary-ovarian-endocrine function.	Low in hypogonadism; cannot differentiate between hypogonadism caused by ovarian disease from that caused by hypothalamic-pituitary disease.	
Serum LH and FSH Normal FSH: <20 IU/L Normal LH: <30 IU/L (except at midcycle = 30–150 IU/L) Postmenopausal Normal FSH: >40 IU/L; and LH >30 IU/L	Hypothalamic-pituitary-ovarian function.	Always evaluate in relation to menstrual function and serum E_2. In hypogonadal female, high values indicate primary ovarian failure, while "normal or inappropriately low" values indicate hypogonadism due to hypothalamic-pituitary disease. High LH/FSH ratio in amenorrheic females points to polycystic ovaries.	Secreted in pulsatile fashion. Draw samples every 20–40 minutes three times and assay LH and FSH in pooled sample. "Low" levels may be found in normal eugonadal females because of insensitivity of assays.
Serum Prolactin Normal, 0–23 ng/ml	Pituitary lactotrophe function.	Hyperprolactinemia is a common cause of hypogonadism; points to hypothalamic-pituitary dysfunction as the cause.	Should be measured in all hypogonadal females. See Hyperprolactinemia and Galactorrhea
GnRH Stimulation Test and Clomiphene Stimulation Test See The Syndrome of Hypopituitarism			
Progesterone Test	10 mg medroxyprogesterone acetate PO for 5 days or 200 mg progesterone in oil IM.	Withdrawal bleeding implies: A. Normal outflow genital tract. B. An intact endometrium exposed to adequate estrogen levels; points, therefore, to anovulation as the cause of amenorrhea.	No withdrawal bleeding can occur in: A. Pregnancy B. Hypoestrogenic state. C. Intrinsic endometrial disease. D. Obstruction of outflow tract.
Estrogen Progesterone Test	Ethinyl estradiol, 0.1 mg or conjugated estrogen, 1.25 mg daily for 20 days followed by medroxyprogesterone acetate, 10 mg PO for 5 days.	Absence of withdrawal bleeding points to a diagnosis of endometrial failure. Presence of withdrawal bleeding points to: (i) Normal outflow tract. (ii) Impaired hypothalamic-pituitary-ovarian axis as the cause of amenorrhea.	Should be done in patients with amenorrhea who have a history suggestive of outflow uterine endometrial impairment.
Buccal Smear	Normal females will have Barr bodies in at least 25% of nuclei and no fluorescent Y.	In an amenorrheic patient, Barr-body negative, Y chromosome negative suggests 45/XO; Barr-body negative, Y positive suggests 46/XY or gonadal dysgenesis mosaics; Barr-body positive, Y negative suggests 46/XX or gonadal dysgenesis mosaics.	
Karyotype	Chromosomal analysis.	Determines chromosomal constitution in tissue studied.	May not show chromosomal abnormalities if present in tissues not studied.

one therapy, endometrial biopsy, and appropriate cultures.

The presence of sexual infantilism implies estrogen lack and denotes either a gonadal or a hypothalamic-pituitary endocrine abnormality. The primary investigation here is measurement of the serum gonadotropins LH and FSH (especially FSH). If the serum FSH is high—hypergonadotropic hypogonadism—the defect is in the gonad. If FSH and LH are normal or low—hypogonadotropic hypogonadism—the defect is in the hypothalamic-pituitary unit. Elevated gonadotropins or the presence of shortness of stature or other stigmata of Turner's syndrome should prompt a karyotype to confirm the diagnosis of gonadal dysgenesis or its variants and indicate the need for gonadectomy if a Y chromosomal mosaicism is present.

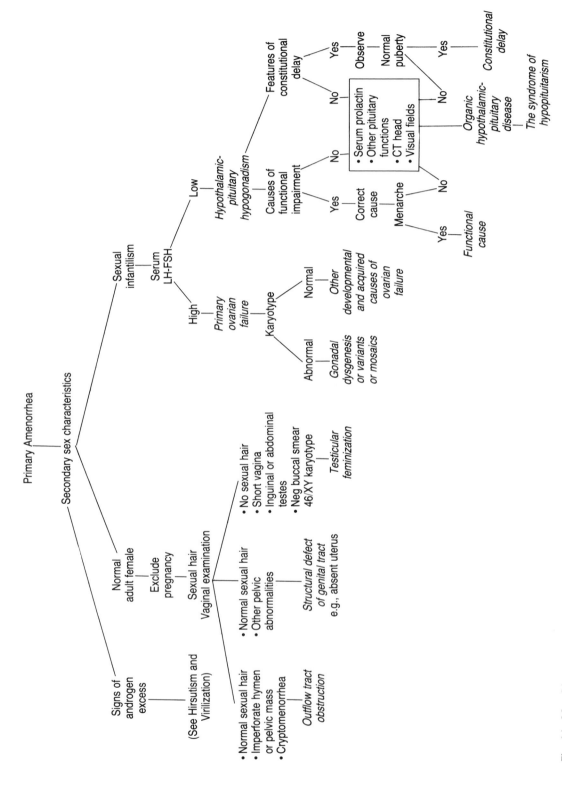

Fig. 11–32. Diagnostic approach to primary amenorrhea.

In hypogonadotropic failure, additional diagnostic steps include assessment of the sense of smell, because hyposmia or anosmia point to Kallmann's syndrome; an attempt to rule out functional causes by a detailed history, examination, and appropriate studies; search for other evidence of anterior pituitary dysfunction especially hyperprolactinemia; and radiologic studies and visual field assessment to rule out a space-occupying lesion in the hypothalamic-pituitary area.

Constitutional delay in puberty may be difficult to differentiate from organic causes of isolated gonadotropin deficiency. Helpful points may include a history of delayed growth and development since early childhood and delayed bone age in relation to chronologic age, maintenance of normal growth velocity for bone age in childhood, signs of puberty appearing when the patient reaches a skeletal age of 11 years with eventual normal development and attainment of secondary sexual development by 18 years of chronologic age, and the frequent family history of a similar pattern of delayed growth in a parent or a sibling.

Presence of evidence of androgen excess should prompt the evaluation outlined in Hirsutism and Virilization.

The diagnostic approach to primary amenorrhea is outlined in Figure 11–32. It is important to remember that approximately 40% of patients will be found to have a form of gonadal dysgenesis, usually Turner's syndrome, another 10% have developmental abnormalities of the müllerian system, uterus, and upper vagina, and the rest will be found to have functional or organic abnormality of the hypothalamic-pituitary axis.

Secondary Amenorrhea. The physician may have to determine if the patient has secondary amenorrhea. In normal women in the reproductive phase of life, menstrual periods occur every 24 to 35 days unless interrupted by pregnancy. There may be some slight abnormality in as many as 20% of the cycles, and an occasional absence of the menstrual period is not uncommon. Secondary amenorrhea is present when there is persistent absence of periods for at least 6 months in a woman with previously established menstrual function.

A careful history and physical examination provide important tools in the differential diagnosis. The physician should obtain information regarding unprotected sexual intercourse, recent D & C and therapeutic abortion, use of drugs such as oral contraceptives, progestational agents, or antidopaminergic agents, recent weight loss or gain, psychopathology of anorexia nervosa, systemic diseases, thyroid or adrenal disease, traumatic childbirth, galactorrhea, signs of androgen or glucocorticoid excess, and family history related to multiple endocrine neoplasia type I, polycystic ovary syndrome, congenital adrenal hyperplasia, or autoimmune endocrinopathies.

In the physical examination, attention is paid to features of pregnancy, hyperandrogenic syndrome, Cushing's syndrome, evidence of hypopituitarism or visual field defects, the presence of a goiter and manifestations of thyroid dysfunction, galactorrhea, nutritional state, Turner's anomalies, and acral changes of acromegaly. Evaluation of secondary sex characteristics, of the external genitalia for evidence of clitoromegaly, and of the pelvis for the presence of pregnancy or ovarian enlargement or mass is important.

The most common cause of secondary amenorrhea is pregnancy. A pregnancy test should be the first step in the laboratory evaluation.

If the patient has manifestations of androgen excess, the workup proceeds according to steps outlined in Hirsutism and Virilization.

Assessment of the anatomic integrity of the uterine endometrium is important if the patient's history, such as history of pelvic infection, trauma (for example, from overzealous D & C), or abnormal pelvic exam, implies endometrial disease as the cause of secondary amenorrhea. The progesterone test and the estrogen-progesterone test will not cause withdrawal bleeding. Gynecologic consultation for hysterosalpingogram and tissue diagnosis are in order.

The next step is an assessment of the function of the hypothalamic-pituitary-gonadal axis by measurements of serum estrogen, LH, and FSH. If the gonadotropins, and especially FSH, are high, a diagnosis of primary ovarian failure is made. Because of the immense implications of primary ovarian failure, a repeat measurement is a wise precaution. If the patient is less than 35 years old, a karyotype is done to rule out a variant of gonadal dysgenesis. The presence of Y chromosome carries a 25% incidence of malignant tumors in the dysgenetic gonad and necessitates gonadectomy. If the patient is over 35 years of age, diagnosis of premature menopause is likely, and further evaluation is not necessary. Other etiologic causes of primary ovarian failure presenting as secondary amenorrhea will be uncovered by a careful history. If autoimmune ovarian failure is suspected, careful assessment for other autoimmune endocrinopathies and other autoimmune diseases and family screening for polyendocrine autoimmune failure is in order.

"Normal" (inappropriately low in the face of hypoestrogenism) or "low" gonadotropins points to hypothalamic-pituitary disease. A careful history and physical examination and appropriate laboratory studies are needed to rule out functional causes of weight loss, anorexia nervosa, exercise, use of drugs, etc.

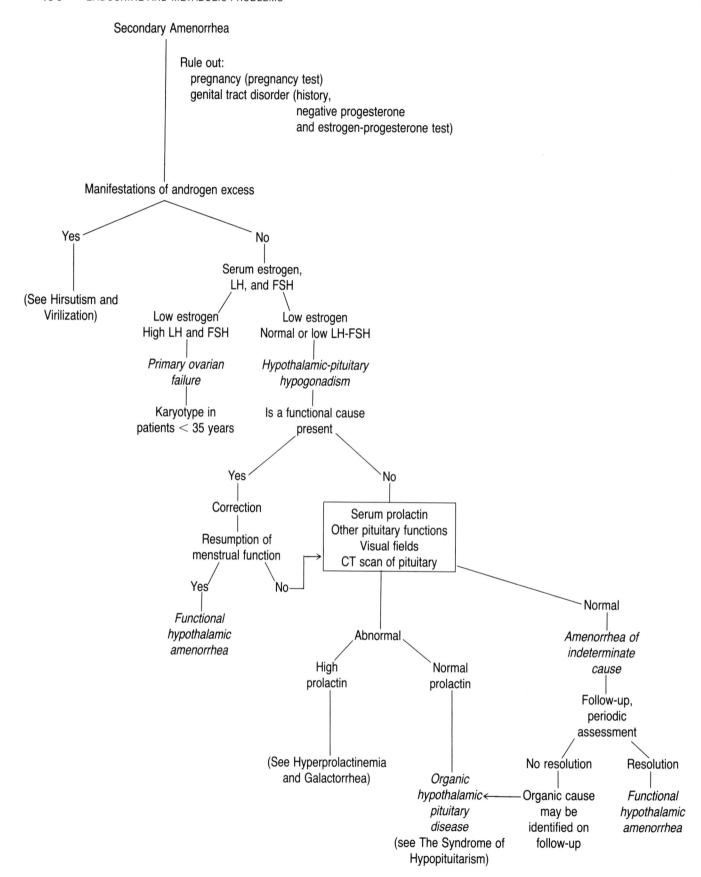

Fig. 11–33. Diagnostic approach to secondary amenorrhea.

Correction of the cause and resumption of menstrual function confirm functional hypergonadotropism.

Consideration of organic hypothalamic-pituitary disease is justified if evaluation is negative for functional causes, amenorrhea persists despite elimination of a recognizable functional cause, and other suggestive symptoms of hypothalamic-pituitary disease are present, e.g., features of hypopituitarism, features of hyperpituitarism, or evidence of a space-occupying lesion in or around the hypothalamic-pituitary area. Serum prolactin, other pituitary function tests, CT scan of the pituitary area, and visual fields are obtained. (For hyperprolactinemia see Hyperprolactinemia and Galactorrhea; for sellar enlargement see Enlargement of the Sella; for hypopituitarism, see The Syndrome of Hypopituitarism; and for functioning pituitary tumors, see Acromegaly and Gigantism, and Hyperprolactinemia and Galactorrhea.) If the investigations are negative, hypogonadotropism is labeled as being of indeterminate cause. Careful follow-up is important if amenorrhea persists. Periodic assessment of the hypothalamic-pituitary unit is in order because an organic lesion may become recognizable at some future date.

The diagnostic approach of secondary amenorrhea is presented in Figure 11–33. It is important to remember that the most common causes of secondary amenorrhea are pregnancy, use of the pill and other functional causes, hyperprolactinemia and other hypothalamic-pituitary disease, and polycystic ovary syndrome.

HIRSUTISM AND VIRILIZATION

DEFINITION

Hirsutism can be defined as androgen-induced excessive hair growth in the androgen-sensitive areas of the body of an adolescent or adult female. Virilization implies the appearance of masculine features in sex organs and secondary sex characteristics and results from a more pronounced increase in androgen stimulation. Virilization includes hirsutism, but hirsutism frequently occurs in the absence of virilization. These entities are important because they are considered disfiguring and cause considerable emotional distress, and they may be an early presentation of a potentially serious and life threatening disease.

Table 11–43. Causes of Hirsutism and Virilization

Endogenous
  Ovarian
    Polycystic ovary syndrome including idiopathic hirsutism
    Ovarian tumors
      Sertoli-Leydig cell (arrhenoblastoma)
      Granulosa-stromal cell
      Gynandroblastoma
      Lipoid cell tumors
      Gonadoblastoma
    Mixed gonadal dysgenesis
  Adrenal
    Late-onset congenital adrenal hyperplasia
      21-hydroxylase
      11-hydroxylase
      3-beta-hydroxysteroid dehydrogenase
    Cushing's syndrome
    Adrenal tumors
      Adenoma
      Carcinoma
Exogenous
  Drugs
    Androgens (Halotestin, danazol)
    Anabolic steroids
    Androgen-related progestins
    Metapyrone

PATHOPHYSIOLOGIC CONSIDERATIONS
(Table 11–43)

There are three general types of human hair. Lanugo hair is the dense, fine hair that covers the entire skin surface of the embryo and that is usually lost during fetal life. Vellus or downy hair is the short (2- to 3-mm), downy-soft, fine nonpigmented hair found widespread over the body and present over apparently hairless areas of the skin. It is present in both sexes in childhood and middle life, tending to disappear in old age. Terminal hair is the longer, thicker, pigmented, coarser hair. According to its site, terminal hair is classified into asexual hair and sexual hair. The growth of asexual hair is not dependent on androgen and therefore occurs in both sexes and in old age. It is present on the scalp, eyebrows, eyelashes, and, to a certain extent, on the arms and legs. The growth of sexual hair is dependent on androgen stimulation and includes sexual hair over the mons pubis, axillae, chest, and face. The degree and extent of sexual hair growth depends on the potency and concentration of the circulating androgens, the sensitivity of hair follicles, and the duration of exposure to androgen. Sexual hair growth is of two types. Ambosexual hair appears at puberty in both sexes; its growth is determined by low concentrations of androgens and comprises the sexual hair growth in the axillae and lower triangle of the pubic area. Male sexual hair, whose growth is determined by high levels of androgen, appears after puberty predominantly in the male, and it affects the face, chest, abdomen, upper triangle of the pubic area, inner thighs and arms, and, to a lesser extent, forearms and legs.

Hirsutism refers to excessive male sexual hair growth. It can be physiologic or pathologic (Table 11–43).

Physiologic Hirsutism. This form includes the mild hirsutism that occurs during pregnancy from androgens secreted by the placenta, and at menopause from the increasing androgen production by the ovaries in response to high levels of gonadotropin.

Pathologic Hirsutism. Since androgens in women are secreted primarily by the adrenals and the ovaries, one or the other of these two glands must be the source of excess androgen, except in cases of factitial hirsutism caused by exogenous androgens.

Idiopathic hirsutism accounts for most cases of hirsutism and results from a mild increase in androgen production of primarily ovarian, and to a lesser extent, adrenal origin. It is most likely a part of the spectrum of the polycystic ovary syndrome. The hirsutism is mild, appears at puberty, and is slowly progressive. Other evidence of hyperandrogenicity is absent. The patient maintains normal menstrual function and fertility. The ovaries are not enlarged, and the patient does not have evidence of adrenal dysfunction. The androgen parameters are normal or mildly elevated, and the ovarian androgen overproduction is gonadotropin dependent and is suppressible by exogenous estrogen therapy.

Polycystic ovary syndrome is the most frequent cause of ovarian androgenicity. Pathologically, the ovaries are either enlarged or normal in size, and they have thickened capsules and very small follicular cysts in various stages of atresia and hyperplasia of stromal cells. The cause is uncertain and may be related to derangement in the interrelationships between the ovary and the hypothalamic-pituitary unit. Increased androgen from any source (for example, congenital adrenal hyperplasia or Cushing's syndrome) may be associated with the characteristic ovarian pathologic changes. The syndrome can occur spontaneously or with a familial pattern (autosomal dominant with variable penetrance). It is characterized functionally by increased androgen production specifically by the ovaries and to some extent also by the adrenals; acyclic secretion of gonadotropins and anovulation with a high LH-FSH ratio; and increased circulating estrogens from peripheral conversion of androgens, uninterrupted and unopposed by progesterone, leading to a proliferative endometrium with adenomatous hyperplasia and increased risk of endometrial carcinoma.

Clinically, polycystic ovary syndrome presents as a chronic, slowly progressive disorder that usually makes its first appearance at or shortly after puberty. The common features include hirsutism, acne, oily skin, menstrual dysfunction usually in the form of oligo- or amenorrhea, and infertility. Most patients are overweight. Virilization is uncommon. The clitoris is usually normal though, rarely, mildly enlarged. Most patients have a normal pelvic exam, but some may have unilateral or bilateral ovarian enlargement. The androgen parameters are mildly elevated and the LH-FSH ratio is >1. The hyperandrogenicity is gonadotropin dependent and estrogen suppressible. Some patients have associated modest hyperprolactinemia and rarely a prolactin-producing pituitary tumor.

Ovarian tumors are a rare cause of hyperandrogenicity. The most common tumors are adrenal rest tumors, hilar cell tumors, and lipoid cell tumors. The presentation is usually with a rapidly progressive severe hirsutism and virilization, hypogonadotropism, and secondary amenorrhea. The androgen parameters are significantly elevated, and the hyperandrogenicity is non-ACTH and nongonadotropin-dependent and, therefore, nonsuppressible by dexamethasone or estrogen. Of patients, 80% have a palpable ovarian mass on pelvic examination. The anatomic diagnosis is by ultrasonography or CT scan of the pelvis, and confirmation is by pathologic examination of the surgical specimen.

Patients with mixed gonadal dysgenesis have an XO/XY chromosomal mosaicism, a streak gonad on one side and a testis on the contralateral side, and a phenotype that ranges from females with or without the characteristics of Turner's syndrome to individuals with ambiguous genitalia to normal phenotypic males. Approximately two thirds of patients are raised as girls; in these, virilization generally occurs at puberty. Diagnosis is made by the clinical setting and a chromosomal analysis.

Acquired adult or late-onset mild congenital adrenal hyperplasia refers to a group of disorders that result from inborn errors of adrenal steroidogenesis caused by mild and partial defects in enzyme activity. Such a level of deficiency of enzyme activity does not produce enough alteration in steroidogenesis to cause manifestations during fetal life and childhood and is not recognized until later in life and more commonly in women than men. Only three defects have been associated with increased production of androgens in later life: 21-hydroxylase, 11-hydroxylase, and 3-beta hydroxysteroid dehydrogenase deficiency (see Ambiguous External Genitalia). In these patients a partial defect in enzyme activity leads initially to a mild decrease in cortisol production and a compensatory increase in ACTH secretion by the anterior pituitary gland. The ACTH hypersecretion results in stimulation of adrenal steroidogenesis, which restores cortisol production to normal but at the expense of an increase in steroidogenic precursors. These precursors are shunted into adrenocortical androgenic pathways, leading to increased adrenal androgen production. The hyperandrogenic state is ACTH dependent. These patients present with virilization of variable degree and with menstrual irregularity. Most of these patients are initially diagnosed as having polycystic ovary syndrome. Those who have 11-hydroxylase deficiency may have hypertension. The diagnosis of late-onset congenital adrenal hyperplasia depends on documentation of the steroidogenic block by assessment of the steroidogenic precursors and on ACTH dependence of the hyperandrogenic state and, therefore, dexamethasone suppressibility.

Patients with Cushing's syndrome caused by Cushing's disease, ectopic ACTH syndrome, or adrenal carcinoma have increased androgen production in addition to the hypercortisol state. Adrenal adenomas causing Cushing's syndrome secrete cortisol almost exclusively and thus do not have the features of hyperandrogenicity. Diagnosis of hyperandrogenic state associated with Cushing's syndrome is based on the finding of evidence of increased cortisol production (increased urinary free cortisol), nonsuppressibility by the standard low-dose dexamethasone suppression test, and on other anatomic abnormalities characteristic of Cushing's syndrome. (See Cushing's Syndrome.)

Adrenal tumors are rare tumors that may be benign or malignant. They may cause a pure hyperandrogenic syndrome, in which the tumor produces androgens exclusively, or a mixed syndrome, in which, in addition to androgens, the tumor produces excess glucocorticoid or mineralocorticoid. These tumors can produce either weak androgens (DHEA-S) or strong androgens (testosterone). In general, they present with rapidly progressive hirsutism and virilization and secondary amenorrhea. The androgen parameters in the blood and urine are significantly elevated, and the hyperandrogenicity is non-ACTH and nongonadotropin dependent and therefore is nonsuppressible by dexamethasone or by estrogen. Diagnosis is made by radiologic documentation of an adrenal tumor and by surgical exploration.

Drugs including androgens, anabolic steroids, some of the androgen-related progestins, and the 11-hydroxylase enzyme blocker metapyrone can lead to hirsutism.

CLINICAL PRESENTATION

Signs

Increased sexual hair is apparent in the upper pubic triangle (male escutcheon), inner thighs, periareolar area, anterior chest, chin, upper lip, cheeks, arms, and legs. The skin may be oily, and acne may be present. Other signs in the more severe cases include frontal balding, temporal hair recession, deep voice, increased musculature, male habitus, and clitoral hypertrophy.

Other clinical manifestations are those related to the cause.

Symptoms

The patient usually presents with a complaint of increased body and facial hair associated with a feeling of disfigurement and consequent emotional distress. In addition, the patient may complain of acne, oiliness of the skin, and menstrual dysfunction ranging from oligomenorrhea to amenorrhea and infertility. In severe cases, the patient may also complain of breast atrophy, deepening of the voice, loss of femininity, an embarrassing increase in libido, and psychologic changes, particularly increased aggression.

DIAGNOSTIC EVALUATION

The complaint of excessive hair requires evaluation because the process has reached a stage abnormal to the patient's body image, and because underlying disease that may be potentially life threatening must be excluded. The two central questions in the diagnostic process are whether hyperandrogenicity is present, and, if present, what is its cause.

Patient History and Physical Examination

In the history and physical examination, attention is directed to determining the age of onset, the duration, and the rate of progress of the hirsutism or virilization; these are of critical importance in the differential diagnosis. The physician must also evaluate menstrual and fertility history; racial background, country of origin, and family history (for idiopathic hirsutism, polycystic ovary syndrome, and congenital adrenal hyperplasia); use of drugs; and physical findings of the type (villus versus terminal), pattern, and extent of hair growth, signs of defeminization, and virilization (including assessment of clitoral size), the presence of galactorrhea, evidence of Cushing's syndrome, and abdominal or pelvic mass. Note is taken of the patient's height (patients with congenital adrenal hyperplasia may be short) and blood pressure (hypertension may occur in Cushing's syndrome and 11-hydroxylase deficiency).

Diagnostic Studies (Table 11–44)

The following laboratory tests are indicated: serum testosterone; free testosterone; DHEA-S; estrogen LH, FSH, and prolactin; and a 24-hour urine collection for

Table 11–44.   Laboratory Tests in Hirsutism and Virilization

Tests	Determinant(s)	Hirsutism/Virilization	Comments
Serum Testosterone Normal, 20–80 ng/dl	Measures total testosterone (bound to SHBG 98%, free biologically active 2%). Serum testosterone is determined by production of T and by SHBG levels. Testosterone is derived equally from adrenal and ovarian sources.	Increased in 50–90% of all hirsute females. Cannot localize the source of the hyperandrogenicity. >200 ng/ml points to adrenal or ovarian tumor.	Fluctuations in serum T occur dependent on those of serum LH and ACTH. Best collect samples every 30–40 minutes three times and assay serum T in pooled sample.
Serum Free Testosterone Normal, 0.3–1.9 ng/dl	Measures free biologically active T. Is derived equally from adrenal and ovarian sources.	Increased in almost all patients with hyperandrogenic states but does not identify source of excess androgen.	Is not influenced by sex hormone–binding globulin levels.
Serum DHEA-S Normal, 200–500 ng/dl	A weak androgen produced almost exclusively by the adrenals. (>90%)	Increased levels are indicative of adrenal source of hyperandrogenicity. Normal levels point to an ovarian source but may be mildly elevated in some patients with PCO. Levels >3 times normal suggest adrenal or ovarian tumor.	Increased DHEA-S in congenital adrenal hyperplasia is dexamethasone suppressible while increased levels in adrenal tumors are nondexamethasone suppressible.
Serum 11-deoxycortisol (Compound S) Normal, 0.3–1.0 µg/dl	11-deoxycortisol is the immediate precursor of cortisol.	Increased in 11-hydroxylase deficiency congenital adrenal hyperplasia (dexamethasone suppressible) and in adrenal tumor (nonsuppressible with dexamethasone).	
Serum Androstenedione Normal, 0.05–0.35 µg/dl	Weak androgen derived from adrenals and ovaries in equal amounts.	Increased in hyperandrogenicity. Increased levels do not localize the source. Marked increase suggests ovarian or adrenal tumor.	Rarely elevated alone. Need not be measured.
Serum 17-hydroxyprogesterone Normal, 60–300 ng/dl	It is a cortisol precursor converted by 21-hydroxylase to 11-deoxycortisol, which is further converted by 11-hydroxylase to cortisol. Measured basally or 30 minutes after 0.25 mg of cosyntropin IV.	Increased basal levels in late-onset congenital adrenal hyperplasia: 21-hydroxylase and 11-hydroxylase deficiency (dexamethasone suppressible). Can also be secreted by certain ovarian and adrenal neoplasms (nondexamethasone suppressible). In late onset congenital adrenal hyperplasia, if basal levels are normal, hyper-responsiveness to cosyntropin documents diagnosis.	
24-hour Urinary Ketosteroids Normal, 4.0–17.0 mg/ 24 hours	Androgenic precursor metabolites: primarily from adrenal source. Accuracy of 24-hour urine collection. Check urinary creatinine, 1 g/50 kg body weight/24 hours.	Good screening test to rule out adrenal tumors and late onset congenital adrenal hyperplasia. >50 mg/24 hours points to adrenal tumor.	Testosterone is not a ketosteroid. Therefore, 17-KS is not an adequate screen for hyperandrogenicity or a reliable estimate of its degree. Normal ketosteroids do not exclude adrenal cause (testosterone-producing adrenal tumor).
Low-dose Dexamethasone Suppression Test	Give dexamethasone, 0.5 mg 4 times a day for 7 days. Test androgen parameters before and on fifth day of dexamethasone administration.	Dexamethasone suppressible hyperandrogenicity points to congenital adrenal hyperplasia and some patients with PCO. Unsuppressible hyperandrogenicity points to Cushing's syndrome or adrenal or ovarian tumors.	
Ovarian Suppression Test	Oral contraceptives in standard cyclic manner. Test androgen parameters before and during the third week of administration of the drug.	Suppressible hyperandrogenicity points to gonadotropin dependent cause, primarily PCO. If nonsuppressible, points to adrenal disease or tumor of the ovary or adrenal.	

urinary free cortisol, ketosteroids, and creatinine. If congenital adrenal hyperplasia is suspected, measurements for plasma 17-hydroxyprogesterone or urinary pregnanetriol (P3) are in order.

Dihydrotestosterone (DHT), the prime androgenic stimulus of the hair follicles, is synthesized intracellularly in the hair follicle from the precursors testosterone (T), androstenedione (AND), and dehydroepiandrosterone (DHEA). Since intracellular DHT levels cannot be measured at present, one has to rely on measurement of the circulating precursors T, AND, and DHEA. Hyperandrogenicity is always associated with increased production of at least one of these precursor androgens.

Plasma Testosterone (T). Plasma testosterone is derived equally from adrenal and ovarian sources. It circulates in two forms: 98% is bound primarily to sex hormone—binding globulin (SHBG); and 2% is a free, biologically active fraction that exerts the androgenic activity. Total testosterone can be affected by testosterone production and clearance and by concentration of SHBG. Free testosterone is independent of SHBG concentration and correlates well with T production. Since androgens can decrease SHBG, total T may not accurately reflect the amount of free T; therefore, free T is the best laboratory parameter of androgen production in the female. Total T is increased in 50 to 70% of all hirsute women, and free T is increased in about 90% of them. Increased testosterone is a measure of the degree of hyperandrogenicity but cannot localize its source. Since plasma T shows fluctuations dependent upon episodic secretion of the trophic hormones LH or ACTH, obtaining hourly plasma samples for 3 hours and assaying testosterone in the pooled sample is preferable. This is the best short-term estimate of 24-hour plasma testosterone level.

Plasma Androstenedione (AND). AND is also derived from the adrenals and the ovaries in equal amounts. Increased plasma androstenedione is another measure of hyperandrogenicity but cannot localize the source. Since plasma AND is rarely elevated alone, it usually need not be measured.

Plasma DHEA/DHEA-S. The adrenals produce 80% of DHEA, the ovaries produce 15%, and the rest is derived from hydrolysis of DHEA-S, which is produced almost exclusively in the adrenals. DHEA-S is the major precursor of urinary 17-ketosteroids. Plasma DHEA-S has replaced the 17-ketosteroids as an indicator of adrenal androgen excess.

Serum 17-Hydroxyprogesterone (17-OH-P) and Serum 11-Deoxycortisol (Compound S). 17-OH-P is a cortisol precursor and is normally metabolized by 21-hydroxylase to compound S, which is then further hydrolyzed by 11-hydroxylase to cortisol. In classic 21-hydroxylase deficiency, basal levels of serum 17-OH-P are increased (normal is 60 to 300 ng/dl); in 11-hydroxylase deficiency, both serum 17-OH-P and serum compound S levels are increased. Since the process in congenital adrenal hyperplasia is ACTH dependent, the elevated 17-OH-P and compound S are dexamethasone suppressible. On occasion the basal levels of these steroid precursors may be normal in patients with partial 21-hydroxylase and 11-hydroxylase deficiencies, but there is hyper-responsiveness to ACTH administration. Cosyntropin, 0.25 mg, given IV, and a plasma sample for 17-OH-P is obtained at 30 minutes. In the normal, the 17-OH-P level rarely exceeds 400 ng/dl. Patients with partial 21-hydroxylase deficiency achieve levels greater than 3000 ng/dl. It is important to remember that 17-OH-P and compound S can also be secreted by certain ovarian and adrenal neoplasms. However, in congenital adrenal hyperplasia, plasma levels of these steroid precursors are dexamethasone suppressible.

Twenty-Four–Hour Urinary 17-Ketosteroids (17-KS). This measures predominantly weak androgens possessing a keto group on C17 as AND and DHEA. They normally provide an index of combined adrenal and ovarian androgenic activity. It is important to remember that testosterone itself is not a ketosteroid although some of its metabolites are; therefore, measurement of 17-KS alone is not an adequate screen or a reliable estimate of the degree of hyperandrogenicity. It is a good screening test to rule out adrenal tumors in patients with hirsutism, because a 17-KS excretion of 50 mg/24 hours or more points to an adrenal tumor. However, 17-KS values should be interpreted with caution because a normal 17-KS does not rule out an adrenal tumor (in the rare testosterone-producing adrenal tumor).

Twenty-Four–Hour Urinary 17-Hydroxysteroids (17-OHCS) and Urinary 17-Ketogenic Steroids (17-KGS). These measure nonandrogenic steroids possessing a hydroxyl group on C17, primarily cortisol and its immediate precursors. The 17-OHCS include metabolites of cortisol, as well as 11-deoxycortisol. The 17-KGS include, as well, 17-OH-P and its metabolite pregnanetriol. These measurements are helpful in the diagnosis of Cushing's syndrome and certain types of congenital adrenal hyperplasia. In 21-hydroxylase deficiency, the 17-KGS are elevated while the 17-OHCS are normal. In 11-hydroxylase deficiency both parameters are increased. Urinary free cortisol (UFC) reflects the nonprotein-bound plasma cortisol and correlates well with the cortisol secretion rate. Increased UFC is the best single test available for the diagnosis of a hypercortisol state. Urinary pregnanetriol (P3) is the metabolic derivative of 17-hydroxyprogesterone; increased values are often helpful in identifying patients with congenital adrenal hyperplasia caused by either 21- or 11-hydroxylase deficiency.

Ovarian Suppression Test. An oral contraceptive is given in a standard cyclic manner. Blood samples for androgen parameters are taken before and during the third week of therapy. Suppression of the androgen parameters indicates a gonadotropin-dependent hyperandrogenic state and points to polycystic ovary syndrome. If no suppression occurs, the hyperandrogenic state is due to a benign adrenal disorder or to an adrenal or ovarian tumor.

Dexamethasone Suppression Test. Dexamethasone is given by mouth in the dose of 0.5 mg, 4 times a day for 7 days, and the androgen parameters are measured before and on the seventh day of dexamethasone administration. This test is designed to test whether the androgen production is ACTH dependent and, therefore, dexamethasone suppressible. Criteria for suppression is a reduction of 50% in the androgen parameters. If the hyperandrogenic state is not dexamethasone suppressible, it raises the question of Cushing's syndrome or an adrenal or ovarian tumor. If suppressible, it points to congenital adrenal hyperplasia, although androgen production by polycystic ovary syndrome can also be dexamethasone suppressible.

Diagnostic Approach

The diagnostic approach to determine the cause is outlined in Figure 11–34. A patient who has a recent onset and rapid progression of severe hirsutism associated with virilization and high androgen levels (greater than two times normal) should be suspected of having a tumor until proven otherwise. Ovarian tumors are best diagnosed by pelvic ultrasonography; adrenal neoplasms, by a CT scan of the adrenal areas. Rarely, laparoscopic visualization of ovarian tumors and selective venous sampling of the adrenal and ovarian veins may be needed for delineation of the tumor. In tumoral hyperandrogenicity, the androgen parameters are neither dexamethasone nor estrogen suppressible. If the diagnostic evaluation reveals an ovarian or adrenal mass, surgical exploration should be undertaken for diagnosis and management.

A high urinary free cortisol, in a patient with or without clinical cushingoid features, should prompt a standard dexamethasone suppression test. Lack of dexamethasone suppressibility confirms the diagnosis of Cushing's syndrome. Additional studies are needed to define its cause (see Cushing's Syndrome).

Hyperandrogenic manifestations dating to puberty associated with modestly elevated androgen parameters, increased urinary 17-KS and urinary P3, and increased serum 17-OH-P points to late-onset 21-hy-droxylase deficiency. Patients with 11-hydroxylase deficiency have hypertension and increased serum compound S. Patients with 3-beta hydroxylase deficiency have an elevated DHEA-S. Borderline steroid precursor levels in a patient with suspected late-onset congenital adrenal hyperplasia should prompt a cosyntropin test to document hyperresponsiveness of the steroidogenic precursor parameters. In all cases of congenital adrenal hyperplasia, the androgen parameters are dexamethasone suppressible.

The presence of hyperprolactinemia should raise suspicion of a prolactin-producing pituitary tumor. (See Hyperprolactinemia and Galactorrhea for Evaluation.)

Mild hyperandrogenicity of long duration dating to puberty with a slow rate of progression and without significant virilization, with modest elevation (less than two times normal), or with normal androgen parameters should raise the suspicion of polycystic ovary syndrome. Idiopathic hirsutism may be a part of the spectrum of polycystic ovary syndrome, and distinguishing between the two entities is not clinically important. Diagnosis is supported by the presence of normal or elevated estrogen levels, an LH-FSH ratio > 1, and estrogen suppressibility of the hyperandrogenic state. Pelvic ultrasonography (which may show normal or enlarged cystic ovaries) and laparoscopic visualization of the ovaries are not needed for diagnosis in the usual case.

Diagnostic Pitfalls

Hypertrichosis is a diffuse excessive lanugo or vellus hair growth occurring in androgen-sensitive as well as nonandrogen-sensitive areas of the skin. The causes of hypertrichosis include a variety of pathologic states, e.g., epidermolysis bullosa, Hurler's syndrome, trisomy, malnutrition from infection or malabsorption, endocrinopathy (such as acromegaly or hypothyroidism), metabolic causes (including starvation), anorexia nervosa, and porphyria cutanea tarda. Drugs such as phenytoin, streptomycin, hexachlorobenzene, penicillamine, diazoxide, glucocorticoids, and minoxidil, local causes such as nerve injury, local skin irritation and nevi, and genetic problems such as Cornelia de Lange's syndrome and congenital hypertrichosis can also cause hypertrichosis.

It is important to remember that the racial and familial background accounts for a wide range of normal variations in sexual hair growth and have to be considered in the evaluation of a complaint of excessive hair growth. Women of Mediterranean heritage origin may have normal downy hair growing on the upper lip and sideburn area, which within that ethnic group is accepted as normal but in another culture may be

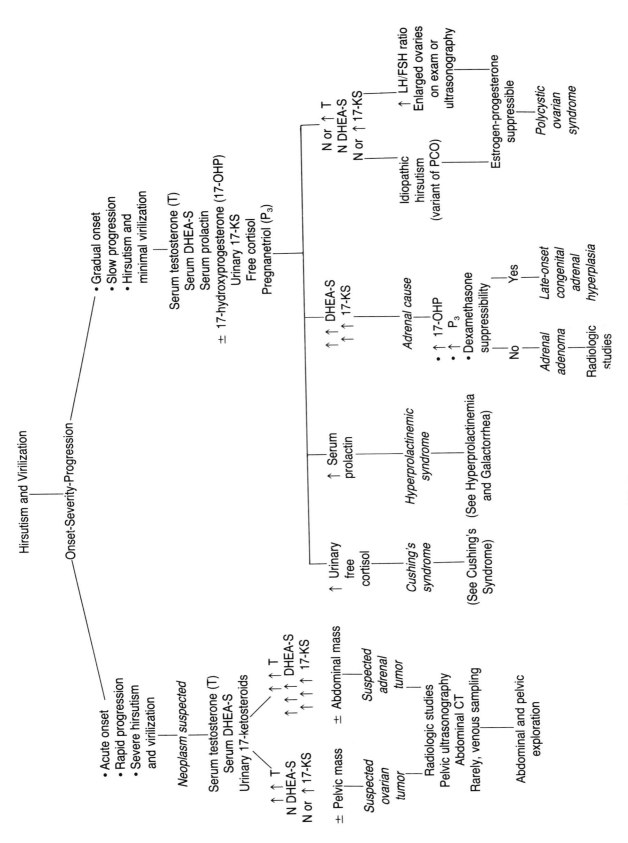

Fig. 11–34. Diagnostic approach to the cause of hirsutism and virilization.

looked upon as excessive. This type of racial or familial prominent hair growth is not androgen dependent, and the androgen production is normal.

HYPOGONADISM IN THE ADULT MALE

DEFINITION

Adult male hypogonadism refers to the symptoms and signs that result from deficiency of testicular function. Such deficiency may affect one or both of the testicular compartments—Leydig's cells and seminiferous tubules—and may present clinically as infertility, potency impairment, or other manifestations of androgen lack. The causes, manifestations, and diagnostic approach to an impaired hypothalamic-pituitary-gonadal axis will be discussed in this chapter. (For discussion of male infertility see Infertility, and for potency impairment, see Impotence.)

PATHOPHYSIOLOGIC CONSIDERATIONS (Table 11–45)

The testis has two anatomical components: the seminiferous tubule and Leydig's cells, each of which has a distinctive physiologic function. The seminiferous tubules contain the germ cells, which are responsible for spermatogenesis and production of mature sperm, and the Sertoli's cells, which subserve the hormonal regulation of spermatogenesis. Leydig's cells, which lie in the peritubular space, synthesize and secrete predominantly the male hormone testosterone and, to a smaller extent, dihydrotestosterone and estradiol. Testosterone plays the key role in male sexual differentiation; in maturation and maintenance of external and internal genitalia, secondary sex characteristics, and masculinity; in the development and maintenance of libido, potency, and ejaculatory capability; and in spermatogenic maturation (through its intratesticular effects).

Testicular function is controlled by the hypothalamic-pituitary unit. The neuroendocrine cells of the hypothalamus secrete a decapeptide, the gonadotropin-releasing hormone (GnRH), which stimulates the synthesis and secretion of the two gonadotropins, luteinizing hormone (LH) and follicle-stimulating hormone (FSH), by the anterior pituitary gonadotrope cells. The gonadotropins control testosterone secretion and sperm

Table 11–45. Causes of Adult Male Hypogonadism

Primary: testicular diseases
  Genetic and developmental
    Klinefelter's syndrome
    Male Turner's syndrome
    Noonan's syndrome
    46/XX male
    47/XYY male
    Functional prepubertal castrate
    Myotonia dystrophica
    Sertoli-cell—only syndrome
  Acquired
    Postpubertal testicular failure
    Cirrhosis
    Castration
      Trauma
      Surgery
    Irradiation
    Chemotherapy
  Male pseudohermaphroditism
    Complete
    Incomplete
      Androgen receptor defect
      5-alpha reductase deficiency
      Enzyme defect in testicular biosynthesis
      Lack of müllerian inhibitor
Secondary: hypothalamic-pituitary diseases
  Functional
    Systemic disease
    Malnutrition
    Anorexia nervosa
    Drugs
    Estrogen-producing tumors
    Thyroid disorders
    Adrenal disorders
  Organic
    Developmental
      Gonadotropin deficiency
        Isolated (Kallmann's syndrome, fertile eunuch syndrome)
        In association with deficiency of other pituitary hormones
    Traumatic
    Inflammatory
      Sarcoidosis
      Histiocytosis
      Granulomatous disease, e.g., TB
    Degenerative, e.g., hemochromatosis
    Vascular, e.g., carotid aneurysm
    Neoplastic
      Pituitary tumors
      Craniopharyngioma
      Glioma
      Other primary and metastatic malignancies

production by the adult testes, with LH regulating testosterone secretion by Leydig's cells, and FSH, in concert with intratesticular testosterone, regulating spermatogenesis. Normal testicular function is maintained by a closed loop negative feedback system that involves testicular hormones and the hypothalamic-pituitary unit. Testosterone is the specific negative feedback signal for the Leydig's cells compartment and modulates LH production by the anterior pituitary.

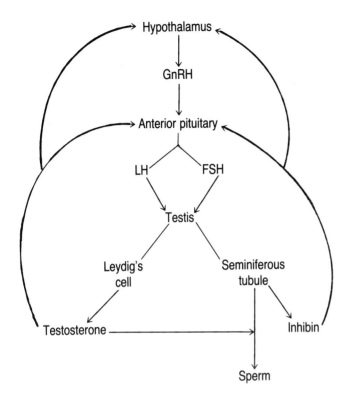

GnRH = Gonadotropin-releasing hormone
 LH = Luteinizing hormone
FSH = Follicle-stimulating hormone

Fig. 11–35. The hypothalamic-pituitary-gonadal axis in the male.

Inhibin, a peptide thought to be produced by Sertoli's cells, is believed to be the specific feedback signal that controls FSH production (Fig. 11–35).

In general, male hypogonadism can be caused by primary testicular disorder, gonadotropin lack because of hypothalamic-pituitary disorders, and peripheral tissue unresponsiveness to the effects of testosterone (Table 11–45).

Primary Testicular Disease. Klinefelter's syndrome is characterized by 47/XXY chromosomal constitution, hyalinization of the seminiferous tubules, clumping of Leydig's cells, small, firm testes and azoospermia, and varying levels of androgen production and masculinization. Buccal smear is Barr-body positive and karyotype shows 47/XXY. The usual presentation of Klinefelter's syndrome is failure of pubertal development. Infrequently and with lesser degrees of testosterone deficiency, the patient may present as an adult for evaluation of male hypogonadism or infertility. Males affected by 47/XYY chromosomal constitution are usually clinically normal and have normal fertility. Occasionally they may have tall stature, pus-

tular acne, antisocial behavior, and impaired gonadal Leydig and tubular function.

In postpubertal testicular failure, the seminiferous tubules and the germ cells are more sensitive to injury than Leydig's cells, and most postpubertal diseases affect spermatogenesis more than testosterone production. Among the causes of postpubertal testicular failure is myotonia dystrophica, a rare neurologic disorder characterized by myotonia, weakness and muscle atrophy, myopathic facies, mental impairment, frontal baldness, cataracts, and diabetes mellitus. Patients with myotonia dystrophica have normal puberty and normal gonadal function; later they develop the progressive hyalinization of seminiferous tubules, clumping of Leydig's cells, and testicular atrophy with infertility and hypogonadism. Another cause is mumps orchitis, occurring in adolescents or young adults, which may lead to tubular damage, hyalinization, fibrosis, small testes, oligo- or azoospermia, and infertility; if severe, Leydig's cell damage and hypogonadism may occur. Other types of orchitis include brucellosis, gonorrhea, and leprosy. Postpubertal testicular failure may also result from testicular damage caused by trauma, surgery, or torsion; and autoimmune primary gonadal failure which may occur as a part of autoimmune polyendocrinopathy (a familial syndrome that can also affect the thyroid, parathyroid, pancreas, and adrenal cortex). Also, irradiation for malignant disease can reduce spermatogenic function temporarily or permanently, though Leydig's cell function is usually preserved. Chemotherapy with chlorambucil, vincristine, vinblastine, and cyclophosphamide can depress spermatogenesis and, if prolonged, can cause permanent seminiferous tubule damage. Leydig's cells may also be affected. Another cause of postpubertal testicular failure is ingestion of toxic substances and chemicals in industrial use (e.g., insecticide). Also, chronic alcohol abuse and liver disease can lead to gynecomastia, impotence, and testicular atrophy caused by enhanced peripheral conversion of androgen to estrogen, by an increase in sex hormone-binding globulin and a decrease in the concentration of biologically active testosterone, and by a decrease in pituitary gonadotropin production and consequent hypogonadism.

Hypogonadism caused by hypothalamic-pituitary disease (hypogonadotropic hypogonadism) is discussed in detail in The Syndrome of Hypopituitarism. Gonadotropin deficiency may be an isolated deficiency in hypopituitarism or may occur in association with other pituitary function impairment. When hypopituitarism affects more than one hormonal axis, hypogonadotropism is usually the first clinical evidence of the disorder. Gonadotropin deficiency usually affects both LH and FSH and rarely one or the other. Gonadotropin deficiency may be caused directly by the disease process or indirectly by the suppressive effect of hyperprolactinemia. Hypogonadotropism may be functional, caused by suppression of the hypothalamic-pituitary unit in the absence of structural disease; this may occur with weight loss, malnutrition, anorexia nervosa, systemic disease, primary thyroid failure, drugs (especially estrogen), and estrogen-producing adrenal tumor. Alternatively, hypogonadotropism may be organic, related to traumatic, inflammatory, degenerative, vascular, or neoplastic processes affecting the hypothalamic-pituitary unit.

CLINICAL PRESENTATION

The clinical manifestations result from the hypogonadism itself and its cause. The usual symptoms are a decrease in libido, potency impairment, a decrease in ejaculate volume, infertility, and a decrease in energy level and stamina. Since adult levels of testosterone must be achieved to stimulate sexual hair growth, but relatively low levels are required to maintain hair growth, decreased hair growth and decreased frequency of shaving are present only in severe or long-standing hypogonadism; if the deficiency is mild or of recent onset, no change in sexual hair growth may be noted. On examination one may see the classic hypogonadal facies with pallor, fine wrinkling in the corners of the mouth or around the eyes, and sparse beard hair growth. Other findings include decreased muscle strength, decreased body hair, testicular atrophy, decrease in prostate size, and the possible presence of gynecomastia. It is important, when evaluating decreased facial and body hair, that the patient's genetic and racial background be taken into account.

DIAGNOSTIC EVALUATION
(Table 11–46) (Fig. 11–36)

The central objectives of the diagnostic approach are to determine whether the patient is hypogonadal, and if he is hypogonadal, to determine whether the hypogonadism is due to a primary gonadal disorder or a secondary hypothalamic-pituitary failure, and to determine the nature of the underlying cause. The diagnosis depends on the clinical assessment, knowledge of the likely differential diagnosis, and selection and interpretation of laboratory and radiologic aids.

Patient History and Physical Examination

In the history and physical examination, important clues to the diagnosis may be discerned. Attention should be paid to pubertal development, its onset and progression; development, extent, and recent change, if any, of secondary sex characteristics; sexual functions, including libido, potency, performance, ejaculation, and previous fertility; previous illness, testicular involvement, or surgery; and general health, with particular attention to the use of alcohol, and drugs, diet, and exercise.

In the physical examination attention is paid to facial appearance; height, body proportions, and span (eunuchoidism implies prepubertal onset of hypogonadism); secondary sex characteristics, body fat distribution, muscle development, hair distribution, and the presence of gynecomastia; genital examination including penile size, scrotal development, testicular size and consistency, and prostate size; and the presence of hyperfunction or hypofunctioning pituitary states, visual field abnormality, other endocrinopathy, and systemic illness.

Diagnostic Studies

The first step in the diagnostic approach is to obtain, if possible, a semen analysis. A normal semen analysis generally implies a normal hypothalamic-pituitary-gonadal axis. If the semen analysis is abnormal or if semen cannot be obtained for analysis, the next step is determination of serum testosterone, LH, and FSH. A low serum testosterone and an elevated LH and FSH point to primary gonadal failure. The cause is usually apparent after a careful history and physical examination. A buccal smear and karyotype may be needed for diagnosis of sex chromosome abnormality. Low serum testosterone and inappropriately low serum LH and FSH indicate hypogonadism caused by hypothalamic-pituitary disease. Investigations to delineate the cause of hypogonadotrophic hypogonadism are outlined in The Syndrome of Hypopituitarism.

The presence of hypogonadotropism should prompt a careful assessment of potential functional causes. If a functional cause is present, an attempt at its reversal is made. Restoration of normal gonadal function as a result of removal of the functional cause points to functional hypogonadotropism. Further testing is indicated if no functional cause is found, a functional cause is found but cannot be reversed, and hypogonadotropism persists after the removal of the functional cause. These additional tests should include an assessment of the other pituitary functions, ophthalmologic evaluation to rule out chiasmal syndrome, and a CT scan of the hypothalamic-pituitary area. Abnormalities in these additional tests point to organic hypothalamic-pituitary disease. If these additional tests are negative, the patient is said to have "hypogonadotropism of an indeterminate origin." Such patients should be followed at regular intervals because an or-

Table 11–46. Laboratory Tests in Male Hypogonadism

Tests	Determinant(s)	Male Hypogonadism	Comments
Semen Analysis	Hypothalamic-pituitary-testicular endocrine function and normal genital duct system.	Abnormal in male hypogonadism. See Hypogonadism in the Adult Male	Normal semen analysis implies normal hypothalamic-pituitary-testicular axis and normal genital ducts.
Serum Testosterone (T) Normal, 300–1200 ng/dl (RIA)	Normal hypothalamic-pituitary-testicular endocrine function. Normal sex hormone-binding globulin. Serum testosterone measures total testosterone: protein-bound T (>98%) and free biologically active T (<2%).	Low in male hypogonadism, but may be normal in hypogonadal patients with increased sex hormone-binding globulin (e.g., hyperthyroidism).	Serum T is secreted normally in pulsatile manner. Best obtain 3 samples at 30-minute intervals and assay T in pooled sample. Serum testosterone may be low in eugonadal patients with decreased SHBG (hypothyroidism, obesity, acromegaly).
Serum Free Testosterone Normal, 9–30 ng/dl (RIA)	Endocrine hypothalamic-pituitary-testicular function. Measures free biologically active fraction.	Low in male hypogonadism.	Not affected by conditions that decrease SHBG.
Serum Estradiol (E$_2$) Normal, 1–5 ng/dl (RIA)	Endocrine testicular function.	Low-normal or increased in primary testicular failure; low in hypogonadism due to hypothalamic-pituitary disease; high in hypogonadism due to estrogen-producing tumor.	
Serum LH and FSH FSH: Normal, <22 IU/L LH: Normal, 4–24 IU/L (RIA)	Hypothalamic-pituitary-gonadal endocrine function.	Always evaluate serum LH and FSH in relation to serum testosterone or semen analysis; in hypogonadal males, high values point to primary testicular disease, while low or normal values point to hypogonadism due to hypothalamic-pituitary disease.	LH and FSH are secreted in pulsatile fashion. Best obtain 3 samples at 30- to 40-minute intervals and assay LH and FSH in pooled sample. Low values may be seen in eugonadal males due to insensitivity of the assay.
GnRH Test Clomiphene Stimulation Tests See The Syndrome of Hypopituitarism			
Serum Prolactin (PRL) Normal, 0–20 ng/ml (RIA)	Endocrine function of the lactotroph of the anterior pituitary.	Hyperprolactinemia may be the cause of hypogonadism due to hypothalamic-pituitary disease.	See Hyperprolactinemia and Galactorrhea
HCG Stimulation Test	HCG has biologic activity similar to LH. The test is used as a stimulation test for testicular function; 4000 IU are given IM daily for 4 days. Serum T is measured before and on the fourth day of administration.	No change in serum T in primary gonadal failure. Qualitatively normal response in secondary gonadal failure.	Used in the differential diagnosis of cryptorchidism (normal response) vs anorchia (no response).
Buccal Smear	Scraping from the buccal mucosa stained with appropriate dyes and examined for Barr bodies (represent inactive X chromosome; number of Barr bodies is 1 < number of X chromosomes) and for Y fluorescence.	Useful in differential diagnosis of primary gonadal failure due to sex chromosome anomalies.	Presence of Barr bodies in 15% or greater of mucosal cells in a male confirms presence of extra X chromosome (Klinefelter's syndrome and its variants). May be negative in Klinefelter's mosaics.
Karyotype	Chromosomal analysis.	Identifies sex chromosomal anomalies, including mosaicism, causing the male hypogonadism.	May not show mosaicism present in tissues other than those examined.

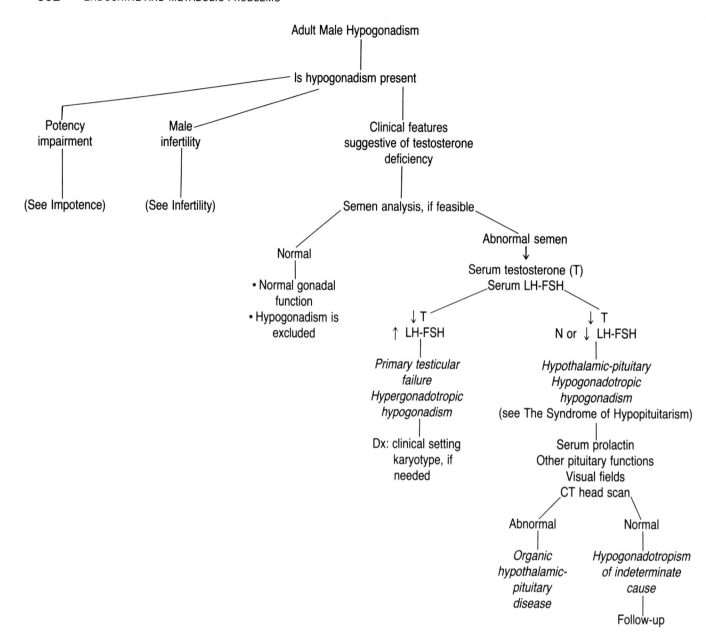

Adult Male Hypogonadism

Is hypogonadism present

Potency impairment

Male infertility

Clinical features suggestive of testosterone deficiency

(See Impotence)

(See Infertility)

Semen analysis, if feasible

Normal

Abnormal semen

• Normal gonadal function
• Hypogonadism is excluded

Serum testosterone (T)
Serum LH-FSH

↓ T
↑ LH-FSH

↓ T
N or ↓ LH-FSH

Primary testicular failure
Hypergonadotropic hypogonadism

Hypothalamic-pituitary
Hypogonadotropic hypogonadism
(see The Syndrome of Hypopituitarism)

Dx: clinical setting karyotype, if needed

Serum prolactin
Other pituitary functions
Visual fields
CT head scan

Abnormal

Normal

Organic hypothalamic-pituitary disease

Hypogonadotropism of indeterminate cause

Follow-up

Fig. 11–36.   Diagnostic approach to adult male hypogonadism.

ganic cause may be identifiable in the course of the follow-up.

IMPOTENCE

DEFINITION

Impotence is defined as the persistent inability to attain or to maintain an erection to conclude coitus successfully. It may be primary, when erectile function has never been established, or, most commonly, secondary, when it occurs in an adult male with previously established potency. Impotence may or may not be associated with impairment of libido or ejaculation.

PATHOPHYSIOLOGIC CONSIDERATIONS

A knowledge of the physiologic events underlying potency and ejaculation is important for understanding the disorder of potency impairment. Erotic stimuli induce an erectile response in normal adolescent or adult males. Two erectile centers are responsible for this response: a cortical psychic erectile center, which is responsive to visual, auditory, and olfactory sensations or to memory of experienced erotic events; and a reflex spinal erectile center in sacral spinal segments 2, 3, and 4, which is responsive to tactile stimulation of the penis and external genitalia via afferent fibers in the pudendal nerves.

The primary efferent innervation of erection is from sacral S2 to S4 segments via the pelvic nerves (nervi erigentes) and parasympathetic outflow. There may be a secondary center in the lower thoracic spinal cord involved in efferent innervation of erection.

Such stimulation induces the vascular component of erection, which consists of dilatation of the arterioles and closure of arteriovenous shunts of the penile corpora leading to turgidity and erection.

Ejaculation is a function of the sympathetic nervous system. Sympathetic outflow from the thoracolumbar spinal cord controls closure of the internal bladder sphincter (to prevent retrograde ejaculation) and transport of secretions of the prostate, vas, deferens, and seminal vesicles into the posterior urethra by smooth muscle contraction (emission). Impulses through the pudendal nerves cause contraction of the bulbocavernous and ischiocavernous muscles and expulsion of the semen from the posterior urethra in an antegrade direction (ejaculation).

Testosterone is essential for the initiation and maintenance of libido, for facilitation of the psychic-neurologic-vascular erectile responses, for the processes of spermatogenesis, and for the secretory function of the internal genitalia.

Hence, the ability to attain and maintain an erection depends on the integrity of the genital apparatus and on complex interrelationships and coordination of psychic, neurologic, vascular, and hormonal factors. Derangement of any of these factors, singly or in combination, can result in potency impairment.

The causes of potency impairment are outlined in Table 11–47.

Among the penile causes are included traumatic injury, usually associated with pelvic and perineal injuries; Peyronie's plaques, causing thickening and contracture of the tunica albuginea surrounding the penile corpora with loss of ability to expand; and destruction of penile sinuses by fibrosis that follows prolonged pathologic erection, priapism. Penile vascular insufficiency can result from aortoiliac vascular disease or sickle-cell disease. Neurologic disorders can cause impairment by effects on the cortical erectile center (anterior temporal lobe lesions), descending pathways, sacral cord erectile centers (e.g., spinal cord lesions, trauma, demyelinating disease, and tumors), and autonomic supply (autonomic neuropathy, as in diabetes

Table 11–47. Causes of Potency Impairment

Psychogenic
Organic
　Penile
　　Trauma to pelvis and perineum
　　Sequela of priapism
　　Peyronie's disease
　Vascular
　　Leriche's syndrome
　　Pelvic vascular insufficiency
　　Sickle-cell disease
　Neurologic
　　Anterior temporal lobe disorders
　　Spinal cord lesions
　　　Trauma
　　　Demyelinating diseases
　　　Tumors
　　Dorsal root lesions (e.g., tabes)
　　Autonomic neuropathy: diabetes mellitus
　　Autonomic injury
　　　Complete prostatectomy
　　　Rectosigmoid operations
　　　Aortoiliac and aortofemoral reconstruction
　　　Lumbar sympathectomy
Endocrine
　Diabetes mellitus
　Testicular failure
　　Primary testicular failure
　　Secondary to hypothalamic-pituitary disorder
　Hyperprolactinemic states
　Thyroid disorders
　　Hypothyroidism
　　Hyperthyroidism
　Adrenal disorders
　　Addison's disease
　　Cushing's syndrome
Systemic disorders
　Cardiac
　Renal
　Hepatic
　Respiratory
Drugs
　Barbiturates
　Phenothiazines
　Butyrophenones
　Tricyclics
　MAO inhibitors
　Antiparkinsonian
　Lithium
　Opiates
　Cocaine
　Alcohol
　Amphetamines
　Spironolactone
　Estrogens
　Guanethidine
　Reserpine
　Methyldopa
　Clonidine
　Beta blockers
　Diuretics
　Antihistamines
　Cimetidine
　Anticholinergics
　Cancer chemotherapeutics

mellitus, or surgical procedures leading to transection of autonomic fibers).

Diabetes mellitus is an important organic cause of impotence due primarily to autonomic neuropathy. It is estimated that one out of four diabetic patients will develop impotence and retrograde ejaculation. Vascular insufficiency may contribute.

Other endocrine causes of impotence include testosterone deficiency, whether caused by primary gonadal or hypothalamic-pituitary diseases; hyperprolactinemia, which is an increasingly recognized cause of impairment of libido and potency through direct CNS effects and through suppression of the hypothalmic-pituitary-gonadal axis; and hypo- or hyperfunction of the thyroid or adrenal cortex acting either directly on the erectile response or through secondary effects on the hypothalamic-pituitary gonadal axis.

Drugs are an important cause of erectile dysfunction, affecting libido or autonomic transmission. Their effects are often unpredictable, may vary from patient to patient, may vary with the dosage and duration of therapy, and are usually reversible by reducing or discontinuing the offending drugs.

CLINICAL PRESENTATION

Signs

Some patients may show evidence of the underlying psychiatric, neurologic, vascular, genital, or endocrine cause. In most patients with psychogenic potency impairment, there are no abnormal physical signs.

Symptoms

The primary symptom is that of potency impairment. It may be gradual or sudden in onset, situational (involving place, time, or particular sexual partner) or global (occurring in all circumstances), and periodic or persistent. The patient may or may not have libido, wet dreams, or nocturnal or early morning erections. It is common for patients to have associated psychiatric symptoms of anxiety, frustration, and fears about masculinity. Other symptoms are related to the primary cause of the potency impairment.

DIAGNOSTIC EVALUATION (Fig. 11–37)

Patient History and Physical Examination

A detailed history and a careful clinical examination will eliminate most of the causes of impotence from the differential diagnosis. The history is critical in the evaluation of potency impairment to determine whether the impairment affects libido, potency, or

ejaculation singly or in combination, and to ascertain the cause of the potency impairment. It is particularly useful in separating psychogenic from organic causes. History should be obtained relative to the use of drugs and alcohol and to relevant psychiatric, medical, neurologic, or surgical problems.

Premature ejaculation is usually related to anxiety in the sexual situation caused by unreasonable expectations about performance or an emotional disorder. It seldom has an organic cause.

Absence of emission may be produced by retrograde ejaculation following bladder neck surgery or spontaneously in diabetes mellitus; by sympathetic denervation (absence of smooth muscle contraction at the time of ejaculation) because of drugs, such as guanethidine and phentolamine; and by androgen deficiency. In retrograde ejaculation and sympathetic denervation, libido and potency are normal. In androgen deficiency, libido and potency are decreased. Diagnosis of retrograde ejaculation is confirmed by demonstration of sperm in postcoital urine. Anorgasmia (absence of orgasm), if libido and potency are normal, is almost always due to a psychiatric problem.

Potency impairment of a sudden onset that is concurrent with a stressful life event, is selective or periodic, is fluctuating or intermittent, and is associated with impairment of libido and psychiatric symptoms is likely to be psychogenic. Impairment that is of more gradual onset and more global character, is persistent, and is associated with normal libido is more likely to be organic.

Any occurrence of erection during the course of the complaint implies intact sexual apparatus, vascular supply, innervation, and endocrine milieu, and strongly suggests that the problem is psychogenic rather than organic. Complete absence of erection during the course does not rule out a psychogenic cause. Even if a psychogenic cause is suspected, the physician has to look for underlying medical problems causing or contributing to the sexual dysfunction. Normal or impaired libido can occur with either psychogenic or organic causes of impotence.

In the physical examination, particular attention is paid to evidence of systemic or endocrine disease; a complete neurologic evaluation seeking any neurologic deficit, including testing for pain sensation in the genital and perianal areas, and assessment of bulbocavernous reflexes; a vascular evaluation that includes palpation of the aortic, femoral, and more distant pulses including the penile pulse, auscultation for bruit over the aortic and femoral areas, and a check for postural hypotension and other evidence of autonomic insufficiency, a careful genital evaluation searching for abnormality of the penis, testicular size and consist-

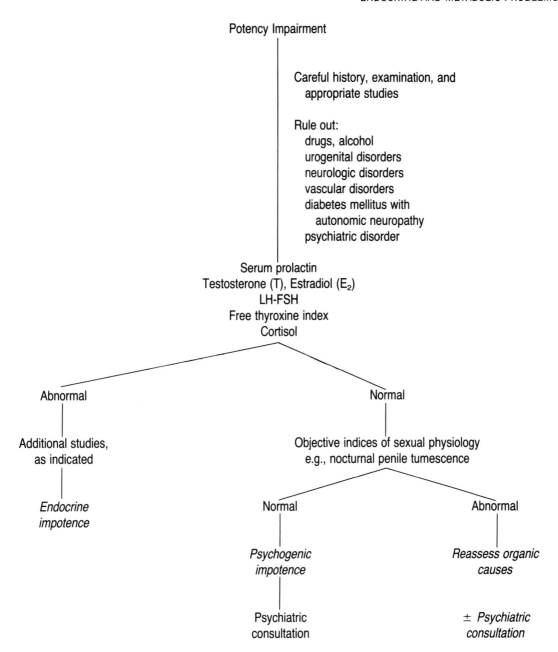

Fig. 11–37. Diagnostic approach to potency impairment.

ency, prostate size and consistency, secondary sex characteristics, or evidence of feminization or gynecomastia.

Diagnostic Studies

If after a detailed history and careful clinical examination the cause of the potency impairment is still not apparent, additional tests are in order. The physician should perform a serum testosterone to assess gonadal axis function. If the serum testosterone is low, serum estrogen, LH, and FSH should be ordered to delineate whether the gonadal failure is primary, tes-

ticular, or secondary to hypothalamic-pituitary disease. (See Hypogonadism in the Adult Male.) Serum estrogen will identify estrogen-producing tumors in the adrenal or testes. (See Gynecomastia.) Also, serum prolactin should be obtained. Hyperprolactinemia is not an uncommon cause of potency impairment and is a marker of hypothalamic pituitary disease.

Fasting plasma glucose, thyroid function tests, and serum cortisol should be obtained to look for other endocrinopathy. In addition, liver function tests, serum creatinine, and other tests should be performed as indicated by suspected systemic disease.

If the history, physical examination, and laboratory tests exclude identifiable organic disease, psychogenic potency impairment becomes very likely. The next step is the evaluation of objective indices of sexual physiology and consideration of psychiatric evaluation.

Examination for nocturnal penile tumescence (NPT) is done by placing a strain gauge behind the glans and at the base of the penis when the patient goes to sleep. From early childhood on, erections occur during sleep, normally 3 to 5 erections per night, associated with rapid eye movement (REM) sleep, adding up to a total time of 100 minutes of erection per night. Alternatively, the penis can be wrapped in gum perforated paper. Failure to break the perforation on 3 successive nights indicates absence of nocturnal erections.

Measurement of penile blood pressure to assess penile blood flow can be performed by using a small pneumatic cuff wrapped around the base of the penis and connected to a manometer with monitoring of the penile blood flow by a Doppler ultrasound device. The average values for the penile blood pressure are 100/55 mm Hg as compared to a brachial blood pressure reading of 120/60.

The bulbocavernous reflex response latency period is used to assess the integrity of innervation of the penis. Electrical stimulation of the dorsal nerves causes contraction of the bulbocavernous muscle with normal latency of 30 to 50 milliseconds.

All the objective indices of sexual physiology are within normal limits in psychogenic impotence. Presence of NPT rules out neurologic, vascular, or sexual apparatus dysfunction and strongly suggests a psychogenic cause. Absence or decreased frequency of NPT strongly suggests an organic cause, but it is important to remember that prolonged, severe psychogenic cause may inhibit nocturnal tumescence.

Only less than 5% of cases of potency impairment will remain undiagnosed after such a diagnostic evaluation. In these patients consideration of psychiatric evaluation and periodic reevaluation are in order.

GYNECOMASTIA

DEFINITION

Gynecomastia refers to enlargement of the male breast resulting from an increase in glandular and stromal tissues. It is the most common disorder of the male breast, accounting for more than 85% of male breast masses.

Table 11–48.   Causes of Gynecomastia

Physiologic
  Newborn
  Adolescence
  Aging
Pathologic
  Decreased testosterone production or action
    Primary testicular failure (see Hypogonadism in the Adult Male)
    Secondary testicular failure due to hypothalamic-pituitary disorder (see The Syndrome of Hypopituitarism)
    Inadequate bioeffects of testosterone
      Congenital
        Androgen insensitivity
        Reifenstein's syndrome
      Acquired
        Drugs
          Spironolactone
          Cyproterone acetate
          Cimetidine
  Increased estrogen production or action
    Tumors producing HCG (e.g., testicular, lung)
    Tumors producing estrogen (testicular)
    Tumors producing estrogen precursors (adrenal)
    Diseases with increased androgen conversion to estrogen
      Liver disease, especially alcohol-induced
      Thyrotoxicosis
      Marked obesity
      Hepatoma
    Exogenous
      HCG
      Estrogens
      Estrogen-like drugs
        Diethylstilbestrol
        Digitoxin
  Refeeding gynecomastia
    Congestive heart failure
    Chronic renal failure
  Hyperprolactinemic states (See Hyperprolactinemia and Galactorrhea)
Uncertain origin
  Drugs
    Methyltestosterone
    Cytotoxic agents
    Amphetamines
    Marijuana
  Idiopathic

PATHOPHYSIOLOGIC CONSIDERATIONS
(Table 11–48)

Gynecomastia is usually a sign of underlying disturbance in androgen-estrogen metabolism resulting in an increased ratio of free estrogen to free testosterone. It may be a consequence of a decrease in testosterone production or action, or an increase in estrogen production. The role of prolactin in the pathogenesis of gynecomastia is not well delineated at present. It may contribute by indirect means through effects on gonadal and adrenal functions. However, prolactin secretion is normal in most patients with gynecomastia, and most hyperprolactinemic men do not develop gynecomastia.

Pubertal gynecomastia occurs in about 60 to 70% of normal boys during puberty, typically in the 12- to 15-year age group. It usually regresses in 1 to 2 years. Although transient increases in plasma estradiol and prolactin levels have been shown to precede development of the breast enlargement, no hormonal abnormalities are discerned in affected patients with established gynecomastia.

Asymptomatic gynecomastia is found in 35% of normal men, and an increase in its prevalence is seen with advancing age. It can often be traced to pubertal gynecomastia. Varying but mild degrees of primary testicular failure and increased incidence of obesity (increased peripheral production of estrogen from androgenic precursors) probably contribute to the increased incidence of gynecomastia with aging.

Hypogonadism resulting from either primary testicular failure or failure secondary to hypothalamic-pituitary disease is frequently associated with gynecomastia. Serum testosterone levels are decreased and estrogen levels are normal or slightly increased. Gynecomastia is seen in the majority of patients with Klinefelter's syndrome, in whom it is associated with increased incidence of breast carcinoma.

Gynecomastia may be an early sign of underlying neoplasia. Tumors alter the androgen-estrogen ratio by several mechanisms: by producing excessive sex steroids or their precursors (tumors of Leydig's cells of the testis or feminizing adrenal tumors); by stimulating Leydig's cells of the testis to produce sex steroids (HCG-producing tumors, e.g., of the testes, lungs, pancreas, or GI tract); or by promoting uptake of sex steroid precursors with subsequent conversion to estrogens (HCG-producing tumors and hepatomas). Gynecomastia is an uncommon association of pituitary tumors.

Hepatic disorders, especially alcoholic cirrhosis, are a frequent cause of gynecomastia; patients with these disorders have reduced testosterone production because of hypothalamic-pituitary-gonadal axis impairment, increased hepatic estrogen production from sex steroid precursors, and increased sex hormone-binding globulin (SHBG) that adds to the decrease in free testosterone concentration.

Prolonged illness of any origin is associated with functional suppression of the gonadal axis. Recovery from such illness leads to resumption of activity of the gonadal axis and the appearance of gynecomastia, a phenomenon known as refeeding gynecomastia. This can occur with treatment of congestive heart failure, with hemodialysis for chronic renal failure, and with management of paraplegia. Refeeding gynecomastia usually regresses within 1 to 2 years.

Gynecomastia occurs in 10 to 40% of men with hyperthyroidism and is related to increased SHBG and increased peripheral production of estrogen from precursors. It usually regresses with restoration of euthyroidism.

Drug-induced gynecomastia is common. Several mechanisms can contribute, such as inherent estrogen activity of the drug (e.g., estrogens, digitoxin), increased endogenous sex steroid production (HCG), competitive displacement of intracellular androgen from receptors (spironolactone, cimetidine), refeeding gynecomastia (e.g., cardiac glycosides, antituberculous therapy), induction of gonadal failure (from cytotoxic agents), production of hyperprolactinemia with consequent suppression of the gonadal axis (e.g., methyldopa, marijuana, phenothiazines, tricyclic antidepressants), or a yet unknown mechanism (androgens and amphetamines).

CLINICAL PRESENTATION

The clinical presentations are those of gynecomastia and its etiologic disorder.

Signs

The increase in glandular and stromal tissues is readily distinguished from adiposity of the breast and other breast masses by palpation. Gynecomastia is identified by its firmness, its fine nodularity, its central location posterior to the areola, from which it spreads radially, and its well-defined outer border. The size can vary from a small subareolar button to a size approaching that of the normal female breast. It is usually bilateral and symmetrical, but there may be pronounced asymmetry. Tenderness may be present. In the early active phase the areola may be swollen. Expressible galactorrhea is rare and denotes a hyperprolactinemic state. Associated features are those of the underlying etiologic disorder.

Symptoms

The patient usually presents with breast enlargement that may be unilateral or bilateral. Tenderness may be noted in about one third of patients. Actual pain is rare. Very rarely the patient may complain of associated galactorrhea.

DIAGNOSTIC EVALUATION (Fig. 11–38)

Gynecomastia may result from a trivial cause or may be an early sign of serious illness. In all cases, the physician has to attempt to identify a specific cause.

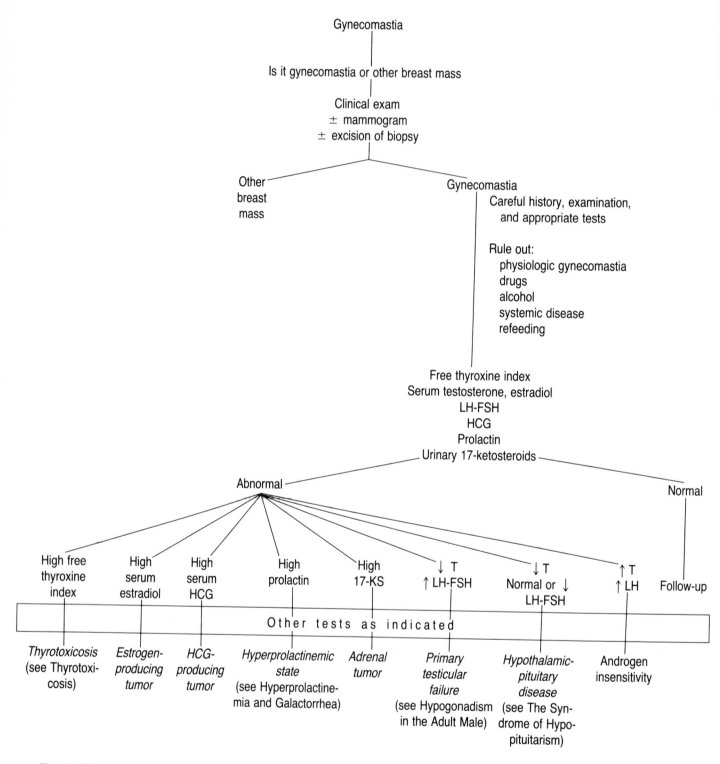

Fig. 11–38. Diagnostic approach to gynecomastia.

Patient History and Physical Examination

In the history and physical examination, attention is paid to the following points, which can be very helpful in differentiation between the various causes of gynecomastia: timing of onset, location, duration, and progression: a detailed inquiry into drug use, including alcohol consumption and marijuana use; stigmata of chronic systemic disease, malignancy, or thyroid dysfunction; changes in libido, potency, ejaculation, secondary sex characteristics, external genitalia, and testicular and prostate size and consistency; evidence of galactorrhea; and evidence of a causative tumor, e.g., abdominal mass, testicular mass, or tumor in or around the sella.

Diagnostic Studies

Laboratory aids are used selectively. These may include β-HCG to exclude an HCG-producing malignancy; 24-hour urinary 17-ketosteroids or serum dehydroepiandrosterone sulfate (DHEA-S) to exclude adrenal carcinoma; serum testosterone, LH, and FSH to assess the activity of the gonadal axis; serum estradiol to evaluate for sources of increased estrogen production, e.g., estrogen-producing tumor or peripheral conversion of androgenic precursors; serum prolactin as an indicator of hypothalamic-pituitary disease or the effect of antidopaminergic drugs; total and free serum thyroxine (or free thyroxine index) to rule out thyrotoxicosis; liver function tests and serum creatinine; appropriate radiologic studies, if a causative tumor is suspected; and buccal smear and chromosomal studies to confirm the diagnosis of Klinefelter's syndrome. Using mammography, a number of radiologic patterns have been identified with gynecomastia, such as the presence of ductlike structures; marked proliferation of the ducts occupying almost the entire breast; homogeneous density occupying subareolar breast tissue; and nonhomogeneous density in the subareolar area. Gynecomastia is symmetrical in relation to the nipple. The presence of a solid, spiculated, more eccentrically located mass in relation to the nipple raises strong suspicion of malignancy.

Diagnostic Approach

The first step in the diagnostic approach, especially in patients with unilateral gynecomastia, is the exclusion of breast malignancy. Carcinoma of the male breast is rare and accounts for 0.2% of all cancers in men. It is also a rare cause of breast enlargement. Aspects of breast enlargement that should arouse suspicion of malignancy include unilaterality, eccentric location relative to the nipple, unusual firmness, fixation, ulceration, bloody discharge from the nipple, and the presence of axillary adenopathy. Mammography shows a solid spiculated or eccentrically located mass. Biopsy should be performed on all suspicious masses and will provide the definitive diagnosis.

The next step is based on an estimate of duration of gynecomastia and the history of associated pain or tenderness. If the gynecomastia is of recent duration and the patient is symptomatic, investigation is necessary.

The two most common causes of gynecomastia in adults are drugs and alcohol-related liver disease. The history and appropriate clinical setting are diagnostic. Drug-induced gynecomastia is associated with recent use of one of the offending drugs and demonstrates regression, at least partially, on the drug's discontinuation. The diagnosis of pubertal gynecomastia is made by recognition of the clinical setting and the onset of breast enlargement in an otherwise healthy pubertal male. In general, no investigations are necessary, although occasionally the initial presentation of Klinefelter's syndrome is with gynecomastia. Patient's with Klinefelter's syndrome, however, also have eunuchoidism and small, firm testes. Their secondary sex characteristics may be normal or deficient. Serum testosterone is usually normal or low and serum LH and FSH are high. The diagnosis is confirmed by a chromatin-positive buccal smear or characteristic karyotype. Because of increased incidence of malignancy of the breast in these patients, periodic breast examination is essential.

The diagnosis of hypogonadism is usually straightforward. The patient has the characteristic clinical presentation and serum testosterone is low. In these patients, serum gonadotropins will differentiate the level of gonadal axis impairment and dictate the need for additional studies; high gonadotropins indicate primary testicular failure, whereas "normal" or low levels, in a hypogonadal patient, indicate hypothalamic-pituitary hypogonadism.

Feminizing adrenal tumors are usually malignant. Most patients will have a palpable abdominal mass at the time of diagnosis. In greater than 75% of patients, 24-hour urinary 17-ketosteroids are increased, and serum estrogen is usually high. A CT scan of the abdomen will outline the adrenal mass.

Testicular tumors producing gynecomastia are of two types: Leydig's cell tumors producing estrogen, which are usually benign, and chorionic germinal tumors producing HCG, which are usually malignant. Testicular tumors are readily palpable in most patients and the level of the secreted hormone is increased. For HCG-producing tumors, serum β-HCG is recommended. (The urinary pregnancy test, which also measures β-HCG, may not be sufficiently sensitive.) Leydig's cell tumors may occasionally be occult, and diagnosis may require testicular thermography, radioisotopic scanning, ultrasonography, or bilateral spermatic vein catheterization with measurement of serum estradiol. Other HCG-producing tumors may be clinically occult. In such cases, β-HCG-levels are elevated, and appropriate radiologic studies such as chest x-ray, CT examination of the chest or abdomen, and gastrointestinal studies are indicated.

Pituitary tumors are recognized by other evidence of pituitary dysfunction (hyper- or hypopituitarism), pituitary mass lesions (skull x-rays and CT scan of the hypothalamic-pituitary area), and visual field dysfunction (perimetry) if suprasellar extension of the tumor is present (see Enlargement of the Sella).

Refeeding gynecomastia is recognized by the clinical setting. It usually regresses in 1 to 2 years. Hyperthyroidism is suspected on the basis of the clinical presentation, the presence of goiter, and the possible presence of other mesenchymal manifestations of Graves' disease (ophthalmopathy or dermopathy). The diagnosis is confirmed by the increased levels of thyroid hormone (T_4, T_3 or both), and in borderline cases by the TRH test or T_3 suppression test (see Thyrotoxicosis).

After all studies, the cause of the gynecomastia will remain undiagnosed in some patients. Follow-up and periodic reassessment are in order.

INFERTILITY

DEFINITION

Infertility is defined as the failure of a couple to achieve conception after 1 or more years of regular sexual intercourse without the use of contraceptive measures. It is estimated that in the U.S. 10 to 15% of couples are infertile. Infertility in a couple that has never had previous pregnancies is referred to as primary infertility, whereas infertility in a couple that has had previous pregnancies but has failed to conceive again after 1 or more years is referred to as secondary infertility.

Pathophysiologic Considerations

For conception to occur, the male partner should have a normal hypothalamic-pituitary-gonadal axis for normal spermatogenesis and normal libido and potency; normal genital ducts for the transport and mat-

uration of sperm and provision of seminal plasma; a normal penis with intact vascular and neurogenic pathways to achieve potency, normal intercourse mechanics, ejaculation, and deposition of semen in the upper vagina; normal sperm motility to penetrate cervical mucus and traverse the uterine cavity to the fallopian tube; and normal sperm fertilizing capacity.

The female partner should have a normal hypothalamic-pituitary-ovarian axis to ensure normal ovulatory cycles, ovulation, and preparation of the genital tract for fertilization and implantation of the zygote into the uterus; and normal genital apparatus to pick up the ovum after ovulation and to transfer the sperm to the fallopian tube, where fertilization normally occurs, and to transport the resulting zygote to the uterus for implantation. For conception to occur, sexual intercourse with deposition of healthy sperm should coincide with ovulation. Infertility can occur as a result of derangement in any of these functions. The causes of infertility are outlined in Table 11–49.

Male Infertility. Varicocele refers to varicose veins of the spermatic cord. It is an important cause of male infertility, present in as many as one third of infertile males, and is the major correctable cause of male infertility. It is associated with impairment of spermatogenesis, manifested by "the stress effect," in which there is an increase in the number of immature and tapering forms and a decrease in sperm motility. Sperm count may also be decreased. The impairment is related to the presence and not necessarily the size of the varicocele. It is almost invariably encountered on the left side because of the long course of the left spermatic vein and its right angle junction with the left renal vein. A right-sided varicocele should prompt investigation to rule out vena caval obstruction caused by tumor. A varicocele should diminish with recumbency. If it does not, the possibility of obstruction must be considered.

Klinefelter's syndrome is characterized by hyalinization of seminiferous tubules and clumping of Leydig's cells; small, firm testes, azoospermia, and varying degrees of androgen deficiency, eunuchoidism, and gynecomastia; and Barr body–positive buccal smear and a karyotype of 47/XXY.

In Reifenstein's syndrome there is partial end-organ resistance to the action of androgen, and the phenotype usually shows a mild defect in virilization with hypospadias, gynecomastia, sparse body hair, eunuchoidism, undescended or scrotal testes, azoospermia, and infertility.

In cryptorchidism, one or both testes are undescended and lie within the abdomen or inguinal canal. Cryptorchidism is present in 10% of males at birth and in 0.3 to 0.4% of males at puberty. Spermatogenesis

Table 11–49. Causes of Infertility

Male Infertility	
Varicocele	35%
Seminiferous tubule disease	25%
Genetic, e.g., Klinefelter's syndrome	
Cryptorchidism	
Sertoli-cell–only syndrome	
Traumatic	
Physical	
Heat	
Irradiation	
Chemical: chemotherapy	
Inflammatory	
Orchitis, e.g., mumps, autoimmune	
Degenerative, e.g., myotonia dystrophica, hemochromatosis	
Idiopathic	
Ductal disease	10%
Congenital: absence of vas and seminal vesicles	
Traumatic: ligation of vas	
Inflammatory	
Prostatitis	
Seminal vesiculitis	
Epididymitis	
Endocrine disorders	10%
Primary testicular (see Hypogonadism in the Adult Male)	
Secondary hypothalamic pituitary disease (see The Syndrome of Hypopituitarism)	
Sexual dysfunction	10%
Potency impairment	
Anatomic defect of the penis, e.g., hypospadias	
Retrograde ejaculation	
Poor coital technique	
Unknown	10%
Female Infertility	
Ovulatory disorders	40%
Anovulation	
Hypothalamic-pituitary disease (see Table 11–41)	
Ovarian disease (see Table 11–41)	
Inadequate luteal phase	
Genital tract disorders	5%
Cervix	
Cervicitis	
Traumatic	
Conization	
Cryosurgery	
Overzealous biopsies	
Uterine	5%
Congenital malformation	
Inflammation	
Infection	
Adhesions (Asherman's)	
In utero exposure to DES	
Neoplasia	
Leiomyoma	
Endometriosis	
Tubal	40%
Congenital	
Acquired	
Salpingitis	
Surgery	
Unknown	10%

is abnormal, leading to infertility, but endocrine function and testosterone production are normal. Cryptorchidism may occur in isolation or in association with other conditions, such as Klinefelter's syndrome, male pseudohermaphrodism, hypogonadotropic hypogonadism, or Sertoli-cell–only syndrome. Cryptorchid testes are at an increased risk of malignant testicular degeneration.

In Sertoli-cell–only syndrome, the seminiferous tubules are lined only with Sertoli cells; germinal cells are absent, leading to azoospermia and infertility. Leydig's cell androgenic function is normal. The testes are somewhat reduced in size, and the karyotype is 46/XY. It may be primary or secondary to ionizing radiation and chemotherapy with cytotoxic agents. Mumps orchitis does not lead to permanent damage in prepubertal children. However, in postpubertal individuals, 15 to 25% develop permanent damage with progressive tubular sclerosis and hyalinization and Leydig's cell damage in severe cases, leading to azoospermia, infertility, a hypoandrogenic state, and small, soft testes.

Myotonia dystrophica is a rare neurologic disorder inherited as an autosomal dominant disease characterized by myotonia, muscle weakness, frontal baldness, cataracts, diabetes mellitus, gonadal atrophy, and mental impairment. In early adult life, testicular function is normal. Later, progressive loss of tubular function occurs with hyalinization of the seminiferous tubule and clumping of Leydig's cells, similar to Klinefelter's histopathology.

Ductal obstruction may be due to congenital absence of the vas and seminal vesicles, surgical ligation of the vas deferens, or postinflammatory scarring. The endocrine causes of male infertility are discussed in detail in Hypogonadism in the Adult Male. Essentially, hypogonadism may be of the primary hypergonadotropic (testicular) or secondary hypogonadotropic (hypothalamic-pituitary) type. Hypogonadotropic hypogonadism may be due to functional or organic disease of the hypothalamic-pituitary unit.

Sexual dysfunction accounts for approximately 10% of cases of male infertility. Such dysfunction includes potency impairment, penile disorders that make penile insertion difficult, poor coital technique, and retrograde ejaculation of semen into the bladder because of damage to the internal bladder sphincter. Infertility is unexplained in about 10% of affected males.

Female Infertility. Ovulatory disorders are among the most frequent causes of female infertility. Anovulation may result from abnormalities of the hypothalamic-pituitary axis or ovarian function (see Amenorrhea). Inadequate luteal phase, found in about 5% of infertile women, is defined as a luteal phase in which the endometrial histology pattern is more than 2 days behind the expected pattern for that day of the cycle. Its cause is multifactorial and may include subnormal FSH levels in the follicular preovulatory phase, suboptimal progesterone production by the corpus luteum, or decreased responsiveness of the endometrium.

Cervical factors account for as much as 10% of cases of female infertility and include cervical incompetence, cervical anatomic abnormalities caused by cervicitis, or cervical surgical procedure, e.g., conization. The role of cervical mucus is little understood. Poor mucus quality from infection, trauma, or estrogen deficiency may be associated with infertility. Uterine problems play a less frequent role. These include congenital abnormalities (e.g., absence or duplication of fundus, and duplication of cervix and uterus), leiomyoma, and intrauterine adhesions from previous endometritis, which can distort or obstruct the uterine cavity. Endometriosis is found in about 8 to 15% of the infertility clinic population. Tubal disorders are also common causes of infertility. Pelvic inflammatory disease (PID) is the most serious problem. It is estimated that after repeated episodes of PID, 50 to 75% of patients will develop tubal occlusion. Other pelvic and abdominal infections or surgery and use of oil-based radiopaque dyes for hysterosalpingography may lead to tubal adhesions.

DIAGNOSTIC EVALUATION

It should be emphasized that infertility is a problem of the couple and not just the female partner; the couple must be evaluated as a unit. It is essential to handle the couple in a careful, considerate manner because the infertility evaluation is time-consuming and tends to place many emotional stresses on the couple, who may be already stressed by the pressures of infertility. Because normal couples have an estimated 50% chance of pregnancy by the third to the fourth month of unprotected intercourse, a 75% chance by the sixth to eighth month, and an 85 to 95% chance in 1 year, the infertility evaluation should begin if more than 1 year has elapsed without conception in a normal couple, at 6 months if the partners are over 30 years of age, or earlier if the cause of infertility is obvious, e.g., if the female has amenorrhea or if the male has small testes.

Patient History and Physical Examination

In the evaluation of the male, a history and physical examination should give information relating to sexual function, libido, potency, mechanics of intercourse, and ejaculation; frequency of intercourse; use of lubricating gel, which may be spermicidal; age (sperm count and mobility gradually decrease with age); occupation—(exposure of the scrotum to factors detrimental to spermatogenesis, e.g., lead, organic chemicals, or excessive heat as experienced by truck drivers, bakers, cooks, and foundry workers); history of cryptorchidism or hypospadias; history of mumps orchitis, genital infections, traumatic damage, or previous surgery on the testicles and inguinal areas; medications such as sex hormones, antihypertensives, cimetidine, or chemotherapeutic agents; and systemic disease. The physician should assess the patient's androgen state, including a clinical evaluation of secondary sex characteristics and of development and size of external genitalia, testes, and prostate; and the physician should make a careful check for the presence of varicocele.

In the female partner, evaluation should include inquiry into gynecologic history including menstrual pattern, age of menarche, cycle interval and duration, and quantity of flow; symptoms of ovulation including mittelschmerz, intermenstrual spotting, increased midcycle discharge, molimina (premenstrual symptoms such as mood changes and breast tenderness), or dysmenorrhea; previous pregnancy, including spontaneous and therapeutic abortion, the interval of coitus without contraceptive measures, and the male partner at the time of previous conceptions; previous genital surgery, septic abortion or D & C, and previous pelvic inflammatory disease; and frequency of coitus, the use of artificial lubricants and douching, and coital techniques and position. During the general exam, particular attention is paid to the thyroid gland and the clinical assessment of thyroid function; to breast examination with attention to possible galactorrhea; to secondary sex characteristics including hyperandrogenic manifestations; and to pelvic examination to rule out congenital anomalies, endometriosis, and masses.

Diagnostic Studies (Table 11–50)

There are four basic analyses that need to be undertaken in the infertile couple: semen analysis, ovulatory function, patency of fallopian tube, and postcoital examination.

Semen Analysis. Semen analysis should be done as the first step in the evaluation of the infertile couple because male factors are common causes of infertility and because the test is relatively simple and inexpensive. Finding male infertility obviates the need for more expensive and prolonged evaluation of the female.

Semen analysis provides information relating to semen volume, viscosity, and pH, and sperm number, motility, and morphology. The normal semen volume is 1.5 to 4 ml. It coagulates immediately after ejaculation because of the coagulation factors normally produced by the seminal vesicles. When the specimen is

Table 11–50.   Tests in the Evaluation of the Infertile Couple

Test	Determinant(s)	Procedure	Comment
Semen Analysis Normal: *Volume*—1.5–4 ml. *Sperm number*—at least >20 × 10⁶/ml. *Sperm motility*—>60% with rapid forward progression (at least 2+). *Sperm morphology*—at least 60% normal. *Coagulation*—prompt *liquefaction* within ½ hour. *pH*—7.3–7.7	Normal hypothalamic-pituitary-gonadal function and normal male ductal genital system.	Collect sample, after 2–4 days of abstinence, by masturbation and put into a glass container. Do not use routinely available condoms, plastic containers, or coitus interruptus. Special condoms available if masturbation is not possible. Keep sample at body temperature and deliver to laboratory within 2 hours.	Volumes >5 ml or <1 ml can be associated with infertility. High % of immature and tapering forms points to presence of varicocele. Lack of coagulation relates to seminal vesicle absence or dysfunction. Lack of liquefaction indicates impaired prostatic function. Low pH suggest occlusion of the ejaculatory ducts. High pH suggest infection with urea splitting organisms.
Serum Testosterone (T), Serum LH, Serum FSH, and Serum Prolactin (PRL). See Table 11–46.	See Hypogonadism in the Adult Male Normal hypothalamic-pituitary-gonadal function.	See Table 11–46.	To determine presence of hypogonadism and delineate the level of hypothalamic-pituitary-gonadal axis impairment.
Basal Body Temperature Normal: Rise in BBT of 0.5–1° F or 0.3–0.6° C occurs after ovulation, attributable to increased progesterone secretion. The rise may be preceded by brief temperature fall. The normal duration of the rise is 14 days.	Ovulation, normal hypothalamic-pituitary-gonadal function.	Chart daily temperature on awakening in a.m.	Absence of rise in BBT in second half of the cycle is evidence of anovulation, but 10–20% of normal ovulating females show no BBT rise. In those with a BBT rise, check for the length of the luteal phase. If <10 days, it suggests inadequate luteal phase.
Serum Estradiol (E₂), LH, and FSH Normal: See Table 11–42	Hypothalamic-pituitary-ovarian endocrine function.	See Table 11–42.	See Amenorrhea
Serum Progesterone (P) Normal: Follicular phase <70 ng/dl. Luteal phase 200–2000 ng/dl. A plasma value >500 ng/dl indicates corpus luteum formation and ovulatory cycle.	Corpus luteum function; implies ovulation.	Blood sample. RIA.	Best laboratory measurement for delineation of ovulation.
Postcoital Test Normal: Normal spinnbarkeit >6 cm and maximal ferning; 5 or more sperm/high power field with good motility and linear progression.	Rising estrogen levels (determine cervical mucus quality), coital technique, and compatibility of semen and cervical mucus.	1–2 days prior to expected day of ovulation (by BBT), intercourse after 2 days of abstinence, examine female partner 2 hours later; for cervical mucus (spinnbarkeit, ferning) and number and motility of sperm/high power field in the mucus.	Normal response indicates adequate coital technique and favorable mucus. If mucus quality is suboptimal, repeat test in the next cycle. If no sperm is found (despite normal semen analysis), evaluate coital technique. If sperm are present with no or low motility, consider immunologic basis for infertility.
Hysterosalpingogram Normal: May show blocked tube(s) and distortion of endometrial cavity due to uterine anomalies, fibroids, endometrial polyps, and synechiae.	Anatomic integrity of an endometrial canal and tubal patency.	Best performed in follicular phase to avoid interference with or irradiation of early pregnancy. A gynecologic procedure.	"Normal" tubes may be present with partial tubal obstruction due to endometriosis and pelvic adhesions.
Laparoscopy	Anatomic integrity of the female internal genital tract	A gynecologic procedure. Allows direct examination of the pelvic organs.	Requires hospitalization and general anesthesia. Does not give information relating to endometrial cavity. It complements but does not replace hysterosalpingography.

allowed to sit, it should liquefy in about half an hour as a result of proteolytic activity by enzymes produced in the prostate. Viscosity is a measure of liquefaction. Semen should flow freely when poured; and if it does not, viscosity is abnormal.

The sperm number should be at least $20 \times 10^6/ml$ but preferably greater than $40 \times 10^6/ml$. A sperm count of less than 20×10^6 carries a less than 15% chance of fertility. Fertility is extremely rare with counts less than $10 \times 10^6/ml$.

Sperm motility should be greater than 60% within 2 hours of collection, with rapid forward progression of the sperm. The sperm velocity is graded on a scale of 0 to 4: 0 = no motility; 1 = tail movement but no forward progression; 2 = sluggish forward progression; 3 = more rapid progression; and 4 = fast forward progression. Normal sperm motility should be at least 2+.

Sperm morphology should show at least 60% normal oval forms. The role of structure in infertility is less clear; however, a high percentage of tapering or immature forms is often a clue to the presence of varicocele.

Zona free hamster eggs can be fertilized by human sperm in vitro. The test is useful in the assessment of the fertilizing capacity of human spermatozoa. The results are expressed as the percentage of ova penetrated. In fertile men, 14 to 100% of ova are penetrated by sperm, whereas less than 10% of ova are penetrated by sperm of infertile men. This test improves the identification of abnormal semen and may be a reliable predictor of fertility potential.

Ovulatory Function Documentation. Documentation of normal ovulatory function should be the first step in the evaluation of the female partner. Ovulation can be detected retrospectively by a number of clinical and laboratory means. Normal regular menstrual function is good presumptive evidence of regular ovulation. Midcycle pain (mittelschmerz) may be a symptom of ovulation but is noticed by only a small proportion of women. Other symptoms that imply prior ovulation are breast swelling and spasmodic dysmenorrhea, because both are related to rising progesterone levels.

The most useful clinical sign of ovulation is a rise of basal body temperature of 0.5 to 1° F (or 0.3 to 0.6° C) that follows ovulation in 80 to 90% of cases and is attributable to increased progesterone secretion. In many cases, the rise is preceded by a brief temperature drop that normally occurs about the time of ovulation. Absence of temperature rise in the second half of the cycle is evidence that ovulation has not occurred, although no rise is seen in 10 to 20% of women shown by other criteria to have ovulation. If the patient is known to be ovulating on the basis of

the basal body temperature, careful attention should be paid to the length of the luteal phase. The normal duration of the luteal phase is 14 days. Temperature elevation for 10 days or less is suggestive of a luteal phase defect.

An endometrial biopsy should not be done routinely. To confirm luteal phase defect, endometrial biopsy is performed in the immediate premenstrual period. If dating of the endometrial tissue is 2 or more days behind the date expected from basal body temperature or from the time of a subsequent period, a luteal phase defect is present.

The most widely used laboratory test to document ovulation is assay of progesterone or its metabolites in the blood or urine. A rise indicates corpus luteal formation and therefore implies prior ovulation. The height of the serum progesterone peak varies considerably, but a plasma value greater than 500 ng/ml or a 24-hour urinary pregnanediol above 2 mg is a reliable indicator of prior ovulation.

The most direct noninvasive assessment of ovulation is visualization by ultrasonography. Follicles greater than 12 mm can be seen easily and followed daily until rupture. Ovulation is likely once the diameter exceeds 20 mm. (This test is reserved for following the ovarian cycle during induction of ovulation by either exogenous gonadotropins or gonadotropin-releasing hormone.)

Postcoital Test. If the male partner has a normal semen analysis, and after ovulatory function has been established in the female partner, the couple is instructed to have intercourse after 2 days of abstinence. The female partner is examined 2 hours later for the quality of cervical mucus and the number and motility of sperm in the mucus. Normally, the rising estrogen level in the follicular phase, as ovulation approaches, leads to an increase in mucus production with increased water content, resulting in a clear acellular mucus with increased elasticity and decreased viscosity. Such mucus can be stretched greater than 6 cm, a phenomenon known as spinnbarkeit. The increased salt level in the mucus leads to enhancement of ferning capacity, which is the formation of crystals in a fern shaped pattern.

If the quality of the mucus is optimal (spinnbarkeit is greater than 6 cm and ferning is maximal) and 5 or more sperm with good motility and linear progression are found per high-power field, the postcoital test is considered adequate. If the mucus quality is not optimal, no definite statement can be made regarding the quality of the sperm; and examination is repeated in the next cycle. If the postcoital test reveals no sperm despite a known normal semen analysis, a careful assessment of coital technique is in order to detect abnormalities in intercourse mechanics. If the postcoital test consistently shows sperm with low or no motility despite a known normal semen analysis, consideration of an immunologic basis for infertility is in order, and sperm agglutinating and immobilizing antibodies are requested. It is important to rule out cervicitis if the preovulatory timing of the tests is good but the mucus is of poor quality. Cervical cultures should be obtained, especially for gonorrhea and Ureaplasma urealyticum.

Tests of Tubal Patency. The hysterosalpingogram gives information regarding tubal patency and distortion of the endometrial cavity caused by uterine anomalies, fibroids, endometrial polyps, and synechia. It is performed in the midfollicular phase to avoid interference with or irradiation of an early pregnancy and to avoid the false impression of tubal obstruction given by the secretory endometrium, which is thick enough to block the cornua. Hysterosalpingogram can miss pelvic adhesions or endometriosis if the tubal blockage is not sufficient to show on the radiologic study.

Diagnostic Approach

The first step in the evaluation in the male partner is the semen analysis. A normal semen analysis indicates a normal male hypothalamic-pituitary-gonadal axis and genital tract, in which case further evaluation of the male partner can be halted.

If the semen analysis is abnormal, repeat analyses (at least 2 to 3 months apart) are in order, because marked variations in several of the parameters may be seen in normal individuals, and normal fertile men can have transient abnormalities in the semen analysis owing to stress, infection, or environmental factors. It is important to remember that approximately 3 months are required for completion of the spermatogenic cycle and movement of the maturing spermatozoa through the ductal system.

Oligospermia refers to a sperm count less than 20 $\times$ 10^6/ml with motility less than 50% and motility grade 2 or less associated with a decreased number of normal forms. Azoospermia refers to absence of sperm in the ejaculate. An abnormal semen analysis may have a normal sperm count but abnormal morphology and motility.

If oligospermia or azoospermia is found, the next step is the evaluation of the hypothalamic-pituitary-gonadal endocrine axis by measurements of serum testosterone, LH, and FSH (Figs. 11–39 and 11–40).

Low serum testosterone and high serum LH and FSH indicates primary testicular failure involving both the Leydig and the seminiferous tubule compartments of the testes. In an azoospermic individual with these findings, a karyotype is justified to rule out Klinefelter's syndrome or its variants.

Normal serum testosterone and LH and a high serum FSH indicate primary seminiferous tubule failure, inhibin deficiency causing the rise in serum FSH, and normal Leydig's cell function.

Low serum testosterone and inappropriately low serum FSH and LH indicate hypogonadotropic hypogonadism caused by hypothalamic-pituitary disease. Additional studies should include a check for anosmia (Kallmann's syndrome), serum prolactin, and other pituitary functions, sellar x-rays and CT scan of the hypothalamic-pituitary area, and evaluation of visual fields (see The Syndrome of Hypopituitarism).

Normal serum testosterone, LH, and FSH in an azoospermic individual point to either seminiferous tubule failure or obstruction of the ejaculatory system. Recognition of obstruction of the ejaculatory system is important because of the potential for surgical correction. Seminal fructose is produced by the seminal vesicles and transported into the vas deferens by the ejaculatory ducts; absence of fructose usually indicates congenital absence of the vas deferens and seminal vesicles (if the vas cannot be palpated) or acquired obstruction of the ejaculatory ducts (if the vas can be palpated). Normal semen fructose levels imply either obstruction of the ductal system proximal to entry of the ejaculatory ducts, or germ cell arrest as a cause of the azoospermia: the definitive diagnostic tool is the testicular biopsy with vasography.

Normal serum testosterone, LH, and FSH seen in the majority of oligospermic individuals should lead to consideration of varicocele, genital infection, or idiopathic oligospermia. Varicocele is confirmed by careful clinical examination; diagnosis of genital infection is established by microscopic examination of the prostatic fluid, examination of the urine passed after prostate massage, and culture of the urine, prostate fluid, and semen.

High-normal or high serum testosterone and serum LH and normal serum FSH indicate partial androgen resistance; this finding is supported by other evidence of male pseudohermaphrodism (for example, hypospadias). Definitive diagnosis is by special studies of tissue androgen receptors.

Patients with a normal sperm count but abnormal structure and motility usually have structural or functional sperm abnormalities or a hostile sperm environment. Presence of inflammatory cells in the semen suggest infection and should prompt appropriate culture. Sperm agglutination may point to the presence of antisperm antibodies, although the relationship of antibodies to infertility is not unequivocally established.

If the semen analysis of the male partner is normal, attention is directed toward assessment of the men-

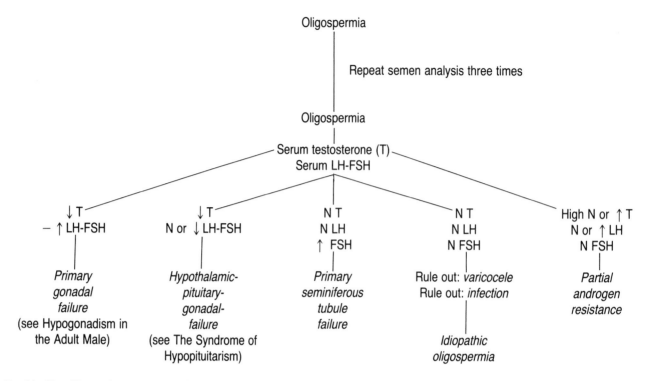

Fig. 11–39. Diagnostic approach to oligospermia.

strual and ovulatory function of the female partner (Fig. 11–41).

If amenorrhea is present, the diagnostic steps are as outlined in Amenorrhea. In the presence of menstrual function, evidence of ovulation is sought. If it is present, the adequacy of the luteal phase can be judged by basal body temperature, endometrial biopsy, or both. If the luteal phase is adequate, attention is paid to the exclusion of pelvic factors by a careful history, hysterosalpingographic study, and, if needed, a laparoscopic study to define cervical, uterine, or tubal factors.

If the patient is amenorrheic, a serum prolactin is determined. Hyperprolactinemia dictates diagnostic steps as outlined in Hyperprolactinemia and Galactorrhea. A normal serum prolactin should prompt a determination of serum estrogen, LH, and FSH. Low serum estrogen and high serum LH and FSH point to primary ovarian failure. Normal serum estrogen and a high LH-FSH ratio strongly suggest the presence of polycystic ovary syndrome. Normal or low serum estrogen, LH, and FSH in an amenorrheic patient should prompt evaluation for hypopituitarism and causative hypothalamic-pituitary disease (see The Syndrome of Hypopituitarism). Presence of hyperandrogenic manifestations dictates the diagnostic steps outlined in Hirsutism and Virilization.

After a thorough evaluation of the infertile couple, 10 to 20% of couples will have no identifiable cause

for their infertility, reflecting our lack of complete knowledge of the cause of infertility.

DELAYED PUBERTY IN MALES

DEFINITION

Any boy 14 years of age or more without signs of pubertal development is considered to have delayed puberty.

PATHOPHYSIOLOGIC CONSIDERATIONS
(Table 11–51)

Normally, in infancy and childhood, the hypothalamic-pituitary-testicular axis functions at a low level because of dominant CNS inhibition, which renders gonadotropin secretion extremely sensitive to negative inhibition by low levels of gonadal steroids. At an age appropriate for the individual, puberty begins, CNS inhibition declines, and gonadotropin levels rise, leading to the development of Leydig's cell and seminiferous tubular testicular compartments. This process results in a progressive rise of testosterone secretion

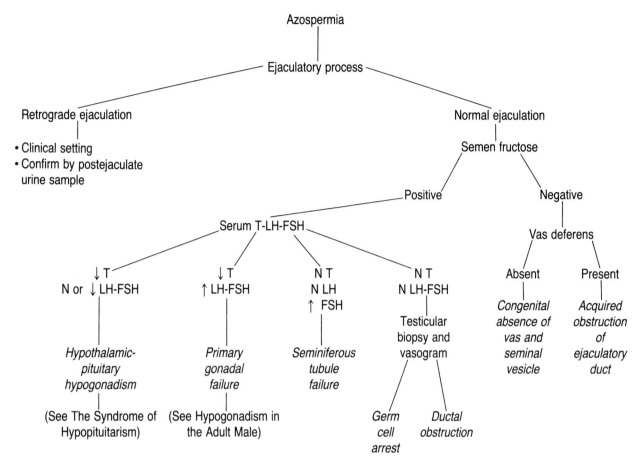

Fig. 11–40. Diagnostic approach to azoospermia.

and initiation of spermatogenic function, enlargement of the testes, and the initiation and completion of pubertal development. Studies in growth and development have shown that the upper age limit in normal boys for the first evidence of testicular enlargement is 13.9 years, for the first appearance of pubic hair is 15.2 years, for enlargement of the penis is 15.5 years, and for peak growth and velocity is 15.9 years. Delayed puberty is caused by failure of pubertal rise in testosterone that may be caused by a lesion at the hypothalamic-pituitary level (hypogonadotropic failure) or at the gonadal level (hypergonadotropic failure).

Constitutional delay in puberty is, by far, the most common cause. This delayed maturation may be genetic, and either parent or a sibling may have experienced a similar delay. The patient shows evidence of delayed growth throughout childhood, a history of always being shorter than age-matched peers, delayed development by bone age and of normal growth velocity for bone age. Generally, signs of puberty will appear after the patient reaches a skeletal age of 12 years, and patients will almost always manifest secondary sex development by 18 years of chronologic age, ultimately progressing through the normal stages of puberty to normal maturation.

Klinefelter's syndrome (seminiferous tubule dysgenesis) is the most frequent sexual chromosomal abnormality. In classic Klinefelter's syndrome, the karyotype is 47/XXY, there is hyalinization of the seminiferous tubules and clumping of Leydig's cells, and the testes are small and firm. The patients have varying degrees of testosterone production and masculinization, azoospermia and infertility, eunuchoid features, except that the ratio of arm span to height is less than 1, gynecomastia with increased incidence of breast cancer, and increased association with diabetes mellitus, varicose veins, and thyroid and mental abnormalities. Klinefelter's variants with chromosomal findings of one to four X and one to two Y chromosomes have comparable clinical features, with increased incidence of somatic abnormalities and mental retardation. Klinefelter's mosaics do occur, e.g., 46,XX/47,XXY; in these patients, the clinical picture is variable, depending on the chromosomal constitution of the testes. If the testes have an XY line, the patient may have normal gonadal functions and be fertile.

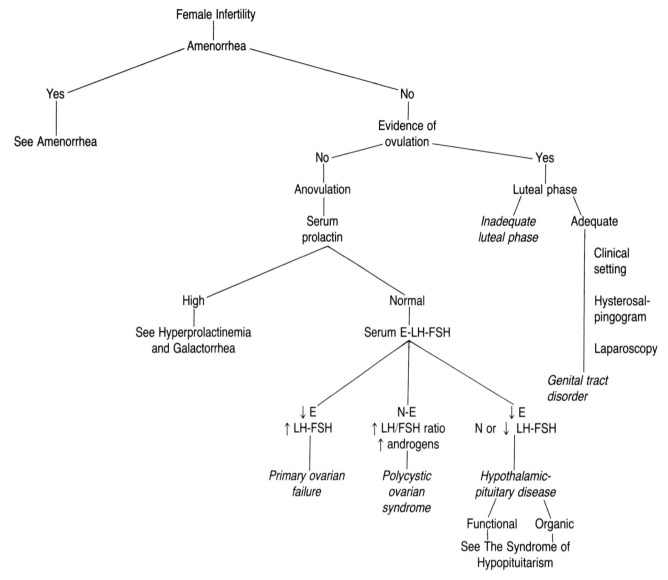

Fig. 11–41. Diagnostic approach to female infertility.

Anorchia is characterized by absence of both testes in phenotypic males with a 46/XY chromosomal constitution. It is rare and its cause is indeterminate. The scrotum is empty, the epididymis is normal or absent, and other internal genitalia are normal. Administration of HCG does not cause a rise in serum testosterone (which helps in the differential diagnosis from bilateral cryptorchid intra-abdominal testes, in which a rise in testosterone does occur). In male Turner's syndrome, the karyotype is 45,XO/46,XY, or other forms of mosaicism. The testes are generally undescended and hypoplastic, and the patient has the same somatic manifestations as the classic Turner's 45/XO (see Amenorrhea). In male Noonan's syndrome the patient usually has a normal male karyotype and phenotype with testes that are normal and descended and normal

pubertal development. Some patients, however, may have undescended and dysplastic testes and consequently may exhibit hypogonadism and azoospermia. Turner's stigmata may be present. Acquired causes of primary testicular failure include traumatic, vascular, and inflammatory causes and the testicular damage that follows radiation and chemotherapy (see Hypogonadism in the Adult Male).

Hypothalamic-pituitary hypogonadotropic hypogonadism may be caused by organic or functional impairment of the hypothalamic-pituitary unit. In organic hypogonadotropism, features may include other pituitary dysfunction and features of the underlying disease. Craniopharyngioma is the most common space-occupying lesion leading to sexual infantilism (see Enlargement of the Sella). Other parasellar tumors such as

Table 11–51. Causes of Delayed Puberty in Males

Constitutional
Testicular disease—primary hypogonadism
  Genetic and developmental
    Klinefelter's syndrome
    Male Turner's syndrome
    Noonan's syndrome
    XX male
    XYY male
    Anorchia
    Male pseudohermaphroditism
  Acquired
    Traumatic
    Vascular
    Infectious
    Irradiation
    Chemotherapy
Hypothalamic pituitary disease—secondary hypogonadism
  Functional
    Systemic disease
    Malnutrition
    Anorexia nervosa
    Drugs
  Organic
    Developmental
      Gonadotropin deficiency
        Isolated
          Kallmann's syndrome
          Fertile eunuch
        In association with deficiency of other
          pituitary hormones
      Prader-Willi syndrome
      Laurence-Moon-Biedl syndrome
    Traumatic
    Inflammatory
      Histiocytosis X
      Granulomatous, e.g., TB
      Sarcoidosis
    Neoplastic, e.g., craniopharyngioma, optic glioma, pituitary tumors

germinoma, glioma, and astrocytoma may occur. Pituitary tumors are rare in children. CNS disorders such as histiocytosis X, sarcoidosis, postinfectious inflammatory lesions, trauma (e.g., stalk section), and developmental defects (e.g., optic dysplasia) may be associated with hypogonadotropism.

Isolated gonadotropin deficiency is most commonly due to Kallmann's syndrome. This is a familial disorder with variable manifestations, classically presenting with anosmia with or without hypogonadotropism. The inheritance pattern varies, being X-linked or autosomal dominant with variable penetrance. The great majority of affected patients are males. Hyposmia or anosmia are caused by hypoplasia or aplasia of the olfactory lobe, and the hypogonadism is due to failure of GnRH production. Other skeletal abnormalities include craniofacial abnormalities, syndactyly, short fourth metacarpal, color blindness, nerve deafness, cryptorchidism, and, frequently, mental re-

tardation. A prepubertal manifestation of the syndrome is microphallus, in which the size of the penis is below the fifth percentile for the age.

Other causes of gonadotropin lack include sporadic or autosomal recessive disorder with associated somatic and genital abnormalities but with normal sense of smell. In the fertile eunuch there is deficiency of LH leading to Leydig's cell hypoplasia, decreased testosterone production, and masculinization; FSH production is normal, and the testes are relatively normal in size with recognizable spermatogenesis. The Prader-Willi syndrome is a sporadic disorder associated with deletion or translocation of chromosome 15. It is characterized by infantile hypotonia, short stature, obesity, characteristic hypotonia, small hands and feet, mental retardation, microphallus, and cryptorchidism. Laurence-Moon-Biedl syndrome is an autosomal recessive disorder characterized by polydactyly, obesity, short stature, mental retardation, retinitis pigmentosa, and hypogonadism, either hypogonadotropic or hypergonadotropic.

CLINICAL PRESENTATION

The clinical manifestations are due to hypogonadism and to its cause.

The features of hypogonadism are related to the failure of sexual and physical maturation. There is failure of growth of the external genitalia and failure of development of male secondary sexual characteristics, libido, potentia, and wet dreams. The pubertal growth spurt does not occur. In some cases, hypogonadism is associated with the development of gynecomastia. On examination, the patient presents with a childish appearance. A eunuchoid habitus is usually present unless there is associated growth hormone lack. Because the androgen-mediated growth spurt fails to occur, the epiphyseal plates of long bones continue to grow under the influence of growth hormone and somatomedins. The long bones of the upper and the lower extremities grow out of proportion to the axial skeleton such that the ratio of the upper to the lower (pubis to floor) segment is less than 1, and the ratio of span to height is greater than 1. In addition there is a high-pitched childish voice, poor muscle development, a female pattern of fat distribution, absence or sparsity of sexual hair, small prepubertal genitalia, and a small prostate. The testes may be scrotal or undescended, and the scrotal testes may be soft or rubbery. Small, firm testes point to Klinefelter's syndrome. It is important to test the sense of smell for hyposmia or anosmia, which, if present, point to Kallmann's syndrome.

DIAGNOSTIC EVALUATION (Fig. 11–42)

The objectives of the diagnostic approach are to determine whether delayed puberty is present, and if present, what is its underlying cause. In the history and physical examination, attention is paid to the following points: previous illness, particularly testicular involvement and surgery; general health and evidence of systemic disease; history of exposure to drugs or hormones; dietary habits and exercise; family history, including the age of pubertal development of siblings and parents and the presence of hypogonadism and infertility; facial appearance, height, body proportions, and growth chart; body fat, sexual hair distribution, and muscle development; the presence or absence of Turner's stigmata and other skeletal malformations; the presence or absence of anosmia, hyposmia, or gynecomastia; evidence of other endocrinopathy; external genitalia development, including penile size and scrotal development; and testicular location, size, and consistency. A check for the presence of epididymis and vas and/or prostate size and consistency should be made.

The first step in the diagnostic approach is a careful assessment of testicular volume. For this measurement one can use the Prader orchidometer, which consists of a series of plastic ellipsoids ranging in volume from 1 to 25 ml. Each testis is compared to the appropriate ellipsoid. Alternatively, testicular volume can be assessed after measuring the length and the width of each testis by calipers. (The volume = $0.52 \times$ length $\times$ width^2.)

A testicular volume greater than 4 ml indicates that the testes are gonadotropin stimulated and that puberty has already started. The patient and his parents are reassured.

A testicular volume less than 4 ml indicates that puberty has not started. The differential diagnosis here is between primary gonadal disease, hypogonadism caused by hypothalamic-pituitary disease, and constitutional delay in puberty. Appropriate tests are serum T, LH, and FSH.

A low serum testosterone and an inappropriately low

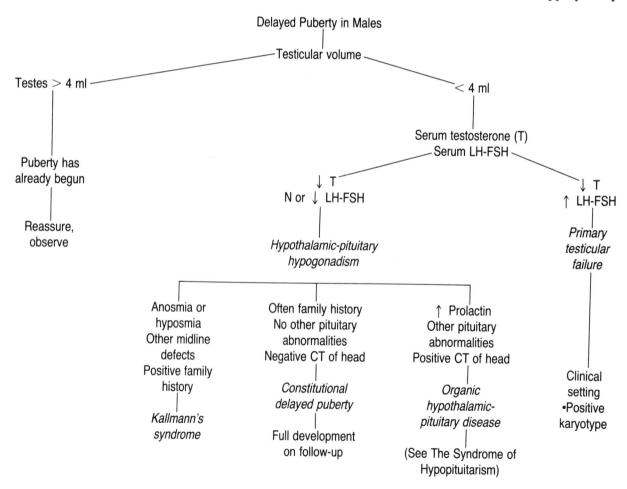

Fig. 11–42. Diagnostic approach to delayed puberty in males.

serum LH and FSH indicate hypogonadism caused by hypothalamic-pituitary disease. Olfactory testing is mandatory because anosmia or hyposmia may not have been noted by the patient. The presence of hyposmia or anosmia, other midline defects, and a positive family history point to Kallmann's syndrome.

Assessment of the clinical setting should be made for evidence of systemic disease, weight loss, the rare anorexia nervosa, and primary thyroid abnormalities to rule out functional hypothalamic hypogonadism. The presence of chronic disease is generally evident on history and physical examination, but occasional disorders, e.g., malabsorption syndrome resulting from Crohn's or celiac disease, may be relatively asymptomatic and go unrecognized. If present, the functional disease should be treated and the cause removed. Restoration of normal gonadal function and the initiation of puberty points to functional hypogonadotropism as the cause.

If the sense of smell is normal and the functional causes have been excluded, the next step is to rule out organic hypothalamic-pituitary disease. Evaluation of other pituitary functions including serum prolactin, ophthalmologic evaluations for chiasmal syndrome, and radiologic examination including skull x-rays and CT scan of the hypothalamic-pituitary area are in order. If these tests are abnormal, they point to organic hypothalamic-pituitary disease, and the diagnosis of its cause is based on evaluation of the clinical setting, on results of laboratory and radiologic studies, and, occasionally, on surgical intervention.

If these studies are normal, the differential diagnosis is between isolated hypogonadotropism and constitutional delay in puberty. Isolated hypogonadotropism is characterized by eunuchoid features and testes of prepubertal size. The presence of microphallus or a family history of hypogonadotropic hypogonadism may be helpful. The features of constitutional delay in puberty are as outlined above. There is no available diagnostic procedure that will allow precise differentiation between these two entities. Follow-up is important. Spontaneous initiation of puberty points to delayed puberty as the cause, whereas lack of spontaneous puberty points to organic hypogonadotropic hypogonadism.

Primary gonadal failure should be considered if the testes are difficult to palpate and if somatic abnormalities are evident. It is confirmed by a low serum testosterone and a high serum LH and FSH. The history and physical examination, buccal smear, and karyotype will point to the cause.

PRECOCIOUS PUBERTY

DEFINITION

In developed countries the onset of puberty in boys, defined by the earliest detectable testicular enlargement, occurs between the ages of 10 and 13 years; onset of puberty in girls, defined by breast or pubic hair development, occurs between the ages of 9 and 12. Puberty is considered precocious if it begins before age 10 in boys and age 9 in girls.

PATHOPHYSIOLOGIC CONSIDERATIONS

Puberty is a dynamic physiologic process that consists of a series of events extending over a period of 3 to 5 years in both boys and girls. These events are somewhat variable in onset, duration, and sequence. Table 11–52 lists the events and the age of onset and is useful for making the distinction between normal individuals and patients with abnormalities of puberty.

Precocious puberty can be classified into true precocious puberty and pseudoprecocious puberty. During childhood there is a central nervous system (CNS) inhibitory influence on the hypothalamic gonadotropin-releasing hormone secretion. At the onset of puberty, this CNS inhibition is reduced, leading to stimulation of secretion in sequence of hypothalamic GnRH, anterior pituitary gonadotropins, and gonadal steroids. In true precocious puberty this reduction of CNS inhibition occurs at an early age, leading to premature activation of the hypothalamic-pituitary-gonadal axis. The maturation of gonadotropin secretion leads to development of endocrine and gameto-

Table 11–52. Pubertal Development

| Sex | Event | Age of Onset | |
		Mean	Range
Boys	Testicular enlargement	11.6	10–13.5
	Pubic and axillary hair growth	13.4	10–15
	Peak growth velocity and growth spurt	14.1	10.5–16
	Adult pubic hair growth	15.2	14–18
Girls	Breast budding	11.2	9.5–13.5
	Pubic and axillary hair growth	11.7	9.5–14.5
	Peak growth velocity	12.1	10–14
	Menarche	13.5	11–16
	Adult pubic hair growth	14.4	12–17
	Adult breast development	15.3	13–18

Table 11–53. Causes of Precocious Puberty

True Precocious Puberty

Both sexes	Females
Idiopathic	Polyostotic fibrous dysplasia
Organic CNS disease	Untreated primary hypothyroid-
Tumors	ism
Gliomas	
3rd ventricular tumor	
Pinealomas	
Hypothalamic hamartomas	
Cysts	

Pseudoprecocious Puberty

Males	Females
Testicular tumors	Ovarian tumors
Adrenal	Adrenal tumors
Congenital adrenal	Estrogen-producing
Hyperplasia	Exogenous
21-hydroxylase	Estrogen
11-hydroxylase	Oral
Tumors	Topical
Exogenous	
Androgen	
HCG	

genic function of gonads; hence these individuals are potentially fertile. True precocious puberty can be idiopathic (when no organic lesion is identifiable) or organic (when related to an identifiable structural lesion of the central nervous system).

Pseudoprecocious puberty results from autonomous extragonadal or gonadal sex-hormone secretion. The high sex steroid levels keep the hypothalamic-pituitary-gonadal axis in its suppressed state. Therefore, the gametogenic function does not develop, and these patients are not fertile. The causes of precocious puberty are outlined in Table 11–53.

Idiopathic true precocious puberty is by far the most common cause of true precocious puberty and underlies the precocity of 80 to 90% of females and 50% of males. The cause is unknown, and there is no identifiable organic disease. Often a family history of early puberty is present. Central nervous system disorders are not uncommon, especially in males with precocious puberty. These include tumors (e.g., optic or hypothalamic gliomas, astrocytomas, and ependymomas), which may cause precocious puberty by interfering with the neuronal pathways that inhibit GnRH secretion. Hypothalamic hamartomas can cause precocity by secretion of GnRH. Among other disorders are infections (e.g., encephalitis), granulomatous inflammatory processes (as in sarcoidosis and histiocytosis X, or suprasellar cyst). Albright-McCune-Sternberg syndrome is a rare disorder characterized by polyostotic fibrous dysplasia of long bones, which tends to be unilateral; irregular café au lait spots

roughly corresponding with the underlying bone lesions; and true precocious puberty, which occurs almost exclusively in girls. Epilepsy and mental retardation have also been associated with true precocious puberty without anatomic lesions of the central nervous system. Severe untreated primary hypothyroidism can be associated with sexual precocity and galactorrhea; the cause is unknown but is postulated to be increased gonadotropin secretion in association with the increase in TSH secretion. Treatment with thyroid hormone will correct the hypothyroidism, precocious puberty, and galactorrhea.

Pseudoprecocious puberty underlies the precocity of 25% of females and 10 to 20% of males. In the male it may be due to stimulation of testicular production of testosterone by excess HCG or LH because of ectopic secretion from hepatomas; from teratoma of the gonads, of the retroperitoneum, and of the mediastinum; or from germinoma of the central nervous system. It may also be due to such stimulation by iatrogenic administration of HCG. In males, pseudoprecocious puberty may also be due to excess androgens as a result either of autonomous secretion of androgens by the testes (e.g., interstitial cell tumors) or adrenal glands (congenital adrenal hyperplasia resulting from 21-hydroxylase or 11-hydroxylase deficiency or virilizing adrenal carcinoma), or of iatrogenic administration of excessive androgens. In the female, pseudoprecocious puberty is due to excess estrogens from either autonomous production of estrogen (follicular cysts, granulosa or theca cell tumors of the ovary, or an estrogen-producing adrenal tumor) or ingestion or topical application of estrogenic compounds.

CLINICAL PRESENTATION

The clinical manifestations are those of precocious pubertal development and its cause. Precocious puberty is more common in females, with a ratio to males of 8 to 1.

In both true precocious and pseudoprecocious puberty, boys exhibit pubertal progressive growth of external genitalia, secondary sex characteristics, erections, and emissions. Precocious girls exhibit early development of secondary sex characteristics and early menses. Regular ovulatory menstrual function and fertility is present in true precocious puberty; however, girls with pseudoprecocious puberty are nonovulatory and nonfertile. Linear growth is initially rapid in both sexes, but adult height is limited by premature closure of the epiphyses.

Clinical manifestations related to the cause of precocious puberty may include features of CNS space-occupying lesions, the triad of Albright-Mc-Cune-Sternberg syndrome, primary hypothyroidism, HCG-producing ectopic tumor, gonadal or adrenal tumors, or congenital adrenal hyperplasia.

DIFFERENTIAL DIAGNOSIS

Precocious puberty should be differentiated from premature adrenarche (growth of sexual hair), which occurs in both sexes but is more common in boys, and from premature thelarche (breast development), which occurs in girls. These premature events occur at an early age as isolated events and are not followed by complete premature pubertal development, in contrast to normal puberty, which develops at the normal age, and to precocious puberty, in which they are very shortly followed by other features of pubertal development. Premature thelarche typically occurs around age 2 or 3 and may last 2 to 3 years before regressing. There is usually little or no stimulation or swelling of the areola and absence of other pubertal changes, in contrast with precocious puberty, in which there is areolar stimulation and swelling and estrogenic changes in the introitus.

DIAGNOSTIC EVALUATION

The diagnosis of precocious puberty is a clinical one supported by the characteristic growth charts and radiologic evidence of accelerated bone age.

Male Precocious Puberty (Fig. 11–43). A careful examination of the testes is important. Boys with true precocious puberty have development of both Leydig's and seminiferous tubule testicular components and have a testicular volume greater than 4 ml associated with normal spermatogenesis and fertility. In pseudoprecocious puberty no tubular development is present and testicular volume is less than 4 ml. In patients with adrenal disease, both testes are unstimulated and small (unless adrenal rests are present in the testes). In testicular tumors there is usually a unilateral testicular enlargement.

Boys with true precocious puberty have uniform bilateral testicular enlargement. Their serum testosterone, LH, and FSH are at the adult levels. If available for examination, a semen analysis will show the presence of sperm. Because these boys have a relatively high incidence of organic CNS disease, a careful search for CNS lesions is in order. Neurologic evaluation should always be undertaken. The diagnosis of causative CNS disease may be supported by the presence of other features of hypothalamic syndrome, including excessive thirst, polyuria, or adipsia, voracious appetite and obesity or cachexia, or disturbances of sleep and temperature; visual abnormalities including visual defect, decrease in visual acuity, optic atrophy, and papilledema; evidence of obstructive hydrocephalus; and evidence of other pituitary dysfunction. The clinical setting and radiologic evaluation, especially CT scan of the head, will point to the causative disorder. The diagnosis of idiopathic true precocious puberty in boys is by exclusion of other causes and is supported by a positive family history.

If the testes are small, less than 4 ml in volume, the differential diagnosis is between congenital adrenal hyperplasia and adrenal tumor. In both entities, the serum testosterone, serum DHEA-S, and 24-hour urinary 17-ketosteroids are elevated. Congenital adrenal hyperplasia is characterized by the presence of elevated steroid precursors (increased serum 17-hydroxyprogesterone or urinary pregnanetriol in 21-hydroxylase deficiency, increased serum 11-deoxycortisol [compound S] in 11-hydroxylase deficiency, and increased 17-ketosteroids and 17-ketogenic steroids in both disorders), and by suppressibility with dexamethasone. Adrenal tumors causing precocious puberty are almost always malignant and are associated with significant elevation in serum testosterone, DHEA-S, and urinary 17-ketosteroids. Urinary pregnanetriol and serum 17-hydroxyprogesterone are normal, the androgenic parameters are not dexamethasone suppressible, and the tumor is identified by anatomic studies (CT of the adrenals).

Unilateral testicular enlargement points to testicular tumor. Serum testosterone is elevated; serum DHEA-S, serum 17-hydroxyprogesterone, 24-hour urinary pregnanetriol, and ketosteroids are usually normal. Alpha-fetoprotein and β-HCG subunit may be increased because of ectopic production by the tumor. The definitive diagnosis is made by surgical exploration and biopsy.

The diagnosis of exogenous administration of HCG or androgen is made by the history.

Female Precocious Puberty (Fig. 11–44). In girls, true precocious puberty is characterized by cyclic menses, adult levels of serum LH and FSH, and evidence of ovulation (biphasic basal body temperature, elevated serum progesterone in the luteal phase, and secretory endometrium during the second half of the cycle by endometrial biopsy). Although idiopathic true precocious puberty is the most likely explanation and structural CNS lesions are very unlikely, it is of utmost importance that structural CNS lesions be looked for in each patient. The clinical setting and the results of the radiologic neuro-ophthalmologic and endocrine studies will usually point to the cause. Albright-McCune-Sternberg syndrome may be recognized clinically by the characteristic skin pigmentations and bony lesions.

Pseudoprecocious puberty in the female presents with irregular menses, absence of ovulation, and an adult level of serum estrogen, but with suppressed serum LH and FSH. In estrogen-producing ovarian tumor, plasma estradiol levels are high; in many cases the tumor is palpable on abdominal, pelvic, or rectal examination. Otherwise, it is identifiable by ultrasonography or CT examination of the pelvis. In estrogen-producing adrenal tumors, 24-hour urinary ketosteroids are significantly elevated, and the parameters are not dexamethasone suppressible. CT scan of the adrenal gland will delineate the presence of the adrenal tumor. The diagnosis of exogenous estrogen administration, either oral or topical, is made by the history.

In both sexes presenting with true precocious puberty, primary hypothyroidism should be excluded by thyroid function tests (total and free serum thyroxine [or free thyroxine index] and serum TSH) (see Hypothyroidism).

AMBIGUOUS EXTERNAL GENITALIA

DEFINITION

Ambiguous external genitalia refers to disorders caused by abnormalities of fetal sexual differentiation, in which the external genitalia cannot be definitely categorized as either a male or female phenotype. It represents a spectrum of abnormalities that includes any combination of male and female components.

PATHOPHYSIOLOGIC CONSIDERATIONS

If disorders associated with ambiguous external genitalia are to be understood, a clear knowledge of events of sexual differentiation is necessary. Sexual differentiation occurs in three stages that normally follow each other in orderly sequence—chromosomal sex, gonadal sex, and phenotypic sex.

Chromosomal sex is determined by chromosomal constitution of female and male gametes at fertilization: 46/XY is male and 46/XX is female.

Gonadal sex is established at about the 40th day of gestation. The H-Y antigen, a product of a gene on the Y chromosome, determines testicular development. If H-Y antigen is present, the gonad will dif-

ferentiate into a testes; if not, and the chromosomal sex is 46/XX, the gonad will become an ovary.

The definitive gonad determines development of internal and external genitalia, i.e., phenotypic sex. The internal genitalia are derived from the wolffian and müllerian duct systems. In the female, the müllerian ducts become the fallopian tubes, uterus, and upper vagina, while the wolffian ducts regress. In the male, the wolffian ducts give rise to the epididymis, vas deferens, and seminal vesicles, while müllerian ducts regress. The external genitalia arise from the urogenital sinus, and the genital tubercle, folds, and swelling. In the female, they form the lower part of the vagina, the clitoris, and the labia minora and majora; in the male, they form the prostate, prostatic urethra, penis, glans penis, and scrotum. The male pattern of development is determined by hormones of the fetal testis; müllerian inhibitory factor (MIF) leads to regression of müllerian ducts, testosterone leads to differentiation of the wolffian duct, and dihydrotestosterone (formed locally from testosterone via 5 alpha-reductase) leads to development of male external genitalia. In the absence of these hormones a female phenotype develops.

In most cases, ambiguous external genitalia reflect an abnormality in fetal sexual differentiation resulting from a hormonal abnormality (in production or in response) or a developmental anomaly; the chromosomal and gonadal sex are clearly male or female—the ambiguity affects the phenotypic sex, resulting in male or female pseudohermaphrodism. A rare cause of an abnormally in fetal sexual differentiation is a disorder of gonadal and chromosomal sex, i.e., mixed gonadal dysgenesis and true hermaphrodism.

Female Pseudohermaphrodism. This results from virilization of an otherwise normal female fetus by androgen. Such infants have 46/XX chromosomal sex, normal ovaries, normal female internal genitalia, and abnormalities of external genitalia consisting of an enlarged clitoris and rugose and bulbous labia with variable degrees of fusion.

The most common cause of female pseudohermaphrodism is congenital adrenal hyperplasia. There are five such syndromes. The two major types are C21-hydroxylase and C11-hydroxylase deficiencies, which are specific for steroidogenesis in the adrenals. The other three are rare and include 17-hydroxylase, 3-beta hydroxysteroid dehydrogenase, and 20, 22 desmolase deficiencies, which affect steroidogenesis in both the adrenals and gonads. The virilizing types of congenital adrenal hyperplasia are the C21-hydroxylase, the C11-hydroxylase, and the 3-beta hydroxysteroid dehydroxygenase deficiencies. These syndromes are inherited as autosomal recessive traits and are characterized by reduced cortisol synthesis, compensatory hypersecre-

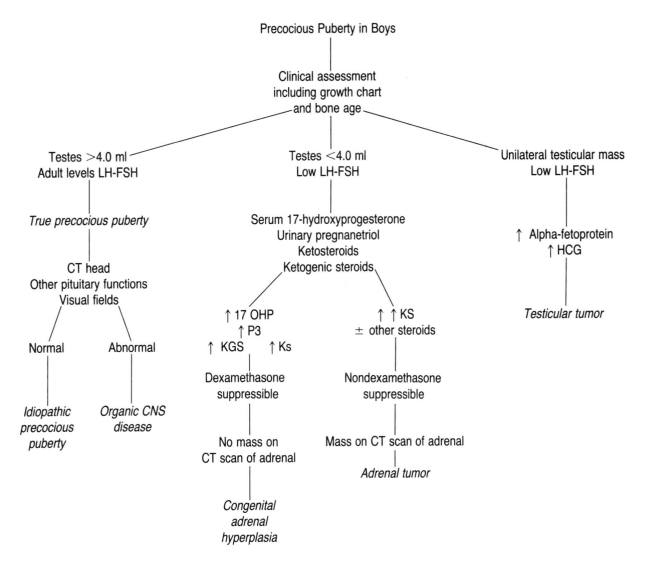

Fig. 11–43. Diagnostic approach to precocious puberty in boys.

tion of ACTH, adrenocortical hyperplasia, increased production of steroid precursors in the biosynthetic pathway proximal to the point of enzyme deficiency, and shunting of these precursors into the steroidogenic pathways that are not affected by the enzyme deficiency. Each enzyme deficiency is associated with a characteristic pattern of steroid deficiency or excess that identifies the defect and forms the basis for expression of a specific clinical syndrome. The steroidogenic pathway is depicted in Figure 11–45 and the various forms of congenital adrenal hyperplasia and their biochemical and clinical effects are outlined in Table 11–54.

Other causes of female hermaphrodism are therapy of threatened abortion with progestogens that have significant androgenic activity; maternal androgen-producing tumor; and idiopathic causes.

Male Pseudohermaphrodism. In affected males,

the chromosomal constitution is 46/XY, the gonads are testes, and the phenotypic sex development is impaired because of lack of müllerian inhibitory factor (MIF), lack of testosterone, lack of conversion of testosterone to dihydrotestosterone, and lack of testosterone and dihydrotestosterone intracellular receptors in the target tissues. The clinical consequences depend on the nature of the defect and the stage of development at which it arises.

Male pseudohermaphrodism can be caused by anorchia or inborn errors of metabolism affecting the enzymes of testosterone synthesis or androgen tissue receptors. Anorchia is caused by dissolution and testicular failure after MIF secretion. In its pure form, the external phenotype is female, the internal genitalia are those of a male, and no testes or müllerian duct structures are identified. Later-occurring or incomplete testicular failure results in incomplete virilization and

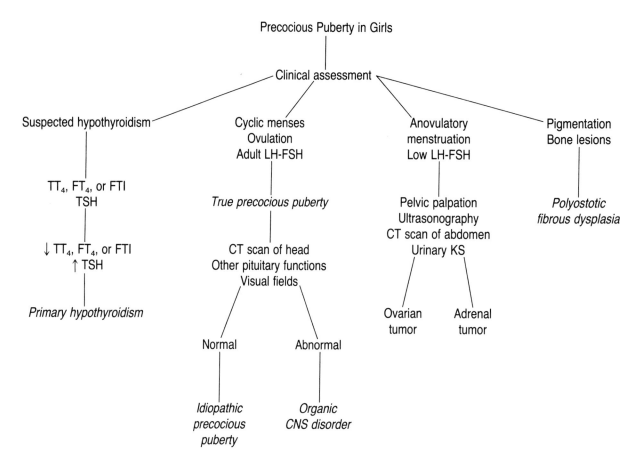

Fig. 11—44.   Diagnostic approach to precocious puberty in girls.

male pseudohermaphrodism. If testicular failure is very mild, the phenotype is clearly male with microphallus and absent testes.

In müllerian inhibitory factor deficiency, testes are present bilaterally, and there are a uterus and bilateral fallopian tubes, normal male external genitalia, and normal male puberty with azoospermia. There may be unilateral cryptorchidism, a contralateral inguinal hernia containing müllerian structures, or testes.

Six autosomal recessive enzyme defects in androgen synthesis have been described (Table 11–55). Depending on the completeness of the defect, the degree of differentiation varies from nearly normal males with hypospadias to nearly normal females. A number of syndromes of androgen receptor deficiency, inherited as X-linked recessive traits, have been described (Table 11–55). The phenotype may be male, female, or indeterminate, depending on the severity of the lesion.

The most important chromosomal and gonadal disorder is mixed gonadal dysgenesis. It is characterized by sex chromosomal constitution usually of 45/XO or 46/XY mosaicism with a testis on one side and streak gonad on the other, or a defect in the degree and timing of testicular MIF and testosterone secretion, müllerian regression, and external genitalia masculinization. The external genitalia may be male, female, or ambiguous. Approximately 60% of such patients are raised as females. One testis, a uterus, a vagina, and at least one fallopian tube are usually present.

True hermaphrodism is characterized by the presence of both ovarian and testicular tissue. The ovaries are histologically normal, but testes do not show spermatogenesis. Sex chromosomal constitution is 46/XX in 60 to 70% of patients, XX/XY mosaic in 20 to 30% of patients, and 46/XY in 10% of patients. Most subjects have ambiguous genitalia and 75% are raised as males. A fallopian tube is almost always found adjacent to the ovary or ovotestis. A uterus is present in approximately 90%. With puberty, there is variable virilization or feminization, and 50% will show evidence of menstrual function. Gynecomastia is present in 80%.

CLINICAL PRESENTATION

The complaint of abnormal genitalia is usually made by parents who have noted the abnormality soon after

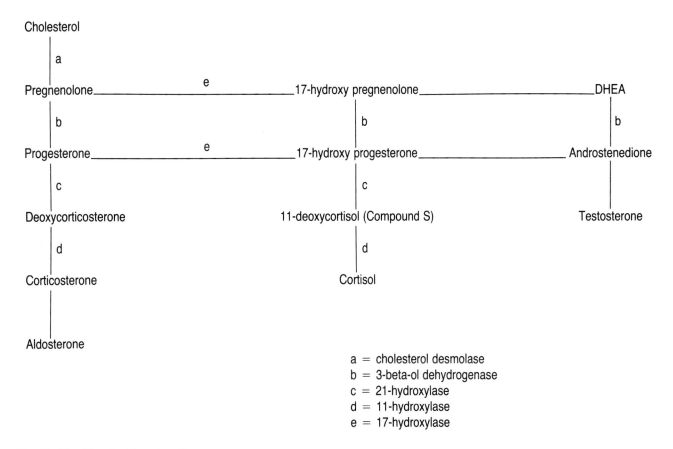

a = cholesterol desmolase
b = 3-beta-ol dehydrogenase
c = 21-hydroxylase
d = 11-hydroxylase
e = 17-hydroxylase

Fig. 11–45. The steroidogenic pathway.

birth, or occasionally, in childhood. Rarely, the abnormality is first noted in adolescence or early adulthood. Patients with congenital adrenal hyperplasia may present with salt-losing crisis.

A detailed assessment of the anatomic abnormality must be carried out including identification of clitoris or penis and labial scrotal folds, the position of urethral and vaginorectal orifices, and the presence of gonads in inguinal areas or the perineum. A probe is passed gently to establish the presence of a vaginalike orifice.

DIAGNOSTIC EVALUATION (Fig. 11–46)

The objectives of the diagnostic approach are to define the anatomic abnormality and to delineate its cause.

Careful documentation of the sexual phenotype by definition of the anatomy of external and internal genitalia is essential. The most important facet of the external genitalia exam is to define whether there is a palpable lower inguinal or scrotal gonad. If palpable, such a gonad almost always is a testis, but it is im-

Table 11–54.   Enzyme Defects in Adrenogenital Syndrome

Enzyme Defect	Steroid Precursor Build-up	Clinical Features Male 46/XY	Female 46/XX	Blood Pressure	Urinary KS	Urinary 17-OHCS	Other Hormonal Studies
Cholesterol desmolase	None	Pseudohermaphrodite—female external genitalia	Normal external genitalia	Salt-losing hypotension	—	—	—
3-beta-ol dehydrogenase	Pregnenolone, 17-hydroxypregnenolone, and DHEA	Pseudohermaphrodite—incomplete male sex differentiation	Partial masculinization	Salt-losing hypotension	High	Low	Increased delta-5 pregnanetriol Increased DHEA
21-hydroxylase	Progesterone, 17-hydroxyprogesterone	Male external genitalia, sexual precocity, small testes	Pseudohermaphrodite	Hypotension	High	Low	Increased pregnanetriol Increased 17-hydroxyprogesterone Decreased compound S
11-hydroxylase	Deoxycorticosterone, 11-deoxycortisol (Compound S)	Male external genitalia, sexual precocity, small testes	Pseudohermaphrodite	Hypertension, hypokalemia	High	High	Increased DOC Increased compound S
17-hydroxylase	Corticosterone, deoxycorticosterone	Female sexual differentiation	Female genitalia	Hypertension, hypokalemia	Low	Low	Increased corticosterone Increased deoxycorticosterone Increased progesterone and pregnanetriol

Table 11–55.   Male Pseudohermaphrodism

Disorder	Pathophysiology	Phenotype	Pubertal Development	
			Feminization	Masculinization
Disorder of androgen biosynthesis				
Swyer's syndrome	Testicular agenesis	Female	No	No
Testicular dysgenesis	Partial dysgenesis	Variable	No	Variable
Leydig's cell agenesis	No Leydig's cells	Female	No	No
Cholesterol 20–22 desmolase hydroxysteroid	Adrenal and gonadal steroidogenesis defect	Female	No	No
3-beta dehydrogenase	Same	Male pseudohermaphrodite	No	No
17-hydroxylase	Same	Female	No	No
17-beta-ol dehydrogenase and 17-keto-steroid reductase	Affects gonads	Female	Variable	Present
Disorders of androgen effect				
5-alpha reductase deficiency (Type II male pseudohermaphrodite)	Peripheral failure of conversion of T to DHT	Female	Absent	Marked virilization at puberty
Partial androgen insensitivity syndrome	Partial lack of androgen receptor and tissue effect	Variable, usually partial masculinization but may be female	Gynecomastia	Variable
Familial incomplete male pseudohermaphrodism Type I				
Reifenstein-Gilbert-Dreyfus-Lubs				
Androgen insensitivity syndrome				
Complete	Lack of androgen receptor	Female	Present—no sexual hair	Absent
Incomplete	Same	Female	Variable	Present

(Adapted from Rabin, D., and McKerra, T.J.: Syndromes of male pseudohermaphroditism. *In* Clinical Endocrinology and Metabolism. Principles and Practice. Vol. 9. The Science and Practice of Clinical Medicine. New York, Grune and Stratton, 1982.)

portant to remember that an ovary may herniate and hence may appear just outside the inguinal ring. Absence of external gonads in the setting of ambiguous external genitalia most often signifies a virilizing syndrome of a female infant but may also imply undescended testes.

In the assessment of the internal genitalia, a urethroscope can be used to identify a cervix. A rectal exam may identify a uterus. Radiologic tools, including ultrasonography, endoscopy, or vaginogram, can be used. An examination under anesthesia or laparotomy with biopsy of any gonad may be necessary.

Delineation of the cause is made by determining the genetic sex and blood steroid levels and, if necessary, by performing a biopsy of the gonads.

In determining genetic sex, buccal smear should not be used because it is unreliable with many false negative chromatin determinations in XX infants, it does not give information about the presence or absence of Y chromosome in the karyotype, and it does not identify mosaics. A complete chromosomal karyotype is essential.

Blood steroid levels are used to determine the presence of steroid biosynthetic defects. Those steroids required as a preliminary screen may include serum deoxycorticosterone, corticosterone, compound S, 17-hydroxyprogesterone, delta-5 pregnenolone, dehydroepiandrosterone, delta-4 androstenediol, testosterone, and dihydrotestosterone. It is important to re-

member that steroid levels may not be diagnostic in affected patients up to 3 weeks of age, that testosterone biosynthetic defects may become apparent only after stimulation with HCG, and that occasional mild congenital adrenal hyperplasia may be apparent only after ACTH stimulation.

In the infant with ambiguous genitalia who does not have a palpable scrotal gonad, the major consideration is that the patient is a female with congenital adrenal hyperplasia, iatrogenic virilization by maternal ingestion of virilizing substances, maternal overproduction of androgen, or idiopathic external genitalia virilization.

In an infant with ambiguous genitalia who has a palpable scrotal gonad, the considerations are asymmetrical or mixed gonadal dysgenesis, true hermaphrodism, male pseudohermaphrodism with partial peripheral insensitivity to DHT, 5-alpha reductase deficiency, or error in the pathway of testosterone biosynthesis, or that the patient is a male with congenital malformations not related to hormone problems.

A diagnosis of congenital adrenal hyperplasia should be suspected in an infant with ambiguous external genitalia, adrenal or salt-losing crisis, hypertension, or hyperpigmentation, in a male with precocious puberty, in a female with heterosexual precocious puberty, and in a patient with a family history of unexplained neonatal death or of documented congenital adrenal hyperplasia. The diagnosis is confirmed by

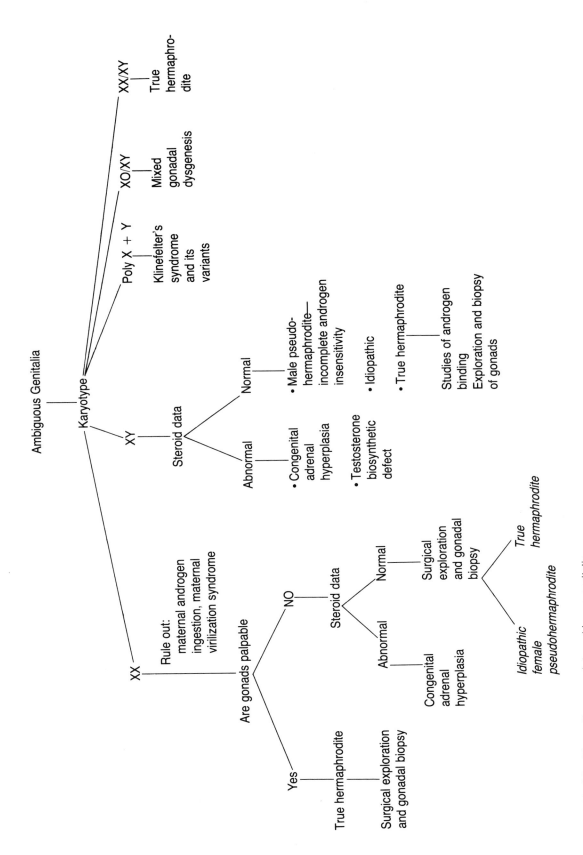

Fig. 11–46. Diagnostic approach to ambiguous genitalia.

appropriate steroid data (Table 11–55). The steroid excess in congenital adrenal hyperplasia is suppressible with dexamethasone. Deficiency of 21-hydroxylase is the most common congenital adrenal hyperplasia; the most accurate, rapid test for its diagnosis is the assay of plasma levels of 17-hydroxyprogesterone. These levels are increased, often to greater than ten times normal. The plasma levels of 17-hydroxyprogesterone are also increased in individuals with 11-hydroxylase deficiency, but so are the plasma levels of compound S and deoxycorticosterone. In patients with 3-beta hydroxysteroid dehydrogenase, the levels of pregnenolone and DHEA are increased. In 17-hydroxylase deficiency, there is increased serum progesterone, deoxycorticosterone, and corticosterone. Once a diagnosis of congenital adrenal hyperplasia is made, a careful family history and evaluation are in order to assess the presence of the disorder in other family members. Measurement of serum 17-hydroxyprogesterone responses to ACTH can demonstrate heterozygosity in patients, siblings, and other relatives.

GENERAL REFERENCES

THE SYNDROME OF HYPOPITUITARISM

Abboud, C.F., and Laws, E.R., Jr.: Clinical endocrinological approach to hypothalamic-pituitary disease. J Neurosurg 51:271, 1979.
Abboud, C.F.: Endocrine laboratory tests in the diagnosis of anterior pituitary diseases in the adult. Clin Lab Annual 4:199–254, 1985.
Abboud, C.F.: Laboratory diagnosis of hypopituitarism. Mayo Clin Proc 61:35–48, 1986.
Brasel, J.A., et al.: An evaluation of 75 patients with hypopituitarism beginning in childhood. Am J Med 38:484, 1965.
Cohen, K.L.: Metabolic endocrine and drug-induced interference with pituitary function tests: a review. Metabolism 26:1165, 1977.
Laws, E.R., Jr., Randall, R.V., Kern, E.B., and Abboud, C.F.: Management of Pituitary Adenomas and Related Lesions With Emphasis on Transsphenoidal Microsurgery. New York, Appleton-Century-Crofts, 1982.
Lieblich, J.M., et al.: Syndromes of anosmia with hypogonadism (Kallmann's syndrome). Clinical and laboratory studies in 23 cases. Am J Med 73:506, 1982.
Purnell, D.C., Randall, R.V., and Ryneaison, E.H.: Postpartum pituitary insufficiency (Sheehan's syndrome). Review of 18 cases. Mayo Clin Proc 39:321, 1964.
Randall, R.V., Scheithauer, B.W., and Abboud, C.F.: Anterior pituitary. In Clinical Medicine. Vol. 8. Edited by J.A. Spittel, Jr. Philadelphia, Harper & Row Publishers, 1983, pp. 1–97.
Randall, R.V., et al.: Transsphenoidal microsurgical treatment of prolactin-producing pituitary adenomas: Results in 100 patients. Mayo Clin Proc 58:108, 1983.
Schwabe, A.D.: Anorexia nervosa. Ann Intern Med 94:371, 1981.

SHORT STATURE

Daughaday, W.H., Hernington, A.C., and Phillips, L.S.: The regulation of growth by the endocrines. Ann Rev Physiol 37:211, 1975.
Preece, M.A.: Diagnosis and treatment of children with growth hormone deficiency. Clin Endocrinol Metab 11:1, 1982.
Rimoin, D.L., and Horton, W.A.: Short stature. J Pediatr 92:697, 1978.
Smith, D.W.: Growth and its disorders. In Major Problems in Clinical Pediatrics. Edited by A.J. Schaffer and M. Markowitz, Philadelphia, W.B. Saunders, 1977, p. 15.
Underwood, L.E., D'Ercole, A.J., and Van Wyk, J.J.: Somatomedin-C and the assessment of growth. Pediatr Clin North Am 27:771, 1980.
Van Wyk, J.J., and Underwood, L.E.: Growth hormone, somatomedins and growth failure. Hosp Pract 13:57, 1978.

TALL STATURE

Costin, G., Fefferman, R.A., and Kogut, M.D.: Hypothalamic gigantism. J Pediatr 83:419, 1973.
Roche, A.F.: Growth assessment in abnormal children. Kidney Int 16:369, 1978.
Smith, D.W.: Growth and its disorders. In Major Problems in Clinical Pediatrics. Edited by A.J. Schaffer and M. Markowitz. Philadelphia, W.B. Saunders, 1977, p. 15.

ENLARGEMENT OF THE SELLA

Abboud, C.F.: Endocrine laboratory tests in the diagnosis of anterior pituitary diseases in the adult. Clin Lab Annual. 4:199–254, 1985.
Cook, D.M.: Pituitary tumors: diagnosis and therapy. Cancer 33:215, 1983.
Crane, T.B., Gee, R.D., Hepler, R.S., and Hallinan, J.M.: Clinical manifestations and radiologic findings in craniopharyngiomas in adults. Am J Ophthalmol 94:220, 1982.
Daniels, D.L., et al.: Differential diagnosis of intrasellar tumors by computed tomography. Radiology 141:697, 1981.
Gharib, H., et al.: Coexistent primary empty sella syndrome and hyperprolactinemia: report of 11 cases. Arch Intern Med 143:1383, 1983.
Scanlon, M.F.: Neuroendocrinology. Clin Endocrinol Metab 12:3, 1983.
Tindall, G.T., and Hoffman, J.C.: Evaluation of the abnormal sella turcica. Arch Intern Med 140:1078–83, 1980.
Valenta, L.J., et al.: Diagnosis of pituitary tumor by hormone assays and computerized tomography. Am J Med 72:861, 1982.
Weisberg, L.A., Zimmerman, E.A., and Franz, A.G.: Diagnosis and evaluation of patients with an enlarged sella turcica. Am J Med 61:590, 1976.

ACROMEGALY AND GIGANTISM

Abboud, C.F.: Endocrine laboratory tests in the diagnosis of anterior pituitary diseases in the adult. Clin Lab Annual 4:199–254, 1985.
Daughaday, W.H., and Cryer, P.E.: Growth hormone hypersecretion and acromegaly. Hosp Pract 13:75, 1978.
Kanis, J.A., Gillingham, F.J., and Harris, P.: Clinical and laboratory study of acromegaly. Assessment before and one year after treatment. Medicine 43:409, 1974.
Melmed S., et al.: Pathophysiology of acromegaly. Endocr Rev 4:271, 1982.
Mims, R.B., and Bethune, J.E.: Acromegaly with normal fasting growth hormone concentrations but abnormal growth hormone regulation. Ann Intern Med 81:781, 1974.
Thorner, M.O., Perryman, R.W., Cronin, M.J., et al.: Somatotroph hyperplasia. Successful treatment of acromegaly by removal of a pancreatic islet tumor secreting growth hormone releasing factor. J Clin Invest 70:965, 1982.

HYPERPROLACTINEMIA AND GALACTORRHEA

Abboud, C.F.: Endocrine laboratory tests in the diagnosis of anterior pituitary diseases in the adult. Clin Lab Annual 4:199–254, 1985.

Abboud, C.F., and Laws, E.R. Jr.: Clinical endocrinological approach to hypothalamic-pituitary disease. J Neurosurg *51*:271, 1979.

Carter, J.N., Tyson, J.E., and Tolis, G.: Prolactin secreting tumors and hypogonadism in 22 men. N Engl J Med *229*:847, 1978.

Frantz, A.G.: Prolactin. N Engl J Med *298*:201, 1978.

Kleinberg, D.L., Noel, G.H., and Frantz, A.G.: Galactorrhea: A study of 235 cases including 48 with pituitary tumors. N Engl J Med *296*:589, 1977.

Koppelman, M.C.S., et al.: Hyperprolactinemia, amenorrhea and galactorrhea. Ann Intern Med *100*:115, 1984.

Randall, R.V., et al. Transsphenoidal microsurgical treatment of prolactin producing adenomas. Results in 100 patients. Mayo Clin Proc *58*:108, 1983.

Randall, R.V., Scheithauer, B.W., and Abboud, C.F.: Anterior Pituitary. Clinical Medicine. Vol. 8. Edited by J.A. Spittel, Jr., Philadelphia, Harper & Row Publishers, 1983, pp 1–97.

Spark, R.F., et al.: Hyperprolactinemia in males with and without pituitary macroadenomas. Lancet *2*:129, 1982.

Tolis, G.: Prolactin physiology and pathology. Hosp Pract *15*:85, 1980.

Tolis, G., and Frank, S.: Prolactin Pathophysiology in Clinical Neuroendocrinology: A Pathophysiologic Approach. New York, Raven Press, 1979, pp. 291–318.

HYPOTHYROIDISM

Blum, M.: Myxedema coma. Am J Med Sci *266*:432, 1972.

Fisher, D.A., et al.: Recommendations for screening programs for congenital hypothyroidism. Am J Med *61*:932, 1976.

Klein, I., and Levey, G.S.: Unusual manifestations of hypothyroidism. Arch Intern Med *144*:123, 1984.

Ladenson, P.W.: Diseases of the thyroid gland. *In* Clinics in Endocrinol. Metab. Investigations of Endocrine Disorders. Vol. 14. Edited by R.L. Ney. Philadelphia, W.B. Saunders, 1985, p. 145.

Pittman, et al.: Hypothalamic hypothyroidism. N Engl J Med *285*:844, 1971.

Postellon, D.C.: Diagnosis and treatment of congenital hypothyroidism. Compr Ther *9*:41, 1983.

Wartofsky, L., and Burman, K.D.: Alteration in thyroid function in patients with systemic illness, "The euthyroid sick syndrome." Endocr Rev *3*:164, 1982.

Wolff, J.: Iodide goiter and the pharmacologic effects of excess iodide. Am J Med *47*:101, 1969.

THYROTOXICOSIS

Amino, N., et al.: High prevalence of transient postpartum thyrotoxicosis and hypothyroidism. N Engl J Med *306*:849–859, 1982.

Borst, G.C., Eli, C., and Burman, K.D.: Euthyroid hyperthyroxinemia. Ann Intern Med *98*:366–378, 1983.

Chopra, I.J., Hershman, J.M., et al.: Thyroid function in nonthyroidal illnesses. Ann Intern Med *98*:946, 1983.

Cooper, D.S., Ridgway, E.C., and Maloof, F.: Unusual types of hyperthyroidism. Clin Endocrinol Metab *7*:199, 1978.

Davis, P.J., and Davis, F.B.: Hyperthyroidism in patients over the age of 60 years. Medicine *53*:161, 1974.

Fradkin, J.E, and Wolff, J.: Iodide-induced thyrotoxicosis. Medicine *62*(1):1–20, 1983.

Ladenson, P.W.: Diseases of the thyroid gland. *In* Clinics in Endocrinol. Metab. Investigations of Endocrine Disorders. Vol. 14. Edited by R.L. Ney. Philadelphia, W.B. Saunders, 1985, p 145.

Nikolai, T.F., et al.: Lymphocytic thyroiditis with spontaneously resolving hyperthyroidism (silent thyroiditis). Arch Intern Med *140*:478, 1980.

Volpe, R. (guest ed): Thyrotoxicosis. Clin Endocrinol Metab *7*:1978.

DIFFUSE AND NODULAR GOITER

Hurley, J.R.: Thyroiditis. Disease-a-Month *24*(3):1–65, 1977.

Lever, E.G., Medeiros-Neto, G.A., and DeGroot, L.J.: Inherited disorders of thyroid metabolism. Endocr Rev *4*:213–239, 1983.

McConahey, W.M.: Hashimoto's thyroiditis. Med Clin North Am *56*:885, 1979.

Studer, H., and Ramelli, F.: Simple goiter and its variants: Euthyroid and hyperthyroid multinodular goiters. Endocr Rev *3*:40, 1982.

SINGLE THYROID NODULE

Ashcraft, M.W., and VanHerle, A.J.: Management of thyroid nodules. I. History and physical examination, blood tests, x-ray tests, and ultrasonography. Head Neck Surg *3*:216, 1981.

Clark, O.M.: Thyroid nodules and thyroid cancer: Surgical aspects. West J Med *133*:1, 1980.

Colacchio, T.A., et al.: Fine needle cytologic diagnosis of thyroid nodules. Review and report of 300 cases. Am J Surg *140*:568, 1980.

Greenspan, F.S.: Radiation exposure and thyroid cancer. JAMA *237*:2089, 1977.

Lowhagen, T., et al.: Aspiration biopsy cytology (ABC) in nodules of the thyroid gland suspected to be malignant. Surg Clin North Am *59*:3–18, 1979.

VanHerle, A.J., et al.: The thyroid nodule. Ann Intern Med *96*:221–232, 1982.

PAINFUL GOITER

Hurley, J.R.: Thyroiditis. Disease-a-Month *24*(3):1–65, 1977.

EXOPHTHALMOS

Dallow, R.L.: Reliability of orbital diagnostic tests. Ultrasonography, computerized tomography, and radiography. Ophthalmology *85*:1218, 1978.

Gorman, C.A.: The presentation and management of endocrine ophthalmopathy. Clin Endocrinol Metab *7*:67, 1978.

Jacobson, D.M., and Gorman, C.A.: Endocrine ophthalmopathy: current ideas concerning etiology, pathogenesis, and treatment. Endocr Rev *5*:200, 1984.

HYPOCALCEMIA

Breslau, N.A., and Pak, C.Y.: Hypoparathyroidism. Metabolism *28*:1261, 1979.

Juan, D.: Hypocalcemia, differential diagnosis and mechanisms. Arch Intern Med *139*:1166, 1979.

Nusynowitz, M.L., Frame, B., and Kolb, F.O.: The spectrum of the hypoparathyroid states. Medicine *55*:105, 1976.

Schneider, A.B., and Sherwood, L.M.: Pathogenesis and management of hypoparathyroidism and other hypocalcemia disorders. Metabolism *24*:871, 1975.

Woodhouse, N.J.Y.: Hypocalcemia and hypoparathyroidism. Clin Endocrinol Metab *3*:323, 1974.

HYPERCALCEMIC SYNDROME

Arnaud, C.D., Tsao, H.S., and Littledike, T.: Radioimmunoassay of parathyroid hormone in serum. J Clin Invest *50*:21, 1971.

Broadus, A.E., and Rasmussen, H.: Clinical evaluation of parathyroid function. Am J Med *71*:457, 1981.

Carney, J.A., Sizemore, G.W., and Hayles, A.B.: Multiple endocrine neoplasia type 2-B. Pathobiol Annu *8*:105, 1978.

Fisken, R.A., Heath, D.A., and Bold, A.M.: Hypercalcemia: a hospital survey. J Med *196*:405, 1980.

Heath, H.H., Hodgson, S.F., and Kennedy, M.A.: Primary hyperparathyroidism: incidence, morbidity, and potential economic impact in a community. N Engl J Med *302*:189, 1980.

Imura, H.: Ectopic hormone syndromes. Clin Endocrinol Metab *9*:235, 1980.

Lee, D.B., Quawadu, E.T., and Kleenan, C.R.: The pathophysiology and clinical aspects of hypercalcemic disorders. West J Med *129*:278, 1978.

Mallette, L.E., Bilezikian, J.P., Heath, D.A., and Aurback, G.D.: Primary hyperparathyroidism: clinical and biochemical features. Medicine *53*:127, 1974.

Marx, S.J., et al.: The hypocalciuric or benign variant of familial hypercalcemia: clinical and biochemical features in fifteen kindreds. Medicine *60*:397, 1981.

Murdy, G.R., and Martin, T.J.: The hypercalcemia of malignancy: pathogenesis and management. Metabolism *31*:1247, 1982.

Purnell, D.C., et al.: Primary hyperparathyroidism: a prospective clinical study. Am J Med *50*:670, 1971.

Sizemore, G.W., Heath, H. III, Carney, J.A.: Multiple endocrine neoplasia type II. Clin Endocrinol Metab *9*:299, 1980.

Symposium on the etiology and management of hypercalcemia. Metab Bone Dis *2*:143, 1980.

Yamaguchi, K., Kameya, T., and Abe, A.: Multiple endocrine neoplasia type I. Clin Endocrinol Metab *9*:261, 1980.

URIC ACID DISORDERS

Bass, G.R., and Seegmiller, J.E.: Hyperuricemia and gout: classification, complications, and management. N Engl J Med *300*:1459, 1979.

Healy, L.A., and Hall, A.P.: The epidemiology of hyperuricemia. Bull Rheum Dis *20*:600, 1973.

Wallace, S.L., et al.: Selected data on primary gout. Bull Rheum Dis *29*:992, 1979.

Wyngeerden, J.B., and Kelly, W.N.: Gout and Hyperuricemia. New York, Grune & Stratton, 1976.

HYPERGLYCEMIA AND DIABETES MELLITUS

Bennett, P.M.: The diagnosis of diabetes. New international classification and diagnostic criteria. Ann Rev Med *34*:295, 1983.

Feig, P.V., and McCurdy, D.K.: The hypertonic state. N Engl J Med *297*:1444, 1977.

Feingold, K.R.: Hypoglycemia. A pitfall of insulin therapy. West J Med *139*:668, 1983.

Foster, D.W., and McGarry, J.D.: The metabolic derangements and treatment of diabetic ketoacidosis. N Engl J Med *309*:159, 1983.

Kereiakes, D.J., et al.: The heart in diabetes. West J Med *140*:583, 1984.

National Diabetes Data Group. Classification and diagnosis of diabetes mellitus and other categories of glucose intolerance. Diabetes *63*:843, 1977.

Raskin, M.D. (guest ed): Symposium on diabetes mellitus. Med Clin North Am Nov *66*:1982.

Ward, J.D.: The diabetic leg. Diabetologia *22*:141, 1982.

HYPOGLYCEMIA

Fajans, S.S., and Floyd, J.C.: Fasting hypoglycemia in adults. N Engl J Med *294*:766, 1976.

Gale, E.: Hypoglycemia. Clin Endocrinol Metab *9*:461, 1980.

Hofeldt, F.D.: Reactive hypoglycemia. Metabolism *24*:1193, 1975.

Johnson, D.D., et al.: Reactive hypoglycemia. J Am Med Assoc *243*:1151, 1980.

Kaplan, E.L., and Lee, C.H.: Recent advances in the diagnosis and treatment of insulinoma. Surg Clin North Am *59*:119, 1979.

Marks, V.: Hypoglycemia. Oxford, Blackwell Scientific Publications, Ltd., 1981.

Scarlett, J.A., et al.: Factitious hypoglycemia: diagnosis and measurement of serum C peptide immunoreactivity and insulin binding antibodies. N Engl J Med *297*:1029, 1977.

Service, F.J.: Hypoglycemic Disorders: Pathogenesis, Diagnosis, and Treatment. Boston, G.K. Hall, 1983.

HYPERLIPIDEMIA

Eder, H.A., and Gidez, L.J.: The clinical significance of the plasma high density lipoproteins. Med Clin North Am *66*:431, 1982.

Goldstein, J.L., and Brown, M.S.: LDL receptor defect in familial hypercholesterolemia. Med Clin North Am *66*:335, 1982.

Itavel, R.J.: The formation of LDL: Mechanisms and regulation. J Lipid Res *25*:1570, 1984.

Kostner, G.M.: Apolipoproteins and lipoproteins of human plasma: Significance in health and disease. Adv Lipid Res *20*:1, 1983.

Kreisberg, R.A.: Lipids, lipoproteins, apolipoproteins, and atherosclerosis. Ann Intern Med *99*:713, 1983.

Murchison, L.E.: Hyperlipidemia. Br Med J *290*:535, 1985.

Schonfield, G.: Disorders of lipid transport: Update 1983. Prog Cardiovasc Dis *26*:89, 1983.

Zimmerman, B.R., and Palumbo, P.J.: Lipid disorders and diabetes. Diabetes Care *6*:417, 1983.

OBESITY

Boisaubin, E.V.: Approach to obese patients. West J Med *140*:794, 1984.

Brownell, K.D.: The psychology and physiology of obesity. J Am Diet Assoc *84*:406, 1984.

Callaway, C.W.: Weight standards, their clinical significance (Editorial). Ann Intern Med *100*:206, 1984.

Horton, E.S. et al.: Symposium on the regulation of energy balance in humans. Am J Clin Nutr *38*:972, 1983.

Simopoulos, A.P.: Health implications of overweight and obesity. Nutr Rev *43*:33, 1985.

Simopoulos, A.P., and Van Itallie, T.B.: Body weight, health and longevity. Ann Intern Med *100*:285, 1984.

Vasseli, J.R., Cleary, M.P., and Van Itallie, T.B.: Modern concepts of obesity. Nutr Rev *41*:361, 1983.

PORPHYRIAS

Del Batlle, A.M. (ed): Porphyrins and porphyria: Etiopathogenesis, clinics, and treatment. Int J Biochem *12*:1, 1980.

Kappas, A., Sassas, S., and Anderson, K.E.: The porphyrias. *In* The Metabolic Basis of Inherited Disease. 5th Ed. Edited by Stanbury, J.B., et al. New York, McGraw-Hill Book Company, 1983.

Schmid, R.: The hepatic porphyrias. Semin Liver Dis *2*:1, 1981.

Stein, J.A., and Tschudy, D.P.: Acute intermittent porphyria. A clinical and biochemical study of 46 patients. Medicine *49*:1, 1970.

CARCINOID SYNDROME

Beaton, H., et al.: Gastrointestinal carcinoids and the malignant carcinoid syndrome. Surg Gynecol Obstet *152*:268, 1981.

Frohlich, J.C., and Margolius, H.S.: Prostaglandins, the Killikrein-Kinin system; Bartter's syndrome and the carcinoid syndrome. *In* Endocrinology & Metabolism. Edited by Felig, P., Baxter, J.D., Broadus, A.E., and Frohman, L.E. New York, McGraw-Hill Book Company, 1981, pp. 1247–1274.

Marks, C.: Carcinoid Tumors, a Clinicopathologic Study. Boston, G.K. Hall, 1979, pp. 1–54.

Zeitels, J., et al.: Carcinoid tumors: A 37-year experience. Arch Surg *117*:732, 1982.

THE OSTEOPOROTIC SYNDROMES

Avioli, L.V.: The Osteoporotic Syndrome: Detection, Prevention and Treatment. New York, Grune and Stratton, 1983.

Baylinch, D.J.: Glucocorticoid-induced osteoporosis (Editorial). N Engl J Med *309*:306, 1983.

Health and Public Policy Committee, American College of Physicians:

Radiologic methods to evaluate bone mineral content. Ann Intern Med *100*:908, 1984.

Leeman, E., et al.: Risk factors for spinal osteoporosis in men. Am J Med *75*:977, 1983.

Riggs, B.L., and Melton, L.J.: Evidence for two distinct syndromes of involutional osteoporosis (Editorial). Am J Med *75*:899, 1983.

Smith, R.: Idiopathic osteoporosis in the young. J Bone Joint Surg (Br) *62*:417, 1982.

Wahner, H.W., Dunn, W.L., and Riggs, B.L.: Assessment of bone mineral. Parts 1 and 2. J Nucl Med *25*:1134, 1241, 1984.

OSTEOMALACIA AND RICKETS

Bickle, D.D.: Calcium absorption and vitamin D metabolism. Clin Gastroenterol *12*:379, 1983.

DeLuca, M.F.: New developments in the vitamin D endocrine system. J Am Diet Assoc *80*:231, 1982.

Frame, B., and Parfitt, A.M.: Osteomalacia, current concepts. Ann Intern Med *89*:966, 1978.

Frame, B., and Potts, J.T., Jr. (eds.): Clinical disorders of bone and mineral metabolism. Excerpta Medica, 1983.

Parfitt, A.M., et al.: Bone histology in metabolic bone disease: the diagnostic value of bone biopsy. Orthop Clin North Am *10*:329, 1979.

MISCELLANEOUS METABOLIC BONE DISEASES

Albright, J.A., and Millar, E.A.: Osteogenesis imperfecta. Clin Orthop *159*:2, 1981.

Altman, R.D.: Paget's disease of bone (osteitis deformans). Bull Rheum Dis *34*:1, 1984.

Altman, R.D., and Singer, F. (eds.): Proceedings of the Kroc Foundation Conference on Paget's disease of bone. Arthritis Rheum *10*(Suppl):23, 1980.

Cowley, M.I.: Complications of Paget's disease of bone. Gerontology *29*:276, 1983.

Grabias, S.L., and Campbell, C.J.: Fibrous dysplasia. Orthop Clin North Am *8*:771, 1977.

THE SYNDROME OF ADRENOCORTICAL INSUFFICIENCY

Irvine, W.J.: Autoimmunity in endocrine disease. Recent Prog Horm Res *36*:509, 1980.

Irvine, W.J., Toft, A.D., and Feek, C.M.: Addison's disease. *In* The Adrenal Gland. Edited by U.H.T. James. New York, Raven Press, 1979, pp. 131–164.

Nekup, J.: Addison's disease—clinical studies. A report of 108 cases. Acta Endocrinol *76*:127, 1974.

Schambelon, M., and Sebastian, A.: Hyporeninemic hypoaldosteronism. Adv Intern Med *24*:385, 1979.

Tyler, F.H., and West, C.D.: Laboratory evaluation of disorders of the adrenal cortex. Am J Med *53*:664, 1972.

Wand, G.S., and Ney, R.L.: Disorders of the hypothalamic-pituitary-adrenal axis. Clin Endocrinol Metab *14*:33, 1985.

CUSHING'S SYNDROME

Aron, D.C., et al.: Cushing's syndrome: problems in diagnosis. Medicine *60*:25, 1981.

Crapo, L.: Cushing's syndrome. A review of diagnostic tests. Metabolism *28*:955, 1979.

Gold, E.M.: The Cushing's syndrome. Changing views of diagnosis and treatment. Ann Intern Med *90*:829–844, 1979.

Liddle, G.W.: Pathogenesis of glucocorticoid disorders. Am J Med *53*:638–648, 1972.

Orth, D.N.: The old and the new in Cushing's syndrome. N Engl J Med *310*:649, 1984.

Streeton, D.M., et al.: Normal and abnormal function of the hypothalamic-pituitary-adrenalcortical system in man. Endocr Rev *5*:371, 1984.

Ward, G.S., and Ney, R.L.: Disorders of the hypothalamic-pituitary-adrenal axis. Clin Endocrinol Metab *14*:33, 1985.

THE SYNDROME OF PRIMARY ALDOSTERONISM

Biglieri, E.G., Stockigt, J.R., and Schambelan, M.: Adrenal mineralocorticoids causing hypertension. Am J Med *52*:623–32, 1972.

Drury, P.L.: Disorders of mineralocorticoid activity. Clin Endocrinol Metab *14*:175, 1985.

Grim, C.E., Weinberger, M.H., Higgins, J.T., and Kramer, N.J.: Diagnosis of secondary forms of hypertension: A comprehensive protocol. J Am Med Assoc *237*:1331–5, 1977.

Weinberger, M.H.: Primary aldosteronism: diagnosis and differentiation of subtypes. Ann Intern Med *100*:300, 1984.

Weinberger, M.H., et al.: Primary aldosteronism: diagnosis, localization, treatment. Ann Intern Med *90*:386–95, 1979.

PHEOCHROMOCYTOMA

Bravo, E.L., and Gifford, R.W.: Pheochromocytoma: diagnosis, localization and management. N Engl J Med *311*:1298, 1984.

Bravo, E.L., et al.: Clonidine suppression test: a useful aid in the diagnosis of pheochromocytoma. N Engl J Med *305*:623, 1981.

Bravo, E.L., Tarazi, R.C., Gifford, R.W., and Stewart, B.H.: Circulating and urinary catecholamine in pheochromocytoma: diagnostic and pathophysiologic implications. N Engl J Med *301*:682–6, 1979.

Cryer, P.E.: Pheochromocytoma. Clin Endocrinol Metab *14*:203, 1985.

Cryer, P.E.: Physiology and pathophysiology of the human sympathoadrenal neuroendocrine system. N Engl J Med *303*:436, 1980.

Mangen, W.M., and Gifford, R.W., Jr.: Hypertension secondary to pheochromocytoma. Bull NY Acad Med *58*:139, 1982.

Remine, W.H., et al.: Current management of pheochromocytoma. Ann Surg *179*:740–8, 1974.

Stewart, B.H., et al.: Localization of pheochromocytoma by computed tomography. N Engl J Med *229*:460–1, 1978.

AMENORRHEA

Davajan, et al.: Symposium on adolescent gynecology and endocrinology: secondary amenorrhea, hirsutism in adolescents and the clinical consequences of stilbestrol exposure in utero. West J Med *131*:516, 1979.

Hall, J.G., et al.: Turner's syndrome. West J Med *137*:62, 1982.

Hirnoven, E.: Etiology, clinical features, and progress in secondary amenorrhea. Int J Fertil *22*:69, 1977.

Jewelewicz, R.: The diagnosis and treatment of amenorrheas. Fertil Steril *27*:1347, 1976.

Kletzky, O.A., et al.: Classification of secondary amenorrhea based on distinct hormonal patterns. J Clin Endocrinol Metab *41*:660, 1975.

Morris, D.V., et al.: The investigation of female gonadal dysfunction. Clin Endocrinol Metab *14*:125, 1985.

Odell, W.D., and Federman, D.D.: Symposium on adolescent gynecology and endocrinology: physiology of sexual maturation and primary amenorrhea. West J Med *131*:401, 1979.

Root, A.W., and Reiter, E.O.: Evaluation and management of the child with delayed pubertal development. Fertil Steril *27*:745, 1976.

Styne, D.M., and Kaplan, S.L.: Normal and abnormal puberty in the female. Pediatr Clin North Am *26*:123, 1979.

HIRSUTISM AND VIRILIZATION

Blankstein, J., et al.: Adult onset familial adrenal 21-hydroxylase deficiency. Am J Med 68:441, 1980.

Farber, M., et al.: Diagnostic evaluation of hirsutism in women. Clin Obstet Gynaecol 20:1, 1977.

Ferriman, D., Gallway, M.: Clinical assessment of body hair in women. J Clin Endocrinol Metab 21:1440, 1961.

Givens, J.R.: Hirsutism and hyperandrogenism. Adv Intern Med 21:221, 1976.

Goldzieher, J.W.: Polycystic ovarian disease. Fertil Steril 35:371, 1981.

Hatch, R., et al.: Hirsutism: implications, etiology, and management. Am J Obstet Gynecol 140:815, 1981.

Kirschner, M.A., Tucker, I.R., and Jespersen, D.: Idiopathic hirsutism, an ovarian abnormality. N Engl J Med 294:637, 1976.

Morris, D.V., et al.: The investigation of female gonadal dysfunction. Clin Endocrinol Metab 14:125, 1985.

Yen, S.S.C.: The polycystic ovary syndrome. Clin Endocrinol 12:177, 1980.

HYPOGONADISM IN THE ADULT MALE

Bunick, E.M., and Rose, L.I.: Testicular syndromes: Part II. Adult abnormalities. Compr Ther 3:69, 1977.

Handelsman, D.J., and Swerdloff, R.S.: Male gonadal dysfunction. Clin Endocrinol Metab 14:89, 1985.

London, D.R.: Medical aspects of hypogonadism. The testis. Clin Endocrinol Metab 4:597, 1975.

Morley, J.E., and Melmed, S.: Gonadal dysfunction in systemic disorders. Metabolism 28:1051, 1979.

Odell, W.D., and Swerdloff, R.S.: Abnormalities of gonadal function in men. Clin Endocrinol 8:149, 1978.

IMPOTENCE

Handelsman, D.J., and Swerdloff, R.S.: Male gonadal dysfunction. Clin Endocrinol Metab 14:89, 1985.

Reckless, J., and Geiger, N.: Impotence as a practical problem. Disease-a-Month 5:1–40, 1975.

Slag, M.F., et al.: Impotence in medical clinic outpatients. J Am Med Assoc 249:1736, 1983.

Sparg, R.F., et al.: Impotence is not always psychogenic: newer insights into hypothalamic pituitary-gonadal function. J Am Med Assoc 243:750, 1980.

GYNECOMASTIA

Carlson, H.E.: Gynecomastia. N Engl J Med 303:795, 1980.

Chandrakant, C.K., and Parekh, N.J.: The male breast. Radiol Clin North Am 21:137, 1983.

Niewochner, C.B., and Nuttall, F.G.: Gynecomastia in a hospitalized male population. Am J Med 77:633, 1984.

Nuttall, F.G.: Gynecomastia as a physical finding in normal men. J Clin Endocrinol Metab 48:338, 1979.

Wilson, J.D., Aiman, J., and MacDonald, P.: The pathogenesis of gynecomastia. Adv Intern Med 25:1, 1980.

INFERTILITY

Davajan, V., and Israel, R.: Infertility: causes, evaluations, and treatment. In Endocrinology. Vol. 3. Edited by W. DeGroot, et al. New York, Grune and Stratton, 1979, pp. 1459–72.

de Krester, D.M.: Endocrinology of male infertility. Br Med Bull 35:187, 1979.

DiZerega, G.S., and Ross, G.T.: Luteal phase dysfunction. Clin Obstet Gynaecol 8:733, 1981.

Dublin, L., and Amelar, R.D.: Etiologic factors in 1294 consecutive cases of male infertility. Fertil Steril 22:469, 1971.

Handelsman, D.J., and Swerdloff, R.S.: Male gonadal dysfunction. Clin Endocrinol Metab 14:89, 1985.

Morris, D.V., et al.: The investigation of female gonadal dysfunction. Clin Endocrinol Metab 14:125, 1985.

DELAYED PUBERTY IN MALES

Hsueh, W.A., et al.: Endocrine features of Klinefelter's syndrome. Medicine 57:447, 1978.

Lieblich, J.M., et al.: Syndrome of anosmia with hypogonadotropic hypogonadism (Kallmann's syndrome): clinical and laboratory studies in 23 cases. Am J Med 73:506, 1982.

Lipsett, M.B.: Physiology and pathology of the Leydig cell. N Engl J Med 303:682, 1980.

Marshall, W.A., and Tanner, J.M.: Variations in the pattern of pubertal changes in boys. Arch Dis Child 45:13, 1970.

Raynor, P.M.W.: Puberty, precocious and delayed. Br Med J 1:1385, 1976.

Root, A.W., and Reiter, E.O.: Evaluations and management of the child with delayed pubertal development. Fertil Steril 27:745, 1976.

Styne, D.M., and Grumbach, M.M.: Puberty in the male and female: its physiology and disorders. In Reproductive Endocrinology, Physiology, Pathophysiology, and Clinical Management. 2nd Ed. Edited by S.S.C. Fen and R.B. Jaffe. Philadelphia, W.B. Saunders, 1986.

PRECOCIOUS PUBERTY

Ducharme, J.R., and Collu, R.: Pubertal development: normal, precocious and delayed. Clin Endocrinol Metab 11:57, 1982.

Marshall, W.A., and Tanner, J.M.: Variations in pattern of pubertal changes in girls. Arch Dis Child 44:291, 1969.

Styne, D.M., and Grumbach, M.M.: Puberty in the male and female: its physiology and disorders. In Reproductive Endocrinology: Physiology, Pathophysiology and Clinical Management. 2nd Ed. Edited by S.S.C. Fen and R.B. Jaffe, Philadelphia, W.B. Saunders, 1986.

Styne, D.M., and Kaplan, S.L.: Normal and abnormal puberty in the female. Pediatr Clin North Am 26:123, 1979.

AMBIGUOUS EXTERNAL GENITALIA

Bunick, E.M., and Rose, L.I.: Testicular syndromes. Part I. Abnormalities of childhood and adolescence. Compr Ther 3:62, 1977.

Dewhurst, C.J.: The etiology and management of intersexuality. Clin Endocrinol Metab 4:625, 1975.

Donahoe, P.K., and Hendren, W.M.: Evaluations of the newborn with ambiguous genitalia. Pediatr Clin North Am 23:361, 1976.

Finkelstein, M., and Shaefer, J.M.: Inborn errors of steroid biosynthesis. Physiol Rev 59:353, 1979.

Griffin, J.E., Leser, M., and Wilson, J.D.: Androgen resistance syndromes. Am J Physiol 243:81–87, 1982.

Imperato-McGinley, J.: Sexual differentiation—normal and abnormal. Curr Top Exp Endocrinol 5:231–307, 1983.

Jaffe, R.B.: Disorders of sexual development. In Reproductive Endocrinology: Physiology, Pathophysiology and Clinical Management. 2nd Ed. Edited by S.S.C. Fen and R.B. Jaffe. Philadelphia, W.B. Saunders, 1986.

Migeon, C.J.: Diagnosis and treatment of adrenogenital disorders. In Endocrinology. Edited by L.J. DeGroot. New York, Grune and Stratton, 1979, p. 1203.

CHAPTER 12

GASTROINTESTINAL AND LIVER PROBLEMS

Graham H. Jeffries, M.D.

Today, clinicians have at their disposal a wide range of new diagnostic procedures and tests that are useful in defining disturbances of structure and function in the gastrointestinal system. The benefits of applying these advances in diagnostic technology may be more accurate and earlier diagnosis, and improved treatment; the disadvantages are an increase in health care costs and the risk of depersonalizing patient care.

A careful analysis of a patient's symptoms and a complete physical examination continue to be of primary importance in diagnosis. This clinical data base is necessary for planning further diagnostic studies in an appropriate and cost-effective manner.

The sections that follow analyze the most important symptoms and signs of gastrointestinal and hepatic disease and discuss approaches to the management of the more common problems confronting the clinician.

DYSPHAGIA

DEFINITION

Dysphagia refers to difficulty in swallowing, either oropharyngeal or esophageal in origin. This symptom is usually described as a "hold-up" or sticking of food, either solid or liquid, during swallowing.

PATHOPHYSIOLOGIC CONSIDERATIONS

Normal swallowing is initiated as a reflex or voluntary act in which the food bolus in the mouth is propelled into the oral pharynx by contraction of the tongue; elevation of the soft palate prevents regurgitation into the nose, while closure of the glottis and elevation of the larynx protect the airway. Simultaneous relaxation of the pharyngoesophageal and gastroesophageal sphincters, followed by sequential contraction of pharyngeal and esophageal muscles (peristalsis), are involuntary motor events coordinated by medullary centers and intramural nerve plexuses.

Dysphagia may be due to mechanical obstruction or may result from disordered neuromuscular function[1] (Table 12–1).

DIAGNOSTIC EVALUATION

Patient History

A careful history in patients with dysphagia often will establish the correct diagnosis. Patients with or-

Table 12–1. Classification of Dysphagia

Mechanical obstruction
  Neoplasm
    Hypopharyngeal
    Esophageal
    Gastric fundal
  Benign stricture
    Reflux esophagitis
    Ingestion of caustic agents
    Radiation injury
    Inflammation
    Congenital lesions
  Esophageal rings and webs
  Extrinsic compression
    Thyroid enlargement
    Neoplasms
    Vascular anomalies
    Aortic aneurysm
    Left atrial enlargement
    Paraesophageal hernia
Disordered neuromuscular function
  Neural lesions
    Central (pseudobulbar lesions)
    Lower motor neuron
    Peripheral nerve lesions
  Myasthenia gravis
  Disorders of muscle
    Primary myopathy
    Myositis
  Disorders of esophageal motor function
    With decreased function
      Scleroderma
      Hypotensive gastroesophageal sphincter
    With increased (disordered) function
      Cricopharyngeal spasm
      Achalasia
      Diffuse esophageal spasm
      Esophageal hyperperistalsis ("nutcracker esophagus")
Inflammatory disease (esophagitis)

opharyngeal lesions usually localize their complaint to the neck, whereas patients with esophageal lesions may indicate the suprasternal or retrosternal region as the site of obstruction. Patients with neurologic disorders, myasthenia gravis, or primary muscle disorders may exhibit oropharyngeal dysphagia with difficulty in initiating swallowing, regurgitation of fluid through the nose, retention of food in the pharynx with the need to swallow repeatedly to clear a single food bolus, or aspiration into the larynx with paroxysmal coughing or laryngeal stridor. In myasthenia gravis, dysphagia typically increases during the course of a meal. Patients with neuromuscular diseases may also have symptoms resulting from involvment of other cranial nerves. Benign strictures are most commonly due to reflux esophagitis; most patients will give a long history of heartburn that preceded their symptom of dysphagia. Progressive narrowing of the distal esophagus is usually associated with a long history of dysphagia initially for solids and later for both solids and liquids. The ingestion of a corrosive acid or alkali is usually an obvious cause for an esophageal stricture; corrosive injury may also be due to retention of pills or capsules in the distal esophagus (aspirin, potassium chloride tablets, and antibiotic capsules). With malignant strictures, there is usually a shorter history of progressive dysphagia with earlier weight loss.

Patients with achalasia, diffuse esophageal spasm, or esophageal hyperperistalsis ("nutcracker eosphagus") often have intermittent dysphagia for solids or liquids; their symptom may be relieved by regurgitating retained food and secretions from the esophagus, by drinking water, or by increasing intrathoracic pressure with Valsalva's maneuver. These motility disorders may also present with retrosternal chest pain that simulates angina; this discomfort, related to increased tension in the wall of the esophagus, may radiate to the neck, to the left forearm, or to the lower interscapular area. Dysphagia in patients with esophageal rings (especially Schatzki's ring, the common lower esophageal membranous ring) is usually intermittent and related to the impaction of a food bolus at a ring with diameter less than 12 mm.

Physical Examination

The more common central nervous system diseases that cause oropharyngeal dysphagia are usually evident on neurologic examination. There may be evidence of peripheral nerve or muscle disease in patients with pharyngeal dysphagia of neuromuscular origin. An examination of the mouth, pharynx, and neck by direct inspection and palpation is a sensitive method for detecting neoplasms, pharyngeal abscesses, thyroid lesions, or a Zenker's diverticulum. Esophageal diseases causing dysphagia may not be associated with physical findings; in scleroderma, eosphageal involvement is usually accompanied by peripheral skin lesions. When dysphagia is due to esophageal compression by intrathoracic lesions (mediastinal tumors, aortic aneurysm, or left atrial enlargement), the primary lesion may be detected by physical examination.

Diagnostic Studies

The studies that are usually necessary to evaluate patients with dysphagia include radiographic studies with barium, esophagoscopy, and esophageal manometry.

Cineradiographic studies with barium are usually necessary to define oropharyngeal swallowing abnormalities in patients without obvious neuromuscular lesions.[2] Impaired pharyngeal contraction or pharyngoesophageal sphincter dysfunction with loss of coordinated sphincter relaxation evident by retention

of contrast material in the pharynx, may be complicated by aspiration of contrast material into the larynx and trachea. Barium studies of the esophagus may suggest a motility disorder when nonperistaltic contractions are observed or when lack of peristalsis impairs esophageal emptying in the supine position. Diverticula, pressure from extrinsic lesions, and obstructing lesions are usually well defined.

Esophagoscopy should be performed in all patients with radiographic evidence of esophageal obstruction. Endoscopic biopsies (preferably multiple) and brushings for cytologic examination provide histologic evidence of benign or malignant disease. Endoscopic evaluation of the distal esophagus must include the gastric cardia and fundus to identify gastric neoplasm that may cause dysphagia by infiltrating the distal esophagus.

Esophageal manometric studies of the lower esophageal sphincter and body of the esophagus are of value in establishing the diagnosis of motility disorders.[3] In diffuse esophageal spasm, repetitive, non-peristaltic contractions are stimulated in the body of the esophagus by swallowing; sphincter relaxation is usually normal. In achalasia, there is not only a loss of normal peristalsis in the body of the esophagus, but also a failure of relaxation of the lower esophageal sphincter with swallowing; sphincter pressure may be normal or increased. Patients with the nutcracker esophagus exhibit peristaltic waves of increased amplitude and duration.

ODYNOPHAGIA

DEFINITION

Odynophagia refers to painful swallowing. This pain may be accompanied by dysphagia.

PATHOPHYSIOLOGIC CONSIDERATIONS

Acute pharyngitis and acute tonsillitis are common causes for pain with the onset of swallowing. Pain relating to cellulitis in the neck, abscesses, acute lymphadenitis, arteritis, or thyroiditis may be accentuated by muscle contraction during swallowing.

Patients with esophagitis caused by candida[4] or herpesvirus infection, acute radiation injury, or caustic injury may suffer from severe retrosternal pain with swallowing; their pain often follows the peristaltic wave down the chest. Although the pain pattern in patients with reflux esophagitis is variable, some patients describe an increase in their pain when they swallow citrus juices. An increased stimulation of afferent nerves from the mucosa is the probable mechanism for pain in patients with esophagitis.

Retrosternal chest pain (esophageal colic) is a common complaint of patients with diffuse esophageal spasm or esophageal hyperperistalsis (nutcracker esophagus). Although spasms of pain are sometimes precipitated by eating or drinking cold liquids, the relationship between pain and swallowing is variable.

DIAGNOSTIC EVALUATION

Odynophagia caused by candida or herpesvirus infection is usually encountered in immunocompromised patients receiving antibiotics or chemotherapy. The diagnosis of Candida esophagitis in susceptible patients with odynophagia can usually be based on the presence of lesions in the mouth; the response to oral antifungal therapy provides clinical confirmation of the diagnosis. Esophagoscopy with mucosal biopsies of macroscopic lesions may be necessary to establish a diagnosis of esophagitis in patients who do not respond to a therapeutic trial of nystatin.[4]

HEARTBURN (PYROSIS)

DEFINITION

Heartburn is a retrosternal burning discomfort that is usually associated with reflux esophagitis. Patients usually feel mild discomfort in the low retrosternal area; with increasing severity, there is radiation to the upper chest and neck.

PATHOPHYSIOLOGIC CONSIDERATIONS

The stratified squamous epithelium of the esophagus is normally protected from prolonged contact with gastric content by the resting pressure of the gastroesophageal sphincter, which limits gastroesophageal reflux; by esophageal peristalsis, which clears the distal esophagus after transient episodes of reflux; and by the intermittent swallowing of alkaline saliva, which neutralizes small amounts of acid that may be retained in the esophagus.

When the esophageal mucosa is exposed to an acid

pH or to bile acids, surface epithelial cells are damaged and are desquamated at an increased rate. The adaptive increase in mucosal cell proliferation from the deep regeneration zone may be insufficient to compensate for cell loss, so that the mucosa becomes shallower or is eroded. The loss of mucosal integrity causes inflammation and local hyperemia and bleeding. Erosive esophagitis is usually maximal just above the junction of the squamous and columnar epithelia at the lower end of the esophagus; with increasing severity, the lesion extends up into the mid-esophagus.[5]

Acid perfusion studies (Bernstein test) indicate that mucosal thinning (possibly with exposure of nerve fibers in exposed dermal pegs that extend to the surface) or erosion causes acid sensitivity; an infusion of 0.1N hydrochloric acid solution usually reproduces the symptom of heartburn.

Mechanisms of Reflux Esophagitis.[6] Continuous pH recordings from the lower esophagus have shown that acid reflux occurs intermittently during periods of sphincter relaxation in normal subjects without heartburn; refluxed acid is usually cleared rapidly by swallowing. Patients with heartburn differ from normal subjects in having more frequent episodes of acid reflux and delayed clearance of acid from the lower esophagus. The major determinants of reflux esophagitis, occurring alone or in combination, include a depressed gastroesophageal sphincter function, impaired esophageal clearance of acid, delayed gastric emptying, increased intra-abdominal pressure, and gastric acid hypersecretion (Table 12–2).

A decrease in the basal gastroesophageal sphincter pressure in response to alcohol and fatty foods may be secondary to the release of peptide hormones; female steroid hormones, cigarette smoking, and anticholinergic drugs lower sphincter pressure by their direct action on esophageal smooth muscle. Patients with scleroderma are likely to develop severe reflux esophagitis that progresses to distal stricture formation; the replacement or separation of esophageal smooth muscle fibers by collagen not only interferes with sphincter function, but also abolishes distal peristalsis and acid clearance from the lumen. In patients with reflux esophagitis, mucosal inflammation is complicated by decreased sphincter function, which may improve with mucosal healing. In many patients with gastroesophageal reflux, depressed sphincter function—lowered basal sphincter pressures, more frequent and prolonged episodes of sphincter relaxation, or a lack of sphincter response to increases in intra-abdominal pressure—is unexplained.

Esophageal clearance of acid depends on peristalsis initiated by swallowing or by distension of the distal esophagus; peristalsis removes the major volume of

Table 12–2. Mechanisms of Gastroesophageal Reflux with Esophagitis

Depressed gastroesophageal sphincter function
  Foods
    Fat
    Alcohol
    Chocolate
  Hormones
    Pregnancy
    Oral contraceptive hormones
  Cigarette smoking
  Drugs
    Anticholinergic agents
    Antidepressants and antihistamines with anticholinergic side-
      effects
    Theophylline
  Esophageal disease
    Scleroderma
    Reflux esophagitis
  Nasogastric intubation
  Cardiomyotomy or sphincter excision
  Idiopathic sphincter dysfunction
Impaired esophageal clearance of acid
  Esophageal aperistalsis: scleroderma
  Decreased secretion of saliva: sicca syndrome
  Depressed secondary peristalsis following acid reflux
Delayed gastric emptying
  Gastroparesis
    Diabetes mellitus
    Truncal vagotomy
    Anticholinergic drugs
  Gastric outlet obstruction
    Pyloric stenosis
    Pyloric channel ulcer
    Pylorospasm
  Impaired small-bowel motility
    Bacterial overgrowth syndromes
    Scleroderma
    Intestinal pseudo-obstruction
  Idiopathic
Increased intra-abdominal pressure
  Obesity
  Ascites
Gastric acid hypersecretion duodenal ulcer, Zollinger-Ellison syn-
    drome

acid from the distal esophagus. Esophageal neutralization may be completed by swallowed saliva. Nocturnal recordings of esophageal pH and swallowing have shown that episodes of acid reflux are less likely to be followed by secondary peristalsis in patients with reflux esophagitis than in normal subjects; the time period of mucosal exposure to acid is thus more prolonged.

Increases in intra-abdominal pressure, either transient with abdominal contraction or sustained in the presence of obesity or ascites, may exceed the lower esophageal sphincter pressure barrier and thus increase reflux of acid. Similarly, delayed gastric emptying in patients with gastric outlet obstruction, gastroparesis,

or impaired small-bowel motility is usually associated with acid reflux. Delayed gastric emptying has been described in the absence of organic gastroduodenal disease in some patients with symptomatic reflux esophagitis; this motility disorder has not been explained.[7]

Esophageal mucosal injury is likely to be more severe when acid hypersecretion is accompanied by reflux. Esophagitis has been described, however, in the absence of acid; the detergent action of bile salts is a likely cause of mucosal injury in patients with bile regurgitation.

DIAGNOSTIC EVALUATION (Fig. 12–1)

When a patient with the complaint of heartburn describes episodic regurgitation of sour (acid) or bitter (bile) liquid into the mouth with changes in posture, the diagnosis is gastroesophageal reflux. When the diagnosis can be established by history alone, it is appropriate to proceed with treatment without further diagnostic studies. If a diagnosis of symptomatic gastroesophageal reflux is uncertain or if symptoms persist in spite of treatment, further evaluation should be considered[8] (Table 12–3).

Barium studies of the esophagus are of limited value in the assessment of patients with heartburn. High-density barium suspensions have a low sensitivity for demonstrating reflux, whereas the water siphon test, in which the subject swallows water in a head-down position while the gastric fundus is filled with barium, is so sensitive that the normal relaxation of the gastroesophageal sphincter with swallowing is demonstrated. A barium swallow is helpful in evaluating the degree of luminal narrowing in patients with strictures complicating reflux esophagitis; the barium study has a low sensitivity in detecting distal esophagitis with mucosal erosions.

In esophageal pH monitoring, a pH electrode, positioned manometrically 2 cm above the gastroeso-

Table 12–3. Diagnostic Procedures to Evaluate Heartburn

To document gastroesophageal reflux
  Barium swallow
  Monitor esophageal pH
  Radioisotopic scanning
To relate symptoms to acid reflux
  Acid/saline infusion test (Bernstein)
  Correlate symptoms with esophageal pH
To evaluate esophageal mucosal injury
  Barium swallow
  Esophagoscopy with mucosal biopsies
To define mechanism for gastro-esophageal reflux
  Esophageal manometry with measurements of sphincter pressure
  Radioisotopic gastric emptying studies

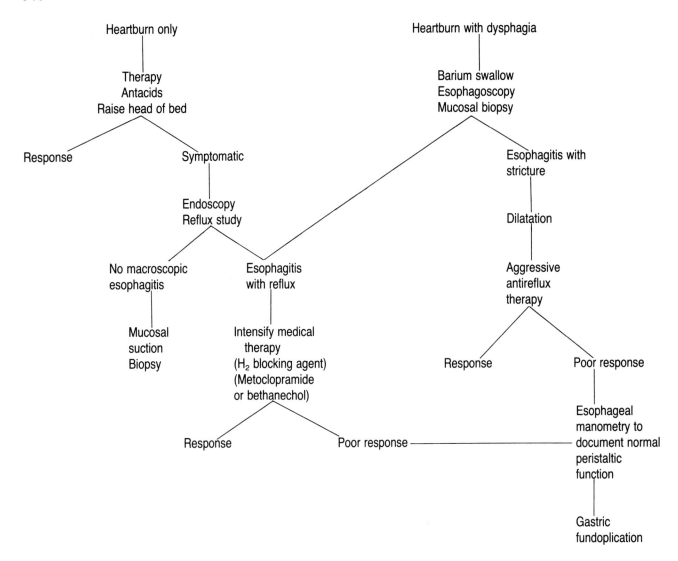

Fig. 12–1. Diagnostic approach to heartburn.

phageal sphincter, provides direct evidence of acid reflux. The sensitivity of pH monitoring is increased by recording pH changes over several hours; the frequency and duration of acid reflux can thus be measured and correlated with symptoms of reflux.[9]

Another study is radioisotopic scanning. Following the ingestion of a 300-ml solution containing ^{99m}technetium sulfur colloid, the distribution of the isotope between the stomach and esophagus can be estimated by surface scanning. The isotope scan is a sensitive, noninvasive test for gastroesophageal reflux.[10]

Sensitivity of the esophageal mucosa to acid can sometimes be demonstrated using the acid infusion test by infusing 0.1N hydrochloric acid or normal saline into the body of the esophagus. If the patient's symptom of heartburn is reproduced by acid infusion only and is relieved during saline infusion, there is a high

probability that the patient's complaint of heartburn results from acid reflux.

Esophagoscopy is the most sensitive method for defining mucosal lesions in the distal esophagus; mucosal hyperemia, increased friability, and linear erosions or ulcerations are typical macroscopic lesions in patients with reflux esophagitis. Esophagoscopic biopsies are usually too small and too difficult to orient for evaluation of early mucosal lesions in reflux esophagitis; well-oriented and sectioned suction biopsies from symptomatic patients with macroscopically normal esophageal mucosae have shown basal cell hyperplasia, infiltration with inflammatory cells; and extension of the dermal pegs close to the mucosal surface.[6]

Esophageal manometry is of limited clinical value in patients with heartburn. Although patients with symptomatic reflux esophagitis have a lower mean basal gastroesophageal sphincter pressure than normal control subjects, a normal pressure recording in an individual patient does not exclude this diagnosis, nor does a low sphincter pressure establish a diagnosis.

ANGINA-LIKE CHEST PAIN OF ESOPHAGEAL ORIGIN

DEFINITION

Retrosternal chest pain with qualities resembling angina pectoris and with radiation into the neck, left arm, or both may have an esophageal origin.[11]

PATHOPHYSIOLOGIC CONSIDERATIONS

Experimental studies have shown that increased tension in the wall of gastrointestinal structures may be appreciated as pain. Clinical studies suggest that patients with abnormal esophageal motility, particularly diffuse esophageal spasm and esophageal hyperperistalsis (nutcracker esophagus),[12] may present with retrosternal chest pain with angina-like features. The segmental distribution of the pain is similar to that of the heart.

DIAGNOSTIC EVALUATION

In patients with recurrent angina-like chest pain, the historical features that may suggest an esophageal rather than a cardiac origin are the lack of relationship to activity, the occasional association with eating (particularly cold liquid or food), and the complaint of episodes of dysphagia. The response to nitrites is of little diagnostic value as these agents cause relaxation of both vascular and gastrointestinal smooth muscle.

When the possibility of a cardiac origin for the chest pain is thought to be likely, the physician should perform a complete cardiac evaluation for coronary artery disease or coronary artery spasm before proceeding with esophageal studies. In the absence of coronary artery disease or spasm, the patient should be evaluated for a motility disorder by esophageal manometry and for reflux esophagitis by a provocative acid infusion test, measurement of esophageal pH, and endoscopy.

ABDOMINAL PAIN

DEFINITION

Abdominal sensations that are perceived by the patient as discomfort are often described as pain. These sensations will differ in their location, quality, and intensity according to the organ involved, the type and intensity of the stimulus initiating the sensation, and the patient's pain threshold.

PATHOPHYSIOLOGIC CONSIDERATIONS[13–15]

Visceral pain from abdominal structures results from stimulation of afferent sympathetic nerves by one or more of the mechanisms of tension, inflammation, ischemia, and neuropathy.

Tension. An increase in tension in the smooth muscle wall of the gastrointestinal tract or ductal structure as a result of either distension or excessive contraction is the most common cause for abdominal pain, either acute or chronic. Increased contraction of visceral smooth muscle may be stimulated by enteric infection (viral, bacterial, or parasitic), by bacterial enterotoxins, by chemical agents (e.g., purgatives), by obstructing lesions (e.g., gallstones in the common bile duct), by mucosal inflammation or ulceration, or by ischemia. The time, course, and intensity of visceral pain caused by smooth-muscle contraction will often correspond to the duration and intensity of the muscle contraction; thus, the patient may describe intermittent waves of cramping or colicky pain resulting from increased peristaltic contractions, or steady pain resulting from continued muscle spasm.

The capsule of the liver, spleen, and kidneys is also sensitive to increases in tension. An acute increase in liver size caused by hepatic venous congestion or acute viral hepatitis stretches Glisson's capsule and causes steady discomfort or pain in the right upper quadrant of the abdomen.

Inflammation. Inflammation involving the peritoneum or retroperitoneal structures may be due to bacterial infection (localized or generalized bacterial peritonitis) or chemical irritation (bile salts, HCl, or proteolytic enzymes). The resulting visceral pain will be less intense and less well localized when inflammation is confined to the visceral peritoneum (i.e., the serosa over an inflamed organ) than when there is involvement of the more sensitive parietal peritoneum that is innervated by somatic sensory nerves.

Ischemia. The pain associated with ischemic injury to the gut, whether caused by strangulation by volvulus, hernia, or adhesive loop or caused by mesenteric vascular disease, initially has a cramping character that may result from altered motility and later becomes steady as tissue injury leads to peritonitis.

Neuropathy. Diabetes mellitus, chronic lead poisoning, acute intermittent porphyria, and tabes dorsalis are diseases that may be associated with acute, recurrent abdominal pain caused by radiculopathy or neuropathy. In patients with retroperitoneal neoplasms, particularly carcinoma of the pancreas, infiltration of sympathetic nerve plexuses by malignant cells appears to be one of the mechanisms for pain.

DIAGNOSTIC EVALUATION

The regional localization of pain arising from different abdominal structures has been evaluated by clinical observations and by experimental studies in which visceral pain from different sites in the gastrointestinal tract has been reproduced by inflating intraluminal balloons. An epigastric distribution of pain is typical of visceral pain from the stomach, duodenum, pancreas, and biliary tree; duodenal pain may be localized to the right of the midline, while pain from the gallbladder, common bile duct, and pancreas usually radiates to the right subcostal area and right scapular area, to the interscapular region, or to the mid-back respectively. A periumbilical distribution of pain is observed from the small bowel, while visceral pain from the colon is classically described as suprapubic or located in the left lower quadrant; studies of colonic pain generated by balloon distension have shown, however, that this pain may be localized to any of the abdominal quadrants.

Acute Abdominal Pain

The causes for acute abdominal pain are classified in Table 12–4.

The approach to a patient with the acute onset of abdominal pain, which may be due to a life threatening condition requiring surgical intervention, differs from the approach to a patient with chronic or recurrent abdominal pain.[15]

Patient History The rate of onset of the pain and its subsequent course provide important diagnostic information. Acute perforation of a viscus (ulcer), acute strangulation by torsion, acute calculous obstruction (biliary colic), or acute infarction (by embolization) causes pain that is usually of more rapid onset than that of inflammatory disease.

The character and severity of the pain will often reflect the underlying mechanism. Pain associated with

Table 12–4. Classification of Acute Abdominal Pain

Pain of sudden onset (within minutes)
  Perforated viscus (e.g., ulcer)
  Strangulated viscus (e.g., by torsion)
  Acute obstruction by calculi (biliary, renal colic)
  Ruptured ectopic pregnancy
  Acute intra-abdominal bleeding (ruptured spleen, ectopic pregnancy, hepatic neoplasm)
  High small-intestinal obstruction
  Mesenteric infarction
  Rupture of aortic aneurysm
  Intrathoracic disease (acute myocardial infarction)
Pain of gradual onset (within hours)
  Acute inflammation of gallbladder, pancreas, liver, appendix, colonic diverticulum, small intestine, peritoneum, urinary system, fallopian tubes
  Distal small-bowel obstruction
  Strangulated hernia
  Intussusception
  Metabolic disease (diabetic ketoacidosis, acute adrenal insufficiency, acute intermittent porphyria)
  Extra-abdominal disease (lower lobe pneumonia, pulmonary infarct, herpes zoster)

increased peristalsis (mechanical obstruction or enteric infection) will have a colicky character, whereas pain associated with inflammation will usually be constant. The site of onset of pain and its subsequent radiation may point to the organ of involvement.

The presence of associated chills and fever, nausea, vomiting, abdominal distension, constipation or diarrhea, urinary symptoms, or gynecologic symptoms is particularly helpful in the interpretation of the pain.

The physician should note factors that may increase or relieve pain. The effect of respiration, movement, position, vomiting, food intake, and bowel or bladder function may be important clues in the diagnosis. Pain in a patient with inflammatory disease is often increased by movement and decreased by rest or by the assumption of a specific posture; by contrast, colicky pain is not aggravated by changes in position.

Additional information such as the history of past illnesses, drug use, or foreign travel, may be particularly relevant. A history of mitral valvular disease or duodenal ulcer increases the risk of embolic phenomena or ulcer perforation, respectively. Prolonged use of oral contraceptive steroids may have been complicated by the development of a hepatic adenoma presenting with acute rupture and intraperitoneal bleeding. Recent foreign travel increases the risk of enteric infection.

Physical Examination. The physical examination should be planned not only to define the cause for the patient's pain, but also evaluate his general condition, to assess the effects of his acute illness on the circulatory system, and to detect any other underlying diseases that may complicate his acute illness. Fever is

Table 12–5. Causes of Hyperamylasemia

Acute pancreatitis
Perforated duodenal ulcer
Mesenteric thrombosis
Small-bowel perforation/obstruction
Ruptured ectopic pregnancy
Diabetic ketoacidosis
Acute parotitis (bacterial, mumps)
Administration of narcotic analgesics
Renal insufficiency
Macroamylasemia

usually suggestive of inflammatory disease; a high fever with shaking chills early in the course of the illness is suggestive of pneumonia, bacterial cholangitis, intra-abdominal abscess, acute bacterial peritonitis, pyelonephritis, or septicemia. Hypovolemia caused by vomiting, blood loss, or loss of fluid from the vascular space in patients with pancreatitis, peritonitis, or bowel obstruction and infarction demands early recognition and treatment with appropriate fluid replacement.

The abdominal examination should focus specifically on localizing of pain and tenderness, the detection of rebound tenderness and muscle guarding, the presence or absence of bowel sounds, distended bowel loops, organ enlargement, or masses, and external hernias. Pelvic and rectal examinations are critical for the evaluation of pelvic structures and the detection of occult gastrointestinal bleeding.

Diagnostic Studies. Laboratory Tests. All patients with acute abdominal pain should have a complete blood count, urinalysis, and serum electrolyte, blood urea and creatinine determinations. An increased white cell count with a shift to the left may indicate an inflammatory process, while examination of the urine will provide evidence of urinary infection or renal calculi. Stool should be examined for overt or occult bleeding, which is a common complication of pancreatitis, intussusception, mesenteric vascular disease, and inflammatory bowel disease.

A serum amylase determination prior to the administration of narcotic analgesics may support a diagnosis of acute pancreatitis; hyperamylasemia, however, is not confined to patients with acute pancreatitis (Table 12–5). In some patients with acute pancreatitis, serum amylase levels may be normal; hypertriglyceridemia, which may precipitate acute pancreatitis, also interferes with serum amylase measurements unless the serum is diluted. When pancreatitis is complicated by a pleural effusion (usually left-sided) or by ascites (caused by a pancreatic-peritoneal fistula), simultaneous measurements of enzyme activity in both serum and effusion usually show higher levels in the effusions. An increase in the renal clearance ratio, the ratio of amylase to creatinine, as well as an increase in urinary amylase levels occurs during an attack of acute pancreatitis. This relative increase in the renal clearance of amylase results from a decrease in the tubular absorption of the enzyme and is also observed in patients with diabetic ketoacidosis, extensive burns, and severe trauma, or following major surgery.

Measurements of serum bilirubin, alkaline phosphatase, gamma-glutamyl transpeptidase, and transaminase activity will provide evidence of hepatitis or biliary tract disease.

Radiologic Studies. Radiologic studies should initially include a chest x-ray and supine and upright views of the abdomen; the abdominal films may show free air under the diaphragm in patients with a perforated viscus, air in the biliary tree in patients with a gallstone ileus, distended loops of intestine with air-fluid levels in patients with obstruction or ileus, or a loss of psoas shadows in patients with retroperitoneal inflammation. In patients with suspected biliary tract disease, an ultrasound examination is the most sensitive test for gallstones. Failure of the gallbladder to fill with isotope following an intravenous injection of ^{99m}Tc–labeled HIDA supports a clinical diagnosis of an obstructed cyclic duct with acute cholecystitis.

Emergency endoscopy, contrast radiography, or arteriography may be indicated in selected patients with acute abdominal pain. Careful sigmoidoscopy without distension of the colon with air will usually establish the diagnosis of acute ulcerative colitis; upper gastrointestinal x-rays with water-soluble contrast material may be helpful in defining an esophageal or gastroduodenal perforation. A barium enema is of value in defining the presence of an obstructing colonic lesion or an area of segmental colonic ischemia and in reducing intussuscepted bowel; and preoperative arteriography is necessary to establish a diagnosis of mesenteric artery occlusion.

Chronic and Intermittent Abdominal Pain

Chronic or recurrent abdominal pain may be due to ulcer disease, inflammation, disordered gastrointestinal motility, recurrent passage of calculi, or obstruction. Somatic pain from the abdominal wall, peripheral nerves, or dorsolumbar spine must also be considered in the differential diagnosis. A classification of chronic or recurrent abdominal pain is presented in Table 12–6.

Patient History. As is the case with acute abdominal pain, the patient's description of the pain—its time course, character, location, and radiation, and associated symptoms and factors that modify it—is of particular importance in the differential diagnosis. The results of previous studies and abdominal operations should be reviewed in detail, and a history of drug use

Table 12–6. Classification of Chronic or Recurrent Abdominal Pain

Chronic peptic ulcer disease
Chronic/recurrent inflammatory disease
　Relapsing pancreatitis
　Chronic cholecystitis
　Chronic inflammatory bowel disease
　Endometriosis
　Chronic pelvic inflammatory disease
Recurrent obstruction
　Choledocholithiasis
　Recurrent intestinal obstruction
　Chronic intestinal pseudo-obstruction
　Recurrent colonic volvulus
Primary motility disorders
　Nonulcer dyspepsia
　Biliary dyskinesia (sphincter of Oddi dysfunction)
　Irritable bowel syndrome
　Withdrawal from narcotic addiction
Somatic pain from the abdominal wall, peripheral nerves, or dorso-
　　lumbar spine
　Incisional pain (e.g., postcholecystectomy)
　Radiculopathy or neuropathy (postherpetic neuralgia, diabetic
　　neuropathy)
　Degenerative arthritis of the spine

should be documented. Evidence of anxiety or depression should be sought during the patient interview; patients with symptoms of irritable bowel syndrome often seek medical care when their adjustment to chronic symptoms is disrupted by emotional problems.

Physical Examination. A complete physical examination, including pelvic and rectal examinations, is necessary in evaluating patients with chronic or recurrent abdominal pain. The absence of physical findings can be as important as positive findings in pointing to a diagnosis. Localized abdominal tenderness is difficult to interpret as it may be present in patients with both inflammatory and functional diseases, but the presence of distended bowel loops, organ enlargement, or a palpable abdominal mass will point to organic disease. If when the patient is first seen pain is not present, arrangements should be made to examine the patient during later attacks of pain.

Diagnostic Studies. The laboratory evaluation of a patient with recurrent or chronic abdominal pain should include a complete blood count, urinalysis, erythrocyte sedimentation rate, and examination of multiple stools for occult blood. An increase in the white cell or platelet count and in the sedimentation rate suggests organic disease (inflammation or neoplasm). Measurements of blood glucose, serum amylase, cholesterol, triglyceride, calcium, phosphate, creatinine, bilirubin, alkaline phosphatase, transaminases, and proteins, particularly during attacks of pain, are of value in the diagnosis. Plain x-ray films of the abdomen may reveal radiopaque gallstones (15 to 20%

of gallstones) and pancreatic calcification associated with chronic pancreatitis.

Endoscopic studies, contrast radiography, and radionuclide, ultrasound, or CT imaging studies should be used selectively in seeking the disease processes suggested by the clinical data.

In patients with suspected ulcer disease, upper gastrointestinal endoscopy is the most accurate diagnostic procedure. Barium studies are of limited value in documenting the presence of a duodenal ulcer in patients with recurrent pain.

In patients with suspected biliary tract disease, ultrasonography is the most sensitive means for detecting gallstones. Pain suggestive of biliary tract disease that persists following cholecystectomy may be due to retained gallstones, spasm of Oddi's sphincter, duodenal or pancreatic disease, or an irritable bowel syndrome; when liver tests are transiently abnormal during attacks of pain, endoscopic retrograde cholangiography and pancreatography should be performed to define lesions in the duodenum, bile duct, or pancreatic ducts.

In patients with suspected pancreatic disease, ultrasound and CT scans provide evidence of organ enlargement or pancreatic pseudocysts, whereas endoscopic retrograde pancreatography defines ductal lesions that may be congenital or caused by pancreatic fibrosis or neoplasm.

In patients with suspected inflammatory bowel disease, colonoscopy with biopsy, and contrast studies of the colon and small bowel usually confirm the diagnosis.

Patients with irritable bowel syndrome should be evaluated with barium and endoscopic studies of the colon to exclude inflammatory and neoplastic disease. The presence of colonic diverticuli in the absence of signs of inflammation, or circular muscular hypertrophy in the sigmoid colon, may be the only objective findings in these patients.

DYSPEPSIA

DEFINITION

The term dyspepsia implies difficulty with digestion but is now used to refer to a spectrum of symptoms that may follow food ingestion. These symptoms include uncomfortable sensations of fullness or bloating, increased eructation of air, a feeling of heaviness in the epigastrium, and epigastric pain of an aching, gnawing, or burning quality.

PATHOPHYSIOLOGIC CONSIDERATIONS

Food in the stomach and duodenum stimulates an increase in secretion and motility either by direct distension or through neurohumoral mechanisms. These physiologic changes postprandially may generate symptoms in patients with organic or functional disease of the upper digestive system. As is the case with abdominal pain, these postprandial symptoms probably relate to changes in pressure or tension in the upper gastrointestinal tract, biliary system, or pancreatic ducts.

DIFFERENTIAL DIAGNOSIS

A wide range of upper gastrointestinal disorders, both organic and functional, must be considered in the differential diagnosis of dyspepsia (Table 12–7). Dyspepsia is a common complaint in patients with ulcer disease, particularly gastric ulcer, with neoplasms of the stomach and pancreas, with biliary and pancreatic inflammatory disease, with superior mesenteric ischemia, and with motility disorders of the stomach, duodenum, and biliary tract.

Table 12–7. Differential Diagnosis of Dyspepsia

Peptic ulcer (gastric, duodenal, or marginal)
Drug-induced gastritis (aspirin, nonsteroidal anti-inflammatory agents, theophylline)
Gastric carcinoma
Pancreatic carcinoma
Biliary tract disease
Chronic pancreatitis
Partial small-bowel obstruction
Motility disorders of the stomach, duodenum, biliary system and colon
Chronic superior mesenteric ischemia (abdominal angina)

DIAGNOSTIC EVALUATION

Patient History

The symptoms of upper gastrointestinal disease are relatively nonspecific. Although "typical" duodenal ulcer pain has been described as a gnawing or burning epigastric pain occurring 1 to 2 hours after a meal, often awakening the patient at night and usually relieved by antacids or food, this pain pattern is variable[16]; many patients with "typical" ulcer symptoms do not have ulcers when examined endoscopically, whereas many patients with ulcers proven by endoscopy remain free of pain. The spectra of upper gastrointestinal symptoms in patients with gastric ulcer, duodenal ulcer, and nonulcer dyspepsia are very similar.[17]

Flatulent dyspepsia, particularly after ingestion of fatty foods, had been considered to be pathognomonic of gallstone disease. Although these symptoms frequently accompany gallstones, they are observed with equal frequency in patients with ulcer disease, nonulcer dyspepsia, and the irritable bowel syndrome.

Physical Examination

There are no specific physical signs in patients with peptic ulcer disease, nonulcer dyspepsia, or motility disorders. Patients with advanced gastric or pancreatic neoplasms may have a palpable epigastric mass, marked weight loss, or evidence of metastatic disease; common bile duct obstruction is an early complication of carcinoma of the head of the pancreas. Localized epigastric tenderness on palpation was once considered to be indicative of duodenal ulcer activity in patients with proven disease; however, endoscopic studies have shown that there is no correlation between epigastric tenderness and ulcer activity. Pyloric obstruction complicating ulcer disease may lead to upper abdominal fullness with visible gastric peristalsis, while a succussion splash may be a sign of obstruction or gastric atony with retained food and secretion in the stomach. Right subcostal tenderness is often elicited in patients with chronic cholecystitis, parenchymal liver disease, or irritable bowel syndrome.

Diagnostic Studies

Acid secretory studies are of no clinical value in the diagnosis of ulcer disease or gastric carcinoma; although acid hypersecretion is important in the pathogenesis of duodenal ulcer, only a third of patients with duodenal ulcer will secrete acid in amounts that exceed the upper limits of normal. In patients with possible Zollinger-Ellison syndrome, measurements of serum gastrin either basally or after provocative stimulation with intravenous infusions of calcium and secretin have replaced secretory studies.

Endoscopy provides direct visualization of lower esophageal, gastric, and duodenal lesions and permits biopsy of suspicious lesions. The decision to proceed with endoscopy (or other diagnostic procedures) must take into account the risks and benefit of the procedure, as well as its cost; endoscopy is unnecessary in the majority of patients whose dyspeptic symptoms respond to a therapeutic trial of antacids, but it may be of particular value in patients whose symptoms persist in spite of treatment.

Double-contrast radiographic studies are both specific and sensitive in detecting mucosal lesions in the stomach but are less sensitive in detecting duodenal lesions, particularly when there is deformity of the duodenal bulb or recurrent marginal ulcers. Endoscopy is unlikely to demonstrate a significant lesion causing symptoms in a patient with a normal double-contrast radiographic study; conversely, a radiographic study is of limited diagnostic value in patients who have been evaluated endoscopically.

NAUSEA AND VOMITING

DEFINITION

Nausea is an unpleasant sensation that is vaguely referred to the epigastrium. It is associated with a loss of appetite or an aversion to food and often precedes vomiting. Severe nausea is usually accompanied by hypersalivation and facial pallor. Vomiting refers to the forceful expulsion of gastric contents from the mouth. Retching describes an unproductive vomiting-like act.

PATHOPHYSIOLOGIC CONSIDERATIONS[18]
(Table 12–8)

Nausea and vomiting are protective physiologic mechanisms that limit the ingestion of potentially harmful materials with a disagreeable appearance, smell, or taste, or that expel such material from the stomach after ingestion. These symptoms commonly reflect psychic, neurologic, or gastrointestinal disturbances.

Nausea is associated with tachygastria (a change in the normal frequency of myoelectric events in the stomach from six cycles per minute to three cycles per minute), a decrease in gastric tone and propulsive contractions, and a delay in gastric emptying. The motor events in vomiting include vigorous and sustained contractions of the abdominal muscles, closure of the pylorus, and relaxation of the esophageal sphincters; gastric content, which is forced up into the body of the esophagus, is then expelled past a closed glottis with additional contraction of the diaphragm and expiratory muscles. With protracted vomiting there may be reverse peristalsis in the upper small bowel and the appearance of bile-stained intestinal secretions in the vomitus.

Neurologically, the medullary vomiting center controls vomiting reflexes through afferent connections from the cortex, through the vestibular system, visual pathways, and the chemoreceptor trigger zone (CTZ) in the floor of the fourth ventricle, from vagal and

Table 12–8.   Pathophysiologic Classification of Nausea and Vomiting

Psychiatric disease
  Psychogenic vomiting
  Bulimia and anorexia nervosa
Vestibular and visual stimulation
  Motion sickness
  Meniere's syndrome
Chemoreceptor zone stimulation
  Drugs (opiates, digitalis, dopaminergic agonists, antineoplastic agents)
  Metabolic and hormonal (ketoacidosis, uremia, pregnancy, acute adrenal insufficiency)
Central stimulation of vomiting center
  Elevated intracranial pressure
  Posterior cranial fossa lesions
Associated with visceral pain
  Myocardial infarction
  Biliary and renal colic
Neuromuscular disorders of the gut with impaired motility
  Vagal denervation (surgical vagotomy, diabetic gastroparesis, anti-cholinergic overdose)
  Sympathetic denervation (visceral neuropathy, Sly-Drager syndrome)
  Spinal shock with ileus
  Myenteric plexus degeneration (amyloidosis, neurogenic chronic intestinal pseudo-obstruction)
  Muscle disease or dysfunction (scleroderma, myogenic intestinal pseudo-obstruction)
Inflammatory disease of the gastrointestinal tract
  Acute enteritis (toxic, bacterial, viral)
  Acute gastritis, pancreatitis, cholecystitis, etc.
  Gastric and duodenal ulcer
  Postoperative ileus
Mechanical obstruction
  Pyloric stenosis
  Small-bowel obstruction
    Luminal (bezoar, stone)
    Intramural (Crohn's disease)
    Extrinsic compression
  Colonic obstruction (luminal, intramural, extrinsic)

sympathetic afferents, and via efferent connections to the vagal motor nucleus and somatic motor pathways.

DIAGNOSTIC EVALUATION

Patient History

The symptoms of nausea and vomiting should be characterized with respect to their time course, their relationship to food intake, and the nature of the vomitus. Evidence of gastric stasis is suggestive of an organic rather than a psychogenic cause. The presence of other symptoms, particularly vertigo, orthostatic fainting, and headache, may point to a central mechanism, whereas abdominal pain may suggest a gastrointestinal problem. Drug ingestion and pregnancy must be excluded. Symptoms suggestive of a psychiatric illness should be noted.

Physical Examination

A complete physical examination should specifically seek evidence of gastrointestinal stasis or obstruction and signs of cranial nerve, vestibular, extrapyramidal, peripheral nerve, or autonomic dysfunction.

Diagnostic Studies

The sequence of diagnostic studies suggested in patients with persistent nausea and vomiting is shown in Table 12–9. A therapeutic trial of oral bethanechol, metoclopramide, or domperidone is appropriate when patient evaluation has failed to define an organic cause for the symptoms.

Additional studies that might be considered in patients with intractable symptoms may provide evidence of a primary or secondary motility disorder involving the stomach or small bowel but are less likely to provide information that is currently of value in treatment.[18] These studies include gastric emptying tests using isotopes incorporated in the solid or liquid phase of test meals[19]; standard esophageal manometry, in which patients with chronic idiopathic intestinal pseudo-obstruction may exhibit disorders of esophageal motility; gastric manometric and electrogastrographic studies to evaluate motor function of the stomach; and laparotomy with full-thickness biopsy of the intestine to evaluate for muscle and myenteric nerve disorder.

FLATULENCE AND GASEOUS DISTENSION

DEFINITION

Patients frequently attribute symptoms of recurrent belching, abdominal fullness, pressure, bloating or distension, and increased passage of flatus to an increase in the volume of gas within the gastrointestinal tract.

PATHOPHYSIOLOGIC CONSIDERATIONS[20]
(Table 12–10)

The intestinal tract normally contains less than 200 ml of gas, which may be eructated, absorbed from the gut to be excreted by the lungs, or passed as flatus from the rectum. A variable volume of gas (200 to 2000 ml, mean 600 ml) is normally excreted daily from the rectum.

Gastrointestinal gas may result from swallowed air, from diffusion of gas from the blood into the lumen, and from bacterial fermentation of intestinal content; nitrogen, hydrogen, carbon dioxide, and methane are the major components. Nitrogen is derived in part from swallowed air and in part from diffusion from the

---

Table 12–9. Diagnostic Studies in Patients with Persistent Nausea and Vomiting

Hematologic and biochemical screening	
Serum electrolytes, BUN, creatinine, glucose, urinalysis	To define metabolic abnormalities that may cause or result from vomiting
Serum calcium	To exclude hypercalcemia
Serum drug levels	To exclude digitalis toxicity
Plasma cortisol levels	To exclude adrenal insufficiency
Catecholamines (supine/erect)	To evaluate sympathetic function
Serum amylase, liver tests	To evaluate pancreatic/biliary disease
Protein electrophoresis	To evaluate for amyloidosis
Radiographic studies	
Supine and erect abdominal films	To evaluate gas pattern of ileus/obstruction
Barium meal and small-bowel study	To define mucosal lesions, obstructive disease, motility
CT scan of head and abdomen	To exclude hydrocephalus and abdominal mass lesions
Endoscopic evaluation	
Panendoscopy (esophagus, stomach, and duodenum)	To exclude mucosal lesions
Tests of sympathetic and labyrinthine function	
Caloric testing	
Psychiatric evaluation	
MMPI test screening	To evaluate for depression or other psychopathology
Psychiatric consultation	

Table 12–10. Classification of Gas-related Symptoms

Increased air swallowing
  Repetitive chewing and swallowing
  Pharyngoesophageal dysfunction with decreased air eructation
  Psychogenic aerophagia
Abdominal bloating
  Irritable bowel syndrome with decreased tolerance to distension
    of small bowel
  Intestinal motility disorders, bacterial overgrowth
Increased flatus
  Carbohydrate malabsorption
  Generalized malabsorption

blood; hydrogen is formed exclusively by bacterial fermentation; carbon dioxide may be produced by neutralization of HCl and organic acids (fatty acid) by secreted bicarbonate and by bacterial fermentation, although the major fraction of this gas produced in the proximal gut is rapidly reabsorbed; methane is produced by bacteria in some normal subjects.

Eructation (belching) is the regurgitation of swallowed air from the body of the esophagus through the pharyngoesophageal sphincter; this air may have come from the stomach bubble or may never have entered the stomach. Recurrent air swallowing (aerophagia) is a common phenomenon in the anxious patient with retrosternal or epigastric discomfort; as the patient attempts to relieve his discomfort by belching he may swallow increasing volumes of air.

Abdominal bloating is a common complaint of patients with functional gastrointestinal disease (irritable bowel syndrome); the discomfort usually increases after meals and may be maximal during the evening hours. Objective studies have not documented excessive intestinal gas in these patients either in the fasting state or after meals. These symptomatic patients differ from normal subjects, however, in that they are less tolerant of intestinal distension during intraluminal infusion of gas and have a low threshold for pain, and they regurgitate infused gas from the small bowel back into the stomach.[21]

Excessive flatus may result from excessive air swallowing or may be due to bacterial fermentation of nonabsorbed nutrients (usually carbohydrate) in the colon. In healthy subjects, lactose malabsorption following milk ingestion may be a source of increased colonic hydrogen and carbon dioxide production.[22] Fruits and vegetables (particularly beans) that contain nonabsorbed carbohydrate provide substrate for bacterial fermentation in the cecum and colon. Recent breath hydrogen studies have suggested that a significant fraction of the starch present with gluten in bread reaches the cecum, where bacterial fermentation produces gas and short-chain fatty acids, which are then absorbed.[23] In patients with malabsorption, an increase in flatus reflects the decreased absorption of fermentable food constituents.

DIAGNOSTIC EVALUATION

Patients with simple repetitive eructation of air may require no evaluation unless there are other symptoms that suggest gastrointestinal disease. In patients with complaints of abdominal bloating or distension, studies should be sufficient to exclude treatable gastrointestinal disease. Absorption studies to document lactase deficiency or a generalized malabsorption syndrome may be indicated in patients with excessive flatus. These studies are more likely to be abnormal if there are other symptoms or signs suggestive of malabsorption.

MALABSORPTION

DEFINITION

Malabsorption refers to impaired intestinal absorption of nutrients, vitamins, or essential minerals. Steatorrhea and creatorrhea refer to increases in fecal fat and nitrogen excretion, respectively. Malabsorption may relate to a single substance (e.g., vitamin B_{12} malabsorption in patients with pernicious anemia) or may involve multiple nutrients.

PATHOPHYSIOLOGIC CONSIDERATIONS AND CLASSIFICATION (Table 12–11)

Malabsorption may be due to one or more of several disturbances of the normal digestive and absorptive process in the intestine.[24]

Intraluminal Digestive Defects. Impairment of the normal intraluminal digestion or processing of food in the small bowel may be the result of impaired acid neutralization. In Zollinger-Ellison syndrome, acid secretion by the stomach exceeds the capacity of the duodenal neutralizing mechanism (HCO_3^- secretion by bile and pancreatic ducts under secretin stimulation); in exocrine pancreatic insufficiency, both pancreatic enzyme and HCO_3^- secretion are depressed.

Decreased pancreatic enzyme secretion may also impair intraluminal digestion. Irreversible denaturation of pancreatic lipase at a pH below 3.0 contributes to steatorrhea in patients with Zollinger-Ellison syndrome. Exocrine pancreatic insufficiency caused by

Table 12–11.   Pathophysiologic Classification of Malabsorption

Intraluminal digestive defects
  Impaired acid neutralization
    Zollinger-Ellison syndrome
    Pancreatic insufficiency
  Deficient pancreatic enzyme secretion
    Pancreatic atrophy
    Chronic pancreatitis
    Pancreatic carcinoma
  Inadequate mixing of food and secretions
    Partial, total gastrectomy
  Decreased intraluminal concentration of conjugated bile salt
    Severe liver disease
    Biliary obstruction
    Ileal resection
    Bile acid sequestrant resins
    Intestinal bacterial overgrowth
Mucosal cell defects
  Specific enzyme deficiency: lactase deficiency
  Specific transport defects: selective vitamin B_{12} malabsorption
  Specific metabolic defects: Abetalipoproteinemia
  Diffuse mucosal disease
    Celiac sprue
    Tropical malabsorption (sprue)
    Giardia lamblia infestation
    Drug injury (neomycin, colchicine)
    Radiation injury
    Mucosal infiltration
      Whipple's disease
      Lymphoma
      Systemic mastocytosis
      Amyloidosis
      Granulomatous disease
  Massive small-bowel resection
Lymphatic obstruction
  Congenital lymphangiectasia
  Lymphangiectasia secondary to fibrosis, neoplasm, or granuloma
  Lymphangiectasia secondary to heart disease
    Constrictive pericarditis
    Congenital heart disease
    Tricuspid insufficiency

chronic pancreatitis or ductal obstruction leads to malabsorption when the secretion of pancreatic enzymes is depressed below 10% of normal.[25]

Another intraluminal digestive defect is inadequate mixing of food with digestive secretions. Steatorrhea following gastric resections, particularly with gastrojejunal anastomosis, is caused by the rapid emptying of gastric content into the jejunum and delayed mixing with pancreatic enzymes and bile.

Also, decreased intraluminal concentrations of conjugated bile salts may impair digestion. Bile salt micelles in the upper small bowel are necessary for solubilization of fatty acids and monoglyceride as well as fat-soluble vitamins (A,D,E, and K) in the aqueous phase. When the intraluminal concentration of conjugated bile salt falls below the critical micellar concentration, the products of triglyceride digestion and

fat-soluble vitamins remain in the lipid phase as fat droplets and are less efficiently transferred to the intestinal epithelium. Low intraluminal concentrations of conjugated bile salts are observed when bile salt secretion is decreased by parenchymal liver disease or biliary tract obstruction; when the bile salt pool is depressed by distal small-bowel resection and interruption of the normal enterohepatic recirculation of bile salt;[26] when intraluminal bile salt is chelated by binding substances, e.g., cholestyramine; and when conjugated bile salts are deconjugated and dehydroxylated by bacterial enzymes in patients with excessive bacterial overgrowth (particularly anaerobic organisms) in the proximal small bowel.

Mucosal Cell Defects. Absorption of specific nutrients by the intestinal epithelial cell may require surface digestion at the brush border (e.g., for disaccharides), active transport across epithelial cell membranes, and intracellular metabolism (e.g., synthesis of apoprotein-B and chylomicron formation). Malabsorption may be due to specific defects or to a general disturbance of absorptive cell function. One cause is specific enzyme deficiency. Lactase deficiency at the brush border causes malabsorption of dietary lactose that is not hydrolyzed by intraluminal digestive enzymes.

Another cause is deficient binding to specific receptors. Vitamin B_{12} malabsorption may result from a lack of intrinsic factor (IF), which is necessary for vitamin B_{12} binding to ileal receptors, or it may result from membrane defects in the ileum (selective vitamin B_{12} malabsorption).

Specific metabolic defects may also cause malabsorption. Abetalipoproteinemia is a rare genetic defect in which lack of apoprotein-B synthesis prevents the formation of chylomicrons in the intestinal epithelium; fat that has entered the cell remains in large fat droplets and passes back into the lumen with cell extrusion from the intestinal villus.

Diffuse mucosal cell disease often leads to malabsorption of multiple nutrients, both fats and water soluble substances that require active intestinal transport.[27] Damage to the absorptive epithelium not only impairs the transport and metabolic functions of individual cells, but also decreases the number of absorptive cells when increased epithelial cell loss causes villous atrophy. Mucosal injury may be due to infectious agents (e.g., Giardia lamblia infestation), may result from bacterial toxins or metabolites (e.g., in tropical malabsorption and intestinal bacterial overgrowth syndromes) or from physical and chemical agents (drugs, radiation therapy), and may be associated with immunologic reactions (celiac sprue, milk protein sensitivity).

Loss of absorptive epithelium is another mucosal cell defect causing malabsorption. The small intestine has considerable functional reserve. The proximal small bowel is normally most active in nutrient absorption, but with proximal disease (e.g., compensated celiac sprue) or proximal gut resection, the distal mucosa may take over more proximal absorptive functions. With massive small-bowel resection or extensive intestinal bypass, the area of absorptive mucosa may be insufficient for normal absorptive function.

Lymphatic Obstruction. Chylomicrons containing absorbed long-chain fats and fat-soluble vitamins are transported from the mucosa via the intestinal lymphatics and thoracic duct. Lymphatic obstruction, either congenital or acquired, leads to dilatation of lacteals in the intestinal villi (lymphangiectasia); rupture of these distended lymphatic vessels through the mucosal epithelium permits leakage of plasma protein, chylomicron fat, and small lymphocytes into the intestinal lumen.

DIAGNOSTIC EVALUATION

Patient History and Physical Examination

Various signs and symptoms are suggestive of malabsorption. The patient may have weight loss unexplained by decreased food intake or increased metabolism (i.e., that caused by hyperthyroidism, or fever). The physicians should note abnormal character of stools, such as stools that are increased in volume, semiformed, or loose, stools that are offensive and floating, or those that contain visible oil.

Abdominal distension with increased bowel sounds (borborygmi) and visible distended loops of small bowel in the absence of overt obstruction may suggest malabsorption. Anemia (iron deficiency or macrocytic) without clinical evidence of an inadequate diet, chronic blood loss, or increased folic acid or iron requirement (as in pregnancy or hemolytic disease) may be another indication. The patient may have protein malnutrition with adequate protein intake and no increased losses (proteinuria). There may be bleeding caused by hypoprothrombinemia in the absence of liver disease.

The patient may also have signs and symptoms of specific deficiency syndromes, such as tetany with hypocalcemia and evidence of osteomalacia; glossitis caused by folate or vitamin B_{12} deficiency; skin lesions of essential fatty acid, zinc, or vitamin B deficiency; or neurologic syndromes caused by vitamin B_{12}, thiamin, or vitamin E deficiency.

The presence of conditions known to cause malabsorption, e.g., gastric surgery, intestinal resection, obstructive jaundice, adminstration of specific drugs (cholestyramine, neomycin), and abdominal radiation, may also suggest malabsorption.

Diagnostic Studies

Studies Documenting the Presence of Malabsorption. D-xylose Absorption Test. A decrease in the urinary excretion of D-xylose, or in the plasma level of D-xylose following a 25-g oral dose, is observed in patients with bacterial metabolism of the sugar (intestinal bacterial overgrowth), short-bowel syndrome (decreased absorptive surface), and diffuse mucosal disease (e.g., celiac sprue); the D-xylose test is of particular value in separating patients with digestive defects (who have normal D-xylose absorption) from those with diffuse proximal mucosal disease (who have markedly impaired absorption).

Quantitative Fecal Fat Measurement. An increased 3-day fecal fat excretion (>7 g daily on a 100-g fat intake daily) is diagnostic of fat malabsorption. Severe anorexia with an inadequate fat intake may invalidate the test. A coefficient of fat absorption (the percentage of dietary fat absorbed) can be calculated from fat intake and fecal excretion. The greatest impairment of fat absorption is usually found in patients with pancreatic insufficiency, massive small-bowel resection, and severe, diffuse mucosal disease. An analysis of triglyceride and free fatty acids in the stool is of limited value in evaluating pancreatic digestion; colonic bacteria may split undigested triglyceride.

^{14}C-Triolein Breath Test. The breath excretion of $^{14}CO_2$ following an oral test dose of labeled triolein reflects fat absorption and metabolism. A decrease in breath $^{14}CO_2$ is observed in patients with fat malabsorption. This test is sensitive and specific and has the advantage of requiring no collection of stool. Its use of ^{14}C isotope is a relative disadvantage, however.

Schilling Test. The Schilling test using radioisotopes of vitamin B_{12} is a sensitive test for vitamin B_{12} malabsorption. Malabsorption of B_{12} alone, corrected by added intrinsic factor, is indicative of IF deficiency (pernicious anemia); malabsorption of IF-B_{12} may be due to pancreatic insufficiency (corrected by pancreatic enzyme), bacterial overgrowth (corrected by antibiotic therapy), or distal mucosal disease.

Studies Defining the Mechanism for Malabsorption and Diagnosing Specific Diseases. In patients with exocrine insufficiency, radiographic studies may show pancreatic calcification. Contrast studies of the small intestine may define multiple diverticula, fistulas, obstruction, or stasis from a pseudo-obstruction that may be associated with bacterial overgrowth.

Tests of pancreatic function consist of analysis of duodenal content following secretin, cholecystokinin (CCK), or test meal stimulation of the pancreas; and of differential Schilling tests. In the latter, patients with pancreatic insufficiency may exhibit malabsorption of vitamin B_{12} in the presence of intrinsic factor; this malabsorption will be corrected by pancreatic enzyme replacement.

Tests to document bile salt deficiency due to malabsorption or bacterial overgrowth involve the bile acid breath test using ^{14}C-glycine-bile acid. Bile acid deconjugation by bacteria in either the small bowel (bacterial overgrowth) or the colon (ileal malabsorption) will increase $^{14}CO_2$ excretion in the breath.

There are several tests to establish a diagnosis of lactase deficiency: the lactose tolerance test with measurement of blood glucose levels; measurement of breath hydrogen excretion following a lactose load; and specific assay of jejunal biopsy for disaccharidase activity.

Per-oral jejunal mucosal biopsy may be useful. Biopsy lesions may be diagnostic of Whipple's disease, agammaglobulinemia, Giardia infestation, lymphangiectasia, and mucosal infiltration by amyloid, lymphoma, or granuloma. Total villous atrophy on jejunal biopsy is suggestive of celiac sprue but may also be seen in severe tropical malabsorption (tropical sprue) and in children with severe protein malnutrition or allergic enteropathy.

Quantitative bacterial cultures (aerobic and anaerobic) of intestinal aspirates may be of value in documenting proximal bacterial overgrowth.

Finally, therapeutic trials should be undertaken. In patients with exocrine pancreatic insufficiency, steatorrhea should respond to treatment with adequate enzyme replacement therapy accompanied by cimetidine (to prevent enzyme inactivation by acid in the stomach). Patients with celiac sprue should respond to a gluten-free diet with symptomatic remission, normal absorption, and improvement in the jejunal biopsy lesion. Antibiotic therapy should decrease intestinal distension, diarrhea, and steatorrhea (at least temporarily) in patients with bacterial overgrowth syndromes.

DIARRHEA

DEFINITION

Diarrhea usually refers to the passage of stools that are more frequent than usual or semiformed or liquid in character. From a more objective viewpoint, diarrhea may be defined as the passage of stools that con-

tain a greater volume of water than normal; stool weight in excess of 200 g daily is abnormal. The term dysentery refers to the passage of liquid stools that contain blood and pus.

PATHOPHYSIOLOGIC CONSIDERATIONS[28,29]
(Tables 12–12 and 12–13)

Under normal circumstances, approximately 9 L of fluid enters the proximal duodenum daily either by ingestion or by secretion from salivary glands, the stomach, the pancreas, and the hepatobiliary system. The major fraction of the fluid is absorbed in the small bowel, so that only about 1 L of ileal effluent enters the colon; in the colon there is further absorption of fluid and electrolytes, so that only 100 ml of water remains in normal stool. In the proximal small bowel there is rapid equilibration of fluid and electrolytes across the mucosa so that the luminal content has the same osmolality as plasma; in the absence of osmotically active organic molecules, the proximal gut fluid has an electrolyte composition close to that of plasma; with passage distally there is an exchange of sodium for potassium and chloride for bicarbonate.

Various pathophysiologic mechanisms may be responsible for increasing the volume of stool water.

Osmotic Effects. The presence of unabsorbed, osmotically active solutes (either organic or inorganic)

Table 12–12. Pathophysiologic Classification of Acute Diarrhea

Osmotic
  Saline cathartics
  Lactulose therapy
  Antacid (Mg^{++}) therapy
  Elemental diets
Secretory
  Without mucosal damage
    Laxatives
    Traveler's diarrhea (enterotoxic E. coli)
    Cholera (enterotoxin)
    Salmonella, Staphylococcal enterotoxin
  With mucosal damage
    Acute allergic reaction to food allergen
    Acute viral enteritis
    Acute bacterial enteritis (with mucosal invasion): salmonella, shigella, clostridia, Vibrio parahaemolyticus, Campylobacter.
    Acute parasitic infection: Giardia lamblia, Cryptosporidiosis, falciparum malaria
Inflammatory exudation
  Antibiotic-related pseudomembranous colitis
  Acute ulcerative colitis
  Acute dysentery: Shigella, E. histolytica, Yersinia enterocolitica
  Acute proctitis (especially in male homosexuals): Gonococci, syphilis, Chlamydia trachomatis
Increased intestinal motility
  Drugs: propranolol, quinidine
  Laxatives

Table 12–13. Pathophysiologic Classification of Recurrent or Chronic Diarrhea

Osmotic
  Chronic laxative abuse
  Lactase deficiency
  Malabsorption
  Postgastrectomy (dumping) syndrome
Secretory
  Without mucosal lesions
    Chronic laxative abuse
    Caffeine, alcohol, drugs
    Bile acid malabsorption: ileal resection, postcholecystectomy,
      idiopathic
    Steatorrhea (fatty acid diarrhea)
    Endogenous secretagogues (hormones)
      Pancreatic cholera
      Medullary carcinoma of thyroid
  With mucosal lesions
    Malabsorption: celiac sprue, tropical sprue, intestinal bacterial
      overgrowth
    Chronic parasitic infestation: Giardia lamblia, Cryptosporidiosis
    Crohn's disease and ulcerative colitis
    Drugs: neomycin
    Radiation injury
    Villous adenoma of the colon
Inflammatory exudation: inflammatory bowel disease
  Increased intestinal motility
  Irritable bowel syndrome
  Chronic laxative abuse
  Diabetic diarrhea
  Hyperthyroidism
  Drugs: quinidine, propranolol, ganglion blocking drugs
  Carcinoid syndrome

in the intestinal lumen increases the volume of intestinal fluid to maintain isotonicity with plasma. A distal increase in sodium reabsorption as well as bacterial metabolism of some organic solutes (e.g., lactose) will decrease the volume of fluid passing through the colon and reduce stool water loss. In the presence of osmotic diarrhea, measurements of electrolyte concentrations in stool water will show a significant osmotic gap with respect to plasma.

Increased Secretion of Fluid and Electrolytes. The volume of fluid remaining in the intestinal lumen at any level represents the balance between the flow of fluid from a more proximal gut segment, and the absorption and secretion of fluid and electrolytes by the intestinal mucosa; an increase in intraluminal volume results from either an increase in mucosal secretion of fluid and electrolytes or a decrease in absorption. Stimulation of ion secretion and inhibition of normal absorption often occur simultaneously in patients with secretory diarrhea.

When secretory stimuli act proximally in the small intestine where there is normally considerable fluid and electrolyte movement, the volume of the intestinal content entering the colon may be markedly increased. In

spite of the absorptive function of the colon (up to 4 L daily), the volume of diarrheal stool with high electrolyte content (isotonic with plasma) will be greatly increased. When secretory stimuli modify colonic mucosal function (e.g., bile salts or fatty acids), the total volume of stool is usually less than that of a small-bowel diarrhea.

Inflammatory Exudation. Diffuse inflammation of the colonic mucosa not only may inhibit the normal absorptive function of the colon, but also will contribute inflammatory exudate containing blood, pus, and mucus. In some patients with distal inflammatory bowel disease, small liquid bowel movements may consist only of inflammatory exudate.

Altered Motility. Changes in intestinal motility may cause diarrhea either by permitting bacterial overgrowth (in conditions causing stasis) or by decreasing the time of contact between the intraluminal fluid and the absorptive surface (increased peristaltic activity).

DIAGNOSTIC EVALUATION IN PATIENTS WITH ACUTE DIARRHEA

Patient History

Historical information that may be of particular value in the diagnosis of patients with acute diarrhea includes recent travel to an area where sanitation is poor or where diarrheal disease is prevalent; the use of drugs that may be complicated by diarrhea, e.g., antibiotics; recent ingestion of pre-prepared foods that might be contaminated with toxins or bacteria; the occurrence of similar episodes of diarrhea recently in the community or household; homosexual contact in males; and associated fever, acute arthritis, skin lesions, tenesmus, or bleeding, which may be suggestive of inflammatory bowel disease.

Physical Examination

In patients with acute diarrhea, the only abnormalities on physical examination may relate to infection (fever, abdominal tenderness) or acute dehydration with electrolyte depletion, particularly in very young and old patients. The presence of perianal inflammation on rectal examnation is suggestive of inflammatory bowel disease.

Diagnostic Studies

Examination of the stool for blood (overt or occult) and pus cells (using Wright's stain or methylene blue) is of particular value in differentiating the acute diarrhea caused by invasive agents (Shigella, Campylobacter, invasive E. coli, salmonella, and E. histolytica), pseudomembranous colitis, and ulcerative colitis from diarrhea caused by viral infection, parasites (Giardia), and bacterial toxins. Also useful is examination of the stained smear and culture of the stool or rectal swabs for pathogenic organisms.

Proctosigmoidoscopy is of particular value in the diagnosis of pseudomembranous colitis, acute ulcerative colitis, and proctitis. Proctosigmoidoscopy should be performed without an initial enema so that mucosal smears can be examined.

DIAGNOSTIC EVALUATION IN PATIENTS WITH CHRONIC DIARRHEA

Patient History and Physical Examination

In patients with intermittent or chronic diarrhea, a careful analysis of the diarrhea may provide important diagnostic clues. The character of the stools may suggest the site of the disease or the mechanism for diarrhea. Large-volume, watery stools are more typical of small-bowel diarrhea caused by secretory stimuli; bulky, semiformed, malodorous stools containing fat may be due to malabsorption; small-volume stools containing blood or pus and accompanied by tenesmus indicate inflammatory disease of the rectum.

The pattern of bowel movements in relation to food intake and activity should be defined. Secretory diarrhea caused by endogenous secretagogues will continue during periods of complete fasting. Food ingestion will stimulate bowel function in many patients either by physiologically releasing digestive peptide hormones that increase colonic motility, or by providing an osmotic load (in lactase deficiency and malabsorption) or secretory stimulus (such as fatty acids or bile salts in the colon). Nocturnal diarrhea, particularly when it is associated with fecal incontinence, is suggestive of diabetic visceral neuropathy.

A long history of diarrhea alternating with constipation or the passage of small pellet-like stools is a common pattern in patients with irritable bowel syndrome; in patients with a short history of constipation and diarrhea, particularly with bleeding, a diagnosis of colorectal carcinoma must be considered.

Psychologic influences are of particular importance in patients with irritable bowel syndrome; in these patients diarrhea may relate to anxiety, depression, or emotional conflict. The abuse of diuretics and laxatives is common in patients who are anxious to lose weight; this drug use may not be volunteered by the patient.

Other signs and symptoms of diagnostic importance include significant weight loss (suggesting malabsorption, neoplasm, inflammatory bowel disease, or thyrotoxicosis), fever (in inflammatory bowel disease), arthralgias or joint swelling (in Whipple's disease and inflammatory bowel disease), lymphadenopathy (in AIDS, Whipple's disease, and lymphoma), postural hypotension and peripheral neuropathy (in diabetic diarrhea and amyloidosis), and skin lesions (flushing in carcinoid and erythema nodosum and pyoderma in inflammatory bowel disease).

Drugs used by the patient should be reviewed; many agents used in the treatment of cardiovascular disease may cause diarrhea. Also, a social history should define the patient's sexual habits. The family history may be positive for similar illness in first-degree relatives of patients with inflammatory bowel disease or endocrine neoplasms.

Diagnostic Studies

Stools should be routinely examined for occult blood, for pus cells (using Wright's stain), and for ova and parasites (examination of a duodenal aspirate is more accurate in the diagnosis of giardiasis). Alkalinization will reveal the presence of phenolphthalein in patients abusing this laxative. Quantitative stool collections are necessary to measure stool volume, to define the response of the patient to complete fasting, and to determine fecal fat content. Stool water, separated by centrifugation, may be analyzed for its electrolyte content and osmolality; this data will provide evidence of secretory or osmotic mechanisms.

Proctosigmoidoscopy may be of value in establishing a diagnosis of laxative abuse; melanosis coli is evidence of use of anthracene cathartics (senna, cascara sagrada). Patients with inflammatory bowel disease causing diarrhea with blood, pus, and mucus usually exhibit overt mucosal lesions on colonoscopy; occasionally, mucosal disease causing diarrhea is not obvious macroscopically and requires colonic mucosal biopsies for diagnosis. Rectal mucosal biopsies should be carefully examined for Cryptosporidia in patients suspected of suffering from AIDS.

When diarrhea is accompanied by other signs or symptoms suggestive of malabsorption, small-bowel and pancreatic function should be evaluated (see section on malabsorption).

Radiographic studies that may be of value in the assessment of patients with diarrhea include a small-bowel series, barium enema, CT scan of the abdomen, and mesenteric arteriography. The small-bowel series may show a malabsorption pattern, motility disorders, structural lesions causing bacterial overgrowth, Crohn's disease, and ileal carcinoid. Barium enema reveals inflammatory bowel disease and colorectal carcinoma; CT scan of the abdomen may show pancreatic disease and endocrine tumor, and mesenteric arteriography provides evidence of mesenteric ischemia.

Hormonal studies should be done in patients with

severe intractable secretory diarrhea. Radioimmunoassay of plasma for the endocrine tumor markers and hormones should be performed; these include VIP, gastrin, calcitonin, prostaglandins, and pancreatic polypeptide.

In a prospective study of 87 patients referred for chronic unexplained diarrhea, detailed evaluation suggested a diagnosis of surreptitious laxative or diuretic use in 20, irritable bowel syndrome in 14, idiopathic secretory diarrhea in 13, bile acid catharsis in 9, malabsorption syndromes in 17, ulcerative colitis in 2, and neuroendocrine tumors in 2. The cause was unidentified in 10.[30]

CONSTIPATION

DEFINITION

The complaint of constipation usually relates to the patient's perception that stool frequency is decreased or that stools are harder in consistency or more difficult to evacuate. Patients may equate constipation with the need to strain at stool or with the sensation of incomplete evacuation of the rectum. In adults, the patient's past bowel function is usually the "normal" point of reference. Not all patients complaining of constipation have an objective abnormality; their stool frequency and consistency may be well within the normal range. Conversely, some patients with fecal retention may have no complaint or may complain of diarrhea when liquid stool passes around an impacted fecal mass in the rectum.

Objectively, there is no precise definition of constipation; healthy subjects usually pass at least three stools each week, but the normal range of stool size and consistency has not been defined. Perhaps the best objective measure of constipation will be derived from studies of colonic transit time using radiopaque markers.

PATHOPHYSIOLOGIC CONSIDERATIONS[31]
(Table 12–14)

Constipation usually results from a change in stool consistency or from an abnormality or change in colonic or anorectal motor functions that delays transit of stool through the large bowel. An increase in colonic transit time will increase mucosal reabsorption of elec-

Table 12–14. Pathophysiologic Classification of Constipation

Changes in diet, physical activity, and habits
  Decreased dietary fiber
  Decreased physical activity (e.g., hospitalization)
Drugs
  Modifying intraluminal content
    Antacids (calcium and aluminum)
    Barium sulfate
    Bismuth
    Bile acid sequestrant resins
  Depressing neuromuscular function
    Anticholinergics
    Antidepressants
    Anticonvulsants
    Antihypertensives
    Muscle relaxants
  Modifying motor function
    Opiates and analgesic agents
    Hormones (oral contraceptive steroids)
Metabolic and endocrine disorders
  Dehydration
  Diabetes mellitus
  Pregnancy
  Hypothyroidism
  Hypercalcemia
Colonic and anorectal disease
  Irritable bowel syndrome (chronic laxative abuse)
  Diverticular disease
  Primary muscle disease (myotonic dystrophy)
  Scleroderma
  Organic obstructing lesions
    Benign strictures
    Malignant lesions
    Extrinsic lesions (neoplasm, endometriosis)
    Incarcerated hernia
    Volvulus
  Anorectal lesions
    Rectocele
    Proctitis
    Rectal prolapse
    Ulcer of the rectum
    Anal fissure
    Painful hemorrhoids
    Anal stenosis
Psychogenic disorders
Neurogenic disorders
  Central
    Meningocele
    Spinal cord trauma
    Multiple sclerosis
    Lesions of lumbosacral cord
    Stroke
    Parkinsonism
    Brain tumor
  Peripheral
    Autonomic neuropathy
    Chagas-Cruz disease
    Hirschsprung's disease
    Idiopathic neurogenic intestinal pseudo-obstruction
    Amyloidosis

trolytes and water and lead to further hardening of the stool.

Colonic and anorectal function is affected by diet, physical activity, habits, hormones (thyroid, peptide, and steroid), emotional factors, visceral and somatic nerve function, drugs, and local influences from the bowel. Thus, constipation may be the result of a change in one or more of these factors.

DIAGNOSTIC EVALUATION

In patients with constipation of recent onset, a change in bowel habit may be the presenting symptom of colorectal carcinoma. In these patients, the colon and rectum must be examined completely by air-contrast barium studies, colonoscopy, or both. Recent changes in medication or metabolic abnormalities (e.g., hypercalcemia due to malignant disease) should also be considered.

Other patients may have a long history of constipation. In children, the possibility of neurogenic disease (either occult spinal lesions or Hirschsprung's disease) must be excluded. The onset of constipation at birth is strongly suggestive of a congenital lesion, but some patients with neurogenic disease may develop constipation insidiously during the first decade of life. Anorectal manometry is of value in patients with suspected neurogenic disease; the presence of normal anorectal reflexes excludes this diagnosis. Rectal suction biopsies at defined distances from the anal sphincter are of value in documenting aganglionic segments in infants and young children.

In adults, the most common cause for chronic constipation is irritable bowel syndrome with or without diverticular disease. In many of these patients, chronic laxative use may have accentuated the problem or resulted in alternating constipation and diarrhea. A dietary and drug history should be obtained, and thyroid function should be evaluated clinically and by hormone assay.

The initial evaluation should include a proctosigmoidoscopy and barium studies of the colon. Follow-up screening studies for the development of colorectal neoplasms should include annual rectal examinations and testing of multiple stool samples for occult blood; endoscopic examination of the distal colon may be indicated at intervals of 1 to 5 years according to the age of the patient or the presence of adenomatous polyps on initial evaluation.

Constipation is a common problem in patients who are confined to bed or chair by chronic debilitating disease. Bowel function should be closely monitored in these patients, and rectal examinations should be performed when a change in bowel function suggests the possibility of incomplete emptying of the rectum.

GASTROINTESTINAL BLEEDING

DEFINITION

Hematemesis refers to vomiting of blood. When blood mixes with acidic gastric juice in the stomach, there is a rapid conversion of hemoglobin to dark, acid hematin; vomitus consisting of altered blood in the gastric content is described as "coffee-ground" in character. Partial degradation of blood by digestive enzymes and bacteria during its passage through the intestine produces a stool that is pitch black, sticky, and typically malodorous; this dark stool is termed melena. Hematochezia refers to the passage of bright blood from the rectum. When blood is present in the stool on chemical testing but is not visible, the bleeding is referred to as occult.

PATHOPHYSIOLOGIC CONSIDERATIONS[32]

Massive upper gastrointestinal bleeding, presenting either as hematemesis or hematemesia and melena, is potentially a life threatening complication of lesions involving the esophagus, stomach, and duodenum. The immediate effect of acute bleeding is a fall in blood volume and cardiac output; this initially may be manifest as postural hypotension or fainting, but with continued blood loss, systemic vasoconstriction and tachycardia will fail to compensate for the decrease in volume and the patient will show signs of shock.

Slow bleeding allows fluid from the extravascular compartment and gut to maintain blood volume by expansion of the plasma volume; this expansion is facilitated by secondary hyperaldosteronism and renal sodium retention. An increase in cardiac output with peripheral vasodilatation maintains tissue oxygenation until anemia is severe.

The passage of bright blood from the rectum usually indicates lower gastrointestinal bleeding. When bleeding from an upper gastrointestinal site is massive and intestinal transit is rapid, the stool may be dark red or maroon; conversely, blood from the cecum or right colon may be altered by intestinal bacteria and have the appearance of melena.

In the upper gastrointestinal tract, mucosal erosions (often drug induced), peptic ulcers, and gastroesophageal varices are the most frequent bleeding lesions. In the lower gastrointestinal tract, inflammatory bowel disease is the most common cause of bleeding in young patients, while carcinoma, angiodysplasia, and bleeding diverticula increase in frequency in elderly patients.

A classification of gastrointestinal bleeding by site and by pathologic lesion is presented in Table 12–15.

DIAGNOSTIC EVALUATION OF SUSPECTED GASTROINTESTINAL BLEEDING

Patient History and Physical Examination

The history and physical examination often provide information from which the nature of the lesion that is bleeding is suggested and the prognosis for continued or recurrent bleeding and complications can be assessed.

A recent history of ingestion of aspirin or nonsteroidal anti-inflammatory agents increases the likelihood of bleeding from acute erosions or acute ulcers in the stomach. Continued or recurrent bleeding from these lesions is unlikely. With chronic ingestion of anti-inflammatory drugs (e.g., for rheumatoid disease), development of a chronic gastric ulcer is highly probable.

Bleeding from a duodenal ulcer is more likely than from other lesions in patients with a history of documented duodenal ulcer disease. Brisk bleeding from an ulcer is often due to erosion of a branch of the gastroduodenal artery and is more likely than bleeding from acute mucosal lesions to be continued or recurrent.

History and physical findings consistent with a diagnosis of cirrhosis (chronic alcoholism, jaundice, cutaneous spider angiomas, hepatosplenomegaly, or ascites) suggest the possibility of bleeding from gastric or esophageal varices. Patients with compensated cirrhosis and portal hypertension are more likely to be bleeding from esophageal varices than from other upper gastrointestinal lesions, whereas those with hepatic decompensation (jaundice, ascites, and coma) often have massive bleeding from ulcers (acute or chronic), gastric erosions, or varices. Hepatic decompensation increases the risk of continued or recurrent bleeding.

When hematemesis is preceded by recurrent retching or vomiting of gastric content without blood, the most likely lesion is a Mallory-Weiss tear in the mucosa at the gastroesophageal junction.

Acute stress ulcers of the stomach often present with massive upper gastrointestinal bleeding in patients requiring intensive care following severe trauma, head injury, severe burns, organ failure, or surgery. The

Table 12–15.   Classification of Gastrointestinal Bleeding

Upper gastrointestinal bleeding[33]
  Esophageal lesions
    Esophageal erosions
    Mallory-Weiss tear
    Esophageal varices
    Esophageal carcinoma
  Gastric lesions
    Gastric erosions (hemorrhagic gastritis)
    Gastric ulcer (benign)
    Gastric varices
    Gastric neoplasms
    Gastric telangiectasia, angiodysplasia
  Duodenal lesions
    Duodenal ulcer
    Duodenal erosion by extrinsic carcinoma (pancreatic, right renal)
    Leaking aortic aneurysm (aortoduodenal fistula)
    Ampullary carcinoma
    Hematobilia
Lower gastrointestinal bleeding
  Jejunal and ileal lesions
    Meckel's diverticulum
    Small-bowel tumors (ulceration, intussusception)
    Ischemic injury to mucosa (mesenteric vascular accident)
    Crohn's disease
    Hemangioma
    Angiodysplasia
    Vasculitis
  Cecal and right colon lesions
    Angiodysplasia
    Neoplasm
    Diverticular bleeding
    Acute ulceration
    Inflammatory bowel disease
  Left colon and sigmoid lesions
    Neoplasm
    Inferior mesenteric ischemia
    Inflammatory bowel disease
    Angiodysplasia
    Diverticular bleeding
  Anorectal
    Neoplasm
    Inflammatory bowel disease
    Solitary ulcer
    Radiation proctitis
    Hemorrhoids
    Anal fissure
Bleeding disorders that may cause gastrointestinal bleeding in the absence of primary mucosal lesions
  Anticoagulant therapy
  Hemophilia
  Vitamin K deficiency
  Thrombocytopenia
  Uremia
  Disseminated intravascular coagulation

frequency of this complication should be reduced by prophylactic therapy with antacids or histamine$_2$-receptor blocking drugs.

The presence of mucosal or cutaneous lesions and an appropriate family history should suggest the diagnosis of hereditary hemorrhagic telangiectasia, Ehler-Danlos syndrome, and Peutz-Jeghers syndrome. Disseminated Kaposi's sarcoma in patients with AIDS may be complicated by bleeding from gastric lesions; when there are gut lesions, skin lesions are usually present.

In patients with a history of progressive weight loss with anorexia, fever, dyspepsia, early satiety, and an epigastric mass, gastric or pancreatic neoplasms are strong diagnostic possibilities.

When there is a history of bleeding from other sites or an increased tendency to bruise, the patient should be evaluated for a generalized bleeding disorder.

Diagnostic Studies (Fig. 12–2)

The goal of diagnostic studies is to define the site and nature of the bleeding lesion so that appropriate treatment can be recommended. A diagnostic study that is unlikely to change patient management should not be performed.

In evaluating the patient with massive upper gastrointestinal bleeding it is critical to assess cardiopulmonary, hepatic, and renal function; the morbidity and mortality in patients with bleeding is increased in patients with cardiovascular, pulmonary, renal, or liver disease. The possibility of a generalized bleeding disorder should be excluded in all patients by a platelet count, prothrombin time, partial thromboplastin time (PTT), and bleeding time measurements.

DIAGNOSTIC EVALUATION OF SUSPECTED LOWER GASTROINTESTINAL BLEEDING

Patient History and Physical Examination

As is the case in patients with upper gastrointestinal bleeding, a complete history and physical examination is necessary and should include a detailed history of gastrointestinal symptoms.

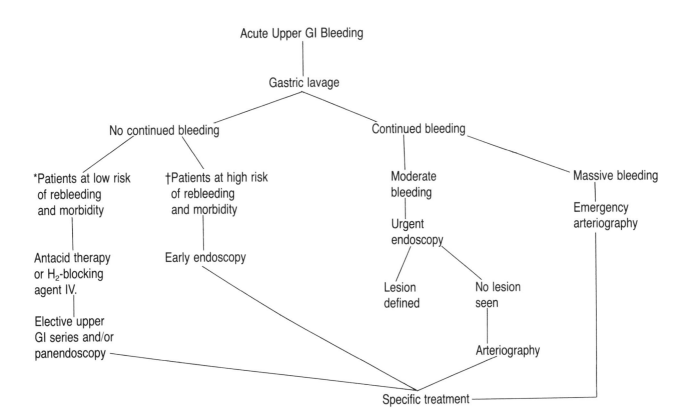

*Young patients without history of ulcer or liver disease and no clinical evidence of cardiopulmonary or renal disease; stable patients with a history of recent aspirin or nonsteroidal anti-inflammatory drug ingestion
†Patients with a history of ulcer or liver disease; patients with clinical evidence of cardiopulmonary disease

Fig. 12–2. Diagnostic approach to acute upper GI bleeding.

The character of the rectal bleeding will sometimes suggest the nature of the bleeding lesion. Patients with arteriolar bleeding from a colonic diverticulum (often right-sided) or a vascular lesion often experience sudden, brisk bleeding with the passage of bright blood or clots. When bleeding is from a prolapsed hemorrhoid, venous blood will frequently continue to drip from the anal area when the anus is contracted. When blood is mixed with mucus and pus, inflammatory disease of the colon is a likely diagnosis; some patients with inflammatory bowel disease may also present with massive arterial bleeding when a submucosal vessel is eroded.

Symptoms that are associated with bleeding should be noted. Abdominal pain and localized tenderness are more suggestive of an inflammatory or ischemic lesion than a vascular lesion without inflammation (diverticular bleeding, angiodysplasia).

When hematochezia is preceded by acute diarrhea with fever and abdominal pain, a diagnosis of enterocolitis should be considered; mucosal ulceration may be due to pathogens or to idiopathic inflammatory bowel disease.

Patients with cardiovascular disease, particularly aortic stenosis, are at risk of developing angiodysplasia in the colon (particularly on the right side) and distal small bowel.

Diagnostic Studies (Fig. 12–3)

Examination of the stool for pus cells will usually separate patients with inflammatory bowel disease (particularly ulcerative colitis, and amebic and bacillary dysentery) from those with noninflammatory bleeding lesions; occasionally, however, bleeding may be more massive and without inflammatory exudate in patients with ulcerative colitis and Crohn's disease. When endoscopic and radiographic studies of the lower bowel fail to reveal a colonic lesion in a patient pre-

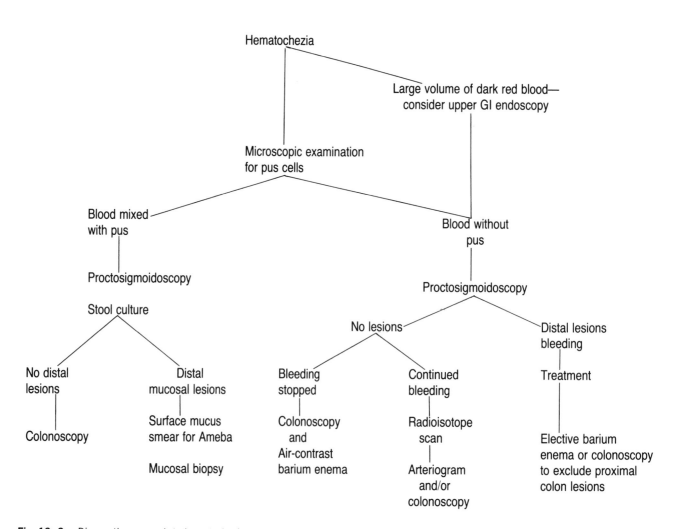

Fig. 12–3. Diagnostic approach to hematochezia.

senting with hematochezia, the diagnostic evaluation should be extended to include an upper endoscopy and small-bowel series to define higher lesions in the gut. When hematochezia is recurrent and previous endoscopic and radiographic studies have been unrevealing, early radioisotopic scanning and selective mesenteric arteriography while the patient is bleeding may reveal vascular lesions in the right colon or distal small bowel.

DIAGNOSTIC EVALUATION OF OCCULT GASTROINTESTINAL BLEEDING

Occult gastrointestinal bleeding is the earliest clinical manifestation of gastrointestinal neoplasms.[34] Unfortunately, tests for occult blood in the stool that are based on the peroxidase activity of hemoglobin (Hemoccult test) do not detect blood that has been modified by bacterial action with conversion of heme to porphyrin; thus, the test is more sensitive for distal blood loss than for more proximal blood loss. False negative tests are produced by reducing substances (e.g., ascorbic acid), and false positive tests occur when the stool is liquid or contains inorganic iron. A more quantitative test of gastrointestinal blood loss estimates both heme and heme-derived porphyrin in the stool; preliminary clinical studies suggest that this test will yield fewer false positive and false negative results than the peroxidase tests that are currently in use.[35]

When stool samples are positive for occult blood, the patient should be evaluated by colonoscopy and barium enema for a colonic lesion; if there is no evidence of a distal bowel lesion, an upper gastrointestinal endoscopy should be performed to evaluate the esophagus, stomach, and duodenum.

JAUNDICE

DEFINITION

Jaundice, or icterus, is a yellow discoloration of the skin and mucous membranes caused by an increased level of bilirubin in the tissue. When there are increased levels of unconjugated bilirubin in the plasma and tissues, the urine remains free of bile pigment; this condition is termed acholuric jaundice. Unconjugated hyperbilirubinemia may be due to an increase in bilirubin production (hemolytic jaundice) or a decrease in hepatic uptake or conjugation of the pigment.

Increased serum levels of conjugated bilirubin (bilirubin diglucuronide) may result from hepatic parenchymal cell dysfunction with depressed hepatic excretion of conjugated pigment, impaired bile flow (cholestasis), or both.

PATHOPHYSIOLOGIC CONSIDERATIONS AND CLASSIFICATION

Bilirubin production, transport, metabolism, and excretion take place in the following sequence:[36]

Production. The major fraction of unconjugated bilirubin (80 to 90%) is derived from the breakdown of senescent red blood cells in the reticuloendothelial system (mainly in the spleen); hemoglobin is degraded with oxidative conversion of heme to the tetrapyrrole pigment, bilirubin. A small fraction of bilirubin (10 to 20%) is produced by the catabolism of heme proteins in the liver, or from ineffective erythropoiesis in the bone marrow (i.e., when heme is not incorporated into circulating red cells).

Transport. Unconjugated bilirubin, a lipophilic molecule with low aqueous solubility, is transported from the spleen to the liver as a complex with albumin. The albumin binding of unconjugated bilirubin and its lipid solubility prevent the renal clearance of the pigment.

Hepatic Uptake. Albumin-bilirubin complexes diffuse from the hepatic sinusoids into the space of Disse, and bilirubin is displaced from albumin by binding proteins on the liver cell membrane.

Intracellular Transport and Metabolism. Unconjugated bilirubin is concentrated in the hepatic parenchymal cell on cytosol binding proteins (Ligandin, Z protein), which have an affinity for many substances. Subsequently, the pigment is conjugated in the smooth endoplasmic reticulum by the microsomal enzyme system, UDP glucuronyl transferase, to bilirubin monoglucuronide (20%) and diglucuronide (80%).

Canalicular Excretion. Water-soluble bilirubin glucuronide is actively secreted into the bile canaliculus by a carrier mediated transport system that is common to several organic anions. The active secretion of conjugated pigment is normally the rate-limiting step in bilirubin clearance from the blood.

Biliary Transport. In the bile, conjugated bilirubin is present in mixed micelles with bile salt.

Bacterial Metabolism in the Gut. In the distal intestine, bilirubin is deconjugated and reduced by bacterial enzymes to form urobilinogens. A small amount of urobilinogen is absorbed in the distal intestine and is re-excreted by the liver. There is an increased urinary excretion of urobilinogen when bilirubin and urobilinogen production increases with hemolysis, or when liver disease impairs hepatic urobilinogen clearance.

A pathophysiologic classification of jaundice is pre-

Table 12–16.   Classification of Jaundice

Increased bilirubin production
  Hemolysis
  Ineffective erythropoiesis: pernicious anemia, thalassemia
Decreased hepatic uptake of unconjugated bilirubin
  Drugs: bunamiodyl, rifamycin SV
  Portal-systemic shunting of blood
Decreased bilirubin conjugation
  Prematurity
  Drugs and hormones: novobiocin, breast-milk jaundice
  Gilbert's syndrome
  Crigler-Najjar syndromes
Decreased liver cell excretion of conjugated bilirubin
  Dubin-Johnson and Rotor's syndromes
  Drugs, ethanol, and toxic agents
    Liver cell injury
    Cholestasis
    Mixed parenchymal cell injury and cholestasis
  Infection: endotoxin, bacteria, viruses, parasites
  Metabolic disorders
  Hepatic circulatory disorders: hypoperfusion, congestion, hepatic
      venous obstruction
  Decompensated cirrhosis
  Space-occupying lesions (abscess, neoplasm, granuloma)
Obstruction to bile flow
  Intrahepatic
    Primary biliary cirrhosis
    Chronic pericholangitis
    Intrahepatic stenosing cholangitis
  Extrahepatic
    Gallstones, ascending cholangitis
    Benign stricture
    Malignant obstruction
      Bile duct
      Pancreas
      Ampulla
      Metastatic neoplasms
    Extrinsic compression
      Pancreatic pseudocyst
      Chronic pancreatitis
      Subhepatic abscess

sented in Table 12–16. Jaundice may result from increased bilirubin production, depressed hepatic uptake, impaired bilirubin conjugation, decreased excretion of conjugated bilirubin, or obstruction to bile flow. In some patients, many factors may be responsible for jaundice; for example, in the postoperative patient there may be hemolysis of transfused blood and impaired pigment excretion because of sepsis, shock, or drugs.

DIAGNOSTIC EVALUATION OF UNCONJUGATED HYPERBILIRUBINEMIA.[37]

Patient History

Severe jaundice from birth, with unconjugated serum bilirubin levels ranging between 6 and 20 mg/dl, and a positive family history of jaundice are typical of the rare type II Crigler-Najjar syndrome. Type I Crigler-Najjar patients, who completely lack hepatic bilirubin glucuronyl transferase, usually die in infancy with kernicterus. Most patients with Gilbert's syndrome, an inherited disorder of bilirubin metabolism in which reduced bilirubin clearance from plasma is associated with depressed hepatic levels of UDP glucuronyl transferase, are not diagnosed until adulthood. The mild unconjugated hyperbilirubinemia in these subjects may become evident only when bilirubin levels increase during periods of fasting, with intercurrent illness, and when the bilirubin load is increased by mild, compensated hemolysis.

Hemolysis should be suspected as a cause for jaundice in patients who have recently received blood transfusions, in patients following drug administration (alpha methyldopa for hypertension and sulfonamides, antimalarials and nitrofurantoin in black patients or Sephardic Jews, in whom glucose-6-phosphate dehydrogenase deficiency is very common), in patients with severe febrile illness (falciparum malaria, septicemia), and in patients with symptoms suggestive of anemia.

A decrease in bilirubin clearance by the liver is relatively common following portocaval shunting in patients with portal hypertension. Jaundice is usually mild.

Physical Examination

Subjects with Gilbert's syndrome will usually be mildly icteric without other physical abnormalities. A palpable spleen tip in some patients will suggest concurrent mild hemolysis. Patients with overt hemolysis may exhibit signs of anemia (pallor of mucous membranes) evidence of an increased cardiac output (tachycardia, precordial ejection systolic murmur, and hyperdynamic peripheral circulation), splenomegaly, or signs of thrombocytopenia (in thrombotic thrombocytopenic purpura, hemolytic uremic syndrome, and disseminated intravascular coagulation). In pernicious anemia, the physician may observe glossitis, mental disturbances, and signs of peripheral neuropathy or subacute combined degeneration.

Diagnostic Studies

The increase in unconjugated bilirubin is the only abnormal liver test in patients with Gilbert's syndrome. A reduction in serum unconjugated bilirubin to normal levels during phenobarbital administration (60 mg three times a day for 2 weeks) and an increase in serum levels with fasting (400 calories daily for 2 days) will support this diagnosis. No additional tests are necessary in these patients.

Unconjugated serum bilirubin levels usually do not exceed 5 mg/dl in patients with hemolysis. When hemolysis occurs in patients with impaired hepatic excretory function, high levels of conjugated hyperbilirubinemia may be observed (e.g., in patients with glucose-6-phosphate dehydrogenase deficiency who develop acute viral hepatitis). When hemolysis is suspected as a cause for jaundice, appropriate hematologic studies may be indicated (see Chapter 4, section on hemolytic disease).

DIAGNOSTIC EVALUATION OF CONJUGATED HYPERBILIRUBINEMIA

Jaundice is a symptom present in a broad spectrum of hepatobiliary diseases, both acute and chronic.

Patient History

The physician should obtain clinical information that may be of value in the differential diagnosis of jaundice. Occupations involving the handling of alcohol increase the likelihood of alcoholic liver disease. A family history of liver disease or jaundice is more common in patients with genetically determined liver disease (Dubin-Johnson syndrome, Wilson's disease) or when several family members are exposed to a toxin (Amanita phalloides) or an infectious agent (hepatitis A virus). The possibility of alcoholism should be carefully evaluated. Patients who admit only to social drinking in moderation may be denying their surreptitious alcohol abuse. All medications taken by the patient should be recorded and checked for their potential to produce acute or chronic liver disease.

Circumstances that increase the risk of transmission of hepatitis viruses include travel to an area of poor sanitation, occupational exposure to blood and blood products (as in high-risk hospital employees), employment in day care centers for preschool children or in institutions for the mentally handicapped (particularly children), receipt of blood transfusions or blood fractions, drug addiction with needle exposure, and male homosexuality.

Symptoms preceding the onset of jaundice or associated with the jaundice often suggest the clinical diagnosis. Jaundice in patients with acute viral hepatitis is usually preceded by prodromal symptoms; the patient with obstructive jaundice from gallstones may describe typical biliary colic (although 10% of patients may be pain free); progressive weight loss with anorexia, pruritus, and epigastric pain radiating to the back will suggest pancreatic carcinoma, particularly in the older patient. In young women with autoimmune chronic active hepatitis, amenorrhea is often an early symptom of chronic liver disease, while a long history of pruritus before the onset of jaundice in a middle-aged woman is suggestive of primary biliary cirrhosis.

Physical Examination

Skin pigmentation is common in primary biliary cirrhosis and hemochromatosis. Cutaneous xanthomata around the eyes, palms, neck, or chest are related to marked elevations of serum cholesterol (high-density lipoprotein X) in patients with chronic cholestasis. Spider angiomas are most prominent in patients with cirrhosis; small lesions may also appear during pregnancy and in patients with acute viral hepatitis or chronic active hepatitis. Hepatitis B may present with a skin rash or urticarial lesions.

In young patients presenting with features of cirrhosis, chronic active hepatitis, or acute liver disease with hemolysis, a diagnosis of Wilson's disease should be considered and Kayser-Fleischer rings should be sought by slit-lamp examination of the cornea.

Breast enlargement (gynecomastia) may result from primary gonadal failure in alcoholic patients, from altered sex hormone metabolism in patients with cirrhosis, or from drug therapy (spironolactone).

The presence of a charcteristic hepatic fetor caused by an increased breath excretion of methylmercaptans is often associated with hepatic encephalopathy, particularly in cirrhotic patients following portal-systemic shunting.

Venous collaterals, or prominent abdominal veins radiating from the umbilical area (caput medusa) are a sign of portal hypertension. Superficial abdominal veins with a normal distribution are often more prominent when abdominal distension by ascitic fluid decreases blood flow through deeper vessels.

Changes in liver size or consistency, splenomegaly, and ascites are of particular importance in the differential diagnosis of liver disease.

A palpable gallbladder in a patient with deep jaundice is strongly suggestive of extrahepatic obstruction caused by pancreatic or ampullary carcinoma.

Diagnostic Studies

The routine laboratory tests that should be performed in all patients with liver disease include a complete blood count, urinalysis, fasting blood glucose, blood urea nitrogen, and serum creatinine and uric acid. Liver tests that are routinely performed are measurements of total and conjugated bilirubin, serum alkaline phosphatase, transaminases, cholesterol, total protein, and albumin. Prolongation of the prothrombin time may be due to vitamin K deficiency in patients with cholestasis or may result from depressed protein synthesis by the liver.

On the basis of clinical data and liver tests, most patients with jaundice will fit into one of the following patterns of disease: acute hepatocellular disease, acute cholestatic disease, acute hepatocellular injury with cholestasis, chronic hepatocellular disease, and chronic cholestatic disease. The further diagnostic evaluation of a patient with jaundice will vary according to the pattern of his disease.

Acute Hepatocellular Disease. In patients with acute hepatocellular disease with or without cholestasis, serum transaminase levels are usually in excess of 500 IU/dl, and serum alkaline phosphatase levels are normal or moderately elevated (< 2 times normal). The most common causes of disease in this category are drugs, toxins, and viral infection. Several tests should be performed, including serologic tests for hepatitis A and B infection. These include HB_sAg, HB_eAg, anti-HB_c, and anti-HA. The presence of IgM antibody to the viral antigens will separate acute infection from the immune response of an earlier infection. Serologic tests for Epstein-Barr virus infection may be indicated if other viral studies are negative. Although these serologic studies do not lead to specific treatment for the patient, their results may determine the need for prophylactic measures for family members or contacts. Also, a liver biopsy is sometimes indicated when the diagnosis remains uncertain.

Acute Cholestatic Disease. Patients with acute cholestasis exhibit minimal biochemical evidence of liver cell injury (serum transaminases show a less than five-fold elevation) with elevation of serum alkaline phosphatase, gamma glutamyl transpeptidase, and serum bile acid levels. The biochemical tests are of limited value in separating patients with intrahepatic disease (intrahepatic cholestasis) from those with extrahepatic biliary obstruction. If a patient has been receiving a drug that typically is associated with intrahepatic cholestasis, no further diagnostic studies are indicated unless the patient's course is subsequently atypical.

When drugs cannot be implicated, several tests may be of value in differentiating intrahepatic from extrahepatic cholestasis. Serologic tests for hepatitis viruses may be useful. Occasionally, viral hepatitis with jaundice follows a predominantly cholestatic course (cholestatic hepatitis), while infectious mononucleosis often causes intrahepatic cholestasis with mild jaundice.

Percutaneous liver biopsy in the presence of extrahepatic obstruction may show bile lakes and acute pericholangitis with edema and polymorphonuclear infiltration of the portal triads.

Imaging techniques that may provide anatomic evidence of biliary obstruction or of the primary disease causing obstruction include ultrasonography and CT scan, percutaneous transhepatic cholangiography, and endoscopy with retrograde cholangiography. These studies should be performed in the sequence suggested in Figure 12–4. Bile duct dilatation may not be seen during the first 2 weeks of jaundice, when ductal obstruction is incomplete. Less expensive, noninvasive tests are usually indicated before expensive invasive tests, which have a higher risk of complications.

Acute Hepatocellular Injury with Cholestasis. (See Acute Hepatocellular Disease)

Chronic Hepatocellular Disease. In patients with chronic hepatocellular disease further diagnostic studies should define the cause and disorder of the liver disease. Serological studies for hepatitis B infection, HB_sAg, HB_eAg, anti-HB_c, and anti-HB_e may be positive in patients with chronic active hepatitis B. Quantitative measurements of immunoglobulin levels and serological tests for antinuclear and anti–smooth-muscle antibodies may support a diagnosis of autoimmune chronic active hepatitis.

In young patients, measurements of plasma ceruloplasmin and serum and urinary copper levels should be performed to establish a diagnosis of Wilson's disease.

Unless contraindicated, a percutaneous liver biopsy should be performed in all patients with chronic hepatocellular disease to establish a pathological diagnosis.

The development of jaundice in a patient with previously documented cirrhosis may be due to a superimposed acute insult (e.g., acute alcoholic hepatitis or viral hepatitis), intercurrent infection, a decrease in hepatic perfusion (shock, heart failure), hemolysis (following transfusion), portal vein thrombosis, or the development of a hepatocellular carcinoma. Further diagnostic studies under these circumstances should be planned on an individual basis.

Chronic Cholestatic Disease. Patients with chronic cholestasis may be suffering from an infiltrative disease of the liver (e.g., granuloma), primary biliary cirrhosis, prolonged cholestatic drug reactions (rarely, after chlorpromazine), stenosing cholangitis, bile duct carcinoma, strictures of the bile duct, or choledocholithiasis. These patients should be studied in the sequence suggested in Figure 12–5.

DIAGNOSTIC EVALUATION OF JAUNDICE IN POSTOPERATIVE PATIENTS[38]

Postoperative jaundice may be a major diagnostic challenge (Table 12–17).

Differential Diagnosis

Postoperative jaundice may occur as a result of decompensation of previous chronic liver disease. A history of alcoholism, signs of chronic liver disease preoperatively, or abnormal liver tests before surgery will usually suggest this diagnosis.

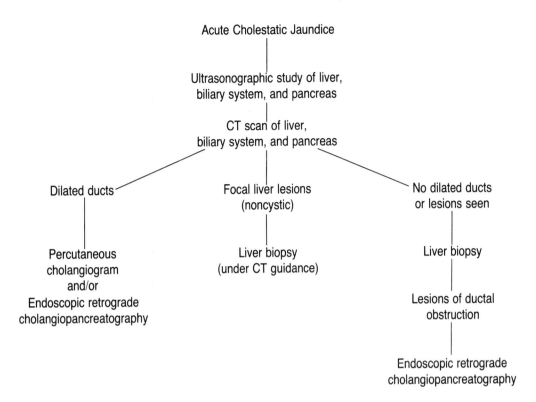

Fig. 12–4. Diagnostic approach to acute cholestatic jaundice.

Acute circulatory liver injury is usually due to a period of hypotension or shock at the time of surgery, particularly in patients with cardiac disease. Striking elevations of serum transaminases prior to the development of jaundice in the immediate postoperative period usually suggest the diagnosis. Jaundice may be accentuated by the increased bilirubin load from transfused blood. No additional diagnostic studies will influence recovery in these patients.

Jaundice may result from halogenated anesthetic agents (especially halothane). Patients with an idiosyncratic reaction to halothane are usually febrile during the first postoperative week and develop jaundice during the second week. Their liver disease is typical of an acute hepatocellular reaction. A history of earlier exposure to halothane is usual. Jaundice may also be related to other drugs.

Jaundice due to hemolysis also occurs. An increase in red cell destruction may be due to mechanical injury (cardiopulmonary bypass, prosthetic aortic valve) or to transfusion of aging red cells; the increase in bilirubin load will contribute to jaundice in patients with impaired liver function. Brisk hemolysis following a transfusion reaction may cause hemolytic jaundice.

Post-transfusion hepatitis is now most frequently of the non-A, non-B type; it occurs insidiously, with a long incubation period (in excess of 6 weeks) following transfusion.

Jaundice may be associated with sepsis. Jaundice associated with severe infections (septicemia) is usually of the cholestatic type; endotoxin impairs hepatic excretory function. Bacterial hemolysins in clostridial and gram-negative infections may also increase red cell destruction. The possibility of a subhepatic abscess or an anaerobic liver abscess should be considered in patients who have had abdominal operations; imaging techniques are most likely to define their presence.

When jaundice follows operations on the biliary tree, the diagnostic possibilities include acute cholangitis, common bile duct injury, retained common bile duct stones, or a subhepatic abscess adjacent to the common bile duct. Postoperative pancreatitis may also cause jaundice by compression of the distal common bile duct.

DIAGNOSTIC EVALUATION OF JAUNDICE DURING PREGNANCY[39]

The more common causes for jaundice during pregnancy should be recognized.

Jaundice Caused by Primary Hepatobiliary Disease

Dubin-Johnson syndrome may present for the first time with jaundice during pregnancy. The patient will have conjugated hyperbilirubinemia without pruritus, serum transaminase levels will remain in the normal

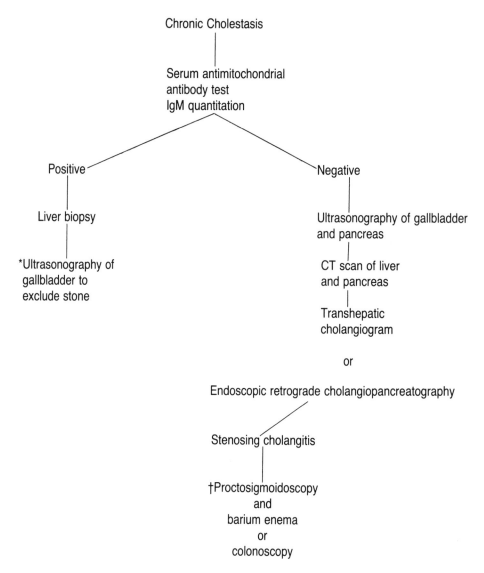

Chronic Cholestasis

Serum antimitochondrial
antibody test
IgM quantitation

Positive

Liver biopsy

*Ultrasonography of
gallbladder to
exclude stone

Negative

Ultrasonography of gallbladder
and pancreas

CT scan of liver
and pancreas

Transhepatic
cholangiogram

or

Endoscopic retrograde cholangiopancreatography

Stenosing cholangitis

†Proctosigmoidoscopy
and
barium enema
or
colonoscopy

*Gallstones are more common in patients with primary biliary cirrhosis.
†Stenosing cholangitis is often associated with inflammatory bowel disease.

Fig. 12—5. Diagnostic approach to chronic cholestatic jaundice.

range, and the serum alkaline phosphatase will be in the normal range for a pregnant patient. The diagnosis should be confirmed by liver biopsy during the postpartum period.

Acute viral hepatitis occurs with equal frequency during the three trimesters of pregnancy. The diagnosis of hepatitis B should be established serologically so that appropriate immune prophylaxis can be provided for the infant during the neonatal period.

Extrahepatic cholestasis caused by gallstones can usually be diagnosed by an ultrasound study to demonstrate residual stones in the gallbladder.

Jaundice Specifically Related to Pregnancy

Intrahepatic cholestasis of pregnancy is an idiopathic condition second only to acute viral hepatitis as a cause for jaundice during pregnancy. Jaundice is usually preceded by pruritus during the second and third trimesters of pregnancy and continues until delivery, at which time symptoms promptly subside. A history in relatives of similar symptoms during pregnancy or a history of symptoms during earlier pregnancies is common. Liver tests show cholestasis without parenchymal cell injury. The prothrombin time may be prolonged because of vitamin K malabsorption; this must be corrected by parenteral vitamin K before delivery.

Acute fatty liver of pregnancy is a rare disorder that usually occurs during the last few weeks of pregnancy. The presenting manifestations are usually abdominal pain and vomiting preceding the onset of jaundice.

Table 12–17. Differential Diagnosis of Postoperative Jaundice

Decompensation of pre-existing chronic hepatobiliary disease
Acute circulatory liver injury (hypotension, shock)
Jaundice associated with drugs
  Halogenated anesthetic agents
  Other agents
Hemolysis
  Transfusion reaction
  Transfusion of aged red cells
  Mechanical injury to red cells (cardiopulmonary bypass)
Post-transfusion hepatitis
  Hepatitis B
  Hepatitis non-A, non-B
  Other viruses
Bacteremia and septicemia
  Endotoxin cholestasis
  Hemolysis
Biliary tract disease (retained stone, cholangitis, bile duct injury, abscesses)

Table 12–18. Pathophysiologic Classification of Ascites

Increased central venous pressure
  Severe congestive heart failure
  Tricuspid insufficiency
  Constrictive pericarditis
Increased portal venous pressure
  Hepatic venous obstruction (Budd-Chiari syndrome)
    Veno-occlusive disease (Bush teas, drugs, irradiation)
    Thrombosis
    Neoplasm
    Valves
  Cirrhosis of the liver
Lymphatic obstruction
  Congenital (primary lymphangiectasia)
  Acquired (trauma, infection, granuloma, neoplasm, heart disease)
Hypoproteinemia
  Nephrotic syndrome
  Severe protein malnutrition
  Protein-losing enteropathy
  Severe hepatic failure
Peritoneal inflammation
  Bacterial infection
    Spontaneous
    Perforated viscus
    Tuberculous
  Bile peritonitis
  Pancreatic ascites
  Malignant ascites
  Eosinophilic peritonitis
  Immunologic (SLE)
Miscellaneous
  Hypothyroidism
  Chronic renal failure

Symptoms, signs, and laboratory features of hepatic encephalopathy, hypoglycemia, and disseminated intravascular coagulation are common features of the illness. An early diagnosis of this disease with immediate termination of the pregnancy may improve maternal survival.

Jaundice is a rare complication of severe hyperemesis gravidarum and toxemia of pregnancy.

ASCITES

DEFINITION

Ascites is a collection of serous fluid within the peritoneal cavity.

PATHOPHYSIOLOGIC CONSIDERATIONS AND CLASSIFICATION (Table 12–18)

The major factors that contribute to the development of ascites, either singly or in combination, include increased central venous pressure, increased portal venous pressure, lymphatic obstruction, hypoproteinemia, and peritoneal inflammation. These factors either increase fluid production within the abdomen or decrease the clearance of fluid from the abdominal cavity.

Increased central venous pressure not only increases the transudation of fluid into serous cavities, but also may retard the return of fluid through lymphatic vessels because of the increase in subclavian vein and thoracic duct pressure. Increased central venous pressure occurs in severe congestive heart failure, tricuspid insufficiency, and constrictive pericarditis.

Increased portal venous pressure (portal hypertension) is most likely to cause ascites when there is an increase in hydrostatic pressure in both hepatic sinusoidal and splanchnic beds. The relative permeability of the hepatic sinusoids causes a marked increase in hepatic lymph flow when there is postsinusoidal venous obstruction, as in cirrhosis and in Budd-Chiari syndrome.[40] In patients with cirrhosis, an increase in aldosterone secretion is triggered by the pooling of blood in the splanchnic circulation; this secondary hyperaldosteronism causes renal sodium retention. Presinusoidal portal hypertension caused by fibrosis within the portal triads (as occurs in schistosomiasis) or portal vein thrombosis may be complicated by ascites only when variceal bleeding stimulates aldosterone secretion. Increased portal venous pressure occurs in cirrhosis of the liver and hepatic vein occlusion (Budd-Chiari syndrome, acute veno-occlusive disease).

Lymphatic obstruction involving the intestinal lymphatic duct or the thoracic duct may be a congenital lesion or may result from trauma (accidental or surgical) and acquired diseases. The increase in lymphatic pressure causes dilatation of intestinal lymphatics (intestinal lymphangiectasia), which may rupture into the intestinal lumen or the peritoneal cavity. The loss of intestinal lymph into the gut (protein-losing enteropathy) may cause severe hypoproteinemia with edema and ascites, and leakage into the peritoneal cavity leads to chylous ascites. Lymphatic obstruction occurs in congenital lymphatic obstruction (primary intestinal lymphangiectasia), surgical trauma to the thoracic duct (especially cardiovascular surgery), constrictive pericarditis and tricuspid insufficiency, filariasis, lymphatic obstruction by tuberculosis and lymphoma, and malignant ascites with peritoneal deposits.

Hypoproteinemia increases fluid losses from the capillary bed by decreasing plasma oncotic pressure. Ascites may be part of a generalized dependent edema in patients with severe hypoproteinemia. Hypoproteinemia occurs in nephrotic syndrome, severe protein malnutrition, protein-losing enteropathy, and hepatic failure.

Peritoneal inflammation causes an increase in capillary permeability with exudation of fluid into the peritoneal cavity. This exudate has a relatively high protein content (as compared to transudates) and usually contains an increased number of inflammatory cells. The peritoneal inflammation may be either chemical or bacterial and occurs in perforated viscus (e.g., perforated ulcer, diverticulitis, perforated appendicitis, and intestinal infarction), bile peritonitis (usually following needle puncture of the gallbladder or a major bile duct), acute pancreatitis or pancreatico-peritoneal fistula causing pancreatic ascites, spontaneous bacterial peritonitis (infection complicating pre-existing ascites in cirrhosis and nephrotic syndrome), tuberculous peritonitis, eosinophilic peritonitis (with eosinophilic infiltration of the intestine), and malignant ascites (ovarian, colonic, gastric, breast carcinoma).

The mechanism for ascites formation is not well defined in hypothyroidism and chronic renal failure.

DIAGNOSTIC EVALUATION

Patient History and Physical Examination

In most patients, a careful history and physical examination will define the primary disease process causing ascites. There are a few particular problems in the differential diagnosis. Constrictive pericarditis causing hepatomegaly, ascites, and abnormal liver tests may closely mimic chronic liver disease. When diagnostic studies include a liver biopsy, measurements of hepatic

and central venous pressure, or both, constrictive pericarditis will become evident. Also, patients with cirrhosis and nephrotic syndrome are at increased risk for developing spontaneous bacterial peritonitis. In the cirrhotic patient, infection may precipitate hepatic coma before signs and symptoms of peritoneal irritation are recognized. A diagnostic paracentesis will avoid errors in diagnosis.

Diagnostic Studies

In addition to undergoing routine urinalysis and hematologic and biochemical studies that may suggest the diagnosis of chronic liver disease, nephrotic syndrome, or acute pancreatitis, all patients presenting with ascites should have a diagnostic paracentesis and ascitic fluid should be examined.

As part of the microscopic analysis, total RBC and WBC counts with differential should be obtained. In the bacteriologic analysis, Gram's stain of centrifuged sediment, aerobic and anaerobic culture of fluid for pyogenic organisms, and culture of centrifuged deposit from a larger volume for M. tuberculosis should be performed. In the biochemical analysis, pH should be measured. In addition, with simultaneous serum analyses, albumin and total protein, and amylase and lactic dehydrogenase should be assessed. To define malignancy, examination of cell block for malignant cells and measurement of carcinoembryonic antigen (CEA) in ascitic fluid and serum should be performed.

In patients with bacterial peritonitis, there is usually an increase in ascitic fluid pH, an increase in white cells ($>1000/mm^3$) or granulocytes ($>300/mm^3$), and an increase in the ascites to serum protein ratio (>0.6).[41,42] Patients with peritonitis caused by perforated viscus will usually have a polymicrobial infection with higher white cell counts in ascitic fluid than patients with spontaneous peritonitis.

In patients with cirrhosis of the liver, the ascitic fluid is a transudate with a low WBC count (usually $<300\ mm^3$) and a low ascites to serum protein ratio. Patients with malignant ascites may have detectable malignant cells in the fluid, increased ascitic CEA levels, high lactic dehydrogenase levels (ascites to serum ratio >1), and an increased protein ratio. In pancreatic ascites, the ascitic fluid will have a high content of amylase. Chylous ascites caused by rupture of intestinal lymphatic vessels may be obviously milky with separation of a cream layer on standing or centrifugation and may have a high lymphocyte count.

A liver biopsy should be performed in patients with clinical evidence of liver disease. The biopsy will usually document cirrhosis or hepatic congestion and centrilobular necrosis caused by Budd-Chiari syndrome or constrictive pericarditis. In selected patients, hepatic venous catheterization with venography and hepatic venous and central pressure measurements will provide diagnostic information.

HEPATIC ENCEPHALOPATHY

DEFINITION

Hepatic encephalopathy, or coma, refers to a spectrum of neuropsychiatric changes that result from metabolic abnormalities in patients with acute or chronic liver disease. Hepatic encephalopathy may be acute, recurrent, or chronic. The disturbance of brain function is usually reversible when the precipitating metabolic abnormality is corrected; occasionally, recurrent episodes of encephalopathy are followed by permanent brain or spinal cord damage. Clinically, hepatic encephalopathy is graded according to the severity of neuropsychiatric dysfunction.

PATHOPHYSIOLOGIC CONSIDERATIONS[43]

The primary metabolic abnormality in patients with hepatic encephalopathy appears to be a disturbance of ammonia metabolism. An increase in blood ammonia is associated with encephalopathy in patients with an acute decrease in hepatic urea cycle enzymes (Reye's syndrome, acute fatty liver of pregnancy), with an increase in protein or amino acid intake or gastrointestinal bleeding in patients with cirrhosis (particularly after portocaval shunting), following ammonium chloride ingestion in cirrhotic patients, and in cirrhotic patients who develop azotemia. Conversely, therapeutic measures that lower blood ammonia levels usually reverse hepatic encephalopathy in these patients. Other agents that may impair brain function in patients with liver disease include short- and medium-chain fatty acids, mercaptans, and changes in amino acid metabolism. Cirrhotic patients exhibit depressed plasma levels of branched-chain amino acids and elevated levels of aromatic amino acids that potentially could lead to the production of false neurotransmitters in the brain.

Patients with cirrhosis and an associated primary metabolic abnormality in brain function are sensitive to a variety of additional metabolic stresses. Thus, hepatic coma may be precipitated in cirrhotic patients not only by changes that increase blood ammonia levels (increased protein intake, bleeding, or azotemia), but also by hypoxia, infection with fever, hypoglycemia, metabolic alkalosis with hypokalemia, hyponatremia, and depressant drugs (sedatives, tranquilizers, and analgesics).

DIFFERENTIAL DIAGNOSIS

In alcoholic cirrhotic patients who present with symptoms suggestive of hepatic encephalopathy, the possibility of delirium tremens, Wernicke's encephalopathy, or head injury must be considered.

DIAGNOSTIC EVALUATION

Patients with stage I encephalopathy may exhibit mood changes, an altered sleep pattern, a shortened attention span, a decrease in higher integrative functions, and muscle incoordination. With progression to stage II, the personality changes are more marked with decrease in memory, inappropriate behavior, an increase in muscle tone and involuntary movements, and ataxia with a flapping tremor (asterixis). In stage III, confusion, disorientation, and somnolence are more severe and may progress to stupor or delirium. There may be muscle rigidity, hyperreflexia, or seizures. Respiration is often stimulated. In stage IV, the patient lapses into coma with varying degrees of responsiveness. In acute coma there may be decerebrate posturing.

It is important to clinically define potentially reversible abnormalities that may have precipitated a change in the patient's mental status. If bleeding is not overt, a rectal examination should be performed to test stool for blood. Pulmonary, peritoneal, or urinary tract infection and septicemia should be considered in febrile patients. Blood glucose, urea, pH, and electrolyte measurements are necessary to exclude hypoglycemia, hyperglycemia, azotemia, disturbances of acid-base balance, and electrolyte metabolism.

Measurements of blood ammonia add little to the clinical evaluation of a patient with known liver disease.

CHANGES IN LIVER SIZE AND CONSISTENCY

DEFINITIONS

The liver normally extends from the fifth intercostal space in the mid-clavicular line to the costal margin.

Table 12–19. Differential Diagnosis of Hepatomegaly

Inflammatory disease
  Viral hepatitis
  Infectious mononucleosis
  Alcoholic hepatitis
  Toxic hepatitis
  Bacterial infections
  Parasitic disease (Schistosomiasis)
Abscesses
  Pyogenic
  Amebic
Hepatic congestion
  Heart failure
  Tricuspid insufficiency
  Constrictive pericarditis
  Hepatic vein obstruction
  Veno-occlusive disease
Cholestasis
  Intrahepatic
  Extrahepatic
Liver cell infiltration
  Fatty liver
  Acute glycogen storage
  Glycogen storage diseases
Reticuloendothelial storage diseases
  Gaucher's disease
  Hurler's disease
Hepatic granulomatous disease
  Tuberculosis
  Leprosy
  Sarcoidosis
  Miscellaneous
Agnogenic myeloid metaplasia
Neoplastic infiltration
  Leukemia and lymphomas
  Primary hepatoma, angiosarcoma
  Metastatic neoplasms
  Hepatic adenoma
Chronic parenchymal disease
  Metabolic
  Alcoholic
  Chronic active hepatitis
  Primary biliary cirrhosis
Cystic disease
  Polycystic disease
  Hydatid cysts

With deep inspiration, the lower border may be demonstrated by light percussion below the costal margin and may be palpable as a soft, sharp edge. Hepatomegaly refers to liver enlargement and should be distinguished from depression of the liver by hyperinflation of the chest (emphysema) or from a normal Riedel's lobe, which extends below the right costal margin.

PATHOPHYSIOLOGIC CONSIDERATIONS AND DIFFERENTIAL DIAGNOSIS (Table 12–19)

Enlargement of the liver may result from diffuse or focal inflammation, venous congestion, cholestasis, liver cell infiltration with fat or glycogen, reticuloendothelial cell hyperplasia or enlargement, granuloma formation, infiltration with bone marrow cells, neoplastic disease (either diffuse or focal), cystic disease, or cirrhosis.

Hepatic tenderness on palpation usually reflects acute processes that cause inflammation (hepatitis, abscess, or tumor necrosis) or that suddenly stretch the liver capsule (venous congestion, acute infiltration).

Nodularity of the liver surface may be caused by cirrhosis, neoplasm, or cystic disease. The infiltrated or cirrhotic liver usually has a firmer consistency than normal.

DIAGNOSTIC EVALUATION

The patient's history and physical examination may provide a complete explanation for the enlargement of the liver. Several studies may be necessary to establish a pathologic diagnosis. A percutaneous liver biopsy can be safely performed in most patients with diffuse or focal liver disease. When there is evidence of a space-occupying lesion in the liver, the liver should initially be evaluated by ultrasound, isotopic, or CT scanning; the imaging study will localize focal lesions and permit directed biopsy or will define lesions on which aspiration rather than biopsy should be performed (e.g., pyogenic or amebic abscesses). When the clinical history is suggestive of a hydatid cyst, aspiration or biopsy should not be attempted.

A decrease in liver size may be due to acute hepatic necrosis in patients with fulminant viral, drug-induced (isoniazid, or acetaminophen overdose), or toxic hepatitis (Amanita poisoning). In patients with macronodular cirrhosis (usually posthepatitic or idiopathic) the liver may be small and shrunken. Displacement of the hepatic flexure between the surface of the liver and the chest wall may decrease hepatic percussion dullness and give the impression of a small liver.

SPLENOMEGALY

DEFINITION

Splenomegaly refers to an enlargement of the spleen. The normal spleen lies deep to the left lower thoracic cage and cannot be palpated. With moderate enlargement, the spleen tip or edge may be palpated on inspiration at the left costal margin. The massively

Table 12–20. Differential Diagnosis of Splenomegaly

Acute infection
  Viral: hepatitis, infectious mononucleosis
  Rickettsial
  Bacterial: septicemia, S. typhae
  Fungal: histoplasmosis
Chronic infection
  Bacterial
    Brucellosis
    Subacute bacterial endocarditis
    Tuberculosis
    Syphilis (secondary, tertiary gumma)
  Parasitic
    Falciparum malaria
    Kala-azar
    Schistosomiasis
Immunologic disorders
  Systemic lupus erythematosus
  Rheumatoid arthritis (Felty's syndrome)
  Serum sickness
  Drug reactions
Granulomatous disease
  Sarcoidosis
Hematologic disorders
  Non-neoplastic
    Pernicious anemia
    Hemolytic disease
  Neoplastic
    Hodgkin's disease
    Lymphoma
    Leukemia
    Myeloproliferative syndromes
Congestive
  Splenic vein thrombosis
  Portal vein thrombosis
  Noncirrhotic portal hypertension
    Vinyl chloride
    Schistosomiasis
    Idiopathic congenital hepatic fibrosis
  Cirrhosis of the liver
  Chronic congestive heart failure, constrictive pericarditis
Infiltrative
  Gaucher's disease
  Niemann-Pick disease
  Hurler's syndrome
  Amyloidosis
Metabolic
  Hyperthyroidism
Miscellaneous
  Splenic cysts
  Abscesses
  Metastatic neoplasms
  Subcapsular hematoma

enlarged spleen may extend to the brim of the pelvis and usually shows a notched medial edge.

PATHOPHYSIOLOGIC CONSIDERATIONS AND DIFFERENTIAL DIAGNOSIS (Table 12–20)

Splenomegaly may be caused by hyperplasia of the normal splenic lymphoid and reticuloendothelial cell populations (e.g., in response to acute or chronic infection or to hemolysis), by sinusoidal congestion (e.g., with splenic vein thrombosis or portal hypertension), by infiltration with abnormal cells (e.g., granuloma, neoplasm, myeloid metaplasia), by reticuloendothelial storage diseases (e.g., Gaucher's disease), by acute or chronic immunologic stimulation (e.g., serum sickness, chronic parasitic infection), or by cysts, abscesses, or hematoma.

Massive splenomegaly is usually seen in patients with neoplastic hematologic disorders, infiltrative disease, parasitic infection, or cirrhosis of the liver. In acute diseases, the enlarged spleen may be tender on palpation and relatively soft (e.g., in typhoid fever). With chronic enlargement and infiltrative disease, the spleen is usually firm and nontender. Splenic infarcts are often associated with massive splenomegaly and present clinically as pain, often pleuritic, in the left upper quadrant. The patient may have tenderness on palpation and a localized splenic friction rub.

DIAGNOSTIC EVALUATION

Clinical information will usually guide the diagnostic evaluation of a patient with splenomegaly. Microbiologic and serologic studies as well as skin tests should provide a diagnosis of acute and chronic infections and immunological disorders. The diagnosis of hematologic disorders may be based on peripheral blood studies but may require bone marrow or lymph node biopsies. The diagnosis of portal hypertension as a cause for splenomegaly can usually be based on the presence of esophageal varices on esophagoscopy; determining the specific cause may require liver biopsy and portal venography. The diagnosis of an infiltrative disease involving the spleen can often be made on liver biopsy, which will show similar disorder (e.g., granuloma, amyloid, Gaucher's disease).

REFERENCES

1. Pope, C.E.: The esophagus: Motor disorders. *In* Gastrointestinal Disease. Edited by M.H. Sleisenger and J.S. Fordtran. Philadelphia, W.B. Saunders and Co., 3rd Ed. 1983, Chapter 26.
2. Seaman, W.: Pharyngeal and upper esopahgeal dysphagia. JAMA *235*:2643, 1976.
3. Castell, D.O.: Achalasia and diffuse esophageal spasm. Arch Intern Med *136*:571, 1975.
4. Kodsi, B.E., et al.: Candida esophagitis. Gastroenterology *71*:715, 1976.
5. Ismael-Beigi, F., and Pope, C.E.: Distribution of the histologic changes of gastroesophageal reflux in the distal esophagus of man. Gastroenterology *66*:1109, 1974.

6. Dodds, W.J., Hogan, W.J., Helm, J.F. and Dent, J.: Pathogenesis of reflux esophagitis. Gastroenterology 81:376, 1981.
7. McCallum, R.W., Berkowits, D.M., and Lerner, E.: Gastric emptying in patients with gastroesophageal reflux. Gastroenterology 80:285, 1981.
8. Behar, J., Biancani, P., and Sheahan, D.G.: Evaluation of esophageal tests in the diagnosis of reflux esophagitis. Gastroenterology 71:9, 1976.
9. Johnson, L.F. and DeMeester, T.R.: Twenty-four-hour pH monitoring of the distal esophagus. Am J Gastroenterol 62:325, 1974.
10. Fisher, R.S., Malmud, L.S., Roberts, G.S., and Lobis, I.F.: Gastroesophageal (GE) scintiscanning to detect and quantitate GE reflux. Gastroenterology 70:30, 1976.
11. Castell, D.O.: Esophageal chest pain. Am J Gastroenterol 79:969, 1984.
12. Benjamin, S.B., Gerhardt, D.C., and Castell, D.O.: High amplitude peristaltic esophageal contractions associated with chest pain and/or dysphagia. Gastroenterology 77:478, 1979.
13. Almy, T.P.: Basic considerations in the study of abdominal pain. In The Differential Diagnosis of Abdominal Pain. Edited by S.M. Melinkoff. New York, McGraw-Hill Book Company, 1959.
14. Holdstock, D.J., Misiewicz, J.J. and Waller, S.L.: Observations on the mechanism of abdominal pain. Gut 10:19, 1969.
15. de Bombal, F.T. et al.: Computer aided diagnosis of acute abdominal pain. Br. Med. J 2:9, 1972.
16. Soll, A.H., and Isenberg, J.I.: Duodenal Ulcer Disease. In Gastrointestinal Disease. 3rd Ed. Edited by M.H. Sleisenger and J.S. Fordtran. Philadelphia, W.B. Saunders Company, 1983, Chapter 40.
17. Edwards, F.C., and Coghill, N.F.: Clinical manifestations in patients with chronic atrophic gastritis, gastric ulcer and duodenal ulcer. Q J Med 37:337, 1968.
18. Malagelada, J.-R., and Camilleri, M.: Unexplained vomiting. A diagnostic challenge. Ann Intern Med 101:211, 1984.
19. Malagelada, J.-R., Rees, W.D.W., Muzzotta, L.J., and Go, V.L.W.: Gastric motor abnormalities in diabetic and post vagotomy gastroparesis: effect of metoclopramide and bethanechol. Gastroenterology 78:286, 1980.
20. Levitt, M.D.: Volume and composition of human intestinal gas determined by means of an intestinal washout technique. N Engl J Med 284:1394, 1971.
21. Lasser, R.B., Bond, J.H., and Levitt, M.D.: The role of intestinal gas in functional abdominal pain. N Engl J Med 293:524, 1975.
22. Bond, J.H., and Levitt, M.D.: Quantitative measurement of lactase absorption. Gastroenterology 70:1058, 1972.
23. Anderson, I.H., Levine, A.S., and Levitt, M.D.: Incomplete absorption of the carbohydrate in all purpose wheat flour. N Engl J Med. 304:891, 1981.
24. Gray, G.M.: Maldigestion and malabsorption: Clinical manifestations and specific diagnosis. In Gastrointestinal Disease. 3rd Ed. Edited by M.H. Sleisenger and J.S. Fordtran. Philadelphia, W.B. Saunders Company, 1983, Chapter 15.
25. DiMagno, E.P., Go, V.L.W., and Summerskill, W.H.J.: Relations between pancreatic enzyme outputs and malabsorption in severe pancreatic insufficiency. N Engl J Med 288:813, 1973.
26. Hofmann, A.F., and Poley, J.R.: Cholestyramine treatment of diarrhea associated with ileal resection. N Engl J Med 281:397, 1969.
27. Trier, J.S.: Celiac sprue. In Gastrointestinal Disease. 3rd Ed. Edited by M.H. Sleisenger and J.S. Fordtran. Philadelphia, W.B. Saunders Company, 1983, Chapter 63.
28. Krejs, G.J., and Fordtran, J.S.: Diarrhea. In Gastrointestinal Disease. 3rd Ed. Edited by M.H. Sleisenger and J.S. Fordtran. Philadelphia. W.B. Saunders Company, 1983, Chapter 16.
29. Gorbach, S.L.: Infectious Diarrhea. In Gastrointestinal Disease. 3rd Ed. Edited by M.H. Sleisenger and J.S. Fordtran. Philadelphia, W.B. Saunders Company, 1983, Chapter 57.
30. Read, N.W., et al.: Chronic diarrhea of unknown origin. Gastroenterology 78:264, 1980.
31. DeVroede, G.: Constipation: mechanisms and management. In Gastrointestinal Disease. 3rd Ed. Edited by M.H. Sleisenger and J.S. Fordtran. Philadelphia, W.B. Saunders Company, 1983, Chapter 18.
32. Peterson, W.L.: Gastrointestinal Bleeding. In Gastrointestinal Disease. 3rd Ed. Edited by M.H. Sleisenger and J.S. Fordtran. Philadelphia, W.B. Saunders Company, 1983, Chapter 12.
33. Zuckerman, G.R., Cornette, G.L., Clouse, R.E., and Harter, H.: Upper gastrointestinal bleeding in patients with chronic renal failure. Ann Intern Med 102:588, 1985.
34. Simon, J.B.: Occult blood screening for colorectal carcinoma: A critical review. Gastroenterology 88:820, 1985.
35. Ahlquist, D.A., et al.: Fecal blood levels in health and disease. A study using HemoQuant. N Engl J Med 312:1422, 1985.
36. Billing, B.H.: Bilirubin Metabolism. In Diseases of the Liver. 5th Ed. Edited by L. Schiff and E.R. Schiff. Philadelphia, J.B. Lippincott Company, 1982, Chapter 11.
37. Berk, P.D., et al.: Unconjugated hyperbilirubinemia. Physiologic evaluation and experimental approaches to therapy. Ann Intern Med 82:552, 1975.
38. Morganstern, L.: Postoperative jaundice. In Diseases of the Liver. 5th Ed. Edited by L. Schiff and E.R. Schiff. Philadelphia, J.B. Lippincott Company, 1982, p. 1581.
39. Krejs, G.J., and Haemmerli, U.P.: Jaundice during pregnancy. In Diseases of the Liver. 5th Ed. Edited by L. Schiff and E.R. Schiff. Philadelphia, J.B. Lippincott Company, 1982, p. 1561.
40. Witte, C.L., Witte, M.H., and Dumont, A.E.: Lymph imbalance in the genesis and perpetuation of the ascites syndrome in hepatic cirrhosis. Gastroenterology 78:1059, 1980.
41. Conn, H.O.: Spontaneous bacterial peritonitis. Gastroenterology 70:455, 1976.
42. Gitlin, N., Stauffer, J.L., and Silvestri, R.C.: The pH of ascitic fluid in the diagnosis of spontaneous bacterial peritonitis in alcoholic cirrhosis. Hepatology 2:408, 1982.
43. Zieve, L.: Hepatic encephalopathy. In Diseases of the Liver. 5th Ed. Edited by L. Schiff and E.R. Schiff. Philadelphia, J.B. Lippincott Company, 1982, Chapter 14.

CHAPTER 13   # JOINTS, MUSCULOSKELETAL, AND CONNECTIVE TISSUE PROBLEMS

Stephen A. Paget, M.D.

INTRODUCTION

Evaluation and treatment of patients with musculoskeletal disorders requires a knowledge of basic anatomy and normal joint anatomy and of the types of diseases that affect the articular structures.

It is important for physicians caring for patients with joint disorders to recognize the two basic articulations: synovial or diarthrodial joints, and synarthroses. Synovial joints are articulations with free movement and with a synovial membrane lining a joint cavity. These are the most common joints in the body and are of particular concern to the rheumatologist. Figure 13–1 is a schematic diagram of a typical diarthrodial joint. Disease states in any of the structures constituting the joint can lead to general joint dysfunction. The synovial membrane is involved in many of the acute and chronic inflammatory joint disorders (e.g., rheumatoid arthritis). The presence or absence of synovitis is often the most obvious and therefore the most important physical finding in the detection of arthritis. Bone, cartilage, and periarticular tissues may also be involved in the inflammatory, traumatic, infectious, neoplastic, metabolic, or hereditary disease states, and the dysfunction of one or more may dominate the clinical picture.

Synarthroses have very little movement. There are four classifications of synarthroses: symphyses, synchondroses, syndesmoses, and synostoses. In symphyses, a fibrocartilaginous disc separates bone ends that are joined by firm ligaments (e.g., in symphysis pubis and intervertebral joints). In synchondroses, bone ends are covered by articular cartilage but there is no synovium or significant joint cavity (e.g., the sternomanubrial joint). Patients with syndesmoses have bones joined directly by fibrous ligaments, with no cartilage involved (e.g., at the union of the distal tibia and fibula). In synostoses, bone bridges the space between bones, producing ankylosis.

The connective tissues are those tissues such as cartilage, ligaments, tendons, and fasciae that support and bind the structural lattice of the bony skeleton and its attachments. They play an important role in regeneration and healing and are involved in inflammation. Connective tissue is the site of a number of inherited malformations (e.g., Marfan's syndrome and Ehlers-Danlos syndrome) and acquired disorders (e.g., rheumatoid arthritis). In many acquired human diseases, the pathologic processes seem predominantly to involve connective tissue, and the resultant destruction or alteration of the tissue plays a significant role in the genesis of the morbid state. Immunity to collagen may play a role in the pathogenesis of chronic inflammation seen in rheumatoid arthritis (RA), and the destructive joint lesions characteristic of RA may be due, at least in part, to degradation of native collagen by collagenase.

Table 13–1 lists nine specific types of musculo-

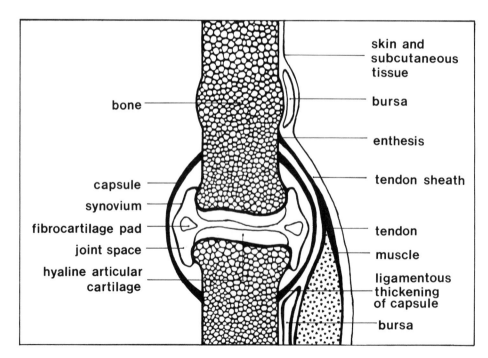

Fig. 13–1. Diagrammatic cross section of synovial joint and its periarticular structures, illustrating some of the structures which give rise to pain and inflammation in rheumatic diseases. Note the synovial lining of the joint, bursae and tendon sheaths.

Table 13–1. Categories of Rheumatic Disease

Disorder	Prototype Disorder(s)	Characteristic Clinical Features	Useful Laboratory Tests
Synovitis Villous hypertrophy Mononuclear cell infiltration Follicles of T-lymphocytes Plasma cell production of immunoglobulin	Rheumatoid arthritis (juvenile rheumatoid arthritis)	Joint disease dominates the clinical picture; systemic disease is the background; symmetrical polyarthritis in the setting of constitutional symptoms; subcutaneous nodules (20%). Women 3:1	Rheumatoid factor in up to 75% Characteristic deformities and erosions on X-ray Moderate anemia Elevated sedimentation rate
Fibrinoid necrosis and degeneration of blood vessels and connective tissue vasculitis	Systemic connective tissue disorders Systemic lupus erythematosus Scleroderma Necrotizing vasculitides Polyarteritis nodosa Wegener's granulomatosis Takayasu's arteritis Giant cell arteritis	Presenting manifestations that may suggest the diagnosis of these disorders Fever of unknown origin Arthralgia or arthritis Pleuritis, pericarditis, peritonitis Skin lesions: nodules, purpura, erythema, ulcerations Raynaud's phenomenon, peripheral vasculitis Pneumonitis, pulmonary infiltration or cavitation Myositis or peripheral neuropathy Glomerulitis or glomerulonephritis Central nervous system disease Ocular involvement including uveitis, keratitis Lymphadenopathy or splenomegaly Hematologic abnormalities including hemolytic anemia, thrombocytopenia, leukopenia, eosinophilia, circulating anticoagulants, disseminated intravascular coagulation False positive serologic test for syphilis	Systemic lupus Antinuclear antibodies Anti-dsDNA and decreased serum complement levels Anti-Sm antibody LE cells Thrombocytopenia, leukopenia, hemolytic anemia, circulating anticoagulant, false positive test for syphilis Kidney biopsy demonstrating nephritis Scleroderma Speckled or nucleolar antinuclear antibody Anemia Increased collagen on skin biopsy Abnormal esophageal motility on UGI series Interstitial pulmonary fibrosis on CXR Vasculitis Necrotizing vasculitis on biopsy of involved tissues Angiographic demonstration of vessel involvement or aneurysm formation Elevated sedimentation rate Leukocytosis Thrombocytosis Anemia
Enthesopathy Inflammation most marked at the transition where ligament attaches to bone	Seronegative spondyloarthropathies Ankylosing spondylitis Reiter's syndrome Psoriatic arthritis Arthritis associated with inflammatory bowel disease	Presenting manifestations that may suggest the diagnosis of these disorders: Synovitis of lower extremity, large joints in an asymmetrical fashion Spondylitis and/or sacroiliitis are prominent articular features; low-back pain or stiffness Psoriasiform skin rash is present; nail pitting Eye involvement including uveitis, conjunctivitis Urethritis, history of nonspecific urethritis or prostatitis, balanitis Mouth or genital ulcers Enteritis or dysentery Heel, Achilles tendon, or plantar fascia inflammation Swollen, sausage-shaped toes (dactylitis) Aortitis, heart block, upper lobe pulmonary fibrosis	Histocompatibility, antigen B27 (B7, BW22, BW40, BW42) Anemia, elevated sedimentation rate X-rays demonstrating sacroiliitis or spondylitis Achilles tendinitis Erosive joint changes

Table 13–1. **Continued**

Disorder	Prototype Disorder(s)	Characteristic Clinical Features	Useful Laboratory Tests
Crystal-induced synovitis	Gout Pseudogout	Gout (males or postmenopausal females) Familial occurrence Podagra and prominent Periarticular inflammation and acute attacks Precipitating factors (drugs, trauma, medical or surgical illness) Tophi, kidney stones Pseudogout (males predominate) Mimics gout, with intense inflammation, especially knees	Gout Increased serum uric acid and uric acid crystals in polys in synovial fluid Tophi and typical erosive disease seen on x-ray Pseudogout Calcium pyrophosphate crystals in polys in synovial fluid Chondrocalcinosis on x-ray
Cartilage degeneration	Osteoarthritis	Absence of inflammatory signs or systemic features Lower extremities predominate DIP (Heberden's nodes) and PIP (Bouchard's nodes) involvement Absence of MCP and wrist disease	X-ray demonstration of bony proliferation with spur formation and irregular joint space narrowing Noninflammatory joint fluid
Joint infection	Bacterial Gonococcal Staphylococcal Streptococcal Gram-negative	Gonococcal Young adults, especially females History of exposure Association with menses or pregnancy After polyarticular onset, often settles in one or two joints; tenosynovitis prominent Association with skin lesions History of shaking chills, genitourinary symptoms Other Organisms Monarticular involvement Presence of predisposing factors (extra-articular source of infection, joint damage, underlying illness)	Isolation of organism from joint fluid, blood, genitourinary tract, skin lesions, rectum, pharynx
Myositis Inflammatory cellular infiltrate in muscle Muscle necrosis or fiber atrophy	Polymyositis/dermatomyositis (PM/DM)	Proximal muscle weakness with or without a characteristic skin rash 25% with muscle pain Dysphagia, arthralgias, and Raynaud's phenomenon in 20% Four times greater incidence of malignancy in elderly patients with PM/DM	Abnormal muscle biopsy Elevated muscle enzymes (CPK, aldolase, SGOT, LDH) Abnormal EMG
Focal conditions	Tendinitis Bursitis Calcific tendinitis Low-back strain	Local site of pain, tenderness, inflammation Pain predominantly on motion and at night; improved with rest Lack of systemic features History of trauma, inciting activities, or overuse	X-ray demonstration of calcium deposits or spurs
Generalized conditions Histologic studies are normal	Fibromyalgia	Diffuse aching, sleep disturbance Localized sites of deep myofascial tenderness (trigger points) No demonstrable inflammation Anxious patient	All laboratory tests are normal Diagnosis of exclusion

(From Fries, James F.: General approach to the rheumatic disease patient. *In* Textbook of Rheumatology. 2nd Edition. Edited by W.N. Kelly, E.D. Harris, S. Ruddy, and C.B. Sledge. Philadelphia, W.B. Saunders, 1985, pp. 361–368.)

skeletal problems and provides a framework for patho-physiologic categorization of disease states.

Inflammation is central to many of the disorders seen by the physician. The components of inflammation and repair may produce widely disparate manifestations. In many disease states, it is those "protective" aspects of inflammation that lead to tissue destruction (e.g., autoantibodies in systemic lupus erythematosus or caseation necrosis in tuberculosis). Conversely, in the physician's rush to control inflammation with the use of strong anti-inflammatory measures (e.g., nonsteroidal anti-inflammatory drugs, corticosteroids, and immunosuppressive drugs), the protective or beneficial effects of inflammation are often neglected or suppressed, and the host becomes more defenseless. The definition of an inflammatory state is important in the differential diagnosis of musculoskeletal disease states. Various clinical and laboratory findings help the clinician separate inflammatory from noninflammatory disorders (Table 13–2). Such differentiation has important diagnostic, prognostic, and therapeutic implications.

DIAGNOSTIC EVALUATION

Patient History and Physical Examination

The diagnosis of most joint, periarticular, or systemic disorders is based primarily on the history and physical examination. Laboratory and radiologic information helps to support the clinical diagnosis but is not in most cases the only way in which the correct diagnosis is made. For example, the diagnosis of rheumatoid arthritis is based on the clinical presentation in a young woman of symmetrical polyarthritis, morning stiffness, and fatigue without typical features of other systemic disorders such as systemic lupus erythematosus. Even if the rheumatoid factor test is negative (as it can be in 20% of patients with typical rheumatoid arthritis), the erythrocyte sedimentation rate is normal, or there is no anemia or thrombocytosis, the diagnosis of RA is certain, especially if the clinical picture remains unchanged with time. Similarly, the tentative diagnosis of ankylosing spondylitis is often made without the characteristic sacroiliac or spinal x-ray abnormalities or the presence of the HLA-B27 antigen (which is not found in 10% of spondylitis cases). Antinuclear antibody–negative systemic lupus is an uncommon entity, whose diagnosis is usually firmly based on the clinical findings of a systemic disorder in young females who present with characteristic features such as a symmetrical polyarthritis with fever, serositis, skin rash, nephritis, central nervous system disease, and hematologic abnormalities.

Patterns of joint or organ involvement are significant guides to the correct clinical diagnosis (Table 13–3. See Table 13–21, Fig. 13–4). While rheumatoid arthritis and systemic lupus usually present as a symmetrical polyarthritis, the seronegative spondyloarthropathies characteristically involve large, lower extremity joints in an asymmetrical fashion. Whereas septic arthritis caused by Staphylococcus aureus or gram-negative organisms is most commonly a highly inflammatory monarticular disorder, gonococcal arthritis and the arthritis associated with rheumatic fever have a migratory pattern despite their relationship to infection.

Systemic diseases often affect various organ systems in a pattern characteristic enough to lead to a definite diagnosis, especially when supported by appropriate laboratory or biopsy information. For example, when the dominant signs and symptoms point to proximal muscle weakness with or without a skin rash, a diagnosis of polymyositis/dermatomyositis (PM/DM) is entertained. Supporting laboratory information (elevated creatine phosphokinase, aldolase, and SGOT, enzymes liberated from muscle by inflammatory, ischemic, or immunologic injury, muscle biopsy and electromyography data) are then sought and the diagnosis is strengthened.

Polyarteritis nodosa is a systemic inflammatory disorder involving small and medium-sized arteries. The clinical pattern of organ involvement relates to those organs affected by the ischemic vasculopathy, and the tentative diagnosis is based on the signs and symptoms of mononeuritis multiplex, bowel infarction, vasculitic skin lesions, and nephritis. Data obtained from biopsy of involved organs (e.g., skin, muscle, testicle, kidney) or angiographic studies finalize the diagnosis. Uncommonly, the diagnosis of both myositis and vasculitis has been made without or with a minimum of supportive biopsy or laboratory confirmation. Usually in these circumstances the clinical diagnosis is strong or the clinical presentation demands a rapid diagnosis and the immediate institution of steroid therapy, immunosuppressive therapy, or both.

Diagnostic Studies

Antibodies reacting with a variety of nuclear and cytoplasmic antigens have been found in the sera of patients with systemic lupus erythematosus as well as a variety of other disease states (Table 13–4 and Table 13–5). Synovial fluid analysis also can provide information about the disorder (Table 13–6).

Although several test abnormalities are common in the rheumatic disorders and some tests are used to follow the activity of disease, they remain nonspecific

Table 13—2.   Examples of Diseases in Various Categories

Inflammatory	*Noninflammatory*
Clinical characteristics	Clinical characteristics
Joint or periarticular disease is inflammatory; associated with redness, warmth, swelling, and decreased function.	Joint disease is *not* inflammatory (save for an intermittent inflammatory component in some disorders).
The joint disease is often part of a more generalized (systemic) inflammatory disorder. Multisystem involvement includes skin rash, serositis, pulmonary and cardiac abnormalities, nephritis, neurologic disorders, and muscle disease. Systemic features include fever, weight loss, fatigue, night sweats, chills, and "failure to thrive."	Although some disorders in this category are systemic, they rarely are associated with the features listed on the left and tend not to be generalized inflammatory disorders.
Characteristic laboratory abnormalities include: Hematologic—anemia (chronic disease, hemolytic, microangiopathic, blood loss), leukocytosis or leukopenia, thrombocytosis or thrombocytopenia, elevated erythrocyte sedimentation rate, circulating anticoagulant, disseminated intravascular coagulation, false positive VDRL, positive Coombs test. Renal—active urinary sediment, renal insufficiéncy, abnormal renal biopsy. SMA-12—elevated gamma globulin, elevated muscle enzymes (CPK, SGOT, LDH, aldolase), abnormal liver function tests (SGOT, SGPT, GGTP, alkaline phosphatase). CXR—pulmonary infiltrates, cavitation, fibrosis; cardiomegaly; pleural reaction or effusions. ECG—conduction abnormalities, coronary ischemia, arrhythmia. Synovial fluid—inflammatory: opaque fluid with low viscosity; > 2000 WBC, primarily polys; high protein and, at times, low glucose; crystals in polys or bacteria in certain disorders. X-ray of joints—characteristic joint changes or effusion. Serologic tests—positive rheumatoid factor, antinuclear antibodies; decreased complement levels; presence of anti-DNA, Sm, Ro, and La antibodies; HLA-B27 positive in some disorders.	Laboratory abnormalities tend to reflect the underlying local or generalized disorder and uncommonly are associated with most of the features listed on the left. Synovial fluid—noninflammatory, clear yellow fluid, WBC < 2000 with low % of polys; normal protein and glucose; negative crystal examination and culture.

Table 13–2. Continued

Inflammatory	Noninflammatory
Disorders	Disorders
Rheumatoid arthritis	Osteoarthritis
Seropositive and negative juvenile rheumatoid arthritis	Isolated
Seronegative spondyloarthropathies	Primary, generalized
Ankylosing spondylitis	Erosive
Reiter's syndrome	Cervical spine syndromes
Psoriatic arthritis	Traumatic arthritis
Colitic arthropathies	Mechanical abnormalities (e.g., torn meniscus, tibial torsion)
Connective tissue disorders	Osteonecrosis
Systemic lupus erythematosus	Neuropathic (Charcot) joint, reflex sympathetic dystrophy
Scleroderma	Amyloid arthropathy
Dermatomyositis/polymyositis	Tumors
Polyarteritis nodosa	Pigmented villonodular synovitis
Wegener's granulomatosis	Synovial cell sarcoma
Temporal arteritis/polymyalgia rheumatica	Metabolic arthropathy
Takayasu's arteritis	Hemochromatosis
Henoch-Schönlein purpura	Acromegaly
Behçet's disease	Hyperparathyroidism
Polychondritis	Ochronosis
Erythema nodosum	Osteoporosis
Cutaneous vasculitides	Osteomalacia
Crystal-induced synovitis	Paget's disease
Gout	Wilson's disease
Pseudogout	Hemophilia
Calcium apatite	Ehlers-Danlos syndrome
Palindromic rheumatism	Sickle-cell disease
Familial Mediterranean fever	
Infectious arthritis	
Bacterial	
Viral	
Spirochetal, including Lyme disease	
Tuberculous	
Fungal	
Rheumatic fever	
Bacterial endocarditis	
Whipple's disease	
Hematologic or malignant disorders	
Leukemia or lymphoma	
Hypertrophic osteoarthropathy	
Cryoglobulinemia	
Sickle-cell disease	
Multicentric reticulohistiocytosis	
Sarcoidosis	
Tenosynovitis and bursitis	
Calcific	
Infectious	
Traumatic	

Table 13–3.   Characteristic Patterns of Joint Pain and Inflammation in Various Types of Arthritis

I	*II*	*III*	*IV*
Monarticular Disease (one joint involved)	Polyarticular Disease with Monarticular Component	Oligoarticular Disease (four or fewer joints involved)	Symmetrical polyarthritis
Any syndrome ordinarily characterized by polyarthritis can present as monarticular disease; most monarticular syndromes are, in practice, oligoarticular	Ankylosing spondylitis	Includes many diseases in Columns I and II	Rheumatoid arthritis
	Psoriatic arthritis	Juvenile rheumatoid arthritis (oligoarticular type)	Juvenile rheumatoid arthritis (polyarticular type)
	Reiter's syndrome	Reiter's syndrome	Systemic lupus erythematosus
	Colitic arthritis	Psoriatic arthritis	Scleroderma
	Whipple's disease	Colitic arthritis	Polyarteritis nodosa
Septic arthritis	Juvenile rheumatoid arthritis	Ankylosing spondylitis	Wegener's granulomatosis
Crystal-induced arthritis	Sarcoid arthritis	Whipple's disease	Polymyalgia rheumatica
Gout	Pseudogout	Pseudogout	Henoch-Schönlein purpura
Pseudogout	Hemophilic arthritis	Gouty arthritis	Hepatitis B polyarthritis
Traumatic arthritis	Hemochromatosis	Sarcoidosis	Dermatomyositis-polymyositis
Mechanical derangement	Septic arthritis (gonococcal and meningococcal)	Erythema nodosum	Serum sickness drug reaction
Localized syndromes (tendinitis, bursitis)	Rheumatoid arthritis	Hypertrophic osteoarthropathy	Sarcoidosis
Neuropathic arthropathy		Type IV hyperlipoproteinemia	Behçet's disease
Gaucher's disease		Rheumatoid arthritis	Polychondritis
Hyperlipoproteinemia			Rubella arthritis
Avascular necrosis			Amyloid arthritis
Pigmented villonodular synovitis			Multicentric reticulohistiocytosis
Synovioma			Leukemia
Sarcoidosis			Carcinomatous polyarthritis
Amyloid arthritis			Hypertrophic osteoarthropathy
Hemophilic arthritis			Hyperlipoproteinemias
Rheumatoid arthritis			
Diabetic osteopathy			

Table 13–3.   Continued

V	VI	VII *Palindromic or Intermittent Patterns (recurrent attacks of polyarticular synovitis that remit without sequelae)*	VIII
Asymmetrical polyarthritis	*Migratory polyarthritis*		*Fever and Polyarticular Arthritis*
Psoriatic arthritis	Rheumatic fever	Short courses (2–3 days)	Sepsis or sepsis-related
Reiter's syndrome	Gonococcal arthritis	Rheumatoid arthritis	Gonococcal arthritis
Ankylosing spondylitis	Meningococcal arthritis	Sarcoidosis	Meningococcal arthritis
Polyarteritis nodosa	Whipple's disease	Familial Mediterranean fever	Lyme disease (spirochete)
Colitic arthritis	Sarcoidosis (acute)	Sickle cell anemia	Rheumatic fever (Streptococcus)
Gouty arthritis	Leukemia	Palindromic rheumatism	Whipple's disease
Sickle cell disease	Type IIa hyperlipoproteinemia	Long courses (7–100 days)	Reiter's syndrome (reactive to enteric infections)
Leukemia		Peripheral synovitis of spondylitis	
Lymphoma		Colitic arthropathy	Connective tissue disorders
Osteoarthritis		Whipple's disease	Systemic lupus
Pseudogout		Intestinal bypass arthritis	Necrotizing, vasculitides
Pancreatic fat necrosis		Behçet's disease	Polyarteritis nodosa
Hemochromatosis		Familial Mediterranean fever	Wegener's granulomatosis
Hemophilic arthritis		Sickle cell anemia	Temporal arteritis/polymyalgia rheumatica
Acromegaly			Henoch-Schönlein purpura
Hypothyroidism			Behçet's disease
Hyperlipoproteinemias			
Familial Mediterranean fever			Rheumatoid arthritis—fever is *not* commonly associated with a flare of joint disease alone. Fever can be seen with RA associated with serositis (pleura and pericardium) or vasculitis or in the setting of an abrupt decrease in steroid dosage
			Erythema nodosum
			Sarcoidosis
			Familial Mediterranean fever
			Juvenile RA or adult onset JRA—Still's variety
			Inflammatory bowel disease
			Reiter's syndrome and ankylosing spondylitis

Table 13–4. Classification of Antinuclear/Anticytoplasmic Antibodies

Antibody	Method of Detection	Disease Association	Clinical Significance
Antinuclear antibody	Fluorescent antinuclear antibody test (FANA)	See Table 13–5.	Sensitive screening test for SLE; nonspecific test
Antinucleoprotein	LE cell test	Highly specific test for SLE but very insensitive (only 40% of SLE patients are +)	*Not* used as a screening or diagnostic test for SLE; insensitive and time-consuming
Anti-DNA Anti-double stranded DNA	FARR assay or immunofluorescent test employing C. Lucilliae	Sensitive and specific tests for SLE; significant binding (> 30%) by the FARR technique is found only in SLE and MCTD	Once an ANA is positive, an anti-DNA test should be performed to confirm a diagnosis of SLE
Anti-single stranded DNA		Much less specific for SLE; found in a wide variety of diseases	Not a routine test
Anti-ENA	All components of ENA give a speckled ANA pattern:		
Anti-ribonucleoprotein	Counterimmunoelectrophoresis	Specific and sensitive test for MCTD	This specific test should follow the finding of a speckled ANA
Anti-Sm	Precipitin test	One of the most specific serologic tests for the diagnosis of SLE; found in only 40% of SLE patients and almost never in other conditions	Not a screening test because of its insensitivity; can be helpful in difficult diagnostic problems
Anti-RO (Anti-SS-A)	Precipitin, C. fixation, immunofluorescent tests	Present in 70% of primary Sjögren's syndrome (SS), 33% of SS + SLE, 1% of SS + RA	Not a screening test; helpful in difficult diagnostic problems involving SS or SLE
		A marker for systemic disease in ANA-negative SLE patients, particularly those with subacute cutaneous lupus or a distinct subpopulation of SLE without skin disease; associated with congenital lupus and congenital heart block in infants of SLE patients	May be an important finding in SLE pregnancy
Anti-LA (Anti-SS-B) (identical antigens SS-B nuclear, LA cytoplasmic)	Precipitin, C. fixation, and immunofluorescent tests	Present in 50% of SS, 70% of SS + SLE, 3% of SS + RA	Not a screening test; sometimes employed in difficult diagnostic problems
Anti-PM-1	Precipitin test or complement fixation	Specific test for polymyositis (> 50%); not found in other diseases so far	Not a routine test
Anti-RNA		Found predominantly in patients with SLE	Not a routine test
Anti-Histone (histones are basic nuclear proteins)	Fluorescent test	A high frequency of this antibody is found among patients with drug-induced lupus	Not a routine test; used in the setting of possible drug-induced lupus

in that many clinically divergent disorders share the same abnormality.

Elevated erythrocyte sedimentation rate and C-reactive protein are nonspecific reflections of the underlying inflammatory state and are rough yet clinically useful guides to the activity of many disease states. An elevated sedimentation rate has its greatest significance in polymyalgia rheumatica and temporal arteritis, in which the diagnosis is based upon this laboratory abnormality in the clinical setting of an elderly patient with proximal muscle soreness, temporal ar-

teritis symptoms, or both. The ESR in this entity is a good guide to disease activity and therapeutic response. ESR elevation can also be seen in malignant and infectious disorders, some of which share clinical features with rheumatic disorders.

Anemia is commonly found in association with various inflammatory rheumatic disorders. Anemia of chronic disease (low hemoglobin, low mean corpuscular volume, and low Fe and TIBC) is probably the most common type, but the physician must consider other causes, including iron deficiency caused by blood

Table 13–5. Patterns of Antinuclear Immunofluorescence

Disease	*Diffuse (homogeneous) (antideoxyribo-nucleoprotein)	Peripheral (RIM) (antinative DNA)	Speckled (anti-Sm or RNP or RO)	Nucleolar	Centromere	% Positive ANA
SLE	+ +	+ +	+ (SM)	±	−	95
MCTD	+	−	+ + (RNP)	±	−	95
RA	+	−	±	±	−	50
Scleroderma	+	±	+ (RNP)	+	+ (CRST)	60
Polymyositis	+	±	±	±	−	20
Sicca syndrome	+	±	+ (RO) (LA)	+	−	70
Drug-induced LE	+	+	±	±	−	90
Chronic liver disease	+	±	±	±	−	20
Aging (> 60 years)	+	±	±	±	−	20

+ + = most common; + = common; ± = uncommon; − = unusual
*Most nonspecific pattern

loss, megaloblastic anemia caused by pernicious anemia, or hemolysis caused by immunologic processes in systemic lupus erythematosus. At times more than one type of anemia may be involved.

Although elevated white blood cell counts with a "left shift" may reflect an underlying infection (related to either the underlying disorder or its therapy), some rheumatic disorders are commonly associated with leukocytosis, unrelated to superimposed sepsis. Examples include diseases as clinically divergent as polyarteritis nodosa, the systemic type of juvenile

rheumatoid arthritis, and Reiter's syndrome. Leukopenia, however, is a more specific abnormality when associated with joint disease and may reflect systemic lupus erythematosus or Felty's syndrome (rheumatoid arthritis with granulocytopenia).

Polyclonal elevation of immunoglobulins is a nonspecific reflection of the overactive inflammatory and immunological state in many rheumatic disorders. Although a monoclonal gammopathy can accompany disorders such as systemic lupus and rheumatoid arthritis, such a gammopathy may reflect multiple myeloma or

Table 13–6. Synovial Fluid Analysis

Classification	Condition	Color	Clarity	Viscosity	WBC/mm³	% polys	Crystals	Glucose (% Serum)	Complement	Culture/ Smear
Normal	Normal	Straw	Translucent	High	200	25%	0	Same	Normal (1/3 of serum)	0
Group I (Noninflammatory)	Osteoarthritis	Yellow	Transparent	High	2000	25%	0	Same	Normal	0
	Trauma	Pink or red	Transparent	High	2000	25%	0	Same	Normal	0
Group II (Inflammatory)	SLE	Yellow	Translucent	Slight	0–9000	25%	0	Same	Normal or low	0
	Gout	Yellow or white	Translucent or opaque	Low	100–160,000	90%	*+	Same	Normal	0
	Pseudogout	Yellow or white	Translucent or opaque	Low	50–70,000	90%	**+	Same	Normal	0
	Rheumatoid arthritis	Yellow or purulent	Translucent or opaque	Low	3,000–75,000	50–75%	0	75–100%	Normal or low	0
Group III (Purulent)	Bacterial arthritis	Purulent	Opaque	Low	50,000–300,000	90%	0	50%	Normal or low	+/+
	Tuberculosis	Purulent	Opaque	Low	2,500–100,000	50%	0	50–75%	Normal or low	+ +/+

* = Negatively birefringent, needle shaped crystals in polys
** = Weakly positively birefringent rhomboid crystals in polys
+ = Culture and Gram's stain are often negative in gonococcal arthritis
+ + = Tuberculous cultures take 6 weeks to become positive. Highest diagnostic yield is through culture of synovial tissue and/or a positive biopsy demonstrating caseating granuloma with or without acid-fast bacteria

amyloidosis, two disorders associated with joint manifestations.

An absolute eosinophilia can be seen in various rheumatic disorders including rheumatoid arthritis and types of necrotizing vasculitis. Eosinophilia can be a prominent diagnostic criterion of Churg-Strauss eosinophilic granulomatous vasculitis with a history of asthma, pulmonary lesions, and a polyarteritis nodosa–type disorder. Eosinophilia can also be seen in Wegener's granulomatosis, polyarteritis nodosa, and eosinophilic fasciitis.

Although thrombocytosis is a common abnormality in diseases of an inflammatory nature and can be followed as a reflection of the activity of the underlying disorder, it is nonspecific.

Since most inflammatory rheumatic disorders are associated with elevated immune complex levels, it is difficult to ascribe specificity or diagnostic significance to them.

The serologic and immunologic tests employed in the rheumatic diseases vary in their sensitivity and specificity. A *specific* test is one in which, when the test is positive, there is a high likelihood that the disease for which the test is done is present *and* that only rarely will the test be positive in patients without the disease. Highly specific tests tend to be less sensitive, so that although when the test is positive the disease usually exists, some patients *with* the disease may have a negative test. A *sensitive* test is one that rarely fails to be positive when the disease for which it is done is present. However, such a test tends to be less specific, and other disorders can have a positive test. An optimal test would be one that has both high sensitivity and specificity. In systemic lupus erythematosus, the fluorescent antinuclear antibody (FANA) test is sensitive but not specific (95% of patients with SLE have a positive FANA test, but so do 52% of patients with rheumatoid arthritis and 55% of scleroderma patients). Antinative deoxyribonucleic acid (DNA) antibodies share *both* specificity and sensitivity (60% of SLE patients have a positive test, while only 3% of RA patients and 5% of controls do). Anti-Sm antibodies are highly specific but less sensitive (28% of SLE patients have antibodies to Sm, as do only 3% of RA patients and 4% of controls).

A diagnostic strategy for musculoskeletal disorders involves both clinical and laboratory data (Fig. 13–2). The clinical facts are collected from a complete history and physical examination. The correct use of laboratory tests, x-rays, radionuclide scanning, and tissue biopsies is guided by an understanding of the underlying pathologic state and the pattern of joint or visceral involvement, the rapidity with which a diagnosis must be made, and prior experience with similar disorders (Tables 13–7 and 13–8).

JOINT PAIN

DEFINITION

Joint pain refers to an unpleasant sensory experience that originates either around or within the structures constituting a joint or from an area distant from the joint itself.

PATHOPHYSIOLOGIC CONSIDERATIONS

Joint pain arises from various types of injury to the joint structures that are highly sensitive to pain, including the fibrous capsule, ligaments, and the periosteum. Menisci, articular cartilage, synovial membrane, and bone are insensitive to pain; however, disease in these areas can lead to pain through eventual deformation of the sensitive structures or through as yet unknown neural pathways.

In disorders such as osteoarthritis, the cause of pain is thought to be multifactorial and includes elevated periosteum, pressure on exposed subchondral bone, trabecular microfracture, intra-articular ligamentous disease, capsule distension, synovitis, periarticular tendon and fascia inflammation, and muscle spasm.

Periarticular tissues (skin, muscles, tendons, and bursae) also can be involved in disease processes and present as joint pain. Pain that is perceived as coming from a joint may actually have radiated to the area of the joint from another musculoskeletal structure. Nerve entrapment syndromes (e.g., herniated lumbar disc) are particularly apt to radiate proximally as well as distally. Hip and back pain may radiate along the hamstring muscles and appear as knee pain. Because of an overlapping neural system, anginal pain can localize in the neck or shoulder, especially if these areas have previously been involved by disease processes. It is important to appreciate such referred pain lest we attribute potentially life threatening, nonmusculoskeletal disease to a less emergent musculoskeletal disorder.

DIFFERENTIAL DIAGNOSIS

The differential diagnosis of joint pain involves all disorders that, by varying disease mechanisms, lead

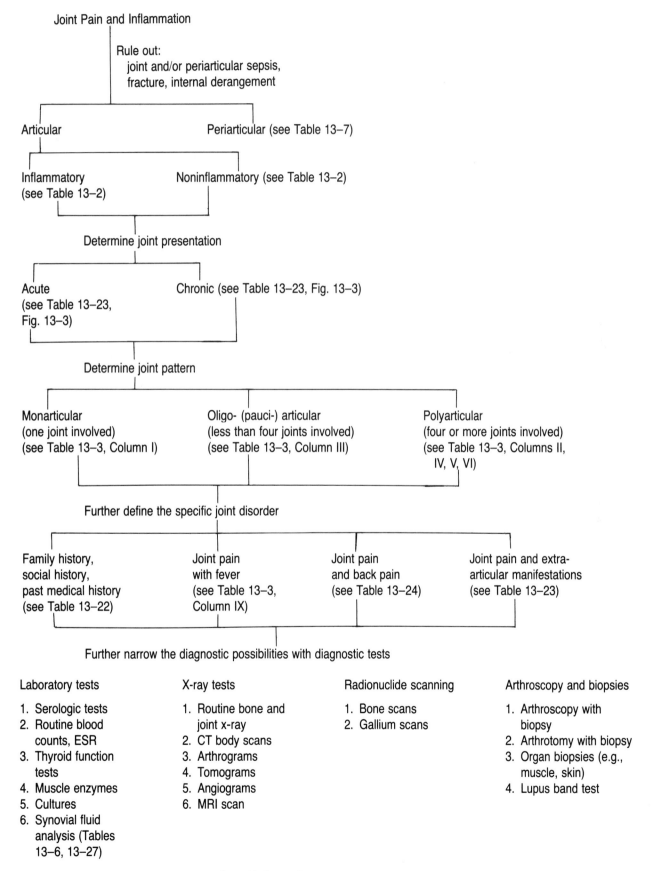

Fig. 13–2. Diagnostic approach to joint pain and inflammation.

Table 13-7.   Diagnostic Tests in Joint, Periarticular, and Systemic Disorders

Test/Procedure	Clinical Significance/Disorder
GENERAL SCREENING TESTS	
Acute-phase reactants	Nonspecific, yet reflect the presence of inflammation and tissue injury
Erythrocyte sedimentation rate	
C-reactive protein	Rough screening tests in which a normal test does *not* rule out disease while an elevated level may reflect an inflammatory or neoplastic disease state
	Can be used as a rough measure of the level inflammation and response to therapy
Complete blood count	
White blood count abnormalities	
Increased white blood cell count	Reflects systemic inflammation in disorders such as juvenile RA, polyarteritis nodosa or joint or other sepsis. Elevated WBC can be secondary to corticosteroid effect. Mild elevation in gout
Decreased white blood cell count	Immunologic destruction; splenic sequestration, or bone marrow suppression in disorders such as SLE or Felty's syndrome or leukemia
Eosinophilia	"Allergic" reaction in disorders such as Churg-Strauss vasculitis, rheumatoid arthritis, and drug reaction to gold
Red blood cell abnormalities	
Anemia (decreased hemoglobin)	Commonly associated with both acute and chronic inflammatory disorders. Improves with disease control
Anemia of chronic disease (decreased Hgb, decreased MCV, decreased Fe + TIBC)	Bone marrow suppression related to the systemic inflammatory state (e.g., RA, SLE, vasculitis, sepsis)
Blood loss anemia (decreased Hgb, decreased MCV, decreased Fe, increased TIBC, decreased % saturation)	Bleeding can occur with organ damage (bowel necrosis in vasculitis), thrombocytopenia (SLE), or related to NSAID use or steroid-related GI irritation
Hemolytic anemia (decreased Hgb, increased LDH, positive Coombs' test)	Related to immunologic factors (SLE), microangiopathy (scleroderma, TTP), hemoglobinopathies (SS disease, thalassemia), pernicious (megaloblastic) anemia (increased MCV)
Polycythemia	Increased cell turnover can be associated with hyperuricemia and gout
Platelet abnormalities	
Thrombocytopenia	Related to immunologic destruction (SLE), splenic sequestration (Felty's syndrome), bone marrow invasion (leukemia, lymphoma), drug effect (gold, penicillamine, immunosuppressive drugs)
Thrombocytosis	Reactive disorder to systemic inflammatory disorders such as rheumatoid arthritis, and polyarteritis nodosa
Serum chemistries	
Increased urea nitrogen, creatinine	Nephritis caused by systemic lupus and vasculitides, amyloidosis, and gout with nephrolithiasis
Increased glucose	Diabetes-associated osteopathy, Charcot's joint, septic arthritis/osteomyelitis; hemochromatosis arthropathy; Cushing's disease/syndrome with myopathy; acromegaly, arthropathy
Increased SGOT	Liver origin: hepatitis B–associated arthritis; dermatitis syndrome or polyarteritis nodosa; chronic liver disease associated with Sjögren's syndrome; hemochromatosis arthropathy; NSAID-associated hepatotoxicity; fatty liver due to corticosteroid; Wilson's disease with chondrocalcinosis
	Muscle origin: dermatomyositis/polymyositis, other forms of myositis
	Cardiac origin: myocardial damage with coronary vasculitis (SLE, PAN), myocarditis
Increased SGPT	As above for liver source of SGOT
Increased LDH	Nonspecific, but elevated levels can reflect hepatic or muscle disorders similar to those noted with SGOT. Helpful sign of hemolysis in hemolytic anemias (e.g., SLE)
Increased CPK	
Positive MM band	Muscle origin: dermatomyositis/polymyositis and other myopathies; hypothyroid myopathy
Positive MB band	Cardiac origin: myocardial damage due to coronary vasculitis (SLE, PAN, Kawasaki disease), myocarditis (SLE, PAN), coronary atherosclerosis with ischemia (hyperlipoproteinemia)
Increased uric acid	Related to primary or secondary gout and hyperuricemia (see Table 13–10)
Increased calcium	Hyperparathyroidism and its associated joint disorders; pseudogout and chondrocalcinosis; sarcoidosis and its joint disorder; neoplastic diseases with associated musculoskeletal disorders

Table 13–7.   Continued

Test/Procedure	Clinical Significance/Disorder
Increased globulin	
Polyclonal	Found in many inflammatory disorders, both acute and chronic (i.e., RA, SLE, vasculitis), seronegative spondyloarthropathies, sarcoidosis
Monoclonal	Found primarily in multiple myeloma and amyloidosis; also found in some patients with RA and SLE
Increased cholesterol	Hyperlipoproteinemias; related to nephrotic syndrome due to lupus- or vasculitis-associated nephropathies; associated with hyperuricemia and gout
Increased amylase	Pancreatic origin: pancreatitis or pancreatic tumor with associated fat necrosis and polyarthritis; pancreatitis due to connective tissue disorders such as SLE, vasculitis, Sjögren's syndrome; pancreatitis associated with hyperparathyroidism Salivary origin: Sjögren's syndrome
Decreased albumin	Associated with nephrotic syndrome due to disorders such as SLE, vasculitis, amyloidosis, diabetes; protein-losing enteropathies; malabsorption syndromes
Increased alkaline phosphatase	Associated with rheumatoid arthritis, polymyalgia rheumatica/temporal arteritis, tuberculosis, sarcoidosis, and neoplasms
Urinalysis	
Proteinuria	Nephritis or nephrotic syndrome due to systemic disorders such as SLE, vasculitides, amyloidosis
Hematuria/red blood cell casts	Nephritis related to SLE, vasculitides
Pyuria	Interstitial nephritis due to SLE, Sjögren's syndrome, drug effect; also seen in urethritis as a component of Reiter's syndrome or gonococcal infection; sterile pyuria seen with tuberculosis

SPECIFIC LABORATORY TESTS

Routine laboratory tests	
Erythrocyte sedimentation rate and C-reactive protein	Screening tests to demonstrate inflammation and tissue damage; rough guide of disease activity
Complete blood count, differential, and platelet count	Screening tests for abnormalities of inflammatory, infectious, or neoplastic disorders
Serum chemistries (e.g., SMA-12, electrolytes)	Screening tests for visceral involvement or metabolic derangement
Urinalysis	Screening test for renal involvement or drug toxicity
Serologic tests	
Rheumatoid factor	Positive in 80% of RA patients but nonspecific appropriate screening tests for RA
Antinuclear antibodies	
Fluorescent antinuclear antibody test (FANA)	Positive in 90% of patients with SLE but nonspecific (see Fig. 13–3); sensitive screening test for SLE
Anti-DNA (double stranded) antibody test	More specific test for SLE; performed after the screening FANA test is positive if a more definitive diagnosis is needed
Anti-Sm antibody	Highly specific test for SLE but insensitive (40%); performed if there is question about the diagnosis of SLE; not a screening test
Anti-RO (also called anti-SS-A)	A marker for systemic disease in ANA-negative SLE patients with cutaneous lupus; not a routine screening test; reserved for diagnostic problems in ANA-negative SLE; associated with congenital lupus and heart block
Antihistone antibodies	A marker for drug-induced lupus, not a routine screening test
Complement (C_3, C_4, CH_{50})	Levels can be low in SLE, cryoglobulinemia, and systemic vasculitis as a result of consumption by circulating or fixed immune complexes; serial measurements may be helpful in guiding therapy of SLE patients, synovial fluid complement levels are *not* routinely performed
Serologic test for syphilis	False positive VDRL (negative FTA-ABS) is present in 20% of SLE patients
Cryoglobulins	Found in SLE and other pathologic states associated with immune complexes; usually reserved for evaluation of mixed cryoglobulinemia and Raynaud's phenomenon
Immune complex (IC) assays	Elevated IC levels are found in many disease states; inappropriate for routine clinical use
Synovial fluid analysis	Important diagnostic test in defining the state of inflammation or noting the presence of crystals or sepsis (see Tables 13–6 and 13–27)

Table 13–7.   Diagnostic Tests in Joint, Periarticular, and Systemic Disorders (Continued)

Test/Procedure	Clinical Significance/Disorder
Diagnostic radiology and nuclear medicine	
X-rays of peripheral and sacroiliac joints and the spine	Acutely, only soft tissue swelling is noted; later, such x-rays can define characteristic abnormalities such as erosions, calcifications, joint destruction and spurs; sacroiliitis can be diagnostic of seronegative spondyloarthropathies
Computed tomography	Particularly helpful in diagnosing neurologic and spinal disorders
Radionuclide bone and joint imaging	Offers documentation of the extent and pattern of early or difficult-to-diagnose joint pain, definition of osteonecrosis, septic arthritis, or osteomyelitis, metabolic bone disease, Paget's disease, neoplasm, and hypertrophic osteoarthropathy
Arthrography	Defines intra-articular anatomy and is particularly helpful in the diagnosis of post-traumatic internal derangement of the knee or torn rotator cuff of the shoulder; also helpful in the diagnosis of a Baker's cyst and pigmented villonodular synovitis
Ultrasonography	Applications include the noninvasive diagnosis of Baker's cyst and pericardial disease and effusions
Magnetic resonance imaging	Early studies demonstrate effective use in the diagnosis of cerebral and spinal disorders
Myelography	Used as a preoperative investigation and as a diagnostic technique; employed in the evaluation of disc herniation and root entrapment, as well as tumors and infection with cord compression
Angiography	Vasculitides can be diagnosed by *arteriography* of specific vascular beds: stenoses and aneurysms of the aorta and its branches are seen in Takayasu's arteritis; aneurysms of renal and mesenteric arteries are characteristic of polyarteritis nodosa; cerebral vessel abnormalities are seen in systemic vasculitides and in isolated angiitis of the brain. Some physicians employ temporal artery angiography to guide the surgeon to an involved area of the vessel for biopsy. *Venography* can diagnose venous thrombosis seen in disorders such as SLE or vasculitides. *Coronary angiography* may help in the diagnosis of coronary angiitis of SLE or polyarteritis. *Pulmonary angiography with pressure measurements* are important tools in defining pulmonary emboli or pulmonary hypertension.
Gallium scanning	This isotope accumulates in collections of polymorphonuclear leukocytes. Thus, this scan may be helpful in defining joint or bone sepsis. Such scanning is also helpful in defining sarcoidosis (lung uptake of isotope) or interstitial nephritis (kidney uptake)
X-rays of the gastrointestinal tract	
Esophagram/cine esophagram, upper GI series, small bowel follow-through	Helpful in defining abnormal esophageal peristaltic activity in diseases such as scleroderma and myositis; also can define lower esophageal stricture due to reflux in scleroderma. Small-bowel studies can characterize a malabsorption pattern seen in Whipple's disease. Crohn's disease of the small bowel can be diagnosed.
Barium enema	Motility disorders of the large bowel as well as colonic sacculations of scleroderma can be defined. Crohn's disease and ulcerative colitis are defined by this procedure. "Thumb-printing" of the bowel is characteristic of vasculitic disorders such as Henoch-Schönlein purpura and is a reflection of bleeding into the wall of the bowel.
Organ biopsies	
Skin	Although the following disorders may be diagnosed by other means, skin biopsy is a simple and safe technique with which to make or support a diagnosis of vasculitis, systemic lupus (band test), scleroderma, sarcoidosis, tumor, or amyloid. Rarely, biopsy must be done on nodules to define rheumatoid or gouty origin. Cholesterol emboli may present as a vasculitis-type disorder and can be diagnosed by skin biopsy.
Temporal artery biopsy	The definitive diagnosis of temporal arteritis is based upon this safe office procedure. At times bilateral biopsy is needed in view of the segmental nature of the vasculitic process. The pathologist should perform multiple sections so as not to miss involved areas. Polymyalgia rheumatica (without temporal arteritis symptoms or signs) is not an indication for biopsy.

Table 13–7. Continued

Test/Procedure	Clinical Significance/Disorder
Muscle biopsy (light microscopy and histochemical staining) are indicated. Special stains (for example, amyloid, AFB, fungal, or bacterial) and cultures may be ordered	The definitive diagnosis of myositis is based upon this safe procedure. Vasculitis can be diagnosed by muscle biopsy (the biopsy performed as a "blind" procedure or directed by muscle weakness or abnormal muscle enzymes). Diagnostic test for myopathy
Nerve biopsy	Sural and other nerve biopsies may be performed as part of the workup of neuropathy. Vasculitis and amyloidosis can be defined in this way. Permanent neurologic deficit can occur after these biopsies.
Kidney biopsy (light microscopy, immunofluorescence, and electron microscopic studies are usually carried out)	Although such a biopsy can be helpful in the diagnosis and treatment of disorders such as systemic lupus, vasculitis, Goodpasture's syndrome and amyloidosis, morbidity is associated with the procedure, and the risks must be weighed against the benefits.
Lung biopsy	Particularly helpful in the diagnosis of vasculitides (e.g., Wegener's granulomatosis), Goodpasture's syndrome, opportunistic infections (e.g., tuberculosis, fungus, Pneumocystis carinii), and tumors. The specific method of biopsy (needle vs bronchoscopic vs open) will depend upon the clinical setting.
Rectal or intestinal biopsy	Rectal biopsy is useful in the diagnosis of inflammatory bowel disease and amyloidosis. Jejunal biopsy is needed for the definitive diagnosis of Whipple's disease.
Ear cartilage	Can diagnose polychondritis
Liver biopsy	Can diagnose tuberculosis, sarcoidosis, chronic hepatitis, and primary biliary cirrhosis
Lymph node biopsy	Can diagnose leukemia, lymphoma, granulomatous disease, and tumors
Synovial membrane (performed by closed biopsy, via the arthroscope or by arthrotomy)	This biopsy should be considered in patients in whom the diagnosis is not clear after clinical evaluation. This procedure may be the only way to make a diagnosis in diseases such as granulomatous infections (TB, fungal), sarcoidosis, malignancy, pigmented villonodular synovitis, hemochromatosis, Whipple's disease, ochronosis, and amyloidosis. Persistent monarticular synovitis is the most common indication for biopsy. The procedure is uncommonly needed for the diagnosis of chronic polyarthritis (such as rheumatoid arthritis).
Bone biopsy	The definitive characterization of the microorganism causing osteomyelitis is by bone biopsy with appropriate cultures. Organisms obtained from a sinus tract or from wound drainage (even if Staph aureus) may not accurately represent the microorganism causing the osteomyelitis.
Other tests Pulmonary function tests (routine volumes, diffusion capacity)	Helpful in defining the restrictive and diffusion capacity abnormalities of the interstitial lung disorders of connective tissue diseases (i.e., scleroderma, systemic lupus).
Esophageal manometry	A combination of manometric and cine radiographic evaluation of the UGI tract is the most sensitive and reliable method for diagnosis of the motility abnormalities of the esophagus seen in scleroderma and dermato- or polymyositis.
Tests employed in the diagnosis of infectious diseases VDRL/STS FTA-ABS or other specific treponeme tests	A false positive VDRL (+VDRL, −FTA-ABS) can be seen in connective tissue disorders (e.g., SLE, RA) or following viral illness (e.g., hepatitis B). Syphilis can always coexist with other medical conditions. A false positive beaded FTA-ABS pattern has been described in SLE but is not common. In general, a positive FTA-ABS represents infection with syphilis.
Serologic tests for Lyme disease (complement fixation and other assays are employed)	A rising antibody titer of 1:256 or more to the offending spirochete helps to characterize this disorder if the clinical picture is consistent with Lyme disease.
Hepatitis B serologies	The definition of an acute (or chronic) infection with hepatitis B can be important information when dealing with the dermatitis-arthritis disorder of hepatitis B or polyarteritis nodosa.
Histocompatibility testing (the HLA-B27 type has a high association with the seronegative spondyloarthropathies and is the most commonly sought type)	Although the associations of certain rheumatic diseases with specific HLA antigens is high, HLA testing remains an expensive test that is employed only in difficult-to-diagnose back and joint disorders. Although it may be helpful in diagnosing seronegative spondyloarthropathies, it should not be considered a routine test.

Table 13–7.   Diagnostic Tests in Joint, Periarticular, and Systemic Disorders (Continued)

Test/Procedure	Clinical Significance/Disorder
SPECIFIC TESTS AND PROCEDURES	
Rheumatoid factor—positive in 75% of patients	Rheumatoid arthritis
Joint x-ray demonstrating erosions, joint space narrowing, or juxta-articular osteoporosis	
Synovial fluid analysis—inflammatory (type 2) fluid	
Antinuclear antibody—positive in 40% (oligoarticular group)	Juvenile rheumatoid arthritis
Rheumatoid factor—positive in 20%, primarily in older age group with nodules and erosions	
Joint x-rays—demonstrating erosions, joint space narrowing, or juxta-articular osteoporosis	
Ophthalmologic examination—especially in the oligoarticular group in which iridocyclitis can be asymptomatic and lead to blindness	
Synovial fluid analysis—inflammatory (type 2) fluid	
X-ray of the sacroiliac joints and spine—characteristic SI joint changes are diagnostic, but may be absent early	Seronegative spondyloarthropathies
HLA-B27—positive in 90%; *not* done routinely, but reserved for difficult diagnostic problems	Ankylosing spondylitis
Synovial fluid analysis—inflammatory (type 2) fluid	
Urinalysis—may demonstrate pyuria and hematuria	Reiter's syndrome
Synovial fluid analysis—inflammatory (type 2) fluid	
X-ray of involved peripheral or sacroiliac joints—peripheral joints can demonstrate destructive changes and/or periostitis; SI joints may show unilateral sacroiliitis in 80% of patients with chronic disease	
HLA-B27—reported in 75% of RS patients; *not* a routine test	
Stool cultures—for enteric organisms in the setting of diarrhea and "reactive arthritis"	
Ophthalmologic examination—in the setting of chronic uveitis or conjunctivitis	
Synovial fluid analysis—inflammatory (type 2) fluid	Psoriatic arthritis
X-ray of involved peripheral and sacroiliac joints—demonstrating characteristic peripheral joint abnormalities and asymmetrical SI joint changes	
HLA-B27—positive in patients with spine disease. *Not* a routine test	
X-ray and/or biopsy—definition of underlying inflammatory bowel disease	Colitic arthropathy
Synovial fluid analysis—inflammatory (type 2) fluid	
X-ray of peripheral, sacroiliac joints, and spine—demonstrating characteristic symmetrical SI or spine disease	
HLA-B27—positive in 75% of patient with back disease. *Not* a routine test	Diffuse connective tissue disorders
Antinuclear antibody testing—most common screening test is the FANA (fluorescent ANA test); this is both very sensitive (found + in 90% of SLE patients) and nonspecific	Systemic lupus erythematosus
The anti-DNA test is both sensitive and specific and should be done if the FANA test is positive. Rarely, *both* tests are negative. If serologic confirmation is still needed, anti-Sm or anti-RO may be sent (see Table 13–4)	
Definition of renal disease—an initial screening urinalysis should be done. If normal, observation is indicated. If proteinuria is found, a 24-hour urine for protein and creatinine clearance is performed. Similar testing is indicated if a screening serum creatinine is elevated. The place of renal biopsy is controversial; is not performed unless persistent proteinuria, abnormal urinary sediment, or renal dysfunction is defined	
Definition of hematologic abnormalities—the presence of the following define the diagnosis, activity, and treatment of SLE: hemolytic anemia, thrombocytopenia, leukopenia, presence of a circulating anticoagulant	
Joint x-rays are rarely needed in view of the nonerosive, nondestructive nature of SLE joint disease. Rarely, an overlap between SLE, RA, and erosive disease may be found	

Table 13–7. Continued

Test/Procedure	Clinical Significance/Disorder
Skin biopsy—histologic and immunofluorescence (lupus band test) studies can help to identify skin lesions as lupus in type. These are not routine tests but are used when the clinical picture is not characteristic of discoid or systemic lupus. 80% of SLE patients with active disease will demonstrate one or more immunoglobulin or complement proteins in uninvolved skin; other diseases (e.g., RA, rosacea), however, also have a positive band test	Diffuse connective tissue disorders Systemic lupus erythematosus (Cont.)
Complement—although not employed as a screening diagnostic test for SLE, the reduction of CH_{50} (total hemolytic complement), C_3 and C_4 levels is often related to renal or CNS disease activity and can be guides to therapy. C_2 levels are not usually decreased except in association with genetic defects (C_2 deficiency).	
VDRL/specific treponeme test—a chronic false positive VDRL (+VDRL X 6 months, -specific treponeme test) is found in 25% of SLE patients and is a useful screening test	
Anticardiolipin antibody—elevated IgM or IgG levels may be predictive of SLE patients at increased risk for problems with pregnancy and vascular complications	
Antinuclear antibodies—an appropriate screening test for scleroderma. Three patterns can be found in scleroderma. The most specific is the nucleolar; a speckled pattern is more specific than the diffuse. Anticentromere antibodies are characteristic of the Crest syndrome.	Scleroderma
Skin biopsy—although skin biopsy may show early, prefibrotic cellular changes or late fibrotic abnormalities, both of which strengthen the diagnosis of scleroderma, this test is *not* routinely performed for diagnosis or followed as a guide to disease progression	
Manometry and cineradiographic studies of the esophagus—sensitive tests that can define hypomotility even in patients without symptoms of dysphagia. They proved early evidence of multisystem disease in patients suspected of having scleroderma	
Pulmonary function tests—as a routine, noninvasive, and available procedure, diffusion capacity remains the single most sensitive indicator of early pulmonary involvement; restrictive defect	
X-rays—joint x-rays may define osteolysis or soft tissue calcifications, but erosive disease is uncommon	
Capillary microscopy—nailfold capillary abnormalities may prove helpful in early, overlapping, or mixed patients by separating the majority, who ultimately develop scleroderma, from the minority with SLE. However, such morphological studies are not widely available and are not a routine screening procedure in most centers	
Muscle biopsy—in those scleroderma patients with proximal muscle weakness, muscle enzymes, and abnormal EMG, a muscle biopsy is appropriate to differentiate between fibrotic and inflammatory changes in the muscle. Such findings have therapeutic significance	
Skeletal muscle enzymes—raised levels of enzymes released into the serum as a result of muscle damage are helpful indicators of the extent and acuteness of the damage. Elevated CPK (MB band negative, MM band positive), SGOT, LDH, and aldolase are seen in virtually all patients at some time in the course of their disease; these are routine screening tests for myopathy/myositis	Dermatomyositis/polymyositis
Antinuclear antibody—anti-Jo-1 is present in 30 to 50% of PM patients but is uncommon in DM; MM/SC 1 antibody is found with high frequency in patients with PM and scleroderma; as many as 80% of DM/PM patients may demonstrate ANA positivity (see Fig. 13–3)	

Table 13–7. Diagnostic Tests in Joint, Periarticular, and Systemic Disorders (Continued)

Test/Procedure	Clinical Significance/Disorder
Electromyography—characteristic changes (increased insertional activity, fibrillation potentials, polyphasic potentials, etc.) are found in most patients with myositis. Only 10% have no abnormality on EMG. This is a routine yet specialized test in the workup of myopathy/myositis	Dermatomyositis (DM)/polymyositis (PM) (Cont.)
Muscle biopsy (with appropriate histochemical staining)—characteristic histologic changes (degeneration of fibers, inflammation, necrosis, variation in fiber size) are found in a majority of myositis patients and are important diagnostically; as many as 20% of patients may have a negative biopsy, an indication of the patchy nature of the pathologic process	
Tissue biopsy—adequate histologic documentation is crucial before instituting therapy	Necrotizing vasculitis Polyarteritis nodosa
Skin biopsy—the simplest procedure, done when the skin is involved (uncommonly); leukocytoclastic angiitis (a nonspecific finding) may be found and further biopsies may be needed	
Muscle biopsy—a low morbidity procedure that is positive for small- to medium-vessel arteritis in 40 to 50% of cases. The yield is higher when there is clinical evidence for muscle disease (elevated CPK, weakness, EMG findings), but "blind" biopsies are appropriate	
Sural nerve biopsy—should be performed if neuropathic signs or symptoms occur	
Renal biopsy—will usually reveal focal necrotizing glomerulonephritis, less commonly arteritis; the nondiagnostic nephritis in the setting of an abnormal urinary sediment and proteinuria and the clinical presentation support the diagnosis of polyarteritis	
Arteriography—most appropriately done when involved organs are not available for biopsy, in the absence of a positive biopsy if the diagnosis is still being strongly considered, and in cases with evidence of intra-abdominal involvement; fusiform or saccular arterial aneurysms can be demonstrated in 60% of patients when the celiac axis, mesenteric, renal, and hepatic circulations are studied	
Nerve conduction studies and electromyography—helpful in diagnosing mononeuritis multiplex	
Tissue biopsy—the definitive diagnosis is based upon demonstrating the typical granulomatous necrotizing vasculitis	Wegener's granulomatosis
Nasal mucosal or sinus tissue biopsy—in those patients with obvious involvement of the upper respiratory tract, biopsy of these areas offers the best and simplest opportunity to secure a histologic diagnosis	
Lung biopsy (generally an open biopsy)—the diagnostic modality in the majority of cases, especially when the above biopsies or skin biopsies are negative or not available	
Renal biopsy—will rarely be distinctive enough to be definitive	
Tissue biopsy—temporal artery biopsy on the symptomatic side of the head is mandatory when the diagnosis of temporal arteritis is made on clinical grounds; empiric high-dose steroid therapy without an attempt to make a histologic diagnosis is *not* appropriate; steroid therapy can be instituted as late as 2 weeks prior to biopsy without masking the presence of arteritis; in patients with classic polymyalgia rheumatica without signs or symptoms of temporal arteritis, temporal artery biopsy is *not* mandatory	Giant cell arteritis/polymyalgia rheumatica
Erythrocyte sedimentation rate (ESR)—although a nonspecific test, in these disorders the clinical diagnoses are based upon characteristic visual, headache, or musculoskeletal complaints in the setting of a markedly elevated (>50 mm/hour Westergren) ESR	
Angiography—diagnosis depends on a compatible clinical picture corroborated by angiographic demonstration of multiple stenoses or occlusions of the aorta and its major branches	Takayasu's arteritis
Tissue biopsy—because of the location of the lesions, biopsy is rarely feasible	

to joint or periarticular injury (that is, noxious insults to the joint).

Two general categories of joint disease include those diseases in which joint inflammation is one of the dominant manifestations, and the noninflammatory disorders in which an inflammatory component is present only intermittently or not at all. These broad categories represent the primary nature of the diseases listed in Table 13–1.

Inflammatory Joint Disorders

These are diseases that lead to inflammatory changes predominantly in the synovial membrane, with secondary changes in other joint and periarticular tissues. Joint pain arises through the development of synovial membrane swelling or the accumulation of large volumes of synovial fluid with secondary involvement of the pain-sensitive joint capsule and ligaments. Aside from well-defined infections or reactive arthritides, the origin of the majority of the disorders in this category is unknown.

Many of the disease entities in this category can present with joint pain alone (arthralgia) or with joint pain associated with signs of inflammation (arthritis), such as joint swelling, tenderness, warmth, and limited range of motion. Although the joint disorder may be the focus in these diseases, many of these diseases are multisystemic, presenting with associated features such as fever, weight loss, weakness, and other symptoms relating to the pathologic process in the involved organs.

The reason for the varied location and pattern of joint involvement in different diseases is unknown, but the physician commonly employs such clinical information in the diagnosis of rheumatologic disorders (Table 13–3).

RHEUMATOID ARTHRITIS

This is a systemic disease that is characterized by a female to male predominance of 3:1, a symmetrical inflammatory polyarthropathy with morning stiffness, and rheumatoid factor positivity in 80% of patients.

Rheumatoid factors (RF) are autoantibodies (of the IgM, IgG, or IgA classes) directed against antigenic determinants on the Fc fragment of an IgG molecule. IgM rheumatoid factors are efficient agglutinators of antigen (IgG)–coated particles (latex beads in the latex fixation test; bentonite particles or sheep red blood cells in other assays), and thus it is this immunoglobulin class of rheumatoid factors that is characterized when a rheumatoid factor test is positive. Rheumatoid factors, especially IgG-RF present in synovial fluid, contribute to the pathogenesis of diseases such as rheumatoid arthritis.

Rheumatoid factors are not specific for rheumatoid arthritis. They are found in a variable proportion of patients with acute and chronic inflammatory disorders, and in some normal individuals (especially elderly individuals).

The rheumatic diseases commonly associated with rheumatoid factor are rheumatoid arthritis (80%), systemic lupus erythematosus (20%), scleroderma (20%), mixed connective tissue disease (25%), polymyositis/dermatomyositis (20%), Sjögren's syndrome (90%), vasculitides such as polyarteritis nodosa, and Wegener's granulomatosis. Acute viral infections with RF are hepatitis B (25%), influenza, and mononucleosis. Chronic inflammatory or infectious disorders include tuberculosis (15%), leprosy (25%), yaws, syphilis (10%), subacute bacterial endocarditis (40%), brucellosis, salmonellosis, sarcoidosis (10%), chronic liver disease (25%), cryoglobulinemia (90%), hyperglobulinemic purpura, and chronic pulmonary disorders. Parasitic infections associated with RF include trypanosomiasis, kala-azar, malaria, schistosomiasis, and filariasis. Neoplasms associated with RF can occur after irradiation or chemotherapy for neoplasms.

In most but not all nonrheumatic conditions, titers of rheumatoid factor are lower than in rheumatoid arthritis. Thus, the specificity of the RF for rheumatoid arthritis increases with serum titer. Titers below 1:160 are considered nonspecific yet may reflect rheumatoid arthritis. (Hence, rheumatoid arthritis can be diagnosed clinically in the *absence* of a positive RF.) It is possible that seropositive arthritis and seronegative rheumatoid arthritis are actually different diseases with overlapping clinical manifestations. Some physicians feel that the seronegative disease is milder than the seropositive.

Once the test is found to be positive, there is no need to repeat it. Although certain drugs (e.g., gold, cyclophosphamide) can lead to a decrease in the RF titer as the disease is controlled, the physician does not use the rheumatoid factor test as a measure of disease activity.

Rheumatoid factor (IgM) may be found in the synovial fluid of patients with rheumatoid arthritis prior to RF's detection in the serum. Such analysis is not routine but can be employed in difficult-to-diagnose joint disorders.

The majority of patients with rheumatoid arthritis manifest a chronic course, and 15% of this group develop a severe progressive crippling arthritis. All joints of the upper and lower extremities can be involved, with characteristic erosive disease in the small joints of the hands and feet. Extra-articular disease manifestations include subcutaneous nodules, pleurisy and pericarditis, neuropathy, vasculitis, and Felty's

Table 13–8. Laboratory Diagnostic Tests in Rheumatic Diseases

Test	RA	JRA	SLE	MCTD	PSS	PAN	DM/PM	WG	PMR/TA	SS	AS	PA	RS	CA	SAR
↑ESR, ↑CRP	++	++	++	+	±	++	+	++	++	+	+	+	+	+	+
Anemia	+	+	+	+	+	+	+	+	+	+	+	+	+	+	+
Chronic disease	+	+	+	+	+	+	+	+	+	+	+	+	+	+	+
Hemolytic	−	−	+	±	±	−	−	+	−	−	−	−	−	−	−
Leukocytosis	±	+	−	−	±	++	−	+	+	−	±	±	±	±	±
Leukopenia	±	−	+	+	−	−	−	−	−	−	−	−	−	−	−
Thrombocytosis	+	+	−	−	−	++	−	++	+	−	±	±	−	−	±
Thrombocytopenia	±	−	+	±	−	−	−	−	−	−	−	−	−	−	−
Circulating anticoagulant	±	−	+	−	−	−	−	−	±	−	−	−	−	−	−
Cryoglobulinemia	±	±	±	−	−	±	−	−	−	±	±	−	−	±	±
↑Cr + BUN	−	−	++	±	+	++	−	++	−	±	−	−	−	−	−
Nephritic/Nephrotic urine	−	−	++	±	±	++	−	++	−		−	−	−	−	−
↑CPK, ↑SGOT, ↑aldolase	±	−	+	+	+	++	++	+	−	±	−	−	−	−	−
Inflammatory synovial fluid	++	++	+	+	+	+	+	+	+	+	+	+	+	+	+
HLA association	DR4	DR5	DR2 DR3	−	−	−	−	−	−	DR3	B27	B27	B27	B27	−
(+) Rheumatoid factor	++	±	+	+	+	+	+	+	−	++	−	−	−	−	+
Antinuclear antibodies															
1) FANA	+	+	++	+	+	+	+	−	−	+	−	−	−	−	−
2) Anti-DNA	−	−	++	+	−	−	−	−	−	±	−	−	−	−	−
3) Anti-Sm	−	−	+	−	−	−	−	−	−	−	−	−	−	−	−
4) Anti-RNP	±	−	+	++	+	−	−	−	−	−	−	−	−	−	−
Serum complement ↓	±	−	++	+	±	+	−	−	−						

RA	Rheumatoid arthritis	AS	Ankylosing spondylitis
JRA	Juvenile rheumatoid arthritis	PA	Psoriatic arthritis
SLE	Systemic lupus erythematosus	RS	Reiter's syndrome
MCTD	Mixed connective tissue disease	CA	Colitic arthropathy
PSS	Progressive systemic sclerosis (scleroderma)	SAR	Sarcoidosis
PAN	Polyarteritis nodosa	G	Gout
DM/PM	Dermatomyositis/polymyositis	PG	Pseudogout
WG	Wegener's granulomatosis	TB	Tuberculosis
PMR/TA	Polymyalgia rheumatica/temporal arteritis	SA	Septic arthritis
SS	Sjögren's syndrome	SBE	Subacute bacterial endocarditis

Table 13–8.   Continued

									Disease									
G	PG	TB	SA	SBE	AM	MR	CP	HPO	PD	RSD	FM	FMF	LD	BD	HEP B	WD	OA	PVNS
+	+	++	++	++	++	+	++	±	−	−	−	+	+	+	+	+	−	−
−	−	+	+	+	+	+	+	±	−	−	−	+	+	+		+	−	−
−	−	+	+	+	+	+	+	±	−	−	−	+	+	+		+	−	−
−	−	+	−	−	−	−	−	−	−	−	−	−	−	−		−	−	−
±	±	+	++	++	−	−	−	−	−	−	−	−	−	±	−	−	−	−
−	−	+	−	−	−	−	±	−	−	−	−	−	−	−	−	−	−	−
−	−	+	−	+	−	−	−	−	−	−	−	−	−	−	−	−	−	−
−	−	−	−	−	±	−	±	−	−	−	−	−	−	−	−	−	−	−
−	−	−	−	−	−	−	−	−	−	−	−	−	−	−	−	−	−	−
−	−	−	−	±	−	−	−	−	−	−	−	−	−	±	±	±	−	−
−	−	−	−	+	±	−	−	−	−	−	−	−	−	−	−	±	−	−
−	−	−	−	+	±	−	−	−	−	−	−	−	−	±	±	−	−	−
−	−	−	−	+	−	−	−	−	−	−	−	−	−	±	−	−	−	−
++	++	++	++	+	−	+	+	−	−	−	−	+	+	+	+	+	−	−
−	−	−	−	−	−	−	−	−	−	−	−	DR2	DR3	B5	−	−	−	−
−	−	+	−	+	−	−	±	−	−	−	−	−	−	−	±	−	−	−
−	−	−	−	−	−	−	−	−	−	−	−	−	−	−	−	−	−	−
−	−	−	−	−	−	−	−	−	−	−	−	−	−	−	−	−	−	−
−	−	−	−	−	−	−	−	−	−	−	−	−	−	−	−	−	−	−
−	−	−	−	−	−	−	−	−	−	−	−	−	−	−	−	−	−	−
−	−	±	+	−	−	−	−	−	−	−	−	−	±	−	−	+	−	−

AM	Amyloidosis	BD	Behçet's disease
MR	Multicentric reticulohistiocytosis	HEP B	Hepatitis B
CP	Carcinomatous polyarthritis	WD	Whipple's disease
HPO	Hypertrophic osteoarthropathy	OA	Osteoarthritis
PD	Paget's disease	PVNS	Pigmented villonodular synovitis
RSD	Reflex sympathetic dystrophy	−	Not present
FM	Fibromyalgia	±	<10%
FMF	Familial Mediterranean fever	+	>10%
LD	Lyme disease	++	>50%

syndrome (rheumatoid arthritis, splenomegaly, granulocytopenia). RA is a classic inflammatory disorder manifested by laboratory features of an inflammatory joint fluid (3–75,000 WBC, mainly polys), an elevated erythrocyte sedimentation rate, and a synovial membrane demonstrating an extensive mononuclear cell infiltrate, nodules, and villous hypertrophy. There is a strong association of the histocompatibility antigen DR4 with rheumatoid arthritis.

JUVENILE RHEUMATOID ARTHRITIS (STILL'S DISEASE)

This group of several different childhood rheumatic disorders is categorized based on the disorders' clinical modes of presentation.

Acute febrile type, or Still's disease, is characterized by a high (104 to 106° F), double quotidian, spiking febrile course, an evanescent salmon colored rash that parallels the fever, lymphadenopathy, hepatosplenomegaly, and polyserositis (pleurisy, pericarditis, or peritoneal inflammation). Although wrist joint fusion can occur, joint inflammation can be mild or absent. In the absence of joint involvement, the patient presents with fever of unknown origin. Laboratory abnormalities include striking leukocytosis, thrombocytosis, elevated sedimentation rate, negative rheumatoid factor, and negative antinuclear antibody.

Polyarticular onset is characterized by progressive, erosive, symmetrical polyarthritis, similar to the adult disease. Systemic features such as rash and splenomegaly are less frequent than in the systemic onset and fever is invariably low grade. A subgroup with polyarticular onset includes teenage girls who have subcutaneous nodules and a positive rheumatoid factor.

Pauciarticular onset (oligoarticular) is the most common presentation (40 to 50%) and is confined to swelling of a single joint, usually a knee, or not more than four joints. Systemic signs are minimal except for chronic iridocyclitis in 20 to 40% of patients. Low titers of antinuclear antibodies are detected most frequently in pauciarticular onset, especially in children with chronic iridocyclitis. A subgroup of this group primarily includes boys nearing their teens who are positive for HLA-B27 tissue antigen but negative for both rheumatoid factor and antinuclear antibody. Most eventually develop ankylosing spondylitis; a few continue to have pauciarticular joint disease only.

SPONDYLOARTHROPATHIES

Features common to all diseases in this group include the presence of spondylitis, sacroiliitis, or both, conjunctivitis and iritis, peripheral joint inflammation (in an asymmetrical pattern with a predominance of large, lower extremity joint involvement), and the histocompatibility antigen HLA-B27 genetic marker. The primary pathologic site is the enthesis (the insertion of ligaments and capsules into bone), where inflammation is followed by fibrosis and ossification.

Ankylosing Spondylitis. The insidious onset of prolonged low-back pain, stiffness, and restricted range of motion in a young patient is the characteristic clinical correlate of the underlying spine and sacroiliac disease. Over one third of patients exhibit peripheral joint involvement, often asymmetrical and more frequently affecting lower-limb joints. Ankylosing spondylitis is a systemic disorder that may lead to anemia, iritis, aortic regurgitation, upper lobe pulmonary fibrosis, and amyloidosis. Characteristic x-ray findings include sacroiliac joint erosion, narrowing, and fusion, and spinal changes such as syndesmophytes, ossification, and ankylosis. Of patients, 90% are HLA-B27 antigen positive.

Psoriatic Arthritis. In the setting of psoriatic skin and nail disease, five broad clinical groups of patients with arthritis have been recognized: Patients in whom distal interphalangeal joints are involved predominantly; patients with a severely deforming, ankylosing, or mutilating type of arthritis; patients with joint disease indistinguishable from rheumatoid arthritis, yet less extensive and more benign and associated with negative rheumatoid factor and no rheumatoid nodules; patients with a single or few joints involved in an asymmetrical fashion; and patients in whom there is spondylitis, sacroiliitis, or both.

Extra-articular diseases, such as conjunctivitis or uveitis, are found in 10% of all patients with arthritis. Typical radiographic features include distal interphalangeal joint involvement with erosions, terminal phalangeal osteolysis giving a pencil-in-cup appearance, asymmetrical nonmarginal syndesmophytes of the spine, and sacroiliitis. Rheumatoid factor is typically negative in all forms of psoriatic arthritis. Of patients with sacroiliitis and spinal involvement, 90% are HLA-B27 positive.

Reiter's Syndrome. In its complete form, Reiter's syndrome presents with an asymmetrical polyarthritis involving predominantly large, lower extremity joints, with conjunctivitis, and with urethritis; a limited form of this syndrome may present with arthritis alone or with only two parts of the classic triad. The complete syndrome may occur in the setting of dysentery, in which enteric organisms (Shigella flexneri, salmonella species, Yersinia enterocolitica, and Campylobacter fetus) lead to a reactive arthritis. Though the disorder can occur just once, a chronic, destructive arthritis can ensue. Uveitis, sacroiliitis, and spondylitis can coexist with sausage shaped digits and the psoriasiform skin lesions of circinate balanitis and keratoderma blennorrhagicum. HLA-B27 antigen is found in as many as 60% of patients, and the disease is typically rheumatoid factor negative.

Enteropathic Arthritis. The common feature in this group of disorders is the association of an abnormality of the gastrointestinal tract (infectious, toxic, inflammatory, or structural) with the development of musculoskeletal disorders such as arthritis, tenosynovitis, spondylitis, and sacroiliitis. The pathogenesis of all of these disorders may involve immune complexes arising from gut mucosa, bacterial antigens, or both.

Arthropathy Associated with Inflammatory Bowel Disease. Peripheral joint arthritis occurs in patients with both Crohn's disease (20%) and ulcerative colitis (10%). Arthritis is more common in patients with extraintestinal manifestations such as erythema nodosum and uveitis, and, at least in ulcerative colitis, flare-ups have a close association with exacerbations of the colitis. Both ankylosing spondylitis (4%) and sacroiliitis (10%) are seen in these patients. In some patients the bowel and spine diseases run separate and autonomous courses; in others the spondylitis is a response to disease in the gut. HLA-B27 is found frequently in patients with inflammatory bowel disease and spondylitis (ulcerative colitis 73%; Crohn's disease 55%) and even more frequently in ankylosing spondylitis alone.

Arthritis with Intestinal Bypass. Over a third of patients undergoing jejunoileostomy for treatment of morbid obesity develop articular symptoms ranging from arthralgia to frank arthritis and tenosynovitis. The joint disease, skin rash, and Raynaud's phenomenon associated with this disorder are probably related to immune complexes containing absorbed intestinal bacterial antigens. A similar type of arthritis has been reported in antibiotic-induced pseudomembranous colitis.

Reactive Arthritis Following Enteric Infections. The term reactive arthritis describes an arthritis caused by an immunologic reaction to a microorganism infecting another organ rather than arthritis caused by direct infection. Whereas the model for such a disease process is rheumatic fever caused by group A streptococcus, four enteric pathogens, Shigella flexneri, salmonella species, Yersinia enterocolitica, and Campylobacter fetus, can also cause a reactive arthritis. These arthritides are associated significantly (60 to 80%) with HLA-B27 antigen. Although patients with enteropathic reactive arthritis frequently develop urethritis, ocular inflammation, or mucocutaneous lesions typical of Reiter's syndrome, the majority manifest only arthritis. The arthritis usually begins 2 to 4 weeks after the enteric infection and persists for 1 to 3 months as a monarthritis, oligoarthritis (less than four joints), or symmetrical polyarthritis. Sacroiliitis or low-back pain can occur during the acute illness.

True septic arthritis can exist (or coexist with reactive arthritis) with Salmonella and Yersinia infections.

Whipple's Disease. This is a systemic, infective process manifested by arthralgia or arthritis and the basic Whipple triad of malabsorption, diarrhea, and weight loss. Joint involvement may precede other disease features by more than 10 years. The characteristic pattern is that of a migratory poly- or oligoarthritis that, along with such nonarticular features as serositis, central nervous system disease, and hepatosplenomegaly, may produce many years of repeated inflammatory episodes. Sacroiliitis alone and ankylosing spondylitis have an association with Whipple's disease approaching that of inflammatory bowel disease. The definitive diagnosis is based upon the finding of PAS-positive inclusions in the macrophages of the jejunum representing bacterial cells. Such microorganisms have been seen in synovial membrane macrophages.

DIFFUSE CONNECTIVE TISSUE DISORDERS

These multisystem disorders of uncertain origin share a number of features. These features include overlapping clinical and laboratory features such as arthritis, serositis. Raynaud's phenomenon, skin rash and antinuclear antibodies, rheumatoid factors, and anemia. Another common feature is immune alterations that correlate with organ injury as a primary or secondary mechanism as indicated by the presence of circulating and tissue-localized immunoglobulins, immune complexes, and complement components. Also, blood vessels are an important target organ in these disorders. Vascular alterations may affect arteries, capillaries, or veins of any size, including a spectrum of changes from noninflammatory intimal responses to acute necrotizing lesions. Finally, similarities in age, sex, and race patterns of these diseases reflect host and genetic predisposition.

Systemic Lupus Erythematosus (SLE), Drug-Induced Lupus, and Overlap Syndromes. As a multisystem disease, SLE predominates in young women and is manifested by nonerosive, symmetrical small and large joint arthritis, fever, skin rash, serositis, nephritis, hematologic disorders (hemolytic anemia, thrombocytopenia, leukopenia), and neurologic disease (seizures, psychosis, central and peripheral nervous system disease). Characteristic laboratory abnormalities include the presence of antibodies to nuclear and cytoplasmic antigens (Tables 13-3, 13-4, and 13-5), complement disorders, a false positive test for syphilis, and circulating anticoagulants.

Many drugs have been implicated in the induction of a lupus-like syndrome with manifestations ranging from an isolated positive antinuclear antibody test to a full clinical lupus syndrome. Hydralazine and procainamide are the most common drugs producing this syndrome. Whereas arthritis, skin rash, serositis, and pulmonary disease are common, central nervous system and renal disease are rarely seen.

Patients with features of more than one rheumatic disease do not fit into traditional classifications and are said to have an overlap syndrome. One of these, the mixed connective tissue disease (MCTD), includes features of systemic lupus erythematosus, scleroderma, and polymyositis in the setting of unusually high titers of a circulating antinuclear antibody with specificity for a nuclear ribonuclear (RNP) antigen (giving a speckled antinuclear antibody test). Features include polyarthralgias and arthritis that can be erosive and deforming (RA-like), Raynaud's phenomenon, puffy hands (sclerodactyly), esophageal dysfunction, myositis, and only rarely renal disease. Some consider this disorder a phase of either systemic lupus or scleroderma.

Scleroderma (Systemic Sclerosis). This is a multisystem disorder of unknown origin characterized by fibrosis and vascular changes in many organs. Although the definitive diagnostic criterion is hidebound fibrosis of skin, the eventual clinical outcome is based on the extent of the vascular involvement of crucial viscera. Clinical characteristics include the classic skin changes (in 95% of patients) from an initial puffy phase to a tight, hidebound phase that limits mobility; a self-limited, nonerosive, symmetrical polyarthritis suggestive of rheumatoid arthritis (10% of patients), Raynaud's phenomenon (90% of patients), esophageal and small-bowel hypomotility (90% of patients); pulmonary fibrosis, hypertension, or both; myopathy; cardiac disease; and renal involvement. The clinical course is extremely variable, ranging from slow progression over 15 years to a rapid clinical deterioration from renal failure, malignant hypertension, or cardiac arrhythmias.

Polymyositis/Dermatomyositis. Polymyositis is an inflammatory disease of striated skeletal muscle. A characteristic skin rash is present in 40% of patients; thus the term dermatomyositis. Both diseases present with symmetrical proximal muscle weakness, elevation of muscle enzymes (CPK, aldolase, SGOT, LDH), an abnormal electromyographic test, and an abnormal muscle biopsy demonstrating inflammation and muscle necrosis. Arthralgia, Raynaud's phenomenon, dysphagia, and pulmonary fibrosis are seen in both disorders. An associated malignancy commonly found in elderly patients with dermatomyositis can be seen in polymyositis as well.

Necrotizing Vasculitis. This term describes multisystem diseases characterized by inflammatory reactions in blood vessels resulting in destruction or necrosis of vessel walls. The differing clinical presentations of these disorders depend on the nature and magnitude of the underlying insult and the size and distribution of affected blood vessels.

Polyarteritis Nodosa. This inflammatory disorder of medium and small muscular arteries presents as an acute or subacute febrile illness with clinical involvement of one or more organ systems including diffuse arthralgias or asymmetrical polyarthritis (in up to 70% of patients), mononeuritis multiplex, intestinal infarction, nodular, purpuric, or ischemic skin lesions, and renal involvement including necrotizing glomerulitis. The diagnosis is supported by the clinical presentation and the presence of an abnormal biopsy of clinically involved tissue (e.g., muscle or skin) or the angiographic demonstration of aneurysms in involved viscera (e.g., kidney, or GI tract). Symptoms related to organ ischemia, rather than joint complaints, are the focus in this disease.

Eosinophilic Granulomatous Vasculitis (Churg-Strauss Vasculitis). This systemic vasculitis is characterized by the combination of asthma, eosinophilia, necrotizing vasculitis of small arteries and veins, and extravascular granulomas. Diagnostically helpful features are noncavitary lung infiltrates, nodular skin lesions, heart failure, and eosinophilia (50% of the white blood count). Arthralgias and arthritis are uncommon. The diagnosis is based on clinical and pathologic features.

Wegener's Granulomatosis. This disease is characterized by necrotizing granulomatous vasculitis of the upper and lower respiratory tract, glomerulonephritis, and generalized focal necrotizing vasculitis involving small arteries and veins in the lungs and organs. Limited forms involving only the respiratory tract have been described. Joint pains and, less commonly, synovitis occur in up to 50% of the cases.

The dominant clinical presentation, however, is referable to the respiratory tract (sinusitis, rhinitis, nasal ulceration, hemoptysis, and cough) and the kidney (proteinuria, red blood cell casts, renal insufficiency). The diagnosis is based upon the clinical features and the histopathologic demonstration of necrotizing granulomas with vasculitis in involved organs (e.g., sinuses, pulmonary infiltrates, or cavities).

Takayasu's Arteritis. This granulomatous vasculitis of unknown cause predominates in young women and manifests as inflammation of the aorta and its major branches, with varying degrees of secondary stenosis or occlusion. The clinical presentation varies from an early prepulseless systemic phase characterized by fatigue, weight loss, fever, and arthralgias and arthritis (in 50% of patients) to a later, pulseless, ischemic phase manifested by absence of peripheral pulse, claudication, or renovascular hypertension. The diagnosis is based on a compatible clinical picture corroborated by the angiographic demonstration of multiple stenoses or occlusions of the aorta or its major branches and/or characteristic vascular disorder on biopsy.

Giant Cell Arteritis (GCA) and Polymyalgia Rheumatica (PMR). Polymyalgia rheumatica is a clinical syndrome of elderly patients (most of whom present after their fiftieth year) characterized by chronic, symmetrical aching and morning stiffness in the shoulder, pelvic girdles, and neck, synovitis of peripheral joints, systemic features such as fever, anemia, weight loss, and fatigue, and an elevated sedimentation rate (usually in excess of 50 mm/hour Westergren, perhaps exceeding 100 mm/hour).

Giant cell arteritis, also known as temporal or cranial arteritis, is a vascular syndrome of elderly patients (peak incidence is from 60 to 80 years of age) that involves giant cell vasculitis of predominantly cranial arteries. With systemic features such as fever, fatigue, and weight loss and a marked elevation of the erythrocyte sedimentation rate (usually between 50 and 100 mm/hour, commonly greater than 100 mm/hour), patients present with symptoms and signs related to involvement of the internal and external carotid branches. These include headache (classically temporal) and physical changes of temporal artery tenderness, beading, and pulselessness, jaw claudication, temporomandibular joint pain, and ocular damage. Visual loss (varying from unilateral to bilateral, incomplete to complete) occurs in up to 50% of patients and is caused by vasculitic involvement of the ophthalmic artery and its posterior ciliary branches. Vasculitis can involve other large arteries including the aorta and its branches.

In view of the fact that as many as 50% of patients with polymyalgia rheumatica have had giant cell arteritis and 60% of patients with giant cell arteritis have had PMR, some physicians consider that these diseases represent different parts of a single disorder. The diagnosis of both is based upon the clinical presentation and, especially in the case of GCA, the temporal artery biopsy.

Cutaneous Necrotizing Vasculitis. The clinical hallmark of this group of disorders is cutaneous vasculitis, with variable amounts of systemic disease. The characteristic cutaneous lesion is that of palpable purpura. The typical histopathologic appearance of skin or visceral lesions consists of infiltration of a postcapillary venule by polymorphonuclear leukocytes, with leukocytoclasis and fragmentation of nuclei ("nuclear dust"). This appearance has led to the term "leukocytoclastic vasculitis," which may be a primary disorder (primary cutaneous vasculitis) or may be associated with a number of other disease processes.

The diagnosis of primary cutaneous vasculitis depends on recognizing the typical recurrent episodes of palpable purpura or other skin lesions (papular, urticarial, or infarctive) occurring in dependent areas. Arthralgias are present in the majority of patients; synovitis is less common. While the predominant manifestation is cutaneous, other organs may be involved, including the kidney, GI tract, and central or peripheral nervous system.

Henoch-Schönlein purpura refers to a syndrome occurring predominantly in children and young adults and characterized by arthralgias or mild arthritis (primarily in the ankles and knees), abdominal pain, gastrointestinal hemorrhage, nephritis, and nonthrombocytopenic (palpable) purpura. Leukocytoclastic vasculitis is found in all organs. IgA is the predominant immunoglobulin found in skin and renal tissue.

Essential mixed cryoglobulinemia consists of palpable purpura, arthralgias, weakness, glomerulonephritis, hepatosplenomegaly, and lymphadenopathy. Mixed cryoglobulins (containing IgM rheumatoid factor and its antigen [IgG]) are present in small amounts and are associated with a positive rheumatoid factor and low levels of serum complement.

The hallmark of hypocomplementemic vasculitis, a disease of young adults, is recurring episodes of an urticarial skin eruption associated with fever, symmetrical small joint synovitis, abdominal pain, and glomerulonephritis. The diagnosis is supported by the clinical picture, the typical leukocytoclastic vasculitis picture on biopsy of the urticarial lesion, and the presence of hypocomplementemia without rheumatoid factor or antinuclear antibodies.

Cutaneous necrotizing vasculitis is also associated with other disorders, including systemic lupus erythematosus, rheumatoid arthritis, Sjögren's syndrome, hematologic malignancies (especially Hodgkin's disease and non-Hodgkin's lymphoma), infectious endocarditis, and drug hypersensitivity reactions.

Behçet's Disease. This is a systemic vasculitic disorder manifested by recurrent aphthous stomatitis, genital aphthous ulcers, uveitis, arthralgias or nondestructive, subacute, or chronic synovitis most commonly affecting knees and ankles, cutaneous vasculitis in the form of pustules, papules, or erythema nodosum-like lesions, and meningoencephalitis. Rarely, sacroiliitis has been noted, and then only in HLA-B27 patients. An HLA-B5 association has been demonstrated in the populations most commonly presenting with this disorder, those of the eastern Mediterranean and Japan.

Erythema Nodosum. This refers to crops of discrete, tender subcutaneous nodules that are erythematous and

Table 13—9.   Diseases Associated with Erythema Nodosum

Infections
  Beta-hemolytic streptococci
  Tuberculosis
  Deep fungal
    Coccidioidomycosis
    Histoplasmosis
    North American blastomycosis
  Lymphogranuloma venereum
  Psittacosis
  Yersinosis
  Lepromatous leprosy
Unknown cause
  Sarcoidosis
  Inflammatory bowel disease
    Regional enteritis
    Ulcerative colitis
  Behçet's disease
Drugs
  Sulfonamides
  Bromides
  Iodines
  Oral contraceptives

Table 13—10.   Classification of Hyperuricemia and Gout

Primary
  Molecular defects undefined
    Underexcretion (90% of primary gout)
    Overproduction (10% of primary gout)
  Associated with specific enzyme defects
    PP-ribose—P synthetase variants— ↑ activity
    Hypoxanthine—guanine phosphoribosyl—transferase deficiency (HGPRT)—partial deficiency (X-linked)
Secondary
  Overproduction of uric acid
    Associated with increased nucleic acid turnover
      Myeloproliferative disorders
      Lymphoma/lymphoproliferative disorders
      Hemoglobinopathies
      Hemolytic anemia
      Psoriasis
      Cancer chemotherapy
      Multiple myeloma
    Associated with specific enzyme defects
      Virtually complete absence of hypoxanthine—guanine phosphoribosyl—transferase—Lesch-Nyhan syndrome (X-linked).
  Underexcretion of uric acid
    Chronic renal failure
    Drugs (diuretics such as thiazides, furosemide, ethacrynic acid; ethambutol, low-dose [<2 g/day] aspirin, pyrazinamide, nicotinic acid, ethanol)
    Lead nephropathy (saturnine gout)
    Lactic acidosis (alcoholism, pre-eclampsia)
    Ketosis (diabetic, starvation)
    Hyperparathyroidism
    Hypertension
  Overproduction and underexcretion
    Glucose-6-phosphatase deficiency or absence (von Gierke's disease, glycogen storage disease type I, autosomal recessive)
  Mechanism unknown
    Sarcoidosis
    Obesity
    Hypoparathyroidism
    Paget's disease
    Down's syndrome

are characteristically located on the shins and ankles. It is thought to be a hypersensitivity reaction to a variety of systemic antigens or diseases and represents an inflammatory disorder of the subcutaneous tissue. Systemic features that can exist include fever, arthralgias, and a picture of periarthritis, especially around the ankles when nodules appear around joints. The presence of this disorder should stimulate a search for an underlying disease process (Table 13–9).

Lobular Panniculitis and Arthritis Associated with Pancreatic Disease. Pancreatitis (acute and chronic) and pancreatic carcinoma have been associated with painful subcutaneous, erythematous nodules and acutely painful asymmetrical arthritis of small and large joints caused by fat necrosis by disseminated pancreatic enzymes. Intramedullary fat necrosis may present as bone pain or cause osteolysis seen on x-ray examinations.

Polychondritis. This is an episodic systemic disorder characterized by recurrent widespread destructive inflammatory lesions involving cartilaginous structures, the cardiovascular system, and organs of sensation such as the eyes and ears. Characteristic clinical manifestations include bilateral auricular chondritis, nonerosive, seronegative inflammatory polyarthritis of peripheral small and large joints and costochondral-manubriosternal articulations, nasal chondritis, ocular inflammation, respiratory tract chondritis, and cochlear and/or vestibular dysfunction. Polychondritis has a significant coexistence with connective tissue diseases such as rheumatoid arthritis and systemic lupus. The diagnosis is based on the clinical

presentation and confirmation by cartilage biopsy of a compatible histologic picture.

CRYSTAL-INDUCED SYNOVITIS

Gout. Gout is a systemic metabolic disease characterized by hyperuricemia, acute or chronic arthritis, and deposition of monosodium urate tophi (Table 13–10). If not controlled, it can lead to chronic destructive arthritis, massive tophaceous deposits, uric acid kidney stones, and renal failure. Joint involvement can take the form of acute self-limited synovitis of a single joint (the first metatarsophalangeal joint being the most common initial site), polyarticular synovitis in 10% of cases, and chronic gouty arthritis mimicking rheumatoid arthritis. The sole diagnostic test for gouty arthritis is the finding of monosodium urate crystals (needle shaped, negatively birefringent) within synovial fluid polymorphonuclear leukocytes.

Elevated serum uric acid, tophus, or kidney stone analyses are supportive diagnostic tests.

Calcium Pyrophosphate Dihydrate (CPPD) Deposition Disease (Pseudogout). Patients with CPPD crystals may present with a variety of clinical syndromes: acute arthritis in one to three joints; chronic polyarticular inflammation of the knees, wrists, and metacarpophalangeal joints mimicking rheumatoid arthritis; destructive arthritis reminiscent of a Charcot's joint; and a coexistence of CPPD crystals with typical osteoarthritis. While a specific diagnosis is made by the demonstration of rhomboid, weakly positively birefringent CPPD crystals within synovial fluid polymorphonuclear leukocytes, CPPD deposition is strongly suggested by linear or stippled calcifications in articular cartilage or menisci.

Apatite Deposition Disease. Apatite, the calcium salt in bone, can be associated with acute self-limited synovitis in one or more joints (including fingers, shoulders, and metatarsophalangeal joints), periarticular inflammation, calcific tendinitis, and polyarthritis with multiple erosions mimicking rheumatoid arthritis. A destructive shoulder arthritis has been seen in dialysis patients and in patients with ruptured rotator cuffs (Milwaukee shoulder). Diagnosis can be made through the presence in synovial fluid of coinlike or irregular clumps of apatite crystals inside or outside of polymorphonuclear leukocytes and by the finding of punctate and periarticular calcification on x-ray.

ARTHRITIS ASSOCIATED WITH INFECTIOUS DISEASES

Rheumatic Fever. This systemic disease is a sequela of group A beta-hemolytic streptococcal pharyngitis and is thought to result from an unusual immunologic reaction of the host (i.e., reactive arthritis) to streptococcal antigens. In the setting of a prior streptococcal infection (determined by throat culture or rising titers of antistreptolysin O [ASLO] antibodies), two or more of the following major manifestations indicate a high probability of acute rheumatic fever: carditis (valvular disease, pericarditis, myocarditis), erythema marginatum, subcutaneous nodules, and arthritis. A migratory polyarthritis of two or more large joints (knees, ankles, elbows, and wrists) in an acute febrile illness is a typical presentation. Polyarthralgias or arthritis can be the only major manifestation in the adult. Minor manifestations include fever, arthralgia, an elevated erythrocyte sedimentation rate or positive reactive protein, a prolonged PR interval, and previous rheumatic fever or rheumatic heart disease.

Septic Arthritis Caused by Bacteria. Compared with many of the previously mentioned noninfectious, inflammatory arthropathies, acute bacterial arthritis is a true medical emergency that requires early recog-

Table 13–11. Causes of Acute Nongonococcal Septic Arthritis

	Adults	Children
Staphylococcus aureus	35%	45%
Streptococcus pyrogenes } Streptococcus pneumoniae	10%	25%
Gram-negative bacilli (E. coli, salmonella, pseudomonas)	5%	15%
Hemophilus influenzae	1%	10%

nition and aggressive treatment. The typical clinical presentation is that of a severe, monarticular synovitis with an inflammatory synovial fluid (>50,000 WBCs) in the setting of a febrile illness and an elevated white blood cell count and elevated sedimentation rate. In gonococcal arthritis polyarticular presentation is common, however, and may *not* be associated with significant fever or elevation of the peripheral synovial fluid leukocyte count. While virtually any organism can produce septic arthritis, several organisms appear to be more common than others. Neisseria gonorrhoea is responsible for an overwhelming proportion of all cases of septic arthritis, especially in younger healthy hosts (in adults, 50% of all acute infectious arthritis; in children, 5%).

Gonococcal arthritis differs from septic arthritis caused by gram-positive and gram-negative organisms in that polyarthritis and monarthritis occur in roughly equal proportions; pustulovesicular skin lesions occur in 40% of cases; tenosynovitis occurs in more than half of cases; synovial fluids show less than 50% growth of the organism, whereas positive cultures are found in the urethra (81%), blood (24%), rectum (13%), and pharynx (17%). In the appropriate clinical setting a positive culture from any site may be considered as confirming the diagnosis. Various organisms can be responsible for acute nongonococcal septic arthritis (Table 13–11). The diagnosis is based on the clinical impression of joint sepsis and an obvious septic source and, most importantly, on the results of synovial fluid Gram's stain and culture. Certain infectious agents can cause a disorder manifested by both septic arthritis and skin rash (i.e., hemophilus, gonococcus, meningococcus).

Septic Bursitis. Acute Staphylococcus aureus olecranon and prepatellar bursal infections usually present with joint pain and inflammation localized to the tip of the elbow and anterior part of the knee, respectively. Diagnosis is based on Gram's stain and culture of bursal fluid.

Osteomyelitis. Although in adults the spine is the most common site of bone infection, juxta-articular (metaphyseal femur or tibia) bone can become infected through hematogenous or local spread and can present as bone or joint pain and swelling with fever and chills. Osteomyelitis can spread from bone to a contiguous joint and present as joint sepsis. Although Staphylococcus aureus is the most common pathogen, gram-negative bacillary infections are becoming more frequent. Drug addicts are particularly prone to Pseudomonas aeruginosa bone infection, and sickle cell patients to Salmonella organisms. The diagnosis is based on the clinical presentation and on cultures of blood and bone aspirate or biopsied material.

Septic Arthritis Caused by Mycobacteria. While Mycobacterium tuberculosis can involve any bone, joint, bursa, or tendon (1.3% incidence of skeletal involvement), infection of the vertebrae (thoracolumbar-cervical spine) and weight-bearing joints (hip, knee, ankle) predominates. Synovitis is usually chronic and monarticular and can lead to osteomyelitis in contiguous long bone; conversely, tuberculous osteomyelitis can lead to a septic joint. Although rare, atypical mycobacteria can lead to similar joint and bone infections as well as to periarticular disease. The diagnosis is based on bacteriologic evidence (synovial fluid is acid fast–stain positive in 20%, culture positive in 80%; synovial tissue culture is positive in 90%) and histopathologic evidence (granulomas with or without caseation).

Septic Arthritis Caused by Fungal Infection. Fungal arthritis usually presents as a chronic monarticular disease but might occur as an acute polyarthritis. Osteomyelitis is the most common type of mycotic skeletal disease, and septic joints may arise by direct extension from such bony foci. The only reliable method of definitive diagnosis is culture of involved tissue.

Viral Arthritis. The most common viral infections associated with arthalgias or arthritis include hepatitis B, rubella, the live attenuated rubella vaccine, and mosquito-borne arboviruses. Typical clinical facts supporting a viral causation include a nonspecific prodrome, a rash, a disease of short duration, and the specific presentations of hepatitis B, rubella, arboviruses, and other viruses.

Hepatitis B arthritis, a presumed immune complex disorder, occurs in the preicteric phase of 30% of patients with hepatitis B infection and presents with a symmetrical or asymmetrical polyarthritis, tendinitis, or bursitis of a few weeks' duration. Half of the patients have a concomitant pruritic, urticarial, or petechial rash. Most important diagnostically is a positive test for HBsAg. The association of hepatitis B infection with the development of polyarteritis nodosa and mixed cryoglobulinemia is noteworthy.

Rubella arthritis, a disorder primarily of adult women, presents with a self-limited, symmetrical stiffness and pain in the fingers, wrists, and knees. The typical morbilliform rash and posterior cervical lymphadenopathy may occur in the company of tenosynovitis and carpal tunnel syndrome. Arthritis like that in the natural infection occurs in 5% of patients within 4 weeks after vaccination with a live, attenuated rubella vaccine. Although most episodes last for less than 1 month, some patients have recurrent attacks in the knees for as long as 3 years.

Joint symptoms with rash are predominant in illnesses caused by mosquito-borne arboviruses; diseases include epidemic polyarthritis of Australia, dengue fever, chikungunya, and Onyong-Nyong.

A low incidence of joint disease is associated with the following viruses: mumps, smallpox, adenovirus type 7, varicella, infectious mononucleosis (Epstein-Barr virus), and echovirus type 6. Viral arthritis is diagnosed clinically and supported by appropriate cultures and serologic testing.

Arthritis Associated with Spirochetal Infection. Lyme disease is a systemic illness that may have dermatologic, neurologic, rheumatologic, and cardiac manifestations. It is caused by the Treponema-like spirochete Borrelia burgdorferi, which is transmitted to humans by the tick Ixodes dammini. Since Steere and associates' original description of the disease in residents of Lyme, Connecticut and the nearby area, Lyme disease has been recognized nationwide. The disease is endemic to Minnesota and Wisconsin, as well as the coastal northeastern and western U.S.

Typically, the course of Lyme disease has three stages, during each of which remissions and different clinical manifestations occur. Stage 1 is characterized by the presence of a circular red rash with central clearing called erythema chronicum migrans and by nonspecific constitutional symptoms including fever, malaise, headache, and fatigue that occur days to weeks after exposure to ticks. During stage 2, which occurs weeks to months after stage 1, cardiac (atrioventricular block, myopericarditis, left ventricular dysfunction) and neurologic (meningitis, encephalitis, chorea, cranial neuritis including facial palsy, motor and sensory radiculoneuritis, mononeuritis multiplex, myelitis, or combinations of these) abnormalities develop. Stage 3, typified by arthritis, occurs in about 60% of cases and may appear weeks to years after the erythema chronicum migrans.

The typical pattern is migratory arthralgia, usually without joint swelling in the early phase. Arthritis does not generally occur until months later. The initial pattern of involvement is pauciarticular, affecting only one or two joints, usually the knee or other large joints. Affected joints are more swollen than painful. Rarely, the small joints of the hands and feet are involved and the pattern of involvement is symmetrical or polyarticular. Synovial fluid white cell counts vary from 500 to 100,000 cells/mm³, averaging 25,000 cells/mm³, most of which are polymorphonuclear leukocytes. In 5 to 10% of patients with arthritis, involvement in large joints becomes chronic, with erosion of cartilage and bone. Synovial biopsies reveal surface fibrin deposits, villous hypertrophy, vascular proliferation, and marked infiltration of mononuclear and plasma cells. Determination of antibody titers against the I. dammini spirochete is the most useful diagnostic test in the appropriate clinical setting. Specific IgM antibody titers usually peak between the third and sixth week after disease onset. Specific IgG antibody titers rise more slowly and are usually highest months after onset, when arthritis is present. A titer of $\geq$ 1:256 is considered diagnostic if accompanied by the clinical pattern noted above. Of great importance is the fact that this disorder in many cases has been found to be responsive to penicillin or tetracycline therapy.

Arthritis and periostitis can occur in primary and secondary syphilis. In late syphilis, granulomatous gumma may involve synovium, bone, or cartilage and may present with large joint inflammation. Neuropathic (Charcot's) arthropathy can be associated with the tabetic neurologic lesion of tertiary syphilis. Congenital syphilis can present as osteochondritis (in the first year of life), dactylitis (at 1 to 3 years of age), and synovitis (Clutton's joints in patients 6 to 16 years old). The diagnosis is supported by associated syphilitic manifestations and a positive Venereal Disease Research Laboratories test.

Arthritis As a Manifestation of Systemic Disease

In systemic disease, musculoskeletal abnormalities, including joint pain and inflammation, can be prominent, secondary manifestations of a more basic, systemic disorder. The underlying disease can cause defects in many organ systems and present as a multisystem disorder. Although the joint symptoms can be the presenting feature of the disease, the diagnosis is usually based on the typical clinical picture of the underlying disorder.

ARTHRITIS ASSOCIATED WITH INFILTRATIVE SYSTEMIC DISEASES

Sarcoidosis. This is a multisystem disorder of unknown origin characterized by the presence of noncaseating granulomas in the involved organs, including the lungs, hilar and other lymph nodes, skin (papules and E. nodosum), and eyes (uveitis). Hepatosplenomegaly, cardiac and skeletal muscle involvement, and central and peripheral nervous system involvement may also occur. An acute, migratory, symmetrical polyarthritis or periarthritis, associated frequently with erythema nodosum and bilateral hilar adenopathy (Lofgren's syndrome), is the most common rheumatic manifestation. Chronic sarcoid arthritis frequently presents in a mono- or oligoarticular pattern involving knees and ankles and may have an insidious onset and produce joint destruction and disability. Osseous sarcoid, often accompanied by chronic lupus pernio skin lesions, is most common in the hands and feet and presents as asymptomatic or symptomatic lytic bone lesions associated with a diffuse "spongy" thickening of the fingers. The combination of characteristic clinical findings and the histologic demonstration of noncaseating granulomas provides the most secure diagnosis. Immunologic (anergy, hyperglobulinemia, and a positive Kveim test), biochemical (elevated serum levels of angiotensin-converting enzyme and lysozyme), and radionuclide (positive pulmonary gallium scan) tests are helpful diagnostically.

Amyloidosis. This is a syndrome characterized by the deposition of an insoluble proteinaceous material in the extracellular matrix of one or several organs. These deposits can produce diverse clinical manifestations including cutaneous and gastrointestinal amyloid, amyloid neuropathy, nephropathy, and cardiomyopathy. Small- and large-joint, rheumatoid-like involvement can occur along with subcutaneous (amyloid) nodules in amyloidosis associated with multiple myeloma and in primary generalized amyloidosis. Infiltration of the glenohumeral joint produces the characteristic shoulder-pad sign. Rheumatoid arthritis is the most frequent predisposing factor in the development of secondary generalized amyloidosis.

Multicentric Reticulohistiocytosis. This is a rare systemic disease of unknown origin characterized by an infiltration of lipid-laden histiocytes and giant cells into various tissues. Clinical presentation includes female predominance (in a ratio to males of 3 to 1), symmetrical polyarthritis (with common involvement of *distal* interphalangeal joints) that leads in 50% of cases to arthritis mutilans, and reddish brown nodules on the dorsum of fingers, face, ears, chest, and mucosal surfaces. Other body parts, including muscle, the stomach, and the pericardium, can be involved. Diagnosis is made by skin or synovial biopsy that demonstrates a ground-glass appearance of multinucleated giant cells and histiocytes.

Arthropathy with Iron Storage Disease (Primary Hemochromatosis). This inherited disorder of increased iron absorption and tissue accumulation presents clinically with symptoms related to cirrhosis, bronze or slate-gray skin darkening, diabetes, congestive heart failure, hypopituitarism, and arthropathy. Joint disease, which can precede or follow the diagnosis, can present with pain, stiffness, and bony swelling of the small joints of the hands (especially the second and third metacarpophalangeal joints), a generalized joint pain and tenderness resembling degenerative osteoarthritis, or acute episodes of inflammatory arthritis caused by pseudogout superimposed on the chronic, progressive arthritis. Secondary hemochromatosis can also be associated with a less well-defined joint disorder. The diagnosis is based on the clinical presentation, an elevated plasma iron concentration with a total iron binding capacity below 300 μg%, and a transferrin saturation greater than 75%. If the latter screening tests are abnormal, the diagnosis is established by a deferoxamine loading test, and by liver or synovial biopsy.

ARTHRITIS ASSOCIATED WITH HEMATOLOGIC AND MALIGNANT DISORDERS

Hemophilia and Other Bleeding Disorders. The term hemophilia refers to two X-linked, recessive disorders, hemophilia A and B, in which a functional deficiency of a clotting factor, Factor VIII and IX, respectively, leads to spontaneous joint and muscle hemorrhage. Hemophilia is the disorder in which recurrent hemarthrosis occurs most frequently, although acute joint hemorrhage can be seen in patients on anticoagulants, or with thrombocytopenia and chronic joint disease in severe cases of von Willebrand's disease. In hemophilia, because of enzymatic and mechanical factors, joint disease can progress from recurrent bouts of acute hemarthrosis, to chronic arthritis (with synovial thickening and limited range of motion), to end-stage disease with loss of joint motion and function. Once hemarthrosis or hemophilic arthritis is suspected, the diagnosis rests on the demonstration of a specific coagulopathy (i.e., using clotting factor level analysis).

Sickle-Cell Disease and Other Hemoglobinopathies. Sickle-cell disease is a systemic disease caused by the sickling of erythrocytes containing an abnormal hemoglobin. Infarction (and expansion) of marrow, cortical bone, periosteum, and periarticular tissues is the cause of the characteristic musculoskeletal manifestations: the hand-foot syndrome of children with severe inflammatory disease of distal extremities; painful crises manifested by bone and joint (primarily knee) pain and joint effusions; bone infarctions; vertebral fractures; and aseptic necrosis. Osteomyelitis (the predominant organisms are salmonellae) must be considered in a prolonged painful crisis with fever. Some joint symptoms can be found in sickle-C, sickle-thalassemia, and sickle trait.

The unstable hemoglobin that results from the inherited disorder thalassemia can lead to severe ankle pain because of microfractures from underlying bone disease with marrow expansion and osteomalacia. Gout, septic arthritis, and transfusion-related hepatitis B polyarthritis can also occur.

The diagnosis of hemoglobinopathies is based on the clinical presentation and the analysis of hemoglobin established by starch or cellulose acetate hemoglobin electrophoresis.

Musculoskeletal Syndromes Associated with Malignancy. Musculoskeletal disorders can arise from the direct involvement of joints, bones, and periarticular tissues by the malignant disease, or from alteration in function caused by but distant from the primary tumor and not related to metastases (i.e., paraneoplastic syndromes).

Direct tumor involvement is associated with primary malignant disease and can affect the synovium, juxta-articular bone, and metastatic disease. The primary involvement of the synovium involves the highly malignant synovial sarcoma, a soft-tissue neoplasm that rarely involves the joint and, when it does, is always from a primary tumor or the adjacent soft tissue that has extended into the joint. This tumor is found on the extremities near large joints (primarily the knee and ankle) and presents as a painless soft tissue mass, or less commonly as a painful, tender mass or joint. Diagnosis is made by tissue biopsy. Epithelioid sarcoma, arising from synovial tissue lining tendons, presents as a mass and only rarely invades the joint.

Another possible synovial disorder is systemic tumor with synovial infiltration. A large percentage of patients with various types of leukemia can present with or develop symmetrical or migratory polyarthritis, arthralgias, and bone pain and tenderness. Such joint manifestations are attributed to leukemic synovial infiltration, hemorrhage into joints, or synovial reaction to periarticular lesions. Diagnosis is based on associated hematologic abnormalities, x-ray demonstration of osteolysis, or periosteal reaction and joint pain disproportional to the degree of arthritis. In lymphoma, both monarticular and polyarticular joint pains are more related to adjacent bone disease than to direct synovial invasion.

In other primary malignant disease, synovial reaction or invasion produced by an adjacent tumor such as chondrosarcoma, osteogenic sarcoma, primary lymphoma, and giant cell tumor should always be considered in the evaluation of patients with monarticular arthritis. Evaluation should include radionuclide scanning or tomograms of radiologic abnormalities.

Metastatic bronchogenic carcinoma, breast carcinoma, and adenocarcinoma of the colon can all spread to the synovium directly or via involvement of juxta-articular bone and present as asymmetrical or symmetrical polyarthritis of large or small joints. The di-

Table 13–12. Paraneoplastic Syndromes

Arthropathy
  Hypertrophic osteoarthropathy
  Carcinomatous polyarthritis
  Amyloidosis
  Secondary gout
Myopathy
  Dermatomyositis-polymyositis
Miscellaneous
  Necrotizing vasculitis
  Cryoproteins
  Lupus syndrome
  Reflex sympathetic dystrophy
  Scleroderma
  Polyarteritis
  Polymyalgia rheumatica—secondary
  Panniculitis
  Polychondritis

agnosis is based on the demonstration of the underlying malignancy, as well as on x-rays, radionuclide scanning, biopsy, study of synovial fluid, and cytology.

Indirect association between malignancy and musculoskeletal syndromes must also be considered (Table 13–12). Carcinomatous polyarthritis, a rheumatoid-like polyarthritis, may be the presenting manifestation of malignancy. This can occur with solid tumors (such as breast) and hematologic neoplasms. Hypertrophic osteoarthropathy (HPO) is defined as a syndrome of clubbing of the fingers or toes, chronic proliferative periostitis, and oligo- or polysynovitis. Various solid and hematologic neoplasms are associated with this disorder, the most common being intrathoracic neoplastic conditions such as bronchogenic carcinoma. Two clinical syndromes are recognized: primary HPO and secondary HPO.

A patient with primary HPO may have pachydermoperiostosis, a familial disorder manifested by the insidious onset of clubbing in adolescence, thickening of the forearms and legs, thickened, furrowed, leonine facial features and mildly symptomatic joint effusions. Primary onset might also be idiopathic.

Secondary hypertrophic osteoarthropathy is most often associated with neoplastic disease (lung tumors, both primary and metastatic, other solid tumors, and hematologic malignancies or lymphomas), infectious disease (e.g., lung infections such as abscess and bronchiectasis), and cardiac disease (congenital heart disease in children). Whenever HPO is diagnosed, it is important to search for an underlying disease. The clinical presentation is one of periostitis with burning pain of the distal extremities, clubbing, and mild to severe symmetrical arthralgias or arthritis in hands, wrists, knees, and ankles. One form of secondary HPO is thyroid acropachy, a disorder associated with previous or current hyperthyroidism that presents with clubbing and painless periostitis of the short bones of the hands. The diagnosis is made on the basis of clinical findings, x-ray demonstration of periosteal new bone formation or radionuclide bone scanning.

ARTHROPATHIES ASSOCIATED WITH ENDOCRINE DISORDERS

Diabetes Mellitus. Patients with diabetes mellitus may have hemochromatosis arthropathy. Diabetic osteopathy, a resorptive osteoarthropathy, presents with hand and foot pain related to radiographic osteopenia, erosions of the phalangeal or metatarsal heads, and, eventually, complete lysis of bone ends with subluxation of metatarsophalangeal joints. These changes can occur in the absence of infection, vascular or neurologic deficit, or severe diabetes. Compromised host defenses in the ischemic and neuropathic foot can lead to osteomyelitis. This is characterized by irregular and progressive bone and joint destruction, sequestrum formation, and periostitis. In the setting of chronic insulin-dependent diabetes and severe peripheral neuropathy, the tarsal and tarsometatarsal joints, the metatarsophalangeal joints, and the ankle joint may develop deformities, subluxation, and destructive changes or an acute inflammatory-like arthritis. Similar changes in the knee, wrist, or spine can appear, radiologically similar to infectious or neoplastic disorders.

Parathyroid Disorders. Patients may have primary or secondary hyperparathyroidism. In primary hyperparathyroidism, the musculoskeletal sequelae of a parathormone level elevated because of parathyroid adenoma or hyperplasia include calcium pyrophosphate deposition disease, which includes chondrocalcinosis and acute or chronic pseudogout, and inflammatory and erosive arthritis. The process of bone softening and collapse of subchondral tissue resulting from localized trabecular fractures can lead to severe periarticular pain and marginal erosions mimicking a polyarthritis. The diagnosis of primary hyperparathyroidism is based on an elevated serum calcium, decreased, or normal PO_4, and an elevated parathormone level. X-ray evidence of endosteal and periosteal resorption and biopsy demonstration of osteitis fibrosa cystica are characteristic.

Secondary hyperparathyroidism occurs in patients with some forms of osteomalacia, pseudohypoparathyroidism, and chronic renal failure (renal osteodystrophy). Subperiosteal and subchondral erosion and resorption can lead to tapering and erosion at the ends of the clavicles and erosion of the sternoclavicular and sacroiliac articulations. Acute periarticular inflammation represents calcium hydroxyapatite-induced soft-tissue inflammatory episodes.

Acromegaly. In acromegaly, a persistent overstimulation of articular cartilage because of excess circulating growth hormone leads to a distinct type of degenerative joint disease in the peripheral joints and the spine. Severe noninflammatory joint pain and swelling is typical, and destructive hip and knee disease can occur. The arthropathy is irreversible despite successful pituitary ablation. Chondrocalcinosis can be present, and acute crystal synovitis is reported. The diagnosis is based on the typical clinical features, elevated growth hormone level, and widened peripheral joint spaces resulting from cartilage hyperplasia.

Thyroid Disease. Patients with thyroid disease may have hypo- or hyperthyroidism. A noninflammatory, painful synovial thickening of the knees and small joints of the hands may be present in certain patients with hypothyroidism. Also, thickening and tenderness of the flexor tendon sheaths of the hands and wrists and, rarely, tibial plateau collapse can be seen. Highly viscous, noninflammatory synovial fluid is characteristic of this generally reversible (with thyroid replacement) arthropathy. Carpal tunnel syndrome, myopathy, and synovitis related to connective tissue diseases (SLE, RA) associated with Hashimoto's thyroiditis are also noted. The diagnosis of this commonly insidious disease is based on a recognition of the clinical features and appropriate thyroid function tests (T_4 and T_3 by radioimmunoassay, free thyroxine index, T_3 resin uptake, and thyroid stimulating hormone assay).

Thyroid acropachy, which rarely may accompany hyperthroidism, presents with clubbing of the fingers and toes and periostitis of the digits with swelling of the overlying tissues.

ARTHRITIS ASSOCIATED WITH HYPERCHOLESTEROLEMIA AND HYPERLIPIDEMIA

Musculoskeletal syndromes related to hyperlipidemia are most likely attributable to defective lipoprotein transport or metabolism within the synovial tissues or joint space. These include type IIa and type IV hyperlipoproteinemia. Homozygous individuals can present with type IIa hyperlipoproteinemia (elevated plasma cholesterol, phospholipid, and low-density lipoproteins), evident in recurrent episodes of migratory, nondestructive polyarthralgias or arthritis of large peripheral joints in the setting of early onset xanthomas and premature atherosclerosis; heterozygous patients present with recurrent bouts of Achilles tendinitis and tenosynovitis with knee arthritis.

In type IV hyperlipoproteinemia (elevated plasma triglycerides, cholesterol, and very low density lipoproteins), episodes of oligoarticular symmetrical or asymmetrical arthritis of large and small joints of the hands and feet occur with moderate joint pain. Juxta-articular osteoporosis associated with metaphyseal cystic lesions is noted.

HERITABLE DISORDERS OF CONNECTIVE TISSUE

The pathogenesis of these rare, heritable disorders of connective tissue is related to a disorder of collagen biosynthesis. A subgroup of patients may present with symptoms that mimic rheumatic diseases.

Marfan's syndrome, the most common heritable (autosomal dominant) disorder of unknown cause, presents with characteristic ocular (ectopia lentis), cardiovascular (aortic dilatation, aortic and mitral regurgitation, and dissecting aortic aneurysm), and skeletal (arachnodactyly, high-arched palate, kyphoscoliosis) abnormalities. The principal rheumatic complaints occur as a consequence of skeletal deformities and include ligamentous laxity with abnormal range of motion, which causes joint effusion (acute or chronic monarthritis) and early degenerative arthritis (arthralgias).

Homocystinuria is an autosomal recessive inherited disease caused by deficiency of the enzyme cystathionine-synthetase and presents, like Marfan's syndrome, with ectopic lentis and a marfanoid habitus. The cardiovascular abnormality is thrombosis of large arteries. Hand contractures with arthralgias present in a scleroderma-like manner. The diagnosis is suspected by detection of urinary homocysteine by the nitroprusside test and is confirmed by direct enzyme assay of fibroblasts or liver.

The Ehlers-Danlos syndromes are a heterogeneous group of inherited disorders of connective tissue biosynthesis. Eight subtypes are currently recognized, each differing in the degree of cutaneous involvement (hyperelastic skin that bruises easily and heals slowly) and visceral involvement (rupture of large artery [type IV], varicose veins, ectopia lentis, mitral valve prolapse). Hypermobility leads to pes plantus (flat feet), kyphoscoliosis, arthralgias from premature osteoarthritis, and joint effusions (acute or chronic monarthritis).

Osteogenesis imperfecta includes four inherited disorders of connective tissue with bony fragility as the cardinal manifestation. The patient may have fractures, blue sclerae, and cardiovascular abnormalities. In addition, joints are hypermobile and dislocate easily, and tendons can rupture.

Pseudoxanthoma elasticum includes four inherited disorders of elastic tissue with clinical manifestations relating to blood vessels (claudication, angina, hypertension), eyes (angioid streaks), and skin (yellow papules of skin and mucous membranes). Rheumatologic complications are uncommon, but joint hypermobility has been described.

Disorders of Cartilage and Bone

The disorders in this group have in common a non-inflammatory degeneration, disintegration, or decrease in bone or cartilage structure. While these disorders do not themselves involve viscera or present with systemic features (such as fever or weight loss), systemic, inflammatory disorders can lead to disorders of bone and cartilage (e.g., rheumatoid arthritis can cause alteration of joint anatomy with the development of secondary osteoarthritis, osteoporosis, or both). Inflammation tends to be a secondary phenomenon in this group of disorders.

OSTEOARTHRITIS (also called degenerative joint disease, osteoarthrosis, and hypertrophic arthritis)

An imbalance between cartilage synthesis and degradation leads to this common progressive joint disorder, which is classified into primary and secondary forms depending on whether the pathogenetic steps are initiated in response to local or systemic factors (Table 13–13). In patients over 40 years of age, characteristic symptoms include joint pain and stiffness most commonly in the distal interphalangeal (DIP) joints, proximal interphalangeal (PIP) joints, first carpometacarpal (CMC) (base of the thumb) joint, knees, hips (often unilateral), spine (cervical and lumbar), and first metatarsophalangeal joint. There are no systemic manifestations. Signs of inflammation are rarely encountered, save for erosive osteoarthritis affecting the DIP and PIP joints. Swelling is minimal or absent and, except in the knees, effusions are infrequently detected. Bony swelling is common in the hands and reflects marginal bony overgrowth (osteophytes). The primary disability is due to hip, knee, and spine involvement.

Primary generalized osteoarthritis is a polyarticular disorder of the DIP, PIP, and CMC joints as well as of the knees, hips, and spine. It is not associated with systemic signs and metacarpophalangeal or wrist joint disease. Diffuse idiopathic skeletal hyperostosis (DISH) is a variant characterized by large osteophytes leading to fusion of the anterior longitudinal ligament of the (primarily thoracic) spine and bony spurs at sites of tendon attachment to bone. Typical laboratory findings exclude evidence of systemic inflammation (evident in erythrocyte sedimentation) or local inflammation (evident in synovial fluid). X-ray of joints demonstrates joint or disc space narrowing, marginal spur formation, and subchondral cysts.

OSTEONECROSIS (formerly called aseptic or avascular necrosis)

This is a focal degeneration of bone, probably secondary to ischemia, that presents with periarticular pain in the area of involvement (all bones can be in-

Table 13–13. Classification of Osteoarthritis

Primary
  Localized (one joint or joint-group)
  Primary generalized osteoarthritis
  Erosive osteoarthritis
  Diffuse idiopathic skeletal hyperostosis (DISH)
Secondary
  Trauma
    Acute
    Chronic
  Inflammatory conditions
    Rheumatoid arthritis
    Seronegative spondyloarthropathies
      Ankylosing spondylitis
      Reiter's syndrome
      Psoriatic arthritis
      Arthropathy associated with inflammatory bowel disease
    Septic arthritis
      Bacterial
      Tuberculous
    Crystal-induced disease
      Recurrent gout
      Pseudogout/chondrocalcinosis
  Congenital or developmental defects
    Hip dysplasias
    Legg-Calvé-Perthes disease
    Slipped capital femoral epiphysis
    Femoral neck abnormalities
  Metabolic
    Hemochromatosis
    Ochronosis
    Paget's disease
    Wilson's disease
  Endocrine
    Acromegaly
    Diabetes
    Hypothyroidism with myxedema
    Iatrogenic hypercortisonism
    Obesity
  Miscellaneous
    Hemarthroses caused by bleeding dyscrasias (e.g., hemophilia)
    Neuropathic joint disease caused by
      Diabetes mellitus
      Syphilis
      Syringomyelia
      Peripheral nerve injury
    Heritable diseases of connective tissue
      Marfan's syndrome
      Ehlers-Danlos syndrome
    Aseptic necrosis
    Chronic intra-articular corticosteroid therapy

volved but the most common are the proximal and distal femur, the proximal tibia, and the proximal humerus). In the majority of patients with osteonecrosis, there is antecedent recognition of an associated condition (Table 13–14). The diagnosis is based on characteristic x-ray and radionuclide bone scan abnormalities. Workup includes the appropriate tests to determine the potential associated conditions.

Table 13–14.   Conditions Associated with Osteonecrosis

High association
   Avascular (traumatic) osteonecrosis
      Proximal femur
         Following subcapital fracture
         Hip dislocation
      Talus
      Proximal humerus
      Distal femoral condyle
   Metabolic disorders
      Excess corticosteroids (steroid therapy, Cushing's syndrome)
      Gaucher's disease
      Hyperuricemia
      Alcoholism
   Hemoglobinopathies—sickle-cell disease, sickle-cell hemoglobin
         disease
   Miscellaneous
      Systemic lupus erythematosus
      Irradiation
      Congenital malformations
      Decompression syndrome (caisson disease)
      Thermal injuries or frostbite
Moderate association
   Diabetes mellitus
   Fat embolism
   Rheumatoid arthritis
Reported but uncertain association
   Hypercholesterolemia
   Hypertriglyceridemia
   Lymphoma
No known association (true idiopathic)
   Proximal femur—Chandler's disease
   Distal femoral condyle
   Carpal lunate—Kienböck's disease

Table 13–15.   Factors Related to Osteoporosis

Immobilization or weightlessness
Endocrine abnormality
   Glucocorticoid excess
      Cushing's syndrome
      Iatrogenic
   Thyrotoxicosis
   Estrogen deficiency
   Diabetes mellitus
   Testosterone deficiency
   Acromegaly
   Postmenopausal
   Hyperparathyroidism
Genetic
   Osteogenesis imperfecta
   Marfan's syndrome
   Homocystinuria
   Ehlers-Danlos syndrome
Nutritional abnormalities
   Scurvy
   Alcoholism
   Metabolic acidosis
   Malabsorption
Hematologic malignancy
   Multiple myeloma
   Leukemia
   Lymphoma
   Metastatic malignancies
Juvenile osteoporosis
Rheumatoid arthritis
Chronic heparin therapy
Liver disease
Systemic mastocytosis

METABOLIC BONE DISEASE

This is defined as a skeletal disorder in which the pathologic process is generalized. Typical signs and symptoms include bone pain, fractures, arthralgias, and radiographic evidence of osteopenia (generalized loss of bone density with thinning of the cortex).

Osteoporosis involves a state of bone loss characterized by a reduction in total bone mass to a level below normal for a patient's age, sex, and race; and it can arise from a variety of underlying pathologic processes (Table 13–15). Diagnosis should emphasize the identification of treatable secondary causes of osteoporosis. Back pain and fractures are the characteristic presenting symptoms. Joint pain can be a manifestation of bone fractures, especially in the hip and distal radius. The diagnosis is based on x-ray, bone scan, bone density, and biopsy studies.

Paget's disease of bone, a disorder of unknown cause, is characterized by increased bone resorption and subsequent reactive bone formation leading to severe skeletal involvement and obvious deformity of individual long bones. Although most patients are asymptomatic (the disease is diagnosed by chance on x-ray), some can present with pain, deformity, or pathologic fracture. Arthritis with joint pain is most commonly seen in the hip and knee. The diagnosis is based on typical x-ray and bone scan abnormalities in the setting of an elevated serum alkaline phosphatase and 24-hour urinary hydroxyproline.

Osteomalacia is characterized by an excess of unmineralized bone resulting from an impairment of bone mineralization. Bone pain and tenderness in the pelvis, spine, ribs, and lower extremities is characteristic. The child with rickets typically manifests the disorder with enlargment of the costochondral junctions and bowing of the lower extremities. The majority of patients will have an abnormality of vitamin D metabolism (malabsorption, renal failure, and use of anticonvulsant drugs), or will have hypophosphatemia. Diagnosis is based on clinical and x-ray abnormalities and bone biopsy and on the definition of an underlying cause.

In renal osteodystrophy, impaired vitamin D metabolism caused by chronic renal failure leads to bone pain and muscle weakness in adults and to skeletal deformities in children. Bone abnormalities are those of either osteomalacia or (secondary) hyperparathy-

Table 13-16. Classification of Traumatic Arthritis

Articular trauma, single episode
  Traumatic synovitis
    Acute, self-limiting synovitis (with or without hemarthrosis)
    Sprains—stretch or tear of a supporting ligament of a joint
  Disruptive trauma (with infarction of the articular cartilage or complete rupture of major supporting structures)
    Fractures through the articular surface
    Dislocations
    Internal derangements (e.g., meniscal tears)
    Major ligamentous ruptures
    Wounds
    Foreign body implantation
  Post-traumatic osteoarthritis
    Disruptive trauma with major residual damage leads to secondary osteoarthritis
Repetitive articular trauma—occupational or sports injuries result in localized chronic osteoarthritis
Induction or aggravation of rheumatic diseases by acute or repetitive trauma
  Neuropathic joint
  Gouty arthritis, pseudogout
  Rheumatoid arthritis
  Septic arthritis, bacterial and tuberculous
  Reflex sympathetic dystrophy
Disorders of extra-articular structures related to trauma
  Tendons
    Tenosynovitis—inflammation of the fibrous sheath through which a tendon moves, caused by a direct blow, abnormal pressure, unusual activity, diseases (RA, gout, Gonococcus); e.g., trigger finger, De Quervain's disease, carpal tunnel syndrome
    Tendon rupture (e.g., Achilles tendon)
  Bursae—closed sacs that facilitate motion of tendons and muscles over bony prominences can, with direct trauma or excessive frictional forces, become inflamed (e.g., subdeltoid bursitis, trochanteric bursitis, olecranon bursitis)
  Muscles—rupture of muscles can occur from sudden stretching force or chronic frictional attrition (e.g., rupture of long head of biceps)
Nonmechanical types of trauma
  Radiation arthropathy—osteoarthritic changes are noted years after joints are exposed to radiation
  Frostbite arthropathy—destructive or hypertrophic changes can occur in fingers and toes
  Decompression (caisson) syndrome—can lead to osteonecrosis

roidism and can present as joint pain, when they occur around joints.

Localized Causes of Joint Pains

TRAUMATIC ARTHRITIS

This term includes a collection of pathologic and clinical states that develop after a single or repeated episodes of trauma and can present as joint pain and swelling (Table 13-16).

TUMOR AND TUMOR-LIKE LESIONS INVOLVING JOINTS

Although there are no proven cases of malignant neoplasms arising within synovial tissue, most tumor-like conditions are of importance in the differential diagnosis and can present with joint pain and swelling. Arthroscopy or surgical intervention is usually needed for diagnosis.

Lipoma arborescens, a benign, fatty, intra-articular mass, is found in the knee or elbow associated with osteoarthritis. It presents with pain, locking, limitation of range of motion, and effusion.

Hemangioma of synovium is rare and is associated with soft-tissue abnormalities such as arteriovenous malformations or skin vascular lesions. Intermittent unilateral joint pain and enlargement with limitation of range of motion, locking, or buckling are the common symptoms, usually occurring in women less than 30 years of age.

In synovial chondromatosis, nodules of metaplastic cartilage within synovial tissue are released into the joint space and as loose bodies, leading to joint pain, swelling, stiffness, and grating with motion. This occurs most commonly in the knee and presents in middle age. X-ray examination may show calcified cartilage or bone in either the synovium or loose bodies.

In pigmented villonodular synovitis, synovial lining-cell proliferation of unknown cause leads to villous and nodular lesions of joints and tendons that are locally aggressive and can invade bone, joint capsules, tendons, and adjacent soft tissues. This disorder most commonly occurs in young adults and presents as unilateral joint pain (predominantly in the knee and also in the hip and ankle) and mild, intermittent, or repeated bouts of swelling over a long period of time. X-ray examination can show a soft tissue mass, bone erosion, or lytic clusters of well-marginated cyst-like lucencies. Arthrogram, arthroscopy, or arthrotomy are common diagnostic tests. Synovial fluid is hemorrhagic, and synovial tissue is red-brown with prominent villous projections and nodules.

REFLEX SYMPATHETIC DYSTROPHY SYNDROME (shoulder-hand syndrome)

An excessive or abnormal response of the sympathetic nervous system in an extremity, caused by injury or another condition (Table 13-17), is thought to be the cause of extremity pain, swelling, trophic skin changes, vasomotor disturbances, and limitation of motion. Typically, this pain involves the shoulder and ipsilateral hand but can also involve lower extremity joints or can be bilateral. Patchy or mottled osteopenia is seen on x-ray, and radionuclide studies demonstrate periarticular uptake of the involved extremity. An event or disorder precipitates the syndrome in two-thirds of patients and should be sought with appropriate tests or from the patient's history.

Table 13–17. Conditions Associated with Reflex Sympathetic Dystrophy Syndrome

Trauma
Neurologic conditions
  Cerebral vascular diseases with hemiplegia
  Hemiplegias of other origins
  Spinal cord lesions
  Cervical spine syndrome
  Herpes zoster and postherpetic neuralgia
  Radiculopathies
  Peripheral nerve lesions
Atherosclerotic cardiovascular disease
  Ischemic heart disease
    Angina pectoris
    Myocardial infarction
  Post coronary artery bypass surgery
Degenerative or calcific lesions of the shoulder
Pulmonary tuberculosis and antituberculous drugs (Isoniazid)
Barbiturates

DISORDERS OF PERIARTICULAR TISSUES

Abnormalities of the tissues surrounding joints can present as joint pain on motion and as swelling with inflammation. Bursae are closed sacs containing a small amount of synovial fluid and lined with a membrane similar to synovium. They are present in areas where tendons and muscles move over bony prominences, facilitating motion. A tendon is a fibrous cord by which a muscle is attached to bone. Since bursae are often located near tendons, the terms tendinitis and bursitis are often used interchangeably to represent the same condition and are the most common causes of soft tissue pain. In both disorders, the causes of inflammation include direct trauma, chronic overuse or irritation, sepsis related to puncture wounds, or surrounding cellulitis or systemic sepsis. The causes could also be a manifestation of a systemic disorder (inflammatory arthritides, e.g., rheumatoid arthritis, gout, and pseudogout).

The clinically important bursae in bursitis are outlined in Table 13–18. In tendinitis, inflammation may occur within the substance of the tendon (as an intratendinous lesion, usually associated with repetitive motion and occurring later in life as the vascularity of the tendon diminishes) or may be associated with the tenosynovial sheath (as tenosynovitis, also associated with diminished vascularity). Since most tendons cross joints, tendinitis must be distinguished from acute inflammatory or septic arthritis. Table 13–18 outlines the most common areas of tendinitis.

Pain originating from muscle can appear as bone or joint pain. The diagnosis of muscle disease is based on the clinical features, elevated creatine phosphokinase and aldolase as signs of muscle necrosis, electromyogram testing, or muscle biopsy. Myonecrosis can occur in circumstances of unusual muscle activity

Table 13–18. Clinical Characteristics of Tendinitis and Bursitis

Tendinitis
  Intratendinous lesions
    Pathology: decreased vascularity with age, microtrauma lead to acute and chronic inflammation and, eventually, calcium salt deposition (i.e., calcific tendinitis)
    Clinical presentation: pain on motion, local swelling, warmth, tenderness, and erythema
    Common areas: tennis elbow (lateral epicondylitis), calcific tendinitis in the shoulder
  Acute or chronic paratendinous inflammation or tenosynovitis
    Pathology: synovial tendon sheath inflammation occurs because of repetitive motion with injury, direct or microtraumatic intratendinous injuries, infection or inflammatory arthritides, or collagen vascular diseases
    Clinical presentation: pain on motion and inflammation, as well as signs of mechanical blocking (e.g., trigger finger, De Quervain's disease)
    Common areas: stenosing tenosynovitis of the abductor pollicis longus and extensor pollicis brevis at the radial styloid (De Quervain's disease), thumb flexor and extensor tendons, and finger flexors; tenosynovitis in the flexor compartment of the wrist leads to carpal tunnel syndrome
Bursitis—the area of pain relates to the site of bursal inflammation
  Shoulder: subacromial, subdeltoid, and subcoracoid bursae
  Elbow: olecranon (tip of elbow), radiohumeral bursae
  Hip: iliopsoas, trochanteric, ischiogluteal
  Knee: prepatellar (housemaid's knee), infrapatellar, and popliteal bursae
  Foot: Achilles and subcalcaneal bursae

such as in postexercise myalgia. Muscle disease can also present as muscle hematoma, related to trauma or coagulopathy. Influenza, echovirus, and other viruses can lead to myalgias, myositis, or both. Also, myalgias may be due to myopathies. Although proximal muscle weakness is the usual symptoms of myopathy, pain in the muscle can exist in disorders such as polyarthritis nodosa and dermatomyositis, myositis caused by trichinosis, acute sarcoid myositis, metabolic myopathies, and other muscle disorders.

Diffuse Musculoskeletal Syndromes

Fibromyalgia (fibrositis) is a noninflammatory pain syndrome characterized by widespread, poorly circumscribed deep pain, stiffness, and aching referred to muscles and bony prominences, by localized sites of myofascial tenderness (so-called trigger points), and by disturbed sleep with morning fatigue and stiffness. In primary fibromyalgia, no underlying systemic disorder is found; all tests are normal and the diagnosis is made by exclusion. Widespread muscle aching and stiffness, when seen in association with viral or other infections and a large variety of rheumatic, endocrine, infectious, myopathic, or malignant disorders, is termed secondary fibromyalgia. The physician must rule out such disorders with appropriate tests, a patient history and a physical examination before making a diagnosis of primary fibromyalgia.

Some patients with psychologic stress or neurosis may present with vague, nonspecific joint, muscle, and bone pain that is greatly out of proportion to objective findings. Bizarre features of the pain facilitate a positive diagnosis of psychopathology. Aside from local tenderness, the physical examination and laboratory tests of psychogenic musculoskeletal syndrome are normal.

Referred Pain Syndromes

Perception of pain at a site remote from the area of irritation is referred pain. The quality of referred pain is determined more by the site to which it is referred than by the nature of the original pain stimulus. Associated with such referred pain are tenderness (deep more than cutaneous), involuntary muscle spasm, inhibition of voluntary motion, increased blood flow, and subjective numbness. When these features are severe or prolonged, the structural changes of reflex sympathetic dystrophy may occur, including restricted range of motion, cutaneous and periarticular fibrosis, and osteopenia.

Reflex sympathetic dystrophy, entrapment neuropathies (nerve entrapment syndromes), and cervical spine syndromes are referred pain syndromes. The term entrapment describes the mechanical irritation by which a specific peripheral nerve becomes injured in a vulnerable anatomic site. This injury can occur at any point where a peripheral nerve passes through an opening in fibrous tissue or through an osseofibrous canal. Pain, numbness, or tingling are the most common presenting features. Table 13–19 lists the most common nerves encountered with entrapment syndromes and the typical clinical involvement. Evaluation of these syndromes includes neurologic examination, electromyography, motor and sensory nerve conduction velocity studies, and appropriate x-rays and laboratory tests (e.g., latex fixation, thyroid function tests).

Not only can cervical spine disorders present at a distance from the cervical spine itself, but many diseases having no relation to the musculoskeletal system can cause neck pain. The examiner should consider the broad range of clinical possibilities in cervical spine disease (Table 13–20). A complete patient history, physical examination, and x-ray evaluation of the cervical spine are the major means of data gathering in the diagnosis and management of cervical pain. Similar referred pain patterns are found in the lumbosacral spine, where distal lower extremity, pelvic, or abdominal pain can reflect disorders of the lower spine, related to radicular disease caused by nerve/spinal cord impingement by disc, spur, or tumor.

DIAGNOSTIC EVALUATION (Fig. 13–3)

The first disorders to consider are those that can cause permanent joint injury unless prompt, specific therapy is instituted. These include infectious arthritis (suggested by monarticular synovitis or migratory polyarthritis in the setting of fever, chills, and leukocytosis), fracture of a juxta-articular bone (suggested by the sudden onset of pain, deformity, or both in the setting of trauma or osteoporosis), and internal derangement of the knee (meniscal or ligamentous tears are suggested by a history of trauma, episodes of joint locking or "giving way," tenderness at the joint margin, or joint instability).

In the appropriate clinical setting, diagnostic tests are indicated to rule out various disorders. In testing for infectious arthritis, joint aspiration is mandatory. The physician should obtain a joint fluid cell count and differential; in sepsis, the white blood cell count is high (usually >50,000/mm³) with a poly predominance. The glucose level is low when compared with a concomitant serum glucose. Also, a Gram's stain should be performed. (Although an important early guide to antibiotic therapy prior to culture results, Gram's stain can be negative despite eventually positive cultures. Hence, a high index of clinical suspicion is needed, and antibiotic therapy may be instituted with a negative Gram's stain, pending culture reports.)

Appropriate joint fluid cultures are indicated, the choice of media guided by the potential pathogens. (Routinely used media include thioglycolate broth, blood agar, MacConkey broth, and chocolate agar. Gonococcal organisms grow best on a Thayer-Martin [selective] medium, whereas anaerobes demand an anaerobic environment [belljar], and mycobacteria and fungi have specific media requirements.) Other cultures include blood, potential sources of joint sepsis (e.g., the skin, the respiratory tract, or the urinary tract), or other areas of infection (in gonococcal disease, the pharynx, anus, cervix, urethra, and skin). X-rays of the joints play a limited role in the acute joint sepsis, though X-ray abnormalities may be seen in more subacute or chronic infections such as those caused by mycobacteria or fungi or related to osteomyelitis. Early changes of joint sepsis can be demonstrated on radionuclide bone scans prior to their appearance on X-rays of the joints.

Whereas most bone fractures (whether or not pathologic) can be demonstrated by x-rays immediately post-trauma, some large bone or stress fractures may not be immediately obvious. Thus, one needs a high

Table 13–19. Peripheral Entrapment Neuropathies

Nerve	Entrapment Syndrome	Clinical Involvement
Upper limbs		
Median	Carpal tunnel	
	Cause: flexor tenosynovitis or swelling at the volar wrist *Diseases:* rheumatoid arthritis, hypothyroidism, amyloid, gout, acromegaly, and other inflammatory reactions involving the tendons and connective tissue at the wrist	Sensory and motor symptoms and signs in first, index, middle, and one half of the ring finger, thenar eminence
Ulnar	Cubital canal	
	Cause: secondary to compression in the cubital fossa of the elbow *Diseases:* rheumatoid arthritis, trauma	Weakness of fourth and fifth finger flexors and intrinsic hand muscles, sensory loss to the dorsum of the ulnar aspects of the hand
Radial	Saturday night palsy	
	Cause: pressure on the radial nerve in the axilla *Diseases:* use of crutches in the axilla, alcoholic, drug addiction	Weakness of triceps, brachioradialis, extensors of the hand, wrist, and fingers; wristdrop; sensory loss in dorsum of the thumb
Brachial plexus	Thoracic outlet	
	Cause: bony, fascial, and muscular structures interfere with functions of the neurovascular bundle located in the thoracic outlet *Diseases:* cervical rib, bifid clavicle, fascial band behind scalenus anticus muscle, fracture of clavicle, subacromial dislocation of humeral head, crush injury to upper thorax	Depends upon characteristic of nerve compression; pain in fingers, hand, forearm, arm, and shoulder; paresthesia and numbness in C8–T1 distribution
Lower limbs		
Sciatic	Piriformis	
	Cause: piriformis muscle entraps the sciatic nerve where it leaves the pelvis through the greater sciatic notch	Distal motor and sensory signs: pain down lateral thigh, footdrop, absent ankle jerk
Posterior tibial	Tarsal tunnel	
	Cause: entrapment of nerve in a flexor retinaculum along the medial malleolus of the ankle *Diseases:* trauma, rheumatoid and other types of arthritis, leprous neuritis, ganglion of subtalar joint	Painful dysesthesias and intrinsic foot weakness; burning feet at night
Common, deep, or superficial peroneal	Pressure palsy	
	Cause: pressure on the nerve where it winds around the neck of the fibula *Disease:* pressure in surgical and medical patients, hereditary compression neuropathy, ganglion, or leprosy	Weakness or paralysis of extension of the foot and toes, and eversion of the foot (footdrop); sensory loss on dorsum of the foot
Lateral femoral cutaneous nerve	Meralgia paresthetica	
	Cause: entrapment at the anterior superior iliac spine at the lateral end of the inguinal ligament *Disease:* trauma, fracture of anterior ilium, pelvic tilt, diabetes, local pressure by tight clothes, obesity	Burning pain and parasthesias with decreased sensation in the lateral thigh

index of suspicion for such fractures; a radionuclide bone scan in most instances will demonstrate the fracture site. Rarely, tomograms of the probable fracture site are needed.

The diagnosis of internal derangement is confirmed by arthrography or arthroscopy. The latter procedure has obviated the need for arthrotomy in many cases.

Once the above disorders have been ruled out, one then must define whether the joint disorder is articular (arising from within the joint) or periarticular (arising from the tissues surrounding the joint, i.e., tendons, bursae, muscles, overlying skin, or surrounding nerve or vascular tissue). Clues pointing to a periarticular origin include localized as opposed to diffuse tenderness or inflammation, the characteristic location of pain and tenderness (e.g., the superolateral aspect of

Table 13–20. Pain Related to the Cervical Spine

Symptoms and Signs Originating in the Cervical Spine	Structures and Disorders Causing Pain in the Neck
Referred pain (from deep cervical structures or by nerve root irritation)	Heart and coronary artery disease
Head pain	Apex of lung, Pancoast's tumor, or bronchogenic carcinoma (C3–C4–C5 nerve roots in common)
Bilateral	Diaphragm muscle (C3–C4–C5 innervation)
Unilateral	Gallbladder
Retro-orbital	Spinal cord tumor
Temporal	Temporomandibular joint
Occipital	Fibromyalgia syndromes
Neck pain	Aorta
Back	Pancreas
Sides	Hiatal hernia, C3–C4–C5
Front	Gastric ulcer
Thoracic spine	
Shoulders	
Scapular areas	
Arms (one or both)	
Fingertips	
Proximal arm and leg pain due to myelopathy	
Paresthesia (numbness or tingling in the segmental distribution of nerve roots)	
Face	
Head	
Tongue	
Neck	
Shoulders	
Arms	
Forearms	
Fingers	
Weakness (signs of anterior radiculopathy are those of a lower motor neuron lesion)	
Headache and occipital neuralgia	
Pseudoangina pectoris	
C6 and C7 lesions can cause neurologic or myalgic pain in the precordium or scapular region	
Eye symptoms	
Irritation of cervical sympathetic nerve supply to eye structures lead to tearing, blurring, or eye or retro-orbital pain	
Ear symptoms	
Gait or balance abnormalities with or without tinnitus or deafness	
Throat symptoms—dysphagia	

the shoulder in tendinitis of the shoulder, the lateral aspect of the thigh in trochanteric bursitis, and the lateral epicondyle of the elbow in tennis elbow), typical inciting events (repetitive activities, athletics), characteristic symptoms and signs (night pain in the shoulder, trochanteric bursitis, limitation of range of motion on internal rotation, and abduction in shoulder tendinitis/bursitis), and supporting laboratory or x-ray data (e.g., calcium deposit in the symptomatic site).

Once periarticular disease is ruled out (at times, the local inflammation is so severe and diffuse that one cannot easily differentiate periarticular from articular disease without arthrocentesis), the next step is to define whether the disease is monarticular, oligoarticular, polyarticular, acute, or chronic in onset. Because joint disorders often can be differentiated on the basis of their pattern of joint involvement, such characteriza-

tion will aid in the differential diagnosis (see Table 13–3, Table 13–21, and Fig. 13–4). It is important to note that in the course of some joint disorders (e.g., rheumatoid arthritis), the presentation can vary from monarticular to polyarticular depending on the characteristics of the joint disease in that patient. At times, after ruling out sepsis by both clinical and laboratory means, the clinician must await the natural disease progression before making a definitive diagnosis. Therapy often remains nonspecific until that time.

The next step is to characterize the joint disorder as inflammatory or noninflammatory, acute or chronic. Table 13–2 lists the clinical and laboratory manifestations of these two categories as well as the disease to consider in each.

As the field of potential diagnoses narrows, further definition can be brought about by using supporting

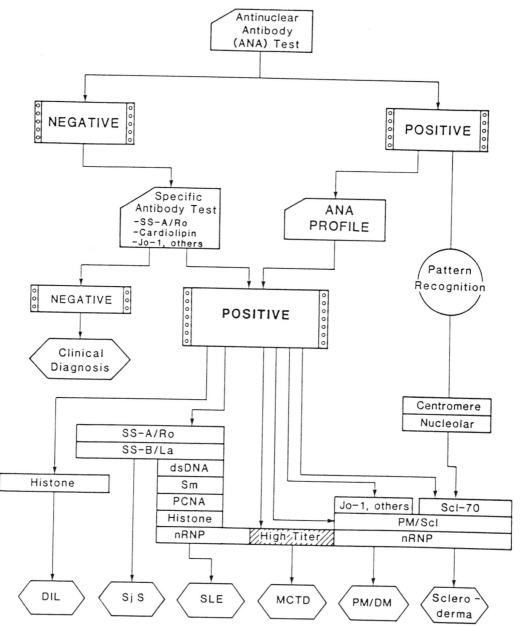

Fig. 13–3. An algorithm to indicate the diagnostic approach to the use of ANA in clinical rheumatology. ANA = antinuclear antibodies; DIL = drug-induced lupus; dsDNA = double-stranded DNA; MCTD = mixed connective tissue disease; nRNP = nuclear ribonucleoprotein; PCNA = proliferating cell nuclear antigen; PM/DM = polymyositis/dermatomyositis; SjS = Sjögren's syndrome; SLE = systemic lupus erythematosus; SS-A, SS-B = Sjögren's syndrome antigens A,B. (Reprinted from Fritzler, M.J.: Antinuclear antibodies in the investigation of rheumatic diseases. Bull Rheum Dis 35:3, 1985. Used by permission of the Arthritis Foundation.)

clinical data from the complete history and physical examination. Pertinent information from the social, family, and past medical history can be very helpful (Table 13–22). Extra-articular manifestations of joint diseases can be important in differentiating one disorder from another (Table 13–23). Back pain of back disease may be helpful because some types of arthritis are characteristically associated with back disorders (Table 13–24).

Eye involvement is commonly associated with systemic rheumatic disorders. Each of the layers of the eye is composed of tissue that can become involved in the pathologic processes leading to the systemic disease. Some parts of the eye share structural characteristics with other parts of the body (e.g., the sclera or uvea and the lining of synovial joints); thus, the eye disorder is a reflection of the generalized nature of the inflammatory process. Although many of the

Table 13–21. Polyarticular Presentation of Joint Pain

Cause	Acute Joint Pain and/or Inflammation	Chronic Joint Pain and/or Inflammation

Infection	Acute bacterial, especially gonococcus and meningococcus
	Haverhill fever (Streptobacillus moniliformis)
	Subacute bacterial endocarditis
	Viral infection, rubella, hepatitis B, other
	Spirochetal disease
	   Lyme disease
	   Syphilis (especially congenital)
		Viral infection, lymphogranuloma venereum
		Spirochetal disease
		   Lyme disease
		   Syphilis (especially congenital)

Sequel to infection	Acute rheumatic fever Whipple's disease	Jaccoud's arthritis (periarticular disease with reducible joint deformities associated with rheumatic fever and systemic lupus) Whipple's disease
Allergic or hypersensitivity disease	Drug reaction, serum sickness Henoch-Schönlein purpura Erythema nodosum Erythema multiforme	Erythema nodosum

Connective tissue disease	Systemic lupus erythematosus
	Necrotizing vasculitis
	   Polyarteritis nodosa
	   Wegener's granulomatosis
	   Churg-Strauss vasculitis
	   Relapsing polychondritis
	   Behçet's disease
	   Polymyalgia rheumatica
	   Henoch-Schönlein purpura
	Scleroderma
	Dermatomyositis
		Systemic lupus erythematosus
		Necrotizing vasculitis
		   Polyarteritis nodosa
		   Wegener's granulomatosis
		   Relapsing polychondritis
		   Behçet's disease
		   Polymyalgia rheumatica

Inflammatory joint diseases, cause unknown	Rheumatoid arthritis
	Juvenile rheumatoid arthritis
	Seronegative spondyloarthropathies
	   Psoriatic arthritis
	   Reiter's syndrome
	   Arthritis associated with inflammatory bowel disease: ulcerative colitis and regional enteritis
		Rheumatoid arthritis
		Juvenile rheumatoid arthritis
		Seronegative spondyloarthropathies
		   Psoriatic arthritis
		   Reiter's syndrome
		   Arthritis associated with inflammatory bowel disease
		   Ankylosing spondylitis

Metabolic and endocrine disorders	Gouty arthritis Pseudogout Hyperlipoproteinemia (type IIa and IV) Hemochromatosis Hyperparathyroidism	Gouty arthritis Pseudogout Ochronosis Hyperlipoproteinemia (type IV) Hemochromatosis–hypothyroidism Acromegaly Hyperparathyroidism

associated ocular lesions are potentially blinding, the presence of an ocular abnormality may be overlooked on careful examination. For example, the uveitis of the oligoarticular type of juvenile rheumatoid arthritis that potentially leads to cataract formation or blindness is usually asymptomatic. Thus, knowledge of such occult eye lesions is needed. Table 13–25 associates musculoskeletal disorders with potential ocular abnormalities.

Fever is an important associated finding because it defines the systemic nature of the disease and narrows the potential diagnosis (Table 13–3, column IX). Specific laboratory or radiologic tests can give strong support for a diagnosis or can define a disorder not previously considered (Tables 13–7, 13–8).

JOINT "NOISE" OR CREPITATION

DEFINITION

Joint crepitation is a palpable or audible grating or crunching sensation produced by joint motion. It may or may not be accompanied by discomfort. It occurs when roughened articular or extra-articular surfaces are rubbed together.

Table 13–22. Clinical Diagnostic Clues in Musculoskeletal Disorders

Historical Facts	Musculoskeletal Disorder to Consider
"Growing pains"	Rheumatic fever, juvenile rheumatoid arthritis
St. Vitus dance	Rheumatic fever
Trauma or accident involving bones, joints, or soft tissue; history of fracture	Post-traumatic osteoarthritis, precipitation of inflammatory arthritis; vertebral compression fracture
Occupation-related injury or repetitive trauma	Tendinitis, bursitis; low-back pain
Sports-related injury	Meniscal or ligamentous tear, internal derangement; lateral epicondylitis (tennis elbow); medial epicondylitis (golfer's elbow)
Sexual activity	Gonococcal arthritis, syphilis, hepatitis B dermatitis/arthritis syndrome, hepatitis B—associated polyarteritis nodosa, Reiter's syndrome (reactive arthritis)
Homosexual, active heterosexual outside of marriage, prostitution, history of venereal disease	
Drug addiction	Hepatitis B—associated dermatitis/arthritis syndrome or polyarteritis nodosa, pseudomonas sternoclavicular joint sepsis, gonococcal arthritis, amphetamine-related vasculitis, infectious arthritis (e.g., Staphylococcus)
Alcohol abuse	Traumatic arthritis, fractures, aseptic necrosis of joints, osteoporosis, gouty arthritis
Exposure to toxins (e.g., vinyl chloride)	Scleroderma-like finger abnormalities
Medications	
Antihypertensives	
Thiazide diuretics	Hyperuricemia, gouty arthritis
Hydralazine	Drug-induced lupus syndrome
Anticonvulsants	
Phenytoin	Drug-induced lupus syndrome
Trimethadione	
Antiarrhythmic	Drug-induced lupus syndrome
Procainamide	
Antibiotic	
Isoniazid (INH)	Drug-induced lupus syndrome
Anticancer drugs	Scleroderma-like disease
Bleomycin	
Hypouricemic drug	Systemic vasculitis
Allopurinol	
Corticosteroids	Osteoporosis with vertebral compression fractures, aseptic necrosis of joints, increased risk of infectious arthritis
Anticoagulant therapy	Hemarthrosis, heparin-related osteoporosis
Heparin	
Warfarin	
Allergy history	Serum sickness, systemic vasculitis
Penicillin, horse serum	
Hives/angioedema	Systemic lupus, angioneurotic edema with joint swelling and pain
Asthma	Churg-Strauss eosinophilic vasculitis
Travel history, with reference to:	
Endemic areas	
San Joaquin Valley, California	Coccidioidomycosis
Ohio Valley	Histoplasmosis
Lyme, Connecticut; other endemic areas for Lyme disease; history of a tick bite followed by a rash and joint pain	Lyme disease
Underdeveloped areas	Hepatitis B, tuberculosis
Dysentery	Reactive arthritis due to Salmonella, Shigella, Yersinia, Campylobacter
Eating of uncooked pork	Trichinosis
Infection, immunization history	
Venereal diseases	Gonoccccal arthritis, syphilis
Enteric infections, dysentery	Reactive arthritis due to Salmonella, Shigella, Yersinia, Campylobacter

Table 13—22.   Continued

Historical Facts	Musculoskeletal Disorder to Consider
Hepatitis B	Hepatitis B—associated arthritis—dermatitis syndrome, polyarteritis nodosa
Tuberculosis—mycobacterium and atypical	Monarticular synovitis, tenosynovitis, osteomyelitis
Fungal infection	Monarticular synovitis, polyarthritis, osteomyelitis, erythema nodosum
History of group A, beta-hemolytic streptococcal pharyngitis or demonstration of a recent infection with an increased ASLO titer, scarlet fever	Rheumatic fever
Rubella infection or recent immunization with rubella vaccine	Rubella arthritis
Recent or active infectious source for an infectious arthritis (sinusitis, pneumonia, endocarditis, otitis, abdominal sepsis, urinary tract infection, skin infection)	Septic arthritis, osteomyelitis
Medical illnesses	
Diabetes mellitus	Diabetic osteopathy, neuropathic (Charcot's) joint, osteomyelitis, finger contractures, peritendinitis of the shoulder, septic arthritis
Hemophilia and other bleeding disorders	Hemarthrosis, secondary osteoarthritis, muscle hematomas, nerve compression disorders due to hematomas
Endocrine disorders	
Hypothyroidism	Myopathy, joint pain and swelling, carpal tunnel syndrome, arthralgias, and myalgias
Acromegaly	Osteoarthritis, carpal tunnel syndrome, Raynaud's phenomenon, crystal-induced synovitis, back pain
Hyperparathyroidism	
Primary	Chondrocalcinosis and pseudogout, hyperuricemia and gout, synovitis, and joint erosions
Secondary	Renal osteodystrophy, subchondral resorption and disruption of joints, hydroxyapatite deposition, and soft tissue inflammation
Psoriasis	Psoriatic arthritis, hyperuricemia, and gout
Inflammatory bowel disease—ulcerative colitis, regional enteritis	Synovitis, sacroiliitis, spondylitis
Neurologic disorders—syphilis with tabes dorsalis, syringomyelia	Neuropathic (Charcot's) joint
Family history	
Gouty arthritis, uric acid kidney stones	
Psoriasis, psoriatic arthritis	
Osteoarthritis	
Connective tissue disorders	
Rheumatoid arthritis	
Systemic lupus erythematosus	
Scleroderma	
Ankylosing spondylitis, seronegative spondyloarthropathies	
Inherited disorders	
Marfan's syndrome	
Ehlers-Danlos syndrome	
Osteogenesis imperfecta	
Pseudoxanthoma elasticum	
Mucopolysaccharidosis	
Hemoglobinopathies—sickle cell anemia, thalassemia	
Amyloidosis	
Psychogenic musculoskeletal conditions	
Rheumatic fever	
Familial Mediterranean fever	

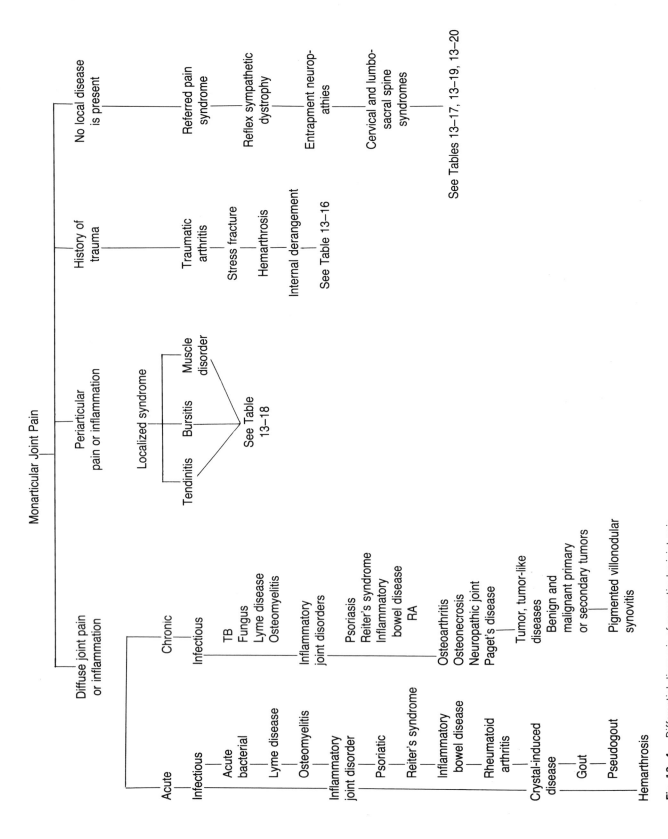

Fig. 13–4. Differential diagnosis of monarticular joint pain.

Table 13–23.   Extra-Articular Manifestations of Acute and Chronic Arthritis

System	Manifestation	Disease Association
Ocular	Conjunctivitis	Reiter's syndrome, relapsing polychondritis, psoriatic arthritis, Wegener's granulomatosis
	Episcleritis or scleritis	Rheumatoid arthritis, polyarteritis, Wegener's granulomatosis, relapsing polychondritis
	Keratoconjunctivitis sicca	Sjögren's syndrome, rheumatoid arthritis, scleroderma, dermatomyositis, polyarteritis nodosa, systemic lupus erythematosus Wegener's granulomatosis
	Uveitis (iridocyclitis)	Juvenile rheumatoid arthritis (oligoarticular type), Reiter's syndrome, ulcerative colitis, regional enteritis, ankylosing spondylitis, sarcoidosis, relapsing polychondritis, Wegener's granulomatosis
	Band keratopathy	Juvenile rheumatoid arthritis
	Ischemic optic neuropathy	Temporal arteritis
	Retinopathy (cotton wool spots, cytoid bodies, hemorrhages)	Systemic lupus erythematosus sarcoidosis, dermatomyositis
	"Heliotrope" eyelid	Dermatomyositis
	Rash	
	Proptosis	Wegener's granulomatosis
	Optic neuritis	Sarcoidosis
Skin	Butterfly malar rash	Systemic lupus erythematosus
	Discoid lupus	Systemic lupus erytematosus, discoid lupus
	Erythema nodosum	Sarcoidosis, ulcerative colitis, regional enteritis, Behçet's syndrome, tuberculosis, deep fungal infections, beta-hemolytic streptococcal infection
	Erythema multiforme, urticaria (hives)	Systemic lupus erythematosus, drug reaction, serum sickness, hypocomplementemic vasculitis
	Erythema marginatum	Rheumatic fever
	Keratodermia blennorrhagica, circinate balanitis	Reiter's syndrome
	Psoriasis, nail pitting	Psoriatic arthritis
	Mouth, nasal ulcers	Behçet's syndrome, Reiter's syndrome, systemic lupus erythematosus, Wegener's granulomatosis
	Nodules	Rheumatoid arthritis, Wegener's granulomatosis, polyarteritis, sarcoidosis, rheumatic fever, systemic lupus erythematosus, Behçet's syndrome, gouty tophi
	Small, red, nonblanching spots on upper extremities (vesiculopustules)	Gonococcal arthritis, rubella
	Infiltrative lesions	Sarcoidosis, amyloidosis, multicentric reticulohistiocytosis
	Nail lesions	Psoriatic arthritis, Reiter's syndrome, systemic lupus erythematosus
	Telangiectasias	Scleroderma, CRST syndrome, systemic lupus erythematosus, dermatomyositis
	Genital ulcers	Behçet's syndrome, Reiter's syndrome
	Palmar erythema	Rheumatoid arthritis
	Raynaud's phenomenon	Scleroderma, CRST syndrome, systemic lupus erythematosus, dermatomyositis, rheumatoid arthritis, cryoglobulinemia, mixed connective tissue disease
	Indurated, puckered, cobblestone skin	Eosinophilic fasciitis
	Positive band test	Systemic lupus erythematosus, mixed connective tissue disease, discoid lupus
	Necrosis of digits	Polyarteritis, systemic lupus, scleroderma
	Violaceous, heliotrope rash of the eyelids	Dermatomyositis
	Calcification	Scleroderma, CRST syndrome, dermatomyositis, polymyositis
	Folliculitis, pustules, furuncles	Behçet's syndrome
	Erythema chronicum migrans	Lyme disease
	Pyoderma gangrenosum	Ulcerative colitis, regional enteritis, rheumatoid arthritis (rare)
	Skin vasculitis (tender red macules, papules, or nodules)	Polyarteritis, Wegener's granulomatosis, rheumatoid vasculitis, systemic lupus erythematosus
	Leg ulcers	Felty's syndrome, rheumatoid arthritis, scleroderma, sickle-cell disease
	Fibrotic, hidebound, thick, taut skin (acrosclerosis)	CRST syndrome, scleroderma, porphyria cutanea tarda, amyloidosis, morphea (local scleroderma), linear scleroderma

Table 13–23.   Extra-Articular Manifestations of Acute and Chronic Arthritis (Continued)

System	Manifestation	Disease Association
Tendon	Livedo reticularis	Systemic lupus, vasculitides
	Tendinitis (tenosynovitis)	*Rheumatoid arthritis*, gonococcal arthritis, psoriatic arthritis, gout, tuberculosis
	Tendon sheath effusions	Rheumatoid arthritis
	Tendon nodules	Rheumatoid arthritis
Muscle	Myositis (myopathy)	*Dermatomyositis/polymyositis*, systemic lupus erythematosus, scleroderma, Sjögren's syndrome, sarcoidosis, rheumatoid arthritis, mixed connective tissue diseases, polyarteritis nodosa, hypothyroid myopathy, acromegalic myopathy
Hematopoietic	Anemia	
	Chronic disease (suppressed bone marrow)	Rheumatoid arthritis, systemic lupus, vasculitides, Reiter's syndrome, psoriatic arthritis, scleroderma, ankylosing spondylitis, juvenile rheumatoid arthritis, ulcerative colitis, regional enteritis, and other inflammatory disorders
	Hemolytic	*Systemic lupus erythematosus*
	Microangiopathic hemolytic anemia	Scleroderma, systemic lupus erythematosus, vasculitides, neoplastic disease
	Blood loss	Polyarteritis nodosa, scleroderma, gastrointestinal erosion due to NSAID and steroids, amyloidosis, neoplastic diseases
	Aplastic anemia	Systemic lupus erythematosus, eosinophilic fasciitis, due to gold salts or penicillamine or immunosuppressive therapy
	Thrombocytopenia	*Systemic lupus erythematosus*, other connective tissue disorders associated with DIC, Felty's syndrome
	Thrombocytosis	Polyarteritis nodosa, rheumatoid arthritis
	Disseminated intravascular coagulopathy	Systemic lupus, polyarteritis nodosa, scleroderma
	Leukopenia	*Systemic lupus*, Felty's syndrome
	Leukocytosis	*Polyarteritis*, Wegener's granulomatosis, Reiter's syndrome, *septic arthritis*, juvenile rheumatoid arthritis (Still's disease), rheumatoid arthritis
	Bleeding disorders	*Hemophilia*, anticoagulant therapy, systemic lupus erythematosus
	Circulating anticoagulant	*Systemic lupus erythematosus*, rheumatoid arthritis
	False positive VDRL	Systemic lupus erythematosus, rheumatoid arthritis, scleroderma
	Lymphadenopathy, splenomegaly	Rheumatoid arthritis, systemic lupus erythematosus, Still's disease, sarcoidosis, rubella, leukemia, lymphoma
Pulmonary	Pleuritis	*Systemic lupus erythematosus*, rheumatoid arthritis, juvenile rheumatoid arthritis (Still's disease), Wegener's granulomatosis, scleroderma
	Pulmonary infiltrates/nodules/cavities	*Wegener's granulomatosis*, systemic lupus, rheumatoid arthritis, *sarcoidosis, Churg-Strauss vasculitis*, scleroderma, dermatomyositis
	Hilar adenopathy	*Sarcoidosis*, erythema nodosum, *lymphoma*
	Pulmonary hypertension	Scleroderma, systemic lupus
	Disorders presenting with both pulmonary hemorrhage or infiltrates and nephritis	Goodpasture's syndrome, Wegener's granulomatosis, systemic lupus
Cardiovascular	Pericarditis	Systemic lupus, juvenile rheumatoid arthritis (Still's disease), rheumatic fever, scleroderma, rheumatoid arthritis (rare), relapsing polychondritis
	Myocarditis (including conduction defects)	Rheumatic fever, systemic lupus, dermatomyositis, scleroderma, sarcoidosis
	Endocarditis (including murmurs)	Rheumatic fever, systemic lupus, bacterial endocarditis, relapsing polychondritis
	Aortitis (aortic regurgitation)	Ankylosing spondylitis, Reiter's syndrome, rheumatoid arthritis (rare), relapsing polychondritis, Marfan's syndrome
	Decreased pulses and bruits	Takayasu's arteritis, giant cell arteritis
	Angina/myocardial ischemia and infarction	Polyarteritis, systemic lupus, giant cell arteritis, Kawasaki disease, relapsing polychondritis
	Aneurysms of the aorta	Relapsing polychondritis, Marfan's syndrome
	Hypertension	Systemic lupus, polyarteritis, Wegener's granulomatosis, Takayasu's arteritis, scleroderma

Table 13–23. Continued

System	Manifestation	Disease Association
Gastrointestinal	Vascular disorders: ischemic arterial disease (necrosis of digits)	Systemic lupus, polyarteritis, scleroderma
	Phlebitis	Systemic lupus, Behçet's disease
	Mouth ulcers	Behçet's disease, Reiter's syndrome, systemic lupus, inflammatory bowel diseases, erythema multiforme
	Tongue swelling	Acromegaly, amyloidosis, hypothyroidism, allergic reactions
	Esophageal motility disorder	Scleroderma, CRST syndrome
	Esophageal motility disorder	Dermatomyositis/polymyositis
	Gastric disorder	Pernicious anemia, ulceration due to vasculitis or medications (NSAIDs, steroids)
	Small- and large-bowel motility abnormality	Scleroderma
	Malabsorption	Scleroderma (bacterial overgrowth), Whipple's disease, amyloidosis, inflammatory bowel disorders, lymphoma, celiac disease, hypogammaglobulinemia, post intestinal bypass for obesity, biliary cirrhosis
	Diarrhea	Scleroderma, diabetic visceral neuropathy, inflammatory bowel diseases, celiac disease
	Bloody diarrhea (dysentery)	Reactive arthritis due to enteric pathogens (Salmonella, Shigella, Yersinia, Campylobacter), arthritis related to pseudomembranous colitis, inflammatory bowel diseases
	Gastrointestinal hemorrhage	Vasculitis of the gastrointestinal tract (systemic lupus, polyarteritis, Henoch-Schönlein purpura), amyloidosis, Ehlers-Danlos syndrome, scleroderma (telangiectasis, esophageal irritation and ulceration due to reflux), ulceration of stomach and duodenum due to NSAID and steroids
	Ileitis/colitis	Inflammatory bowel diseases (ulcerative colitis, regional enteritis), Behçet's disease, ischemic colitis due to vasculitis, infectious colitis due to enteric organisms
	Ischemic bowel disease/bowel infarction	Polyarteritis, systemic lupus
	Colonic disease/constipation	Scleroderma
	Pancreatitis	Systemic lupus, polyarteritis, polyarthritis and skin nodules due to fat necrosis
	Cholecystitis	Polyarteritis
	Splenomegaly	Felty's syndrome (RA with splenomegaly), juvenile RA of the systemic type (Still's disease), systemic lupus, serum sickness, drug reaction
	Splenomegaly	Endocarditis, acute infections (bacterial, viral, rickettsial), lymphoma, leukemia, metastatic neoplasms
	Organ rupture	Polyarteritis (gallbladder, hepatic), systemic lupus (spleen)
	Diverticular disease and rupture	Systemic lupus, polyarteritis
	Peritonitis	Systemic lupus, familial Mediterranean fever, tuberculosis
	Abdominal pain	Systemic lupus, polyarteritis, Henoch-Schönlein purpura, juvenile rheumatoid arthritis (Still's type), inflammatory bowel diseases, reactive arthritis associated with enteric infections, Behçet's disease, lymphoma, leukemia, intra-abdominal neoplasm, hyperparathyroidism
	Hepatitis	Arthritis-dermatitis syndrome, associated with hepatitis B infection, chronic active hepatitis with arthritis, polyarteritis associated with hepatitis B infection, systemic lupus, Sjögren's syndrome, scleroderma, gonococcal disease, sarcoidosis (granulomatous hepatitis), due to anti-inflammatory drugs and acetaminophen
Genitourinary/renal	Urethritis, prostatitis, vaginitis, cervicitis, pelvic inflammation	Reiter's syndrome, gonococcal arthritis
	Genital ulcers	Behçet's disease, Reiter's syndrome
	Genital rash	Reiter's syndrome, psoriasis
	Renal calculi	Hyperparathyroidism, inflammatory bowel disorders, gout

Table 13–23.   Extra-Articular Manifestations of Acute and Chronic Arthritis (Continued)

System	Manifestation	Disease Association
	Renovascular hypertension	Scleroderma, systemic lupus, polyarteritis, Takayasu's arteritis
	Glomerulonephritis	Systemic lupus, polyarteritis, Wegener's disease, Henoch-Schönlein purpura, Goodpasture's syndrome, endocarditis
	Nephrotic syndrome	Systemic lupus, amyloidosis, multiple myeloma, sickle cell anemia, Goodpasture's syndrome, Henoch-Schönlein purpura, syphilis, diabetes
	Hematuria	Nephritis due to systemic lupus, polyarteritis, Goodpasture's syndrome, Henoch-Schönlein purpura, thrombotic thrombocytopenic purpura, endocarditis, thrombocytopenia due to systemic lupus
Neurologic	Loss of proprioception, deep pain	Neuropathic (Charcot's) joint due to syphilis (tabes dorsalis), syringomyelia, diabetes mellitus
	Neuropathy (sensory, sensorimotor, motor, or mononeuritis multiplex)	Systemic lupus, polyarteritis, Wegener's disease, rheumatoid arthritis, amyloidosis, sarcoidosis, diabetes, multiple myeloma and macroglobulinemia, cryoglobulinemia, carcinoma
	Cerebrovascular accident	Systemic lupus, polyarteritis, giant cell arteritis, Wegener's disease, thrombotic thrombocytopenic purpura, Takayasu's arteritis, hypertension secondary to systemic disorders, thrombocytopenia secondary to systemic lupus and leukemia, hemorrhage due to hemophilia, septic embolism or ruptured mycotic aneurysm due to endocarditis
	Transverse myelitis	Systemic lupus, multiple sclerosis
	Spinal cord compression	Cervical, thoracic, or lumbar spondylosis caused by degenerative joint and disc disease, atlantoaxial and subaxial subluxation caused by rheumatoid arthritis, vertebral compression fracture caused by osteoporosis
	Seizure disorder	Systemic lupus, drug-induced lupus caused by anticonvulsants
	Meningitis (aseptic, septic)	Systemic lupus, polyarteritis, sarcoidosis, Lyme disease, syphilis, related to drugs (ibuprofen) given for systemic lupus
	Psychosis	Systemic lupus, caused by steroid medication
	Headache	Giant cell arteritis, related to cervical spondylosis, related to sinusitis due to systemic disorders, related to meningitis
Ear, nose, and throat	Temple pain, swelling and tenderness; temporal artery tenderness, nodularity or decreased pulsations	Giant cell arteritis
	Jaw claudication	Giant cell arteritis
	Blindness (transient, fixed, monocular, binocular)	Giant cell arteritis, Takayasu's arteritis, systemic lupus
	Tongue pain or swelling	Acromegaly, amyloidosis, hypothyroidism, Sjögren's syndrome, giant cell arteritis
	Sinusitis (sinus pain, drainage, sinus abnormalities on x-rays, history of sinusitis)	Wegener's granulomatosis
	Nasal septal ulcers, perforation or collapse (saddle nose deformity)	Wegener's granulomatosis, systemic lupus, relapsing polychondritis
	Ear abnormality	
	1. External ear inflammation or deformity	Relapsing polychondritis, connective tissue disorders associated with chondritis
	2. Otitis media, sensorineural hearing loss, serous otitis media	Wegener's granulomatosis, relapsing polychondritis, serous otitis media associated with polyarteritis
	3. Ossicle arthritis	Rheumatoid arthritis
	Salivary gland swelling, pain, tenderness; dry eyes and dry mouth	Sjögren's syndrome and the diseases associated with it
	Temporomandibular joint pain	Due to arthritis such as rheumatoid arthritis, due to jaw claudication related to giant cell arthritis
	Tracheal pain and/or tenderness, tracheal stenosis	*Relapsing polychondritis,* rheumatoid arthritis, ankylosing spondylitis
	Hoarseness	Cricoarytenoid disease due to rheumatoid arthritis, recurrent laryngeal nerve damage due to vasculitis, hypothyroidism, relapsing polychondritis

Italicized associations are common or characteristic.

Table 13–24. Disorders Involving Peripheral Joints and the Spine

Disease	Peripheral Arthritis	Area of Spine Involved	X-Ray Changes	Systemic Features	Other Features
Ankylosing spondylitis	Asymmetrical, large joint—hips, shoulders; 30% peripheral joint	Entire spine often begins at T12-L1 and ascends and descends	Obliteration of sacroiliac joints, sclerosis of apophyseal joints, kyphosis, fusion and ligamentous CA^{++}	Occasional	Iritis 15% HLA-B27 in 90%; negative rheumatoid factor (RF)
Reiter's syndrome	Asymmetrical, large, lower extremity joints, knees, ankles; heels, asymmetrical small joints of the hands; sausage shaped digits in toes	Sacroiliac joints asymmetrical and spotty spine disease	Extensive fusion uncommon except in sacroiliac joints; asymmetrical ligamentous CA^{++}	Frequent	Conjunctivitis or iritis; psoriasiform skin lesions, urethritis, HLA-B27 (75%); negative RF
Psoriatic arthritis	Asymmetrical DIP hand or toe disease, an RA-like disease, a mutilans picture, or an asymmetrical large-joint disease	Same as Reiter's syndrome	Same as Reiter's syndrome	Common	Psoriasis HLA-B27 (50%); negative RF
Colitic arthropathy	Asymmetrical, large, lower extremity joints; same as ankylosing spondylitis	Same as ankylosing spondylitis	Same as ankylosing spondylitis	Common	Bowel involvement may be subtle or strongly correlated with peripheral arthritis; erythema nodosum; HLA-B27 (50%); iritis; negative RF
Rheumatoid arthritis	Symmetrical polyarthritis small and large joints of upper and lower extremities	Upper cervical segments	Erosion, fusion rare, atlantoaxial subluxation (C1-C2) and subaxial subluxation	Common	(+) Rheumatoid factor (80%), nodules (20%), HLA-DR4; HLA-B27 not found; extra-articular manifestations
Degenerative arthritis (osteoarthritis)	Noninflammatory asymmetrical large- and small-joint disease; DIP disease—Heberden's nodes; PIP disease—Bouchard's node	Cervical and lumbar segments, no sacroiliitis	Sclerosis and spur formation, spondylosis	Never	Nerve root compression
Tuberculosis	Subacute or chronic monarthritis or tenosynovitis	Thoracic and lumbar segments	Destructive lesion in disc space with anterior collapse	Common	Tuberculosis elsewhere
Other infections	Monarthritis—highly inflammatory	Disc space apophyseal joints; unilateral sacroiliac	No change, or destructive lesion of bone	Common	Acute bacterial; IV drug abuse, brucellosis; other primary infection
Ochronosis	Same as degenerative arthritis	Diffuse	Disc degeneration and calcification; secondary degenerative changes	Never	Hereditary alkaptonuria; black sclerae and ear cartilage

PATHOPHYSIOLOGIC CONSIDERATIONS

A coarse crackle in the joints of some normal people is thought to come from tendons snapping over bony prominences and is of no pathologic significance. Generally, the finer the crepitus, the more significant it is clinically.

Crepitus may arise from the grating of roughened cartilages against one another, or from the rubbing of bone against bone, as in osteoarthritis. This crepitus is coarse. Local crepitus may be found over the patella in chondromalacia patellae.

Fine crepitus can be felt or heard when a chronically involved rheumatoid load-bearing joint (hip and knee) is moved. This crepitus is thought to be due to friction between severely destroyed articular cartilages. In-

Table 13–25. Ocular Manifestations in Rheumatic Diseases

Musculoskeletal Disorder	Clinical Characteristics	Associated Ocular Abnormalities
Rheumatoid arthritis	Symmetrical polyarthritis; subcutaneous nodules (20%), systemic disease; rheumatoid factor positive in 80%	*Keratoconjunctivitis sicca* (Sjögren's syndrome) (30%) Scleritis and episcleritis; necrotizing scleritis with scleromalacia perforans; uveitis secondary to scleritis
Juvenile rheumatoid arthritis	Oligoarticular type of arthritis (4 joints), systemic disease, ANA positive, rheumatoid factor negative	**Iridocyclitis (anterior uveitis) with secondary band keratopathy and cataract* (17%)
Ankylosing spondylitis	Spondylitis and sacroiliitis predominate with back pain; 30% with asymmetrical, large-joint, peripheral arthritis; HLA-B27 positive in 90%, men predominate	*Iridocyclitis (anterior uveitis)* (20%), conjunctivitis less commonly
Reiter's syndrome	Asymmetrical, large-joint polyarthritis and spondylitis common (20%); keratoderma blennorrhagia and circinate balanitis; urethritis. HLA-B27 positive in 80%	*Conjunctivitis* (a classic part of the triad of arthritis and uveitis and conjunctivitis) (50%); iridocyclitis (anterior uveitis) with intraocular hemorrhage and optic neuritis
Psoriatic arthritis	Asymmetrical large and small-joint polyarthritis; psoriasis with nail involvement; sacroiliitis and spondylitis (30%); HLA-B27 positive with back involvement	*Conjunctivitis*, uveitis (10%); scleritis (2%)
Systemic lupus erythematosus	Symmetrical polyarthritis; serositis; fever; skin rash; nephritis; CNS disease; cytopenias; positive ANA and anti-DNA; female predominance	Retinopathy, ischemic and hypertensive 　*Cotton wool patches* 　Cytoid bodies 　Hemorrhages Conjunctivitis Keratoconjunctivitis sicca (Sjögren's syndrome)
Polyarteritis nodosa	Polyarthritis, fever, mononeuritis multiplex, skin vasculitis, nephritis; WBC and platelets; positive. HBsAG in 20%	Toxic retinopathy with retinal hemorrhages or exudates Exudative retinal detachment Keratitis Conjunctivitis; scleritis Keratoconjunctivitis sicca (Sjögren's syndrome)
Scleroderma	Tight, hidebound skin, Raynaud's phenomenon, polyarthritis, dysphagia, hypertensive renal crisis, pulmonary fibrosis and hypertension; speckled ANA	*Tightness of the eyelids* Keratoconjunctivitis sicca (Sjögren's syndrome)
Polymyositis/dermatomyositis	Proximal muscle weakness due to myositis; skin rash in dermato patients; elevated muscle enzymes and abnormal EMG and muscle biopsy	*Violaceous "heliotrope" suffusion about the eyelids* Weakness of eye muscles Conjunctivitis, episcleritis, iritis Keratoconjunctivitis sicca (Sjögren's syndrome)
Giant cell arteritis	Headaches, visual loss, temporal artery swelling and tenderness, polymyalgia rheumatica symptoms, systemic disease, ESR positive, temporal artery biopsy	*Ischemic optic neuropathy* of the ophthalmic artery supplying the optic nerve; visual loss Central retinal artery occlusion
Wegener's granulomatosis	Granulomatous necrotizing angiitis of the upper or lower respiratory tract, focal necrotizing glomerulonephritis and arteritis; polyarthritis, skin vasculitis; elevated ESR, elevated WBC	*Proptosis* (18%) Conjunctivitis, scleritis, episcleritis, or corneoscleral ulcer (16%) Vasculitis of retina or optic nerve Tear sac inflammation (3%) Uveitis (2%)
Relapsing polychondritis	Chondritis of the ears, nose, and tracheobronchial tree; inner ear involvement; cardiovascular disease; positive cartilage biopsy	*Scleritis/episcleritis* (38%) Conjunctivitis (33%) Iritis/chorioretinitis (22%)
Sarcoidosis	Systemic granulomatous disease, lung, heart, muscle, and nodal involvement; acute or chronic arthritis; erythema nodosum; positive biopsy of skin, lung, lymph node. Elevated angiotensin-converting enzyme; positive Kveim test.	*Uveitis* (iris and ciliary bodies granulomatous in nature) Retinal perivasculitis Optic neuritis Scleritis and episcleritis—rare Eyelid involvement Conjunctival nodules

Italicized associated anomalies are most common.
*Can be asymptomatic and yet lead to blindness.

flamed, thickened synovial tissue can also give rise to a fine crepitation. This general type can be seen in rheumatoid arthritis and other inflammatory diseases associated with destructive joint disease and synovial inflammation.

Tendon crepitus, related to extensive fibrin deposition, occurs in certain kinds of trauma (such as the repeated use of tendons as occurs in sports or certain occupations) or inflammatory diseases (such as scleroderma). In scleroderma, crepitus produced by a rubbing together of the roughened surfaces of articular membranes or periarticular tendons and tendon sheaths gives a peculiar coarse, creaking, leathery sound that may be palpated or heard around the knees, wrists, and ankles. This friction rub may best be appreciated by auscultating the tendons with a stethoscope. Tendon crepitus is prominent after rest and diminishes with repetitive movement.

Knuckle cracking is due to mechanical subluxation of the joint, with gas formation in the joint caused by the accompanying decrease in intra-articular pressure. The vaporization of joint fluid produces an audible crack.

Finally, crepitus of various types can be seen in osteochondritis, ochronosis, and hemochromatosis.

DIAGNOSTIC EVALUATION

Crepitation from within the joint should be differentiated from cracking sounds caused by the slipping of ligaments or tendons over bony surfaces during motion. The characteristic clinical features of the causes of crepitus should be considered in the diagnostic process. Appropriate clinical features, laboratory tests, and x-rays should be used as needed.

JOINT OR MORNING STIFFNESS

DEFINITION

Stiffness implies a sense of relative immobility, disability, or restriction of the joints. When it occurs in rheumatic diseases, it is most prominent after inactivity of the joints and is notably worse in the morning. Whereas the duration of morning stiffness is a reliable parameter of disease activity in inflammatory disorders such as rheumatoid arthritis, the severity of stiffness is not a reliable symptom. Some patients equate stiffness with pain, others with fatigue, soreness, aching,

Table 13–26. Causes of Joint or Morning Stiffness

Systemic inflammatory disorders
  Rheumatoid and juvenile rheumatoid arthritis
    Peripheral joint stiffness
  Seronegative spondyloarthropathies
    Back and peripheral joint stiffness
      Ankylosing spondylitis
      Reiter's syndrome, psoriatic arthritis, colitic arthropathies
  Connective tissue disorders
    Systemic lupus erythematosus
    Scleroderma
    Polymyalgia rheumatica/temporal arteritis
Noninflammatory joint diseases
  Osteoarthritis
  Ochronosis
  Mucopolysaccharidoses (Hurler's and Morquio's syndromes)
  Stiff-man syndrome (stiffness in proximal distal muscles, abdomen, and back manifested by walking with a straight back and turning en bloc)
  Hemochromatosis
  Hypothyroidism (manifested by stiffness on cold exposure)
Miscellaneous
  Serum sickness and other edema-producing disorders
  Systemic infections (e.g., influenza)
  Neurologic disorders (e.g., Parkinson's disease)

tightness, swelling, or weakness, while others cannot describe clearly what they feel. When stiffness is mild, the patient can become limber in minutes; when severe, stiffness may improve in hours or not at all. In systemic disorders (such as rheumatoid arthritis), stiffness can be generalized and long-lasting; in noninflammatory disease (such as osteoarthritis) it is of shorter duration, more localized to the involved joints, and less severe. Changes in environmental temperature, humidity, and barometric pressure can influence stiffness or its symptomatic onset of duration.

PATHOPHYSIOLOGIC CONSIDERATIONS

The basic process leading to joint stiffness is not well defined but may involve an alteration, with inactivity, in the sol-gel characteristics of synovial fluid, a rise in intra-articular friction caused by disruption of the normally smooth cartilaginous surface, cross-linking of articular cartilage, transudation of fluid into para-articular tissues because of the loss of pumping action at rest, or a combination of these factors.

Among disorders that typically are associated with joint stiffness are systemic inflammatory disorders and noninflammatory joint disease (Table 13–26).

DIAGNOSTIC EVALUATION

Most of the disorders can be diagnosed on the basis of clinical criteria. Laboratory tests may reveal the pathologic processes causing stiffness. Rheumatoid factor, antinuclear antibody, complete blood count with differential, erythrocyte sedimentation rate, and thyroid function tests are appropriate screening tests. The clinical impression, supported by these tests, should elucidate the cause of joint stiffness. X-rays and radionuclide bone scanning may be needed in some cases. Histocompatibility antigen HLA-B27 is used only in cases of spondyloarthropathies that are difficult to diagnose.

JOINT EFFUSION (FLUID)

DEFINITION

Intra-articular collection of fluid, with or without associated synovial thickening, causes mild to marked distension of the joint capsule that can be palpated throughout the circumference of a joint or in a particular area. Ballotability or a bulge sign (the ability to push the fluid from one side of a knee joint to the other and observe a fluid wave) is caused by intra-articular fluid, while a doughy feeling is attributed to synovial thickening (in many instances both features are present).

PATHOPHYSIOLOGIC CONSIDERATIONS

Nearly any intra-articular disorder can alter the characteristics of synovial fluid by the disorder's effect on the synovial membrane itself or on other intra-articular structures. Any injury or irritation to the synovial membrane can lead to an increased production of synovial fluid and thus to the development of an effusion. The associated synovial fluid characteristics (glucose, protein, or complement levels; the white blood cell or erythrocyte count; the presence of bacteria or tumor cells; or the presence of rheumatoid factors or immune complexes) are dependent on the underlying disorder and its pathogenesis. The volume of the effusion varies greatly, from as little as 4 ml to as much as 250 ml. The amount of effusion is one measure of the severity of arthritis and can be used for comparison with previous arthrocenteses. Low effusion volumes do not mean absence of an important intra-articular process.

Disorders leading to effusions fall into several broad categories. They may be noninflammatory, such as trauma or osteoarthritis; inflammatory, such as rheumatoid arthritis, or crystal-induced disease (gout and pseudogout); infectious, such as bacterial or tuberculous infections; or hemorrhagic, such as disorders leading to a bloody effusion such as fractures, hemophilia, or pigmented villonodular synovitis.

DIAGNOSTIC EVALUATION

A complete history and physical examination are indicated to determine the clinical diagnosis of the joint disorder leading to the effusion (e.g., a history of trauma, hemophilia, or anticoagulation therapy, or clinical and physical clues supporting a diagnosis of rheumatoid arthritis or gout).

Analysis of joint fluid should be performed as part of the diagnostic evaluation in any patient with joint disease with an effusion. Some common or therapeutically important diseases (rheumatoid arthritis, gout, septic arthritis) can be quickly and definitively diagnosed in this manner. Even with a well-established diagnosis, one might demonstrate a superimposed joint disorder that is altering the clinical presentation (e.g., the coexistence of gout and pseudogout), or the superimposition of bacterial sepsis on a chronic inflammatory disorder (such as rheumatoid arthritis, or systemic lupus). The most commonly performed evaluations of synovial fluid include gross examination to define color, clarity, and viscosity; cell count and differential; crystal examination using polarizing microscopy; Gram's stains and cultures; and biochemical and serologic tests including glucose. Protein analysis provides little information. Complement levels, which are decreased in some SLE, rheumatoid arthritis, and septic joint fluids, are rarely helpful for diagnosis. Rheumatoid factor can be positive in the synovial fluid of some rheumatoid patients prior to its presence in the serum.

Tables 13–6 and 13–27 tabulate the various joint disorders by fluid group based upon the degree of inflammation. The final diagnosis is based on these synovial fluid findings in the clinical setting defined by the history and physical examination. Because of the overlap in synovial fluid WBC counts, the physician bases a diagnosis on the clinical criteria, the general synovial fluid profile, and other specific synovial fluid characteristics, such as the characteristic crystals in gout and pseudogout and a positive Gram's stain or culture in septic arthritis. Septic arthritis can be diagnosed only by appropriate cultures in the correct clinical setting, and it can coexist with crystal-induced arthritis (gout or pseudogout) or other types of inflammatory joint disorders.

Table 13–27.   Joint Disorders Associated with Various Synovial Fluid Groups

Noninflammatory Joint Effusions	Inflammatory Joint Effusions	Hemarthrosis (bloody joint fluid)
GROUP I (WBC < 2000/mm³)	GROUP II (WBC > 2000/mm³)	GROUP III
Osteoarthritis	Rheumatoid arthritis	Trauma, with or without fractures
Traumatic arthritis	Juvenile RA	Pigmented villonodular synovitis
Mechanical derangement	Seronegative spondyloarthropathies	Synovioma, other tumors
Aseptic necrosis	Ankylosing spondylitis	Hemangioma
Paget's disease	Psoriatic arthritis	Neuropathic (Charcot's) joint
Charcot's joints	Reiter's syndrome	Hemophilia and other bleeding disorders
Hypertrophic osteoarthropathy	Colitic arthritis	Anticoagulant therapy
Ochronosis	Diffuse connective tissue diseases	Thrombocytopenia
Ehlers-Danlos syndrome	Systemic lupus erythematosus	Scurvy
Wilson's disease	Scleroderma	Ruptured aneurysm
Hyperparathyroidism	Polymyositis	Arteriovenous fistula
Acromegaly	Necrotizing vasculitis	
Sickle-cell disease	Polyarteritis nodosa	
Amyloidosis	Wegener's granulomatosis	
Hemochromatosis	Polychondritis	
Pigmented villonodular synovitis, tumors	Behçet's disease	
Erythema nodosum	Henoch-Schönlein purpura	
	Polymyalgia rheumatica/temporal arteritis	
	Churg-Strauss angiitis	
	Crystal-induced arthritis	
	Gout	
	Pseudogout	
	Hydroxyapatite arthritis	
	Infectious arthritis	
	Bacterial	
	Spirochetal, including Lyme disease	
	Tuberculous	
	Viral	
	Fungal	
	Parasitic	
	Bacterial endocarditis	
	Enteropathic disorders	
	Postileal bypass arthritis	
	Postsalmonella, Shigella, Yersinia, Campylo- bacter arthritis	
	Whipple's disease	
	Systemic disorders	
	Infiltrative disease	
	Sarcoidosis	
	Multicentric reticulohistiocytosis	
	Leukemia	
	Hyperlipoproteinemias	
	Agammaglobulinemia	
	Serum sickness	
	Palindromic rheumatism	
	Familial Mediterranean fever	

LIMITATION OF JOINT RANGE OF MOTION

DEFINITION

Disease in the joint or periarticular tissues (tendons, bursae) can lead to a decrease in the normal arc of motion of a particular joint. Active motion is that produced by voluntary movement of the joint; passive motion is that achieved by the observer moving the joint for the patient. In any painful joint, passive motion will be greater than active motion. Passive motion, then, is a more reliable indication of joint disorder. When the degrees of limitation of active and passive motion are about equal, intra-articular disorder is likely. Limited active motion may be produced by periarticular disorders such as bursitis, tendinitis, and tendon rupture. Muscle weakness, such as that seen in polymyositis, inhibits active motion.

PATHOPHYSIOLOGIC CONSIDERATIONS

Limitation of range of motion of a joint may be caused by intra-articular factors such as destruction of the articulating surfaces which itself is caused by destructive joint disorders such as rheumatoid arthritis, juvenile rheumatoid arthritis, seronegative spondyloarthropathies (ankylosing spondylitis, Reiter's syndrome, psoriatic arthritis), osteoarthritis, septic arthritis, severe traumatic arthritis or fracture, severe chronic gout and pseudogout, multicentric reticulohistiocytosis, malignancy, or neuropathic (Charcot's) joint.

Other intra-articular factors limiting joint range of motion are impingement by hypertrophic spurs, which is caused by primary osteoarthritis and the many causes of secondary osteoarthritis (Table 13–13); subluxation (displacement beyond normal movement of a joint but with persistent cartilage to cartilage contact), which can be caused by destructive disorders such as rheumatoid arthritis or can occur in post-traumatic disorders; fibrous adhesions, which are related to intra-articular inflammatory or septic lesions or can occur in the healing phase of post-traumatic arthritis or following surgical procedures; bony ankylosis, which can occur in the setting of chronic inflammatory joint diseases (particularly rheumatoid arthritis, juvenile rheumatoid arthritis, and the seronegative spondyloarthropathies) or after surgical (ankylosis) fusion in the

treatment of types of inflammatory joint disorders or septic arthritis; joint effusion or synovial hypertrophy, which can be caused by most of the inflammatory joint diseases and noninflammatory disorders such as osteoarthritis, pigmented villonodular synovitis, and traumatic arthritis; loose bodies, which are caused by the breaking off of osteoarthritic spurs or by osteochondromatosis; and meniscal tears, which are due to trauma or degenerative meniscal disease.

Extra-articular factors can also limit joint range of motion. Capsular contracture is due to inflammatory joint disorders or occurs after surgery. Tendon shortening results from inflammatory, traumatic, or surgical causes. Tenosynovial adhesions are related to inflammatory tenosynovial disorders (Table 13–18) or occur after surgery. Muscle spasm is related to pain or occurs as a response to local disorder. Finally, pain or fear of pain is one of the major causes of failure to move a joint (see the section on joint pain).

DIAGNOSTIC EVALUATION

A complete history and physical examination will define the cause of limitation of range of motion in most situations. Laboratory tests such as latex fixation, HLA-B27, and uric acid levels may be needed to define the joint disorder leading to limited range of motion.

Specific x-rays of the involved joint will define both bony tissue changes (fracture, the typical changes of osteoarthritis with spur formation or rheumatoid arthritis, and loose bodies) and soft tissue changes that may be associated with motion abnormalities.

An arthrogram, which is an x-ray of a joint that has been injected with contrast dye and air and stressed to better define anatomic abnormalities, is particularly helpful when seeking a structural defect such as meniscal tear, a ligamentous disorder, or a loose body. Arthrogram can also define the presence of a Baker's (popliteal or calf) cyst or pigmented villonodular synovitis.

A bone scan can be helpful when the patient history, physical examination, and laboratory and x-ray information are nondiagnostic. Characteristic bone scan patterns can be seen in inflammatory joint disorders, septic arthritis or osteomyelitis, osteonecrosis, osteoarthritis, fractures (stress, traumatic, pathologic resulting from malignancy, or osteomalacia), and malignancy.

Certain internal derangements such as meniscal tears or ligamentous abnormalities can be viewed directly or treated through the arthroscope. This technique is not commonly used for the diagnosis of inflammatory joint disease, save for some cases of monarticular arthritis in which sepsis (primarily tuberculosis) or pigmented villonodular synovitis is considered. Using this procedure can, in some situations, preclude arthrotomy, a more extensive surgical procedure.

JOINT SWELLING

DEFINITION

Joint enlargement is reliable, objective evidence of a disease process.

PATHOPHYSIOLOGIC CONSIDERATIONS AND DIFFERENTIAL DIAGNOSIS

A swollen joint may be the result of either an intra-articular or an extra-articular process.

Intra-articular processes include effusion, synovial hypertrophy, combinations of effusion and synovial hypertrophy, and bony enlargement. Effusion is an accumulation in a joint of synovial fluid, purulent material, or blood that can be easily palpated or balloted. Common causes of effusions include inflammatory joint disorders (especially rheumatoid arthritis, systemic lupus erythematosus, juvenile rheumatoid arthritis, crystal-induced disorders, septic arthritis, seronegative spondyloarthropathies, and other disorders); disorders of cartilage and bone (especially osteoarthritis and Paget's disease), and localized causes of joint disease (especially hemarthrosis related to trauma such as fracture, internal derangement, traumatic arthritis, or hemophilia or to pigmented villonodular synovitis).

Synovial hypertrophy, thickening of synovial tissue, usually has a doughy feeling and is associated with diffuse extra-articular swelling. Swelling of synovial tissue can be caused by infiltration by tissue fluid, mononuclear or malignant cells, or polymorphonuclear leukocytes, and by the development of hypervascularity and villous hypertrophy. Disorders that lead to such synovial membrane changes include rheumatoid and juvenile rheumatoid arthritis, seronegative spondyloarthropathies, diffuse connective tissue disorders, septic arthritis, arthritis associated with infiltrative disorders and malignancy, benign joint tumors, and pigmented villonodular synovitis.

Bony enlargement is commonly associated with bone hypertrophy caused by primary or secondary osteoarthritis. It may or may not be associated with an effusion and tends to be more firm and irregular in shape. Causes include the many disorders that lead to

osteoarthritis (Table 13–13). Osteophytes, which produce a swollen appearance, are called Heberden's nodes when in the DIP position and Bouchard's nodes in the PIP position. A new or healed fracture of a juxta-articular bone can also lead to a bony abnormality and appear as joint swelling.

Extra-articular processes include bursal effusions, tenosynovial hypertrophy, interstitial edema, and nodular swellings. Accumulations of fluid in bursae are sharply defined, fluctuant in a confined area, and closely associated with bony prominences such as the olecranon, greater trochanter, and first metatarsal head and in the prepatellar area. The disorders that typically lead to bursal swelling (bursitis) include rheumatoid arthritis, gouty arthritis, traumatic bursitis, septic bursitis, and about bony prominences caused by osteoarthritis (bunion, first metatarsophalangeal joint). A popliteal (Baker's) cyst, which can result from many joint disorders, can protrude from the posterior knee and reflect bursal or capsular swelling and fluid accumulation.

In tenosynovial hypertrophy, synovial tissue surrounding tendons can become inflamed and swollen, leading to joint swelling and fine crepitation on physical examination. Such extra-articular synovial hypertrophy is most prominent in the tendon sheaths of the ankle and dorsum of the hand, where the hypertrophy is confined and demarcated by retinacula. This finding is most commonly associated with rheumatoid arthritis, seronegative spondyloarthropathies, tuberculosis or gonococcal tenosynovitis, gouty arthritis, and traumatic tenosynovitis.

Interstitial edema, a collection of tissue fluid, is characterized by a diffuse, ill-defined border, distal swelling, and absence of an intra-articular effusion, joint tenderness or pain, warmth, or erythema. Causes include congestive heart failure.

Nodular swellings can be felt over joints or areas exposed to repeated trauma (such as the olecranon, back of head or heel, ischiatic tuberosity, external ear, or bridge of the nose in patients wearing eyeglasses) and may be due to rheumatoid nodules, gouty tophi, xanthomata, or amyloid masses. Tendon nodules occur in rheumatoid arthritis, systemic lupus, and rheumatic fever. Some nodular swellings over rheumatoid joints are due to a reducible synovium herniated through defects in the joint capsule. A ganglion is a cystic swelling on the dorsum of the hand that may be found near and often attached to a tendon sheath or joint capsule; it is believed to be derived from these structures. Ganglia are also noted on the fingers and dorsum of the foot.

DIAGNOSTIC EVALUATION

The evaluation should include the clinical diagnosis, laboratory testing (e.g., ANA, latex fixation), and x-ray evaluation for localization and evaluation of the cause of joint swelling. At times an arthrogram is needed to define potential defects in intra-articular structures or to demonstrate a Baker's cyst.

JOINT DEFORMITY

DEFINITION

A misalignment of a joint results in deformity of the limb.

PATHOPHYSIOLOGIC CONSIDERATIONS AND CLASSIFICATION

Misalignment is caused by various joint disorders, leading to ligament destruction, bony enlargement, collapse of bone from erosive disease, subluxation (displacement beyond normal alignment with maintained cartilage-to-cartilage contact), and contractures of surrounding soft tissues.

Flexion Deformity (Contracture). This is an inability to passively move a joint to the fully extended position. The knee, hip, elbow, wrists, and fingers are joints with frequent flexion contractures. The inability to dorsiflex (extend) the ankle to neutral is termed an equinus deformity. An extensor lag is the difference between passive extension by the examiner (which can be normal) and active extension from the flexed position by the patient (which is less than normal). Such a lag can be seen in chronic joint disease, especially after reconstructive surgery.

Flexion deformities can be found in any joint that causes pain but need not be associated with active pain or inflammation. The patient assumes the flexed position as a pain-reducing mechanism, or the position occurs concomitant to the joint disease. A pillow under the knee is one of the commonly used (and inappropriate) methods by which a patient attempts to diminish joint pain. Such positioning can lead to a flexion deformity. The faulty mechanics caused by this deformity can increase the energy expenditure necessary for ambulation and accelerate the destruction of the involved and surrounding joints beyond the destruction caused by the disease process itself.

Disease processes most commonly associated with flexion deformities are those that cause chronic pain and joint destruction because of an underlying inflammatory disorder (with its associated synovial hypertrophy, effusions, and periarticular soft-tissue inflammation), and neuromuscular disorders that lead to spasticity and muscle atrophy with altered mechanics around the joint.

Joint disorders include rheumatoid and juvenile rheumatoid arthritis as well as seronegative spondyloarthropathies, most specifically psoriatic arthritis and ankylosing spondylitis. Whereas many patients develop a wet, inflammatory type of synovitis manifested by redness, warmth, and swelling, others develop a dry, ankylosing type of disease with a propensity for contractures. Neuromuscular causes of flexion deformities include cerebral palsies and other spastic disorders.

Valgus and Varus Deformities. These skeletal deformities refer to the distal segment; lateral deviation is called valgus, and medial deviation is called varus. For example, in the knee, lateral deviation of the leg below the knee (knock-knees) is called genu valgum; medial deviation (bow legs) is called genu varum. In the wrist, deformities are referred to by the long bones (e.g., radial deviation, ulnar drift, volar subluxation).

Destructive joint disorders lead to such deformities and include inflammatory diseases (rheumatoid arthritis, juvenile rheumatoid arthritis, and seronegative spondyloarthropathies) and noninflammatory diseases (osteoarthritis). Although varus and valgus deformities at the knee can be caused by various joint disorders, genu varum is most commonly associated with osteoarthritis, and genu valgum with rheumatoid arthritis. Ulnar deviation of the fingers and volar subluxation of the wrist are deformities associated with rheumatoid arthritis and other inflammatory joint disorders. Jaccoud's syndrome (postrheumatic fever syndrome) is an uncommon condition characterized by flexion deformities of the metacarpophalangeal joints with ulnar deviation caused by recurrent episodes of soft-tissue, periarticular inflammation. Such changes are seen in both rheumatic fever and systemic lupus erythematosus.

DIAGNOSTIC EVALUATION

Misalignment can be defined clinically or on x-ray by the determination of the juxtaposition of bony structures constituting a joint. Laboratory tests are helping in defining the type of systemic or local disease causing the deformity (e.g., latex fixation for rheumatoid arthritis, or antinuclear antibody for systemic lupus).

However, the clinical diagnosis is usually the most helpful one.

POPLITEAL (BAKER'S) CYST

DEFINITION

This is a fluctuant swelling in the popliteal area, occasionally extending into the calf and presenting superficially at the medial border of the gastrocnemius muscle. Typical symptoms include swelling, fullness, and pain. Rupture and dissection of the cyst is not uncommon and presents as a classic picture of thrombophlebitis (so-called pseudothrombophlebitis).

PATHOPHYSIOLOGIC CONSIDERATIONS

Popliteal cysts may form from three processes. They may result from posterior herniation of the joint capsule caused by increased intra-articular pressure. The pressure is related to a knee joint lesion and its concomitant accumulation of fluid or synovial membrane thickening. Distension of one of the six bursae (most commonly the gastrocnemius-semimembranous bursa) associated with the posteromedial knee by fluid originating as a result of the knee lesion may also cause popliteal cysts. Finally, the cysts may result from accumulation of fluid in a noncommunicating bursa. A ball-valve mechanism is often found through which fluid freely passes from the knee to the cyst but not in the opposite direction.

In half of the cases, some abnormality of the knee joint is present. Almost any inflammatory or noninflammatory joint disorder can lead to the development of physical conditions (i.e., synovial fluid production) that result in the formation of the cyst. The most commonly associated disorders include osteoarthritis, rheumatoid arthritis, cartilage tears, or trauma.

Synovial cysts, in rheumatoid arthritis, can be seen in other joints (e.g., a cyst connecting with the hip joint may present anteriorly as a mass in the groin or posteriorly with sciatic pain).

Dissection or rupture of these cysts can simulate thrombophlebitis (including a positive Homans' sign, redness, warmth, and swelling of the calf). The inflammation generated by the ruptured popliteal cyst is caused by the release, into calf tissues, of hydrolytic enzymes and inflammatory fluid. Baker's cysts, especially in rheumatoid arthritis, rarely can entrap the lower sciatic nerve with the associated neurologic abnormalities.

The differential diagnosis includes aneurysms, benign neoplasms, varicosities, and thrombophlebitis.

DIAGNOSTIC EVALUATION

Patient History and Physical Examination

The presence of the cyst is usually defined by the patient's complaint of a swelling in the popliteal fossa and its recognition on physical examination. At times, the patient presents with acute knee or calf pain, and the physician must differentiate between thrombophlebitis and a cyst that has dissected or ruptured into the calf. If the patient has past or present history of knee disease, the physician must have a high index of suspicion and perform a detailed joint history and examination to define the presence of a knee disorder. Other causes of posterior knee and calf pain and swelling should be ruled out.

Diagnostic Studies

The diagnosis of a popliteal cyst should be made as definitively as possible because specific therapy will be based on the presence or absence of a cyst. If a cyst is present, therapy will be aimed at the cause of the joint or bursal disorder (e.g., local cortisone injection and aspiration of joint fluid in inflammatory joint disease or osteoarthritis, and repair of cartilage tears or immobilization for traumatic arthritis). If a disorder such as phlebitis is present, anticoagulation therapy is indicated.

Diagnostic Approach

If a popliteal cyst is strongly considered (i.e., knee disease is present and phlebitis is unlikely), an arthrogram of the involved knee or a sonogram or CT scan of the calf is performed. The former test involves knee arthrocentesis with the aspiration of fluid and injection of a contrast medium and air. In most cases, a lateral x-ray of the knee will demonstrate the popliteal or calf cavity filled with contrast medium and air. In some patients, the cyst does not communicate with the joint and the arthrogram is negative.

If the arthrogram is negative, a sonogram of the knee, calf, or both can be performed to define the cystic area within the semimembranous muscle or posterior knee. If an arthrogram is not easily available, an initial sonograph is an appropriate and sensitive diagnostic test. Radionuclide injection into the knee or directly into the cyst with subsequent scanning is another test, though not commonly performed.

If phlebitis is as likely to be the cause of the symptoms and signs as a popliteal cyst, one may need to rule out the most clinically important disorder first and do a venogram. An arthrogram or sonogram can then be done with some leisure in view of the lack of phlebitis. Rarely, a popliteal cyst can coexist with thrombophlebitis. If a ruptured, dissected popliteal cyst is the cause of the calf pain, anticoagulation therapy (for presumed, but not demonstrated, thrombophlebitis) can lead to massive bleeding into the bed of the ruptured, inflamed cyst. Thus, one can appreciate the need for the definitive diagnosis of the popliteal cyst or thrombophlebitis.

FELTY'S SYNDROME (FS)

DEFINITION

This is a variant of seropositive rheumatoid arthritis with splenomegaly and granulocytopenia (<2000 granulocytes/mm³). Although the complete triad (rheumatoid arthritis, decreased white blood cell count, splenomegaly) is required for a diagnosis, some patients may be considered for the diagnosis when only two features are present; the third appears after a period of observation. Rheumatoid arthritis patients with Felty's syndrome typically have severe articular disease, profound immunologic abnormalities (positive, high-titered rheumatoid factor [98%], positive granulocyte-specific antinuclear antibodies [60%], hyperglobulinemia, hypocomplementemia, and cryoglobulinemia), extra-articular manifestations (rheumatoid nodules, lymphadenopathy, leg ulcers, pleurisy, neuropathy, scleritis, and Sjögren's syndrome), an increased risk of infections, and hematologic abnormalities (anemia of chronic disease and anemia associated with shortened survival time because of splenomegaly and thrombocytopenia).

PATHOPHYSIOLOGIC CONSIDERATIONS

Felty's syndrome is uncommon, occurring in the 1% of patients with rheumatoid arthritis who are severely involved, and immunologically active. Splenomegaly represents both that hyperimmune state and the sequestration function of the spleen. Granulocytopenia appears to be multifactorial in origin and involves ingestion and surface-coating of immune complexes which leads to impaired granulocyte functions and facilitates the removal of granulocytes by the mon-

ocyte-phagocyte (RES) system; granulocyte-specific antinuclear and cell surface antibodies; sequestration in the spleen with or without premature destruction of granulocytes; and bone marrow suppressant factors.

Splenomegaly and granulocytopenia may be caused, in patients with rheumatoid arthritis, by superimposed illnesses such as drug reactions, myeloproliferative disorders and reticuloendothelial malignancies, cirrhosis, amyloidosis, sarcoidosis, tuberculosis, and chronic infections. These disorders must be considered and excluded before a diagnosis of Felty's syndrome is certain.

DIAGNOSTIC EVALUATION

The diagnosis is based on the above-mentioned clinical criteria and is definitive only after other potential causes of splenomegaly and granulocytopenia are ruled out using the pertinent clinical and laboratory facts.

Appropriate laboratory tests include complete blood count with differential and close examination of the peripheral smear, platelet count, sedimentation rate (usually very high), rheumatoid factor, antinuclear antibody, complement levels (CH_{50}, C_3, and C_4), and bone marrow aspiration and biopsy. The bone marrow aspiration and biopsy is needed to rule out other causes of granulocytopenia and splenomegaly, for example, malignant or infectious causes. Liver-spleen scanning is sometimes done to define the size and anatomic characteristics of the spleen and associated hepatomegaly (mild hepatomegaly is common in FS).

RAYNAUD'S PHENOMENON (RP)

DEFINITION

Raynaud's phenomenon is recurrent attacks, usually related to cold exposure or emotional stress, consisting of sequential pallor extending from the distal digits proximally, followed by cyanosis and finally by rubor, often associated with pain or tingling. Attacks last from minutes to hours, can involve the lower extremities in 40% of patients, and may be associated with only one or two of the classic color changes.

PATHOPHYSIOLOGIC CONSIDERATIONS

This disorder, related to episodic ischemia of the digits, can take the form of a primary, idiopathic proc-

Table 13–28. Causes of Raynaud's Phenomenon

Primary
  Idiopathic disorder—50 to 90% of patients
Secondary
  Collagen vascular disease
    Scleroderma—90% have RP
    Systemic lupus erythematosus—70% have RP
    Rheumatoid arthritis—5% have RP
    Polymyositis—25% have RP
    Vasculitis
  Traumatic vasospastic disease
    Repetitive local trauma
    Frostbite
  Peripheral vascular disease
    Atherosclerosis
    Arteriosclerosis obliterans
    Arterial emboli
    Digital artery thrombosis
    Aneurysms of the ulnar artery
  Nerve compression
    Thoracic outlet and carpal tunnel syndromes
  Drugs/chemicals
    Ergot alkaloids
    Methysergide
    Polyvinyl chloride
    Arsenic
    Beta blockers (unopposed α tone)
    Bleomycin
  Hematologic abnormalities
    Cryoglobulinemia
    Cold agglutinin disease
    Polycythemia
    Macroglobulinemia
  Others
    Malignancy
    Hepatitis

ess (accounting for over 50% of patients with the phenomenon) or may be associated with an underlying disease and designated as secondary Raynaud's phenomenon. (Some call the primary disorder Raynaud's disease and the secondary one Raynaud's phenomenon.) In both disorders, unknown mechanisms, triggered by cold exposure or emotional stress, lead to digital pallor caused by the pooling of blood in digital capillaries and to rubor related to decreased vasospasm and reactive vasodilatation.

One of the diagnostic criteria for the designation of primary Raynaud's phenomenon is the presence of symptoms for at least 2 years without the appearance of an underlying cause. Although the primary disease accounts for 50 to 90% of cases that manifest the syndrome, some patients examined for presumed primary RP have been noted to develop systemic disease many years after the onset of symptoms. Several disease states have been associated with secondary RP and need to be ruled out by appropriate clinical and laboratory evaluation both at the presentation of RP and over the course of the disorder (Table 13–28).

DIAGNOSTIC EVALUATION

The diagnosis is based on a history of the classic sequential color changes in the fingers and toes on cold exposure or emotional stress. The differentiation of primary from secondary RP is carried out by a thorough history and physical examination to rule out the above-mentioned disorders and medications.

Patient History

Symptoms related to atherosclerosis are supported by the finding of abnormal peripheral pulses and a history of coronary artery disease and hypertension; malignancy is suspected by adenopathy or hepatosplenomegaly. Thoracic outlet syndrome and carpal tunnel syndrome are diagnosed by appropriate maneuvers (Adson's test for the thoracic outlet syndrome, Tinel's and Phalen signs for the carpal tunnel syndrome). Allen's test makes it possible to determine whether the radial and ulnar arteries are supplying the hand to their full capacities. Collagen vascular disorders (scleroderma, systemic lupus, dermatomyositis), blood dyscrasias and malignancy, vascular or anatomic abnormalities, occupational factors, and drug exposures should be sought.

Physical Examination

The presence of sclerodactyly (tightened skin from the MCP joints distally), calcinosis (calcium deposits under the skin), telangiectasias, and digital ulcers supports a diagnosis of scleroderma, whereas typical rheumatoid joint changes support a diagnosis of rheumatoid arthritis.

Diagnostic Studies

An appropriate screening laboratory evaluation for patients with RP should include complete blood cell count with differential, platelet count, urinalysis, erythrocyte sedimentation rate, antinuclear antibody, rheumatoid factor, serum protein and immunoelectrophoreses, cryoglobulin, and a chest x-ray. Abnormalities in these tests should stimulate further evaluation with appropriate studies such as cervical spine films, anti-DNA antibody and complement studies, electromyogram, and nerve conduction studies. Neurologic examination and vascular consultation with Doppler studies of vessels may be needed in more complicated cases (such as thoracic outlet or cervical spine disorders or, possibly, severe peripheral vascular disease caused by atherosclerosis or embolus). Angiography is rarely needed. Discontinuation of medications thought to contribute to RP is commonly employed.

SJÖGREN'S SYNDROME

DEFINITION

This is a chronic, inflammatory, autoimmune syndrome associated with lymphocytic infiltration of salivary, lacrimal, and other exocrine glands (minor salivary, upper and lower respiratory, gastrointestinal, vaginal, pancreatic, and skin glands) and is defined by two elements of the diagnostic triad of keratoconjunctivitis sicca (or dry eyes) with or without salivary gland enlargement; xerostomia (or dry mouth) with or without salivary gland enlargement; or the presence of a connective tissue disease (Table 13–29). The remainder of patients (without an associated connective tissue disorder) are said to have primary, or first degree, sicca syndrome.

Extraglandular involvement in SS includes hepatic disease, such as primary biliary cirrhosis, chronic active hepatitis, and cryptogenic cirrhosis; renal disease, such as renal tubular acidosis, nephrogenic diabetes insipidus, chronic interstitial nephritis, and immune complex glomerulonephritis; pulmonary involvement, such as pulmonary infiltrates (pseudolymphoma), and fibrosing alveolitis; myositis; neurologic disorders (central and peripheral); vasculitis and hyperglobulinemic purpura; and hematologic and malignant disorders, such as cryoglobulinemia, macroglobulinemia, and lymphoproliferative disorders with a spectrum from benign lymphadenopathy to pseudolymphoma to malignant lymphoreticular neoplasm.

PATHOPHYSIOLOGIC CONSIDERATIONS

The cause of Sjögren's syndrome is unknown but is thought to involve genetic (HLA-DW3, HLA-B8), humoral (antibodies against salivary duct antigens or soluble acidic nuclear antigens [Ro, La]), viral, and immune complex mechanisms. Lymphocytic infiltration of exocrine glands with acinar destruction is the final factor and leads to the characteristic clinical picture.

Salivary and lacrimal gland enlargement (with or without "sicca" symptoms) caused by other conditions may be confused with Sjögren's syndrome. Salivary gland enlargement may result from viral, bacterial, fungal, or tuberculous infection; from sarcoidosis; from infiltrative disorders (primary benign and malignant parotid gland neoplasms, leukemia, lymphoma, Burkitt's lymphoma, and pseudolymphoma); from systemic diseases (cirrhosis, diabetes mellitus, or hyperlipidemic states); from nutritional or mineral abnormality (malnutriton, deficiency of vitamins B_6, C, and A, and hypersensitivity to iodide, lead, or copper), and from drugs associated with dry mouth (sedatives, hypnotics, narcotics, phenothiazines, atropine, anti-Parkinson's drugs, antihistamines, ephedrine, and amphetamines).

Lacrimal gland enlargement can be caused by inflammation or tumors. Inflammation, which can be unilateral or bilateral, may result from acute infection (e.g., gonococcal infections or mononucleosis); chronic infection (e.g., trachoma, tuberculosis, leprosy, and actinomycosis); sarcoidosis; and Sjögren's syndrome. Tumors, which are usually unilateral, may be cystic; lymphoreticular (e.g., in Hodgkin's disease, lymphosarcoma, leukemia, or Waldenström's macroglobulinemia), or angioma or melanoma.

DIAGNOSTIC EVALUATION

In evaluating the patient with Sjögren's syndrome, the physician must demonstrate the presence of sicca complex—dry eyes and dry mouth with or without glandular enlargement. One must rule out an associated connective tissue disorder and other potential causes of enlargement of the salivary or lacrimal gland and/or the sicca complex.

An ophthalmologic evaluation should be performed, employing Schirmer's test (to demonstrate a decreased rate of tear wetting of filter paper) and a slit lamp examination using rose bengal dye (to demonstrate characteristic filamentary keratitis). Keratoconjunctivitis sicca is diagnosed when both decreased tear production and keratitis are found.

Although the diagnosis is usually made on the basis of the above clinical findings, additional studies can be undertaken if there is any diagnostic doubt. A lip biopsy showing the minor salivary glands reflects the histologic abnormalities found in the larger glands. Because of potential hazards (i.e., facial nerve palsy), biopsy of the major salivary gland is recommended only when there is a suggestion of intraparotid malignancy or when serious diagnostic doubts are present.

Table 13–29. Connective Tissue Disorders Associated with Secondary Sjögren's Syndrome

Connective Tissue Diseases in SS (%)	Diseases	SS in Connective Tissue Diseases
55%	Rheumatoid arthritis	30%
10%	Systemic lupus erythematosus	50%
8%	Scleroderma	40%
4%	Dermatomyositis	—

Histologic abnormalities include lymphocytic infiltration and destruction and epimyoepithelial "islands."

Routine rheumatologic laboratory testing may show elevated ESR (80%), anemia (40%), hypergammaglobulinemia (50%), positive rheumatoid factor (70%), and positive antinuclear antibody (60%). Less commonly, antibodies to soluble acidic nuclear antigens extracted from lymphoid cell lines can be tested. SS-A or Ro antibodies are present in primary Sjögren's syndrome (70%); Sjögren's syndrome with rheumatoid arthritis (1%), and Sjögren's syndrome with SLE (33%). SS-B or La antibodies are present in primary Sjögren's syndrome (50 to 70%); Sjögren's syndrome with rheumatoid arthritis (5%); and Sjögren's syndrome with SLE (73%). Finally, parotid studies, such as parotid salivary flow rate, radionuclide scanning of the parotid gland, and parotid sialography, may be performed.

CARPAL TUNNEL SYNDROME (CTS)

DEFINITION

This is a common entrapment syndrome in which compression of the median nerve at the wrist leads to the characteristic symptoms of numbness and paresthesias of the thumb, index finger, middle finger, and one half of the ring finger, and eventually to weakness and atrophy of the thenar muscles. The patient is often awakened at night by these symptoms and has to shake or knead out the hand(s). Carpal tunnel syndrome is frequently bilateral and can lead to retrograde pain in the forearm or shoulder. Examination of the patient may demonstrate a positive Tinel's sign (percussion of the entrapped median nerve at the volar wrist causing paresthesias in the distribution of that nerve) or Phalen sign (reproduction of pain and paresthesias on flexion of the hand at the wrist for over 1 minute). Hypoesthesia (for touch more than pain) in the median nerve distribution and thenar weakness and atrophy may be present later. Opposition strength and two-point sensory discrimination abnormalities may also be found.

PATHOPHYSIOLOGIC CONSIDERATIONS

As the median nerve passes through the unyielding carpal tunnel in company with flexor tendons of the fingers, it is at risk for compression by the transverse carpal ligament. Disorders leading to swelling of the tendons (e.g., tenosynovitis associated with rheumatoid arthritis) or the surrounding connective tissue in the wrist can lead to median nerve compression and the characteristic clinical presentation.

The differential diagnosis of the causes of carpal tunnel syndrome includes the several disorders that by different mechanisms lead to tissue swelling or infiltration and eventual median nerve entrapment.

Idiopathic disorders are the most common group, responsible for CTS in 60% of cases. While no specific cause can be determined, thickening and proliferation of the peritendinous synovium are seen.

Disorders leading to synovitis or tenosynovitis of the wrist include connective tissue disorders such as rheumatoid arthritis, systemic lupus erythematosus, scleroderma, and necrotizing angiitis–polyarteritis nodosa; seronegative spondyloarthropathies such as Reiter's syndrome, psoriatic arthritis, ankylosing spondylitis, and colitic arthropathies; crystal-induced arthritis such as gout, pseudogout, and calcium apatite; and infectious arthritis caused by bacteria, virus (hepatitis B), Lyme disease, tuberculosis, and other infections around the wrist.

Disorders leading to infiltration of abnormal tissue or overgrowth of local tissue include hypothyroidism, amyloidosis, multiple myeloma, and acromegaly.

Finally, trauma, fracture, or both can cause carpal tunnel syndrome.

DIAGNOSTIC EVALUATION

Rapid clinical diagnosis is important to prevent further nerve damage and motor abnormalities (weakness and atrophy are not as responsive to decompression therapy as sensory changes are). Electrodiagnostic testing including electromyography (EMG) of the thenar and upper limb muscles and motor and sensory nerve conduction studies should be done to diagnose a prolonged distal median nerve motor latency (found in the majority of cases), delayed sensory latency across the wrist (found in 90% of patients and the most reliable indicator of the CTS), and denervation of thenar musculature. Such studies may show that CTS-like symptoms are caused actually by cervical radiculitis (of the C5, C6, and C7 roots) or by thoracic outlet syndrome. Further, such studies can define the presence of both carpal tunnel syndrome and cervical radiculopathy (the so-called double-crush syndrome).

It is appropriate to screen for the potential causes of CTS, especially if one is guided by the clinical facts gathered in the history and physical examination. Appropriate tests include complete blood count, erythrocyte sedimentation rate; rheumatoid factor, antinuclear antibody test, and thyroid function test to rule out hypothyroidism. X-ray of the wrist (AP and lateral) with special carpal tunnel views may show a fracture or erosive disease typical of rheumatoid arthritis or amyloidosis. Protein electrophoresis and immunoelectrophoresis are needed only if amyloidosis or multiple myeloma are considered. Growth hormone assay is not routine and should be done only if there is a high index of suspicion for acromegaly. Gouty arthritis is usually defined clinically and by synovial fluid crystal examination; a serum uric acid level is an appropriate screening test to rule out gout. Pseudogout can be defined by x-ray examination and the demonstration of triangular ligament or other calcifications.

THE PAINFUL SHOULDER

DEFINITION

Pain perceived by the patient as originating in the shoulder can arise from intrinsic lesions of the glenohumeral joint or periarticular tissues (e.g., tendons, capsule, bursae, and muscles) or as referred pain from extrinsic lesions of neither joint nor periarticular origin. When shoulder pain persists for days, weeks, or months, it becomes more diffuse and poorly localized and can be present in the neck, down the arm, or across the back. Because the shoulder is a complex joint, whose function involves the interplay of many tissues, including joints, tendons, and muscles, painful lesions often lead to limitation in range of motion as the patient attempts to diminish pain or compensate for impaired joint function. Diminished ability to perform active range of motion is highly suggestive of an intrinsic shoulder disorder, whereas a normal range of motion without pain indicates an extrinsic source.

PATHOPHYSIOLOGIC CONSIDERATIONS AND DIFFERENTIAL DIAGNOSIS

Intrinsic Lesions of the Shoulder

TENDINITIS/CALCIFIC TENDINITIS

Injury leads to the deposition of calcium around the rotator cuff and can lead to recurrent or chronic shoulder pain and inflammation. Shoulder x-rays usually demonstrate calcium deposition in the tendon insertion at the greater tuberosity. Subdeltoid or subacromial bursal inflammation (i.e., bursitis) often accompanies tendinitis and, in the absence of a bursal effusion, is clinically indistinguishable from tendinitis.

BURSITIS

The most common cause of subacromial or subdeltoid bursitis is inflammation secondary to adjacent tendinitis. Bursitis unassociated with tendinitis is uncommon, and the differential diagnosis must always include bursitis secondary to infection. This latter diagnosis is made by aspiration of fluid from the bursa and subsequent analysis and culture.

BICIPITAL TENDINITIS

Tendinitis and tenosynovitis of the long head of the biceps tendon can cause acute shoulder pain. The diagnosis is confirmed by Yergason's sign (direct tenderness to palpation in the bicipital groove and pain referred to this area with resistance to flexion and supination of the elbow). The clinical setting is often the onset of pain associated with lifting or strenuous activity.

ROTATOR CUFF TEAR

The rotator cuff (formed by the confluence of the teres minor, infraspinous, supraspinous, and subscapular muscles) can tear acutely as a result of trauma or sports injuries or insidiously either spontaneously or related to chronic humeral joint inflammation (caused by diseases such as rheumatoid arthritis). Definitive diagnosis requires arthrography, which can demonstrate the characteristic abnormal extra-articular accumulation of contrast media in the subacromial bursa.

IMPINGEMENT SYNDROMES

Impingement of the rotator cuff beneath the coracoacromial arch can lead to chronic recurrent shoulder pain. The impingement may cause subacromial bursitis or tears, primarily in the supraspinous portion of the rotator cuff.

ADHESIVE CAPSULITIS ("FROZEN SHOULDER")

Contraction of the capsule of the shoulder joint by adhesions is the hallmark of this condition, which presents with increasing pain and decreasing shoulder mobility over weeks or months. The exact cause of this disorder is unknown, but theories suggest stress, tendinitis, impaired circulation, and effects secondary to autonomic dysfunction and immobilization. Physical examination demonstrates a limitation in abduction and internal rotation; these clinical findings are shared with rotator cuff tear, hemarthrosis, and anterior capsular tear.

TRAUMA/HEMARTHROSIS

Hemarthrosis can occur in the setting of trauma (e.g., in apparent sports injury), anticoagulant therapy, or both, and can present with pain and limited range of motion.

SHOULDER PAIN CAUSED BY ARTHRITIS

The shoulder can be involved in forms of inflammatory and noninflammatory disorders including rheumatoid arthritis, juvenile rheumatoid arthritis, seronegative spondyloarthropathies (ankylosing spondylitis, Reiter's syndrome, psoriatic arthritis), systemic lupus, crystal-induced disorders (gout, pseudogout, and calcium apatite disease), infectious arthritis, osteoarthritis, and osteonecrosis. Polymyalgia rheumatica (or giant cell arteritis) must always be considered in view of its potential for blindness in the setting of shoulder and neck pain in an elderly patient with an elevated ESR.

Extrinsic Lesions

Diaphragmatic irritation can cause stimulation of the phrenic nerve, which can be perceived as pain in the C5 to C6 dermatome level (i.e., the scapulodeltoid area). The major nonarticular conditions that can present as such referred shoulder pain include pulmonary embolus, myocardial infarction, cholecystitis, and subphrenic abscess.

Cervical root compression caused by osteoarthritis and brachial neuritis may produce pain in the shoulder region by irritation of C4, C5, and C6 nerve roots. The diagnosis is confirmed by nerve conduction studies and x-rays of the cervical spine (anteroposterior and lateral, and oblique-foraminal views).

Impingement on nerve and vascular structures at the thoracic outlet by a neoplasm at the apex of the lung (Pancoast's tumor) can lead to shoulder pain. Chest x-ray can define the presence of this tumor.

Reflex sympathetic dystrophy (shoulder-hand syndrome), which presents as shoulder pain with limited range of motion associated with redness, pain, and swelling of the ipsilateral hand, is thought to be due to overactivity of the sympathetic nervous system and related to myocardial infarction, cerebrovascular lesions, and prolonged immobilization.

Occult metastatic breast, lung, and prostatic carcinoma can present as shoulder pain caused by bone involvement. Appropriate x-rays, radionuclide bone scanning or both can define the abnormality in bone.

Musculoskeletal involvement by amyloidosis can present with shoulder pain, limitation of range of motion, and markedly enlarged shoulders with a rubbery consistency (shoulder-pad sign).

DIAGNOSTIC EVALUATION

Patient History and Physical Examination

Initially, the physician must distinguish whether the cause of the shoulder pain is intrinsic or extrinsic. This can be defined on clinical grounds. If the problem is intrinsic (i.e., if there are local tenderness or pain and restricted range of motion), the history and physical findings will guide the physician toward one of the diagnostic possibilities. If the problem is extrinsic, referred pain sources should be sought with the appropriate clinical and laboratory inquiries.

Diagnostic Studies

LABORATORY TESTS

An elevated erythrocyte sedimentation rate may define an inflammatory process, (e.g., synovitis, or sepsis), although a normal test does not rule out this possibility. The most important disorder characteristically causing shoulder pain and a markedly elevated ESR is polymyalgia rheumatica. The presence of a positive rheumatoid factor in the correct clinical setting may be helpful in diagnosing rheumatoid arthritis.

Aspiration of the glenohumeral joint with synovial fluid analysis and arthrography (to assure entry into the joint itself) is helpful in defining inflammatory disorders (e.g., rheumatoid arthritis, crystal-induced disease with characteristic diagnostic crystal findings), infectious disorders, or hemorrhagic disorders. Appropriate synovial fluid analysis is indicated in each instance (e.g., cell count and differential, crystal analysis, serum glucose analysis, and Gram's stain and culture). Aspiration is performed in those instances of intrinsic lesions associated with marked or persistent inflammatory findings (redness, warmth, tenderness) with joint effusion where there is clinical evidence of joint (not periarticular) involvement.

Electromyography and nerve conduction studies are employed only in those situations in which brachial neuritis, cervical radiculopathy, or carpal tunnel syndrome is considered as a cause of shoulder pain.

RADIOLOGIC STUDIES

An anteroposterior x-ray with the arm in internal and external rotation is almost always mandatory in cases of shoulder pain or restricted range of motion. This test can define tendon calcium deposits of calcific tendinitis, the erosions or the glenohumeral joint space narrowing characteristic of rheumatoid arthritis, chondrocalcinosis with pseudogout, subchondral collapse of osteonecrosis, spur formation in osteoarthritis, lytic or blastic lesions of neoplasm, or fracture related to trauma. The absence of these radiologic abnormalities does not rule out any of the disorders mentioned. In cases of suspected trauma, an axillary view should be done to better define the relationship of the humeral head to the glenoid.

The injection of contrast medium and air into the glenohumeral cavity is, at present, the only way to establish the diagnosis of adhesive capsulitis or a rotator cuff tear without surgical exploration. Arthrography is indicated for patients with persistent diminished range of motion of unknown cause.

Radionuclide bone scan is not commonly used for the diagnosis of shoulder pain except in those instances in which one suspects neoplasm, osteonecrosis, sepsis, fracture, or synovitis not well defined by clinical or x-ray evaluation.

LOW-BACK PAIN

DEFINITION

Pain in the area of the spine inferior to the L1 level can be caused by disorders of any of the diverse components of the lumbosacral complex.

Back pain is usually categorized as local, referred, radicular, or spasmotic. Local pain, presumably from a pathologic process stimulating a sensory nerve ending, is usually steady although occasionally intermittent, it changes with position, it is sharp or dull, and it is felt in the affected part. It most often causes reflex paravertebral muscle spasm. Referred pain from pelvic or abdominal viscera is referred to dermatomal areas and takes on a deep and aching quality. Referred pain from spinal sources is noted in the sacroiliac area, buttocks, and posterior thigh. Radicular pain is related to a spinal nerve root distribution, worsens with root stretching maneuvers (e.g., the straight leg raising sign of Lasègue, bending, and sitting), and usually improves with rest. The pain has neurologic characteristics of paresthesias and numbness, and there may be associated motor weakness. Spasmotic pain has a cramping, achy character.

DIFFERENTIAL DIAGNOSIS

The source of low-back pain should be diagnosed according to the site of involvement and the presence or absence of radiculopathy.

Low-back pain without radiculopathy occurring in the vertebrae may result from primary or metastatic tumor; from fracture (traumatic or osteoporotic); from coccydynia (pain in the coccyx); or from congenital or developmental abnormalities. The latter include spondylolysis (defect in the pars interarticularis); spondylolisthesis (forward displacement of one vertebra over a lower one); and transitional vertebra, with complete or incomplete sacralization of L5 or lumbarization of S1.

Nonradiculopathic pain in the intervertebral disc may come from disc herniation, degenerated disc, or infection, most commonly Staphylococcus aureus and gram-negative organisms.

Nonradiculopathic pain in the apophyseal joints may come from osteoarthritis; rheumatoid arthritis (mostly in the cervical spine); or ankylosing spondylitis and other seronegative spondyloarthropathies.

Visceral causes of nonradiculopathic pain include aortic aneurysm; uterine disorders (fibroids, sacral menstrual pain, uterine malposition and prolapse, endometriosis, or carcinoma); renal stones or bladder cancer, retroperitoneal bleeding, lymphoma, or sarcoma; colonic tumors; gastric or pancreatic tumors; or prostatic tumor and prostatitis.

Low-back pain may also occur with radiculopathy. Radicular pain is aggravated by coughing, sneezing, and straining and is characterized by paresthesias in a dermatomal distribution and associated with numbness or weakness and bowel or bladder dysfunction. Signs of nerve root compression include a positive straight leg raising sign, diminished reflexes, an abnormal sensory examination, muscle weakness, and poor rectal tone.

Spondylolisthesis and spondylolysis can produce radicular pain in the vertebrae (usually without neurologic deficit) by applying tension on the nerve root. Herniation or degeneration of the intervertebral disc often causes symptoms and signs of nerve root compression. Patients with hypertrophic apophyseal joints secondary to osteoarthritis may develop stenosis of the neural foramina, which can cause radicular pain or neurologic deficit. The patients are generally elderly and the pain is increased with walking (pseudoclaudication). The general term for this group of disorders is spinal stenosis. The ligaments rarely cause radicular symptoms. In scoliosis, low-back pain with leg radiation stimulates disc-type symptoms in some patients.

DIAGNOSTIC EVALUATION

Patient History and Physical Examination

The patient history is important and may provide information about a history of trauma (accident, fall, lifting), inflammatory joint disease (rheumatoid ar-

Table 13–30.   Erythrocyte Sedimentation Rate as a Diagnostic Guide in Back Pain

Normal or Variable Sedimentation Rate	Elevated Sedimentation Rate
Lumbosacral sprain	Infections of the spine
Lumbar degenerative joint and disc disease	Bacterial
Spondylolisthesis	Tuberculous
Diffuse idiopathic skeletal hyperostosis (DISH)	Fungal
Kyphoscoliosis	Seronegative spondyloarthropathies
Paget's disease	Ankylosing spondylitis
Ochronosis	Reiter's syndrome
Neuropathic spine	Psoriatic arthritis
Psychoneurotic back pain	Ulcerative colitis
Osteoporosis	Regional enteritis
Vertebral fracture	Multiple myeloma
Referred pain	Polymyalgia rheumatica
	Neoplasms, mostly metastatic (e.g., lung, breast, prostate, kidney)

thritis, seronegative spondyloarthropathies), a visceral source (gastrointestinal, pelvic, retroperitoneal), previous malignancy, or present symptoms consistent with malignancy or a metabolic bone disorder (osteopenia, Paget's disease). The mode of onset and timing, localization of pain, and aggravating and relieving factors are all important facts to be gathered.

Several maneuvers can be performed to stretch the sciatic nerve and elicit pain. The straight leg raising sign is a test that stretches the roots of the lumbosacral plexus by putting tension on the sciatic nerve, a tension that increases as the leg is raised higher. The knee is held extended and the leg is raised gradually from the table by the heel until the point of pain is reached. The angle at which the pain begins is recorded and the patient is questioned about radicular (sciatica) pain.

Lasègue's test is done by flexing the hip and knee and then slowly extending the knee until the point of pain is reached.

Diagnostic Studies

An erythrocyte sedimentation rate test can be a good screening evaluation to differentiate between benign and inflammatory, infectious, or neoplastic causes of back pain (Table 13–30). Routine laboratory tests including calcium, alkaline phosphatase, appropriate cultures, and purified protein derivative may be useful.

Anteroposterior, lateral, and oblique x-ray views of the lumbosacral spine may help to define various potential causes of back pain and should be done in patients with persistent low-back pain. Intervertebral disc space narrowing can indicate a longstanding degenerative process. Complete disc space obliteration with vertebral end-plate destruction may indicate a septic spondylitis or a discitis caused by ankylosing spondylitis. Calcification of the disc is consistent with ochronosis. Congenital or developmental defects revealed by x-rays include spondylolysis, spondylolisthesis, transitional vertebra, and scoliosis. Also, de-

generative changes and spondyloarthropathies may be noted in apophyseal joints. Finally, destructive lesions of the vertebral body revealed on x-ray suggest a metastatic or septic process. Large anterior spur formation will define diffuse idiopathic skeletal hyperostosis (DISH); syndesmophytes will support a diagnosis of one of the seronegative spondyloarthropathies. Sacroiliac joint x-rays (AP of the pelvis or specific sacroiliac joint x-rays) may be needed to demonstrate the characteristic and diagnostic joint changes (i.e., erosions, widening and narrowing, and sclerosis) of the seronegative spondyloarthropathies.

Radionuclide bone scanning is useful if a malignant lesion or infection is suspected and routine x-rays are normal. Paget's disease can also be diagnosed with this test. A CT scan is employed to evaluate patients in whom spinal stenosis or disc disease may be the cause of back pain. Malignant and infectious disorders are sometimes diagnosed with this test. At times, myelography is combined with CT scanning to better define the anatomy of a defect.

Myelography is indicated when symptoms are severe and do not resolve with conventional treatment. Both intra- and extradural abnormalities may be seen. Injecting dye into the disc (discography) may reveal evidence of disc degeneration. This test is reserved for patients with persistent symptoms and an equivocal or negative myelogram. Electromyogram may identify nerve root disease not detected by clinical examination. A nuclear magnetic resonance scan can add useful information to the workup of back pain without the use of x-rays or the need for myelography.

GENERAL REFERENCES

Ansell, B.M. (ed.): Clinics of Rheumatic Diseases. Inflammatory Disorders of Muscle. London, W.B. Saunders Co., 1984.

Beary, J.E. III, Christian, C.L., and Sculco, T.P. (eds.): Manual of Rheumatology and Out-Patient Orthopaedic Disorders. Boston, Little, Brown and Company, 1981.

Cohen, A.S. (ed.): Laboratory Diagnostic Procedures in the Rheumatic Diseases. Boston, Little Brown & Company, 1979.

Forrester, D.M., and Brown, J.C. (eds.): Clinics in Rheumatic Diseases. Radiological Investigation in Rheumatology. London, W.B. Saunders Co., 1983.

Fritzler, M.J.: Antinuclear antibodies in the investigation of rheumatic diseases. Bull Rheum Dis 35:1–10, 1985.

Holt, P.J.L. (ed.): Clinics in Rheumatic Diseases. Endocrine and Metabolic Aspects of Rheumatic Disease. London, W.B. Saunders Co., 1981.

Hoppenfeld, S.: Physical Examination of the Spine and Extremities. New York, Appleton-Century-Crofts, 1976.

Jeffrey, M.S., and Dick, W.C. (eds.): Clinics in Rheumatic Diseases. The Role of the Laboratory in Rheumatology. London, W.B. Saunders Company Ltd., 1983.

Kelley, W.N., Harris, E.D. Jr., Ruddy, S., and Sledge, C.B. (eds.): Textbook of Rheumatology. 2nd Ed. Philadelphia, W.B. Saunders Company, 1985.

McCarty, D.J. (ed.): Arthritis and Allied Conditions. Philadelphia, Lea & Febiger, 1985.

Polley, H.F., and Hunder, G.G. (eds.): Rheumatologic Interviewing and Physical Examination of the Joints. Philadelphia, W.B. Saunders Company, 1978.

Stevens, M.B.: Rheumatic disease. In The Principles and Practice of Medicine. Edited by A.M. Harvey, et al. Connecticut, Appleton-Century-Crofts, 1984.

CHAPTER 14

CONSTITUTIONAL AND NONSPECIFIC PROBLEMS

A.H. Samiy, M.D.

Disease processes alter normal physiologic body functions, and these dysfunctions are manifested by signs and symptoms. Signs are those alterations noted by patients or detected by physicians during examination. Symptoms, categorized as specific, constitutional, or nonspecific, are subjective experiences noted by patients alone.

In this chapter we have arbitrarily included several common constitutional complaints, such as fatigue, weakness, flushing, diaphoresis, hypothermia, and hyperthermia. Other constitutional and nonspecific symptoms are discussed in other chapters of the book. Specific symptoms frequently are manifestations of disease in a particular organ system and more commonly are associated with a specific disease entity. Fever, however, usually a nonspecific symptom occurring with a wide variety of disease entities and with disorders of various organ systems, could also be considered a specific symptom or sign of infectious disease. Nonspecific and constitutional symptoms tend to be more subjective and vague. They are not usually localized and cannot be objectively quantified. Psychologic factors often significantly modify and influence the way patients perceive and report these symptoms.

Very little is known about pathophysiologic disturbances associated with constitutional symptoms. The difficulty in quantifying these symptoms, in part, may account for lack of scientific investigations of their basic or cellular mechanisms.

For instance, although more than ten million office visits are precipitated by a complaint of fatigue annually, very little is known about fatigue's pathophysiology. It is known, however, that fatigue is associated with a wide range of diseases (Table 14–1).

Interpretation of constitutional symptoms is often difficult because of the subjective and vague nature of the complaint. The clinician should obtain a detailed description of the symptoms, rather than simply report the patient's terminology. Many patients use complaints of weakness, fatigue, lack of energy, or tiredness interchangeably. Occasionally, the real complaint of patients seeking medical help because of fatigue may be shortness of breath.

The patient's history is the key to the diagnostic evaluation. Constitutional symptoms, as a single complaint, may occur with a wide range of diseases. The concomitant presence of other symptoms, particularly a specific symptom or sign, may further reduce the diagnostic possibilities. For instance, whereas fatigue may occur with endocrine disorders, malignancy, hematologic diseases, cardiopulmonary problems, and a variety of other chronic diseases, the coexistence of

dyspnea with fatigue may reduce the diagnostic possibilities to cardiopulmonary diseases.

In contrast to specific symptoms, constitutional symptoms such as fatigue, lassitude, and weakness are more frequently associated with functional and psychologic disorders. A psychologic evaluation of patients with nonspecific symptoms may reveal chronic depression or anxiety.

It is also important to review patients' use of medication. A number of commonly used drugs such as antihypertensive, psychotropic, antihistaminic, and weight-reducing drugs may produce nonspecific and constitutional symptoms. The use of nonprescription over-the-counter drugs should also be explored.

FATIGUE

DEFINITION

Fatigue or lassitude is a physical or mental weariness or exhaustion from effort or activity. Patients may complain of being unable to do what they used to perform without becoming fatigued. They may also complain of being tired, listless, and exhausted and of "getting old."

PATHOPHYSIOLOGIC CONSIDERATIONS AND DIFFERENTIAL DIAGNOSIS

Fatigue is one of the most common complaints presented by ambulatory patients who do not have major recognizable diseases. Patients with chronic diseases such as heart disease and neoplasms often expect to be fatigued and only mention this symptom if asked. It is estimated that more than ten million office visits were precipitated by the complaint of fatigue in 1975, and fatigue was the seventh most common initial complaint.[1] Patients with fatigue can usually be classified as belonging in one of two groups after the initial evaluation: patients with chronic diseases, e.g., heart disease or malignancies, anemia, and chronic inflammatory disorders; and patients who frequently have no obvious cause for the complaint of fatigue. The latter group of patients frequently proves more frustrating to the physician. About half of patients with fatigue have functional or nonorganic disorders.[2-4] The National Ambulatory Care Survey suggested that one fourth of patients presenting with fatigue have serious disease, over one third have slightly serious disease, and one

Table 14–1.   Diseases Associated with Fatigue

Cardiovascular	Neurologic
Heart failure of any cause	Dementia
Valvular heart disease	Parkinsonism
Arrhythmias	Neuropathy
Hypertension	Physiologic
Pharmacologic	Environmental stress
Alcohol excess	Noise
Drugs	Heat
Antihypertensives	Cold
Antihistamines	Increased physical activity
Anticonvulsants	Sedentary life-style
Tranquilizers	New major disease
Toxins and heavy metals	Recent illness, surgery, or trauma
Caffeine excess	Too little scheduled sleep
Other drug abuse	Sleep disruption (travel, etc.)
Endocrine-Metabolic	Aging
Hyperthyroidism—patient can be apathetic	Psychosocial
Hypothyroidism	Anxiety
Addison's disease	Depression
Pituitary insufficiency	Stress
Hematologic-Neoplastic	Pulmonary
Anemia	Insufficiency of any cause
Occult malignancy	Sleep apnea
Infection	Renal
Any body system	Insufficiency
Hepatitis	
Endocarditis	
Tuberculosis	
Infectious mononucleosis	

third have no serious disease.[1] In patients in whom the cause of fatigue is undiagnosed after the first visit, physical causes are eventually found in 39%, psychologic origins seem to be the cause in 41%, the causes are mixed in 12%, and causes are undetermined in 8%.[4]

A symptom like fatigue or lassitude has a broad differential diagnosis that could include a large number of diseases discussed in this book. The rapidity of onset of the symptom, its duration, and its severity all play a major role in directing the medical decision-making process. Many of the diseases known to be associated with fatigue are listed in Table 14–1.

DIAGNOSTIC EVALUATION

Patients presenting with a complaint of fatigue are usually concerned that they may have cancer, anemia, or thyroid disease. The possibility of the presence of any of these can be assessed by reviewing the history and noting the physical findings. Organic diseases are much less apt than functional disorders to be stress related; the fatigue often gets worse as the day goes on, it usually shows little fluctuation and it frequently has been present less than 2 months before the individual seeks medical attention. In contrast, psychologic illnesses or functional disorders often have been

present for many months or even years before the patient seeks treatment (Figs. 14–1, 14–2, and 14–3).

Some individuals present with preconceived ideas about their fatigue or self-diagnoses such as hypoglycemia,[5,6] food allergies,[7] and fungus allergies.[8] An aggressive and ridiculing response by physicians to these beliefs will only guarantee that the patient will not cooperate in the diagnostic evaluation of what may be a treatable and even serious condition. Some patients do have hypoglycemia, usually a reactive type. Empathy and reassurance by the physician can be very helpful in the management of these patients. Everything from depression to mitral valve prolapse syndrome may be found in this group of patients.[9] It should also be remembered that individuals can have dysfunctions causing considerable symptoms in the absence of recognizable disease.

A commonly missed source of fatigue and irritability is excessive consumption of alcohol. The executive who has never missed a day's work but has slipped into a pattern of having a drink before dinner—often a double—then wine with dinner and a little nightcap to sleep may not associate the alcohol with poor sleep, poor appetite, fatigue, and irritability the next day. Amounts smaller than those consumed in the described pattern also can contribute to symptoms. When one remembers that alcohol consists of totally ''empty''

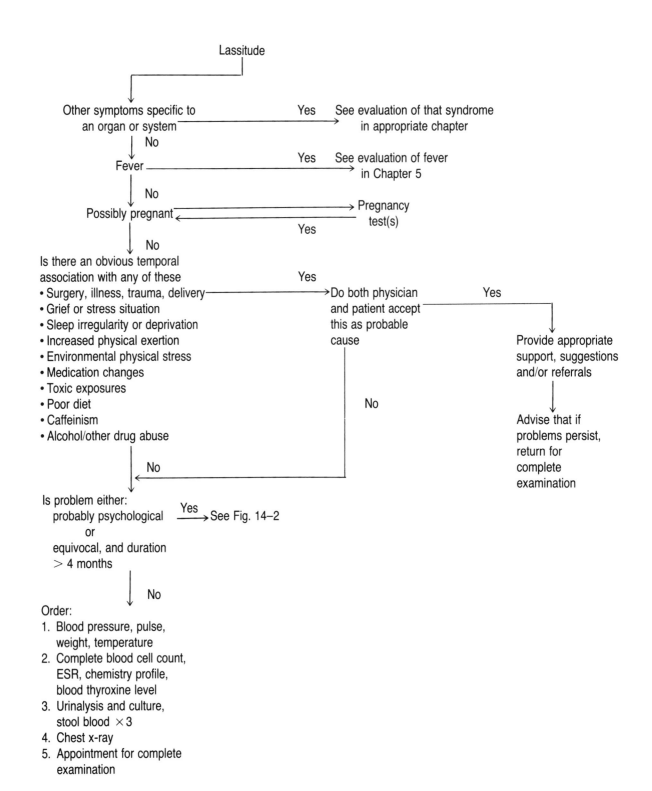

Fig. 14–1. Diagnostic approach to lassitude. (Adapted from Solberg, L.I.: Lassitude, a primary care evaluation. JAMA *251*:3272, 1984.)

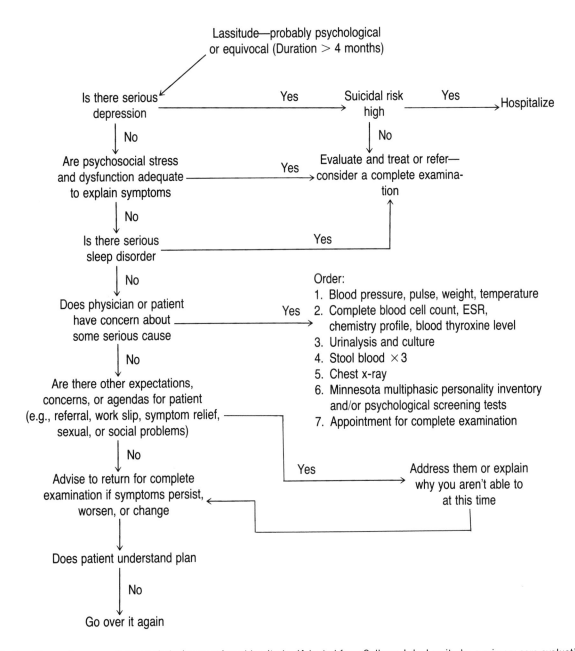

Fig. 14–2. Diagnostic approach to psychologic or equivocal lassitude. (Adapted from Solberg, L.I.: Lassitude, a primary care evaluation. JAMA *251*:3272, 1984.)

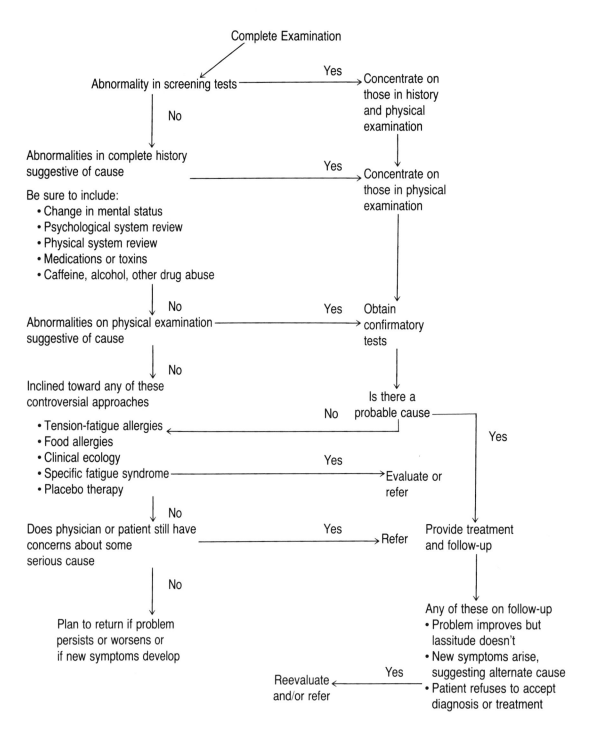

Fig. 14–3. Diagnostic evaluation of lassitude. (Adapted from Solberg, L.I.: Lassitude, a primary care evaluation. JAMA *251*:3272, 1984.)

calories, falling between carbohydrates and fats with regard to caloric content, the poor appetite is quickly understandable. Even small doses of alcohol result in significant changes in REM sleep.[10]

When initial screening studies are nonproductive, more sophisticated but simple psychologic testing can be helpful. Self-administered tests to screen for alcoholism and depression are often very helpful.[11,12] Treatments for depression can be successful, but certainly not all patients require medication.[13] The beneficial role of the supportive physician in caring for the patient who has symptoms for which an organic disease cannot be found was beautifully addressed by Francis Peabody more than 5 decades ago, and his lecture is still timely.[14]

WEAKNESS

DEFINITION

Weakness represents a reduction in the peak strength of muscular contraction.[15] Patients frequently complain that they are weak, though they tend to confuse complaints of fatigue, weakness, and tiredness. The clinician must be very careful to determine exactly what the patient means. Commonly, fatigue, weakness, and tiredness are present simultaneously, although they can occur separately. Any weakness or loss of strength may be persistent or episodic, localized or generalized.

PATHOPHYSIOLOGIC CONSIDERATIONS

Objective or real weakness occurs when muscle contraction is impaired as a result of inadequate nutrition and oxygenation in muscle cells, impairment of nerve stimulation, or inadequate time for recuperation during repetitive contraction (i.e., exhaustion). These dysfunctions may result from disorders of the nervous system, exposure to toxins that damage the nervous system, impaired circulation with its resultant decreased oxygen and energy source, and a wide array of metabolic derangements.

DIFFERENTIAL DIAGNOSIS

By careful questioning, the physician can differentiate weakness from fatigue. Whereas fatigue is a subjective sense of loss of energy, true weakness or loss of strength often can be demonstrated objec-

tively.[16] The patient's complaints must be categorized with regard to date of onset, nature, and severity. Specific questions about what the patient is unable to do now that he used to be able to do are helpful in assessing the severity. The differentiation of weakness from fatigue is complicated by the fact that many patients admit to both complaints on further questioning. Also, while weakness has been defined by physicians as a diminution in the force of contraction with repetitive effort, most patients mean something else when they complain of fatigue or weakness. The true definition of disease-related fatigue, i.e., easy fatigability or premature fatigue, has been discussed in an earlier section. All three complaints (fatigue, tiredness, and weakness) could occur as normal phenomena under the proper circumstances.

The differential diagnosis is complicated even more by the fact that complaints of weakness, tiredness, and fatigue are commonly voiced by depressed and emotionally disturbed patients. Assessing whether there are objective findings to support weakness and whether the weakness is localized or involves the whole body is important. Severe pain in muscles or joints that inhibits mobility is often misinterpreted as weakness. Furthermore, chronic pain contributes to the confusing overlapping symptoms of fatigue and tiredness.

DIAGNOSTIC EVALUATION

Considerable effort must be made to establish whether the failure to sustain required force is due to psychologic factors and disorder of the nervous system rather than diseases of the muscle.[17] Usually, a careful history and examination will suffice, but additional special techniques for studying muscle such as dynamometry, which measures strength, electrical stimulation, which permits force measurements under brief tetanic contraction, and needle biopsy may need to be employed.

Patients often use the word "weakness" when they talk about light-headedness, giddiness, dizziness, or faintness. These episodes may represent problems associated with cardiac and circulatory events, such as syncope, transient ischemic attacks, and arrhythmias. Obviously, with reduced cardiac output or decreased cerebral perfusion, real weakness may occur. Impaired or altered consciousness accompanying these events and systemic metabolic disturbances such as uremia, hypothyroidism, and hyperthyroidism may help to differentiate them from other causes of weakness not accompanied by mental changes, such as myasthenia gravis and hypokalemia. Many of the disorders associated with weakness are listed in Table 14–2.[18]

It is helpful to categorize the weakness as either

Table 14–2. Causes of Weakness

Episodic
  Cardiovascular
    Impaired vasoconstriction mechanisms
      Vasovagal
      Postural from neuropathy and drugs
      Cardiac sinus syncope
    Arrhythmias
    Reduced cardiac output
      Obstruction
      Pump failure
      Embolism
      Cardiac tamponade
    Hypovolemia
      Hemorrhage
      Dehydration
  Central nervous system
    Transient ischemic attacks
    Hypertensive encephalopathy
    Anxiety attacks
Persistent or chronic
  Carcinomatosis
  Cardiovascular
    Heart failure
    Heart valve obstructions
    Heart valve insufficiency
    Electrolyte disturbances
  Endocrine
    Hyperthyroidism
    Hypothyroidism
    Hypercalcemia of any cause
    Hypercortisolism (Cushing's syndrome)
    Hypoadrenalism (Addison's disease)
    Hypopituitarism
    Hypoglycemia
    Hyper- and Hypo-aldosteronism
  Hematologic
    Anemia
    Hemochromatosis
  Infection (e.g., infectious mononucleosis, influenza, hepatitis)
  Nutritional
    Starvation
    Malabsorption
    Illness
  Pulmonary
    Insufficiency of any cause
  Renal failure
  Toxic
    Drugs
    Alcohol
    Carbon monoxide

episodic or persistent, although obviously overlap in this classification is possible. Even more confusingly, in a disease such as early Addison's disease, a patient may be chronically weak and have intermittent episodes of severe weakness.[19,20] Each group of disorders and diseases has its own differential diagnosis and specific workup. In characterizing the weakness, it is important to emphasize the duration. Acute onset of

muscle weakness, lasting hours to days, can represent a life threatening medical emergency.[21]

FLUSHING

DEFINITION

Flushing is transient erythema or evanescent vasodilatation that can be violaceous or bright red.

PATHOPHYSIOLOGIC CONSIDERATIONS

In certain instances, the manifestations of flushing are similar to the vasodilatation associated with intravenous histamine injection. Systemic manifestations include headache, malaise, vascular dilatation, tachycardia, weakness, dizziness, nausea, vomiting, diarrhea, hypotension, and shock. Many of these more severe manifestations are due to a substantial drop in peripheral vascular resistance.

DIFFERENTIAL DIAGNOSIS

A large number of disorders are associated with flushing (Table 14–3). Anxiety, exercise, extreme pain, emesis, and defecation can lead to transient vasodilatation or flushing. Mastocytosis and other neoplasias, such as carcinoid syndrome, ganglioneuromas, and neuroblastomas may be associated with flushing. Ganglioneuromas and neuroblastomas are most commonly seen in early infancy or childhood. These tumors arise from the sympathetic ganglia or the adrenal medulla. Carcinoid syndrome is usually manifest in the malignant phase after metastatic implantation in the liver. These tumors originate from the argentaffin cells of the intestine, stomach, or bronchial tree.

The toxicologic differential diagnosis is broad. Ethanol by itself is a common cause of flushing in Orientals and American Indians. Ethanol ingestion associated with acetaldehyde dehydrogenase inhibition, an Antabuse-type reaction, is a common cause. Drugs such as disulfiram, chlorpropamide, metronidazole, and other antibiotics can inhibit acetaldehyde metabolism. Chloral hydrate yields a similar reaction, as do monoamine oxidase inhibitors ingested concomitantly with products containing tyramine (Chianti wine and aged cheeses). Other drugs such as boric acid, dinitrophenol, reserpine, beryllium, gold, and cobalt may

Table 14–3. Causes of Flushing

General
  Anxiety
  Exercise
  Extreme pain
  Defecation
  Headaches (migraine and cluster)
Mastocytosis syndrome
Malignancy
  Carcinoid
  Ganglioneuromas
  Neuroblastomas
Toxicologic
  Acetaldehyde flush (Orientals/American Indians)
  Antabuse reaction (disulfiram, metronidazole, chlorpropamide)
Anticholinergic agents
    Belladonna alkaloids
    Tricyclic antidepressants
  Beryllium
  Boric acid
  Carbon monoxide
  Chloral hydrate
  Cobalt
  Cyanide
  Dinitrophenol
  Ethanol (withdrawal and intoxication)
  Gold
  Iodide
  Loxoscelism
  Monosodium glutamate
  Niacin, nicotinamide
  Reserpine
  Scombroid fish poisoning
  Sympathomimetic agents
    Cocaine
    LSD
    Amphetamines
  Tyramine reaction (associated with MAO inhibitors)
  Yohimbine

also be associated with flushing. Anticholinergic agents may cause marked persistent vasodilatation. Sympathomimetic agents such as cocaine, lysergic acid diethylamide (LSD), and amphetamines may produce a persistent flush response.

Other causes of flushing include scombroid poisoning. The fish in the scombroid family include the marine tuna, albacore, bonito, mackerel, and skipjack. The dark meat of these fish has a very high concentration of histidine, and when the catch is not chilled appropriately, the proteus species on the fish skin, which contain a histidine decarboxylase, transform the histidine to histamine and saurine. The large quantities of ingested saurine and histamine lead to a dramatic flush. Another flush syndrome associated with eating is related to ingestion of monosodium glutamate (MSG). The typical Chinese restaurant syndrome may be associated with flush as well as the more common

symptoms of diaphoresis, weakness, dysesthesias, and headache.

CLINICAL PRESENTATION

Flushing may be the sole symptom of vasomotor instability or may be associated with diverse manifestations of a syndrome. Flushing may be confined to the face; it may be transient and frequent, or it may be protracted, covering large parts of the body from face to trunk. Associated physical findings in the most severe forms of carcinoid syndrome may be periorbital edema, wheezing, hypoactive bowel sounds, and hypotension. Flushing of the face in carbon monoxide or cyanide poisoning, if present, is associated with grave prognostic implications unless treatment is initiated immediately. Flushing in association with anticholinergic agents such as the belladonna alkaloids or the tricyclic antidepressants is commonly associated with dry skin, dry mucosae, decreased bowel sounds, urinary retention, alteration of consciousness, tachycardia, and hyperthermia. The clinical presentation of sympathomimetic agent overdose is similar to that of the anticholinergic agents and includes flushing, tachycardia, and dilated pupils; the patient with this syndrome lacks dry skin, however, and frequently has associated diaphoresis and active bowel sounds without urinary retention.

DIAGNOSTIC EVALUATION

A careful patient history emphasizing any symptoms prior to the acute event is particularly valuable for diagnostic consideration of mastocytosis, migraine and cluster headaches, carcinoid syndrome, ganglioneuromas, and neuroblastomas. Determining the events immediately preceding the onset of flushing is important, especially the events related to anxiety, exercise, extreme pain, emesis, and defecation. What the patient has recently eaten and where it was done may be important with respect to causes of food poisoning (such as ingestion of an anticholinergic agent), an acetaldehyde flush, Chinese restaurant syndrome, an Antabuse reaction, or a tyramine reaction associated with monoamine oxidase inhibitors. In the case of an altered level of consciousness, any information provided by family, friends, or paramedics is essential. One must always consider toxins, such as cyanide and carbon monoxide.

A meticulous physical examination is essential to differentiate sympathomimetic agent toxicity from toxicity of the anticholinergic agents. A careful search for cutaneous manifestations related to the desquamation associated with boric acid or for bullae associated with carbon monoxide is important. Loxoscelism may be manifested solely by the necrotic lesion of a spider bite. Mastocytosis may be manifested by urticaria pigmentosa, isolated mastocytomas, or generalized or multiple red-brown plaques or nodules.

Laboratory studies may be helpful in determining carboxyhemoglobin levels, oxygen saturation, or specific toxins such as ethanol or acetaldehyde. Blood and urine toxic metabolites such as 5-hydroxy indoleacetic acid (carcinoid syndrome) and histamine or saurine (scombroid poisoning) may be helpful in diagnosis. Skin biopsy may be valuable in the assessment of mastocytosis. Other substances such as anticholinergic agents and sympathomimetic agents may be determined by urine or blood toxicologic studies. Electrocardiogram is of value in determining the extent of myocardial damage related to carbon monoxide and cyanide poisoning as well as the potential risk associated with tricyclic antidepressant toxicity, or in evaluating supraventricular or ventricular arrhythmias found with anticholinergic and sympathomimetic agent overdose.

DIAPHORESIS

DEFINITION

Diaphoresis is generalized excessive perspiration or the production of large amounts of sweat.

PATHOPHYSIOLOGIC CONSIDERATIONS

There are two types of sweat glands: eccrine and apocrine. The apocrine glands open directly into the hair follicle or onto the skin. These glands are controlled by sex hormones and begin functioning at puberty. The excretion of apocrine glands, located in the axilla, mons pubis, and perineum, results in the production of pheromones. These glands normally have a limited role in evaporative heat loss.

Eccrine sweat glands cover the entire surface of the body and are the major source of the sweat volume. These glands are under the influence of sympathetic nerve and acetylcholine release. They produce a plasma ultrafiltrate, the concentration of which is controlled by reabsorptive processes in the duct, normally yielding a hypotonic sweat. The eccrine glands also function more broadly as excretory organs for varied macromolecules (protein and polysaccharides), heavy

metals, and organic compounds (lactate, urea, ammonia, and amino acids).

The evaporation of sweat is an essential part of the body's thermoregulatory control. The eccrine sweat glands can produce large volumes of a solution of varying degrees of hypotonicity, depending on the individual's neuroendocrine control and the state of acclimatization. The rate of sweating and the concentration of sweat are also determined by serum osmolality.

Hypohidrosis is inadequate production of sweat in response to a stimulus; anhidrosis is the absence of sweat production. These conditions are associated with heat stroke, hypothalamic lesions, anticholinergic and ganglionic blocking agents, ectodermal dysplasia, and Sjögren's syndrome. Sweat is invariably hypotonic, except in the presence of cystic fibrosis or Addison's disease.

DIFFERENTIAL DIAGNOSIS

Diaphoresis may be due to certain nonspecific conditions such as anxiety, extreme pain, and emesis. Endocrinologic disorders such as hyperthyroidism, hypoglycemia, and pheochromocytoma and infectious diseases such as tuberculosis and sepsis may also lead to diaphoresis. Various toxicologic agents that lead to the stimulation of the sympathetic nervous system, such as amphetamines, lysergic acid diethylamide (LSD), and cocaine, are common causes of diaphoresis. Those agents with muscarinic or anticholinesterase manifestations such as carbamates, organophosphates, or physostigmine will lead to diaphoresis. Less common causes for diaphoresis include rare fish-related toxins such as tetrodotoxin or ciguatera poisoning, plant related toxins such as the death camas, and snake bites (Table 14–4).

CLINICAL PRESENTATION

The entities considered in the differential diagnosis such as pain, anxiety, hyperthyroidism, pheochromocytoma, or ingestion of amphetamines or cocaine are associated with a sympathetic drive. These entities may also be associated with warm, moist skin.

Hypoglycemia may also be manifested by diaphoresis, but usually, a low body temperature and cool, moist skin are noted. The typical clinical presentation of those individuals ingesting mushrooms with muscarinic characteristics or anticholinesterases is diffuse diaphoresis, salivation, lacrimation, urination, and defecation associated with myofasciculations.

DIAGNOSTIC EVALUATION

The diversity of entities associated with diaphoresis mandates a meticulous history and physical exami-

Table 14–4. Causes of Diaphoresis

General
    Anxiety
    Emesis
    Exercise
    Pain
Endocrinologic
    Hyperthyroidism
    Hypoglycemia
    Pheochromocytoma
Infectious diseases
    Tuberculosis
    Sepsis
Toxicologic agents
    Amphetamines
    Anticholinesterases (carbamates, organophosphates, physostig-
        mine)
    Ciguatera
    Cocaine
    Death camas (Zygadenus)
    Fluoroacetate
    Hexachlorobenzene
    Jessamine
    Lobeline
    Lysergic acid diethylamide (LSD)
    Mushrooms—muscarinic
    Naphthalene
    Nicotine
    Perchloroethylene
    Picrotoxin
    Snake bites
    Tetrodotoxin

nation. The general assessment of the patient's recent health and close observation of the patient's behavior will be helpful in the evaluation. A careful history with regard to the common associated findings of hyperthyroidism, hypoglycemia, and pheochromocytoma is necessary to determine whether any of these endocrinologic disorders is present. A careful history is especially important in determining whether infection or drug ingestion is a consideration. If the patient's mental status is abnormal, the likelihood of poisoning becomes greater. Patient utilization of unknown preparations and the possibility of ingestion of fish, plants, or mushrooms should be assessed. The possibility of an occupational or accidental exposure to anticholinesterases should be considered.

Determination of pulse, blood pressure, respiratory rate, and temperature may aid in the differentiation of many of these disorders. Because of the overactivity of the sympathetic nervous system, most of these entities may be accompanied by hypertension, tachycardia, hyperthermia, and tachypnea. In contrast, hypoglycemia is usually associated with hypothermia. Sepsis manifests itself with either hypo- or hyperthermia and usually is associated with hypotension. Some of the more severe toxic ingestions such as am-

phetamines, cocaine, and LSD may result in severe hypertension. On the other hand, the toxicity associated with anticholinesterases, snake bites, and tetrodotoxin may be manifested by hypotension and life threatening respiratory emergencies.

Endocrinologic assessment includes the determination of serum T_4 and T_3 as well as the free thyroxine index (hyperthyroidism), serum glucose (hypoglycemia), urinary catecholamines, metanephrines, and vanillylmandelic acid (VMA). Studies for tuberculosis should include acid-fast sputum examination and cultures of suspected involved tissues. Bacterial cultures of appropriate fluids should be performed when sepsis is a major consideration. Relevant signs and symptoms suggestive of toxicologic agents should be followed by examination of blood, urine, and gastric contents.

HYPOTHERMIA

DEFINITION AND CLASSIFICATION

Hypothermia has been arbitrarily defined as a rectal or body core temperature below 95° F (or 35° C). A normal individual's temperature varies from 1 to 2° F during a 24-hour period. Among normal individuals, temperatures may range from 96 to 100° F. Note that most clinical thermometers are not designed to detect hypothermia and do not record temperatures below 94° F.

Hypothermia is classified as accidental or induced. The latter term is used to identify patients in whom hypothermia has been deliberately produced under controlled conditions for therapeutic purposes. Considerable valuable information has been obtained from studies of these carefully controlled hypothermic patients, but this review will deal primarily with the accidental hypothermia a practicing physician encounters.

Experimental studies and clinical experiences have suggested that it is useful to divide hypothermic patients into three groups[22]:

1. Responsive range (95 to 90° F). In this stage, uncompromised patients shiver. Cutaneous vasoconstriction occurs to conserve heat, blood pressure and pulse rate increase, and diuresis occurs as a result of expansion of the intravascular volume.

2. Slowing phase (89 to 75° F). The ability to generate heat diminishes, probably from slowing of enzyme kinetics and decreasing metabolism. Basal met-

abolic rates fall 50% at 82° F.[23] The muscles grow stiffer and shivering subsides to little more than a fine tremor. Blood pressure, pulse rate, and respiratory efforts may fall.

3. Poikilothermic phase (below 75° F). Patients are strikingly cold and are often presumed dead.

Hypothermia develops so slowly that it may be hardly noticeable to either the victim or observers. The individual may feel that he is just tired while gradually slipping into semicoma. Alcohol directly causes peripheral vasodilatation and inhibits gluconeogenesis, which disturbances overwhelmingly contribute to the pathogenesis of hypothermia. The victim of hypothermia should not be pronounced dead until rewarming has been accomplished. Even dilated pupils do not confirm death.[24]

PATHOPHYSIOLOGIC CONSIDERATIONS

Humans can adjust to hot weather much better than to cold. Whereas physiologic changes including increased sweating and decreased blood viscosity aid in heat acclimatization, the two major mechanisms for maintaining body heat are peripheral blood vessel constriction and shivering. The thermogenesis of exercise and eating plays a major role in generating body heat above that produced by the basal metabolic rate.

Individuals most likely to present with severe losses of body heat are sportsmen and campers exposed to adverse cooling environments, individuals who have abused alcohol and fallen asleep or become unconscious in an exposed area, individuals who have been accidentally immersed in cold water, and thin, elderly, or other malnourished people who live in poorly heated homes; hypothermia occurs in very elderly patients exposed to indoor temperatures as high as 65° F. The three most important contributors to hypothermia are alcohol abuse, hypoglycemia, and infection. Frequently, two or all three of these factors are found in the same patient. The requisite exposure can be very mild if the hypothalamic thermal regulatory factors are impaired, if body shivering is reduced because of medications or aging, and if vasoconstriction is compromised. The cause of hypothermia can be judged from where the patient is being observed. Sepsis is probably the most common cause in patients in the intensive care unit, while environmental exposure in association with excess alcohol consumption is the most common presentation in most emergency departments. Although many factors can contribute to the development of hypothermia, environmental exposure always plays a role.

Table 14–5.   Factors Contributing to Hypothermia

Impaired muscle movement
  Drugs
    Alcohol
    Phenothiazines
    Barbiturates
    Most sedatives
  Age
    Very young and very old
  Paralysis of major muscle groups
  Hypothyroidism
Impaired vasoconstriction
  Drugs
    Alcohol
    Phenothiazines
    Antihypertensives
  Sepsis
  Erythroderma
Metabolic and endocrine factors
  Starvation
  Hypothyroidism
  Adrenal insufficiency
  Hypopituitarism
  Hypoglycemia
  Uremia
  Hepatic failure
  Thiamine deficiency
Central nervous system
  Brain tumors
  Brain injuries

DIFFERENTIAL DIAGNOSIS

A large number of patients are at potential risk of developing hypothermia. The diagnosis can be overlooked if the clinical mercury thermometer is not shaken down adequately. There is so much emphasis on increased temperature that examiners are often satisfied when they have shaken the thermometer to only the normal temperature reading. The diagnosis must be considered in any patient who is obtunded, who presents with cardiac arrhythmias, and who is exposed to contributing factors (Table 14–5).

Although a careful patient history is vital to alert the clinician to the contributing factors of drugs or other illnesses, which often threaten the survival of the patient more than the degree of hypothermia does, the history is often not helpful. Therefore, in patients with hypothermia alone, mortality occurs in up to 10%, but in the presence of an underlying disease, mortality is often between 75 and 90%.[25] Hypothermia should always be suspected in a patient in wet clothing, for wetness reduces the clothing insulation to almost zero. Actual immersion results in heat loss in the patient 25 to 30 times faster than standing in ambient air of the same temperature. Wind chill has a dramatic effect on environmental temperature. For example, 10° F becomes nearly −10° F with a 10 mph wind.

DIAGNOSTIC EVALUATION

Victims of hypothermia usually complain of cold only during the early stages, when the body temperature is between 95° F and 90° F. Mentation is often severely impaired and the patient may be unconscious as body temperature falls below 90° F. Although many ill patients have cold extremities, the hypothermic patient feels strikingly cold, even on covered areas, where body heat is usually preserved. Swelling and ecchymoses occur in association with poor circulation and sustained pressure from immobility. The patient may demonstrate muscular rigidity suggesting an acute systemic drug reaction, parkinsonism, or even the stiff neck of meningitis. The tendon reflexes are depressed and plantar reflexes are sometimes abnormal. The pupils may be dilated and react sluggishly to light. Lateralizing focal neurologic signs can occur.

Many of these patients will be volume depleted because of cold diuresis and poor intake. Although cold initially stimulates the heart, heart rate and contractility are depressed as hypothermic temperatures are reached. Myocardial creatinine phosphokinase and lactic dehydrogenase may be elevated. Electrocardiographic changes include increases in the PR interval, QT prolongation, nodal rhythms, and the classic "J" (Junctional) or Osborne wave, which is a positive deflection in the left ventricular leads at the junction of QRS and ST segments. A fine baseline oscillation from muscle rigidity should not be disregarded as electrical interference. Patients are particularly prone to atrial fibrillation and ventricular fibrillation when body temperature reaches 86° F.[25] The cold heart can survive unusual episodes of ventricular fibrillation.

Bowel function is frequently depressed, and slowed peristalsis may result in distension and depressed bowel sounds. Pancreatitis may be asymptomatic and remain unsuspected until rewarming is accomplished. Pneumonia from aspiration or infection is often present initially, and the patient must be followed closely for the possibility of pneumonia throughout the evaluation and treatment.

The initial laboratory data should include a hemogram, platelet count, evaluation of electrolytes, glucose, BUN, creatinine, amylase, liver enzymes, urinalysis, stool guaiac test, blood cultures, blood gases, electrocardiogram, and chest x-ray. Although hypoglycemia can cause hypothermia, serum glucose will usually be elevated rather than low if the hypothermia is the initial event.

The physician should administer 50 ml of 50% glucose in water IV and 100 mg of thiamin as a diagnostic test because of the high incidence of alcoholism and its associated hypoglycemia in hypothermic patients.

Placement of any central lines must be done with great caution since the myocardium is irritable. Endocrine function seems to parallel the depressed metabolic activity. One must always look carefully for the telltale goiter or thyroidectomy scar on the neck suggesting the possibility of thyroid deficiency. In case of a real emergency, the patient should be treated for adrenal insufficiency before the evaluation is completed.

Hypothermic patients who develop ventricular fibrillation are resistant to atropine, electric pacing, and countershock. Countershock should be attempted, but it is important to remember the protection afforded by the hypothermia to the myocardium and to proceed with prolonged cardiopulmonary resuscitation. In this setting, rapid core temperature warming may be essential, even during evaluation.

HYPERTHERMIA

DEFINITION

Hyperthermia is elevation of the body temperature as a single manifestation of disease. The thermoregulatory set point may not be readjusted in hyperthermia by itself. Temperature regulation may be so impaired that the temperature elevation itself can be fatal. Heat dissipation may also be impaired. In the adult, temperatures in excess of 105° F should be considered life threatening.

PATHOPHYSIOLOGIC CONSIDERATIONS

Hyperthermia occurs when an imbalance results between the heat generated and retained and the heat dissipated. There are five basic mechanisms of heat loss: radiation, conduction, convection, respiration, and evaporation. The relationship between heat storage, excretion, metabolism, and heat loss is defined by the equation

$$S = M \pm C_1 \pm C_2 \pm R_1 \pm R_2 - E_1 - E_2$$

where S = Heat storage

M = Basal metabolic rate—65 to 85 Kcal/hour, it increases dramatically with any substantial motor activity or exercise

C_1 = Conduction—the direct transfer of heat to cooler objects or receipt of heat from warmer objects when direct contact is made; heat transfer is proportional to the thermal gradient

Table 14–6. Causes of Hyperthermia

Environmental exposure (temperature, humidity)
Chronic systemic diseases
    CNS
    Heart
    Lungs
    Kidneys
    Diabetes mellitus
Nutritional deficiencies
Acute and chronic motor disorders
Trauma
Impaired environmental perception
Psychiatric disorders
Dermatologic disorders
Psychotropic agents
    Tricyclic antidepressants
    Phenothiazines
    Lithium
Toxins
    Cocaine
    Salicylates
    Amphetamines
    Phencyclidine
    Ethanol
    Ethanol and sedative hypnotic withdrawal
Drugs causing thermoregulatory interference
    Antihistamines
    Atropine
    Inhalational anesthesia
    Succinylcholine
    Pancuronium bromide

C_2 = Convection—the transfer of heat is dependent on the wind velocity, humidity, and ambient air temperature

R_1 = Respiration—heat exchange is determined by the amount needed to warm inhaled air to body temperature or the amount absorbed from the air

R_2 = Radiation—the transfer of heat to those cooler parts of the environment not in contact with the body, or receipt of heat from external sources

E_1 = Evaporation—water is evaporated from the body surface, depending on the temperature, air velocity, and humidity; and

E_2 = Excretion—heat loss derived from feces and urine

One of the most common environmental stresses placed on humans is hot, humid weather. When the humidity and environmental temperature increase convection, radiation and evaporation decrease dramatically and the patient must adapt substantially to dissipate heat. Elderly and neonatal individuals have the smallest capacity to adapt to thermal stress and experience frequent heat-related disorders.

DIFFERENTIAL DIAGNOSIS

Causes of hyperthermia include exposure to the environment, dermatologic impairment of heat loss, spinal cord injuries, extensive surgical wrappings, burns, obesity, chronic diseases of the heart, lungs, and kidney, and diabetes (Table 14–6). Nutritional deficiencies (particularly thiamine), acute and chronic motor disorders, utilization of psychotropic agents, possibly associated with malignant neuroleptic syndrome, diverse toxicologic agents, inhalational anesthesia, pyrogenic stimuli, and drug interactions may also cause temperature elevation.

Malignant hyperthermia frequently associated with inhalational anesthesia is another important cause of hyperthermia. This syndrome occurs only in the operating room or in the postoperative period. Pyrogenic stimulation usually involved in the treatment of neoplastic disease may also be associated with hyperthermia.

Heatstroke is the most severe and life threatening of heat-related disorders, and is manifested by headache, weakness, confusion, delirium, coma, and death. Patients with heatstroke usually have an altered consciousness, hot, dry skin, and a temperature in excess of 105° F. Certain patients present with heat exhaustion or prostration in hot, humid weather. These individuals have salt and water depletion and an inadequate cardiovascular response to these disturbances. Patients have anorexia, nausea, vomiting, faintness, weakness, occasional muscle cramps, and myalgias, as well as postural hypotension. Occasionally they may have an altered mental status, even with mildly elevated temperature.

DIAGNOSTIC EVALUATION

It is important to elicit a history of chronic diseases of the heart, lungs, kidney, pancreas, or central nervous system, and, in particular, a history of psychiatric, neurologic, and dermatologic disorders that predispose patients to hyperthermic states. Toxicologic assessment should include evaluation for drug dependency and abuse, as well as for use of psychotropic agents such as tricyclic antidepressants, lithium, phenothiazines, butyrophenones, and MAO inhibitors. A careful physical examination must search for dermatologic and neurologic disorders.

Diagnostic studies including serum electrolytes, glucose, BUN, liver function studies, and a coagulation profile should be carried out. These tests will help in the diagnosis of impending acute renal failure associated with rhabdomyolysis and acute hepatic necrosis with a resultant coagulopathy. Muscle breakdown is assessed by an increase in serum creatine phosphokinase and myoglobin. Specific toxicologic studies should be performed on blood and urine.

MALIGNANT HYPERTHERMIA

DEFINITION

Malignant hyperthermia (MH) is an inherited life threatening syndrome characterized by marked temperature elevation (hyperthermia) during or following surgical procedure in response to inhalational anesthetic agents such as halothane or to muscle relaxants such as succinylcholine. Involuntary muscle contraction, marked rigidity, autonomic dysfunctions, and metabolic acidosis are other major clinical features of the syndrome (see Table 14–8).

PATHOPHYSIOLOGIC CONSIDERATIONS

A number of agents may precipitate MH in a susceptible individual (Table 14–7). Most commonly the syndrome occurs with the use of a halogenated anesthetic agent and succinylcholine. MH usually develops only during the second exposure to general anesthesia, although MH has also been reported during local anesthesia. Many studies support the hypothesis that MH is an autosomal dominant disorder; in the majority of patients, however, the pattern of inheritance is obscure. It is likely that MH can occur by more than one genetic pattern.

In normal muscle contraction, calcium is released from the sarcoplasmic reticulum into the intracellular space; the calcium ion activates ATPase to convert ATP to ADP, phosphate, and heat. During relaxation, calcium ions are returned to the sarcoplasmic reticulum. It is believed that in susceptible individuals with MH there is a defect in the outflow of calcium from the sarcoplasmic reticulum to the intracellular space, as well as a disturbance in calcium re-uptake. This phenomenon results in a persistent elevation of myoplasmic calcium concentration and sustained muscle contraction, thus explaining muscle rigidity and hyperthermia.

In MH, temperature elevation should not be considered as fever. Fever, in contrast to hyperthermia, results from an upward adjustment of the hypothalamic thermostat in response to pyrogens or other factors. Fever usually responds to antipyretic agents and has diurnal variation. In contrast, patients with hyper-

Table 14–7. Agents Implicated in Malignant Hyperthermia

Caffeine
Succinylcholine
Halothane
KCl
Lidocaine (local)
Carbocaine (local)
Curare
Gallamine
N-alkyl Nortoxiferine
Spinal analgesia
Enflurane
Trichloroethylene
Methoxyflurane
Diethyl ether
Cyclopropane
Ethylene
Nitrous oxide (meperidine)
Thiopentone
D-tubocurarine
Stress

(From Schvaneveldt, J.A., et al.: Malignant hyperpyrexia: an update for the otolaryngologist. Otolaryngology 88:921, 1980.)

thermia have a persistent elevation of temperature without much fluctuation and with no significant response to antipyretic agents.

In MH, severe muscle contraction results in myonecrosis with an accompanying increase in serum myoglobin and myoglobinuria. Thus, acute renal failure is not an uncommon complication.

Table 14–8. Comparison of Neuroleptic Malignant Syndrome (NMS) and Malignant Hyperthermia (MH) Manifestations

	NMS	MH
Premorbid exhaustion as a risk factor	+	+
Sex	Predominantly males	?
Age	Young adults	Young adults
Length of syndrome	5–30 days*	1–3 days*
Drug metabolism	Several weeks	Several hours
Sialorrhea	+	?
Dyskinesia	+	+
Dysphagia	+	?
Rigidity	+	+
Akinesia	+	?
Tachypnea/dyspnea	+	+
Tachycardia	+	+
Hypertension (labile)	+	+
Arrhythmia	+	+
Febrile	+	+
Creatine phosphokinase	+	+
Liver function tests	+	+
Potassium	?	+
Myoglobinuria	?	+
Respiratory acidosis	+	+
Heritable	?	Autosomal dominant

*This perhaps reflects the longer half-life of the neuroleptic drugs.

DIFFERENTIAL DIAGNOSIS

MH and neuroleptic malignant syndrome (NMS) share many common signs and symptoms (Table 14–8). The history of neuroleptic therapy and the characteristic clinical and laboratory findings readily differentiate NMS from MH.

DIAGNOSTIC EVALUATION

Muscle rigidity during anesthesia and marked temperature elevation in the postoperative period should arouse the suspicion of MH. The physician should also consider MH when patients undergoing anesthesia demonstrate cyanosis, instability of blood pressure, tachycardia, arrhythmias, and tachypnea. In particular, rigidity following a sufficient dose of a muscle relaxant such as succinylcholine should raise the possibility of MH.

Several diagnostic studies are helpful. Arterial blood gases will demonstrate hypoxemia, metabolic or respiratory acidosis, and hypercapnia. The serum level of potassium, CPK, and myoglobin will often be elevated, and accompanying myoglobinuria will give a red pigmentation to the urine.

The most accurate method of diagnosing susceptibility to MH is a skeletal muscle biopsy. The muscle fibers are subjected to increasing doses of triggering agents such as caffeine and caffeine with halothane. A positive diagnosis of susceptibility to MH is established when muscle fibers respond with greater contraction than muscle fibers of nonsusceptible individuals respond with.

Surgery should be performed only if absolutely indicated in susceptible patients or in individuals with known malignant hyperthermia. In these cases, inhalational agents and muscle relaxants should be avoided.

REFERENCES

1. The National Ambulatory Medical Care Survey: 1975 Summary. Hyattsville, Md., National Center for Health Statistics, 1978, p. 22.
2. Berris, B., and Racklis, A.: Investigation of fatigue. Can Fam Physic 23:465, 1977.
3. Morrison, J.D.: Fatigue as a presenting complaint in family practice. Fam Pract 5:795, 1980.
4. Solberg, L.I.: Lassitude, a primary care evaluation. JAMA 251:3272, 1984.
5. Johnson, D.D., et al.: Reactive hypoglycemia. JAMA 243:1151, 1984.
6. Hofeldt, F.D., Adler, R.A., and Herman, R.H.: Postprandial hypoglycemia, fact or fiction. JAMA 223:1309, 1975.
7. Rea, W.J.: Diagnosing food and chemical susceptibility. Cont Educ (Sept) 47, 1979.
8. Randolph, T.G.: The scope of food and chemical allergy/addiction. Cont Educ (Sept) 63, 1979.
9. Gonzalez, E.R.: The 'non-neurotic' approach to mitral valve prolapse. JAMA 246:2113, 1981.
10. Stone, B.M.: Sleep and low doses of alcohol. Electroencephalogr Clin Neurophysiol 48:706, 1980.
11. Swenson, W.M., and Morse, R.M.: The use of a self-administered alcoholism screening test (SMAST) in a medical center. Mayo Clin Proc 50:204, 1975.
12. Berndt, S.M., Berndt, D.J., and Byars, W.O.: A multi-institutional study of depression in family practice. J Fam Pract 16:83, 1983.
13. Swenson, W.M.: Automated personality assessment in medical practice. Med Clin North Am 54:835, 1970.
14. Peabody, F.W.: The care of the patient. JAMA 88:877, 1927. Republished in JAMA 252:813, 1984.
15. Harvey, A.M., Bordley, J., and Barondess, J.A.: Differential Diagnosis, the Interpretation of Clinical Evidence. 3rd Ed. Philadelphia, W.B. Saunders Co., 1979, p. 650.
16. Kraytam, M.: Weakness. In The Complete Patient History. Edited by M. Kraytam. New York, McGraw-Hill Book Co., 1979.
17. Edwards, R.H.T.: Physiologic analysis of skeletal muscle weakness and fatigue. J Sci and Mol Med 54:463, 1978.
18. Lazzaro, R.P., and Kirshner, H.S.: Proximal muscle weakness in uremia. Arch Neurol 37:555, 1980.
19. Ludmer, K.M., and Kissane, J.: Wasting in a 33 year-old woman. Am J Med 76:302, 1984.
20. Cutler, P.: Hematologic problems. In Problem Solving in Clinical Medicine, from Data to Diagnosis. Edited by P. Cutler. Baltimore, Williams and Wilkins Co., 1979, p. 79.
21. Campbell, W.W., and Swift, T.R.: Differential diagnosis of acute weakness. South Med J 74:1371, 1981.
22. Fitzgerald, F.T., and Jessop, C.: Accidental Hypothermia: A Report of 22 Cases and Review of the Literature. Chicago, Yearbook Medical Publishers, Inc., 1982.
23. Reuler, J.B.: Hypothermia: pathophysiology, clinical settings, and management. Ann Intern Med 89:519, 1978.
24. Fell, R.H., Gunning, A.J., Bardham, K.D., and Triger, D.R.: Severe hypothermia as a result of barbiturate overdose complicated by cardiac arrest. Lancet 1:392, 1968.
25. Goldfrank, L., and Kirstein, R.: Emergency management of hypothermia. Hosp Physic 1:47, 1979.
26. O'Keefe, K.M.: Accidental hypothermia: a review of 62 cases. J Amer Coll Emer Physic 6:491, 1977.

GENERAL REFERENCES

FLUSHING

Adamson, A.R., Peart, W.S., Grahame-Smith, D.G., and Starr, M.: Pharmacological blockage of carcinoid flushing provoked by catecholamines and alcohol. Lancet 2:293, 1969.
Oates, J.A., and Sjoerdsma, A.: A unique syndrome associated with the secretion of 5-hydroxytryptophan by metastatic gastric carcinoid. Am J Med 32:333, 1962.
Schaumburg, H.H., Byck, R., Gerstl, R., and Mashman, J.H.: Monosodium, L Glutamate: Its pharmacology and role in Chinese Restaurant syndrome. Science 163:826, 1969.

DIAPHORESIS

Sato, K.: The physiology, pharmacology and biochemistry of the eccrine sweat gland. Rev Physiol Biochem Pharmacol 79:52–131, 1977.

HYPERTHERMIA

Granoff, A.L., and Davis, J.M.: Heat illness syndrome and lithium intoxication. J Clin Psychiatry 39:103–107, 1978.

Greenblatt, D.J., and Gross, P.L.: Fatal hyperthermia following haloperidol therapy of sedative hypnotic withdrawal. J Clin Psychiatry 39:673–675, 1978.

Gronert, G.A.: Malignant hyperthermia (MH). Anesthesiology 53:395–423, 1980.

Knochel, J.P.: Environmental heat illness. Arch Intern Med 133:841–863, 1974.

MALIGNANT HYPERTHERMIA

Adriani, J., and Sundin, R.: Malignant hyperthermia in dental patients. JADA 108:180, 1984.

Gronert, G.A.: Malignant hyperthermia. Anesthesiology 53:395, 1980.

Marchildon, M.B.: Malignant hyperthermia: Current concepts. Arch Surg 117:349, 1982.

Rodgers, I.R.: Malignant hyperthermia: A review of the literature. The Mt Sinai J Med 50:95, 1983.

Tollefson, G.: A case of neuroleptic malignant syndrome: In vitro muscle comparison with malignant hyperthermia. Clin Psychopharmacol 2:266, 1982.

Willner, J.: Malignant hyperthermia. Pediatric Ann 13:128, 1981.

CHAPTER 15

NEUROLOGIC PROBLEMS

John J. Caronna, M.D.

HEADACHE

DEFINITION

Head pain is the most common pain syndrome encountered in clinical practice and in one form or another affects almost all of the population. Headaches may arise from extracranial or intracranial sources.

Almost all extracranial tissues are pain sensitive. By contrast, most intracranial structures, including the parenchyma of the brain, most of the dura and pia-arachnoid, the ependyma lining the ventricles, and the choroid plexus, are insensitive to pain. The intracranial pain-sensitive structures include the dural and cerebral arteries, the great venous sinuses and cortical veins, the fifth, seventh, ninth, and tenth cranial nerves, and the upper two cervical nerves.

The first division of the fifth cranial nerve (CNV_1) innervates pain-sensitive intracranial structures located on or above the superior surface of the tentorium. Therefore, pain arising from supratentorial structures is experienced in the cutaneous distribution of CNV_1, that is, the eyes, forehead, and vertex.

The ninth and tenth cranial nerves and the upper two cervical nerves innervate pain-sensitive structures on or below the inferior surface of the tentorium. Pain of infratentorial origin, therefore, is experienced in the posterior parietal and occipital regions and the dermatomes corresponding to the cutaneous distribution of the upper cervical nerves.

PATHOPHYSIOLOGIC CONSIDERATIONS

Head and face pain arising from extracranial structures usually is due to one or more of the following conditions: painful dilatation and distension of extracranial arteries; sustained contraction (spasm) of skeletal muscles about the face, scalp, and neck; disease of the eyes, ears, nose, teeth, and sinuses; neuralgias and neuritides involving CNV, IX, and X and the upper cervical nerves; inflammation of the extracranial arteries; and trauma, infection, or neoplasms of the extracranial tissues.

Headache from intracranial sources can result from one or more of the following conditions: displacement of, or traction on, and dilatation or distension of intracranial arteries; displacement of, or traction on, the cerebral venous sinuses and their tributary veins; inflammation of any intracranial pain-sensitive structure; and direct pressure by mass lesions on intracranial pain-sensitive structures.

CLINICAL PRESENTATION AND DIFFERENTIAL DIAGNOSIS
(TABLE 15–1)

Headaches from Extracranial Sources.

Vascular or Migraine Headaches. These headaches are due to painful distension of extracranial and sometimes of intracranial arteries. The headaches are periodic and vary in intensity, duration, and frequency. Frequently, headache begins in the morning just after arising, and symptoms may last for hours or even days. Severe vascular headaches are accompanied by nausea, vomiting, photophobia, and sometimes diarrhea. Young women are affected more than men, and migraine headaches frequently accompany or precede menstrual periods. Various foods, drinks, and allergens have been implicated in the genesis of these headaches, which often have a familial incidence.

Migraine headaches are of several types. Classic migraines are preceded by a variety of visual disturbances and other neurologic abnormalities. These prodromes or auras occur for minutes to an hour and may take the form of scintillating scotomas, visual field defects including bilateral blindness, hemisensory deficits, and hemiplegia. Neurologic dysfunction is attributed in part to cerebral ischemia caused by constriction of intracranial arteries and by depression of cerebral electrical activity by a potassium mediated mechanism. As the prodrome recedes, a vasodilator headache begins, usually unilaterally, then becoming generalized.

Common migraines are vascular headaches without a striking prodrome. At onset, common migraines (or "sick headaches") are more likely to be generalized or bilateral rather than unilateral.

Cluster headaches are predominantly unilateral headaches that affect men, especially in middle age,

Table 15–1. Differential Diagnosis of Headache

Headache from extracranial sources
  Vascular or migraine headaches
  Classic migraine
  Common migraine
  Cluster headache
  Muscle contraction or tension headaches
Headache from intracranial sources
  Brain tumor headache
  Headache due to increased intracranial pressure
  Headache associated with increased cerebral blood volume
  Headache associated with inflammation of intracranial tissues
  Headache associated with low cerebrospinal fluid pressure

much more than women. The headaches typically begin at night, usually 1 or 2 hours after bedtime, and generally are brief, lasting minutes to hours rather than days. Cluster headaches are associated with unilateral flushing, sweating, rhinorrhea, increased lacrimation, ptosis, and miosis. The name cluster refers to the fact that headaches occur in groups or clusters lasting days to weeks, separated by long remissions.

Muscle Contraction or Tension Headaches. These headaches are associated with steady, nonpulsatile, occipitofrontal pain. Additional symptoms include tightness, pressure, or constriction about the head. Headaches may occur daily and last for weeks or months. Unlike migraine headaches, tension headaches often begin late in the day and usually respond to over-the-counter analgesics.

The cause of muscle spasm or tension headaches is long-sustained contraction of skeletal muscles about the face, scalp, and neck. Concurrent vasodilation of extracranial arteries may also contribute to the pain. Neurologic examination is normal in patients with tension headaches, but palpation of the muscles of the scalp, neck, and face may reveal localized painful areas or nodules. The points of insertion of the involved muscles are especially likely to be tender.

Tension headaches usually can be differentiated from vascular headaches by the historical features mentioned above. Sinus headaches caused by congestion, inflammation, and edema of nasal and paranasal mucous membranes usually present as anterior headache associated with nasal stuffiness and rhinorrhea. Head pain caused by dental disease occasionally occurs without toothache. In eyestrain headache, caused by errors of refraction, headache usually starts around and over the eyes and subsequently radiates to the occiput, mimicking muscle contraction headache. The pain of increased intraocular pressure begins in the eyeball, then extends throughout most of the dermatome supplied by the ophthalmic division of CNV. In each kind of headache, a detailed clinical history and careful examination of the head, neck, oral cavity, and eyes will identify the source of headache. Sinus roentgenograms, measurement of intraocular pressure, refraction, or other studies can be used as confirmatory tests.

Headaches from Intracranial Sources

Brain Tumor Headache. Head pain from mass lesions is deep and aching, steady and dull, rather than the excruciating and throbbing pain of migraine headaches. Headache usually is noted in the morning before arising and diminishes as the patient assumes a vertical posture. Caffeine and nonprescription analgesics usually relieve brain tumor headaches not associated with increased intracranial pressure. Mass lesions in the supratentorial compartment cause unilateral or bilateral pain in the dermatomal distribution of the first division of CNV. Subtentorial lesions are associated with occipital or suboccipital headache and stiffness or aching of the neck muscles.

Headache from Increased Intracranial Pressure. Brain tumors, intracerebral hemorrhages, acute hydrocephalus, and acute obstructions of cerebral venous drainage lead to sudden increases in intracranial pressure. Such headaches may be excruciating and generalized. Vomiting may occur because of severe pain or as a result of medullary compression. In the latter case, the vomiting, which occurs without nausea or warning, tends to be projectile.

The initial headaches of brain tumor result from displacement of intracerebral arteries, veins, and cranial nerves. Increased intracranial pressure per se does not cause pain unless distension, displacement, or inflammation of intracranial structures occurs, as in acute intracerebral hemorrhage and bacterial meningitis. Chronically increased intracranial hypertension, as occurs in benign intracranial hypertension or chronic communicating hydrocephalus, may not be associated with headache.

A history of progressively severe daily headaches in association with lethargy, focal neurologic deficits, and unilateral or bilateral papilledema serves to identify the patient with a progressively enlarging intracranial mass.

Apoplectic onset of headache and paralysis or coma is the hallmark of intracerebral hemorrhage. Subacute onset of signs and symptoms in the setting of fever and stiff neck identifies bacterial meningitis. A CT scan usually will identify the abnormality suspected on physical exam.

Headache Associated with Increased Cerebral Blood Volume. Headaches associated with fever, generalized sepsis, nitrite and carbon monoxide inhalation, anoxia, and epileptic seizures are due to distension of intracranial arterial structures. A similar mechanism causes the headaches that accompany sudden rises in arterial blood pressure such as occur in patients with pheochromocytoma or acute hypertensive encephalopathy.

Headache Associated with Inflammation of Intracranial Tissues. The headache of chronic or acute meningitis is related to the lowered pain threshold of inflamed tissues. Inflammation usually is most marked at the base of the brain. In cases of cerebral arteritis, as occurs in the syndromes of giant cell arteritis and other collagen vascular diseases, the inflammation of extracranial and intracranial vessels causes the usually painless arterial dilatation during cardiac systole to become painful, hence the characteristic throbbing headache.

Headache Associated with Low Cerebrospinal Fluid Pressure. Dull, pulsating, occipital headache develops in one fourth to one fifth of patients undergoing lumbar puncture. The headache begins within hours after the procedure and is orthostatic i.e., it occurs when the patient is in the erect position and subsides if he lies flat. The headache usually disappears within days to 2 weeks.

The cause of postlumbar puncture headache is leakage of cerebrospinal fluid (CSF) through a hole in the dural sac. The consequent loss of fluid buoyancy in the skull results in downward movement of the brain and traction on pain-sensitive intracranial structures.

Postlumbar puncture headaches are more common and more prolonged after a difficult lumbar puncture requiring several passes with the spinal needle or after an accurate lumbar puncture with a large-bore needle. Surgical or post-traumatic tears in the dural sac may lead to prostrating and prolonged headache symptoms. Occasionally, surgical repair or "blood patching" of a persistent dural fluid leak is required.

DIAGNOSTIC EVALUATION

Each headache patient deserves a careful history and a complete physical and neurologic examination. Even if the medical history suggests a specific diagnosis, the physician should not omit a complete examination.

The general examination may reveal systemic illnesses that can cause headache, for example, abnormalities of the cervical spine and paranasal sinuses. The mental status examination may reveal anxiety, depression, or agitation. Aphasia in a right-handed person indicates a lesion of the left hemisphere. Impairment of memory, if accompanied by chronic headache, requires an intensive search for brain tumor, subdural hematoma, or hydrocephalus. Focal motor and sensory deficits may indicate the presence of a cerebral infarct or mass lesion.

Headache can be the first symptom of organic disease. If the patient is being seen for the first time for headache, some laboratory tests are indicated. The erythrocyte sedimentation rate (ESR) if elevated may indicate the presence of malignancy, infection, or arteritis. A CT scan should be used when focal disease is suspected, when the pattern of headache attack changes, or if screening tests suggest the presence of an abnormality. A CT scan with contrast can identify most intracranial tumors, angiomas, hematomas, and some cerebral aneurysms. A lumbar puncture with careful measurements of opening and closing CSF pressures is indicated when intracranial hypertension,

chronic meningitis, or hydrocephalus is suspected on the basis of a prior CT scan.

SYNDROMES OF PAIN AND SENSORY DISTURBANCES

FACE PAIN

Trigeminal Neuralgia (Tic Douloureux)

Trigeminal neuralgia is characterized by sudden paroxysms of pain in the distribution of one or more divisions of the trigeminal nerve, usually the second or third divisions.

The pathogenesis of trigeminal neuralgia is unknown because the pain is usually unassociated with recognizable structural disease of the central nervous system. Occasionally, tic douloureux may be a symptom of multiple sclerosis, a tumor of the gasserian ganglion, or a brain stem infarct involving the pathways (descending root or quintothalamic tract) of the trigeminal nerve.

The patient history is diagnostic in typical trigeminal neuralgia. The pain occurs as brief, lightning-like stabs and is frequently precipitated by touching a trigger point around the lips or buccal cavity. At times, talking, eating, or brushing the teeth serves as a trigger. Although the pains rarely last longer than seconds, they often occur in clusters so that the pain seems to last for minutes or hours. Pain rarely occurs at night. In typical idiopathic trigeminal neuralgia, the neurologic exam is normal. The dramatic response of face pain to carbamazepine is almost diagnostic of idiopathic tic. In atypical face pain, there may be sensory changes in the distribution of the trigeminal nerve; such a finding should prompt a careful search for structural disease of the nervous system, including a CT scan.

Glossopharyngeal Neuralgia

Glossopharyngeal neuralgia is characterized by pain similar to that of trigeminal neuralgia, but in the distribution of IX and X. The condition, usually idiopathic, is occasionally the presenting complaint in a patient with a tonsillar tumor.

The trigger zone in glossopharyngeal neuralgia usually is in the tonsil or posterior pharynx, and the pain spreads ipsilaterally toward the angle of the jaw and the ear. Patients may experience cardiac slowing or arrest during attacks as a result of the intense afferent discharge over the glossopharyngeal nerve. The response to carbamazepine may be less dramatic than in cases of tic douloureux and is not diagnostic of idiopathic glossopharyngeal neuralgia. A careful examination of the nasopharynx by a specialist is mandatory in each case.

PAIN IN THE TRUNK AND EXTREMITIES

Tabes Dorsalis

The lightning pains of tabes dorsalis in the trunk and lower extremities are analogous to trigeminal and glossopharyngeal neuralgias. This pain, caused by luetic damage to the dorsal roots, results in a sensory ataxia such that the patient manifests Romberg's sign (loss of balance when the feet are together and the eyes are closed).

Tabes dorsalis develops in less than 5% of patients with untreated syphilis. Symptoms become manifest after a latent period of 10 to 30 years. Mentation is normal, unless general paresis coexists with tabes. The gait is broad-based, there is hypotonia, and the deep tendon reflexes are absent or diminished. Pupillary abnormalities include miosis, irregularity, and poor response to light; retained reaction to accommodation (Argyll Robertson pupils), however, is present in most cases. Lightning pains develop in 75% of tabetic patients and may appear in any area of the body, including the viscera, but are most common in the lower extremities. Variable degrees of hypoesthesia and hypalgesia in a radicular distribution are found in the lower extremities. Involvement of sacral nerve roots leads to impotence, overflow incontinence of urine, and constipation. The course of tabes is unpredictable and the response to therapy is variable.

Lightning pains are not pathognomonic of tabes dorsalis because they occur in other diseases affecting dorsal roots, especially diabetic neuropathy. Early in the course of tabes dorsalis, the serologic tests for syphilis are strongly positive. The CSF may reflect a meningeal inflammatory process with pleocytosis, an elevated total protein, and positive VDRL. Late in the disease, especially after antisyphilitic treatment, the serologic tests may be negative (in 25 to 50% of cases) and the CSF negative (in 20% of cases).

Herpetic and Postherpetic Neuralgia

Herpetic and postherpetic neuralgia refers to severe and prolonged burning pain in the involved dermatome after an attack of herpes zoster. Herpes zoster is an acute viral infection of sensory ganglia. The disease, caused by the same virus that causes chickenpox (varicella) and that has remained latent in the sensory ganglia since the primary attack of chickenpox, produces an acute localized recrudescent infection. In most patients, immunity to the virus has declined with age, allowing activation of the virus. In some cases, however, activation is associated with the development of malignancy, local x-ray irradiation, immunosuppressive therapy, trauma, or tumor entrapment of the dorsal root ganglion or nerve root. When the virus multiplies in the ganglion, a ganglionitis develops, causing pain along its sensory distribution. Virus particles then pass down the nerve and multiply in the skin, causing characteristic clusters of vesicles. Localized herpes zoster lesions are most common over the face and trunk corresponding to the areas of major eruption during the antecedent chickenpox infection. (The rash of chickenpox has been described as centripetal, whereas that of measles tends to be centrifugal—that is, affecting the limbs more than the torso.)

The eruption of herpes zoster is often preceded by malaise and fever for 2 to 4 days. Pain and dysesthesias along the involved dermatome also precede the rash. The acute pain of herpes zoster varies in quality and intensity and usually persists for 1 to 4 weeks. Approximately 30% of patients over the age of 40 develop postherpetic neuralgia that persists for months to years.

The pain of herpes zoster has been mistaken for pruritus, appendicitis, cholecystitis, and pleurisy. Painful zoster without characteristic vesicles may resemble trigeminal neuralgia or facial palsy (Bell's palsy) when occurring on the face.

The treatment of postherpetic neuralgia with carbamazepine, amitriptyline, or nerve block is not always successful, but in many patients the pain disappears spontaneously after 1 or 2 years.

Causalgia (Reflex Sympathetic Dystrophies)

Causalgia refers to pain and autonomic changes that occur after an injury to a peripheral nerve. The exact mechanism of the pain and sympathetic changes is not understood. It has been postulated that injury to sensory and sympathetic fibers results in the formation of an abnormal synapse (ephaptic transmission) such that descending sympathetic impulses to a limb will excite painful afferent impulses.

The pain of causalgia is severe and continuous and exacerbated by touching or moving the involved limb. Along with the pain are vasomotor changes, first vasodilatation (warm and dry skin) but later vasoconstriction (cool, cyanotic skin). Other autonomic disturbances include osteoporosis and trophic changes in the skin, subcutaneous tissue, and muscles. Treatment by surgical sympathectomy often gives permanent relief.

THALAMIC SYNDROME

The combination of pain and sensory impairment may be encountered in lesions at a number of sites along the ascending sensory pathways, from the sensory nerve ending to the parietal cortex. A distinctive clinical syndrome accompanies complete lesions of the hemithalamus. Unilateral thalamic injury, usually caused by an ischemic stroke, causes loss of all forms of sensation on the opposite side of the body, as well as spontaneous pain in the same distribution.

Thalamic pain may be severe and burning. Application of noxious stimuli to the affected side of the body induces unpleasant sensations, often with radiation of pain beyond the point of stimulation. Thermal and tactile stimuli may cause the same type of painful over-reaction or dysesthesia. Dysesthesia refers to perversion of sensation, that is, experiencing one form of stimulation as another form, usually unpleasant or painful. The combination of hemibody sensory loss, spontaneous pain, and dysesthetic sensations is characteristic of the thalamic syndrome.

CORTICAL SYNDROMES OF PAIN AND SENSORY LOSS

Hemibody sensory disturbances resulting from involvement of the parietal or sensory cortex typically manifest a loss of discriminatory function more severe than the loss of superficial or crude sensation. Usually there is a loss of position sense, impairment of two-point discrimination, difficulty in appreciating differences in texture or weight, reduced ability to recognize figures written on the skin (agraphesthesia), and impairment of the ability to recognize the shape of an object placed in the hand (astereognosis). The loss of basic sensations such as pain, touch, and temperature, which are appreciated at the thalamic level, is inconsistent. At times, there is spontaneous pain like that encountered in lesions of the thalamus; in addition, focal painful sensory seizures may appear.

The parietal lobe syndrome of the nondominant hemisphere is also characterized by the occurrence of agnosia and certain forms of practic disorders such as constructional and dressing apraxias. In addition, disturbances of body image such as unilateral neglect, denial of hemiparesis (anosagnosia), or denial of the entire half of the body (hemisomatopagnosia) may be present.

In patients with thalamic or parietal lobe syndromes, CT scanning usually will identify an infarct, tumor, or hemorrhage. In cases of ischemic infarction, a thorough search must be made for a cardiac or intra-arterial source for cerebral emboli. If no cardiac source for cerebral embolism is identified by echocardiography or other means, a cerebral arteriogram may be required. Thromboembolic occlusion of the thalamogeniculate branches of the basilar artery accounts for thalamic infarction. By contrast, parietal lobe infarction is due to occlusion of middle cerebral artery branches of the internal carotid artery. Electroencephalography (EEG) may identify a cortical seizure focus in patients with paroxysmal episodes of hemibody pain.

PAIN FROM LESIONS OF THE DORSAL ROOT OF THE SPINAL NERVES

The spinal cord is divided into segments. Nerve roots exit the spinal cord at each segmental level and are numbered according to the level at which they exit. There are 8 cervical, 12 thoracic, 5 lumbar and 5 sacral nerves. The C5 to T1 segments innervate the upper extremity; T2 to T12 innervate the trunk; L1 to S4 innervate the lower extremity; and S2 to S5 innervate the bladder and anus.

Each spinal nerve has a dorsal sensory root and a ventral motor root.

The dorsal root syndrome is characterized particularly by pain. Pain radiates along the affected root or roots and may be increased with maneuvers that increase intraspinal pressure, such as coughing or straining. Pain increased in this manner probably results from sudden distension of the subarachnoid sheath surrounding the irritated root or from compression of the affected root by the sudden wave of spinal fluid.

Demonstrable sensory disturbances are also found in root disease. These consist of hyperesthesia with irritative lesions and, with destructive lesions, loss of sensation to superficial pain, temperature, and light touch in the appropriate root distribution.

Disorders affecting the spinal cord and nerve roots produce signs and symptoms in the trunk and extremities according to the specific levels involved. These levels can usually be diagnosed clinically because each level of injury has its own characteristic pattern of denervation.

Evaluation of the integrity of spinal cord levels depends on a knowledge of the dermatomes (areas of sensation on the skin supplied by a single spinal segment), the myotomes (groups of muscles innervated by a single spinal segment), and the deep tendon reflexes (the stretch reflex arc, composed of a muscle spindle, an afferent peripheral nerve, a synapse at a single spinal cord segment, an efferent peripheral nerve, and a muscle). A thorough clinical evaluation of sensation, motor power, and reflexes will determine level of neurologic involvement.

Evaluation of Nerve Root Lesions of the Upper Extremity

Cervical Roots 1 to 4:

The innervation of the upper three cervical nerves has been discussed above. The fourth cervical nerve has a dermatome that corresponds to the so-called football shoulder pad area. C4 is the major innervation of the diaphragm via its contribution to the phrenic nerve.

Cervical Root 5:

1. Sensation—C5 supplies sensation to the lateral arm from the summit of the shoulder to the elbow via the axillary nerve.

2. Muscle testing—The deltoid and biceps are the two most easily tested muscles with C5 innervation. The deltoid is almost a purely C5-innervated muscle; the biceps is innervated by both C5 and C6. (Standard texts should be consulted for specific directions on how to test and grade muscle power.)

3. Reflex testing—The biceps reflex is innervated predominantly by C5 but also has a smaller C6 component.

Cervical Root 6:

1. Sensation—C6 supplies sensation to the lateral forearm, thumb, index finger, and one half of the middle finger.

2. Muscle Testing—The biceps muscle, in addition to its C5 innervation, is partially innervated by C6. The radial wrist extensors, extensor carpi radialis longus and brevis, are innervated by C6 via the radial nerve. The extensor carpi ulnaris is innervated primarily by C7. If C6 innervation is absent and C7 is present, the wrist will deviate to the ulnar side on extension.

3. Reflex Testing—The biceps reflex may be used as an indicator of C6 neurologic integrity as well as of C5. The brachioradialis muscle is innervated by the radial nerve (C6) and therefore is the preferred reflex for indicating integrity of the C6 level.

Cervical Root 7:

1. Sensation—C7 supplies sensation to the middle finger. Since middle finger sensation occasionally is supplied by C6 and C8, there is no conclusive way to test C7 sensation.

2. Muscle testing—The triceps (radial nerve), flexor carpi radialis (median nerve), and finger extensors (radial nerve) are predominantly C7-innervated muscles.

3. Reflex testing—The triceps reflex is innervated by the C7 component of the radial nerve.

Cervical Root 8:

1. Sensation testing—C8 supplies sensation to the ring and little fingers of the hand and the distal half of the forearm.

2. Muscle testing—The flexor digitorum profundus, which flexes the distal interphalangeal joint, and the lumbricals, which flex the metacarpophalangeal joint, receive innervation from the ulnar nerve on the ulnar side of the hand and from the median nerve on the radial side. The flexor digitorum superficialis, which flexes the proximal interphalangeal joint, has only median nerve innervation.

3. Reflex testing—None.

Thoracic Root 1:

1. Sensation—T1 supplies sensation to the upper half of the medial forearm and the medial portion of the arm.

2. Muscle testing—The finger abductors (dorsal interossei and the abductor digiti quinti) are innervated by T1 via the ulnar nerve.

3. Reflex testing—None.

The most common causes of nerve root compression in the cervical region are cervical spondylosis and protrusion of an intervertebral disc, but extramedullary tumors (neurofibroma, meningioma) and metastatic cancer and epidural abscesses also occur. Cervical disc herniations occur most frequently at the fifth and sixth interspaces. The symptoms caused by an intervertebral disc protrusion must be differentiated from those caused by arthritis of the spine and other bone and joint diseases, including tumors and infections. Neuropathies caused by entrapment or systemic disease may be confused with radicular syndromes because they also present with localized pain and with motor and sensory deficits. Patients with cervical disc protrusions rarely and patients with tumors commonly present with cord compression. In such patients, long motor and sensory tract signs develop below the level of the lesion.

Evaluation of Radicular Syndromes Involving T2 to T12

Thoracic radiculopathy is associated with pain along the distribution of intercostal roots.

1. Sensation—The sensory areas for each thoracic nerve root are available in dermatomal charts in standard text books. The sensory area for T5 crosses the nipple line, T10 the umbilicus, and T12 the groin.

2. Muscle testing—The intercostal muscles are segmentally innervated but difficult to evaluate individually. The rectus abdominis muscles are segmentally innervated by the anterior divisions of T5 to T10 above the umbilicus and T11 to T12 (L1) below it. To test the integrity of the segmental innervation of the rectus abdominis muscles, have the patient do a partial sit-up and observe the umbilicus. Normally, the umbilicus should not move. If, however, it is drawn up or down

or to one side or the other, there is asymmetrical dysfunction of the anterior abdominal muscles. In cases of spinal cord compression at a lower thoracic level, weakness of the lower rectus abdominis muscles will be revealed by a positive Beevor's sign (the umbilicus will be drawn rostrally).

Thoracic neuralgic pains may be due to compression of nerve roots by neoplasms or infections. Herniated discs are uncommon in the thoracic region. Herpetic neuralgia has been discussed above. Painful diabetic neuropathy may involve the intercostal nerves and their roots.

Evaluation of Nerve Root Lesions of the Lower Extremity

L1 to L3:

1. Sensation—Nerve roots from L1 to L3 provide sensation over the anterior thigh between the inguinal ligament and the knee.

2. Muscle testing—There is no specific muscle test for each upper lumbar spinal cord level. The iliopsoas (T12 to L3, femoral nerve) is the main flexor of the hip. The quadriceps muscle (L2 to L4, femoral nerve) extends the knee. The hip adductors (L2 to L4, obturator nerve) remain strong when a femoral nerve lesion causes weakness of the iliopsoas and quadriceps muscles.

3. Reflex testing—The patellar reflex, although mediated through nerves arising at L2 to L4, is predominantly an L4 reflex.

L4:

1. Sensation—The L4 dermatome covers the medial side of the foot and leg. The knee joint divides the L3 dermatome above from the L4 dermatome below. The sharp crest of the tibia divides the L4 dermatome on the medial side of the leg from the L5 dermatome on the lateral side.

2. Muscle testing—The tibialis anterior (deep peroneal nerve) is predominantly innervated by L4, but also receives L5 innervation. The tibialis anterior inverts the foot.

3. Reflex testing—The patellar tendon reflex or knee jerk is considered to be an L4-mediated reflex.

L5:

1. Sensation—The L5 dermatome covers the dorsum of the foot and the lateral leg.

2. Muscle testing—The extensors of the foot and the gluteus medius muscle, which abducts the leg, are innervated by the L5 foot.

3. Reflex testing—The tibialis posterior reflex is difficult to elicit but represents an L5 reflex. To elicit the reflex, the foot is held in slight eversion and dorsiflexion, and the tendon of the tibialis posterior muscle

on the medial side of the foot is struck. The reflex consists of a slight plantar inversion response.

Sacral 1:

1. Sensation—The S1 dermatome covers the lateral side and a portion of the plantar surface of the foot.

2. Muscle testing—S1-innervated muscles include the peroneus longus and brevis (superficial peroneal nerve, S1), the gastrocnemii-solei muscles (tibial nerve, S1-S2), and the gluteus maximus (inferior gluteal nerve, S1). The peronei are everters of the ankle, the gastrocnemii-solei muscles plantar flex the foot, and the gluteus maximus extends the hip.

3. Reflex testing—The Achilles tendon reflex is mediated predominantly by nerves originating from the S1 root.

A herniated intervertebral disc is the most common cause of lumbar and sacral root compression. The L5 and S1 roots are commonly affected. Symptoms include low backache and pain radiating into the buttocks, thigh, and lower leg. Pain may be spontaneous but usually is increased or provoked by straight leg raising on the side of the compression. Pain is usually unilateral when the disc protrudes laterally but may occur in both lower extremities when there is a central disc protrusion.

Compression of several roots of the cauda equina by a central disc protrusion may give rise to bilateral pain, to sensory and motor changes, and even to loss of sphincter control. Nerve root compression caused by intervertebral disc disease must be differentiated from that caused by bone disease such as arthritis, infection, and tumor, and from neuropathies caused by entrapment or systemic disease such as diabetes.

Investigation of the patient with symptoms of spinal root compression should begin with x-rays of the suspected site of spinal cord or root compression. Frontal, lateral, and oblique views are required for examination of the cervical spine. Frontal and lateral views generally are satisfactory for visualization of the thoracic, lumbar, and sacral spine.

Plain films may indicate the presence of certain specific conditions. Degenerative arthritis or spondylosis may cause narrowing of the anteroposterior diameter of the spinal canal with compression of the spinal cord or roots. Enlargement of an intervertebral foramen may indicate the presence of a neurofibroma. Vertebral bone destruction may indicate tumor metastases.

Bone scanning after radioisotope injection may identify metastases as a cause of bone destruction; fractures, infection, and arthritic areas may also cause increased uptake of radioisotope.

Computerized tomography of the spine often is useful for the investigation of lesions in the spinal canal and surrounding tissues.

At present, the definitive technique for precise localization of intraspinal masses is metrizamide myelography by lumbar or cisternal injection. Myelography should be performed before surgical treatment of a herniated disc or unknown tumor is carried out and when radiation therapy of a known metastatic tumor is planned.

Magnetic resonance imaging (MRI), a new and promising technique, may replace both CT scanning and myelography for examination of the spine.

Electromyography is useful for the localization of intraspinal lesions affecting anterior horn cells or nerve roots.

DIZZINESS

DEFINITION

Dizziness is one of the most common medical complaints. Patients use the term "dizzy" to describe several different sensations: a rotational sensation (vertigo), a feeling of faintness (near-syncope), and a sensation of disequilibrium (fear of falling).

Vertigo is a false sense of movement of the individual or of the environment and indicates a disorder of the vestibular system, either of the peripheral labyrinth or its central connections (Table 15–2).

PATHOPHYSIOLOGIC CONSIDERATIONS

Functional Anatomy

The vestibular system takes its name from the vestibule of the inner ear, in which lie the utricle and saccule and into which open the three semicircular canals. The vestibular system is involved in equilib-

Table 15–2. Causes of Vertigo

Peripheral causes of vertigo
  Benign positional vertigo
  Acute peripheral vestibulopathy
  Meniere's syndrome
  Toxic damage to the labyrinths
Central causes of vertigo
  Cerebrovascular disease
  Multiple sclerosis
  Cerebellopontine angle tumors
  Vertiginous migraine

rium and spatial orientation and the regulation of posture and muscle tone.

The semicircular canals (anterior, posterior, and lateral) on the two sides are sensitive to rotational movements. The lateral semicircular canal is vertical, and its ampulla is uppermost when the individual is in the supine position with the head tilted forward 30°. This position is important in performing caloric tests (see section on coma). The semicircular canals are particularly concerned in vestibulo-ocular reflexes, which help maintain the direction of gaze when the head is moved. The utricle registers the position of the head in relation to gravity and to linear acceleration. It is particularly concerned in the coordination of body posture and head position. The vestibular nerve innervates the hair cells of the semicircular canals and the utricle and saccule.

Afferent fibers of the vestibular nerve pass centrally with the cochlear nerve as the eighth cranial or acoustic nerve. The eighth nerve passes centrally, with the facial nerve, through the internal auditory meatus, across the cerebello-pontine angle, to reach the lateral brain stem at the junction of the pons and medulla. Most of the vestibular fibers end in the vestibular nuclei.

The vestibular nuclei have extensive and reciprocal connections with various brain stem and spinal cord nuclei as well as with the cerebellum. There are also connections with the reticular formation and the nuclei subserving ocular movement via the medial longitudinal fasciculus, as well as connections between the vestibular nuclei and autonomic centers in the brain stem reticular formation, particularly the dorsal vagal nuclei. These connections are responsible for the nausea, vomiting, sweating, salivation, hypotension, and faintness that can occur in severe vestibular disturbance.

Peripheral Causes of Vertigo

Benign positional vertigo is the most frequent type of vertigo. The patient experiences a sensation of spinning with a change of position. The cause is obscure, but the vertigo may follow a head injury, in which case the likely explanation is shaking loose of otoliths. Clinically, the vertigo is paroxysmal, with a brief latency following head movement, and with transient (seconds to minutes) nystagmus. There are no auditory or central neurologic deficits; the caloric responses may be normal in 50% of patients or may reveal depressed labyrinthine function in one ear. Symptoms subside spontaneously within weeks.

Acute peripheral vestibulopathy is defined as a single episode of spontaneous vertigo lasting hours to days. Attacks occasionally follow infections, especially viral involvement of the upper respiratory tract, but the relationship is not clear. On examination, the patient appears acutely ill and resists motion of the head. Nystagmus invariably accompanies the vertigo. Unilateral impairment of vestibular function is present in about one half of patients. As with benign positional vertigo, there are no auditory or brain stem signs, and the condition runs a self-limiting course of days or weeks. Repeated bouts of vertigo occur in 50% of patients over a period of months or years. The absence of auditory impairment distinguishes recurrent peripheral vestibulopathy from Meniere's syndrome.

Meniere's syndrome accounts for only about 10% of cases of vertigo. It usually occurs in adults and consists of recurring episodic vertigo, hearing loss, and tinnitus. The diagnosis depends on the characteristic history and the audiometric findings (low frequency hearing loss and loudness recruitment). Hearing loss is unilateral in 80 to 90% of patients. Overdistension of the membranous labyrinth with endolymph is the immediate cause of symptoms, but the explanation for the excess of endolymph is unknown.

Aminoglycoside antibiotics (e.g., streptomycin and gentamicin) may damage the labyrinths in a dose-related manner. Patients with impaired renal function can develop labyrinthine dysfunction with ordinary doses of these drugs. Tinnitus, hearing loss, or vertigo may be the presenting symptom. Vertigo continues for days to weeks. If the ototoxic drug is discontinued immediately, damage to the labyrinth is arrested. Following the acute stage of vertigo, loss of balance and blurring of vision with motion (oscillopsia of Dandy) are present as a result of loss of the vestibulo-ocular reflexes. Adaptation to the loss of vestibular function occurs within months. Diagnosis is based on the history of the exposure to ototoxic drugs. Clinically, Romberg's sign is present, and caloric responses are hypoactive bilaterally.

Central Causes of Vertigo

Cerebrovascular disease may cause vertigo. Ischemia in the distribution of the vertebrobasilar artery damages the vestibular nuclei and their connections. Vertigo caused by cerebrovascular disease is accompanied by signs of injury to adjacent brain stem motor and sensory pathways. Isolated vertigo rarely occurs as a manifestation of stroke or transient ischemic attack.

Multiple sclerosis can produce vertigo in young patients. Vertigo may be the presenting symptom of the condition.

Tumors of the cerebellopontine angle are a rare cause of vertigo. The majority are benign tumors that arise from the eighth cranial nerve (acoustic neuromas). These tumors develop in middle-aged patients who experience mild dizziness and unilateral hearing loss progressing over a period of years. Vertigo is rarely spontaneous or acute, but usually is positional. In addition to hearing loss, tinnitus, facial weakness and numbness, nystagmus, and cerebellar ataxia may be present. Von Recklinghausen's disease (neurofibromatosis) is associated with unilateral or bilateral acoustic neuromas.

Vertigo may occur before and during migraine headaches or may occur without headache as a migraine equivalent.

CLINICAL PRESENTATION

In general, peripheral causes of vertigo are marked by direction-fixed nystagmus that is horizontal or rotatory, never vertical. The vertigo and nystagmus follow head movements with a latency of a few seconds and manifest adaptation or habituation to repeated movements. Brain stem signs are absent, and the sensation of movement is severe, with marked systemic symptoms of nausea, vomiting, pallor, and sweating.

Central causes of vertigo are marked by the onset of vertigo and nystagmus immediately upon movement. Nystagmus persists and often is direction-changing or vertical. Ataxia, multiple cranial nerve deficits, and hemiparesis are present, and systemic symptoms are mild.

DIAGNOSTIC EVALUATION

The history may distinguish between peripheral and central syndromes of vertigo. The pattern of neurologic involvement demonstrated on physical examination may also indicate the site of the lesion responsible for vertigo. The Nylen-Bárány maneuver, in which the examiner carries the patient's head backward from an upright position, so that it is hanging 45° below the horizontal and turned 45° to one side, may produce vertigo and nystagmus with the distinguishing features of the peripheral or central types described above.

Electronystagmography (ENG), in which the amplitude, speed, and duration of ocular movements is recorded during a series of eye and head movements, may also identify the locus of dysfunction.

Caloric testing, which mimics rotational stimulation of each semicircular canal, provides information on the function of the vestibular apparatus. Audiometric tests are used to evaluate lesions of the middle ear, labyrinth, and cochlea, particularly in cases of Meniere's syndrome and acoustic neuroma. Brain stem auditory-evoked responses (BAERs) is a sensitive test for distinguishing between brain stem and peripheral disorders, although up to 50% of patients with peripheral disorders will have abnormal BAERs. In cases of suspected central vertigo, CT scanning of the posterior fossa is required to identify the type and location of the lesion.

CONFUSION, DELIRIUM, AND COMA

DEFINITION

The human nervous system undergoes daily cycles of sleep and wakefulness characterized by striking changes in sensitivity to environmental stimuli and in motor activity. These global changes in level of consciousness depend upon a brain stem regulatory system called the reticular activating system (RAS).

Anatomically, the RAS consists of the paramedian regions of the tegmentum of the mesencephalon and the pons that are not associated with cranial nerves or specific ascending or descending pathways. Included in the RAS are the functionally related medial, intralaminar, and reticular nuclei of the thalamus. By its location, the RAS has access to incoming sensory information and widespread connections to the cortical and subcortical motor systems.

Consciousness has two aspects: arousal and awareness. Mutually sustaining areas of both the RAS and the cerebral hemispheres are required to maintain full consciousness.

Arousal is a crude function (i.e., wakefulness) and reflects activation of the RAS by somatosensory stimuli or innate motivational systems such as hunger. Natural sensory stimuli activate not ony specific sensory relays to cortical sensory areas appropriate to the stimulus modality, but also the nonspecific projection system (RAS) that produces cortical arousal. Clinically, arousal is indicated by eye opening, either spontaneously or in response to stimuli. In some cases arousal may occur in spite of complete destruction of the hemispheres.

Awareness is manifested by cognition of self and environment and implies functioning cerebral hemispheres. Clinically, awareness is marked by goal-directed or purposeful motor behavior and the use of language.

Confusion and delirium are characterized by disturbances in the content of consciousness rather than in the level of arousal. They probably reflect disturbances mainly in the cerebral hemisphere or higher cortical function.

Confusion is marked clinically by disorientation of time and place and by impairment of perception, comprehension, concentration, attention, memory, and abstract thinking.

Delirium includes all of the above disorders, as well as hallucinations, delusions, and agitation. The hallucinations in organic brain disorders, as opposed to those in psychiatric conditions, are more commonly visual than auditory. Sleep frequently is disturbed and hypervigilance or restlessness may be extreme. Excitement, anger, and fear may lead to assaultive or self-destructive behavior.

The causes of confusion and delirium are many and include febrile and toxic states caused by systemic infection or metabolic derangements. Other causes include encephalitis, meningitis, head injury, and abstinence following prolonged abuse of alcohol or sedative drugs.

Coma is a state of pathologic unconsciousness in which neither arousal nor awareness is present. Coma is the product of a wide spectrum of life threatening conditions that damage or depress brain functioning.

PATHOPHYSIOLOGIC CONSIDERATIONS

All types of coma may be divided into three pathophysiologic categories: metabolic encephalopathy, supratentorial lesions, and infratentorial lesions. Metabolic processes such as sedative drug poisoning, or uremia and hepatic failure affect consciousness by diffusely impairing the metabolism of both hemispheres and the brain stem. A unilateral supratentorial lesion such as a brain tumor or hematoma produces coma by herniating beyond the confines of the supratentorial compartment and compressing the brain stem RAS. Two types of infratentorial lesions produce coma: lesions intrinsic to the brain stem that destroy the reticular formation, e.g., pontine hemorrhage or paramedian infarction of the midbrain or pons; and lesions extrinsic to the brain stem that compress and distort it, e.g., cerebellar tumor or hematoma.

CLINICAL PRESENTATION

The comatose patient maintains a sleeplike unresponsiveness from which he cannot be aroused; eye opening does not occur, no comprehensible speech is detected, and the extremities move neither to commands nor appropriately to localize or ward off noxious stimuli. No purposive reflex movements such as decorticate or decerebrate posturing may be present. Stupor resembles coma, except that the patient is arousable if strong external stimulation is provided.

In some cases, particularly after cardiac arrest or

head trauma, both hemispheres are severely damaged, but the brain stem is preserved. After a period of coma lasting hours to days, wakefulness returns without evidence of cognition or purposive behavior. This functionally decorticate state of "vigilant" or "eyes-open coma" is termed the vegetative state.

In evaluating an unconscious patient, the physician should distinguish coma from the vegetative state. The distinction is important because lay people ordinarily equate eye opening with consciousness. Therefore, the physician who terms a vegetative patient "comatose" will confuse and upset the patient's family.

DIFFERENTIAL DIAGNOSIS

In metabolic encephalopathy, symmetrical neurologic abnormalities usually are difficult to attribute to a regionally restricted lesion. Pupillary light reflexes generally are preserved (except in patients who have ingested glutethimide, atropine-like agents, or barbiturates in high doses) even with signs of lower brain stem depression such as apnea, absent caloric responses, and motor unresponsiveness. In severe sedative drug poisoning, nearly all central nervous system functions may be absent, including electrocerebral activity. Failure to appreciate the presence of depressants can lead to an erroneous diagnosis of brain death.

With supratentorial lesions, an expanding mass in or adjacent to one cerebral hemisphere may displace the medial portion of the temporal lobe (uncus) over the edge of the tentorial opening and compress the third cranial nerve, the adjacent midbrain, and the posterior cerebral artery. The earliest sign of uncal herniation is unilateral pupillary dilatation with a preserved or sluggish reaction to light. As the uncus continues to compress the midbrain, the patient becomes deeply comatose and manifests an ipsilateral third cranial nerve palsy and contralateral decerebrate posturing. Bilateral decerebrate rigidity develops when the contralateral cerebral peduncle is compressed against the tentorial edge opposite from the side of herniation. If treatment cannot halt brain displacement at this point, the pons and then the medulla will fail in an orderly rostral-caudal progression.

Pontine hemorrhage destroys the reticular formation and produces a distinctive clinical pattern of infratentorial lesions. Coma occurs abruptly and death usually follows within hours to days. The pupils are pinpoint but often reactive, horizontal eye movements are impaired although vertical eye movements may be preserved, and ocular bobbing may occur. Decerebrate rigidity or flaccid quadriplegia, hyperthermia, and progressive slowing of respiration are characteristic.

Compressive lesions of the brain stem such as cer-

ebellar hemorrhage often are difficult to distinguish from intrinsic lesions and clinically may mimic brain stem stroke. In other cases, the caudal-to-rostral evolution of neurologic signs may resemble the patchy brain stem depression of sedative drug intoxication. Asymmetrical motor signs and hypertension caused by Cushing's reflex usually serve to identify brain stem compression.

DIAGNOSTIC EVALUATION

In the acute situation it is not unusual for a physician to be uncertain whether a coma is due to an expanding intracranial mass requiring surgery and immediate decompression by osmotic agents, or to a metabolic encephalopathy for which supportive measures may suffice. When faced with such a patient, the physician must apply diagnostic and therapeutic efforts concurrently to avert death or prolonged disability.

The physician must first ensure that the patient has a patent airway and stable vital signs. If the patient is deeply unconscious, a cuffed endotracheal tube should be inserted and ventilation supported if spontaneous respirations are ineffective. An intravenous line should be inserted and blood samples drawn to assess glucose, complete blood count, arterial blood gases, electrolytes, calcium, liver and kidney function, and the presence of toxins. After the blood is drawn, 25 or 50 g of glucose should be given intravenously to prevent hypoglycemic brain damage while the results of laboratory tests are awaited. An arterial blood sample should be obtained for pH, $Paco_2$, and Pao_2. Concomitant administration of thiamine 100 mg IV in malnourished patients will prevent precipitation or worsening of Wernicke's encephalopathy. If repetitive convulsions are present, they should be treated immediately with diazepam 10 to 20 mg IV, and then phenytoin 1 to 1.5 g IV to maintain seizure control. Naloxone hydrochloride 0.4 to 0.8 mg should be administered intravenously to any comatose patient in whom the diagnosis is not clear, regardless of whether a narcotic overdose is suspected. Because the duration of action of naloxone is brief, usually 20 minutes to 2 hours, patients who have taken an overdose of a long-acting narcotic such as methadone may relapse after an initial period of improvement.

Increased intracranial pressure from an expanding mass lesion or cerebral edema should be lowered immediately by passive hyperventilation until $Paco_2$ is 25 to 30 mm Hg. Hypocapnia leads to cerebral vasoconstriction, decreased cerebral blood volume, and lowered intracranial pressure. In addition, mannitol 50 g in a 20% solution should be given over 10 to 20 minutes intravenously. The cerebral dehydrating effects of mannitol begins immediately and lasts several hours. Corticosteroids decrease cerebral edema associated with brain tumors and may be useful in maintaining the reduced intracranial pressure obtained at first by hyperventilation and osmotic agents. Steroids begin to act after several hours.

In coma caused by drug ingestion, gastric aspiration and lavage with normal saline within 4 hours of ingestion may remove unabsorbed intoxicants. Salicylates and anticholinergic drugs (tricyclic antidepressants, phenothiazines, scopolamine) that induce gastric atony may be recovered from the stomach many hours after ingestion. The following agents should not be lavaged: caustic materials (regurgitation may cause further esophageal damage and perforation); analeptic toxins, e.g., strychnine, picrotoxin (lavage may provoke uncontrollable seizures and cardiac arrhythmias); and petroleum distillates (lethal pneumonia may result if these hydrocarbons are accidentally aspirated). When the gag reflex is depressed, the airway must be protected by a cuffed endotracheal tube prior to lavage to prevent aspiration. Emesis induced by ipecac (30 ml with one L of water, effective in 30 minutes) or apomorphine (0.07 to 1 mg/kg subcutaneously, effective in 4 minutes) should be reserved for alert patients. Concurrent with other diagnostic and therapeutic efforts, a history should be obtained and the patient rapidly examined for signs of trauma to the head and elsewhere.

In every case it is important to determine the circumstances in which coma occurred and, if possible, the details of the medical history. These facts must be obtained from relatives, friends, police, ambulance attendants, or anyone who may have observed the patient prior to admission. A history of psychiatric illness, depression, drug abuse, previous head injury, seizures, or underlying chronic illness may point to the cause of coma. If there is a history of alcoholism, a diagnosis of coma resulting from drunkenness should not be made until an intracerebral hematoma has been ruled out.

The general examination of the comatose patient may give important clues to the cause of coma. The scalp should be checked for contusion, laceration, and edema; the nares and ear drums for blood and CSF; and the head and face for subperiosteal blood (Battle's sign and raccoon eyes). A stiff neck may mean meningitis, subarachnoid hemorrhage, or cerebellar tonsillar herniation. The remainder of the general and neurologic examinations, not discussed here, should not be neglected.

In the unconscious patient it is useful to consider the brain in terms of its hierarchic, longitudinal organization and divide it into cortical and brain stem

functions. Clinical neurologic signs can be corrected with specific levels of brain function to establish the depth of coma. For example, any form of speech, even if only unintelligible grunts and groans, denotes the preservation of some cortical function, since alone the brain stem cannot produce speech. By contrast, apnea not affected by higher than normal levels of $Paco_2$ indicates medullary failure, which, in coma caused by structural disease, often means brain death.

The following neurologic examination has been derived from the practical scale developed for head injury by Teasdale and Jennett and from the techniques for evaluating brain stem function described by Plum and Posner. It consists of an assessment of the level of consciousness as determined by eye opening, verbal responses, and reflex or purposive movements in response to noxious stimulation of the face, arms, and legs; neuro-ophthalmologic function as indicated by pupillary size and response to light, spontaneous eye movements, oculocephalic (doll's eyes) and oculovestibular (ice-water caloric) responses; and vegetative function as reflected by blood pressure and respiratory pattern.

Level of Consciousness. The level of consciousness is best determined by the ease and degree, if any, of behavioral arousal. Attempts should be made to elicit a behavioral motor response by verbal stimulation alone. If no response follows even shouted commands, noxious stimulation can be applied to the face by digital supraorbital pressure, and individually to the arms and legs by compression of distal interphalangeal joints with a tongue blade or pen.

The significance of eye opening as an indication of activity of the RAS, and the correlation between verbal responses and hemisphere function, have been discussed above. Lack of motor response to stimulation, especially if flaccidity and areflexia are present, indicates severe brain stem depression and frequently is found in terminal coma. Damage may be reversible, however, if the patient is intoxicated with sedative drugs.

Decerebrate or extensor responses correlate with destructive lesions of the midbrain and upper pons but may also be present in reversible metabolic states such as hepatic coma and anoxic-ischemic encephalopathy. Decorticate or flexor responses occur following damage to the hemispheres or diencephalon, and in metabolic depression of brain function. Withdrawal and localizing responses imply purposive or voluntary behavior. Obeying commands is the best response and marks the return of consciousness.

Neuro-ophthalmologic Assessment. The size, equality, and light reactivity of the pupils should be noted. In coma caused by metabolic brain disease the pupils are generally small but reactive to light. Similar pupils are present in normal people during sleep, in the diencephalic phase of central herniation, and in the initial stages of brain stem compression by a cerebellar mass. Pinpoint pupils occur in pontine hemorrhage. Midposition, fixed pupils indicate midbrain failure caused by metabolic or structural disease.

Deeply comatose patients usually have no spontaneous eye movements. Spontaneous, roving, horizontal eye movements indicate only that the midbrain and pontine tegmentum are intact and do not require the preservation of the occipital or frontal cerebral cortex. Roving eye movements can return despite complete destruction of the supratentorial cerebral gray matter. In coma after cardiac arrest, however, a good outcome is likely if roving eye movements return within the first 12 hours following resuscitation.

Doll's eyes and ice-water caloric responses can be used to determine the integrity of the eighth, sixth, and third cranial nerves and their interconnecting brain stem pathways. The physiology of these reflexes is presented in detail elsewhere.

Oculocephalic Response (Doll's Eyes). When cortical influences are depressed, as in normal sleep or coma, if the head is lifted up and rotated horizontally to one side, the eyes will deviate conjugately to the opposite side. Doll's eyes require the integrity of proprioceptive fibers from the neck structures that enter the spinal cord through the dorsal roots of C2 to C4, then ascend to reach the vestibular nuclei. The remainder of the central pathway, which includes the medial longitudinal fasciculus and the nuclei of the third and sixth cranial nerves, is the same as that for oculovestibular response. Doll's eyes are particularly brisk in certain types of metabolic coma, especially hypoglycemic and hepatic encephalopathy.

Oculovestibular Response (Ice-Water Calories). The oculovestibular response is elicited with the patient supine with the head elevated 30° by irrigating the tympanum with 5 ml of ice water; if there is no response, 20 ml is used. In this position the lateral canal is approximately vertical and the ampulla is uppermost. Water against the tympanum at a temperature different from body temperature sets up convection currents in the lateral canals, since they are closest to the surface. Cold water produces a downward, ampullofugal current that inhibits the normal, spontaneous firing of the vestibular nerve. Warm water produces an upward, ampullopetal current and is excitatory. The caloric test is very selective in that one canal on one side of the body can be stimulated to excite or depress the ipsilateral vestibular nerve.

In coma, when the central pathways of the oculovestibular reflex are intact, cold caloric stimulation produces conjugate, tonic deviation of the eyes to the side of irrigation. Disconjugate ocular deviation implies a structural or metabolic brain stem lesion. If one or both eyes fails to adduct, the lesion is in the medial longitudinal fasciculus of CNIII. The distinction between the two can be made by examining the pupillary responses. Failure of abduction indicates a CNVI lesion. In deep coma, the doll's eyes usually disappear before the ice-water caloric responses, the latter being a much stronger stimulus. Absence of the oculovestibular response, therefore, correlates with severe depression of brain stem function and connotes a poor prognosis, except in coma caused by depressant drugs, or when ophthalmoplegic drugs have been administered.

Vegetative Function. In many cases of coma the spontaneous respiratory pattern is obscured by therapeutic measures such as intubation and mechanical ventilation. Nevertheless, disordered respiration, when it can be evaluated, is one of the best indicators of brain dysfunction. Severe hyperventilation occurs when brain damage or hemorrhage produces a lactic acidosis in CSF that stimulates medullary receptors. Periodic respiration implies bilateral hemisphere dysfunction, while ataxic breathing heralds impending medullary failure and apnea.

Elevated blood pressure can be a reflex response to increased intracranial pressure or brain stem ischemia. Hypotension may indicate myocardial infarction, hemorrhagic shock, sepsis, or sedative drug depression.

CT Scan. In coma, the CT scan is of great value in the diagnosis of intracranial hemorrhage, tumors, and infarcts. At certain stages in its evolution, a subdural hematoma may be isodense with the brain. In such cases, the presence of a subdural hematoma may be indicated by ventricular shift. Ventricular shift may be absent if subdural hematomas are bilateral, but bilateral signs of ventricular compression or obliteration of the cerebral cisterns and sulcal marking of the hemispheres will indicate the presence of subdural hematomas. MRI can identify subdural hematomas missed by CT scanning.

Lumbar Puncture. Lumbar puncture in the presence of increased intracranial pressure carries risks of inducing transtentorial or foramen magnum herniation. When meningitis is the suspected diagnosis, however, the advantage of lumbar puncture is likely to exceed the danger.

Cerebral Arteriography. The need for cerebral arteriography in cases of coma has been reduced by the use of CT scanning. Nevertheless, cerebral arteriography may give both localizing and diagnostic information of occluded, abnormal, or displaced cerebral vessels.

Electroencephalography. The EEG has little diagnostic value, except when coma is caused by nonconvulsive epilepsy or a metabolic encephalopathy. Certain encephalopathies, notably hepatic, give rise to an EEG pattern of triphasic slow waves that is highly suggestive of the diagnosis. Sedatives and tranquilizers may increase the amount of beta wave activity. An isoelectric or flat EEG, in the absence of sedative drugs and hypothermia, indicates irreversible, generalized cerebral damage.

Plain x-rays. Plain x-rays of the skull usually are unnecessary when CT scanning is available. However, if there is a question of trauma, radiography of the cervical spine is important. Care must be taken not to aggravate any damage to the spinal cord, and the neck should be held in a fixed, neutral position until the presence of a cervical fracture has been excluded.

DISTURBANCES OF GAIT

Gait refers to the manner of walking. A normal gait requires the coordinated interaction of joints and muscles. Every level of the nervous system, including the cerebral cortex, basal ganglia, cerebellum, spinal cord, and peripheral nerves, participates in the act of locomotion. Therefore, disturbances of gait may be due to non-neurologic conditions such as arthritis and myopathy, or may result from neurologic diseases as diverse as stroke, parkinsonism, and peripheral neuropathy (Table 15–3).

HEMIPARESIS

In mild hemiparesis, the abnormality of gait may be limited to failure of the arm to swing on the affected side and of the lower limb to advance smoothly. In more severe, chronic hemiparesis, the upper limb is held in flexion at the elbow, wrist, and metacarpophalangeal joints, and the lower limb is advanced stiffly, the knee in extension, and the ankle plantar flexed so that circumduction at the hip is necessary for the foot to clear the ground.

Table 15–3. Disturbances of Gait

Hemiparesis
Spastic paraparesis
Apraxia of gait
Parkinsonism
Senile gait disorder
Ataxic gait
   Cerebellar gait
   Sensory ataxia
Choreic gait
Gait in proximal muscle weakness
Steppage gait

SPASTIC PARAPARESIS

In spastic paraparesis, the impairment of gait increases with the degree of spasticity. In severe cases, the step is short and the patient tends to stumble. The causative lesion may be in the parasagittal cortex of both hemispheres or in the spinal cord.

APRAXIA OF GAIT

Apraxia is a disorder characterized by the inability to perform a movement in the absence of any motor or sensory impairment. In apraxia of gait, the legs may appear normal when examined in bed, but when the patient tries to walk, the feet seem to be glued to the floor. The patient walks with a broad-based, halting gait, taking short steps (marche à petits pas), or he may shuffle tentatively in one place (the slipped clutch phenomenon). Most cases of apraxia result from degenerative disorders of the frontal lobes, especially senile dementia of the Alzheimer type. Other causes include frontal lobe tumors, multiple cerebral infarcts, normal pressure hydrocephalus, and subdural hematomas.

PARKINSONISM

Patients with parkinsonism manifest various gait disturbances. They may have slowness and difficulty in initiating gait (bradykinesia) and paucity of associated movements; stooped posture with the body held in a posture of forward flexion of the neck, trunk and limbs; shuffling, short steps (marche à petits pas) or feet that slide forward, gathering speed (festinating or hurrying); or lateral pulsion or retropulsion, which may be induced when the patient looks up. Patients with parkinsonism have a pronounced increase in tone of the axial muscles that accounts for much of their postural and gait disturbances. In progressive supranuclear palsy (Steele-Richardson-Olszewski syndrome), axial dystonia is marked and is associated with progressive gaze palsies, especially affecting vertical movements, and with pseudobulbar signs.

SENILE GAIT DISORDER

Some elderly patients have a gait that resembles that of parkinsonism. The gait disorder cannot be attributed to a regionally restricted lesion and reflects a combination of factors: diffuse forebrain damage, labyrinthine dysfunction, chronic myelopathy resulting from cervical spondylosis, and diminished joint position sense caused by peripheral neuropathy.

ATAXIC GAIT

Ataxia or unsteady gait can be caused either by cerebellar disease or by the loss of proprioception in the legs.

Cerebellar Gait

Restricted disease of the midline or vermal portion of the cerebellum causes disorders of stance and gait without other signs of cerebellar dysfunction such as nystagmus and limb ataxia. This pattern is typical of nutritional or alcoholic cerebellar degeneration. Unilateral lesions of the cerebellar hemispheres produce ipsilateral disorders of limb movement as well as ataxia of gait. This pattern is typical of cerebellar infarction, tumor, and hemorrhage.

Patients with bilateral cerebellar hemisphere disease display an ataxic gait similar to that seen in vermal disease, as well as signs of bilateral incoordination of limb movements. This picture is seen in pancerebellar degeneration resulting from the remote effects of malignancy, or in diffuse disease of the cerebellar inflow and outflow tracts as occurs in multiple sclerosis.

Patients with cerebellar disease stand with the legs farther apart than normal. Often they cannot stand with their feet together and fall whether their eyes are open or closed. They lurch from side to side when walking and in severe cases may not be able to walk without support.

Clinical evaluation of patients with ataxia of gait includes testing the ability to stand with the feet together and to tandem walk in a straight line. Limb movements should be evaluated for dysmetria, incoordination of rapid movements, and hypotonia. A CT or MRI scan in most cases will define the locus and cause of cerebellar dysfunction.

Sensory Ataxia

Lesions of the afferent fibers in peripheral nerves, dorsal roots, dorsal columns of the spinal cord, or medial lemnisci cause loss of proprioception in the limbs.

Patients with sensory ataxia are unaware of the position of their limbs and therefore have difficulty standing or walking. Like patients with cerebellar ataxia, they stand with their legs spread widely apart. Unlike patients with cerebellar disease, they can stand with feet together and eyes open. However, when the eyes are closed, they sway and fall (Romberg's sign).

Evaluation of the patient with sensory ataxia includes a careful examination of sense of joint position and all other sensory modalities in the upper and lower extremities. Patients with an acute inflammatory sensory polyradiculoneuropathy complain of painful dysesthesias with an elevated threshold for sensation in the affected dermatomes. When the threshold for sensation is exceeded, discomfort (hyperpathia) is excessive. The lower limbs are affected more than the upper limbs, and sense of joint position is severely impaired. In chronic inflammatory polyradiculoneuropathy, the neurologic deficit progresses slowly over months or years. The process tends to affect motor, autonomic, and sensory peripheral neurons in varying proportions. Ataxic neuropathy in diabetic patients is a diffuse distal neuropathy especially affecting the lower limbs. The neuropathy affects afferent fibers as well as motor and autonomic fibers. Joint position, vibration, and touch pressure sensation are most affected. Pain and temperature discriminations tend to be spared. Severe cases with gait ataxia are referred to as pseudotabes diabetica.

Patients with tabes dorsalis have a slowly progressive course of sensory loss resulting from syphilitic involvement of the dorsal roots and dorsal columns of the spinal cord. Variable degrees of diminished pain sensation and position sense loss are present. Involvement of sacral nerve roots leads to bladder and bowel dysfunction.

Patients with gait ataxia should have blood tests for an underlying endocrine abnormality (diabetes, hypothyroidism), infection (serologic tests for syphilis), and dysimmunity (serum protein electrophoresis). A search for an underlying malignancy should be made in patients with subacute sensory ganglioradiculoneuropathy. The determination of nerve conduction and electromyography may indicate the type of neuropathic involvement. Examination of the CSF for pleocytosis, elevated protein, and VDRL may indicate the cause of symptoms.

CHOREIC GAIT

Choreic gait refers to the gait disorder seen in children with Sydenham's chorea or adults with Huntington's disease. Both conditions cause continuous rapid movements of face, trunk, and limbs. Facial grimacing occurs with flexion, extension, and rotary movements of the neck and twisting movements of the trunk and limbs. Walking accentuates these movements. In an adult, the presence of dementia and a characteristic CT scan showing bilateral caudate nucleus atrophy serve to identify Huntington's disease as the cause of chorea.

GAIT IN PROXIMAL MUSCLE WEAKNESS

Patients with weakness of the proximal muscles of the legs walk with legs spread widely apart and have a characteristic waddling motion of the pelvis that results from weakness of the gluteal muscles. In attempting to rise from a seated position, patients put hands on knees and push the trunk upward by working the hands up the thigh (Gowers' sign). Such a pattern of weakness is seen in patients with muscular dystrophy or severe steroid-induced myopathy.

STEPPAGE GAIT

Disease of the motor neurons or peripheral nerves causes distal weakness and footdrop. In peroneal nerve palsy or chronic intervertebral disc herniations, the footdrop is unilateral. In motor neuron disease or in peripheral neuropathies, the disorder may be bilateral. In either case, the patients cannot dorsiflex the foot in walking, so that the toes are scuffed along the ground. To prevent this, the patient raises the knee higher than usual, resulting in a "steppage' gait.

DISEASES OF THE CRANIAL NERVES

CNI (OLFACTORY NERVE)

Dysfunction of the olfactory nerve causes a loss of sense of smell (anosmia). Anosmia often results from local disease of the nose, head trauma, skull fracture, meningitis, or brain tumor. The pathogenesis of anosmia in cases of head trauma appears to be shearing of the nerve fibers as they enter the cranial cavity via perforations in the cribriform plate of the skull.

Patients with anosmia may be unaware of loss of smell and report only that their sense of taste has diminished. (See also Chapter 22.)

Anosmia caused by disease of CNI must be differentiated from olfactory hallucinations. The latter are brief occurrences of bad odors not noticed by others and are part of the syndrome of partial complex epilepsy, or "uncinate fits," caused by disease of the temporal lobe of the brain.

Evaluation of the patient with anosmia should include a careful history of antecedent trauma and infection and a detailed neurologic examination to identify signs of an underlying frontal lobe tumor. A careful

examination by an otolaryngologist, as well as CT scanning of the brain, is mandatory.

CNII (OPTIC NERVE AND VISUAL SYSTEM)

Visual loss may be due to refractive error; intraocular disease; disease of the retina, optic nerve, optic tract, and optic radiation; and disease of the visual cortex. (See also Chapter 20.)

Visual loss caused by refractive errors and opacities of the ocular media will not be discussed here. From the neurologist's point of view, there are several common and important causes of loss of vision.

Retinal Vascular Disease. Embolic occlusion of the central artery or a branch retinal artery produces sudden monocular visual loss. Because of the vertical orientation of the retinal vesels, loss of vision may be described in terms of a shade lowering that blocks vision. Occlusion may be transient, lasting minutes, and produce a brief episode of monocular blindness (transient monocular blindness or *amaurosis fugax*). Persistent retinal artery occlusion produces infarction of the retina. With infarction, the inner layers of the retina become opalescent, except over the fovea, which remains as a cherry-red spot.

Embolic disease of the retinal arteries usually indicates the presence of extracranial carotid vascular disease as a source for emboli.

The retinopathies of hypertension, diabetes, and vasculitis may all cause visual loss, but without a sudden onset. Exudates, microaneurysms, hemorrhages, and retinal edema usually are present. Central retinal vein occlusion produces a hemorrhagic retinopathy with variable visual loss.

Optic Nerve Disease. Visual loss generally is characterized by dimness, an afferent pupil defect if unilateral, color vision disturbance, and later, atrophy of the optic disc.

In acute optic neuritis, unilateral visual loss develops rapidly over hours to days. The disc may appear normal (retrobulbar neuritis) or swollen (papillitis). Pain may be present on eye movement. Most patients recover in weeks to months, but often incompletely. Optic neuritis may be idiopathic or represent a first attack of multiple sclerosis. Multiple sclerosis develops in approximately 50% of all optic neuritis patients, especially in women aged 20 to 40 years. Other causes of optic neuritis include demyelination following vaccination or viral infection, sarcoidosis, systemic lupus erythematosus, diabetes mellitus, and syphilis.

In ischemic optic neuropathy, visual loss develops over hours to days, associated with a pale, swollen disc. The two major causes of ischemic optic neuropathy are arteriosclerotic vascular disease and giant cell arteritis. Patients with giant cell arteritis usually are over age 65 and have a markedly elevated erythrocyte sedimentation rate. Headache, systemic signs (anemia, polymyalgia rheumatica), and tenderness over the superficial temporal artery may be present. If giant cell arteritis is suspected, high-dose corticosteroid therapy should be started and biopsy should be performed on a generous length of temporal artery.

The syndrome of optic nerve compression by a neoplasm is characterized by slowly progressive loss of vision, acquired disturbance of color vision, an afferent pupillary defect, and a normal or pale optic disc. In cases of compression of the optic chiasm, a bitemporal hemianopia develops. The lesions responsible include meningioma, pituitary adenoma, metastatic tumor, craniopharyngioma, and aneurysm. CT scanning of the head has greatly enhanced the potential for early diagnosis of neoplastic optic nerve compression. Other causes of optic nerve disease include optic nerve gliomas, frontal head trauma, glaucoma, meningeal carcinomatosis, and B_{12} deficiency.

Papilledema. Papilledema, or edema of the optic disc, is characterized by swelling of the head of the optic nerve with engorgement of the retinal veins, and, in severe cases, by hemorrhages in the nerve and adjacent retina.

Papilledema is due to increased intracranial pressure that is transmitted in the sheaths of the optic nerves from stagnation of the venous return from the retina and nerve head. Bilateral papilledema is common in patients with intracranial tumors. The nature and location of the tumor are important factors in the development of papilledema. Papilledema appears early in patients with a tumor that, because of its location, interferes with the circulation of CSF. Tumors that occlude the outlets of the ventricles produce papilledema early in their course. Such tumors include gliomas of the thalamus, cysts of the third ventricle, pinealomas, and posterior fossa tumors in general. Intracranial tumors confined to a cerebral hemisphere do not produce hydrocephalus and hence do not cause papilledema until they grow large enough to cause increased intracranial pressure and brain shift. Such tumors include pituitary adenomas, slowly growing cerebral astrocytomas, meningiomas, and pontine gliomas.

It is not always possible to differentiate papilledema caused by intracranial tumor from papilledema caused by swelling of the optic nerve head associated with optic neuritis and ischemic optic neuropathy. In general, papilledema caused by intracranial hypertension is almost always bilateral and not associated with a loss of vision, except for enlargement of the blind spot. The pupils are normally responsive to light. Optic nerve head swelling caused by optic neuritis or ischemic optic neuropathy usually is unilateral and is accompanied by visual loss and an afferent pupillary defect. In addition, patients with brain tumor practically always have other signs of cerebral dysfunction including stupor, limitation of eye movements, and perhaps focal motor and sensory deficits.

Evaluation of the patient with papilledema includes a careful history and physical examination and CT scanning. CT scanning after intravenous injection of contrast material usually gives an accurate localization of the lesion and frequently indicates its histologic type. If the CT scan is normal, the CSF should be examined. An elevated CSF pressure in the absence of any other abnormalities indicates the presence of benign intracranial hypertension or pseudotumor cerebri.

Disease of the Optic Tract and Optic Radiations. Lesions of the optic tract between the optic chiasm and lateral geniculate body cause a noncongruous (asymmetrical) homonymous hemianopia with greatest involvement in the ipsilateral eye. Neoplasms and infarcts are the most common causes. Lesions of the optic radiation between the lateral geniculate body and the visual cortex produce a congruous contralateral homonymous hemianopsia. Temporal lobe lesions affect the inferior portion of the visual radiation and usually produce a visual defect that is more dense superiorly ("pie in the sky"). Parietal lobe tumors may compress the superior portions of the visual radiation and cause denser involvement inferiorly. Parietal lobe infarction caused by atherothrombotic or embolic disease of the middle cerebral artery causes a homonymous hemianopia that is equally dense superiorly and inferiorly. Patients with parietal lobe lesions usually are unaware of any visual deficit because of the syndrome of parietal neglect.

Visual Cortex Disease. Unilateral disease of the occipital cortex produces a contralateral homonymous hemianopia of which the patient may be aware. Bilateral disease causes cortical blindness, that is, blindness with preserved pupillary reactivity to light. Embolic occlusion of one or both posterior cerebral arteries causes hemianopia and cortical blindness, respectively. Transient cortical blindness sometimes is noted in patients resuscitated after cardiac arrest. The mechanism is disproportionate ischemia in the occipital pole border zones between the middle and posterior cerebral arteries.

Evaluation of Patients With Visual Loss

The evaluation of a patient with visual loss should include measurement of visual acuity, testing of color vision, ophthalmoscopic examination, determination of pupillary reactivity to light, and testing of the visual fields.

Visual acuity at a distance of 20 feet should be determined if possible. If the patient has glasses, they should be worn; if they are unavailable, viewing through a pinhole will improve vision reduced by refractive causes.

Color vision may be tested with a standard book of color plates. Loss of color vision with preserved acuity suggests optic nerve disease.

In the ophthalmoscopic examination, the fundus of each eye should be examined for papilledema, optic atrophy, vascular occlusions, hemorrhages, exudates, or other retinal abnormalities.

In pupillary testing, the pupils are observed while a flashlight is shone alternately into each eye. A symmetrical response is normal. An abnormal response, indicating an afferent pupillary defect (reduced acuity), occurs when one pupil fails to constrict as briskly as the other, or even dilates when exposed to light.

In testing visual fields, each eye should be tested separately by confrontation techniques. Finger wiggling in the periphery is useful for detecting large hemianopias such as occur in patients with strokes. Use of colored objects will detect subtle hemianopias because the color in the involved field will appear less bright to the patient.

On the basis of the findings on the above tests, the physician should be able to localize the site of disease along the visual pathway and other more detailed tests such as visual-evoked cortical responses, and CT scan, or MRI scanning. The former test is an objective means of detecting optic nerve damage. Visual-evoked responses detect prolonged latencies and lowered amplitudes of cortical responses to a focused retinal image. A CT scan will identify and localize tumors and infarcts in the visual pathways. The MRI scan has the additional capacity to detect plaques of multiple sclerosis.

CNIII

The size of the normal pupil results from the opposing forces of the parasympathetic or cholinergic fibers of the third nerve that cause constriction and the sympathetic fibers that cause dilatation. Normal pupils should be round, regular, central, and of equal size. Anisocoria, or unequal pupils, is present in nearly 20% of healthy individuals.

The pupils constrict to light and dilate in darkness both directly and consensually. The pupils constrict in accommodation (increased convexity of the lens), that is, when the patient focuses on a near object. The pupils dilate when the skin of the neck is pinched (ciliospinal reflex).

Afferent pupillary fibers travel with the visual fibers in the optic nerve, chiasm, and tract, but instead of proceeding to the lateral geniculate nuclei, they leave the optic tracts to pass to the pretectal nuclei. Fibers from each pretectal nucleus pass to the Edinger-Westphal nucleus on the same and the opposite side.

There are two types of efferent fibers to the pupil. Parasympathetic fibers originate in the Edinger-Westphal nucleus of CNIII and pass via the oculomotor nerve to the ciliary ganglion and then to the sphincter muscle of the pupil. Sympathetic fibers originate in the contralateral cerebral cortex and pass to the ipsilateral hypothalamus. From the hypothalamus, fibers pass through the brain stem and cervical spinal cord to reach the lateral gray matter of the upper thoracic region. Preganglionic sympathetic fibers leave the cord via the T1 and T2 motor roots and pass via the cervical sympathetic chain to the superior cervical ganglion, where they synapse. From there, postganglionic fibers pass via the carotid artery plexus and along ciliary nerves to the dilator muscle of the pupil. The normal pupillary light reflex requires an afferent limb that includes the ipsilateral optic nerve, both optic tracts, and both pretectal nuclei, and an efferent limb that includes both oculomotor nerves. The cerebral visual cortex is not involved in this reflex; hence, a patient with cortical blindness will have an intact light reflex.

Clinical Syndromes (Neurologic Causes of Abnormal Pupillary Reactions)

Although pupillary disorders caused by neurologic disease are our main concern in this chapter, non-neurologic conditions, such as iridectomy, trauma, iritis, glaucoma, and drugs, commonly alter pupillary function. (See also Chapter 20.)

SYNDROMES ASSOCIATED WITH MIOSIS (TABLE 15–4)

Horner's syndrome (unilateral sympathetic paralysis) is characterized by miosis from paralysis of the dilator muscle of the pupil, from ptosis, and from narrowing of the palpebral fissure from paralysis of the tarsal smooth muscle. In addition, it is characterized by apparent enophthalmos caused by the associated ptosis; loss of sweating on the same side of the face or body, depending upon the level of the lesion; dilatation of the conjunctival vessels; and retained pupillary reactions to light and accommodation.

The sympathetic pathways may be interrupted at various levels from the hypothalamus to the orbit. Locating the site and level of the lesion causing sympathetic paralysis is aided by the presence of ''neighborhood'' signs. For example, unilateral Horner's

Table 15–4.   Causes of Miosis (Constricted Pupil)

Unilateral
  Topical use of miotic drugs such as physostigmine and pilocarpine
  Sympathetic paralysis, as in Horner's syndrome
  Parasympathetic overactivity
  Constricted phase of Adie's pupil
  Unilateral Argyll Robertson pupil
Bilateral
  Central effect of drugs such as opium and its derivatives
  Sympathetic underactivity, as in sleep or certain stages of coma
  Sympathetic paralysis, as in pontine hemorrhage
  Old age (senile miosis)
  Bilateral Argyll Robertson pupil also seen in diabetic pseudotabes

Table 15–5.   Causes of Mydriasis (Dilated Pupil)

Unilateral
  Topical use of mydriatics such as atropine
  Local contact with belladonna preparations or plants such as jimson weed
  Parasympathetic paralysis, as in early uncal herniation or ophthalmoplegic migraine
  Sympathetic stimulation
  Dilated phase of Adie's pupil
Bilateral
  Internal use of drugs such as atropine
  Parasympathetic paralysis
  Botulism
  Neuropathy (diphtheria, diabetes)
  Thyrotoxicosis
  Asphyxia
  Alcoholic intoxication (may be normal or dilated)

syndrome associated with vertigo, ipsilateral cerebellar signs, and ipsilateral loss of pain and temperature sensation on the face with contralateral loss of pain and temperature sensation in the limbs indicates the presence of a lesion in the ipsilateral lateral medulla (Wallenberg's syndrome). Similarly, "neighborhood" signs will indicate the site of the lesion as being the spinal cord (syringomyelia or tumor), paraspinous region (Pancoast's tumor), or carotid plexus (occluded carotid, carotid-cavernous fistula, etc). Horner's syndrome may also be intermittent when associated with cluster headache, which is characterized by recurring, often nocturnal pain in one eye or one side of the face and head, accompanied by nasal congestion, conjunctival injection, facial flushing, and Horner's syndrome, all on the same side as the pain.

The Argyll Robertson pupil is small and unreactive to light but retains the reaction to accommodation. It is usually bilateral but may be unilateral. The site of the lesion is pretectal, involving the connections between the pretectal and Edinger-Westphal nuclei but sparing the connections with the brain stem center for convergence. Miosis is caused by involvement of the adjacent sympathetic fibers. The Argyll Robertson pupil has been described in association with CNS syphilis but also has been noted in diabetes, old age, and compressive lesion of the pretectum.

Bilateral pinpoint pupils, smaller than in Horner's syndrome, occur in pontine hemorrhage. In addition to sympathetic paralysis, an irritation of the parasympathetic outflow to the pupil causes maximal constriction of the pupils. The differential diagnosis includes bilateral miosis caused by opiate drugs.

SYNDROMES ASSOCIATED WITH MYDRIASIS (TABLE 15–5)

Adie's Pupil (Tonic Pupil). Adie's Pupil is usually dilated and apparently fixed to light and accommodation. It is seen most often in young women and may be unilateral or bilateral. On careful patient testing, the pupil contracts slowly to strong illumination and to convergence.

The lesion responsible for the tonic pupil may be in the ciliary ganglion. The tonic pupil may exist alone as an incidental finding or may be part of a wider syndrome of dysautonomia (absent sweating, orthostatic hypotension, and absent deep tendon reflexes).

CNIII Palsy. A unilateral, dilated, fixed pupil occurring in the absence of other evidence of third nerve palsy may be due to ipsilateral compression of the nerve by tumor, aneurysm, or uncal herniation. The parasympathetic fibers are paralyzed selectively because they are located on the periphery of the nerve trunk and hence are most vulnerable to trauma. The differential diagnosis of unilateral mydriasis includes the topical use of mydriatics either intentionally or inadvertently.

Diplopia and Abnormal Eye Movements. Diplopia or double vision is caused by extraocular muscle imbalance. Separation of images is greatest in the direction of action of the weak muscle.

In evaluating the patient with diplopia, one must first determine whether the patient's diplopia is binocular or uniocular. Unilateral diplopia persists if the normal eye is covered, whereas binocular diplopia disappears. In cases of binocular diplopia, physical examination may enable the physician to localize the cause of diplopia to a nuclear or infranuclear lesion of a cranial nerve. The history and collateral findings may suggest a diagnosis (e.g., bilateral sixth nerve palsy and papilledema suggest a brain tumor with increased intracranial pressure; a unilateral CNIII palsy in a patient with depressed consciousness and a stiff neck suggests a ruptured aneurysm). Following the neurologic examination, special studies are likely to yield a diagnosis. CT scan may show evidence of a tumor or bleeding. Examination of the CSF obtained by lumbar puncture may show evidence of meningitis. Arteriography may show an aneurysm.

CNIII (Oculomotor Nerve) Paralysis. In paralysis of the third cranial (oculomotor) nerve, all the external ocular muscles are affected except the lateral rectus and superior oblique. The unopposed actions of these unaffected muscles turn the eye outward and downward. The patient does not complain of diplopia because of the complete ptosis. In complete CNIII palsies, there is also internal ophthalmoplegia; the pupil is dilated and unreactive to light or accommodation. Since the pupillary fibers occupy a peripheral position in the third nerve, they often are initially involved by a compressing lesion such as occurs in uncal herniation. Vascular lesions of the third nerve, as occur in diabetes, usually spare the pupillary fibers.

CNIV

Trochlear or fourth cranial nerve palsy produces vertical diplopia and weakness or depression of the adducted eye (superior oblique muscle). The patient usually tilts his head to the opposite side to reduce the separation of images.

CNVI

Sixth cranial nerve palsy causes failure of abduction (lateral rectus muscle) and horizontal diplopia.

The functions of CNIII, IV, and VI may be disrupted by lesions anywhere along their courses, from the brain stem to the neuromuscular junction in the eye.

In the brain stem, vascular disease, neoplasms, demyelinating disease, and inflammatory disease may affect the nuclei and intramedullary fibers of these nerves. After the nerve fibers leave the brain stem and enter the subarachnoid space, they may be damaged by meningitis, compression by aneurysms (especially CNIII by aneurysms of the carotid-posterior communicating artery junction), and compression by tumors. In the cavernous sinus, all three nerves and the first division of CNV may be involved by carotid-cavernous fistula, intracavernous carotid aneurysm, and pituitary tumor. Various inflammatory, neoplastic, and traumatic conditions can involve the ocular nerves in the orbit. In addition, the peripheral fibers of the cranial nerves may be involved by various diseases, including alcoholism (Wernicke- Korsakoff's syndrome), diabetes (ischemic demyelination), giant cell arteritis, sarcoidosis, herpes zoster, syphilis, and diphtheria, Guillain-Barré syndrome (Fisher variant), and ophthalmoplegic migraine.

Diplopia as a result of injury to the oculomotor nerves must be differentiated from the external ocular palsies of myasthenia and other conditions that affect the neuromuscular junction (botulism), and from ocular muscle disease.

Myasthenia gravis may present with unilateral or bilateral ptosis with external ocular muscle palsies. The ptosis and pareses typically fluctuate and may undergo periods of remission. Improvement in diplopia following the administration of edrophonium can be diagnostic.

The neuromuscular junction also is affected in botulism, in which bilateral ptosis, dilated pupils (internal), and external ophthalmoplegia accompany general muscle weakness.

The ocular muscles may be involved by myopathies such as the Kearns-Sayre syndrome and by endocrine disorders such as dysthyroid exophthalmos. Diplopia may also be uniocular as a result of local eye disorders, such as irregularities of the cornea, astigmatism, subluxation of the lens, detachment of the retina, or development of cataracts.

CNV AND CNVIII

Disorders of CNV and CNVIII have been considered earlier.

CNVII

The facial or seventh cranial nerve is predominantly a motor nerve to the muscles of facial expression. In addition, it carries parasympathetic secretory fibers to the salivary and lacrimal glands and to the mucous membranes of the oral and nasal cavities. It conveys taste sensation from the anterior two thirds of the tongue and innervates the stapedius muscle, which increases the tension of the middle ear ossicles and the tympanic membrane. Facial weakness may result from an upper motor neuron lesion, namely, above the facial nucleus in the brain stem, or from a lower motor neuron lesion of the nucleus or of the nerve itself. Because the portion of the facial nucleus that supplies the muscles to the upper third of the face receives bilateral supranuclear innervation, a unilateral upper motor neuron lesion produces an incomplete weakness that affects the lower part of the face more severely than the upper part.

An incomplete facial weakness indicates an upper motor neuron lesion usually in the contralateral motor cortex. In such lesions, there may be a discrepancy between the extent of volitional and emotional movements. Volitional contractions under the control of the damaged motor cortex will be less than those that occur when the patient smiles or laughs. The innervation of the muscles involved in emotional contractions comes from the limbic cortex.

Complete unilateral facial paralysis (Bell's palsy), caused by a peripheral lesion, is accompanied by decreased tearing in the ipsilateral eye, loss of taste sensation in the ipsilateral side of the tongue, and increased sensitivity to sounds in the ipsilateral ear.

Differential diagnosis between a facial paralysis from a cortical lesion and that from a lesion of the nucleus or nerve usually can be made without difficulty. Sparing of the muscles of the forehead and upper lid, signs of cortical involvement such as expressive aphasia when the dominant hemisphere is damaged, and preservation of electrical reactions indicate an upper motor neuron lesion. CT scanning of the brain may indicate an infarct, hemorrhage, or neoplasm in such cases.

Lesions in the brain stem are accompanied by paralysis of lateral gaze caused by concomitant injury to the nucleus of CNVI, and by hemiparesis caused by involvement of the corticospinal tract. Lesions of the seventh nerve at the point of emergence from the brain stem caused by meningitis and neoplasms are accompanied by paralysis of adjacent nerves, namely, the fifth, sixth, and eighth.

Sudden complete facial paralysis unassociated with other neurologic deficits (Bell's palsy) is due to injury to the nerve caused by virus. Occasionally, it is caused by herpes zoster. Traumatic injury to the seventh nerve caused by surgery or basal skull fracture should be obvious on the basis of history and examination.

Bilateral facial weakness accompanies disease of muscles (muscular dystrophy), disease of the neuromuscular junction (myasthenia gravis), and disease of nerves (Guillain-Barré syndrome).

CNIX AND X

The glossopharyngeal and vagus nerves are closely related. Injury to these nerves results in hoarseness, dysphagia, a depressed or absent gag response ipsilaterally, and depressed or absent sensation in the pharynx on the same side.

CNXII

Injury to the hypoglossal nerve results in weakness and atrophy of the ipsilateral half of the tongue. When the tongue is protruded, it deviates toward the weak side.

TRANSIENT ALTERATIONS OF CONSCIOUSNESS

SYNCOPE

Definition

Syncope, or fainting, is a temporary loss of consciousness. The onset of syncope may be sudden, and without warning or may be preceded by symptoms of lightheadedness, weakness, and graying of vision. The duration of loss of consciousness is brief if the patient is allowed to remain supine, usually lasting only seconds to a few minutes at most. During a syncopal spell, a significant number of patients will have convulsive movements, but the motor activity is less than in a generalized convulsion if the patient is supine. Individuals who are kept upright during a syncopal episode may have a generalized seizure as a result of cerebral ischemia. Following an uncomplicated syncope, the patient is alert and without the postictal signs that follow generalized seizures.

Pathophysiologic Considerations

The cause of syncope is a generalized decrease in cerebral blood flow as a result of a sudden loss of vasomotor tone in the systemic circulation. Hence, syncope usually occurs when the patient is standing or sitting and seldom when the patient is lying down.

Clinical Presentation (Table 15–6)

A vasovagal syncope or common faint is precipitated by emotional stress, injury, or pain. A decrease in peripheral vascular resistance causes hypotension. Because of increased vagal tone, bradycardia is present. Premonitory symptoms include nausea, giddiness, weakness, and perspiration. Consciousness returns immediately when the patient is placed supine.

Cardiac syncope follows a sudden decrease in cardiac output caused by a sudden arrhythmia. When cardiac syncope is due to an atrioventricular conduction block, it is called a Stokes-Adams attack. The

Table 15–6.   Causes of Syncope

Vasovagal syncope
Cardiac syncope
Carotid sinus syncope
Cough syncope
Micturition syncope
Orthostatic syncope

onset of cardiac syncope is sudden, frequently without warning. The duration of unconsciousness is variable, depending on the type and duration of the arrhythmia.

Carotid sinus hypersensitivity may cause syncope through a mechanism of increased vagal tone. Compression of the carotid sinus by head turning or a tight collar can evoke the hypersensitive reflex and syncope. The clinical features are similar to those of vasovagal syncope.

Tussive or cough syncope occurs during a prolonged bout of coughing. Reduction in venous return to the heart because of increased intrathoracic pressure during coughing is the probable cause of syncope.

Syncope following micturition is rare. Syncope occurs predominantly in men and is usually associated with micturition at night. The mechanism of syncope appears to be vagal stimulation.

Syncope upon standing occurs when normal homeostatic mechanisms fail to maintain adequate venous return to the heart. Susceptibility to orthostatic hypotension and syncope is increased by diseases of the autonomic nervous system, blood volume depletion, anemia, prolonged recumbency, and the use of drugs that are vasodilating or ganglion blocking. In elderly individuals, orthostatic mechanisms are likely to be impaired so that syncope may follow getting out of a hot bath or out of a chair after a big meal, especially one including alcohol. In pregnancy, orthostatic syncope may result from pressure of the gravid uterus on the inferior vena cava. Orthostatic syncope occurs in various neuropathies (diabetic, alcoholic) and degenerative diseases (parkinsonism, olivopontocerebellar atrophy). Hypotension complicates the Guillain-Barré syndrome, syringomyelia, tabes dorsalis, and lumbar sympathectomy.

Differential Diagnosis

Several points differentiate syncope from seizures. Vasovagal syncope starts with the patient in a standing or sitting position and often has specific precipitating causes. Seizures occur from any body position and often have no immediate precipitating cause. The patient with syncope is pale with a slow, weak pulse, whereas the epileptic patient often is cyanotic during a seizure and has a normal pulse. Tongue biting and urinary incontinence are common during seizures but rare in syncope. The prodrome of a syncopal spell usually involves only lightheadedness and nausea; the prodrome of an epileptic attack may involve complex sensory and psychologic experiences. Syncope usually has no postictal residua, while epilepsy is marked by postictal sleep, confusion, and headaches. The interictal EEG is frequently abnormal in epilepsy, but is normal in syncope.

Diagnostic Evaluation

A careful history of the circumstances in which loss of consciousness occurred often will indicate the correct diagnosis. If the episodes are associated with a situation conducive to fainting, further studies may not be necessary. The physical examination is unlikely to be helpful unless the patient is examined during an episode.

Laboratory studies should include an electrocardiogram with Holter monitoring if cardiac syncope is suspected. Carotid sinus massage with ECG monitoring may be diagnostic in some cases but should be carried out only if resuscitative equipment is available. Fasting blood glucose and a glucose tolerance test should be obtained in patients with suspected hypoglycemia. A CT scan of the head, EEG, and lumbar puncture are rarely diagnostic in cases of syncope, unless the history and physical examination indicate an abnormality of the CNS. In general, despite extensive laboratory investigations, a specific diagnosis is reached in only 50% of patients with syncope.

SEIZURES

Definition

A seizure is a sudden, usually transient episode of disturbed central nervous system function caused by an uncontrolled discharge of cerebral neurons. Epilepsy is a disorder characterized by recurrent convulsions (seizures). The incidence of seizures in the general population is estimated to be 1 in 200. However, not everyone who has seizures suffers from epilepsy. Generalized tonic-clonic seizures can occur as a transient complication of systemic disorders, such as febrile illnesses of childhood, or withdrawal from alcohol or sedative drugs. Persons who suffer such provoked, nonfocal seizures should not be termed "epileptic."

Pathophysiologic Considerations and Classification (Table 15–7)

Several classifications of epilepsy are based upon the cause, anatomic or physiologic substrate, the clin-

Table 15–7. Classification of Seizure

Generalized seizures
  Tonic-clonic seizures
  Simple seizures with impairment of consciousness only (petit mal)
Partial seizures
  Partial motor and sensory seizures
  Partial complex seizures (psychomotor or temporal lobe seizures)
Status epilepticus

ical manifestations, or a combination of features. Basically, seizures are either generalized or partial.

Generalized Seizures

Tonic-Clonic Seizures. Generalized tonic-clonic seizures occur at all ages and arise from a diffuse epileptogenic state of the cerebral cortex. Tonic-clonic seizures without a focal onset occur from metabolic causes such as encephalitis, hypoglycemia, anoxia, and alcohol withdrawal, as well as from genetically inherited factors. By contrast, tonic-clonic seizures that begin with an "aura" or focal onset and then become generalized are caused by a localized epileptogenic focus such as a tumor, infarct, or contusion.

Tonic-clonic seizures are characterized by an initial loss of consciousness, together with a phase of generalized muscle contraction during which there is apnea. After a tonic phase lasting less than a minute is a tonic-clonic phase, which is typically associated with incontinence of urine (but rarely of feces), tongue biting, hypertension, and tachycardia. Most seizures terminate spontaneously in 2 to 5 minutes and are followed by a period of postictal lethargy, confusion, muscle weakness and soreness, and headache. In patients with structural brain lesion, transient, focal abnormalities on neurologic examination, such as Todd's (postictal) palsy, may be observed. These help to localize the site of cerebral damage.

Simple Seizures with Impairment of Consciousness Only (Petit Mal). Petit mal epilepsy is a convulsive disorder of childhood and adolescence. The age of onset of this form of epilepsy is between 5 and 12 years. These seizures cease by the age of 20 years in approximately three fourths of patients. Of patients with petit mal seizures, 50% develop major motor seizures during adolescence. The clinical pattern of petit mal seizures is characteristic and should not be confused with the complex symptoms of psychomotor seizures. In petit mal, there are typically brief "absences" or losses of consciousness, sometimes associated with blinking of the eyelids. Often, a blank stare is the only sign of seizure because there are neither prodromal nor postictal signs or symptoms. Petit mal seizures have a genetic origin; these absence seizures have not been associated with neoplasm, degenerative disease or metabolic derangements. The electroencephalogram is diagnostic when the characteristic symmetrical 3 cycles/second spike and wave pattern is identified. No further work up is usually indicated.

Partial Seizures

Partial Motor and Sensory Seizures. Focal motor seizures result from an epileptic focus near the motor strip, i.e., the precentral gyrus of the frontal lobe. Focal sensory seizures stem from a similar focus in the parietal lobe or, less commonly, the occipital cortex. For example, an irritable focus near the cortical motor representation of the upper extremity can produce focal tonic-clonic movements of the contralateral hand and arm. If the electrical discharge spreads to involve contiguous areas of motor cortex, a progression of involuntary movements that involve the hand, arm, face, leg, and foot is observed. This progression of movements is known as a jacksonian march.

Partial continuous epilepsy (epilepsia partialis continua) is a form of focal epilepsy in which there are repetitive, often continuous, movements, usually of the face, arm, and hand. An underlying structural lesion may be present, but frequently there is a metabolic cause such as hyperosmolality.

Partial Complex Seizures (Psychomotor or Temporal Lobe Seizures). These focal seizures with complex symptoms usually arise from epileptogenic foci in the temporal lobes. The clinical expressions of these seizures are protean and include purposive but irrelevant motor movements (automatism) together with psychic phenomena including hallucinations, illusions, emotions of fear, intense feelings of recognition (déjà vu) or strangeness (jamais vu), distortions of vision, and bizarre visceral sensations.

Partial complex seizures usually begin before age 20. Causes include asphyxial injuries at birth, head trauma, and tumors. The most common lesion found in the surgically resected temporal lobes of intractable epileptics is mesial temporal sclerosis caused by gliosis of the hippocampus, amygdala, and uncus. This scarring is attributed to an acquired lesion caused by a hypoxic episode during childhood. In one surgical series, nearly one half of epileptic patients with mesial temporal sclerosis gave a history of prolonged febrile seizures.

Interictally, the standard electroencephalogram (EEG) is abnormal in less than 50% of patients with partial complex seizures, but sensitivity may be increased to 80% if the EEG is recorded during sleep and with nasopharyngeal electrodes.

Status Epilepticus. The repetitive occurrence of any type of seizure without recovery between attacks is called status epilepticus. Although status epilepticus sometimes begins spontaneously or in response to acute brain injury, most attacks follow sudden withdrawal from anticonvulsant medication. Generalized tonic-clonic status epilepticus requires emergency treatment because of the danger of cerebral ischemic anoxia and of cardiac failure.

Diagnostic Evaluation

In analyzing an episode of unconsciousness, the physician's goals are to determine whether the spell was a seizure or a syncopal episode, and, if it was a seizure, whether there was a focal onset.

PATIENT HISTORY

A detailed history obtained from the patient or an observer of the seizures is the most important clinical information for establishing a diagnosis of epilepsy and determining its causes. Observers should be questioned about the onset, pattern, and duration of attacks. The patient should be questioned concerning any premonitory symptoms, aura, or postictal weakness, which indicate the area of the brain in which the seizure originates. Depending on the age at onset of the seizures, the physician should seek information about a family history of epilepsy or degenerative disease; any prenatal or birth injury or delayed development; a history of childhood encephalitis, meningitis, and febrile seizures; head trauma; headaches; any alteration in intellect, personality, vision, or motor strength and coordination; and the use of alcohol, barbiturates, phenothiazines, or street drugs.

Differentiating seizures from syncope usually is not difficult (Table 15–8). In vasodepressor syncope (common faint) the subject may appear pale and sweaty and have bradycardia. Most faints occur in the erect or upright position. As soon as the patient becomes recumbent, there is rapid, complete recovery of consciousness without postsyncopal symptoms. However, if the syncopal subject is maintained in the upright position, a generalized seizure may result from cerebral ischemia.

Table 15–8. Differences Between Syncope and Seizure

	Syncope	Seizure
Position at onset	vertical	any
Tongue biting	no	yes
Incontinence	no	yes
Skin	cold and wet	hot and wet
Breathing	normal	apnea
Duration	short	long
Confusion after	no	yes
Headache after	no	yes
Myalgia after	no	yes
Abnormal EEG after	10%	60%

PHYSICAL EXAMINATION

Evaluation of developmental achievement and measurement of head circumference are important parts of the examination of the infant or child. The examination of the skin may suggest the cause of seizures; café au lait spots are a sign of neurofibromatosis, and facial hemangioma identifies the Sturge-Weber syndrome of epilepsy, hemiparesis, mental retardation, and intracranial calcifications.

In the adult patient, in whom acquired lesions such as brain tumors and strokes assume greater importance, the examination of the optic fundus for papilledema, arterial narrowing, hemorrhages, and exudates may provide diagnostic findings.

DIAGNOSTIC STUDIES

A complete blood count, urinalysis, fasting blood sugar, serum calcium, serum electrolytes, and blood urea nitrogen should be ordered. The desirability of additional tests for the diagnosis of systemic disease such as acute intermittent porphyria and collagen disease and for drug withdrawal seizures will be suggested by the history and the results of physical examination.

The EEG should be performed on all patients with seizures and is an excellent diagnostic and screening test. Nevertheless, a diagnosis of epilepsy is in most cases based on the history and physical examination, independent of the EEG. The CT scan is helpful for the detection of cerebral tumors and hemorrhages and for evaluation of ventricular size. A lumbar puncture is mandatory only when meningitis is suspected. It is an important procedure for the evaluation of febrile seizures of neonates and children. In the adult, lumbar puncture usually does not provide specific information and may be dangerous if a mass lesion is present.

TRANSIENT ISCHEMIC ATTACKS

Definition

Transient ischemic attacks (TIAs) are ischemic episodes of focal cerebral dysfunction lasting less than 24 hours, and usually only a few minutes, followed by complete recovery with absence of evidence of neurologic deficit on neurologic examination. TIAs provide a warning of a possibly impending permanent neurologic deficit and are a risk factor associated with both stroke and myocardial infarction.

Pathophysiologic Considerations and Classification

Whenever the cerebral blood flow (CBF) of a region declines to a point low enough to impair neuronal function, clinical symptoms of focal ischemia can appear. If the supply of oxygen and glucose is restored before permanent damage has occurred, the focal neuronal dysfunction is reversible and the associated clinical symptoms are transient.

The term TIA comprises a diverse group of pathologic conditions that result in intermittent focal interruptions of CBF. The causes of TIAs can be divided into three pathophysiologic categories: abnormalities of the blood vessels themselves, including the heart and extracranial and intracranial vessels; alterations in

Table 15–9. Conditions Associated with Generalized Cerebral Ischemia

Abnormalities of blood vessels
  Atherosclerosis of extracranial or intracranial arteries
  Fibromuscular dysplasia
  Inflammatory disorders
    Giant cell arteritis
    Systemic lupus erythematosus
    Polyarteritis nodosa
    Meningovascular syphilis
    Granulomatous angiitis
    Takayasu's disease
  Dissection of extracranial arteries
    Spontaneous
    Traumatic
  Multiple progressive intracranial arterial occlusions (Moya Moya syndrome)
Cardiac abnormalities leading to embolic phenomena
  Ischemic heart disease
    Myocardial infarct with mural thrombus
    Arrhythmia
  Rheumatic heart disease (including prosthetic valves)
  Infective endocarditis
  Atrial myxoma
  Mitral valve prolapse
Hematologic abnormalities
  Platelet disorders
    Thrombocytosis
    Intrinsic platelet hyperactivity
  Red blood cell abnormalities
    Polycythemia
    Anemia
  Serum hyperviscosity syndromes (paraproteinemia)
  Abnormalities of hemoglobin
  Sickle cell anemia (Hg SS)
Altered cerebral circulation
  Hypotension
    Cardiac arrest or arrhythmias
    Orthostatic hypotension
  Cervical spondylosis with vertebral artery compression
  Abnormal shunting of blood
    Cerebral arteriovenous malformations, carotid cavernous fistula (following repair)
    Subclavian steel syndrome
    Hereditary hemorrhagic telangiectasia (Rendu-Osler-Weber syndrome) with pulmonary AV shunt
    Patent foramen ovale
Miscellaneous conditions
  Migraine headache with transient ischemic accompaniments
  Use of oral contraceptive agents
  Complications of cerebral angiography
  Chiropractic manipulation-induced stroke

the composition of the circulating blood; and changes in the manner in which the blood circulates (Table 15–9).

The major theories advanced to explain TIAs are vasospasm, hemodynamic factors, and thromboembolism.

Vasospasm of an intracerebral or extracerebral artery is now considered unlikely as a cause of transient ischemia, except in cases of hypertensive encephalopathy, subarachnoid hemorrhage, or migraine.

Hemodynamic factors such as reduced perfusion pressure distal to a severely stenotic or occluded cerebral artery account for a small proportion of TIAs.

The most common mechanism producing alterations in CBF is probably platelet emboli originating from atherosclerosis of the extracranial or intracranial cerebral arteries. The evidence for this mechanism is mainly clinical. In patients with transient monocular blindness, the passage of emboli through the retinal circulation has been witnessed. Cerebral arteriography has demonstrated occlusion of small intracranial arteries in the vascular distribution of diseased carotid arteries of patients with TIAs. Pathologic examination of carotid arteries obtained at the time of endarterectomy from patients with TIAs has shown ulcerated atheromatous plaques with an adherent fresh thrombus. TIAs often cease when the source of microemboli is removed by carotid stenosis progressing to complete occlusion. Surgical elimination of carotid stenosis reduces the incidence of TIAs. TIAs often cease in patients treated with anticoagulants or antiplatelet aggregation drugs.

TIAs can occur in the carotid and vertebrobasilar territories. The history of a TIA in the carotid artery territory is generally quite typical. The most common symptom experienced by the patient is a sudden onset of weakness, paralysis, or clumsiness of one or both extremities on the same side. Sensory symptoms may be present, including a feeling of numbness or paresthesias involving one or both extremities on the same side. If the TIA involves the hemisphere dominant for language function, dysphasia will be present. Another potential component of a carotid system TIA is transient loss of vision in one eye or part of one eye.

In vertebrobasilar TIAs, the most common symptom is a motor defect such as weakness, clumsiness, or paralysis of any combination of extremities up to quadriplegia. Sensory phenomena include numbness, loss of sensation, or paresthesias in any combination of extremities. The patient may complain of unsteady gait, disequilibrium, and vertigo. Loss of vision may occur, varying from complete blindness to partial blindness in homonymous fields. Diplopia is another common visual symptom in vertebrobasilar TIAs.

Differential Diagnosis

The differential diagnosis of TIAs is not large but includes classic migraine with scintillating scotomas, hemiplegic migraine, focal convulsive events, Meniere's disease, and peripheral vestibulopathy.

TIAs may be distinguished from migrainous accompaniments by the fact that, whereas TIAs are generally maximal at onset or come all at once, migrainous phenomena generally "build up" or progress for several minutes. Headache may accompany TIAs, but it generally is brief and not severe. Focal seizures generally march or progress from the distal to the proximal portions of an extremity and produce persistent neurologic deficits on physical examination (Todd's postictal paralysis). Isolated vertigo without other motor and sensory phenomena rarely is caused by a TIA.

Diagnostic Evaluation

PATIENT HISTORY

The most valuable part of the evaluation of a patient with TIAs is the history of the attack. Rarely does a physician actually observe a patient during a TIA and therefore must rely on the patient's account of the attack.

PHYSICAL EXAMINATION

Because TIAs are closely linked with atherosclerotic vascular disease, the evaluation of such patients is directed toward detecting evidence of cardiovascular disease. Attention should be given to heart rate, rhythm, and size, heart sounds, blood pressure in both upper extremities, and peripheral pulses. There should be a search for atherosclerotic vascular disease elsewhere in the body and a search for audible bruits over various arterial sites.

The physician should perform a neurovascular examination. Cranial arteritis, an unusual cause of TIA, may be detected by palpating the involved temporal artery. Absence of temporal artery pulses may also indicate occlusive disease of the ipsilateral external carotid artery. It is virtually impossible to accurately palpate the internal carotid artery in the neck; what one feels is the common carotid or the bifurcation of the internal carotid. Absence of carotid pulse that had been present is associated with significant carotid artery disease.

Bruits often can be heard by auscultating over the carotid artery as it passes up the neck, or they can be heard over the vertebral artery just above the clavicle and sometimes over the back of the neck or head. When present in an individual with TIAs, a bruit strongly suggests that the cerebral vessels are involved with atherosclerosis.

DIAGNOSTIC STUDIES

By scanning the region of the carotid artery with an ultrasonic probe, it is possible to identify the outline of the carotid bifurcation and to give a reasonably accurate picture of the degree of stenosis of the artery. B-mode scanning, when coupled with Doppler techniques to estimate velocity of blood flow in the vessel under study, adds to the accuracy of this noninvasive technique.

Cerebral arteriography remains the most definitive test in the evaluation of a patient with TIAs. Currently, cerebral angiography is done by catheterization of the femoral artery and then selective identification of each cerebral arterial tree by placement of the catheter. The aortic arch, the carotid, and the vertebrobasilar circulations, both extracranial and intracranial, may be studied. Although digital intravenous subtraction angiography has been substituted for cerebral arteriography in some cases, this technique does not have the same accuracy as arteriography in delineating the extracranial or intracranial vessels.

CT brain scanning is rarely useful in patients with TIAs but may identify unsuspected intracranial lesions such as a tumor, subdural hematoma, or previous stroke.

DISORDERS OF COGNITIVE FUNCTION

DEMENTIA

Dementia is a common disorder that affects nearly 5% of all persons over age 65. The most common type of dementia is Alzheimer's disease, now known as senile dementia of the Alzheimer type (SDAT). SDAT is a progressive disease that accounts for nearly two thirds of all cases of dementia.

Definition

Dementia is defined as a deterioration of intellectual function and cognitive functions without disturbance of perception. Dementia is manifested by impairment in orientation, memory, intellectual functions, and judgment and by lability and shallowness of affect.

Pathophysiologic Considerations

Recent research has identified a genetic contribution in SDAT. A first-degree relative has a three or four times greater risk for SDAT than the general population. Studies of twins with dementia, especially if autopsy is performed, have shown a high degree of concordance. The age differentials in onset in twins suggest an environmental factor, as well. The occurrence of SDAT changes in Down's syndrome also supports the genetic hypothesis. Autopsy studies of patients in Guam, where a disease complex of parkinsonism, amyotrophic lateral sclerosis, and dementia is common, have found most nonaffected Guamanians to have similar neuropathologic changes. This finding suggests an environmental cause with a widespread subclinical effect.

The lesion of SDAT is senile plaques and neurofibrillary tangles. These changes are distributed throughout the cerebral hemispheres, although there may be a concentration in certain areas. The recent findings of decreased cholinergic neurons and neuronal endings in the hemispheres has stimulated new research. The nucleus basalis of Meynert is the origin of most of the cholinergic fibers in the cortex, and this area shows neuronal loss in SDAT. Noradrenergic systems also may be involved. Deficiencies of the neuropeptides, somatostatin, and substance P also are present. Atherosclerotic cerebrovascular disease plays no part in the cause of SDAT.

Differential Diagnosis and Diagnostic Evaluation

The differential diagnosis of dementia requires first that dementia be separated from pseudodementia caused by depression. Dementia is derived from depression in 10 to 30% of affected individuals. In such patients, memory difficulties may be prominent, perhaps accompanied by difficulty with naming objects as well as with complaints of depression and anxiety. Disorientation and other signs of cognitive dysfunction tend to be less marked than in patients with SDAT. Pseudodementia shows a fluctuating or nonprogressive course and may respond dramatically to antidepressant treatment.

There is no specific diagnostic test for SDAT. The typical patient will have a slowly progressive and global loss of intellectual function without focal features. Each patient must be screened for drug toxicity, hypothyroidism, B$_{12}$, folate, or thiamin deficiency, and syphilis. The CT scan is used to rule out intracranial tumors, multiple infarcts, hydrocephalus, and subdural hematomas. There is no specific CT appearance in SDAT. Atrophy with enlargement of the sulci and ventricles can be marked but correlates poorly with the clinical picture. Positron emission tomography (PET) studies show normal oxygen extraction but reduced metabolism of glucose in most cortical areas, although the primary motor and sensory cortical areas are relatively unaffected.

Other diseases that can present as dementia include occult normal pressure hydrocephalus (NPH), Huntington's disease (HD), parkinsonism, spinocerebellar degeneration, progressive supranuclear palsy, multiinfarct dementia, chronic subdural hematoma, and brain tumor. The CT scan is helpful in detecting NPH, multi-infarct dementia, subdural hematoma, and tumor.

Occult normal pressure hydrocephalus is much less common than previously thought. The typical presentation is with the triad of dementia, urinary incontinence, and gait disturbance. The CT scan may show panventricular enlargement with small sulci, but commonly a mixed picture of ventriculomegaly and atrophy is present. Ventricular drainage by a shunt is most successful in patients who have incontinence and gait disturbance more marked than their degree of dementia.

Huntington's disease is a dementing movement disorder, inherited as autosomal dominant, that usually presents in the fifth or sixth decade. A negative family history is not always reliable. CT, PET, and MRI studies of patients with symptomatic and presymptomatic HD have shown decreased glucose metabolism in the caudate nucleus, whether normal or atrophied. This change is not diagnostic of HD because PET studies have shown decreased metabolism in the caudate nuclei of patients with benign chorea. The gene responsible for HD has recently been traced to the short arm of chromosome four.

Creutzfeldt-Jakob (CJ) disease is a rapidly progressive, dementing disorder with myoclonus that is caused by an as yet unidentified submicroscopic transmissible agent resistant to formalin fixation. CJ is a familial disorder in about 15% of cases.

Dialysis dementia is a progressive dementia preceded by a peculiar progressive language disturbance. The sudden onset of hesitant nonfluent speech is the characteristic and usually the earliest sign. Both dysarthric and dysphasic elements are found. Myoclonus, seizures, and gait difficulty also are seen in the majority of these patients. Dialysis dementia may be associated with increased aluminum content of the dialysate and local water supply, but aluminum toxicity has not been a consistent epidemiologic association. Treatment is unsatisfactory.

Multi-infarct dementia is characterized by a stepwise course caused by many small strokes. The diagnosis depends on assessing the history of abrupt onset, fluctuating course, focal neurologic signs and symptoms, and a past history of stroke or hypertension.

Mild dementia may be apparent in patients with Parkinson's disease and may progress with the disease. Conversely, patients with SDAT may experience movement disorders, including tremor and bradykinesia, characteristic of parkinsonism.

AMNESTIC SYNDROMES

Definition

Memory is a faculty of mind by which experiences, such as facts, events, ideas, and sensations, are acquired, stored, and retrieved. Memory has at least three categories: immediate, recent or short-term, and remote or long-term.

Immediate memory refers to and is tested by the ability to repeat immediately, or within a few moments, a series of numbers or other data. The ability to remember the seven digits of an unfamiliar telephone number from the directory long enough to dial it is an example of immediate memory.

Recent memory refers to the ability to recall events that occurred minutes to an hour before. Short-term memory is tested by asking the patient to remember a list of unrelated objects (e.g., red, table, and Broadway) for 15 or 30 minutes.

Remote memory refers to the ability to recall experiences that happened hours, days, or years before. Remote or long-term memory can be divided into personal and nonpersonal memories. Personal memories such as the date and place of birth and names of parents and spouses are "over-learned" and tend to be preserved in amnestic states, even when nonpersonal remote memories, such as the names of presidents, are lost.

Pathophysiologic Considerations

At least three processes are involved in memory: registration, retention, and recall. Attention, concentration, and interest are required for memory registration or acquisition. Therefore, memory mechanisms are influenced by the reticular formation of the brain stem, which maintains alertness. Memory is also affected by emotions, which are influenced by the limbic system. An emotional context tends to fix an event in memory; conversely, stress, anxiety, and depression help to exclude events without immediacy.

Memory is related to intelligence, but not directly, because some people of modest or low intelligence have photographic memories.

Registration or acquisition of new memories requires full consciousness. Thus, in a cerebral concussion or an epileptic fit, the period of unconsciousness may be succeeded by a stage of consciousness in which the patient appears rational but for which he subsequently has no memory. This period between the regaining of consciousness and the restoration of memory registration is termed the period of antegrade amnesia. Retrograde amnesia is a loss of memory for events preceding the onset of illness or injury.

All three types of memory may be impaired in neurologic disease. Immediate memory may be impaired in dementia, states of confusion, or delirium as a hysterical reaction or resulting from drug use.

Impaired recent memory commonly is associated with diseases of the limbic system (hippocampus, for-

nix, mamillary bodies, thalamus, and angulate gyrus). Bilateral resection of the hippocampus permanently and severely impairs recent memory. Unilateral resection or destruction of the hippocampus of the dominant hemisphere transiently impairs recent memory. Other causes of impaired recent memory include cerebrovascular disease, hypoxia, ischemia, ingestion of drugs or alcohol, and hysteria.

Remote memory is the most resistant to disruption and commonly is the last type of memory to be impaired or lost. Seldom is remote memory loss encountered without a disturbance of immediate and recent memory.

Clinical Presentation

The amnestic syndromes (Table 15–10) are those in which memory is affected out of proportion to the other components of mentation and behavior. The amnestic syndrome seen in Korsakoff's psychosis is prototypical. Korsakoff's psychosis is characterized by an impaired ability to acquire new information or to form new memories (antegrade amnesia) and an impaired ability to recall events and other information that had

Table 15–10. Amnestic Syndromes

Amnestic syndromes with gradual complete or incomplete recovery
  Clinical: sudden or subacute onset
  Pathology: injury to the diencephalon and temporal lobes
  Causes and prognosis
    Occlusion of both posterior cerebral arteries (incomplete recovery)
    Occlusion of the posterior cerebral artery supplying the dominant hemisphere (recovery)
    Severe cerebral trauma (incomplete recovery)
    Anoxia-ischemia due to cardiac arrest, profound hypotension, or carbon monoxide poisoning (prognosis varies)
    Inflammatory disease (herpetic or other temporal lobe encephalitis) (incomplete recovery)
    Wernicke-Korsakoff syndrome (usually incomplete recovery)
    Metabolic encephalopathy (meningitis, uremia) (prognosis varies)
    Electroconvulsive therapy (recovery)
    Surgical trauma (incomplete recovery)
Amnestic syndromes of transient duration and complete recovery
  Clinical: sudden onset
  Pathology: unknown or nonspecific
  Causes
    Transient global amnesia
    Temporal lobe seizures
    Postconcussive states
    Hypoglycemia
    Drug-induced (scopolamine poisoning)
Slowly progressive amnesias without recovery
  Clinical: amnesia as part of global dementia
  Pathology: destruction or degeneration of the diencephalon
  Causes
    Alzheimer's disease and other degenerative disorders
    Infiltrating tumors and those involving the floor and walls of the third ventricle.

been learned before the onset of the illness (retrograde amnesia). Other cognitive functions that do not depend on memory may also be impaired, but to a relatively minor degree.

The amnestic patient, as a rule, is apathetic and lacks insight into his disability. Confabulation, the filling-in of memory gaps with fictitious responses, is not present consistently.

Korsakoff's amnestic syndrome is seen most commonly in chronic alcoholism but also occurs in other disorders associated with deficiency of B-complex vitamins. Other causes of the amnestic syndrome are listed (Table 15–10).

Transient global amnesia (TGA) is a disorder of short-term memory. Immediate memory is spared and remote memory is only mildly affected. TGA occurs in middle-aged and elderly adults. The onset is abrupt and the attack lasts several hours. During an attack, the patient acts bewildered and may repetitively ask ''where am I?'' Personal identification is intact, as are consciousness, motor, sensory, and reflex functions. As soon as the attack has ended, no abnormality can be detected, although the patient remains amnestic about the events of the attack. The pathogenesis of TGA is unknown, but possibly it represents a transient ischemic attack or an unusual type of temporal lobe epilepsy.

Differential Diagnosis

The main differential diagnosis in an amnestic patient is between organic and psychogenic amnesia. The distinction usually is not difficult because in hysterical amnesia, remote memory is impaired but immediate and recent memory are spared. In psychogenic amnesia, the memory loss tends to be absolute, and the patient characteristically disclaims all knowledge of self, including name, age, religion, and past history. He often shows remarkable unconcern about memory loss. In some cases, there may be frank malingering to avoid criminal prosecution for past deeds.

Diagnostic Evaluation

The diagnosis of isolated amnesia can be made readily on the basis of the history and the mental status examination. The cause of amnesia usually will be obvious from the history alone. In cases of suspected infarction or tumor, CT scanning can be diagnostic. Examination of the CSF is mandatory in cases of suspected meningitis or encephalitis. An electroencephalogram should be performed to rule out partial complex epilepsy as a cause of amnesia.

APHASIA AND APRAXIA

Definition

Aphasia refers to the loss or impairment of language caused by brain damage. Disturbances in speech and language are usually caused by lesions in the region of the sylvian fissure of the dominant hemisphere. Almost all right-handed people and most left-handed people are left-hemisphere dominant for language.

Pathophysiologic Considerations

In the classic view of aphasia, the front half of the brain is devoted to motor functions and the back half to sensory functions, with the two regions connected by pathways in the white matter. Therefore, lesions of the frontal regions cause motor or expressive aphasia, lesions affecting the posterior regions cause sensory or receptive aphasia, and lesions interrupting the pathways between the motor and sensory regions cause conduction aphasia.

Interruption of the intrahemispheric and transcallosal pathways to the motor and sensory speech areas cause what is called a transcortical aphasia. In transcortical motor aphasia, words can be repeated and copied, but no spontaneous communication by speech or writing occurs. In transcortical sensory aphasia, words are repeated or copied without comprehension.

Other disconnection syndromes have been postulated. Disconnection of pathways bearing visual information causes pure alexia; disconnection of pathways conveying auditory information causes pure word deafness; disconnection of efferent pathways from motor speech areas causes pure word mutism.

Motor Aphasias (nonfluent aphasias). Lesions involving the opercular cortex from the anterior inferior frontal region to the anterior parietal region disrupt speech and cause motor aphasia. Speech may be absent (acute mutism), or, if present, may be uttered slowly, with great effort and poor articulation. Characteristically, the speech of such patients lacks the small grammatical words and endings and so may sound telegraphic.

Lesions of the inferior frontal region (Broca's area) produce a nonfluent aphasia in which comprehension of words heard or read is intact. Patients with Broca's aphasia also have a hemiparesis with weakness of the contralateral face and arm, more than the leg, because of involvement of the adjacent motor cortex.

Sensory Aphasia (fluent aphasias). Large posterior lesions (posterior temporoparietal lobes and lateral occipital lobe) produce fluent aphasia. Patients with fluent aphasia effortlessly produce well-articulated, long phrases or sentences with a normal grammatical skeleton, having normal rhythm and melody. The speech is abnormal, however, since it is remarkably devoid of content. In fluent aphasias, the patient fails to use the correct word, instead substituting circumlocutory phrases, nonspecific words, or incorrect words or paraphrases. In some cases, neologisms are substituted for the correct word. The patient with a fluent aphasia does not suffer from hemiplegia, but may have a hemianopia or hemisensory deficit.

There are several forms of fluent aphasia. In Wernicke's aphasia, the patient fails both to understand words and to repeat them. The patient with conduction aphasia has normal comprehension of spoken language, but repeats words incorrectly. In some cases, a massive lesion destroys both Broca's area and Wernicke's area, so that the patient has global or total aphasia, that is, a nonfluent aphasia combined with a loss of comprehension and repetition. The patient also almost invariably has a severe contralateral hemiplegia, hemianopia, and hemisensory defect.

Alexia. A focal lesion that damages the posterior parietal and lateral occipital regions causes impairment of reading comprehension (alexia) because of disconnection of the visual cortex from the speech areas. If writing to dictation also is impaired, the syndrome is known as alexia with agraphia.

Anomia. Anomia, the term applied to errors in tests of naming, is common in all varieties of aphasia. Anomic aphasia describes a fluent aphasia with essentially normal comprehension and repetition. Such a syndrome occurs in lesions restricted to the angular gyrus of the parietal lobe as well as in cases of Alzheimer's disease and of metabolic encephalopathy.

Thalamic Aphasia. An acute lesion involving the posterior thalamic nuclei that has reciprocal connections with the language zones can cause aphasia. Language behavior fluctuates from normal to abnormal, and the syndrome of thalamic aphasia may be mistaken for delirium. Complete recovery is the rule in thalamic aphasia caused by a hematoma.

Diagnostic Evaluation

Evaluation of aphasia begins with the monitoring of spontaneous speech by the patient. Aphasic output is nonfluent or fluent.

Nonfluent aphasia is characterized by decreased output, usually fewer than 50 words/minute and sometimes fewer than 10/minute. A second feature is effortful articulation. In addition, pronunciation is dysarthric. Phrase length is decreased, producing so-called telegraphic speech. The combination of all of the above features produces an unmelodic, nonrhythmic output that is termed dysprosody. In nonfluent aphasia, the words produced are usually nouns, action verbs, or adjectives. Absence of syntactic filler words produces a nongrammatical sentence structure (agrammatism).

Fluent aphasia is characterized by low-normal to super-normal levels of speech. Speech production is effortless and articulation is normal. Phrases are of normal length and are melodic. Specific, meaningful words often are absent, however, and descriptive phrases or circumlocution are substituted. Fluent aphasic patients therefore may produce long sentences with few substantive words, so that their output can be called empty speech, devoid of information. Paraphasias, that is, substitutions of a syllable (literal paraphasia), a word (verbal paraphasia), or a nonsense word (neologism), are present in fluent aphasia. The ability to repeat words presented by the examiner exactly is a simple clinical test that aids in the classifi-

Table 15–11. Aphasia with Impaired Repetition

Type	Speech	Comprehension Spoken/Written	Writing	Naming	Lesion	Mechanism	Associated Deficits
Broca's	Nonfluent	+/+, −	−	+	Inferior frontal region	Embolus to branch of superior division left MCA, tumor, carotid stenosis	Right hemiparesis, facial and left upper extremity ideomotor dyspraxia, literal alexia
Wernicke's	Fluent	−/−	−	−	Inferior parietal, superior temporal region	Embolus to inferior division left MCA, tumor, putamenal hemorrhage	Right hemisensory, right homonymous hemianopia
Total	Nonfluent	−/−	−	−	Frontal and parietal perisylvian territory	Embolus to trifurcation of the left MCA, tumor, carotid stenosis, putamenal hemorrhage	Right hemiparesis, hemisensory, facial paresis, ideomotor dyspraxia left upper extremity
Conduction	Fluent	+/+	+, −	+	Inferior parietal region	Embolus to branch of inferior division left MCA	Right hemisensory, ideomotor dyspraxia left upper extremity

Table 15–12. Aphasia with Intact Repetition

Type	Speech	Comprehension Spoken/Written	Writing	Naming	Lesion	Mechanism	Associated Deficits
Anomic	Normal	+/+	+,–	–	Temporal region	Tumor, trauma, otitic abscess, encephalitis, Alzheimer's disease	Right homonymous hemianopia
Alexia without agraphia	Normal	+/–	+	+	Left occipital cortex, splenium of corpus callosum	Embolus to left PCA, tumor	Right homonymous hemianopia
Alexia with agraphia	Normal	+/–	–	–	Left angular gyrus	Embolus to inferior division left MCA	Right hemisensory

cation of the aphasic patient (Tables 15–11, 15–12). Additional tests of aphasia include the comprehension of spoken language, word finding or naming, reading, and writing.

The neurologic examination is of considerable value in localizing the lesion causing aphasia (Tables 15–11, 15–12). CT scanning provides the most accurate anatomic localization of aphasia-causing lesions. Cerebral angiography frequently demonstrates the site of major vessel or branch vessel occlusion responsible for an aphasic-producing infarct.

WEAKNESS

Weakness can result from a lesion at any one of the following anatomic sites: the motor cortex and corticospinal tracts, the motor nuclei of the brain stem and spinal cord, the cranial and spinal nerves, the neuromuscular junction, and skeletal muscle.

UPPER MOTOR NEURON WEAKNESS

Weakness caused by involvement of the motor cortex or the corticospinal tracts is called upper motor neuron weakness. The characteristic features are weakness without atrophy of the affected muscles, unless there has been prolonged paralysis and disuse; spasticity and hyper-reflexia, except in the acute stages; and Babinski's sign if the leg is involved.

Monoplegia, hemiplegia, paraplegia, and quadraplegia refer to paralysis of one limb, one side of the body, both lower limbs, and all four limbs, respectively. The term paresis rather than plegia is used if there is weakness rather than total paralysis.

In upper motor neuron weakness, the level of the lesion is indicated by the pattern of weakness and by neighborhood or collateral signs, such as associated cranial nerve palsy or sensory disturbance. For example, in a spastic hemiplegia involving the face, arm, and leg, the associated lesion must be in or above the upper brain stem. If a right hemiplegia of the face, arm, and leg has an associated language disturbance (aphasia), the lesion must involve the cerebral hemisphere.

In the brain stem, a unilateral lesion may cause an alternate or crossed hemiplegia; that is, motor cranial nerve nuclei or their intramedullary fibers are involved, as are the still uncrossed corticospinal fibers. The result is an ipsilateral motor cranial nerve palsy (for example, extraocular, facial, or hypoglossal) and a contralateral upper motor neuron-type weakness of the limbs.

Paraplegia may be of upper or lower motor neuron type. In cases of spinal paraplegia, such as occurs in compression of the spinal cord by tumors of the vertebral bodies or in transverse myelitis, the level of the lesion is determined by the dermatomal level of sensory loss. A band of hyperesthesia may indicate the upper level of the lesion.

Lower Motor Neuron Weakness

Weakness caused by lesions of the motor nuclei of nerves is called lower motor neuron weakness. The characteristic features are flaccidity and atrophy of the affected muscles; possible fasciculations in muscles innervated by damaged neurons; and impairment or loss of deep reflexes mediated by the involved segment.

Lesions of the motor nuclei result in weakness and atrophy of the muscles they innervate. Involvement of the motor nuclei of the cranial nerves produces discrete clinical syndromes. At the spinal level, because the motor neurons do not form discrete nuclei, loss of function isolated to a single segment is unusual. In addition, because the limb muscles are innervated by several segments, discrete weakness caused by a single segmental lesion is unusual. Injury to the spinal motor neurons by trauma, tumor, or vascular disease can be localized by neighborhood signs of sensory loss caused by injury to adjacent tracts in the spinal cord. Diseases affecting the motor nuclei selectively, such as amyotrophic lateral sclerosis (ALS) and poliomyelitis, cause widespread deficits not restricted to a single segment.

ALS is a progressive degenerative disease of adults that occurs in sporadic and familial forms. Clinically, the disease is confined to the motor system, with sparing of the extraocular muscles. Involvement of cortical and cranial motor neurons, as well as of spinal motor neurons, results in both upper motor neuron and lower motor neuron weakness in limb and bulbar muscles. The usual course of ALS is relentlessly progressive, with death by 3 years after diagnosis in 50% of patients.

LESIONS OF PERIPHERAL NERVES

Peripheral nerve involvement, or neuropathy, may be generalized (polyneuropathy) or restricted to a single nerve (mononeuropathy). The most common cause of mononeuropathy is trauma, including pressure. Pressure-caused neuropathies involve the ulnar nerve at the elbow, the median nerve at the wrist, and the peroneal nerve below the knee. Distal symmetrical polyneuropathies have a metabolic or toxic cause, as in diabetes, uremia, malnutrition, and vitamin deficiency states.

Since peripheral nerves contain both sensory and motor fibers, the symptoms of neuropathy usually are both sensory and motor. In some polyneuropathies, such as the Guillain-Barré syndrome, motor symptoms predominate.

Motor findings in neuropathies are characterized by flaccid weakness and atrophy of the distal muscles and by subsequent involvement of more proximal muscles.

Sensory symptoms of polyneuropathy include pains, paresthesias, and sensory loss.

WEAKNESS CAUSED BY DISORDERS OF THE NEUROMUSCULAR JUNCTION

Neuromuscular junction disorders usually are generalized, purely motor, and have no associated sensory abnormality.

Myasthenia gravis is characterized by weakness and fatigability that is usually most severe in the extraocular, buccofacial, and pharyngeal muscles. In this condition, postsynaptic sensitivity to the transmitter acetylcholine is decreased because of an autoimmune reaction directed against the postsynaptic acetylcholine receptors. The weakness associated with myasthenia gravis fluctuates during the day and is associated with preserved deep tendon reflexes despite profound weakness. Improvement of muscle strength following the administration of edrophonium or other acetylcholinesterase inhibitors is diagnostic.

The myasthenic syndrome, or Eaton-Lambert syndrome, is characterized by weakness predominantly in the proximal limb muscles. Less common symptoms are impotence in males and paresthesias. There is usually little involvement of extraocular or bulbar muscles, and the tendon reflexes are reduced or absent. The diagnosis of the myasthenic syndrome is made by EMG testing.

Botulism results from intoxication by botulin. The toxin is produced anaerobically by the bacterium Clostridium botulinum and occurs most commonly in incompletely sterilized preserved food. When ingested, the toxin produces generalized paralysis caused by blockage of acetylcholine release from synaptic endings.

Diagnosis is based on the history and the laboratory demonstration of the toxin in the food consumed or in the patient's serum.

Tick paralysis is caused by the bite of a wood tick that remains embedded in the skin of the victim. The neurotoxin released causes rapidly progressive generalized paralysis. Diagnosis is made by discovery of the tick.

WEAKNESS CAUSED BY DISEASE OF SKELETAL MUSCLE

Diseases of the skeletal muscles are called myopathies and are of two general types, genetic and acquired. The genetic muscle diseases are rare and are identified by generalized weakness and hypotonia at birth or soon afterwards. They are nonprogressive or slowly progressive and are diagnosed on the basis of muscle pathology. Muscular dystrophies are present in childhood or adolescence and progress slowly. The diagnosis is based on clinical findings.

Acquired muscle diseases, by contrast, have a relatively rapid progression and present as weakness of the proximal limbs. They may be of unknown origin, as in polymyositis, have an endocrine cause such as hyper- or hypothyroidism, or be related to collagen vascular disease or cancer. Laboratory tests (serum enzymes, EMG, muscle biopsy) reflect destruction of muscle.

INVOLUNTARY MOVEMENTS

Movements that cannot be controlled voluntarily are classified according to their clinical characteristics. These include the portion of the body involved, the frequency and rhythm of the movements, and the effects of sleep on the movement. Evaluation to determine the cause differs among the diagnostic categories. Often, no laboratory tests are needed because the diagnosis is made by history and observation of the movements.

TREMORS

A tremor is a rhythmic oscillation caused by alternate contraction and relaxation of opposing groups of muscles. Tremors are graded as fine or coarse, as slow or fast, and as occurring at rest, during maintenance of a posture, or on movement of the affected part.

Physiologic Tremor. Physiologic tremor is a postural or action tremor occurring at a rate of approximately 10/second. Such tremors occur in febrile states and states of nervousness and excitement, as well as in hyperthyroidism. The consumption of coffee, alcohol, sympathomimetic drugs, tricyclic antidepressants, and lithium can cause similar tremors.

The mechanism of physiologic tremor is unknown, but the most likely cause is central synchronization of motor neuron activity at about 10 impulses each second, whether motor neurons are activated by descending motor pathways or by segmental reflexes. The similarity in frequencies between physiologic tremor and the alpha rhythm of the EEG is striking, but no link between cortical and tremor rhythms has been proven.

The diagnosis of physiologic tremor is established from the history and collateral findings. For example, tremor caused by hyperthyroidism may be accompanied by tachycardia, exophthalmos, and abnormal thyroid function tests.

Essential Tremor. Essential tremor, also called familial or senile tremor, is a postural or action tremor with a frequency of eight to ten per second. The hands are usually involved, and there also may be a nodding ("yes") or a rotary ("no") shaking of the head. The jaw may be involved and the voice quavering. The tremor usually constitutes the sole neurologic disturbance and tends to increase with age. Sometimes a family history of tremor is obtained; families harboring the trait seem to have unusual longevity. There is no

known pathology, and the pathophysiology is not fully understood.

The patient typically seeks medical help because of embarrassment over spilling liquids when attempting to hold a glass or cup. Patients often report that the tremor is more severe when they get up in the morning. Many patients note that the tremor is temporarily suppressed by drinking alcoholic beverages.

A similar postural tremor of the hands often is present in patients with spasmodic torticollis; it is also seen in association with torsion dystonia.

Essential tremor frequently is misdiagnosed as parkinsonism. Differentiation can be made by the absence of bradykinesia, muscle rigidity, and the postural features of parkinsonism. The patient with essential tremor has a large, irregular handwriting, in contrast to the micrographia of the parkinsonian patient. Severe tremor of the hands, head, and diaphragm and the positive family history occasionally may suggest Huntington's disease. Differentiation can be made by the absence of chorea and dementia of Huntington's disease.

Tremor of Parkinsonism. The tremor of parkinsonism begins in the fingers and hands but may spread proximally to involve the rest of the upper limb, jaw, tongue, trunk, and lower limbs. It typically occurs at rest as a 3/second to 6/second pill-rolling tremor and is suppressed by action of the involved limb or by conscious attention to the tremor. The tremor disappears during sleep and increases when the patient is tense.

The loss of pigmented neurons, particularly in the substantia nigra, locus ceruleus, and brain stem nuclei, is a pathologic feature of parkinsonism. The exact mechanism by which this selective damage occurs is unknown.

Parkinsonism may be defined biochemically as a dopamine-deficient state resulting from disease, injury, or dysfunction of the dopaminergic neuronal system.

Parkinson's disease usually begins between the ages of 50 and 65, although there is a rare juvenile form. There is no evidence to indicate a hereditary factor. The classic triad of symptoms is tremor, rigidity, and akinesia. In addition, symptoms caused by dysfunction of the autonomic nervous system are encountered. There is a tendency toward hypotension, with a poor baroreceptor mechanism that sometimes causes orthostatic syncope. Dementia, frequently a feature of parkinsonism, increases in severity as the disease progresses.

Parkinsonism is a progressive disorder leading over a period of years to considerable motor disability. Although no current therapy alters the underlying progressive pathologic process, therapy with levodopa and other agents prolongs survival time and improves functional capacity.

The diagnosis of parkinsonism can be made when other features such as cog-wheel rigidity and mask-like facies are present. The differential diagnosis includes drug-induced parkinsonism following therapy with dopamine antagonists and the tremor of Wilson's disease (hepatolenticular degeneration). In Wilson's disease and in other hepatic encephalopathies there may be asterixis (liver flap), which is best demonstrated by having the patient extend the arms with the wrists dorsiflexed and the fingers spread. The flapping tremor may be limited to the fingers or wrists or may involve the whole arm. Asterixis may be present in other metabolic encephalopathies such as uremia and anoxia.

Intention Tremor. Intention tremor, a coarse oscillation of the limbs, is seen in the performance of delicate precise movements. It is best elicited in the finger-to-nose test, increasing as the movement nears completion. In severe cases, the tremor interferes with writing, eating, and drinking.

Intention tremor occurs in diseases of the cerebellum or its connections. The tremor is indicative of the site rather than the nature of the cerebellar lesion.

Diagnosis involves the radiographic demonstration of the causative lesion. The differential diagnosis includes cerebellar disease caused by stroke, tumor, intoxication, and multiple sclerosis. Iatrogenic causes include phenytoin, lithium, and cancer chemotherapeutic agents.

CHOREA AND BALLISMUS

Choreiform movements are brief, irregular, non-rhythmic, and unpredictable contractions of muscles. The jerks affect individual muscles at random. Ballismus is a form of chorea in which the choreic jerks are of large amplitude and produce a flinging movement of the affected limb.

Chorea is related to disorders of the caudate nucleus but also must involve other structures. Sydenham's chorea, also called acute or rheumatic chorea, is an infectious disease of spring and fall, affecting children between the ages of 5 and 15. There is frequently history or signs of rheumatic disease such as nodules or acute endocarditis. Huntington's disease is a slowly progressive chorea of dominant inheritance that usually appears after age 40. Mental deterioration may precede, accompany, or follow the onset of chorea. Ballismus is related to lesions of the subthalamic nucleus of Luys or its connections. Ballismus is com-

monly one-sided (hemiballismus), but it may be confined to one arm or, rarely, a leg.

The differential diagnosis of acute chorea in children includes restlessness or fidgeting, and psychiatric disorders. The differential diagnosis of late-onset chorea includes senile chorea (chorea unassociated with dementia), Wilson's disease, intoxication with anticonvulsant or antipsychotic drugs, chorea gravidarum, and conditions causing presenile dementia such as Alzheimer's and Pick's diseases.

ATHETOSIS

Athetosis is a continuous slow, writhing movement of the limbs, trunk, head, face, and tongue. The movements are slower than those of chorea, but they may be brief and similar to choreiform jerks (choreoathetosis).

Athetosis indicates disordered basal ganglia function and accompanies various disorders, including kernicterus, tuberous sclerosis, and Wilson's disease, as well as vascular and neoplastic lesions.

The diagnosis of the cause of athetosis is made on the basis of the history, aided by a CT scan of the brain in cases of gross structural damage to the basal ganglia.

DYSTONIA

The term dystonia is applied to a number of slow involuntary movement disorders, including torsion spasm or movements of a continual twisting nature; sustained contractions of both agonist and antagonist muscles; overflow involuntary contractions on attempted voluntary movement; action dystonia, or inappropriate and opposing contractions during specific voluntary actions; and dystonic tremor or rhythmic interruptions of involuntary, sustained contractions when the patient attempts to oppose them.

Torsion dystonia (dystonia musculorum deformans) is a rare disease of childhood that sometimes has a hereditary factor. Dystonia is also seen in postencephalitic parkinsonism and Wilson's disease and as a complication of neoplastic and vascular disease of the striatum and globus pallidus. Dystonia is diagnosed on the basis of history aided by CT scanning of the brain. In the differential diagnosis, acute dystonic movements of the face, limbs, and trunk may follow treatment with neuroleptic drugs, prochlorperazine, and levadopa.

TICS

Tics are patterned sequences of coordinated movements that appear suddenly and intermittently. The movements may be simple, like a myoclonic jerk, or complex, such as eye blinking, facial distortions, jumping movements, or arm waving. In addition to motor tics, vocalizations ranging from sounds such as barking or throat-clearing to the utterance of obscenities (coprolalia) can occur.

Tics may occur in encephalopathies, as mannerisms in the mentally retarded, and in otherwise normal individuals. The distinction between mannerisms, habit spasms, and pathologic tics often is not clearly made. The trend now is to consider tics a neurologic disorder.

Motor and vocal tics are essential features of Gilles de la Tourette's syndrome. In other cases of pathologic tics, the patient history may reveal a remote history of encephalitis, head trauma, antipsychotic and street drug use, or a family history of tic. A search for collateral signs on neurologic examination may reveal evidence of CNS dysfunction. The CT scan usually is normal in patients with tics.

GENERAL REFERENCES

HEADACHE

Dalessio, D.: Wolff's Headache and Other Head Pain. 4th Ed. New York, Oxford University Press, 1980.
Lance, J.W.: Mechanism and Management of Headache. 4th Ed. London. Butterworths, 1982.
Moskowitz, M.: The neurobiology of vascular head pain. Ann Neurol 16:157–168, 1984.
Olesen, J., Larsen, B., and Lauritzen, M.: Focal hyperemia followed by spreading oligemia and impaired activation of CBF in classic migraine. Ann Neurol 9:344–352, 1981.

SYNDROMES OF PAIN AND SENSORY DISTURBANCES

Dyck, P.J., Thomas, P.K., and Lambert, E.H. (eds.): Peripheral Neuropathy. Philadelphia, W.B. Saunders, 1975.
Hoppenfeld, S.: Physical Examination of the Spine and Extremities. Norwalk, Appleton-Century Crofts, 1976.
Martin, J.J.: Thalamic syndromes. In Handbook of Clinical Neurology. Edited by P.J. Vinken and G.W. Bruyn. Vol 2. Amsterdam, North-Holland, 1969, pp. 469–496.
Plum, F., and Posner, J.B.: Neurology. In Pathophysiology—The Biological Principles of Disease. Edited by L.H. Smith and S.O. Thiers. Philadelphia, W.B. Saunders, 1985.
Swanson, P.D. (ed.): Signs and Symptoms in Neurology. Philadelphia, J.B. Lippincott, 1984.

DIZZINESS

Baloh, R.W., and Honrubia, V.: Clinical Neurophysiology of the Vestibular System. Philadelphia, F.A. Davis, 1979.

Brandt, T., and Daroff, R.B.: The multisensory physiological and pathological vertigo syndromes. Ann Neurol 7:195–203, 1980.
Drachman, D.A., and Hart, C.W.: An approach to the dizzy patient. Neurology 22:323–334, 1972.
Leigh, R.J., and Zee, D.S.: The Neurology of Eye Movements. Philadelphia, F.A. Davis, 1983.

CONFUSION, DELIRIUM, AND COMA

Bates, D., et al.: A prospective study of nontraumatic coma: methods and results in 310 patients. Ann Neurol 2:211–220, 1977.
Caronna, J.J.: Diagnosis, prognosis and treatment of hypoxic coma. In Advances in Neurology. Edited by S. Fahn, J.N. Davis, and L.P. Rowland. Vol 26. New York, Raven Press, 1979, pp 1–15.
Caronna, J.J., and Simon, R.P.: The comatose patient: a diagnostic approach and treatment. Int Anesthesiol Clin 17:3–18, 1979.
Levy, D.E., et al.: Prognosis in nontraumatic coma. Ann Intern Med 94:293–301, 1981.
Plum, F., and Posner, J.B.: The Diagnosis of the Stupor and Coma. 3rd Ed. Philadelphia, F.A. Davis, 1980.

DISTURBANCES OF GAIT

Gilman, S., Bloedel, J., and Lechtenberg, R.: Disorders of the Cerebellum. Philadelphia, F.A. Davis, 1981.
Herman, R.M., et al. (eds.): Neural Control of Locomotion. New York, Plenum Press, 1976.
Smith, B.H.: Differential Diagnosis: Neurology. New York, Arco, 1979.
Stein, R.B., et al. (eds): Control of Posture and Locomotion. New York, Plenum Press, 1973.

DISEASE OF THE CRANIAL NERVES

Cogan, D.G.: Neurology of the Ocular Muscles. Springfield, Ill, C C Thomas, Co., 1956.
Cogan, D.G.: Neurology of the Visual System. Springfield, Ill, C C Thomas Co., 1966.
Glaser, J.S.: Neuro-ophthalmology. New York, Harper & Row, 1978.
Graham, M.D., and House, W.F. (eds.): Disorders of the Facial Nerve: Anatomy Diagnosis and Management. New York, Raven Press, 1982.
Rowland, L.P. (ed.): Merritt's Textbook of Neurology. 7th Ed. Philadelphia, Lea & Febiger, 1984.
Rush, J.A., and Younge, B.R.: Paralysis of cranial nerves III, IV and VI: cause and prognosis in 1000 cases. Arch Ophthalmol 99:76–79, 1981.
Swanson, P.D. (ed.): Signs and Symptoms in Neurology. Philadelphia, J.B. Lippincott, 1984.

TRANSIENT ALTERATIONS OF CONSCIOUSNESS

Day, S.C., et al.: Evaluation and outcome of emergency room patients with transient loss of consciousness. Am J Med 73:15–23, 1982.
Kapoor, W.N., et al.: A prospective evaluation and follow-up of patients with syncope. N Engl J Med 309:197–204, 1983.
Silverstein, M.D., et al.: Patients with syncope admitted to medical intensive care units. JAMA 248:1185–1189, 1982.
Simon, R.P.: Syncope and transient loss of consciousness: differential diagnosis and treatment. West J Med 123:164–170, 1975.

SEIZURES

Delgado-Escueta, A.V., Ferrendelli, J.A., and Prince, D.A.: Basic mechanisms of the epilepsies. Ann Neurol 16:51–158, 1984.

Lesser, R.P. (ed.): Diagnosis and treatment of epilepsy. Cleve Clin Q *51*:193–332, 1984.
Solomon, G.E., Kutt, H., and Plum, F.: Clinical Management of Seizures: A Guide for the Physician. 2nd Ed. Philadelphia. W.B. Saunders, 1983.
Tharp, B.R.: Recent progress in epilepsy: diagnostic procedures and treatment. Calif Med *119*:19–48, 1973.

TRANSIENT ISCHEMIC ATTACKS

Dyken, M.L., et al.: Cooperative study of hospital frequency and character of transient ischemic attacks: I. Background, organization, and clinical survey. JAMA *237*:882–886, 1977.
McDowell, F.H., Sonnenblich, E.H., and Lesch, M. (eds.): Current Concepts in Cerebrovascular Disease. New York, Grune and Stratton, 1980.
Price, T.R., et al.: Cooperative study of hospital frequency and character of transient ischemic attacks: VI. Patients examined during an attack. JAMA *238*:2512–2515, 1977.
Ross Russel, R.W. (ed.): Vascular Disease of the Central Nervous System. 2nd Ed. Edinburgh, Churchill Livingstone, 1983.
Warlow, C., and Morris, P.J. (eds.): Transient Ischemic Attacks. New York, Marcel Dekker, 1982.

DISORDERS OF COGNITIVE FUNCTION

Benson, D.F.: Aphasia, Alexia, and Agraphia. New York, Churchill Livingstone, 1979.

Folstein, M., Folstein, S., and McHugh, P.: The mini-mental state examination. J Psychiatr Res *12*:189–198, 1975.
Geschwind, N.: Disconnection syndromes in animals and man. Brain *88*:237–252; 585–602, 1965.
Geschwind, N.: Language and the brain. Sci Am *226*:76–83, 1972.
Victor, M.: The amnestic syndrome and its anatomical basis. Can Med Assoc J *100*:1115–1125, 1969.
Victor, M., Adams, R.D., and Collins, G.H.: The Wernicke-Korsakoff Syndrome. Philadelphia, F.A. Davis, 1971.
Wells, C.E.: Dementia. 2nd Ed. Philadelphia, F.A. Davis, 1977.

WEAKNESS

Brooke, M.H.: A Clinician's View of Neuromuscular Diseases. Baltimore, The Williams & Wilkins Co., 1977.
Rowland, L.P. (ed.): Merritt's Textbook of Neurology. 7th Ed. Philadelphia, Lea & Febiger, 1984.
Swanson, P.D. (ed.): Signs and Symptoms in Neurology. Philadelphia, J.B. Lippincott, 1984.
Walton, J. (ed.): Disorders of Voluntary Muscle. 4th Ed. Edinburgh, Churchill Livingstone, 1981.

INVOLUNTARY MOVEMENTS

Denny-Brown, D.: The Basal Ganglia and Their Relations to Disorders of Movement. London, Oxford University Press, 1962.
Lance, J.W., and McLeod, J.G.: A Physiological Approach to Clinical Neurology. 3rd Ed. London, Butterworths, 1981.
Marsden, C.D., and Fahn, S. (eds.): Movement Disorders. London, Butterworths, 1982.

CHAPTER 16

PSYCHIATRIC AND BEHAVIORAL PROBLEMS

Charles A. Shamoian, M.D., Ph.D.

INTRODUCTION

Symptoms thought to be psychiatric in origin are ubiquitous in our present high pressure society. Many of these symptoms inappropriately labeled psychiatric are actually normal experiences of daily living, such as sadness, blueness, irritability, and anger. These and other symptoms may, however, be manifestations of bona fide medical syndromes or illnesses. For example, anxiety, depression, or difficulties with recent memory may be secondary to prescribed medications, drug toxicity, metabolic disorders, or endocrinopathies[1]; the very same symptoms may be the cardinal presentation of major syndromes such as anxiety states, a major depressive episode, Alzheimer's disease, or schizophrenia. Not infrequently, and especially in the geriatric patient, these syndromes are accompanied by a major medical problem and the patient's personal emotional reaction to the illness or the psychiatric syndrome. A typical clinical situation is the patient with rheumatoid arthritis, hypertension, diabetes, and depressive symptoms. The physician is confronted with the diagnostic dilemma of whether this is a major depressive episode requiring intensive somatic intervention; whether it is secondary to the prescribed medications; whether it is secondary to the medical illness(es); or whether it is the patient's reaction (i.e., a coping mechanism) to the overwhelming medical illnesses.

Probably the most common psychiatric disorders seen by physicians are those related to the affective, perceptual, and cognitive spheres. These disorders are, respectively, major depressive episode, schizophrenia and anxiety disorders, and the reversible and irreversible dementias. Anxiety may be a prodromal symptom or may be the predominant presentation of depression, schizophrenia, dementia, or anxiety states.[2] The effective treatment of each disorder is quite different, and a working knowledge of the various syndromes is required for an accurate diagnosis. In psychiatry as in medicine, an accurate diagnosis depends on a comprehensive history including the psychiatric examination. The latter includes not only a history of the current illness but also a personal and family history and a mental status exam. The focus of the examination is on affect, thought content and form, motor activity, and memory-intellectual processes.[2] The mental status exam in psychiatry is the equivalent of the baseline laboratory studies of medicine. The findings of the comprehensive medical and psychiatric evaluations will determine the laboratory studies to be conducted.

Motor disorders, probably more common than is suspected in patients treated with antipsychotic drugs, include extrapyramidal syndrome, tardive dyskinesia, and the life threatening neuroleptic malignant syndrome.[1] Not uncommonly, however, schizophrenics during the psychotic phase may manifest stereotypic movements that are not secondary to the prescribed antipsychotic but rather an integral component of the functional disorder. The distinction is usually made by the history and the association or lack of association with the use of tranquilizers. In elderly patients a more common differential diagnostic problem is that of Parkinson's disease and pseudo-Parkinson's disease (i.e., Parkinson's disease secondary to the antipsychotic).

For many years the symptoms of anorexia and bulimia were not considered as major syndromes, but rather as symptoms of medical or psychiatric illnesses, which in fact they may be; not uncommonly, anorexia or bulimia are symptoms of syndromes such as depression, anxiety states, schizophrenia, or medical illnesses such as a malignancy or endocrinopathies.[2,3] However, anorexia and bulimia may be the predominant manifestations of major syndromes that can be clearly elucidated by history. A comprehensive medical evaluation may be needed to rule out the possibility of undiagnosed underlying medical causes or secondary consequences.

Sexual dysfunctions are usually not openly discussed by either the patient or the physician. Many patients with sexual dysfunctions will seek a medical evaluation on some other pretense. Only by direct, open questioning will sexual difficulties be made clear. Sexual dysfunctions may be psychiatric or medical in origin. Cardiovascular problems such as a recent myocardial infarction, cerebrovascular accident, or angina can induce a fear of sexual activity. Many prescribed medications may cause impotence or retrograde ejaculation, and the use or abuse of alcohol or illicit drugs may induce sexual dysfunctions. Psychiatric syndromes such as depression, schizophrenia, or anxiety may contribute to or be the sole cause of the presenting sexual dysfunction. Prescribed medications for such syndromes may initiate or exacerbate sexual difficulties. A comprehensive psychiatric exam including a sexual and drug history will assist in determining the cause of the dysfunction.[2,4]

Alcohol and drug abuse are common phenomena in our society. While the 1960s saw the peak of the hallucinogen culture, use and abuse of alcohol, cocaine, and heroin and addiction to prescribed medications (meperidine, benzodiazepines, etc.) continue. These drugs are used frequently by individuals with underlying psychiatric illnesses such as depression, mania, schizophrenia and anxiety. Patients with personality disorders (i.e., borderline personality, antisocial personality) frequently abuse drugs, prescribed or nonprescribed. Unfortunately, drug abusers have multiple medical complications that require treatment; moreover, many of these patients need inpatient treatment to monitor and treat withdrawal. Treatment does not end with the withdrawal phase. Rehabilitation programs are critical for successful abstinence. Not infrequently, a history of drug abuse will be obtained during an acute psychotic episode. The patient may require detoxification prior to institution of psychopharmacotherapy. Upon complete withdrawal from the toxic agent a comprehensive psychiatric evaluation is critical.[2,4]

A number of studies have demonstrated that "emotionally loaded" life events often precede the onset of medical illness.[5] Also, the mental state of the patient may influence the course and prognosis of the medical disorder. The corollary, that the presence of medical illnesses can affect the psychologic state of the patient, has been documented in a variety of pathologic states, including cardiovascular disease.[3]

The clinician often approaches patients presenting with psychiatric symptoms with the notion that they have a functional, i.e., psychiatric, disorder. Studies have demonstrated that patients with bona fide psychiatric illnesses also have concomitant undiagnosed medical illnesses that often contribute to the psychiatric clinical presentation. The true incidence of medical problems in patients with psychiatric symptoms is equivocal, with figures ranging from 5% to 40%. In one study, approximately 10% of patients had medical disorders thought to be the primary cause of psychiatric symptoms.[3] Cardiovascular and endocrine disorders were the most frequent etiologic factors, followed by infections, pulmonary disease, gastrointestinal and hematological disorders, central nervous system diseases, and malignancies.[3]

A variety of physical illnesses such as cardiac arrhythmias, respiratory insufficiency, head injury, subarachnoid hemorrhage, and cirrhosis are associated with or can present with psychiatric symptoms.[3,4] To illustrate the point, anxiety often heralds the beginning of a medical or psychiatric illness; the medical causes of anxiety are numerous and must be ruled out prior to labeling the symptom a manifestation of a psychiatric disorder.[4]

The evaluation of any psychiatric symptom or syndrome proceeds as with any typical medical problem. A comprehensive history, both past and present, and psychiatric assessment will assist in determining the possibilities of a psychiatric illness.[3] A thorough physical examination will assist in delineating the diagnosis, as will appropriate laboratory testing. The latter should be pursued thoughtfully rather than in a haphazard manner. At this point most diagnostic problems will be resolved. However, in certain conditions, such as suspected Alzheimer's disease, a CT scan is appropriate. The routine use of CT scans, magnetic resonance imaging, and the dexamethasone suppression test is not justified. For example, while the latter may assist in confirming the presence of a depression, it will not make the diagnosis any more than the presence of abnormal thyroid functions. Unfortunately, many patients with psychiatric disorders are unnecessarily exposed to a variety of procedures, many of which are not without morbidity or mortality risks. The absence of a medical illness does not necessarily substantiate the presence of psychopathology, however.

DISORDERS OF PERCEPTION

INTRODUCTION

Disturbances in perception are pathologic experiences of reality. Abnormalities range from the purely perceptual disorders, such as experiences of depersonalization, derealization, and illusion, to those that include a pathologic cognition or knowledge of reality, such as hallucinations and delusions. The disorders range from the distortion of an actual sensation (illusion) to the production of a frankly false percept (hallucination). Although no type of disorder has diagnostic specificity, the type and content of the disturbance along with the associated clinical findings can help the physician arrive at an accurate and precise diagnosis. Types of perceptual disorders and their respective causes will be considered separately, but all of these disturbances can be considered as arising from conditions on a spectrum between the functional and the organic (Table 16–1).

DEPERSONALIZATION AND DEREALIZATION

Definition

These states represent disturbances in the relationship to and perception of reality without disturbances in the patient's ability to assess the validity of these distortions.[6,7] The patient recognizes the altered perception as abnormal.

Table 16–1. Classification of Conditions Causing Disordered Perception Along a Functional-Organic Spectrum

Type of Condition	Examples
Primary psychiatric disorder with clear sensorium	Schizophrenia Depersonalization disorder
Organic hallucinosis with clear sensorium	Amphetamine abuse Hallucinogen abuse Focal CNS lesions

Episodic neurologic disorder
    With clouded consciousness
    With clear consciousness
	
	Complex partial seizures
	Migraine

Acute brain syndrome (delirium)	Delirium tremens Atropine psychosis

Depersonalization is marked by a feeling of detachment from the self, the external world, or both. It is frequently associated with the sense of strangeness and unreality present in derealization, in which the predominant sense is that objects in the external world or the world itself are unreal. In depersonalization the focus is on an altered perception of oneself. In both cases, the disturbed sense of reality is usually experienced with profound anxiety.

Pathophysiologic Considerations

Psychoanalytic theory has explained these disturbances in terms of their defensive functions.[8] A patient overwhelmed with forbidden sexual or aggressive impulsiveness experiencing depersonalization is considered as detaching the rational observing self from the body experiencing the impulses. Derealization can represent a more profound distortion in which the patient's emotional investment in the real world is temporarily withdrawn.

Alternative psychologic and neurophysiologic mechanisms hypothesize an excess of internal stimulation relative to external.[9,10] In these models, sensory isolation associated with stress causes a disruptive effect on cortical processing of perceptions similar to that of an acute brain syndrome. This explanation has also been used to explain the pathogenesis of hallucinations.

The finding of depersonalization and derealization in patients with temporal lobe disease suggests that disturbances of the limbic system can play a causative role.[11,12]

Differential Diagnosis

Isolated instances of depersonalization and derealization have been found in over 50% of college students.[13] They can be seen in normal individuals exposed to sensory deprivation and stress.[14,15] Persistent and intense symptoms are pathologic and usually indicative of a psychiatric or neurologic disorder.

Depersonalization disorder is a specific psychiatric entity in which depersonalization dominates the clinical picture.[16] In this disorder, depersonalization recurs with a rapid onset and disappearance. Each episode lasts for minutes to hours and is associated with a feeling of loss of control, usually with profound anxiety. Symptoms of depersonalization can also occur in depression, in schizotypal, hysterical, and schizoid personality disorders and in schizophrenia. Examination for associated phenomenologic and historical features of these disorders assists in accurate diagnosis.

Derealization can occur as an associated feature of depersonalization disorder or can exist independently. Derealization can also occur as a symptom in other psychiatric disorders such as schizotypal personality or schizophrenia. When derealization exists alone or is the dominant symptom, the diagnosis of a more malignant withdrawal from reality and an incipient schizophrenic illness should be considered.[16]

Depersonalization and derealization can be present as features of an acute brain syndrome. Disturbances in memory, cognition, and level of consciousness should lead to an accurate diagnosis of a generalized dysfunction of the CNS.[11,17]

An altered experience of reality can be indicative of a focal CNS disorder, most often involving the temporal lobe.[11,12] Such an experience can represent the aura of a temporal lobe seizure. The occurrence of this phenomenon in the absence of other seizure manifestations is sometimes referred to as a psychic aura.[11] Accurate diagnosis in patients with symptoms of depersonalization and evidence of temporal lobe disease is rendered especially complex by the frequent finding of schizophrenia-like psychoses in patients with lesions in this area.[18,19]

Information regarding age of onset can be useful because depersonalization and derealization are most often seen in both depersonalization disorder and schizophrenia, syndromes that usually begin before age 30.[16]

ILLUSIONS

Definition

The misrepresentation of a real external sensation is an illusion. Such experiences are more likely to occur at times of heightened anxiety and diminished sensory acuity.

Pathophysiologic Considerations

The psychologic explanation for an illusion is the projection of one's internal feelings and concerns onto an ambiguous and therefore easily distorted external object. Such phenomena are common and not inherently pathologic. A child's distortion of an inert night-time shadow on the bedroom wall into a threatening monster represents such a benign illusion. Factors such as a high level of anxiety, diminished cognitive integrity, and impaired sensory acuity contribute to the formation of an illusion.

Distortions of reality such as déjà vu and jamais vu combine elements of derealization with illusion. In the former case, a novel percept is experienced as strangely familiar, whereas in the latter, a familiar percept is experienced as new. The perceptual disturbance is illusionary, while the accompanying sense of strangeness arises from a feeling of unreality.

Differential Diagnosis

Evaluation of the patient's cognitive functioning as well as the sensory and emotional context within which an illusion takes place will clarify the diagnosis. A paranoid schizophrenic patient with intact cognition and excellent vision can distort a passerby's glance into a threatening gaze. A patient with delirium tremens can produce the same misrepresentation, but with clouding of consciousness rather than a functional psychosis as the cause.

Accurate differential diagnosis of an illusion occurring in the absence of sensory deprivation relies on evaluation for an organic confusional syndrome. Periodic experiences of illusions or disturbances of familiarity, such as depersonalization and derealization, can comprise the aura of temporal lobe seizures. The episodic and abrupt nature of such phenomena, the usual presence of features of a complex partial seizure, and a normal level of consciousness associated with the event assist in making the diagnosis.

HALLUCINATIONS

Definition

Hallucinations are false sensory perceptions of the external world in the absence of real external stimuli. The false percepts can be attributed to any sensory modality including auditory, olfactory, tactile, and visual. Unlike illusions, hallucinations do not involve the distortion of genuine sensations; rather, they occur in the context of a sensory vacuum. The hallucinating individual cannot appreciate the unrealistic aspect of the perception or subject its validity to logical analysis. Organic hallucinosis refers to recurrent or persistent hallucinations of an organic cause that occur with intact higher cortical functioning and a normal level of consciousness and without the disturbed thought processes or other features of schizophrenia.[20]

Pathophysiologic Considerations

The causes and mechanisms of hallucination are more varied than those of any other form of perceptual disturbances. Psychiatric diagnosis, organic factors, individual psychology, and cultural background interact in determining the type and content of hallucinatory experiences. Hallucinations that are not influenced by organic factors are thought to be caused by the use of the defense mechanism of projection.[8] Unacceptable internal conflicts are projected and experienced as part of the external world. Most hallucinations cannot be subjected to reality testing and are therefore psychotic. Patients with hallucinations caused by an organic process that has not caused impaired intellectual functioning can often recognize the unreality of their perceptions.

Hallucinations occurring as part of a functional or nonorganic psychosis disappear when that condition responds to treatment or remits spontaneously. Because most antipsychotic drugs block dopamine, and the antipsychotic potency of these agents is proportional to their ability to block this neurotransmitter, the neurophysiologic mechanism is considered to result from excess dopamine activity in specific locations of the CNS.[21] The fact that the visual and auditory hallucinations of many toxic/metabolic states also respond to dopamine blocking medications suggests that excess dopamine activity plays a causative role in these conditions as well.

Differential Diagnosis

Hallucinations vary in their diagnostic specificity. The particular sensory modality and the form and content of the hallucination must be considered. The same hallucination can be associated with very different disorders, and different individuals can suffer different types of hallucinations from the same causative factor.

Hallucinations are not necessarily pathologic. Situations of extended sleep loss and sensory deprivation contribute to normal hallucinatory experiences.[14] Hallucinations occurring after prolonged night-time driving or while falling asleep (hypnagogic) or awakening (hypnopompic) are examples of these phenomena. Reflex and kinesthetic hallucinations are additional types of nonpathologic hallucinations. A toothache stimulating an auditory hallucination can produce a reflex

700 PSYCHIATRIC AND BEHAVIORAL PROBLEMS

Table 16–2. Classification of Hallucinations by Type and Diagnostic Considerations

Sensory Modality	Diagnostic Considerations
Auditory	Least diagnostically specific
	Primary psychiatric disorders (schizophrenia more than affective illness)
	Organic hallucinosis (especially alcoholic hallucinosis)
	Drug withdrawal (delirium tremens)
	Acute brain syndromes
	Focal cerebral lesions (acoustic neuroma, temporal lobe lesions)
	Diffuse cerebral disease (postencephalitis)
Visual	Usually indicative of organic brain disease
	Occurs in primary psychiatric illness
	Organic hallucinosis (especially due to hallucinogens)
	Drug withdrawal (delirium tremens)
	Acute brain syndrome (common, terrifying, worse at night)
	Focal cerebral defects (occipital tumors)
	Sensory deficit
	A symptom of migraine
Gustatory and olfactory	As temporal lobe aura, especially if sensation is unpleasant
	Schizophrenia (associated with personal significance and bizarre delusion)
	Temporal lobe tumors, migraine
Tactile	Occurs in schizophrenia in association with other modalities of hallucinations and as part of a bizarre delusional system
	Drug withdrawal (delirium tremens)
	Drug abuse (formication in cocaine users)
	Temporal lobe tumors, migraine

hallucination; a phantom limb experience is an example of a kinesthetic hallucination. Nonpathologic hallucinations are transient and accessible to reality testing, whereas hallucinations that are sustained, are recurrent, or occur in a fully awake state with normal sensory input are indicative of underlying disorder.

Table 16–2 classifies hallucinations according to sensory type and provides diagnostic considerations. Auditory hallucinations are the most common and least specific form. They are commonly seen in schizophrenia, usually in association with a complementary delusion. Classic features of schizophrenia including onset in young adulthood, poor premorbid history, chronicity, and clinical findings of blunted or inappropriate affect, impaired interpersonal relatedness, and disturbed thought processes assist in the diagnosis. Auditory hallucinations are also frequent in other functional psychotic disorders such as mania and major depression. Affectively ill patients are more likely to hallucinate only when they are alone.[22] Auditory hallucinations also accompany the cognitive dysfunction

of an acute brain syndrome, but they occur only rarely in an uncomplicated dementia.[23]

Visual hallucinations continue to be considered suggestive of organic disease.[11,23–25] Controversy over this question persists based on reports that a high percentage of schizophrenic patients have visual hallucinations.[22,26,27] Because of the extremely high prevalence of visual hallucinations in patients with organic disease and the prominent nature of these hallucinations in delirium, the physician should strongly suspect an organic process when visual hallucinations are part of the clinical picture.[28]

The characteristics of visual hallucinations can be of diagnostic value. Halos are seen around dark objects (white vision) in digitalis toxicity,[29] and objects are typically perceived as having a yellow or green hue. Lilliputian hallucinations of small objects are usually indicative of organic disease and can result from toxicity to drugs such as atropine[30] or in the aura of a temporal lobe seizure.[11] Visual hallucinations caused by withdrawal from drugs such as alcohol and benzodiazepines are usually more intense at night and are especially terrifying. Hypnagogic hallucinations are part of the clinical picture of narcolepsy and also are found in patients suffering from sleep apnea.[26] Hallucinations of flashing lights, lines, or complex geometric patterns are usually indicative of temporal lobe epilepsy or migraines.[31] Similar perceptions can be caused by hallucinogens (organic hallucinosis).[31] Visual hallucinations caused by psychiatric or diffuse cerebral disease occur in the context of intact visual acuity. A change in the clarity of visual perception in association with a visual hallucination suggests a focal CNS cause.[32]

Tactile (haptic) hallucinations, when occurring in schizophrenia, are usually associated with hallucinations in other sensory modalities and form part of a complex and bizarre delusional system.[30] Specific forms of haptic hallucinations are drug related. Formication, the hallucination of tiny bugs creeping under the skin, occurs in cocaine abuse. The withdrawal state of delirium tremens can be associated with the hallucination of small animals crawling on the skin. Unpleasant gustatory and/or olfactory hallucinations (such as the smell of burnt rubber) are highly suggestive of temporal lobe epilepsy (uncinate fits). Such auras are often accompanied by other disorders of perception (e.g., depersonalization or déjà vu) and alteration in state of consciousness (the dreamy state).[11,33]

Organic hallucinosis was initially described as a feature of chronic alcoholism.[34] The use and abuse of new classes of drugs has broadened the classes of agents known to cause this disorder. Psychostimulants (amphetamines, cocaine, methylphenidate) and hallucinogens (LSD, psilocybin, mescaline) can cause hallucinosis without impairment in arousal. Levodopa and bromocriptine can produce the same state, presumably through the excitation of hypersensitive postsynaptic dopamine receptors.[35] The hallucinosis of chronic alcoholism is usually auditory, in contrast to the predominantly visual syndrome caused by hallucinogens.[34] Although auditory hallucinations are usually prominent in the hallucinosis caused by psychostimulants, visual hallucinations are frequently present.[26] Less commonly, diminished perception caused by lesions to sensory organs, and diffuse cerebral disease that disrupts CNS sensory pathways, cause this disorder.[31,33]

DELUSIONS

Definition

Delusions are fixed false beliefs that cannot be validated by the laws of logic and that are not consistent with an individual's cultural background. They are the result of a medical or psychiatric illness. Delusions are by definition pathologic and psychotic. They are not true disorders of perception. Delusions are indicative of a false processing of information about reality and an inability to assess the validity of such knowledge.

Pathophysiologic Considerations

The psychoanalytic explanation for delusions involves withdrawal from external reality to internal mental life with a secondary restitutive false knowledge of reality developed in an attempt to resolve inner mental conflicts.[36] The patient has denied external reality and has projected the internal world onto it. The boundary between the self and the external world has been broken. Organic conditions that disrupt higher intellectual functioning sufficiently to prevent reasoning and reality testing can contribute to the development of delusions. The responsiveness of the delusions of both primary psychiatric and organic illnesses to dopamine-blocking medications suggests that increased CNS activity of this neurotransmitter is part of the pathogenetic mechanism.

Differential Diagnosis

Delusions can be conceptualized as occurring across a spectrum of disease states from the entirely psychiatric to the medical (Table 16–3). Differential diagnosis through examination of the delusion and of the overall picture is most easily carried out at the extremes. The relative contributions of an underlying psychiatric predisposition as opposed to an organic

Table 16–3. Classification of Disorders Associated with Delusions Across a Psychiatric-Medical Spectrum

Class of Disorder	Examples
Primary psychiatric illness	Schizophrenia, affective illness

Possible mixed pathogenesis	Drug related: alcoholic paranoia
	CNS disease
	    Interictal behavior of epilepsy (especially temporal lobe)
	    Huntington's chorea
	    Brain tumors
	Systemic medical illness
	    Endocrine disease
	    Systemic lupus erythematosus

Medical (organic) causes	Drug induced: amphetamine psychosis Organic brain syndromes: delirium, dementia

factor are more difficult to discern in the many intermediate conditions. In these situations, the very existence of a causal relationship between the delusions and organic factors remains controversial.[34]

The primary psychiatric delusion is classically fixed and well defined. In schizophrenia, the delusion is often elaborate and bizarre. In affective illness, it is usually, but not necessarily, congruent with the patient's primary mood disorder. In both cases, the delusions are central to the patient's presenting psychopathology and experience of the world.

The delusions of a chronic organic brain syndrome are characteristically transient and poorly defined.[11] They can occur in dementia when real or imagined losses resulting from a failing memory are projected onto the environment. A demented patient may accuse a staff member of stealing a toothbrush that has been misplaced or forgotten. The delusions of dementia are usually fleeting and reactive. The delusions of a delirium syndrome are contributed to by an acute and diffuse cerebral dysfunction, an altered level of consciousness, and specific effects of the causative organic factor. The associated anxiety and visual hallucinations give rise to transient and terrifying paranoid delusions. Capgras' syndrome is a delusion in which the patient believes certain persons in the environment, usually close family members, are not their real selves but imposters. This type of delusion can be seen in a variety of psychiatric illnesses but is most common in organic brain disease,[37] in which impaired cognition contributes to the misidentification of the familiar. The delusion serves an explanatory function.

Paranoid delusions play a prominent role in amphetamine psychosis. Clinical features of delusions and hallucinations in the absence of the associated clinical features of schizophrenia aid in making the correct diagnosis. The diagnosis is corroborated by a history of psychostimulant abuse, a prompt response to neuroleptics, and, when necessary, drug screening.[26]

In the delusional jealousy of chronic alcoholism (alcoholic paranoia) and the schizophreniform psychoses seen in patients with epilepsy and endocrine disorders, the nature of the organic mechanism remains poorly understood.[25] The differentiation of schizophreniform disorders secondary to medical or CNS disease from primary schizophrenia can be especially difficult. Although the former conditions often lack the thought disorder and feelings of passivity seen in primary schizophrenia,[38] a definitive diagnosis relies on the identification of specific signs and symptoms of the underlying disorder and the pursuit of an appropriate laboratory workup.

DIAGNOSTIC EVALUATION

Patient History and Physical Examination

Diagnostic precision in evaluating perceptual disorders relies on clinical signs and symptoms, historical information, and laboratory evaluation. In all instances special attention must be paid to identifying evidence of organic brain disease. Such evidence includes an abnormal level of arousal (can be increased or decreased); fluctuations in the level of arousal; impaired recent memory; disorientation and the inability to become oriented when accurate information is provided; impairment in other higher intellectual functions such as insight and abstract reasoning; and a clinical picture worse at night or at times of diminished external stimulation. In examining patients with episodic perceptual disorders, the focus must be on evidence of organicity at times of abnormal sensation.

The absence of evidence of organic brain disease essentially limits the diagnosis to primary psychiatric illnesses, organic hallucinosis, and organic delusional syndromes. Nevertheless, the physician must remember that some organic causes of psychiatric disturbance can occur with little early evidence of organic brain disease (Cushing's disease, hyperthyroidism, frontal lobe tumors).

The patient must be examined for associated features of possible primary psychiatric disorder. Phenomena such as blunted affect, lack of interpersonal relatedness, thought disorder, and auditory hallucinations associated with a bizarre delusion system are consistent with schizophrenia. In primary affective disorders, hallucinations or delusions are associated with affective disturbances with perceptions that are usually mood congruent. Signs and symptoms of primary psychiatric illness may fluctuate, but in response to ex-

Table 16–4. Medications Known to Cause Perceptual Disturbances*

Class of Agents	Examples and Comments
Cardiac glycoside	Digoxin (sign of toxicity)
Antiarrhythmic	Propranolol (especially visual, often hypnagogic)
Antitubercular	Isoniazid (INH) (as part of toxic psychosis)
Anticholinergic	Atropine
Antihistamines	Chlorpheniramine maleate
Antiparkinsonian	Levodopa, bromocriptine
Amantadine	Especially in patients with renal disease
Penicillin	Parenteral penicillin G

*Many other medications can cause perceptual disturbance as part of a psychosis that is usually, but not always, marked by features of an acute organic brain syndrome. These include anticonvulsants, indomethacin, methyldopa, steroids, and sulfonamides.

ternal stress and not autonomously. Dramatic changes in clinical phenomena, which appear to occur independent of external reality, are suggestive of an episodic internal biologic process.

Historical information can be critical. This is especially evident in cases of drug abuse or withdrawal, when the patient has suffered recent head trauma, and when prescribed medication has recently been changed. Medication history can reveal whether the patient has been prescribed a new medication with possible psychiatric side effects[26,39] (Table 16–4). In other cases, a new medication can interact with a previously administered agent to increase CNS levels to the point of causing toxicity (e.g., cimetidine and diazepam, hydrochlorothiazide and lithium). Premorbid history is helpful in supporting the diagnosis of specific psychiatric illnesses. Schizophrenic patients classically have a history of marginal premorbid functioning since adolescence, whereas patients with affective episodes can be expected to have had previous episodes of a similar kind if not always of severity. Information about age of onset can also be helpful in that both schizophrenia and manic depressive illness (bipolar type) have their peak onsets in young adulthood.

Diagnostic Studies

Laboratory workup in a patient with a perceptual disorder depends on the results of clinical and historical investigations. Patients with evidence of organic brain disease should receive the appropriate investigations.

An electroencephalogram (EEG) will show diffuse slowing in most cases of acute brain syndrome,[23,40] but the sensitivity of this test is limited by lack of data on any particular patient's baseline. Thus, a patient with a high-normal baseline frequency may have a slower recording resulting from a toxic metabolic state yet still fall within the normal range. In patients with clinical features of temporal lobe epilepsy, an EEG is strongly indicated. Negative findings on a routine examination should be followed by specialized recordings including temporal leads when clinical findings indicate temporal lobe epilepsy. A CT scan may reveal a silent temporal lesion when an episodic perceptual disturbance occurs in association with impaired consciousness.

Electrolyte levels are indicated in all cases of unexplained organic brain syndrome. Signs and symptoms of endocrine disease should also lead to appropriate laboratory procedures. Drug screening is indicated in cases of organic hallucinosis and organic delusional syndrome when a careful history fails to identify the causative factor.

Elderly patients with perceptual disturbances in association with confusion are too often diagnostically dismissed as suffering from dementia. The risk of missed diagnosis is increased by the frequent presentation in this population of medical illness such as acute organic brain syndromes[41] or treatable dementias.[41,42] Finally, the fact that patients with primary psychiatric disease often have concurrent medical illnesses and that these conditions can contribute to the presenting phenomena must be remembered.[43]

DISORDERS OF COGNITION

DEMENTIA

Definition

Dementia is a clinical entity characterized by loss of several intellectual functions severe enough to interfere with social or occupational function or both. Memory dysfunction is always present. Other functions, including the learning of new tasks, orientation in time, place, and person, abstract thinking, judgment, problem solving, and language functions, are frequently compromised. While dementia has been described as a global loss of function, a more accurate conceptualization is of a disturbance in several distinct, yet often related, intellectual functions. Depending on the underlying disease, dementia may present with prominent impairment in some intellectual functions with other functions relatively preserved, at least during the initial stages. For example, patients with dementia caused by chronic communicating hydrocephalus or Huntington's chorea present with marked memory impairment and motor retardation, while the remaining high intellectual functions are less affected.

Dementia must be distinguished from mental retardation, a state in which normal intellectual ability has not been achieved and which can by diagnosed only after brain maturation, which occurs at about 15 years of age. In dementia the state of consciousness remains unaffected; a characteristic that differentiates dementia from delirium.

Usually the course of dementia is that of slow deterioration. The earliest symptoms, which may be subtle and remain unrecognized, include lack of initiative, irritability, distractibility, reduced general comprehension, perseveration, inability to perform at usual capacity, occasional forgetfulness, misplacing of objects, and name-finding problems. Difficulty in coping with new tasks, especially under time pressure, and avoidance of such situations are often observed in the early stages. Forgetfulness sometimes occurs with normal aging but is benign and does not interfere with activities of daily living. In dementia, however, forgetfulness soon becomes qualitatively different. The patient forgets not only minor details, but also important events. Mental status examination is abnormal, with short-term memory and ability to spell words backward affected primarily.

During the early stages of dementia, personality change is frequently encountered. Premorbid personality traits are accentuated, impulses are expressed with little regard to their consequences, and there is a lability of emotional expression, with rapid change from sadness to anger or cheerfulness. Many patients present symptoms of depression; approximately 20% develop major depression.[44] Patients may deny intellectual dysfunction and appear euphoric.

As dementia progresses, language difficulties may appear. The individual is unable to use words appropriately and begins to depend on habitual expression forms. Speech becomes vague and repetitive and the patient is unable to separate essentials from details. Apathy frequently develops and further compromises the already poor performance. Appropriate social behavior is maintained for extended periods, even in the presence of relatively severe intellectual deterioration. In many cases, however, socially maladaptive behavior such as abrupt language, neglect of personal appearance, disregard of the needs and feelings of others, and unusual sexual behavior may occur quite early.

Behavioral changes aimed at compensating for the loss of intellectual ability often are observed even in states of fairly advanced deterioration. For example, some patients may withdraw socially, while others may keep developing strict routines as a way of coping with their affliction. Short-lived sudden outbursts of anger, anxiety, and sadness may occur when a patient is confronted with a failure at a simple task, probably catastrophic reactions to the realization of "losing one's mind." Paranoid ideas and delusions may occur, taking the form of jealousy directed at the patient's spouse or angry accusations of others for withholding money or information or for misplacing objects. Paranoid ideas and delusions may even cause the patient to perform criminal acts. Violence occurs sometimes when the patients act on their delusions.

As deterioration progresses, particularly in dementias with degenerative causes almost all intellectual functions are lost. Dysarthria, aphasia, sphincter incontinence, reduced ability to respond, and impaired locomotion occur. These changes are followed by general physical deterioration, and the patient dies, usually from pneumonia or some other intercurrent infection. The course of dementia depends on the underlying causes. Dementia is neither invariably progressive nor irreversible. Cognitive dysfunction may remain relatively stable, as is the case in head trauma or hypoxia, or may improve, as in metabolic disorders (e.g., hypothyroidism or B_{12} deficiency).

Pathophysiologic Considerations

The mechanisms leading to dementia remain unclear. With the exception of the reversible dementia syndrome secondary to psychiatric disorders, dementia results from an organic condition affecting the brain. The extent of brain damage appears to be as important as the site of the lesion. Most diseases that produce dementia are extensive and affect the frontal lobes more often than other parts of the brain. Neuronal degeneration confined to the thalamus may cause dementia.[45] Recent positron emission tomography (PET) studies have shown that dementia may develop from lesions located primarily in subcortical areas while the cortical metabolism is normal as in supranuclear palsy, normal pressure hydrocephalus, and Huntington's chorea[46]; in Alzheimer's disease, cortical metabolism is usually reduced.[46]

Neurochemical studies cast doubt on the concept that diffuse cerebral cell degeneration is a necessary and sufficient condition for the development of dementia. Specific neuropathologic lesions and specific biochemical dysfunctions seem to be particularly important in the pathogenesis of certain dementias. In Alzheimer's disease, for example, a correlation has been found between intellectual impairment and senile plaques,[47] one of the microscopic brain changes in these disorders, whereas dementia does not seem to correlate with cortical atrophy.[48] Poor cognitive performance and the number of senile plaques are strongly correlated with reduced cerebral levels of choline acetyltransferase, the enzyme involved in the synthesis of acetylcholine.[49] Most brain cholinergic neurons have

Table 16–5. Causes of Dementia

Most frequent causes of dementia
Alzheimer's disease
Multi-infarct dementia
Mixed Alzheimer's disease and multi-infarct dementia
Other causes of dementia
Normal pressure hydrocephalus
Alcoholic dementia
Intracranial masses
Huntington's chorea
Other degenerative diseases
Drug toxicity
Metabolic disorders
Jakob-Creutzfeldt disease
Other CNS infections
Head trauma
Epilepsy

their cell bodies at the nucleus basalis of Meynert, which appears to be particularly affected in Alzheimer's disease.[50] Drugs enhancing cholinergic neurotransmission have failed to improve dementia consistently, however, and deficiencies in some other brain neurotransmitters have been reported in Alzheimer's disease.[51-53] These findings suggest that complex mechanisms are involved in Alzheimer's disease and raise the possibility that dementia may have different pathogeneses even in individuals suffering from the same illness.

Vascular dementia was originally attributed to a diminished blood supply to the brain. It now appears that dementia correlates not with the degree of cerebral arteriosclerosis but with the extent of damage to cerebral hemispheres by multiple strokes. Damage of 50 to 100 g of cerebral hemisphere tissue is sufficient to cause dementia regardless of whether the damage is due to thrombosis, emboli, or hemorrhage.[54] Hypertensive patients with dementia often have multiple small lacunae in the basal ganglia resulting from infarcts. In Binswanger's disease, multiple lacunae, cysts, and demyelination occur primarily in the white matter. This dementia has been attributed to changes in brain arterioles caused by hypertension.

Classification and Differential Diagnosis

Dementia may be produced by a wide variety of diseases (Table 16–5).[55] The most frequent cause of dementia, Alzheimer's disease, accounts for 50 to 60% of cases.[55a] The second most common cause of dementia, multi-infarct dementia, is responsible for 20 to 24% of cases, while 5 to 15% of cases are caused by the combination of Alzheimer's and vascular dementias.[55a] With the exception of patients with Alzheimer's disease and multi-infarct dementia, dementias occur most frequently in patients younger than 70 years.[56]

The diagnosis of Alzheimer's disease can be made only by brain biopsy. This procedure is rarely recommended unless a treatable cause of dementia is suspected. Alzheimer's disease may be suspected in otherwise healthy patients with insidious onset of dementia after age 65 and a uniformly progressively deteriorating course. Multi-infarct dementia frequently occurs in patients with other evidence of vascular disease. It usually has abrupt onset followed by stepwise deterioration. Early in its course some intellectual function may remain relatively unaffected and localizing neurologic symptoms are found frequently. As in Alzheimer's disease, the diagnosis of multi-infarct dementia can be confirmed only by biopsy or autopsy. Clinical criteria systematically applied as part of Hachinski's ischemic rating scale appear to correlate strongly with a diagnosis of multi-infarct dementia, however.[57]

Early dementia should be differentiated from benign forgetfulness of senescence. If cognitive dysfunction is minimal and a diagnosis cannot be made with mental status examination and neuropsychologic tests, follow-up examinations will establish the diagnosis as forgetfulness of senescence, a relatively stable condition in contrast to most dementias, which deteriorate with time.

Another diagnostic problem may be the identification of patients with reversible dementia secondary to psychiatric disorders. Patients with depression, mania, schizophrenia, and personality disorders may present with a reversible cognitive dysfunction.[58] A considerable percentage of demented patients develop depression or other psychiatric manifestations as part of the dementing process, and it may be difficult to distinguish these patients from those whose dementia is due to their psychiatric condition. Some clinical characteristics may be helpful in differentiating patients with reversible dementia secondary to depression. These patients frequently have a previous history of depression, and their dementia is mild, has acute onset, and is usually preceded by depressive symptoms. Neuropsychologic tests may be atypical for dementia, and the majority of patients have a normal EEG. In some cases, however, the clinical picture does not permit differentiation, and an adequate trial of antidepressant treatment may be the only way to make the diagnosis.

Approximately 5% of cases of dementia may be due to space-occupying lesions without localizing neurologic signs.[55] The majority of these cases can be diagnosed by brain CT scan and treated readily.

Normal pressure hydrocephalus is responsible for approximately 1 to 5% of cases of dementia.[55,56] This disorder often follows head injury, meningitis, or intracranial hemorrhage, but it may also be idiopathic. Gait disturbance and ventricular enlargement in the CT scan may point to the diagnosis, although none of these findings is specific. Unsteady gait occurs in several dementing diseases including Korsakoff's psychosis, Jakob-Creutzfeldt disease, and hereditary ataxias. Ventricular enlargement on the CT scan is difficult to distinguish from enlargement caused by atrophy.

Huntington's chorea may be responsible for as many as 3% of cases of dementia.[55,56] This diagnosis is suspected in patients with early-onset dementia with prominent memory impairment and motor retardation who present with choreic movements and have a family history of Huntington's chorea.

Drug toxicity may cause a clinical picture indistinguishable from dementia. Chronic use of sedatives is the most frequent cause of this problem. The patient history obtained from the patient and family and the patient's blood levels of drugs may establish the diagnosis.

Metabolic dementias are important to recognize because they are easily treated. Hypothyroidism and B_{12} deficiency are probably the most frequent causes. A minority of cases with B_{12} deficiency present with dementia before anemia or spinal cord damage is established. B_{12} deficiency must be suspected in demented patients with a history of gastrectomy.

Korsakoff's psychosis usually occurs in chronic alcoholics and is attributed to thiamin deficiency. In contrast to dementia, high intellectual function impairment is circumscribed in Korsakoff's psychosis. These patients are unable to retain new information, although immediate recall and long-term memory are relatively preserved. Wernicke's encephalopathy manifested by confusion, nystagmus, ophthalmoplegia, and ataxia sometimes precedes Korsakoff's psychosis.

The infection that most commonly causes dementia is Jakob-Creutzfeldt's disease, which produces a rapidly progressing dementia with cortical symptoms, myoclonus, and gait disturbance.[54] Fungal meningitis and neurosyphilis are rarer causes of dementia.

A considerable percentage of patients with Parkinson's disease develop dementia. The differential diagnosis in these patients is rarely complicated because they present with bradykinesia, rigidity, tremor, and gait disturbance.

Diagnostic Evaluation

The diagnosis of dementia depends on the patient history and the physical and mental status examination. Use of brief rating scales of high intellectual functions, including the scale of Blessed, et al.[47] and the mini-mental state examination,[59] may help to identify patients with early dementia and possibly differentiate patients with benign forgetfulness of senescence, who usually give normal responses.[56] Neuropsychologic tests are often required, and repeated evaluations may be needed in order to establish that the illness is worsening. Particular attention should be given to the pattern of cognitive deficits of demented patients. In certain diseases (e.g., Huntington's chorea, normal pressure hydrocephalus, and progressive supranuclear palsy) there is a subcortical dementia—memory impairment and motor retardation—while in others (e.g., neurosyphilis and Alzheimer's, Pick's and Jakob-Creutzfeldt diseases), cortical functions also are affected.

Neurologic examination may reveal signs and symptoms diagnostic of a variety of diseases causing dementia, including parkinsonism, normal pressure hydrocephalus, Huntington's chorea, Jakob-Creutzfeldt's disease, hereditary ataxias, and space-occupying lesions.

A previous psychiatric history or presence of psychiatric symptoms should raise the possibility of reversible dementia secondary to psychiatric disorders, most often depression. The dexamethasone suppression test (DST) has been thought to help in the differential diagnosis of these dementias[60,61]; however, a recent study demonstrated that an abnormal DST cannot predict the outcome of dementia following antidepressant treatment in patients with mixed cognitive and depressive symptoms.[62] Psychiatric consultation, the presence of a normal EEG, and adequate treatment with antidepressant drugs or electroconvulsive therapy are often necessary in patients with depression and dementia. In several patients a trial of antidepressant therapies may be the only way to arrive at the diagnosis.

Blood tests including complete blood count, blood chemistry, thyroid function tests, B_{12} and folate blood levels, drug screening, VDRL are essential in order to diagnose toxic, metabolic, or infectious causes of dementia.

The majority of patients with Alzheimer's disease show a generalized background slowing of EEG greater than that of normal aging. This finding has been shown to be diagnostically reliable.[56] Patients with Jakob-Creutzfeldt's disease present a characteristic EEG picture. Dementias caused by focal lesions may present focal EEG findings, although the CT scan is a more reliable diagnostic tool in such cases.

Brain CT is important in the diagnosis of tumors, subdural hematomas, and normal pressure hydrocephalus. High-resolution CT scans can aid in the diagnosis of multi-infarct dementia by revealing areas of focal attenuation resulting from old infarcts.

Examination of the cerebrospinal fluid is especially helpful in the diagnosis of fungal meningitis, a treatable cause of dementia. Brain biopsy, though rarely obtained, is particularly useful in younger patients, who have a higher probability of suffering from a treatable dementia that cannot be identified by other means. Recently, the twist drill brain biopsy technique has been used in some cases. This procedure requires local anesthesia, has reduced morbidity and mortality, and may be used in outpatients.

DELIRIUM

Definition

Delirium is a clinical state that presents with a characteristic clouding of consciousness and inattention to internal or environmental stimuli. Memory and orientation are impaired to various degrees. Perceptual disturbances are common and take the form of illusions, misinterpretations, and hallucinations. The most frequent perceptual disturbances are visual, but sometimes other sensory modalities are affected. Misinterpretations may be simple and uniform or highly complex. In most cases the patients are convinced of the reality of their hallucinations and behave accordingly. Thinking appears incoherent, nongoal directed, and fragmented. Thought disorder in delirium may range from mild acceleration or slowing of thinking to complete disorganization of thought. Perseveration of speech is frequent. The sleep-wakefulness cycle is almost always impaired. Drowsiness during the day and hypervigilance and insomnia during the night are present. Vivid dreams and nightmares are common. Most patients have behavioral disturbances ranging from motor agitation to retardation. Some patients are restless, pick on their clothes, strike at nonexisting objects, and change position frequently. Others are lethargic and sluggish. A rapid shift from retardation to agitation is sometimes observed.

Frequently, delirious patients are fearful. Fear is usually related to the frightening perceptual experiences and can be so intense that the patient may attack or flee without concern for the consequences. Depression may lead to suicidal attempts or self-mutilation. Anxiety, irritability, anger, and euphoria are also common. The patient may maintain one emotional state during the course of delirium or change from one emotional state to another unpredictably; as early as 1935, Wolff and Curran observed that the emotional manifestations of delirium are much influenced by previous experience and personality.[63] Abnormal autonomic signs such as tachycardia, elevated blood pressure, perspiration, flushed skin, and dilated pupils occur frequently.

With the exception of movement disorders, localizing neurologic signs are relatively uncommon in delirium. The characteristic movement disorders in delirium are tremor, asterixis, and multifocal myoclonus.[64] The tremor is coarse and irregular, occurring at a rate of approximately 8 to 10/second. It is usually absent at complete rest. Asterixis is an abnormal, involuntary jerking movement of the hands elicited at dorsiflexion of the wrist with extended fingers. These movements are nonrhythmic and are not synchronized in the two hands. Asterixis may involve the feet and tongue. Bilateral asterixis occurs in almost all patients with metabolic delirium. Multifocal myoclonus occurs at rest and presents as sudden nonrhythmic gross muscle contractions that are most common in the face and shoulders. If not present at rest, myoclonus can be elicited by passive movement of the shoulder and upper arm. Multifocal myoclonus occurs most frequently in uremia, anoxia and hypercapnia, and penicillin overdose, although it can develop in any severe metabolic delirium. Generalized seizures, symmetrical muscular weakness, and hyper-reflexia often occur in severe delirium. Focal seizures or unilateral paresis may also develop. The latter is usually mild and transient. Disorders of cortical function including dysnomia and dysgraphia occur in some patients.

The onset of delirium is usually abrupt. Sometimes, however, delirium is preceded by prodromal symptoms including restlessness, thinking difficulty, sensory hypersensitivity, insomnia, daytime somnolence, vivid dreams, and nightmares. Fluctuation of symptoms is an important characteristic in delirium; patients may be out of contact one moment and lucid the next. Lucid intervals appear unpredictably and last for minutes or hours. Some of the fluctuation may be a response to environmental changes. Characteristically, delirious patients become disoriented at night, in unfamiliar surroundings, and when restrained. The duration of delirium is usually short.

Until recently the term acute organic brain syndrome was used by the American Psychiatric Association to denote delirium.[65] The problem with this designation has been that ''acute organic brain syndrome'' implies its cause and assumes that the syndrome is reversible. Some acute organic brain syndromes, however, are associated with irreversible diseases. The 1980 Diagnostic and Statistical Manual (DSM III) of the American Psychiatric Association reintroduced the term delirium and defined it by its clinical presentation, rather than its cause.[66] Adams and Victor have suggested that the term delirium should be used to denote a special transient confusional state characterized by acute onset, gross disorientation, heightened alertness, illusions and vivid hallucinations, agitation, nightmares,

and increased activity of the autonomic nervous system.[45] They distinguished this syndrome from confusional states with depressed consciousness. Because neither syndrome is characteristic of distinct pathophysiologic disturbances, however, the term delirium presently includes all confusional states.

Pathophysiologic Considerations

Since the seventeenth century it has been known that many pathophysiologic entities can produce delirium.[67] In their classic paper, Engel and Romano reported that impairment in the level of consciousness correlated with generalized slowing of the EEG.[68] Moruzzi and Magoun described the role of the brain stem reticular formation in regulating the activity of EEG.[69]

Presently, the disturbance of consciousness found in delirium is thought to be caused by dysfunction in the reticular activating systems in the brain stem that maintain and modify arousal and consciousness. These neurons are probably the most susceptible to metabolic change, and, at least initially, the cortical neurons malfunction only because they lose their reticular stimulation. This theory is supported by animal experiments in which anoxia, hypoglycemia, anesthesia, and cyanide poisoning blocked electrical conduction at the reticular formation before they interfere with the function of the lemniscal system, which permits the cortex to receive information from afferent pathways.

While the brain stem reticular activating system function is the most vulnerable to metabolic changes, the first anatomic changes appear in the cortex.[64] As the process becomes more severe, subcortical structures are affected caudally. The phylogenetically oldest structures seem to be the most resistant to metabolic insults.

Posner has pointed out that these concepts provide only a limited explanation of the process by which pathophysiologic changes occurring during disease lead to the clinical state of delirium.[64] In the same metabolic condition, early dysfunction may differ from patient to patient or even from attack to attack in the same patient. This fact is demonstrated in hypoglycemia. Some patients first suffer loss of consciousness and have bilateral synchronous waves in the EEG, suggesting an initial involvement of the reticular formation. Others initially show cerebral motor or sensory disturbances without impaired consciousness or EEG abnormalities. It is likely that regional factors such as energy needs and blood flow may vary over time and thus predispose different parts of the brain to malfunction.

Delirium is usually caused by extracerebral diseases (Table 16–6). Cerebral disorders arising from failure of neuronal or glial metabolism usually begin insidi-

Table 16–6. Disorders Leading to Delirium

Extracerebral disorders
  Systemic infections
  Hypoxia
  Hypoglycemia
  Electrolyte disturbances
  Postoperative states
  Substance intoxication and withdrawal
  Hepatic failure
  Renal failure
  Thiamin deficiency
  Collagen diseases
  Blood dyscrasias
Cerebral disorders
  Encephalitis
  Meningitis

ously, progress slowly, and give the clinical picture of dementia. The distinction between encephalopathies caused by cerebral disorders and encephalopathies caused by extracerebral disorders is not sharply defined, however. Some systemic metabolic encephalopathies, e.g., vitamin B_{12} deficiency or hypothyroidism, may lead to a clinical picture resembling dementia that may be reversible with treatment. Conversely, some primary disorders of the brain, i.e., encephalitis, meningitis, and seizures, have a clinical presentation similar to that of delirium and may be reversed with treatment.

Pathologic changes in delirium depend on the nature and severity of the underlying disease. The brains of some delirious patients are entirely normal at post-mortem examination. In other cases, microscopic changes occur if the process causing delirium lasted for hours or days. Pathologic changes are usually bilateral and are distributed diffusely in the hemispheres and, in more severe cases, in the midbrain and subthalamus. Depending on the nature of the underlying condition, the neurons, the white matter, or the glia may be affected.

The most common pathologic changes are observed after anoxia, hypoglycemia, or ischemia. If mild insult occurs, cytoplasmic microvacuoles appear in the neocortex and the hippocampus. These changes are reversible. In more severe disturbances, there is a dissolution of the Nissl granules, the nuclei may become shrunken and hyperchromatic, and granules and basophilic rings may appear in the cytoplasm. These changes are irreversible. After very severe and prolonged insults, the third cortical layer may degenerate completely. Anoxia may also affect the basal ganglia. The brain stem and the spinal cord are spared unless the process has been very severe. In hepatic enceph-

alopathy, characteristic ballooned glial cells with lobulated nuclei are observed in the cortex and the basal ganglia. In viral or bacterial inflammation of the brain or meninges there is a perivascular infiltration by leukocytes and lymphocytes.

The mechanisms by which systemic diseases cause delirium are only partly understood. Glucose is the brain's only source of energy under normal conditions. Reduction of brain glucose to levels below 30 mg/dl leads to confusion, and reduction below 10 or 15 mg/dl leads to coma. Hypoxia with arterial oxygen levels below 50 mm Hg causes delirium, and levels below 20 mm Hg, coma. In addition to glucose and oxygen, the brain requires other substances, e.g., electrolytes, vitamins, and aminoacids, for its metabolism and its function. Abnormalities in any of these substances may lead to delirium. Neurotransmission depends on energy from oxidative processes and requires a delicate balance of intra- and extracellular electrolytes. Hyper- or hyponatremia, for example, may interfere with the propagation of the action potential and lead to delirium. An overdose of psychotropic drugs may cause delirium by changing the activity of brain neurotransmitters. Hallucinogenic drugs may produce delirium by acting as "false neurotransmitters." Disturbances in substance inactivation in the liver may permit an excessive amount of substances to enter the circulation and, acting as false neurotransmitters, lead to hepatic delirium or coma.

Diagnostic Evaluation and Differential Diagnosis

PATIENT HISTORY AND PHYSICAL EXAMINATION

Delirium is a medical emergency. Systematic diagnostic evaluation is necessary because the same clinical picture may result from various causes but may require different management. Past medical history may reveal essential information. Recent head trauma, kidney, liver, or cardiac disease, diabetes mellitus, use of insulin, alcoholism, drug abuse, or history of suicidal behavior may direct the clinician in pursuing further diagnostic studies.

The onset and clinical presentation of delirium may orient the physician to its underlying causes. For example, in elderly patients with respiratory infection, delirium may present as a quiet confusion and lethargy. In contrast, delirium tremens is marked by agitation, hyperactivity, vivid frightening hallucinations, and increased autonomic activity including tachycardia and fever. The onset of delirium tremens is usually abrupt and occurs 24 to 48 hours after discontinuation of chronic alcohol use.

Physical and neurologic examination can be revealing. Hypertension raises the question of hypertensive encephalopathy, cerebral hemorrhage, or subarachnoid hemorrhage as the underlying cause of delirium. Hyperventilation may result from metabolic acidosis caused by diabetes, uremia, adrenal insufficiency, or drug poisoning, although it may occur in alkalosis as a result of pulmonary or cardiac disease, liver failure, or hysteria. Hypotension in a delirious patient may indicate hemorrhagic or septic shock, dehydration, myocardial infarction, or poisoning with CNS depressant drugs. Bradycardia may be due to myocardial infarction or bradyarrhythmias. Supraventricular tachycardia may lead to anoxic delirium as a result of lowered cardiac output. Kussmaul's respiration raises the question of metabolic acidosis. Dyspnea may be indicative of respiratory failure. Fever suggests infection or neoplasm. Hypothermia can be a result of hypoglycemia, drug poisoning, or insult at the brain stem.

Examination of the skin may reveal signs of nutritional problems, jaundice and spider angioma, petechiae, or ecchymoses. Cardiac murmurs may be associated with bacterial endocarditis and brain embolism. Lung examination can reveal obstructive pulmonary disease. Hepatomegaly may be found in delirium caused by hepatic failure. Splenomegaly occurs often in blood dyscrasias and infectious mononucleosis. Both conditions can lead to encephalopathy and present with delirium. Fundoscopy is particularly helpful because it may reveal a picture suggestive of hypertensive vascular disease, diabetes, collagen vasculitis, increased intracranial pressure, leukemia, tuberculosis, embolism, and cryptococcosis.

Neurologic examination must always include a mental status examination in order to establish the presence of delirium. Intellectual impairment, obvious when the delirium is florid, may be missed in early cases unless the patient is examined systematically. Mental status examination includes orientation in time, place, and person; assessment of remote, recent, and immediate memory; concentration, tested by spelling a word backwards; abstract thinking, examined by asking the patient to interpret proverbs; and judgment. The most sensitive of these functions appear to be short-term memory, concentration, and orientation to time. Language examination covers disorders such as dysphasia, constructional apraxia, right-left disorientation, inability to carry out complex commands, unilateral neglect, or inattention on double stimulation. Language disorders occur primarily in primary brain disease but may also be found in delirium from extracerebral causes.

DIAGNOSTIC STUDIES

Laboratory tests are almost always required to establish the cause of metabolic delirium. Blood glucose, BUN, electrolytes, and calcium may be diagnostic in delirium caused by hypoglycemia, diabetes, uremia, osmolar abnormalities, or hypocalcemia. Arterial blood gases should be determined because they can reveal anoxia, acidosis or, alkalosis. Rapid diagnosis and treatment are essential in delirium caused by anoxia or hypoglycemia because anoxia and hypoglycemia may rapidly lead to irreversible brain damage. Lumbar puncture should be obtained if CNS infection or hemorrhage is suspected. Liver function tests and drug blood levels can establish the diagnosis in hepatic or drug-induced delirium.

The CT brain scan is normal in delirium but can be useful in excluding structural brain diseases. The EEG is almost always abnormal in severe delirium. The most frequent picture is that of bilateral symmetrical slowing. The background activity ranges between 5 and 7 Hz with bursts of delta waves (1 to 3 Hz). The degree of EEG slowing correlates roughly with the severity of delirium.[70] A minority of patients, however, may present rapid EEG rhythms. These patients are usually suffering from delirium caused by drug withdrawal.[64]

It is essential to establish that delirium is due to metabolic encephalopathy and does not result from structural brain lesions. Supratentorial masses may affect the diencephalon and suppress the level of consciousness. Most supratentorial lesions, however, present focal motor and sensory signs and sometimes focal or generalized seizures before they affect the level of consciousness. These localizing signs persist even after the patient becomes delirious or stuporous. They are usually replaced by bilateral decorticate or decerebrate rigidity late in the course, when transtentorial herniation occurs. The EEG usually shows focal slowing over the area of the mass or over the whole hemisphere, whereas in patients with metabolic delirium, the EEG presents diffuse slowing. CT brain scan is the most reliable laboratory test for the identification of brain space-occupying lesions and should be performed in all delirious patients with unclear diagnoses. Subtentorial masses usually present as early signs of cranial nerve involvement that persist even after consciousness is affected. The pupils are almost always unequal, and the pupillary light reflexes are unilaterally pathologic in subtentorial lesions, whereas they are spared in metabolic delirium. Other brain stem signs, including disconjugate eye movements, ocular bobbing, rotating ocular deviations, eye deviation toward the paralyzed arm and leg, and unilateral facial anesthesia, suggest a subtentorial lesion.

AMNESTIC SYNDROME

Definition

The cardinal symptom of amnestic syndrome is memory disturbance. Sensorium is clear and cognitive functions that do not depend on memory remain relatively unaffected. Memory for events learned before the onset of illness (retrograde amnesia) and the ability to register new events in memory (antegrade amnesia) are deficient. Remote memories are better preserved than recent ones, although when the disease has progressed there may be no difference. Orientation is affected because it depends on memory. Confabulations, which are fabrications of fictitious events or improper sequencing of events, are present in most patients with amnestic syndrome. They are not, however, pathognomonic for this condition, and they tend to disappear when the syndrome progresses into chronicity. Immediate recall is intact. Concentration is relatively unaffected and the patient is able to make spatial and visual abstractions and solve problems that do not require memory.

Patients with amnestic syndrome are usually unaware of their disability or, if they acknowledge it, they appear unconcerned. They seem complacent and lack spontaneity and initiative. Their emotional tone is bland and shallow although they may be superficially engaging. As a rule, socially acceptable behavior is maintained.

The Wernicke-Korsakoff syndrome is the most common amnestic syndrome. It is usually observed in malnourished chronic alcoholic patients, but it can develop in the context of thyrotoxicosis, gastric carcinoma, hyperemesis gravidarum, prolonged intravenous therapy, or chronic hemodialysis.

Wernicke's disease typically has acute or subacute onset. Diplopia and ophthalmoplegia with predominant weakness or paralysis of the external recti muscles bilaterally and paralysis of lateral conjugate gaze are common early symptoms. Horizontal nystagmus is always present, and frequently, vertical nystagmus is observed. In some cases, complete third, fourth, and sixth nerve ophthalmoplegia is observed with ptosis, complete paralysis of eye movements, and lack of pupillary responses to light.

Ataxia occurs in all cases. It may be mild, requiring tests of cerebellar function in order to be detected, but if severe it interferes with the gait to the point that some patients are unable to walk. Intention tremor occurs sometimes and is more prominent in the legs. The speech is rarely affected. Polyneuropathy affecting both the sensory and motor neurons is found in approximately half of patients with Wernicke's disease.

The mental status is characteristic. The patient is apathetic, shows little interest in his surroundings, is disoriented, and has severe memory dysfunction. If thiamin treatment and appropriate diet are provided, ophthalmoplegia, ataxia, and polyneuropathy are com-

Table 16–7. Disorders Leading to Amnestic Syndrome

Thiamin deficiency
  Wernicke-Korsakoff syndrome
Vascular disorders
  Subarachnoid hemorrhage
  Thrombosis or embolism of posterior cerebral arteries bilaterally
  Transient global amnesia
Head trauma
  Diencephalon
  Medial aspects of temporal lobes
Intoxication
  Carbon monoxide
CNS infections
  Herpes simplex encephalitis
  Basal meningitis
Space-occupying lesions
  Tumors of third ventricle
  Tumors of temporal lobes

pletely reversed in most cases. Cognitive disturbances, however, may persist, and the patient develops the characteristic picture of amnestic syndrome that is known as Korsakoff's psychosis. It should be noted that some patients with Korsakoff's psychosis do not have a history of Wernicke's disease.

Pathophysiologic Considerations

Memory depends on the integrity of certain structures located in the diencephalon and the temporal lobes. More specifically, the medial aspects of the dorsomedial thalamus, the hippocampus, and the adjacent white matter are of particular importance for memory functions. Bilateral lesions in any of these areas lead to a pronounced memory dysfunction while the remaining cognitive functions remain relatively intact.[71] Unilateral lesions of these structures on the dominant side lead to a milder memory disturbance, whereas damage on the nondominant side is not sufficient to produce significant memory problems. It appears that these structures participate in the registration of information, along with the brain stem reticular formation, a structure necessary to maintain alertness, and the cortex, where verbal and spatial information is integrated.

The amnestic syndrome may develop from vascular, traumatic, infectious, toxic, neoplastic, or other diseases (Table 16–7). The most frequent amnestic syndrome is Wernicke-Korsakoff syndrome, caused in part by lack of vitamin B_{12}.[72] While the syndrome occurs most frequently in alcoholic patients, continuous intake of alcohol is not followed by exacerbation of symptoms if adequate nutrition is provided. Administration of thiamin reverses apathy, inattentiveness, and ophthalmoplegia and reduces nystagmus and ataxia in a few days, although the memory dysfunction remains. Selective administration of various other vitamins of the B complex does not change the clinical picture of the syndrome.[2]

Cell culture experiments have shown that the ability of neurons and glia to synthesize fatty acids and cholesterol is impaired if the neurons and glia are grown in a low-thiamin environment.[73] Chronic thiamin deprivation in animals leads to decreased utilization of glucose, predominantly in brain areas that develop histologic abnormalities in Wernicke-Korsakoff syndrome.[74] This selective vulnerability to lack of thiamin probably explains the distribution of brain lesions in Wernicke-Korsakoff syndrome and the subsequent mental status changes. In vitro experiments have shown a decrease of serotonin re-uptake in cerebellar synaptosomes of animals with thiamin deficiency, suggesting that the cerebellar symptoms of Wernicke-Korsakoff syndrome may be caused predominantly by selective dysfunction of serotoninergic neurons.[73] Patients suffering from Wernicke-Korsakoff syndrome have a genetic red blood cell and fibroblast abnormality in transketolase. Abnormalities in this enzyme result in weak binding with the active thiamin cofactor and therefore in interference with the utilization of thiamin. It has been proposed that this genetic abnormality predisposes to Wernicke-Korsakoff syndrome. Symptoms become evident when supplies of thiamin are inadequate, as in malnutrition, or when a combination of inadequate supplies and increased need for thiamin exists, as in alcoholism.

Diagnostic Evaluation and Differential Diagnosis

The first task when approaching a patient with memory disturbance is to establish whether an amnestic syndrome exists and to differentiate it from the more frequently occurring syndromes of dementia and delirium. Patients with amnestic syndrome have a considerable antegrade and retrograde memory dysfunction with a secondary disturbance in orientation. In contrast, patients with dementia have a more global intellectual dysfunction. Impairment of abstract thinking, demonstrated as inability to find similarities between related words, difficulty in defining concepts, and concrete interpretation of proverbs, is almost always present in dementia. Judgment is impaired, and, in most demented patients, high cortical dysfunction includes aphasia, apraxia, and agnosia. Delirium, on the other hand, presents a characteristic clouding of consciousness that is not found in amnestic syndrome.

In patients with an amnestic syndrome, a detailed patient history may give crucial diagnostic information. Chronic alcoholism and a history of Wernicke's disease orient the clinician toward the diagnosis of Korsakoff's psychosis. Cerebrovascular disease or generalized arteriosclerosis raises the possibility of amnestic syndrome caused by occlusion of posterior cerebral arteries or their lower temporal branches. A history of tuberculosis may lead the clinician to consider basal exudative meningitis resulting in amnestic syndrome. Head trauma or carbon monoxide poisoning may be other underlying causes of amnestic syndrome.

Acute onset and rapid, complete recovery suggest either transient global amnesia or epilepsy as the underlying cause of amnestic syndrome. Epileptic patients may present with amnesia either during the postictal phase or during the seizure period if the epileptic focus is in the temporal lobes. Sudden onset with a course of gradual but incomplete improvement occurs in amnestic syndromes of vascular, traumatic, or toxic origin. Finally, subacute or insidious onset with a chronic course is usually observed in patients with Wernicke-Korsakoff disease, herpes simplex encephalitis, tuberculosis, meningitis, or neoplastic disease.

Neuropsychologic tests are helpful in localizing the lesions and in following the course of the memory disturbance. Brain CT scan may be diagnostic in amnestic syndrome caused by neoplastic or vascular diseases. Electroencephalogram can establish the diagnosis of epilepsy, although a normal record does not exclude this disorder. Lumbar puncture is diagnostic in subarachnoid hemorrhage but may reveal helpful findings in other disorders leading to amnestic syndrome. Cerebrospinal fluid is bloody in all cases with subarachnoid hemorrhage, in 85% of cases with cerebral hemorrhage, and in 15% of cases with embolism. Opening pressure is elevated more than 200 mm in the majority of patients with cerebral or subarachnoid hemorrhage. CSF pressure is increased in proportion to the amount of blood in the cerebrospinal fluid. In tuberculosis meningitis the cerebrospinal fluid has a clouded or ground-glass appearance with formation of a clot on standing. The pressure is elevated as a rule, and there is moderate pleocytosis with a predominance of lymphocytes. Glucose is decreased and the protein content is increased, while serologic tests are negative for syphilis. In Korsakoff's psychosis a minority of patients have increased cerebrospinal fluid pressure, slight pleocytosis, and a mildly increased protein content. Moderate anemia is present in 50%, and severe anemia is seen in about 10% of cases. A leukocytosis is present in one third of patients. Carbon monoxide poisoning may be confirmed by demonstration of carboxyhemoglobin in the blood using a spectroscope.

MOVEMENT DISORDERS

DYSKINETIC MOVEMENTS

Definition

Dyskinetic movements are abnormal, involuntary movements that may affect almost any part of the body. They may take various forms, ranging from the irregular, jerky, brief movements characteristic of choreiform motion to very complex stereotypic activity. Although the spectrum of these movements is extremely wide, there are characteristic features of some movement disorders that are usually related to a specific disease entity (Table 16–8).

Pathophysiologic Considerations

The pathophysiology of dyskinetic movements is complex. The path leading to movement involves the motor cortex, basal ganglia, brain stem, spinal cord, peripheral nerves, and muscle. Dyskinetic movements are involved largely with disorders of basal ganglia structures that lead to abnormal motor tone, an excess or paucity of movement, and, in some cases, difficulty in performing complex motor tasks. The basal ganglia appear to be organized into parallel cortico-striato-pallido-thalamo-cortical feedback loops. Disruption of these pathways through biochemical, anatomic, or pharmacologic means leads to abnormalities in movement. Dopaminergic systems are critical to the functioning of this system. Heightened activity of dopamine receptors has been implicated in disorders such as tardive dyskinesia, while decreased activity is responsible for akinetic and parkinson-like states. The functioning of the basal ganglia interconnections is known to be more complex than dopaminergic activity as ongoing research reveals varying integral roles for other neurotransmitters such as acetylcholine and gamma-aminobutyric acid.

Differential Diagnosis and Diagnostic Evaluation

The diagnosis of a dyskinetic movement disorder is based on the patient history, including careful documentation of past and present drug use, precise characterization of the type of abnormal movements, and evaluation for underlying medical and psychiatric illness. Within a psychiatric patient population the most common cause of dyskinetic movements is neuroleptic medicine. Tardive dyskinesia is a hyperkinetic movement disorder that occurs after prolonged use of neu-

Table 16–8. Classification of Dyskinetic Movements

Neuroleptic induced
  Tardive dyskinesia
  Withdrawal dyskinesia
  Akathisia
  Rabbit syndrome
Drug induced
  Amphetamines
  L-dopa
  Tricyclic antidepressants
  Lithium
  Anticholinergics
  Oral contraceptives
  Phenytoin
  Chloroquine
  Amodiaquine
  Methadone
  Monoamine oxidase inhibitors
Disease states
  Huntington's disease
  Chorea gravidarum
  Sydenham's chorea
  Wilson's disease
  Systemic lupus erythematosus
  Encephalitis (Jakob-Creutzfeldt)
  Hepatic encephalopathy
  Uremic encephalopathy
  Hyperthyroidism
  Hypoparathyroidism
  Postanoxic state
  Temporal lobe epilepsy
  Brain neoplasm
Idiopathic
  Gilles de la Tourette's syndrome
  Tic disorders
Functional
  Stereotypies and mannerisms of schizophrenia
  Spontaneous
  Edentulous state and poorly fitting dentures

roleptics, drugs that block dopamine receptors. These include drugs such as phenothiazines, butyrophenones, and thioxanthenes, which are usually prescribed for psychiatric reasons, although tardive dyskinesia may be seen in nonpsychiatric patients who are chronically treated with prochlorperazine and metoclopramide for gastrointestinal disturbances. Older patients and women may be at higher risk. Orofacial dyskinesia, the most characteristic feature, is marked by protruding and twisting tongue movements, pouting and twisting lip and cheek movements, and various chewing jaw motions. Vermicular movements of the tongue on the floor of the mouth are a very early sign. Unlike in Huntington's disease, upper portions of the face are usually spared. In more severe cases, choreiform movements of the extremities, tapping motions of the feet, rocking movement of the trunk, and rotatory pelvic movements may be seen. Disturbances of respiratory rhythm and grunting vocalizations can also occur. As with most movement disorders, dyskinetic movements disappear with sleep and worsen with anxiety.

Tardive dyskinesia usually begins after a minimum of 3 months of exposure to neuroleptics but frequently occurs after a much longer exposure. Movements begin while the patient is on a steady dosage of neuroleptics or when the dosage is decreased, and they are frequently ameliorated by increasing the dosage, though this practice is discouraged as movements will eventually occur at the higher dosage. After neuroleptics are withdrawn, the dyskinesia does not progress as do degenerative CNS disorders; it either remains permanently unchanged or gradually improves, and in some cases it disappears completely. The many cases that resolve within 6 to 12 weeks of drug discontinuation are called withdrawal dyskinesia.

Akathisia is a disorder of motor restlessness that, unlike tardive dyskinesia, occurs following early administration of neuroleptics or upon augmentation of the dosage. The severity varies from a shuffling or tapping movement of the feet to incessant pacing and agitation. There is a marked sense of inner tension and a need to resist inactivity. The patient is intensely aware of and stressed by this movement disorder, unlike the patient with tardive dyskinesia, who may be relatively unconcerned about his movements. Akathisia usually responds to a decrease in the neuroleptic dosage, although rare cases have been reported of increasing severity after drug discontinuation, perhaps indicative of a worsening psychiatric condition.

Rabbit syndrome, like tardive dyskinesia, is a perioral movement disorder associated with prolonged use of neuroleptics. It is manifested by quickly alternating, regular movements of the jaw and perioral area that resemble a rabbit's munching. The rapidity of the movements and the absence of lingual involvement distinguish this syndrome from the slower, more irregular movements of tardive dyskinesia. Also, rabbit syndrome typically responds well to treatment with anticholinergic agents, whereas tardive dyskinesia may be exacerbated by such agents.

Dyskinetic movements are occasionally seen in patients taking other drugs. Patients with amphetamine psychosis frequently exhibit stereotyped behavior such as purposeless, repetitive actions, pacing, twisting movements, and grimacing. Transient orofacial dyskinesias have been reported in patients taking chloroquine and amodiaquine for malaria. Rarely, tricyclic antidepressants, lithium salts, and monoamine oxidase inhibitors cause myoclonic jerks, though this is more likely following toxic doses. Persistent choreic movements have been reported following lithium intoxication. Intoxication with phenytoin and antihistamines may also cause dyskinetic reactions. Rarely, methadone may induce choreic movements. Infrequently, choreic movements will be seen in young women receiving estrogen-containing contraceptives. It has been suggested that dyskinetic movements caused by methadone, oral contraceptives, and phenytoin require an underlying abnormality of the basal ganglia that becomes apparent when the patients are placed on a medication regimen. A large percentage of patients receiving L-dopa for treatment of parkinsonism will develop oral dyskinesias and choreic movements of the extremities. These abnormal movements are related to the dose of L-dopa and frequently improve on a reduced dosage.

Dyskinetic movements of various types frequently occur secondary to an underlying disease process. Though these illnesses are not usually thought of as psychiatric disorders, they frequently exhibit dramatic psychiatric symptoms. Huntington's disease is a disorder with an autosomal dominant inheritance pattern with three types of presentation: dyskinetic movements, dementia, and emotional disturbance. The emotional disorder may present as a psychotic or affective disorder and may occur before any obvious manifestations of dementia or chorea arise. Choreiform movements are most commonly seen in the extremities but also occur frequently in the orofacial area. The differential diagnosis may be complicated by the fact that Huntington's patients may have been treated with neuroleptics and may also have tardive dyskinesia. Unlike tardive dyskinesia, with Huntington's disease there is usually a strong family history for a similar movement disorder, the disease is progressive and results in death, and CT scan may show atrophy of the caudate nucleus.

Chorea gravidarum is a disorder that appears during pregnancy and is manifested largely by choreic movements in the hands that disappear after delivery but may be seen again in later pregnancies. In such patients there is often a history of rheumatic fever or chorea before pregnancy.

Sydenham's chorea is a common cause of choreic movements in young adults who have had rheumatic fever; generally the chorea tends to follow rheumatic arthritis and carditis by several months. Tests for group A streptococci will help confirm the diagnosis and differentiate Syndenham's chorea from chorea that follows infection with diphtheria, rubella, pertussis, and the encephalitides. As with tardive dyskinesia, neuroleptics suppress the dyskinetic movements in Huntington's disease, chorea gravidarum, and Sydenham's chorea. Choreic movements have also been observed in patients with diffuse CNS disease secondary to systemic lupus erythematosus. Patients with this disorder may present with signs of seizures, confusion, and dementia; a significant number will also become psychotic at some point.

Jakob-Creutzfeldt disease, a rare illness thought to be caused by a slow virus infection, frequently produces changes in mood and intellect. With progression, signs of parkinsonism and choreoathetoid movements develop. The EEG demonstrates a characteristic pattern of biphasic and triphasic waves. Wilson's disease is a rare illness of autosomal recessive inheritance with age of onset between 10 and 40 years, frequently occurring in patients of Jewish parentage. Patients may present with emotional instability, impaired intellect, and psychotic disorders. A movement disorder marked by incoordination, tremor, and dyskinetic movements of the extremities develops, occasionally becoming severe and consisting of wild, flinging movements. The illness is based on a disorder of copper metabolism that results in degenerative changes in the basal ganglia and liver. The diagnosis is based on increased urinary copper, low serum levels of ceruloplasmin, and development in the eye of Kayser-Fleischer rings.

Other rare causes of dyskinetic movements are hyperthyroidism, hypoparathyroidism, brain neoplasm, and postanoxic states. In hepatic and renal encephalopathy the patient may develop asterixis, a myoclonic twitching, prominent about the face and upper extremities and accentuated by auditory or tactile stimuli. During seizures, patients with temporal lobe epilepsy may develop automatisms such as lip-smacking, chewing, swallowing, and other stereotyped repetitive motions. During these episodes consciousness is clouded and the patient is not related to the environment, a condition very different from the intact relatedness seen in patients with dyskinetic movements from other causes. A sleep-deprived EEG with nasopharyngeal leads and a detailed seizure history delineating discrete episodes is helpful in making the diagnosis.

There is a group of idiopathic movement disorders manifested by tics for which no specific biologic cause has been identified (although increasingly clinicians believe that a neurologic lesion underlies them). Tics are brief and unsustained involuntary movements of functionally related groups of skeletal muscles; they occur suddenly, intermittently, and irregularly, in contrast to the more continuous, rhythmic movements seen in tardive dyskinesia. Tics occur most commonly in the face, head, and neck regions; arms are less involved and legs are affected least often. The patient often has an irresistible urge to execute the tic, though he is usually able to resist this urge for brief periods of time. Tic disorders usually begin in childhood or adolescence and either remit spontaneously or remain unchanged and chronic. In recent years much attention

has been paid to a disorder called Gilles de la Tourette's syndrome, a tic disorder with age of onset between 2 and 13 years manifested by motor and vocal tics. The syndrome is more frequent in males. A family history will often reveal tic disorders in first-degree relatives. In most children the initial tic is motor and usually involves the face. Motor tics are expressed as blinking, shoulder shrugging, and explosive movements of the extremities. Vocal tics such as grunts, coughs, and snorts usually begin later. Coprolalia, the involuntary uttering of obscenities, occurs in a large percentage of patients. Tics usually show a waxing and waning over time, and the pattern of specific tics changes. The majority of patients seem to have a lifelong disorder that frequently improves in adult life. As many of these people are treated with neuroleptics, especially haloperidol, the possibility always exists that tardive dyskinesia will be superimposed on their basic movement disorder.

Dyskinetic movements are sometimes seen in patients with no identifiable or presumed CNS dysfunction. Occasionally patients with chronic schizophrenia who have no history of neuroleptic treatment will preset with spontaneous, involuntary movement disorders with a predominant orofacial distribution. In these patients, careful examination for poorly fitting dentures or an edentulous state must be made, as these conditions may simulate spontaneous or tardive dyskinesia. More commonly, stereotypies and mannerisms are found in chronic schizophrenia. A stereotypy is a purposeless movement carried out in a uniform and repetitive way; a mannerism is a stereotypic act incorporated into a goal-directed movement. The semblance of volitional activity and the complex nature of the movement serve to distinguish these movements from those seen in neurologic disorders.

TREMORS

Definition

The term tremor refers to involuntary, rhythmic, oscillating movements caused by alternating contractions of opposing agonist and antagonist muscles. Tremor may affect any part of the body, is exacerbated by anxiety, and ceases during sleep. Tremor is usually classified as static, postural, or intention (Table 16–9). Static tremor occurs when the affected part of the body is at rest; postural tremor is present when a posture such as extending the arms in front of the body is sustained; and intention tremor is present only during active movement directed toward an object.

Pathophysiologic Considerations

These tremors have various underlying pathophysiologic mechanisms that may involve central and pe-

Table 16–9. Classification of Tremors

Static
  Parkinson's disease
  Neuroleptics
  Encephalitis
  Manganese
  Carbon disulfide
  Carbon monoxide
  Reserpine
  Vascular lesion
  Tumor
  Trauma
Postural
  Essential
  Lithium
  Tricyclic antidepressants
  Neuroleptics
  Thyrotoxicosis
  Anxiety
  Severe fatigue
  Alcohol
  Uremic encephalopathy
  Hepatic encephalopathy
  Wilson's disease
Intention
  Multiple sclerosis
  Tumor
  Degenerative disease
  Phenytoin toxicity

ripheral structures. Dysfunction of the dopaminergic nigroneostriatal fibers typically causes the static tremor associated with Parkinson's disease. Postural tremors, like thyrotoxic tremor, are generally thought to be caused by increased sympathetic activity. Intention tremor is frequently regarded as resulting from a lesion of the brachium conjunctivum, which consists of the major outflow from the cerebellum; this type of tremor occurs typically in multiple sclerosis. Though these discrete, specific mechanisms exist, the physiology of any specific tremor may be more complex, as in toxic, metabolic, and infectious cases, which affect various areas of the CNS. In addition, normal people have a subtle physiologic tremor that appears to involve the lower motor neuron, muscle, and afferents back to the spinal cord.

Differential Diagnosis and Diagnostic Evaluation

Probably the most common cause of static tremor is parkinsonism, a disorder composed of tremor, rigidity, bradykinesia, and postural instability. Parkinson's disease, the idiopathic form, is frequently associated with dementia and depression. The tremor, which has a frequency of 4 to 6 Hz, is more often present in the hands and fingers than in the feet, and usually begins on one side of the body before spreading to the other side. It is a regular and coarse tremor; the term ''pill-rolling tremor'' has been used to describe the movement when the index finger flexes and extends in contact with the thumb. Actively moving the affected part will usually diminish or abolish the tremor. This tremor may be seen in other types of parkinsonism caused by encephalitis, manganese, carbon disulfide, carbon monoxide, reserpine, vascular lesions, tumor, and trauma. Neuroleptics frequently cause a parkinsonian state, with bradykinesia and rigidity being early and prominent signs that may persist, in some cases, weeks after drug cessation. While a resting tremor commonly occurs early in the course of Parkinson's disease, it occurs infrequently and late in neuroleptic-induced parkinsonism. A postural tremor is more commonly found. Also, while Parkinson's disease usually produces asymmetrical rigidity and akinesia in early stages, neuroleptic-induced parkinsonism is almost always symmetrical.

A common postural tremor is essential tremor, sometimes referred to as familial tremor, or, when it begins in old age, senile tremor. It frequently begins in early adulthood, though the prevalence increases with advancing age. The tremor is usually inherited in an autosomal dominant pattern and has a frequency in the range of 6 to 11 Hz and increasing amplitude with age. It is a progressive illness but may remain stable for prolonged periods of time. The tremor eventually becomes coarse and usually involves the hands and fingers, though the legs, lips, tongue, jaw, and head may become involved. It is accentuated by extending the arms; when the tremor is severe it may persist when limbs are at rest. Essential tremor can be differentiated from Parkinson's disease by the absence of bradykinesia, postural instability, rigidity, and micrographia. Alcohol ingestion will frequently cause a transient reduction of essential tremor, and some physicians have suggested that people with essential tremor have a higher incidence of alcoholism. Tricyclic antidepressants and lithium may increase tremor amplitude in essential tremor.

Other causes of postural tremor that cause a fine, rapid tremor include thyrotoxicosis, anxiety, severe fatigue, tricyclic antidepressants, and lithium. Lithium frequently causes a fine tremor of the hands that occurs at therapeutic levels. The tremor worsens with outstretching the arms, writing, and bringing food to the mouth, but it may also be present at rest. The incidence of lithium tremor decreases with time during lithium maintenance but may persist for years in some patients who continue to take lithium. A coarsening of the tremor may indicate that the lithium has reached toxic levels; other neurotoxic indicators are vomiting, diarrhea, weakness, ataxia, dysarthria, and muscle twitching. Rarely, severe lithium intoxication will produce persisting neurologic sequelae including resting tremor and cogwheel rigidity. Also, lithium at therapeutic levels may potentiate the parkinsonian tremor in people being treated with neuroleptics. A postural, irregular tremor may be found in alcoholic patients as a withdrawal phenomenon during an abstinent period or as a permanent tremor in a chronic alcoholic. The effects of ataxia and peripheral neuropathy may also affect this tremor. Other causes of postural tremor are uremia, hepatic failure, and Wilson's disease.

Disease of the cerebellum and brachium conjunctivum can cause intention tremors. The tremors begin and worsen progressively as the limb gets closer to its target, as in the finger-to-nose test. The tremor whose frequency is 3 to 5 Hz, needs to be distinguished from limb ataxia, which is a dysmetria rather than a rhythmic oscillatory tremor. Tremor is common in patients with multiple sclerosis and tumors and in degenerative diseases of the cerebellum and tegmentum of the midbrain. Intention tremor is also a common sign of phenytoin toxicity; ataxia and nystagmus may also be seen.

DYSTONIA

Definition

Dystonic movements are sustained, involuntary, twisting movements that affect muscles in the limbs, neck, trunk, or face. The movements may be generalized, segmental (occurring in contiguous body parts), or focal (occurring in a single body part) and are usually not present during sleep. They are usually slow movements and in some cases may present as a spasm resulting in a fixed posture.

Clinical Presentation

There are many common manifestations. Sustained, forced closure of the eyelids through contraction of the orbicularis oculi, called blepharospasm, is the most common dystonia of the upper face. Involvement of the lower face, jaw, and tongue is called oromandibular dystonia. Blepharospasm and oromandibular dystonia occurring together in a patient is referred to as Meige syndrome. Extension to the pharynx, tongue, and larynx may lead to dysphagia, dysarthria, and dysphonia. In torticollis, involvement of neck muscles leads to tilting of the head and elevation of the shoulder. When the trunk is affected, lordosis, scoliosis, kyphosis, tortipelvis, and opisthotonos with severe arching of the back may be seen. Various twisted postures may be observed in the arms and legs.

The dystonias are usually divided into primary and secondary forms. The primary dystonias are hereditary or have no known cause. The secondary dystonias are associated with other neurologic disorders, infections, toxins, injuries, drugs, and emotional disorders. The origin of dystonic movements is largely unknown, though involvement of the basal ganglia-thalamo-cortical circuits is likely.

Differential Diagnosis and Diagnostic Evaluation

In a psychiatric population, the secondary dystonias are more common. Neuroleptics, drugs that block dopamine receptors, frequently cause dystonic reactions. These reactions are more likely with the use of high-potency neuroleptics like haloperidol. Other agents such as metoclopramide and prochlorperazine, used for their gastrointestinal and antiemetic properties, cause similar reactions.

Acute dystonia may appear within hours of a single dose of a neuroleptic, and most reactions will occur within several days of initiating treatment; such reactions may reappear when the dosage is increased or as serum levels increase after administration of parenteral long-acting depot preparations. These dystonic reactions can be quickly relieved by administering parenteral anticholinergic agents such as benztropine. The incidence of dystonia has been estimated to be 2.5% to 5% following use of neuroleptics. Patients with hypoparathyroidism and hypocalcemia may be more sensitive to developing this reaction. These acute dystonic reactions are frequently very frightening and painful. Severe dystonic reactions may cause rhabdomyolysis resulting in increased serum creatine phosphokinase levels and, rarely, myoglobinuria. As dystonic reactions sometimes can be affected by suggestion, they may be mistaken for hysterical reactions.

In adults, common dystonic reactions following neuroleptics are blepharospasm, opisthotonos, trismus, twisting of the jaw, protrusion or twisting of the tongue, glossopharyngeal contractions, and torticollis. Forced upward deviation of the eyes, called oculogyric crisis, is a common reaction but may also be seen as a consequence of encephalitis. While adults tend to have dystonic movements restricted to the neck, face, tongue, and upper extremities, children tend to have more generalized involvement of the trunk and extremities, resembling the pattern of distribution of dystonic movement seen in primary dystonia of children and adults.

Prolonged use of neuroleptics can lead to tardive dystonia, a persistent dystonic reaction, similar to tardive dyskinesia in that it occurs while taking a neuroleptic or soon after discontinuation of the drug and may be ameliorated by increasing the dosage. The dystonia may persist unchanged for months or years and may coexist with movements of tardive dyskinesia. Patients with Parkinson's disease may develop dystonic postures as part of their illness or as a result of medicine taken for treatment of parkinsonism.

There are other, less common diseases that also need to be ruled out. Wilson's disease can be evaluated with serum ceruloplasmin and copper levels, 24-hour urinary copper excretion, and slit-lamp examination. Genetic diseases such as lipidosis, hexosaminidase deficiency, gangliosidosis, and Hallervorden-Spatz disease need to be considered. Toxins such as manganese and carbon monoxide may result in dystonic reactions. Other causes include encephalitis, head trauma, focal cerebrovascular injury, and brain tumor.

Dystonic movements are commonly misdiagnosed as hysteria for several reasons: they may seem bizarre; they may appear only with certain actions, while other acts using the same muscles may be carried out normally; they may be relieved by trick actions; they are made worse by stress and fatigue and lessened with relaxation; there may be evidence of psychopathology; and there is no apparent physical cause. All of these features may be seen in dystonia of any type. Hysterical dystonia appears to be relatively rare but may be diagnosed with clear evidence such as resolution of symptoms with psychotherapy. Dystonia of organic origin does not usually improve spontaneously. Other suspicious signs of hysterical dystonia are inappropriate weakness, unusual sensory complaints, self-inflicted injuries, and multiple somatic complaints. The diagnosis should be made with extreme caution as primary and secondary dystonias may present in an idiosyncratic way. Also, as various CNS disorders may lead to psychopathologic symptoms as well as dystonic movements, having emotional symptoms does not exclude an organic cause. In addition, it is well known clinically that conversion reactions may occur concomitantly with and be similar to organically caused symptoms in the same patient.

The primary dystonias include those with hereditary patterns, called hereditary torsion dystonia or dystonia musculorum deformans, and those without any known cause. Three varieties of hereditary dystonia have been proposed: autosomal dominant, sex-linked recessive, and autosomal recessive. The only neurologic abnormality is dystonic movement. Any associated neurologic deficits should suggest a secondary dystonia. Laboratory tests are usually normal, and any abnormality in the EEG, CSF, or CT scan may also indicate a secondary dystonia. There is no laboratory test to diagnose primary dystonia; the diagnosis depends on lack of evidence of any environmental or disease process that could cause the symptoms. The primary dystonias are slowly progressive, persistent disorders that may plateau at any point. They almost always begin

as an action dystonia, the dystonic movement occurring with certain voluntary motor activity. With time, dystonic postures may develop. By contrast, secondary dystonias usually begin at rest or with sustained postures. Children frequently develop generalized dystonia, whereas adults more commonly develop focal dystonias involving the neck, face, and upper extremities. With progression of the illness, dystonia commonly spreads contiguously from one body part to another.

NEUROLEPTIC MALIGNANT SYNDROME

Definition

Neuroleptic malignant syndrome (NMS) is a potentially lethal disorder consisting primarily of hyperthermia and rigidity in patients taking neuroleptics. Once the syndrome occurs, it may progress rapidly, with development of diffuse muscular rigidity, akinesia, tremors, and dystonic reactions either before or concomitant to the onset of fever. Body temperature may reach 42° C. Abnormal autonomic function is manifested by tachycardia, labile blood pressure, severe diaphoresis, sialorrhea, and incontinence. Altered levels of consciousness range from mild unresponsiveness and agitation to stupor and coma. Dysphagia, dysarthria, and dyspnea may also occur. Catatonic behavior with mutism and posturing may dominate the clinical picture.

Until recently, NMS had been considered a rare disorder; now it has gained attention and is being reported more frequently. It is likely that partial NMS syndromes with moderate symptoms exist, and in other cases incipient forms are terminated by the immediate cessation of neuroleptics prompted by the increasing awareness of this disorder. All neuroleptics have been implicated in NMS but high-potency neuroleptics as well as long-acting depot preparations seem to present a greater risk. Further predisposing factors may include an excited manic state, prior physical exhaustion and dehydration, high doses of neuroleptics, and, possibly, concomitant use of lithium. Withdrawal of dopaminergic drugs has also been reported to cause NMS. Asymptomatic exposure to neuroleptics during prior courses of treatment has been reported in patients who develop NMS. In addition, the syndrome may develop hours to months after the initial drug exposure. After resolution of NMS, in some cases neuroleptics may be restarted without return of symptoms, while in others the same florid syndrome will recur.

Pathophysiologic Considerations

After the cessation of oral neuroleptics, NMS typically lasts 5 to 10 days; after long-acting depot injections, the course may be weeks, reflecting persistently elevated neuroleptic levels. The mortality rate has been estimated as high as 20%, though this figure may be artificially high because only the worst cases tend to be reported in the literature. Fatality can result from respiratory or renal failure, arrhythmias, and cardiovascular collapse. Important causes of morbidity include thromboembolism, aspiration pneumonia, and acute renal failure. Occasionally, persistent, residual neurologic disorders will occur. Postmortem histopathologic examinations of the CNS have failed to demonstrate specific structural changes.

The cause of NMS is complex and probably involves several factors. There is evidence that neuroleptics, through dopamine blockade in the hypothalamus and possibly the limbic system, alter thermoregulatory control and lead to hyperthermia. Thermodetection in the hypothalamus may involve noradrenergic, serotoninergic, and cholinergic pathways, but central dopaminergic neurons are also involved. Other autonomic derangements such as tachycardia, labile blood pressure, and diaphoresis are also thought to be caused by disregulation of hypothalamic centers. Also, through basal ganglia mechanisms, neuroleptics cause profound rigidity and tremor. The resulting intense muscle contractions liberate large quantities of heat, contributing to the hyperthermic state. Elevations of serum CPK occur from myonecrosis from this sustained muscular contraction. A peripheral defect in calcium migration at the sarcoplasmic reticulum has been hypothesized but not proven. It remains unclear what predisposing factors enable this syndrome to develop in some patients while so many people use neuroleptics without adverse effects.

Differential Diagnosis (Table 16–10)

Though NMS typically occurs while the patient is on neuroleptics, other causes must be ruled out. Fever and CNS abnormalities present a wide differential diagnosis that includes infectious, neurologic, toxic, and metabolic causes. Encephalitis, tetanus, strychnine

Table 16–10.   Disorders with Similar Presentation

Psychogenic catatonia
Heatstroke
Malignant hyperthermia
Withdrawal from anti-parkinsonian medication
Dopamine-depleting agents
Viral encephalitis
Lithium toxicity
Tetanus
Monoamine oxidase inhibitor overdose
Strychnine poisoning
CNS mass lesions
Hypocalcemia

poisoning, and hypocalcemia need to be considered. All of these possibilities must be explored because psychiatric patients frequently have concomitant medical illness.

Any abnormality on examination of CSF or brain scan should alert the physician to an alternative diagnosis, as these tests are typically normal in NMS. Recent use of inhalation anesthetics or depolarizing muscle relaxants may indicate the development of malignant hyperthermia, a pharmacogenetic disorder affecting skeletal muscle that leads to rigidity, hyperthermia, shock, and death in a high percentage of susceptible individuals (see Chapter 14). Muscle relaxation can be achieved with pancuronium bromide and curare in NMS but not in malignant hyperthermia. Patients on neuroleptics are also susceptible to the development of heat stroke. Unlike NMS, heat stroke usually presents with lack of sweating and an absence of rigidity. Finally, acute catatonia in patients untreated with neuroleptics may present with a syndrome identical to NMS. When such patients are also on neuroleptics, it is not possible to determine whether the psychiatric disorder alone or the neuroleptic treatment is the cause of the syndrome. In such cases, withdrawal of neuroleptics and consideration of other therapeutic interventions becomes necessary.

Diagnostic Evaluation

Several laboratory abnormalities are commonly found in NMS, though none is diagnostic of NMS. Leukocytosis with a shift to the left is seen frequently. Serum creatine phosphokinase (CPK) may be markedly elevated, reflecting a state of myonecrosis, and serum aldolase may be increased. Elevated serum CPK is also seen frequently in agitated patients and in those receiving intramuscular injections. Myoglobinuria may result from progression of rhabdomyolysis, with acute renal failure resulting in some instances. Raised serum transaminases, lactic dehydrogenase, and alkaline phosphatase levels can be seen. Because dehydration is common, BUN is frequently elevated. CSF, CT scan, isotope brain scan, and EEG are usually normal, though EEG may show nonspecific slowing.

AFFECTIVE DISORDERS

DEPRESSION

Definition

Dysphoric mood, i.e., sadness, low spirits, or "feeling blue," is experienced transiently by healthy indi-

Table 16–11. Diagnostic Criteria for Major Depression (DSM III)[74a]

Dysphoric mood or loss of interest or pleasure in all or almost all usual activities and pastimes

At least four of the following present nearly every day for a period of at least 2 weeks:

Poor appetite or significant weight loss (when not dieting), or increased appetite or significant weight gain

Insomnia or hypersomnia

Psychomotor agitation or retardation (but not merely subjective feelings of restlessness or being slowed down)

Loss of interest or pleasure in usual activites, or decrease in sexual drive not limited to a period when patient is delusional or hallucinating

Loss of energy; fatigue

Feelings of worthlessness, self reproach, or excessive or inappropriate guilt (either may be delusional)

Complaints or evidence of diminished ability to think or concentrate, such as slowed thinking, or indecisiveness not associated with marked loosening of associations or incoherence

Recurrent thoughts of death, suicidal ideation, wishes to be dead, or suicide attempt

Table 16–12. Classification of Major Depression

Chronology
  Primary
  Secondary
Polarity
  Unipolar (major depression single episode; recurrent)
  Bipolar disorder
By signs and symptoms of episode
  Melancholic, nonmelancholic
  Psychotic, nonpsychotic
Other proposed categories
  Chronicity
  Family history

viduals. It is also identified in others through their speech, facial expression, posture, or movement. When it occurs in the setting of life's problems, it is accepted as normal by the individual and others, and it takes a predictable course of lessening over a period of days to weeks.

When dysphoric mood is persistent and intense and is accompanied by other characteristic signs and symptoms, a syndrome of major depression is present (Table 16–11). The individual may seek medical attention himself, feeling that something is wrong, or he may be brought by family or friends. An explanation for the symptoms and signs may or may not be offered.

Depressed patients frequently have low self-regard. They are characteristically pessimistic; they may feel unable to help themselves and think that there is no hope of improvement. Thoughts of death occur and may be followed by suicidal ideas, plans, and behavior.

Depressed patients often complain of impaired mental efficiency. They report difficulty concentrating and slowed thoughts. Symptomatic depressive patients, especially older ones, may perform poorly on intellectual tasks and may appear confused. These difficulties remit when the depression abates.

Depressed patients demonstrate abnormalities in physiologic function including disruption in the sleep pattern. There may be marked slowing of speech and movement to the point of mute immovability; such patients also may be agitated and restless. Taste and other perceptions may be dulled. Appetite is often decreased and the patient may lose weight. Constipation can develop. Sexual interest may diminish, and indeed there may be no enjoyment of any activities.

Some severely depressed patients have a psychotic

mental content, that is, delusions (fixed false beliefs), hallucinations, or both. The delusional ideas are generally consistent with feelings of worthlessness and self-contempt; the patient may have delusions of guilt or of deserved persecution and punishment. Other common delusional themes are personal poverty and ruin or catastrophe involving loved ones or possibly the entire world. When hallucinations occur they are usually auditory and consist of voices describing the patient as evil and worthless, deserving of suffering or death.

Anxiety and its physical concomitants may be part of the depressive syndrome. Depressed patients may further complain of fatigue and of a variety of vague aches and pains. Such physical complaints may be what brings the patient to medical attention. Sometimes delusional ideas about bodily malfunction are expressed.

Depression is an episodic disorder. Illness episodes last for a period of months. Patients usually regain apparent normal mental health between episodes, although in some cases only partial remission of symptoms occurs. Whereas some have single episodes, most patients have recurrences of illness. Depression may occur throughout life.

Classification

Many ways of subtyping depression have been proposed. Early categories referred to the circumstances of the episode, including presumptions about cause, and to the kinds of signs and symptoms and their severity. Various terms were used, defined vaguely. Systems such as DSM III that have developed recently in this country incorporate operational definitions and longitudinal history and have attempted to avoid etiologic connotations.[65]

Two subtypes of depression based on signs and symptoms of the episode have received some validation from empirical studies. One subtype is defined by the presence of features considered melancholic in DSM III (Table 16–12). This category has also been referred to as "endogenomorphic." Neither term connotes constitutional or biological origin, as did the older word, "endogenous," which was contrasted with the terms "neurotic" or "reactive," the reliability and validity of which are uncertain at this time. The other subtype is defined by the presence of psychotic phenomena in the narrower sense (Table 16–12). This usage contrasts with earlier uses of the term, in which "psychotic" referred merely to severity and was contrasted with "neurotic," which implied, among other things, mild intensity of signs and symptoms.

Unipolar versus bipolar illness is a distinction based on longitudinal history.[74a] By convention, the term unipolar affective disorder (major depression in DSM III) is applied to patients with one or more (recurrent) depressive episodes. Bipolar affective disorder denotes any patient with an episode of mania. Patients initially considered to have unipolar illness may be reclassified as bipolar during the course of their illness. Unipolar illness is more prevalent.

Another dichotomy based on longitudinal history is primary versus secondary illness, a distinction introduced by Feighner and associates.[74b] Primary depression is that which occurs without other antecedent major psychiatric syndromes. Secondary depression is that which occurs after such a condition, or a life threatening medical illness, is already established. For clinicians and investigators the implications are that treatment and prognostication begin with consideration of the primary disorder, and that pathophysiologies to be discerned will probably be related to that of the primary disorder.

Other subgroupings of depression may be useful for investigators and clinicians. While depression is predominantly an episodic disorder, chronic major depression, which has a poorer prognosis, occurs in some patients; chronicity is conventionally defined as an episode lasting for more than 2 years. Some validity has been demonstrated for classifying depressive illness based on the age at onset of the first episode. Further, Winokur and co-workers proposed subgrouping primary unipolar affective illness based on family history of major syndromes in first-degree relatives— familial depression, in which relatives have depression; sporadic depression, in which they do not have psychiatric disorders; and depressive spectrum disorders, in which relatives have alcoholism or sociopathy.[74c]

Pathophysiologic Considerations

Neither the pathophysiology nor the etiology of depressive illness is understood. As McHugh and Slavney have pointed out, since the time of Sydenham the characteristic sequence of progress in medicine has been from describing syndromes, to defining morbid anatomies and pathophysiologies, and finally to determining etiologies.[74d] For depressive illness, as with most other disorders dealt with in psychiatry, physicians still work at the level of the identification of syndromes. Interestingly, this limitation has led to a developing rigor in syndrome definition and classification, as described above, that is in the forefront among medical specialties.

Patients often offer or seek explanations for episodes of depressive illness in terms of the circumstances of their lives. Physicians may come to appreciate individual patients' styles and vulnerabilities that are understandably problematic in the face of particular events. However, patients also present with degrees or kinds of signs and symptoms that are not understandable, with or without a reasonable story associated with them. Hence, general theories of causation for depressive illness that have focused solely on apparent or obscure meaningful connections have limited use in clinical practice.

Various medical and neurologic disorders have been known to be associated with depressive syndromes, and some medications may produce depression; these considerations and others further support the role of constitutional processes in the origin of some depressions.

Indirect evidence for the influence of abnormal brain neurotransmitter function in the pathophysiology of major depression has been suggested by the effect of drugs in animals and man. Reserpine can produce a suppression of behaviors in animals and a depressive syndrome in man. This drug depletes brain monoamine neurotransmitters. Monoamine oxidase–inhibiting and monoamine re-uptake–inhibiting drugs have antidepressant properties and reverse the behavioral and neurochemical effects of reserpine.

Early formulations of the neurotransmitter dysfunction hypothesis focused on deficits of synaptic release of norepinephrine or serotonin in depression. More recently, indirect measurements in patients have implicated other neurotransmitters such as dopamine and acetylcholine in subgroups of patients. With advances in neurobiology, more complex formulations have been proposed that take into account our understanding of neurotransmitter and drug receptors; some evidence for synaptic hyperfunction in depressive patients has emerged from clinical investigations.

Abnormalities of neurovegetative regulation have been described during depressive episodes. Hypercortisolemia, representing hyperfunction of the hypothalamic-adrenocortical axis, occurs in a large proportion of depressive patients and is revealed by the dexamethasone suppression test. Abnormalities of other neuroendocrine challenge tests have also been described, including a blunted thyrotropin response to TRH. Abnormalities in sleep patterns, including shortened REM latency, have been demonstrated in depressed patients; it is interesting that antidepressant drugs suppress REM, and that REM deprivation has an antidepressant effect.

A variety of other new investigative tools, including brain imaging techniques, are being used in an effort to elucidate the pathophysiology of depression. Abnormalities in CT scans in depressed patients, for example, have been correlated with the patient's age at onset of illness and the presence of reversible cognitive impairment.

Depressive illness occurs in families, suggesting heredity or familial environment as causal components. Monozygotic versus dizygotic twin concordance ratios support a hereditary factor, as do adoption studies of twins. There is a familial link with alcoholism and sociopathy, as well. Neurotransmitter abnormalities may be an expression of this genetic predisposition; in normal subjects without a personal history of depression, those with and those without family history of depression were differentiated in one report on the basis of cerebrospinal fluid concentrations of monoamine neurotransmitter metabolites.

Presumably, a variety of pathophysiologies and etiologies will be elucidated within what is already a heterogeneous disorder at the syndrome level.

Diagnostic Evaluation and Differential Diagnosis
(Table 16–13)

Physicians seeing patients with depressive complaints should consider whether the severity of the signs and symptoms indicates that evaluation and management in a psychiatric hospital is necessary. If such questions arise, psychiatric consultation is appropriate. Patients with depression are at greater risk for suicide than patients with other psychiatric disorders; older patients and male patients are at especially high risk. Such patients need not be delusional or hallucinating. Depressed patients, especially if delusional, may also commit homicide. Physicians need to ask depressed patients about thoughts of injury to self or others throughout their illness. Patients who are profoundly anorexic may develop severe, life threatening weight loss and dehydration—another indication for hospitalization. Finally, the presence of psychotic symptoms alone may be an additional general indication that outpatient management will not be adequate.

The possibility that depressive signs and symptoms may be iatrogenic should be considered. Various drugs used in the treatment of cardiovascular disease have been associated with depressive symptoms or side ef-

Table 16–13. Differential Diagnosis of Major Depression

Other affective disorders
  Dysthymic disorder
  Cyclothymic disorder
  Atypical depression
  Atypical bipolar disorder
Other psychiatric syndromes
  Dementia
    Primary degenerative dementia
    Multi-infarct dementia
  Organic affective syndrome
  Chronic schizophrenia
  Schizoaffective disorder
  Somatization disorder
  Bereavement
  Substance abuse (e.g., alcohol, sedative hypnotics)
Other medical disorders
  Drug induced
  Infectious
  Endocrine
  Neoplastic
  Collagen
  Neurologic
  Nutritional

fects. The historical use of reserpine was mentioned above, and other antihypertensive agents such as alpha methyldopa and beta blockers have also been implicated. In addition, quinidine and related antiarrhythmic agents and calcium channel blockers can have similar effects. Antiparkinsonian agents such as levodopa and dopamine receptor agonists may exacerbate or produce depressive symptoms in these patients. Withdrawal from chronic d-amphetamine use may precipitate depression. Treatment with major tranquilizers may also lead to new depressive symptoms in some psychiatric patients.

Certain infectious diseases are often accompanied by depressive symptoms. Viral pneumonia and hepatitis are among these, as are general paresis and tuberculosis.

Endocrine dysfunction should be ruled out on the basis of the patient history, physical examination, and laboratory tests. Hypothyroidism, hyperparathyroidism, and Cushing's and Addison's diseases need to be considered. Specific treatment of these underlying disorders may be associated with remission of depressive symptoms. The postpartum state is a time of rapid endocrine change, when depressive symptoms may appear or recur.

Various nutritional deficits are associated with depressive signs and symptoms. These include niacin, folate, and B_{12} deficiencies.

Depression can occur in the setting of brain disease with known neuropathology. Alzheimer's disease can be complicated by secondary depression. Stroke patients, particularly those with cortical lesions of the left hemisphere near the frontal lobe, are at risk for depressive syndrome. Frontal lobe brain tumors also may produce depressive symptoms. Depressive symptoms are a frequent concomitant of Parkinson's disease and may be an early manifestation of Huntington's chorea. Demyelinating illness should also be considered.

Life threatening physical illness may be accompanied by depression. Among the group of malignant disorders, carcinoma of the pancreas may be especially likely to have depressive symptoms associated with it.

Depressive illness may sometimes be hard to differentiate from other psychiatric disorders (Table 16–2). When there is uncertainty in the differential diagnosis between depression and other disorders with poorer prognosis, such as schizophrenia and degenerative dementia, efforts should be made to treat the more benign disorder adequately. The diagnosis will eventually be clarified by following the course of the illness.

Depressive syndromes may also occur superimposed on other established psychiatric disorders (secondary depression), such as schizophrenia or substance abuse. Acute efforts are first directed at adequate treatment of the primary disorder. The course and prognosis are those of the primary psychiatric illness.

ELATION

Definition

Elation (euphoria) is a normal human emotion. It is recognized in ourselves and others in relation to happy events.

Some patient's euphoria is intense and persistent and is accompanied by other signs and symptoms of the manic syndrome (Table 16–14). Many of these features are the opposite of the features of depression. In contrast to depressed patients, for example, their attitude toward themselves is one of self-satisfaction, and they are pompous and grandiose concerning their talents. Manic patients, however, are not always predominantly or consistently elated; irritability, in particular, may be prominent.

When psychotic phenomena are part of the manic syndrome, their content usually is consistent with the patient's elevated mood and inflated self-regard. The patient may have grandiose delusions, saying, for example, that he has superhuman powers or is himself a divine being. A manic patient may express persecutory delusions that less talented and jealous people are attempting to frustrate his plans.

Manic patients experience increased mental and physical energy. They speak rapidly and often. They

Table 16–14. Diagnostic Criteria for Mania (DSM III)

One or more distinct periods with a predominantly elevated, expansive, or irritable mood. The elevated or irritable mood must be a prominent part of the illness and relatively persistent, although it may alternate or intermingle with depressive mood

Duration of at least 1 week (or any duration if hospitalization is necessary), during which, for most of the time, at least three of the following symptoms have persisted (four, if the mood is only irritable) and have been present to a significant degree:

Increase in activity (either socially, at work, or sexually) or physical restlessness

More talkative than usual or feeling pressure to keep talking

Flight of ideas or the subjective experience that thoughts are racing

Inflated self-esteem (grandiosity, which may be delusional)

Decreased need for sleep

Distractibility, i.e., attention too easily drawn to unimportant or irrelevant external stimuli

Excessive involvement in activities whose high potential for painful consequences is not recognized, e.g., buying sprees, sexual indiscretions, foolish business investments, reckless driving

feel that their thoughts "race." Their speech can become difficult or impossible to follow; they jump from one idea to another, and in severe cases they may be totally incoherent. They are restless and overactive. Sometimes their movements may include periods of bizarre posturing. Their need for sleep may be reduced and they may go without sleep for days. Concomitant physical exhaustion can pose a health risk to frail individuals. Manic patients display increased interest in the environment; they are socially intrusive and their sexual drive is increased.

Patients with manic illness do not realize the abnormality of their feelings, thoughts, and behavior. They generally do not bring themselves to physicians and they are poorly compliant with treatment efforts. Their lack of judgment may lead to physical harm provoked from others, to social embarrassment, and to financial difficulty.

Bipolar illness is characterized by symptomatic episodes, manic or depressed, with intervals of normal functioning in between. Patients may have their first episode of illness between childhood and old age; bipolar patients tend to be younger than unipolar patients at the time of their first illness episode. Bipolar illness tends to be more severe in that there are more frequent symptomatic episodes and more social impairment. The rate of suicide may also be higher in bipolar patients.

Classification

Current nomenclature treats manic episodes as more homogeneous than depressive episodes. Like depressions, they are denoted as having or not having concomitant psychotic symptoms. The presence of psychotic symptoms may be related in part to overall syndrome severity.

Further distinctions within mania have been proposed. Kraepelin described grades of severity in mania from "hypomanic" to a "delirious mania" in which patients are incoherent and near stuporous.[74e] Some have suggested that predominant euphoria or predominant irritability has predictive validity. Others point to subgroups in which the manic syndrome is chronic, in which, with depressive episodes, mania is frequently recurrent (rapid cyclers), or in which manic episodes apparently occur alone—so-called unipolar mania. The validity of these distinctions remains to be assessed further.

Pathophysiologic Considerations

The pathophysiology and etiology of bipolar illness is unknown compared to major depression. It is regarded as a more homogeneous disorder with stronger biologic determinants. The fact that manic-like signs and symptoms can be manifestations of drug intoxication, metabolic abnormalities, and brain disease with definable neuropathologies is one argument for applying the illness model to bipolar disorder.[74f]

Studies of biologic measurements related to neurotransmitter activity have indicated differences between bipolar and unipolar patients during depressive episodes. These differences include monoamine metabolite concentrations in body fluids, degradative enzyme activity, and neuroendocrine parameters. Abnormal calcium ion metabolism has also been proposed. Bipolar patients generally differ from control subjects more than unipolar patients do, although this has not always been found.

Studies of bipolar patients have implicated increased dopaminergic neurotransmission in the pathophysiology of the manic syndrome. Drugs that enhance dopaminergic neurotransmission can elicit manic signs and symptoms, and drugs that block dopamine receptors are therapeutic in mania. However, evidence for dysfunction of the brain neurotransmitters norepinephrine and acetylcholine in bipolar patients has also been presented.

Family history studies and twin studies have supported a genetic contribution to the origin of bipolar illness; this contribution appears stronger than for unipolar illness. The prevalence of affective illness in first-degree family members is higher for bipolar than for unipolar patients. The concordance rates for monozygotic and dizygotic twin pairs is higher for bipolars. Evidence for chromosomal X-linkage in some bipolar pedigrees has been reported.

Treatment studies have indicated differences between bipolar and unipolar patients. Lithium carbonate

Table 16–15. Differential Diagnosis of Bipolar Disorder, Manic

Other affective disorders
  Bipolar disorder, mixed
  Cyclothymic disorder
  Atypical bipolar disorder
Other psychiatric disorder
  Chronic schizophrenia, especially paranoid type
  Schizoaffective disorder
  Organic affective syndrome
  Substance abuse or intoxication
Other medical disorders
  Drug-induced
  Infectious
  Endocrine
  Collagen
  Neurologic

may be more effective in relieving depressive symptoms in bipolar than in unipolar patients. Lithium may also be more effective than tricyclic antidepressants in preventing further episodes in bipolar patients in particular.

Diagnostic Evaluation and Differential Diagnosis
(Table 16–15)

Patients with apparent acute mania will often require psychiatric hospitalization even if they are not psychotic. As noted above, the potential adverse consequences of their behavior, if uncontrolled, are serious, and adequate medical assessment and treatment can often be achieved only in a hospital.

The cornerstone of evaluation is a thorough history, taken from family or friends as well as the patient, who may be unreliable and uncooperative. The history is combined with careful physical and neurologic examination and mental status examination.

Drug-induced states can have a manic form, and the history and examination may direct attention to substances of abuse or to medication prescribed for other disorders. D-amphetamine or phencyclidine have been described as producing manic signs and symptoms; the use of laboratory drug detection tests may assist the clinician. Treatment with oral steroids has also been associated with manic-like states. Treatment with antidepressant drugs or convulsive therapy may induce manic symptoms.

Endocrinopathies may be accompanied by mania. Examples are hyper- and hypothyroidism, Cushing's disease, and Addison's disease. Infectious disorders such as influenza and general paresis may induce a manic syndrome.

Brain disease with demonstrable structural abnormality or known neuropathology may produce manic-like syndromes and must be excluded on the basis of the history and examination. Frontal lobe dysfunction can produce affective lability and an uninhibited social behavior that must be distinguished from mania. Tumors in the diencephalic and third ventricle areas have been reported in association with manic syndromes. Cerebrovascular and demyelinating disease also need to be excluded. Patients with Huntington's chorea may develop a manic syndrome as the earliest feature.

Patients presenting with some but not all features of mania may also have several depressive signs and symptoms. In this instance the category bipolar disorder ''mixed type'' is used.

Other idiopathic psychiatric disorders need to be considered in the differential diagnosis of mania (Table 16–15). Patients with schizophrenia, particularly of the paranoid type, may appear manic if they are irritable, grandiose, and excited; here the history of premorbid functioning and family history are most important. In some patients with relatively acute onset and brief duration of illness, both manic and schizophrenic features may be present and the diagnosis is not clear. In such ''schizoaffective'' patients the family history and the course of illness are often those of affective disorder.

Other residual categories to be considered in the differential diagnosis are characterized by incomplete or mild syndromes. Cyclothymic disorder denotes recurrent partial or mild manic and depressive syndromes, while atypical bipolar disorder denotes mild or incomplete manic syndromes and a history of full major depressive episodes. The relationship of these categories to bipolar disorder remains to be explored.

ANXIETY

Definition

A feeling of apprehension and dread, anxiety is also a common part of normal human experience. Fear, a closely related emotion, is an apprehension concerning something that is immediate and dangerous, while anxiety is a sense of tension concerning possible difficulty and distress anticipated in the future.

When anxiety is very high, intellectual performance may be impaired. This state contrasts with mild anxiety, which may improve performance. People avoid situations that produce marked anxiety.

Patients complain to physicians about anxiety that is intense and prolonged. They also complain if their anxiety seems out of keeping with their situation. Anxiety syndromes seen by physicians include recurrent brief episodes of panic and persistent, less severe signs and symptoms (Table 16–16). Some patients experience both syndromes.

Anxiety, when intense, is typically accompanied by

Table 16–16. Diagnostic Criteria for Anxiety

Generalized anxiety disorder (DSM III)
  Generalized, persistent anxiety is manifested by symptoms from three of the following four categories:
    Motor tension: shakiness, jitteriness, jumpiness, trembling, tension, muscle aches, fatigability, inability to relax, eyelid twitch, furrowed brow, strained face, fidgeting, restlessness, easy startling
    Autonomic hyperactivity: sweating, heart pounding or racing, cold, clammy hands, dry mouth, dizziness, light-headedness, paresthesias (tingling in hands or feet), upset stomach, hot or cold spells, frequent urination, diarrhea, discomfort in the pit of the stomach, lump in the throat, flushing, pallor, high resting pulse and respiration rate
    Apprehensive expectation: anxiety, worry, fear, rumination, and anticipation of misfortune to self and others
    Vigilance and scanning: hyperattentiveness resulting in distractibility, difficulty in concentrating, insomnia, feeling "on edge," irritability, impatience
  The anxious mood has been continuous for at least 1 month.
Panic Disorder (DSM III)
  At least three panic attacks within a 3 week period in circumstances other than during marked physical exertion or in a life threatening situation. The attacks are not precipitated only by exposure to a circumscribed phobic stimulus.
  Panic attacks are manifested by discrete periods of apprehension or fear, and at least four of the following symptoms appear during each attack:
  Dyspnea
  Palpitations
  Chest pain or discomfort
  Choking or smothering sensations
  Dizziness, vertigo, or unsteady feelings
  Feelings of unreality
  Paresthesias (tingling in hands or feet)
  Hot and cold flashes
  Sweating
  Faintness
  Trembling or shaking
  Fear of dying, going crazy, or doing something uncontrolled during an attack

a variety of autonomic manifestations. Patients with anxiety accompanied by these somatic complaints may seek medical attention because of them; for example, they may be concerned about possible cardiac disease.

Anxiety disorders usually have their onset between the mid-teens and early thirties. The course is usually one of waxing and waning of symptoms, and the degree of disability is often mild.[74g] Patients often report both the occurrence of symptoms in settings that would be expected to produce mild anxiety, suggesting oversensitivity, and the occurrence of symptoms in the absence of apparent provocation.

Classification

Current nomenclature distinguishes two categories within anxiety disorders (Table 16–5). Generalized anxiety disorder is a syndrome consisting of chronic signs and symptoms. Panic disorder is marked by recurrent brief episodes of acute symptoms.

Pathophysiologic Considerations

Certain kinds of situations produce anxiety, such as when an important decision is required and the correct choice is ambiguous. The amount of anxiety elicited by the same situation varies in normal individuals. Apparently, states of extreme anxiety can be produced in all normal subjects by sufficiently extended exposure to severely stressful conditions. For example, "battle fatigue" can be produced in increasing percentages of infantry by increasing the duration of participation in combat.

Vulnerability to anxiety may be increased by various factors including fatigue and physical debility. A variety of medical illnesses may be associated with anxiety symptoms. Brain diseases with known neuropathology or brain injuries that impair intellectual capacity may render individuals susceptible to anxiety in relatively benign circumstances. Drugs such as hallucinogens that distort perception may have the same effect.

Persistent anxiety states may also follow severely frightening events. Learning may play a role in these cases and in other types of anxiety syndromes.

The anxiety syndromes defined above run in families. Family studies and twin studies suggest a genetic contribution to these disorders.

Certain somatic changes regularly accompany anxiety, mediated by hyperactivity of the sympathetic autonomic nervous system, via norepinephrine, and by adrenal medullary secretion of epinephrine. These changes include tremor, increased heart rate and blood pressure, perspiration, dilation of pupils, and reduced salivation and gastric acid secretion. Some physicians have argued that the cardiorespiratory changes themselves enhance anxiety. The beta receptor blocking agent propranolol can be effective in reducing somatic symptoms.[74h]

Certain signs and symptoms that accompany panic attacks can be exacerbated by hyperventilation. Respiratory alkalosis can produce light-headedness and vertigo, tingling in the fingertips, and even tetany.

Despite the prominence of somatic symptoms, patients with these disorders do not have a reduced life span. Furthermore, they do not have increased risk of disorders such as peptic ulcer and asthma that have been termed psychosomatic.

There is evidence that individuals with anxiety disorders differ in some physiologic measures from normal individuals. Also, in such patients, anxiety symptoms can be elicited by infusion of sodium lactate or

Table 16-17. Differential Diagnosis of Generalized Anxiety Disorder and Panic Disorder

Other anxiety disorders
　Phobic disorder
　Obsessive-compulsive disorder
Other psychiatric disorders
　Major depression
　Somatization disorder
　Substance abuse
　　Intoxication
　　Dependence, withdrawal
　Schizophrenia
　Dementia
Other medical disorders
　Cardiovascular
　Endocrine
　Neoplastic
　Neurologic

the noradrenergic drug yohimbine, or by administration of caffeine.[74i]

Diagnostic Evaluation and Differential Diagnosis

Patients suffering from anxiety generally do not require hospitalization. Evaluation and treatment in the clinic setting begins with thorough patient history and physical and mental status examination.

History-taking should include information concerning the amount of caffeinated beverages ingested as well as a drug history. Withdrawal from alcohol and sedative and hypnotic barbiturates or benzodiazepines can cause signs and symptoms of anxiety.

Medical illness must be considered when anxiety is chronic and unexplained. Cardiovascular disorders including arrhythmia—particularly paroxysmal atrial tachycardia, angina pectoris, and mitral valve prolapse—should be excluded. Endocrine disorders such as diabetes mellitus and parathyroid disease may be considered. Occult neoplasm, including pheochromocytoma, should be ruled out.

Certain brain diseases with known neuropathology may produce anxiety. The postconcussion syndromes are examples. Elderly patients with early dementia may show anxiety as an initial sign.

These anxiety disorders need to be differentiated from other psychiatric disorders, for which other treatment may be indicated (Table 16-17). Major depressive illness is often overlooked, and the clinician needs to be sensitive to affective symptoms, particularly when anxiety presents for the first time relatively late in life. Phobic disorders are distinguished by the specific stimuli that elicit the anxiety symptoms. Obsessional ideas and compulsive behavior are distinct phenomena that suggest other diagnoses, including obsessive-compulsive disorder.

EATING DISORDERS

ANOREXIA NERVOSA

Definition

Anorexia nervosa is characterized by a preoccupation with food and body weight, with behavior directed toward losing weight. The patient has a disturbance of body image and an intense fear of becoming fat despite a weight loss that can become severe. Refusal to maintain a minimally acceptable body weight for age and height is the essential diagnostic criterion for anorexia nervosa. Amenorrhea is present and may precede the loss of body weight.

Pathophysiologic Considerations

Most of the metabolic and physiologic changes found in anorexia nervosa are also present in starvation states and thus do not provide clues for the cause of this disorder. The metabolic aberrations caused by starvation revert to normal with nutritional rehabilitation and weight restoration.

Hematopoietic changes seen in anorexia nervosa include a leukopenia with a relative lymphocytosis. Leukopenia is associated with a hypocellularity of the bone marrow that reverses with clinical improvement. Although the granulocyte bactericidal capacity is reduced in anorectic patients, the risk of infection seems to be no greater in anorectics than in control subjects. However, the morbidity risk in an anorectic patient who does develop an infection may be much greater than in a healthy person because the anorectic patient has a reduced bactericidal capacity.

Impaired water diuresis is associated with a decreased glomerular filtration rate (GFR), which varies directly with the duration of malnutrition.

Elevation of serum enzymes reflecting liver dysfunction is not unusual in anorexia nervosa. Serum glutamic oxaloacetic transaminase (SGOT), lactic dehydrogenase (LDH), and alkaline phosphatase are the enzymes most frequently elevated. The elevation of these enzymes most likely reflects some fatty degeneration of the liver and can be found in both emaciated patients and in patients undergoing refeeding.

Cardiovascular abnormalities such as bradycardia, hypotension, tachycardia, and electrocardiographic changes are observed in malnourished patients with anorexia nervosa. ECG changes usually consist of flattened or inverted T waves and a depression of the ST segments. While there may be many mechanisms to explain the cardiac abnormalities in anorexia nervosa, such as decreased myocardial contractility or reduced muscle mass, these cardiac changes improve with weight gain.

Growth retardation observed in patients with anorexia nervosa may be due to aberrations of growth hormone or, in those patients with a long history of the illness, particularly those patients who engage in purging behaviors, to osteoporosis.

Brain CT scan in emaciated anorectic patients has shown enlargement of the cortical sulci and ventricles. These atrophic changes revert to normal with nutritional rehabilitation.

Most of the changes in the endocrine system may be understood as secondary to a malnourished state. These include the changes seen in thyroid function such as low serum triiodothyronine (T_3) and delayed TSH response to TRH. The reduced clearance rate of cortisol and the incomplete suppression of ACTH and cortisol by dexamethasone are seen in protein calorie malnutrition as well as in anorexia nervosa. The low 3-methoxy-4-hydroxyphenylglycol excretion seen in anorexia nervosa is related to weight loss.

Some of the physiologic changes observed in anorexia nervosa are not readily explained as a consequence of emaciation or diet and may represent a primary hypothalamic impairment or vulnerability. With regard to the hypothalamic-pituitary-ovarian axis, amenorrhea is found to occur in one fifth to one third of patients with anorexia nervosa before a substantial weight loss occurs; therefore, the amenorrhea cannot be attributed solely to the patient's emaciation. Also, after nutritional rehabilitation the return of the normal menstrual cycle lags behind the return of body weight and is associated with marked psychologic improvement. Prepubertal luteinizing hormone (LH) secretion patterns, absence of estrogen feedback on LH, and failure of LH response to clomiphene can persist despite normalization of weight.

Hypothalamic anatomic structures regulating feeding, sexual behavior, and menstrual activity, all of which are disturbed in anorexia nervosa, are strongly influenced by dopaminergic activity. The failure of L-dopa to induce normal growth hormone response in anorectic patients restored to normal weight suggests an impairment at postsynaptic dopamine receptors.

Clinical Presentation

Of all patients with anorexia nervosa, 95% are female. The incidence of anorexia nervosa has increased in the last ten years, based on the number of patients being treated in various hospitals and clinics. The age

Table 16–18. Diagnostic Criteria for Anorexia Nervosa

Intense fear of becoming obese, which does not diminish as weight loss progresses

Disturbance of body image, e.g., claiming to "feel fat" even when emaciated

Weight loss of at least 25% of original body weight; if the patient is under 18 years of age, weight loss from original body weight plus projected weight gain according to growth charts may be combined to make the 25%

Refusal to maintain body weight over a minimal normal weight for height and age

No known physical illness that would account for the weight loss

of onset follows a bimodal pattern of distribution, with peaks at 14½ and 18 years of age.

The term "anorexia" is a misnomer. Actual loss of appetite is rare unless the patient is emaciated. Patients with anorexia nervosa think about food constantly and may collect recipes and cook for the family and others. Anorectic adolescents lose weight by drastically decreasing their total food intake, particularly intake of high-carbohydrate and fat-containing foods. Commonly, these adolescents refuse to eat with their families or in public places. Some patients are unable to continuously restrict their intake and have episodes of binge eating. These binge eating episodes occur usually in secret and frequently at night. Binges are often followed by purging activities such as self-induced vomiting or laxative abuse.

Anorectic patients exhibit peculiar behaviors around food, such as hiding food in their rooms, cutting food into small pieces, rearranging the food on their plates, and surreptitiously disposing of food when in public places or at the family meal.

Extensive exercising regimens as well as a generalized increase in activity are commonly seen. As emaciation progresses, patients may lose the ability to sustain such a rigorous level of activity.

The body image distortion seen in anorexia nervosa reflects the patients' perceptions that they are at a normal weight or overweight. They fail to recognize their degree of emaciation and describe themselves as feeling fat. Severe body image distortion in the presence of profound weight loss may indicate a poorer outcome to treatment. The fear of gaining weight and becoming obese contributes to these patients' resistance to therapy.

Differential Diagnosis

The diagnosis of anorexia nervosa should be made only if the patient meets the diagnostic criteria, with the exception of the 25% loss of body weight (Table 16–18); there is no consensus of opinion or data as to the degree of weight loss required for the diagnosis of anorexia nervosa. The patient's refusal to maintain a

body weight over a minimum normal weight for age and height should be considered the essential criterion for the diagnosis of anorexia nervosa. Because patients often steadfastly deny the presence of symptoms, it is important that the physician speak with family and friends who have had an opportunity to observe the patient's behavior.

Anorexia nervosa can be distinguished from medical illnesses involving a true loss of appetite in that anorectic patients will lose their appetites only after they have become emaciated. Also, patients with a loss of appetite are not preoccupied with food or cooking, nor are they obsessed with a slender body image or involved in exercise programs to lose weight. Patients suffering from depression may report a loss of appetite and experience weight loss but do not become preoccupied with the calorie content of foods or spend an inordinate amount of time cooking and preparing foods. Patients with schizophrenia may have delusions about food but are seldom concerned with calorie content. Although these distinctions may be helpful in differentiating patients with anorexia nervosa from patients with a medical or psychiatric illness resulting in weight loss or loss of appetite, on occasion a patient may have both anorexia nervosa and a medical illness or another psychiatric illness; in these situations, both diagnoses should be made and treated.

Diagnostic Evaluation

If a physician suspects the diagnosis of anorexia nervosa, a consultation with a psychiatrist or a psychiatric clinic experienced in the diagnosis and treatment of eating disorders should be obtained. Prompt initiation of treatment is essential in order to prevent a prolongation of the disorder. A physical examination and some basic laboratory work should be performed, with particular attention to serum electrolytes and the electrocardiogram. Physical changes commonly seen in anorexia nervosa include amenorrhea, which may actually precede the weight loss, bradycardia, hypotension, and electrolyte disturbances, particularly in those patients who vomit or abuse laxatives or diuretics. In those patients who meet the diagnostic criteria, extensive workups are unnecessary and in fact delay effective treatment.

BULIMIA

Definition

Bulimia is an eating disorder characterized by episodic binge eating, i.e., the rapid consumption of high-calorie, easily ingested food in a short period of time. The patients are aware that the eating pattern is abnormal and may be filled with self-deprecating thoughts following a binge eating episode. Patients may express a fear of not being able to stop eating voluntarily. Bulimic patients, unlike those with anorexia nervosa, maintain their weight within a normal range but may have frequent fluctuations of 10 to 15 pounds. Anorexia nervosa patients may also binge and purge and should be distinguished from the normal-weight bulimic patients.

Pathophysiologic Considerations

Unlike anorexia nervosa, in which most of the physiologic and metabolic changes observed are due to the emaciated state, changes seen in bulimia are less well understood.

Both anorexia nervosa and bulimic patients who engage in self-induced vomiting or abuse purgatives and diuretics are susceptible to developing hypokalemic alkalosis. A metabolic acidosis may be seen in laxative abusers.

The severe dental attrition and erosion of tooth enamel may be due to binging on carbohydrates and to chronic vomiting of the acid contents of the stomach. Parotid gland enlargement is another common physical sign. Elevated serum amylase levels are often observed in patients who binge and purge. The underlying pathophysiologic basis for these changes is unclear.

Sudden deaths resulting from cardiac disturbances have been reported in those eating-disorder patients who binge and purge whether they are emaciated or within a normal weight range. Undoubtedly, multiple mechanisms for cardiac arrhythmias exist in these patients. Recent investigations have found cardiac rhythm disturbances despite normal serum electrolytes in normal-weight bulimia patients. A possible cause may be the stimulation of sympathetic centers within the hypothalamus.

Patients who have practiced self-induced vomiting for years are at greater risk for developing osteoporosis.

Electroencephalographic abnormalities such as epileptiform arrhythmias, a 6/second spike and wave, and 6 to 14/second spikes have been described in association with the malnourished state of anorexia nervosa and in association with binging and purging behaviors irrespective of weight status. EEG abnormalities in the bulimia subgroup may represent a constitutional predisposition to the illness.

With regard to endocrine functioning of the hypothalamic-pituitary-ovarian axis, some normal-weight bulimic patients have low FSH and LH levels compared with normal controls. Postpubertal bulimic patients of normal weight can have a loss of menstrual cycling and show an age-inappropriate secretion pattern for gonadotropins.

Most bulimic women show an abnormal response of growth hormone to thyroid-releasing hormone (TRH). In one study, normal-weight bulimics demonstrated a blunting of the TSH response to TRH; in another they responded normally. The meaning of these findings in bulimic patients is unclear at this time.

As for the adrenocortical axis, one half to two thirds of normal-weight bulimics fail to suppress to dexamethasone.

Clinical Presentation

The incidence of bulimia among adolescent girls has increased in the last few years. A recent survey of a college population revealed an incidence of about 15% in women.

Many bulimic patients purge following a binge by either inducing vomiting or abusing laxatives. Since bulimic patients try to keep the behavior secret, the disorder may first come to the attention of a dentist because of the severe tooth erosion that accompanies the vomiting behavior. Chronic vomiting and laxative abuse can lead to electrolyte imbalance and a metabolic alkalosis. These patients are susceptible to the development of cardiac arrhythmias that might lead to sudden death. Recent evidence suggests that these arrhythmias may be unrelated to low serum potassium and develop secondary to the purging behavior itself. The binge/purge cycle, once established, takes on an addictive quality, with some patients spending every waking moment planning binges, shopping for food, consuming the food during the binge, and afterwards, engaging in purging behaviors.

Differential Diagnosis

The diagnosis of bulimia should be made in those persons fitting the diagnostic classifications as suggested by the DSM III (Table 16–19). For the diagnosis of bulimia the patient should be in a normal weight range, although the bulimic patient's weight may fluctuate frequently because of alternating fasts and binges. The patient with anorexia nervosa may exhibit bulimic behaviors, such as binge eating and purging activities, but the degree of weight loss in the anorectic patient is more marked and indicates that anorexia nervosa be cited as the diagnosis. Some of the symptoms of bulimia may be present in certain neurologic diseases, but rarely does one see the entire syndrome. Neurologic disease such as epileptic equivalent seizures, tumors of the central nervous system, Klüver-Bucy syndromes, and the Kleine-Levin syndrome is distinguished from bulimia by the presence of the neurologic signs and symptoms and the absence of the

Table 16–19. Diagnostic Criteria for Bulimia

Recurrent episodes of binge eating (rapid consumption of a large
      amount of food in a discrete period of time, usually less than 2
      hours)
At least three of the following:
  Consumption of high-calorie, easily ingested food during a binge
  Inconspicuous eating during a binge
  Termination of such eating episodes by abdominal pain, sleep,
      social interruption, or self-induced vomiting
  Repeated attempts to lose weight by severely restrictive diets,
      self-induced vomiting, or use of cathartics or diuretics
  Frequent weight fluctuations greater than 10 pounds due to alter-
      nating binges and fasts
Awareness that the eating pattern is abnormal and fear of not being
      able to stop eating voluntarily
Depressed mood and self-deprecating thoughts following eating
      binges
The bulimic episodes are not due to anorexia nervosa or any known
      physical disorder

full psychiatric syndrome of bulimia. In the rare event that both a neurologic disease and bulimia are present, both diagnoses need to be made and appropriate treatment instituted.

Diagnostic Evaluation

The evaluation of the bulimic patient begins with a history and physical examination. Since bulimia is a secretive syndrome accompanied by much shame on the part of the patient, a sensitive and nonjudgmental approach to the history will help put the patient at ease and yield the most information. The clinician should be alert to the possibility of bulimia in those patients who present with complaints of fatigue, lethargy, and various gastrointestinal symptoms such as esophageal reflux, chronic "heartburn," or abdominal discomfort after eating. Questions regarding dental history, eating habits, and purging behaviors, specifically the use of laxatives, enemas, and diuretics and the self-induction of vomiting should be asked. On physical exam, the condition of the teeth and oral cavity should be noted. Enlargement and tenderness of the parotid glands and calluses on the dorsum of the hands may indicate chronic self-induced vomiting.

Laboratory investigation should include blood chemistries with particular attention to serum electrolytes, which may indicate a hypokalemic alkalosis or, in the case of laxative abuse, a metabolic acidosis. Also indicated is an electrocardiogram.

Once the diagnosis of bulimia is made, the patient should be referred to a therapist for treatment or to a psychiatric clinic experienced in the treatment of eating disorders.

ALCOHOL AND OTHER SUBSTANCE ABUSE

INTRODUCTION

Alcoholism and substance abuse are increasingly recognized as medical problems with complex biopsychosocial interactions. Myers reports that 6.3% of the population has had a substance abuse problem in the past 6 months, and Robins reports an 18% lifetime risk.[75,76] Over 200,000 deaths per year are alcohol related; these include death by accident, suicide, homicide, and medical complications.[77] In spite of a recent report by the beverage industry that total alcohol consumption has declined slightly, alcohol remains the most used and abused psychoactive chemical with the average annual consumption per person over age 14 being 2.77 gallons of absolute alcohol.[78] One third of the population hardly drinks at all; one third consumes an average of 14 drinks per week; and one tenth consumes half the alcohol sold. The ratio of alcoholism in males to females has been measured at 3:1 or more, depending on the population and culture studied.[79] Alcoholism begins in the teenage years and is a progressive and relapsing illness. Over 90% of high school students drink, 60% use drugs, and 9% of seniors use marijuana daily. One third of seventh graders have tried an illicit drug. With costs declining, cocaine use and abuse has spread rapidly, with 14% of high school students reporting use.[80]

The medical problems associated with substance abuse leading to morbidity and mortality include the effects of intoxication and overdose, withdrawal, and chronic use. Every organ system can be affected by alcoholism. Gastritis, ulcers, pancreatitis, liver disease, cardiomyopathy, anemia, neurologic complications, sexual dysfunction, and fetal alcohol syndrome are among the major complications. Cancer is increased in the mouth, tongue, larynx, esophagus, and liver. Though less than 10% of alcoholics develop cirrhosis, 11,000 die from liver disease annually. Withdrawal syndromes are often most dangerous when accompanied by medical illnesses such as pneumonia, liver failure, and subdural hematomas.

The medical and dental complications of drug abuse relate to poor personal care surrounding addictive drug abuse in addition to the drugs themselves. The use of unsterile needles, injection of mixtures of unknown quantities of impure substances, and the psychosocial problems associated with addiction to legal or illegal drugs are causes of these problems. Hepatitis occurs frequently in IV addicts and may be exacerbated by additional use of alcohol. The addict is more prone to lung diseases including pneumonia and tuberculosis. Other infections commonly experienced are cutaneous abscesses, endocarditis, mycotic aneurysms, septic arthritis, AIDS, osteomyelitis, meningitis, and brain abscess. Antigen antibody immune complexes resulting from these infections can lead to renal disease. Hypertension, tachycardia, and arrhythmia can result from stimulant use and may be a factor in sudden deaths that occur with cocaine use. Chronic drug use can reduce sexual performance and desire. Studies indicate that tetrahydrocannabinol decreases serum testosterone in males. Poor nutrition and vitamin deficiency contribute to illness and lowered resistance to illness. Perinatal effects of drug addiction include teratogenicity, prematurity, withdrawal symptoms after birth, and maternal neglect.[81]

SUBSTANCE ABUSE

Definition

As with many other chronic illnesses, while it is easier to make the diagnosis of alcoholism or substance abuse late in the course of the illness, prevention and treatment are easier and more effective when the diagnosis is made early. One major problem in making the diagnosis early is that one of the hallmarks of the illness is the tendency for the patient to deny that there is a problem until he has been confronted by others or is seriously impaired.

Early diagnosis is enhanced by a high index of suspicion, an awareness of the defensiveness that often surrounds the addictive process, and attention to the signs and symptoms of substance abuse. One of our major problems is that, while 18% of the U.S. population has a lifetime incidence of substance abuse, only a small percentage of those with a problem ever deals with it, whether by seeing a doctor or attending Alcoholics Anonymous.[76] In an era of increased public attention, alcoholism remains the most underdiagnosed, undertreated, and under-researched major medical problem. The vast cost of alcoholism to the country is estimated at 116.7 billion dollars and is heavily felt by industry, families, the legal system, physicians, and the affected patients.[82]

In the DSM III, the distinction is made between *abuse* and *dependency* for alcoholism and other psychoactive substances.[83] In order to qualify as being an abuser, an individual must have had a pathologic pattern of use of a substance on a regular basis for at least the past month, in addition to psychosocial problems in the family, work, legal, or health area. The diagnosis of dependency is made when, in addition to having psychosocial problems, the individual either tolerates a substance or suffers withdrawal symptoms when discontinuing use. Recently there has been controversy about the distinction between abuse and dependency. It is hard to delineate at what point tolerance or withdrawal symptoms are a problem and withdrawal symptoms may be mild, moderate, or severe, with individual variation. People's tolerance to substances varies a great deal, and tolerance is difficult to measure. The ability of a 180-pound man to consume five drinks in an hour and not develop signs of intoxication is evidence of considerable tolerance to alcohol and might be considered evidence of dependency. Similarly, use of one quart of spirits, one gallon of wine, or one case of beer per day, or a finding of a blood level over .15% (150 mg/ml), is almost pathognomonic for alcoholism.

In recent discussions, a committee of consultants on substance use disorders meeting to develop a revision of the DSM III decided to broaden the definition of substance dependency (making it more like the World Health Organization concept of dependence) to include individuals who have a pattern of pathologic use, tolerance, or withdrawal. At this point in the discussion of the DSM III, most who formerly would have been diagnosed as abusers would be diagnosed as dependent. Those who do not qualify for dependence but have problems associated with intoxication would be diagnosed as abusers. The consultants developed a code for mild, moderate, and severe dependency. The presence of three of the following items would be diagnostic for dependence:

1. The patient has made repeated efforts to cut down or control substance use.
2. The patient is often intoxicated or impaired by substance use when expected to fulfill social or occupational obligations (e.g., he doesn't go to work because he is hung over or high, goes to work high, or drives when drunk).
3. *Tolerance:* The patient needs increased amounts of a substance in order to achieve intoxication or the desired effect, or he experiences diminished effect with continued use of the same amount.
4. *Withdrawal:* The patient experiences a substance-specific syndrome following cessation or reduction of intake of a substance.
5. The patient has frequent preoccupation with seeking or taking the substance.
6. The patient has given up some important social, occupational, or recreational activity in order to seek or take the substance.
7. The patient often uses a psychoactive substance

to relieve or avoid withdrawal symptoms (e.g., takes a drink or uses diazepam to relieve morning shakes).

8. The patient often takes the substance in larger doses or over a longer period than intended.
9. The patient continues to use a substance despite a physical or mental disorder or significant social problem that he knows is exacerbated by the use of the substance.
10. The patient has a mental or physical disorder or condition that is usually a complication of prolonged substance use (e.g., cirrhosis, Korsakoff's syndrome, or perforated nasal septum).

Field trials will be necessary to determine the validity of these items. In this system, it would be possible to make the diagnosis of cocaine dependency on the basis of psychosocial symptoms and without entering the controversy of whether there is a physical cocaine withdrawal syndrome.

Alcoholism and drug abuse can both mimic and interact with a wide variety of medical and psychiatric conditions. Adverse drug responses from psychoactive substances of abuse can, for example, look like schizophrenia, an affective disorder, a panic disorder, or other organic conditions.

A high degree of alertness to subtle signs of a problem is important. Early signs and symptoms of substance use disorders include loss of communication in a marriage, frequent temper flare-ups, belligerent demands, a general loss of interest in the marital relationship, and personality change. Substances may be used either to allow a person to enjoy sex or as a way of avoiding a sexual life. Disruption of a parent's ability to relate to children and unrealistic demands and expectations placed on the child may occur, as may parental abuse, either aggressive or sexual.

The person's ability to drive a car may be affected long before a person has gotten into a severe accident or lost a driver's license because of driving while intoxicated. Lateness and absence from work, inability to complete projects on time, and irritability at work may be clues. Drinking or drug use may accompany early signs of a depressed mood or increased anxiety and may be used as a sleep aid. Gastrointestinal symptoms such as morning vomiting, abdominal pain, diarrhea, gastritis, and an enlarged liver may be present. Increased proneness to accidents and bruises, blackouts, and seizures, increased episodes of infection, and cigarette-burned fingers are other symptoms. Evidence of a family history of alcoholism should be sought; patients may be vulnerable on a genetic basis.

Pathophysiologic Considerations

Various theories explain the mechanisms of tolerance, physical dependence, and the addictive process in substance dependence. Most of these relate to the fact that withdrawal phenomena are opposite phenomena or counteradaptive responses to the action of the drug, and that with tolerance, there is a need to maintain use in order to maintain homeostasis. The counteradaptive response has been postulated as resulting from intracellular enzyme activity, redundancy of receptors, redundancy of normal pathways, or disuse supersensitivity.[84]

At first, use is aimed at producing positive reinforcement through a euphoric state, a change in mood, or anxiety reduction; however, with tolerance and dependence, continued use becomes a required way of controlling the highly aversive anxiety and uncomfortable dysphoria accompanying withdrawal states. For example, chronic opiate use leads to supersensitivity in the dopaminergic, cholinergic, and serotoninergic transmitter systems. In addition, inhibition at the level of the locus ceruleus involving the noradrenergic neurons may be the basis of clonidine's reduction of opioid withdrawal symptoms. Morphine can also act at the cellular level through the adenylate cyclase system.

Alcoholism has biologic, psychologic and social contributing factors, though the pathophysiology of the problem is not well understood. The mechanism for risk factors such as a positive family history of alcoholism, sex, and hyperactivity in childhood is not known. Adoption studies in men by Goodwin and others indicate that alcoholism runs in families even when children are separated from their parents and raised by nonalcoholic adoptive parents.[85] Two twin studies found the incidence in monozygotic twins to be substantially higher than in fraternal twins, supporting the existence of genetic factors.[86,87] Those alcoholics who do have familial alcoholism have early onset, more antisocial features, more severe medical problems, and a poorer prognosis.[88,89]

It is not known exactly what is inherited or what effects of alcohol at biochemical levels lead to tolerance, dependency, and an addictive cycle. Several current hypotheses are being explored. First, alcohol might lead to increased activity and then depletion of a neurotransmitter such as serotonin or other substances such as prostaglandins. In this model, susceptible individuals would be drinking at first to correct a deficiency, then overshooting and making the problem worse. A second theory is that alcohol could lead to increased activity of morphine-like substances such as tetrahydroisoquinalones (products of acetaldehyde and monoamines) or endorphins. Third, alcohol might lead to increased relaxation in susceptible individuals such as sons of alcoholics, as measured by increased slow alpha wave activity on EEG. Fourth, factors such as unpleasant physiologic reactions to alcohol such as the oriental flush might be protective against alcoholism. A high percentage of orientals and a smaller percentage of white people react to alcohol with a cutaneous flush, queasiness, tachycardia, and decreased blood pressure. This reaction has been associated with atypical forms of alcohol dehydrogenase, aldehyde dehydrogenase, and elevated acetaldehyde. This biologic deterrent, along with cultural factors, contributes to a low frequency of alcoholism in orientals. Mechanisms of interactions of biologic protective factors with psychologic and sociocultural variables need to be further researched.[90]

The effects of alcohol itself on various organ systems are also not well understood. The question of whether alcohol has direct toxic effects on the liver, the cortex, and the fetus, or whether these effects are due to malnutrition or other variables, has not been fully answered. Most likely, the combined effects of alcohol, diet, and heredity play a role. Some baboons given a nutritious diet and chronically force-fed with alcohol developed cirrhosis; however, it is not possible to rule out an alcohol-induced malabsorption syndrome that might contribute to a nutritional intervening variable.[90] Wernicke-Korsakoff psychosis is marked by nystagmus, ataxia, confusion, short-term memory loss, and sometimes confabulation, which clinically affects 2% of alcoholics. Wernicke-Korsakoff psychosis is most probably caused by a thiamin deficiency; early signs are removed by thiamin. Blass reports a familial transketolase deficiency that causes vitamin deficiency in a subgroup at risk for Korsakoff's psychosis.[91]

Diagnostic Evaluation

Laboratory tests provide a direct evaluation of the level of intoxication or overdose. Patients' reports of the exact drugs they have taken and the amount they have used tend to be distorted by unconscious denial, outright lying, and organicity. Obtaining the blood directly from the patient or supervising urine samples can provide identification and quantification of drugs. Breathalyzers are widely used to measure blood alcohol level although false positives are possible if alcohol-containing substances such as mouthwash have been used recently. Blood levels are the best measure of intoxication. Some drugs, like cocaine, which has a half-life in plasma of half an hour, will require either blood or urine levels of its metabolite benzoylecgonine.

Thin-layer chromatography (TLC) is the most widely used inexpensive form of drug screen, and it recently has had some improvement in sensitivity (down to 2 mg/ml). A qualitative method, it is ideal for use in the emergency room or in methadone programs in which drugs taken are unknown and quick assessment of the toxic drug is the task. Marijuana, PCP, and LSD are not identified by TLC, and cocaine will be missed unless high doses were used. TLC is 100 to 1000 times less sensitive and has more false positives than antibody-based radioimmunoassay (RIA), enzyme immunoassay (EIA), and gas chromatography mass spectrometry (GCMS). Because of false positives and false negatives, TLC is not generally admissible as forensic evidence.[92]

Many laboratories split samples and screen first with a TLC or EIA. In order to then get a highly sensitive and accurate quantitative level in the nanogram to picogram range, a GCMS can be run on the remaining sample. GCMS blood testing is the most expensive test; however, it is useful when accurate correlation of blood concentration with behavioral effects is important, such as in forensic cases. The GCMS has become so sensitive that drugs may be detected in small amounts weeks after they have been used. Even exposure to smoke-filled rooms can lead to trace levels of tetrahydrocannabinol (marijuana). GCMS is especially needed in children and adolescents, in whom an accurate and sensitive test is especially important. In inpatient and outpatient treatment of substance abuse, laboratory testing has an important role in early diagnosis of relapses and in helping to keep the patient honest.[93]

Routine laboratory workup of patients with substance abuse, including a sequential multiple analyzer (SMA) test and complete blood count and along with hepatitis antigen and antibody screening is also useful. Blood gamma-glutamyltranspeptidase (GGT) is increased in more than 50% of alcoholics.[94] Increased mean corpuscular volume, uric acid, triglycerides, aspartate aminotransferase, and urea can also be found in alcoholism. Quadratic discriminant analysis of commonly available blood chemistry tests produce a fingerprint specific for recent heavy drinking; however, its usefulness in detecting alcoholism is limited by both false negatives and false positives.[95] EEG will show nonspecific slowing in intoxication and overdose with sedative hypnotics. Additional testing is needed as indicated to diagnose the presence of complications of substance abuse.

INTOXICATION AND OVERDOSE

Definition

Intoxication involves the recent ingestion of quantities of a psychoactive substance sufficient to produce

Table 16–34. Diagnostic Criteria for Barbiturate or Similarly Acting Sedative or Hypnotic Withdrawal*

Prolonged, heavy use of barbiturate or similarly acting sedative or hypnotic, or more prolonged use of smaller doses of a benzodiazepine

At least three of the following due to recent cessation of or reduction in substance use:

Nausea and vomiting

Malaise or weakness

Autonomic hyperactivity, e.g., tachycardia, sweating, elevated blood pressure

Anxiety

Depressed mood or irritability

Orthostatic hypotension

Coarse tremor of hands, tongue, and eyelids

Not due to any physical or mental disorder, such as barbiturate or similarly acting sedative or hypnotic withdrawal delirium

*From American Psychiatric Association: Diagnostic and Statistical Manual of Mental Disorders. 3rd Ed. Washington, D.C., American Psychiatric Association, 1980. Used with permission.

The criteria for diagnosis of opioid withdrawal are described in Table 16–35.

SUBSTANCE ABUSE IN SPECIAL GROUPS

Substance Disorders in Psychopathologic Patients

Substance disorders may occur along with other psychopathology. In 1972, alcoholic men constituted 37% of male inpatient admissions to psychiatric hospitals.[98] The superimposition of alcoholism and other substance abuse on other psychiatric illnesses is common. Many chronic mentally ill patients will self-medicate with alcohol or drugs or will use symptoms of substance abuse to explain their psychiatric illness to themselves

Table 16–35. Diagnostic Criteria for Opioid Withdrawal*

Prolonged, heavy use of an opioid (or administration of a narcotic antagonist following a briefer period of use)

At least four of the following symptoms due to the recent cessation of or reduction in opioid use:

Lacrimation

Rhinorrhea

Pupillary dilation

Piloerection

Sweating

Diarrhea

Yawning

Mild hypertension

Tachycardia

Fever

Insomnia

Not due to any other physical or mental disorder.

*From American Psychiatric Association: Diagnostic and Statistical Manual of Mental Disorders. 3rd Ed. Washington, D.C., American Psychiatric Association, 1980. Used with permission.

or others. Differentiating drug toxic effects from preexisting psychiatric disorders is difficult.

Often, many psychiatric inpatient units, psychiatric halfway houses, outpatient clinics, and other support systems in the community are unable to treat alcohol abusers who are also chronic mental patients. On the other hand, severely disturbed alcoholics are shunned by alcohol rehabilitation facilities, which are generally not equipped to handle them. In addition, a total abstinence model involving a preference for confrontational methods found in therapeutic communities and self-help groups rather than use of prescribed psychotropic medication may not be appropriate for some mentally ill patients.

Though few, facilities that combine psychiatric treatment with substance use rehabilitation techniques, are increasingly important. Recently attention has been focused on the interaction of alcoholism with other psychiatric disorders. Longitudinal studies, adoption studies, and family studies raise questions concerning the primary or secondary role of substance abuse, the clustering of psychiatric disorders with substance abuse, and interactions of other diagnoses with substance abuse. As a result of the implementation of the DMS III multiaxial diagnostic system, patients who present with substance abuse concomitant with other psychiatric disorders receive more careful assessment.

For both clinicians and researchers it is difficult to separate primary traits and disorders from symptoms secondary to acute and chronic intoxication, toxicity, idiosyncratic reactions, withdrawal, and the psychosocial effects of the addiction process. The work of McCord and McCord, Vaillant, and Pettinati, Sugarman, and Maurer would indicate that the majority of psychopathology is secondary.[99–101] Still, the prevalence of additional psychiatric problems in patients with addiction points to the need for careful psychiatric assessment in all patients with substance abuse. The important role of psychiatry in the assessment and treatment of substance abuse should be stressed both inside and outside the profession. Because alcoholism and substance abuse both mimic and interact with all mental illnesses, to know substance abuse is to know all of psychiatry.

A small percentage of patients with alcoholism (5 to 15%) have a primary affective illness, though a high percentage of alcoholics appear to be depressed.[102] It is not clear yet whether alcoholism and affective disorder are inherited discretely, as Goodwin's data might indicate, or whether there is a familial interaction between alcoholism and affective disorders, as Winokur thinks.[85,103]

There has been no single personality or Axis II diagnosis that is thought to be specific for addiction.

However, using research diagnostic criteria, 10 to 20% of male and 5 to 10% of female alcoholics requiring admission can be diagnosed as having "antisocial personality."

The frequency with which diagnosed personality disorders are secondary to the organic and psychosocial effects of substance abuse is not clear; nor is it clear whether, as Pettinati found, there is likely to be an improvement over time with complete abstinence.[101] Wender, in 1971, described minimal brain dysfunction (MBD) in children and its persistence as attention deficit disorder of the residual type in adults.[104] A number of writers have found an increase in MBD in alcoholics and their relatives. Tarter has found this to be the case especially in essential alcoholism.[105] There have been reports of a relationship between anxiety disorder and post-traumatic distress disorder in alcoholism, as well.

Several controversial questions need to be raised in research on interaction between alcoholism and other psychiatric disorders: 1) Is substance abuse inherited distinctly, or does it interact with a broad-based, genetic vulnerability to psychiatric illness? 2) To what degree is familial substance abuse predictive of psychiatric illness? 3) To what degree can substance abuse be secondary to psychiatric illness? 4) What is the contribution of substance abuse in exacerbating or causing other psychiatric symptoms? 5) In what ways can substance abuse mask, treat, or alter the expression of other psychiatric illness? The use of multiaxial diagnosis and reliable diagnostic criteria are steps forward in improving our ability to classify and study patients.

Substance Disorders in Multidisabled Patients

Rehabilitation centers that work with the multihandicapped patient report that 25 to 30% of their clients abuse alcohol alone or in combination with other drugs.[106] Disabled individuals are at a high risk of becoming substance abusers for several reasons. They often have easy access to alcohol and to other drugs because staff and families, out of guilt or a sense of futility, often will not object to their use. Disabled people often feel frustrated and angry at being dependent, socially isolated, and discriminated against by the rest of society. As a group, they have a high vulnerability to feelings of depression, anxiety, self-hatred, low motivation, and low self-esteem—feelings that are often self-medicated with alcohol and other substances.

Blind and deaf individuals have special problems that may include denial of the existence of alcohol and substance problems within their community, fear of being stigmatized, and lack of adequate signs in sign language to symbolize drunkenness or sobriety. Treatment facilities generally do not have counselors or professionals trained in sign language. Alcoholism in patients with spinal cord disability is common, probably because many sustained their injuries while intoxicated and continue to use alcohol to cope with their situations. Patients with spinal cord injury may have physical problems that are aggravated by substance abuse, including decubitus caused by immobility, poor nutrition, and sexual dysfunction.

The developmentally disabled alcoholic, mentally retarded patients with IQs of 60 to 85 are concrete and easily manipulated and have difficulty learning from experience. Since deinstitutionalization, many mentally retarded people, living in the community and lacking necessary skills for positive socialization, turn to alcohol and substance abuse as an easy solution. It is hard for them to learn about alcohol in programs with a strong emphasis on education, and they therefore need special support and help as well as a high degree of acceptance, warmth, and emotional support.

Substance Abuse in Adolescents

Adolescent experimentation with and use of alcohol and drugs is normal in western society. Of high school seniors, 90% use alcohol; alcohol is often a first step to other substance use, and familial alcoholism begins in adolescence. This is a population that requires more work in terms of treatment and prevention than has been previously thought.

Peer influence is also considered an important factor. Programs stress the importance of finding nonalcohol and nondrug-using friends. Alienation, poor self-esteem, depression, promiscuity, poor academic performance, truancy, and a greater tendency toward antisocial and aggressive acts can be both predisposing factors and consequences of substance abuse.

Adolescents may require treatment programs tailored to their needs and special problems, including lack of motivation and distrust of adults. The adolescent may need to be pushed into treatment because few adolescents seek treatment voluntarily. Once in treatment, these youngsters tend to test limits by running away, breaking the rules, and smuggling alcohol into a program. The staff needs to be knowledgeable of developmental problems in adolescence to be able to deal with issues of transference and countertransference.

Substance Dependency in Geriatric Patients

One third of elderly alcoholics have developed that problem late in life. The organic effects of alcohol and drugs, including clouding of consciousness, disturbances of equilibrium, withdrawal reactions, and tolerance and psychologic dependence, increase with each decade. Because of loss of tolerance and greater neuropsychiatric impairment that is age-related, use of lower doses of alcohol and drugs may be abusive. The interaction of alcohol and medications contributes to problems requiring treatment in the elderly.

Substance Abuse in Women

Alcoholism is increasing in women; programs report that approximately 30% of patients with alcoholism are female. Addiction to prescription drugs and cocaine are as high in women as in men. Most studies in substance abuse have been in men, and more work needs to be done studying the problems among women. Though many of the problems are similar, women often will have had later detection of a problem, more depression, and less sociopathy, will have faced greater social stigma, and are more likely to have had a telescoped course and greater severity. Women are more likely to be left by a spouse, physically abused, and less able to afford treatment.

SUMMARY

The prevalence of alcoholism and substance abuse problems and the high degree of denial in patients with these problems require that the clinician be alert to signs and symptoms, take the patient history carefully, and use laboratory tests in all patients. Patients will frequently be abusing several chemicals at once and may also be suffering from other psychiatric disorders, further complicating diagnosis. Intoxication and withdrawal may exacerbate or mimic other medical and psychiatric disorders. Special populations may need specific tailored approaches to diagnosis and treatment.

SEXUAL DISORDERS

Human sexual behavior does not conform to any single pattern. People have variable sexual drives and activities, and societies differ in their attitudes toward sexual activities. The last 25 years has seen a liberalization of legal and cultural sanctions concerning sexual behavior. Although medical interest in sexual disorders dates to the time of Hippocrates, such disorders were not the subject of scientific investigation until Kinsey's pioneering work on human sexual response and the therapeutic labors of Masters and Johnson.[107,108]

Table 16–36. Classification of Sexual Disorders

Sexual dysfunctions
  Affecting sexual desire
    Low libido
    Hyperactive sex drive
  Impaired sexual arousal
    Erectile impotence
    Failure of arousal in women
  Affecting orgasm
    Premature ejaculation
    Retarded ejaculation
    Anorgasmia and premature orgasm in women
  Others
    Painful ejaculation in men
    Vaginismus
    Dyspareunia
    Sexual phobia
Sexual deviations
  Disorders of sexual orientation
    Homosexuality
    Pedophilia
    Fetishism
    Exhibitionism
    Sadomasochism
    Voyeurism
    Bestiality
    Neurophilia
  Gender role abnormality
    Simple transvestism
    Transsexualism

It is difficult to draw a line where normal sexual behavior ends and abnormal behavior starts. Sexual behavior exists on a continuum, and establishing clear boundaries is difficult. DSM III and International Classification of Diseases-9 (ICD-9) have tried to establish diagnostic criteria. A particular sexual behavior may lack a diagnostic criterion and yet may be a source of great distress for the patient. Physicians should be aware of these variations of sexual activities and attitudes and should not impose their own values on their patients; instead, they should work within the patient's values and cultural attitudes.

Sexual disorders are of two kinds: sexual dysfunctions and sexual deviations (Table 16–36).

SEXUAL DYSFUNCTIONS

As a background for discussing various dysfunctions, it is important to understand the normal physiologic response cycle. There are four phases: excitement, plateau, orgasm, and resolution. The first two phases are a parasympathetic response; the second two phases are a sympathetic response.

Sexual dysfunction may be an absolute or relative deficit in sexual performance. It may be global or restricted to certain situations. The terms primary and secondary refer, respectively, to life-long conditions and to those that develop after a period of successful performance.

Disorder of Sexual Desire. Complaints of low libido are common in females. Low libido often reflects problems in the relationship between the partners. Occasionally it may be due to a long-standing inhibition about sex, to a biologic variation of sexual drive, to a low capacity to fantasize, or to low curiosity. Low libido may be related to commitment to marriage or to childbirth.

Disorder of Sexual Arousal. Erectile impotence is the inability to reach an erection or to sustain it long enough for satisfactory coitus. It may be primary, i.e., poor at the first attempt at intercourse, or may be secondary, i.e., it may develop after a period of normal function. Impotence is more common among older men. It may be global, that is, occurring with all sexual partners, or it may be restricted, that is, occurring with only one partner.

Failure of genital response in women or failure of vaginal lubrication is often secondary to lack of sexual interest. Other causes of inadequate genital response are anxiety about intercourse and inadequate sexual foreplay. From menopause onward, hormonal changes often lead to reduced vaginal lubrication.

Disorder of Orgasm. Premature ejaculation is defined as habitual ejaculation before penetration or ejaculation so shortly after penetration that the woman has not gained pleasure. It is more common among younger men. Retarded ejaculation is less common and is defined as serious delay in ejaculation or complete absence of ejaculation. It is associated with general psychologic inhibition about sexual relations. It is also seen in patients taking antipsychotic, antidepressant, or ganglion blocking drugs. Orgasmic dysfunction in women depends on both partners. Many women do not regularly achieve orgasm during intercourse. About 25% of women have no orgasm during intercourse for the first year of marriage.

Other Disorders. Vaginismus is a spasm of the vaginal muscles that causes pain when intercourse is attempted. There may also be spasm of the muscles in the surrounding area. The spasm is usually associated with fears about penetration; occasionally it is associated with painful scarring after episiotomy. It is made worse by an inexperienced partner. The spasm starts as soon as the attempts to penetrate. Extreme cases of vaginismus may lead to nonconsummation of marriage.

Dyspareunia is described as pain on intercourse. Pain after partial penetration may result from impaired lubrication of the vagina, from inflammation, or from the muscle spasm of vaginismus. Pain on deep penetration suggests a pelvic disorder such as endometriosis, tumors, infection, or ovarian cyst.

Sexual phobias may range from fear of being touched to specific aspects of the sexual act such as being touched on the genitalia or being kissed.

Pathophysiologic Considerations

Several causal factors are common to various kinds of sexual dysfunctions, and it is impossible to discuss each disorder individually (Table 16–27). However, the distinction between organic and psychologic causes of sexual dysfunction is paramount. Although there are no substantiating studies, it is often stated that 90% of sexual dysfunction is psychogenic.

Organic factors influence sexual functioning and may produce different patterns of disorders of desire, arousal, and orgasm. Some organic causes affect specifically the arousal and orgasm phase; for example, through metabolic imbalance and autonomic neuropathy, diabetes may affect sexual arousal and orgasm. Such sexual dysfunctions are chronic and may be the presenting problem in diabetic patients. There are many drugs that affect sexual functioning (Table 16–36); sympatholytic drugs, for example, guanethidine, produce a dissociated erectile dysfunction; ganglion blocking agents may lead only to failure of ejaculation.

Sexual dysfunction in postmyocardial infarction and postcerebrovascular accident (CVA) has been a cause for concern. Sexuality is restricted in patients with a history of recent myocardial infarction. About 12% of the patients stop sexual intercourse completely, about 60% reduce their sexual activity, and the rest resume normal sexual activities.[109] CVA may affect sexual activities by causing physical limitations such as paralysis. In some cases of CVA, altered perception of the partner may cause difficulties in sexual relationship.

Diagnostic Evaluation

A detailed history should be obtained from the patient and the partner. Sexual dysfunction should not be labeled psychogenic merely by exclusion of organic factors; rather, a full history and complete examination should be performed. To establish the nature and contingency of sexual dysfunction, it must be established whether the dysfunction is partial or total, episodic or constant, restricted or global. Quite frequently certain findings are suggestive of the psychogenic cause of impairment; for instance, the retained ability to obtain a firm erection in response to a full bladder on waking indicates an intact vascular and neurologic mechanism.

A detailed history of the patient's physical health and drug usage must be followed by a clinical examination. Clinical findings direct further appropriate

Table 16–37. Organic and Psychiatric Causes of Sexual Dysfunction

Chromosomal
  Klinefelter's syndrome
  Turner's syndrome
Genetic
  Testicular feminization
Congenital
  Local anatomic abnormalities, e.g., hypospadias
Endocrine
  Acromegaly
  Addison's disease
  Primary and secondary hypogonadism
  Thyroid imbalance
  Diabetes
Drugs
  Alcohol (abuse)
  Guanethidine
  Beta adrenoceptor antagonists
  Methyldopa
  Tricyclics
  MAO inhibitors
  Benzodiazepines
  Barbiturates
  Thioridazine
  Propantheline
  Bendrofluazide
  Steroids
  Possibly oral contraceptives
  Cyproterone
  Antabuse
  Methadone
  Opiates
Surgery and radiotherapy
  Perineal
  Prostatectomy
  Aortofemoral bypass
  Sympathectomy
  Irradiation of pelvis
  Oophorectomy
Trauma
  Cord fracture
  Castration
  Pelvic fracture
  Penile trauma
Cardiovascular
  Angina pectoris
  Previous myocardial infarction
Gynecologic
  Vaginitis
  Endometriosis
  Infections
Neurologic
  Epilepsy, particularly of temporal lobe
  Multiple sclerosis
Psychiatric
  Depression
  Anxiety states
  Obsessional neurosis
  Sexual deviations

investigations, although some routine laboratory investigations, including testing blood glucose should always be performed. Other investigations for hormone levels, karyotyping, and a vascular test should be based on the clinical findings. In some cases both psychogenic and organic causes contribute to the dysfunction. Additional assessment of several areas is necessary in most cases of dysfunctions. These include the extent of sexual knowledge of each partner; the level of anxiety related to sexual performance; the feelings and attitudes of each toward sexual activity; any problems with technique; the level of the subjects' social skills; and the nature of the relationship between the partners.

Some of the special investigations available are measurement of penile blood pressure and strained gauge assessment of nocturnal erection.

SEXUAL DEVIATION

Disorder of Sexual Orientation

HOMOSEXUALITY

The term homosexuality denotes erotic thoughts and feelings toward a person of the same sex, whether or not they are associated with overt sexual behavior. People cannot be divided sharply into those who are homosexuals and those who are heterosexual. Sexuality exists on a continuum, with exclusively homosexual and heterosexual behavior at each end, and between them are varying degrees of both homo- and heterosexual relationships.

Kinsey, in study of 4108 adult American males, showed that 4% were exclusively homosexual. Of the men, 10% were homosexuals for at least 3 years.[107] Kanyon reported that about 2% of the female population is predominantly homosexual.[111]

Heredity has long been supposed to be one of the causative factors of homosexuality. In some studies a high concordance for male homosexuality has been found in monozygotic twins.[112] There is no convincing evidence of an abnormality of sex chromosomes or the neuroendocrine system in either male or female homosexuals.[111,113]

Many studies have been made of the psychologic and social causes of homosexuality. Patients with schizophrenia and brain damage (mania) may sporadically engage in homosexual activity. Other possible factors include the absence of the father during childhood, an overprotective and unduly intimate mother, unresolved castration complex, and anxiety.[114] Homosexuality as a learned behavior has been proposed as a cause, especially in the absence of self-confidence and other social relationships.[113]

DSM III includes ego dystonic homosexuality as a mental illness. In such a disorder, the individual complains that persistently absent or weak heterosexual arousal significantly interferes with initiating or maintaining a wanted heterosexual relationship. Also, the individual explicitly mentions a sustained pattern of homosexual arousal.

Some homosexuals adopt an effeminate style of life, preferring work and leisure activities that would usually be undertaken by females. Some adopt exaggerated feminine mannerisms, and a small number like to dress in women's clothes. Most homosexual men do not behave in this way. Many homosexual men live as happily as those who are heterosexual, forming a stable relationship with a partner.

Homosexual women usually do not show unusual social behavior, but some prefer a dominant sexual role and seek the kind of work and leisure activities usually associated with men. As a group, homosexual women are less promiscuous than homosexual men; they are usually able to form lasting relationships and consequently are less likely to suffer loneliness and depression in middle life.

SEX ROLE DISTURBANCE

Transsexualism is a condition in which a person is convinced that he or she is of the sex opposite that indicated by his or her normal external genitalia. The transsexual individual feels estranged from his or her body, has an intense desire to live as a member of the opposite sex, and seeks to alter bodily appearance and genitalia to conform to those of the opposite sex.

Transsexualism occurs in approximately 1 man in 35,000. It is less frequent among females. The cause remains unknown, despite numerous theories to explain this condition. There is no convincing genetic cause. The sex chromosomes are normal in transsexuals, and there is no evidence of upbringing in the wrong sex role. A hormonal hypothesis suggests that transsexualism might result from hormonal abnormalities during intrauterine development. There is some evidence that when pregnant rhesus monkeys are given large doses of androgens their female infants behave more like males during play.[115] Female children with the adrenogenital syndrome have been reported to show rather boyish behavior in childhood, but they do not become transsexuals.[116]

The diagnosis is made from the patient history and description of feelings. Male patients report a strong conviction of belonging to the opposite sex usually dating back from the prepubertal period. Their parents sometimes report that in childhood they preferred the company of girls. They dress as women to feel like women and not for sexual excitement. Commonly they wear makeup and arrange their hair in feminine style. They try to adopt feminine gestures and attempt to alter the pitch of their voices. They lack maternal instincts and their sex drive is low. Unlike transvestites, transsexuals turn from their sex organs in disgust. They seek surgery for sex change and pursue hormonal treatment for development of breasts.

The diagnosis of transsexualism can be made only if the disturbance has been persistent for over 2 years and there is no evidence of illness like schizophrenia, physical intersexuality, or genetic abnormality; if the patient has a sense of discomfort and inappropriateness about his anatomic sex; and if the patient has a wish to be rid of his own genitalia and to live as a member of the other sex (DSM III).

The other sexual disorders are encountered in psychiatric practice but have not been studied extensively. There are few follow-up and family studies of these disorders and no universally accepted treatments of these disorders.

REFERENCES

1. Bernstein, Jerrold G.: Handbook of Drug Therapy in Psychiatry. Boston, John Wright—PSG Inc., 1983.
2. Ludwig, A.M.: Principles of Clinical Psychiatry. New York, The Free Press, 1980.
3. Hall, C.W. (ed.): Psychiatric Presentations of Medical Illnesses: Somatopsychic Disorders. New York, SP Medical & Scientific Books, 1980.
4. Jefferson, J.W., and Marshall, J.R.: Neuropsychiatric Features of Medical Disorders. New York, Plenum Medical Book Co., 1983.
5. Holmes, T.H., and Rahe, R.H.: The social readjustment rating scale. J. Psychosom Res. *11*:213–218, 1967.
6. Beres, D.: Ego deviation and the concept of schizophrenia. Psychoanal Study Child *2*:164–235, 1956.
7. Frosch, J.: The psychotic character: clinical psychiatric considerations. Psychiatr Q *38*:81–96, 1964.
8. Fenichel, O.: Psychoanalytic Theory of the Neuroses. New York, W.W. Norton and Company, Inc, 1945.
9. West, L.J.: A general theory of hallucinations and dreams. *In* Hallucinations. Edited by L.J. West. New York, Grune and Stratton, 1962.
10. Fischer, R.: The perception-hallucination continuum. Diseases of the Nervous System *30*:161–171, 1969.
11. Lishman, W.A.: Organic Psychiatry: The Psychological Consequences of Cerebral Disorder. Oxford, England, Blackwell Scientific Publications, 1978.
12. Kenna, J.C., and Sedman, G.: Depersonalization in temporal lobe epilepsy and the organic psychoses. Br J Psychiatry *111*:293–299, 1965.
13. Dixon, J.: Depersonalization phenomena in a sample population of college students. Br J Psychiatry *109*:371–375, 1963.
14. Schultz, D.P.: Sensory Restriction: Effects on Behavior. New York, Academic Press, 1965.
15. Noyes, R., and Kletti, R.: Depersonalization in the face of life-threatening danger: a description. Psychiatry *39*:19–27, 1976.
16. Nemiah, J.C.: Dissociative disorders. *In* Comprehensive Text-

book of Psychiatry. 3rd Ed. Edited by H.I. Kaplan, A.M. Freedman, and B.J. Sadock. Baltimore, Williams and Wilkins, 1980.

17. Lipowski, Z.J.: Organic brain syndromes: overview and classification. *In* Psychiatric Aspects of Neurologic Disease. Vol. 1. Edited by D.F. Benson and D. Blumer. New York, Grune and Stratton, 1975.

18. Slater, E., and Beard, A.W.: The schizophrenia-like psychoses of epilepsy. Br J Psychiatry *109*:95–150, 1963.

19. Waxman, S., and Gerschwind, N.: The interictal behavior syndrome of temporal lobe epilepsy. Arch Gen Psychiatry *32*:1580–1586, 1975.

20. Lipowski, Z.J.: Organic mental disorders. *In* Comprehensive Textbook of Psychiatry. 3rd Ed. Edited by H.I. Kaplan, A.M. Freedman and B.J. Sadock. Baltimore, Williams and Wilkins, 1980.

21. Peroutka, S.P., and Snyder, S.H.: Relationship of neuroleptic drug effects at brain dopamine serotonin, α-adrenergic and histamine receptors to clinical potency. Am J Psychiatry *137*:1518–1522, 1980.

22. Goodwin, D.W., Alderson, P., and Rosenthal, R.: Clinical significance of hallucinations in psychiatric disorders. Arch Gen Psychiatry *24*:76–80, 1971.

23. Stub, R.L.: Acute confusional state. *In* Psychiatric Aspects of Neurologic Disease. Vol. 2. Edited by D.F. Benson, and D. Blumer. New York, Grune and Stratton, 1982.

24. Slade, P.D.: Hallucinations. Psychol Med *6*:7–13, 1976.

25. World Health Organization: International Pilot Study of Schizophrenia. Vol 1. Geneva, WHO, 1973.

26. Jefferson, J.W., and Marshall, J.R.: Neuropsychiatric Features of Medical Disorders. New York, Plenum Medical Book Company, 1981.

27. Lowe, G.R.: The phenomenology of hallucinations as an aid to differential diagnosis. Br J Psychiatry *123*:621–633, 1973.

28. Klein, D.F., Gittelman, R., Quitkin, F., and Rifkin, A.: Diagnosis and Drug Treatment of Psychiatric Disorders: Adults and Children. 2nd Ed. Baltimore, Williams and Wilkins, 1980.

29. Hoffman, B.F., and Bigger, J.T. Jr.: Digitalis and allied cardiac glycosides. *In* The Pharmacological Basis of Therapeutics. 6th Ed. Edited by A. Goodman and A. Gilman. New York, MacMillan, 1980.

30. Linn, L.: Clinical manifestations of psychiatric disorder. *In* Comprehensive Textbook of Psychiatry. 3rd Ed. Edited by H.I. Kaplan, A.M. Freedman, B.J. Sadock. Baltimore, Williams and Wilkins, 1980.

31. DeVaul, R.A., and Hall, R.C.: Hallucinations. *In* Psychiatric Presentations of Medical Illness: Somatopsychic Disorders. Edited by R.C. Hall. New York, Spectrum Publications, Inc., 1980.

32. Benson, D.F., and Gerschwind, N.: Psychiatric conditions associated with focal lesions of the central nervous system. *In* American Handbook of Psychiatry. Vol. 4. Edited by M. Reiser. New York, Basic Books, 1975.

33. Blumer, D., and Benson, D.F.: Psychiatric Manifestations of Epilepsy. *In* Psychiatric Aspects of Neurologic Disease. Vol. 2. Edited by D.F. Benson and D. Blumer. New York, Grune and Stratton, 1982.

34. Lipowski, Z.J.: Organic Mental Disorders. *In* Comprehensive Textbook of Psychiatry. 3rd Ed. Edited by H.I. Kaplan, A.M. Freedman and B.J. Sadock. Baltimore, Williams and Wilkins, 1980.

35. Moskovitz, C., Moses, H., and Klawans, H.L.: Levodopa-induced psychosis: A kindling phenomenon. Am J Psychiatry *135*:669–675, 1978.

36. Freud, S.: Psycho-analytic notes in an autobiographical account of a case of paranoia (dementia paranoides) Part III, on the mechanism of paranoia. 1911. *In* Standard Edition of the works of Sigmund Freud. Vol. 12. Edited by J. Strachey. London, Hogarth Press, 1955.

37. Christodolulu, G.N.: The Syndrome of Capgras. Br J Psychiatry *130*:556–564, 1977.

38. Davison, K., and Bagley, C.R.: Schizophrenia-like psychoses associated with organic disorders of the central nervous system: A review of the literature. *In* Current Problems in Neuropsy-

chiatry. Edited by R.N. Herrington. Ashford, Kent, Authority of the Royal Medical-Psychological Association (Br J Psychiatry, Special Publication, No. 4), 1969.

39. Hall, R.C., Stickney, S.K., and Gardner, E.R.: Behavioral toxicity of nonpsychiatric drugs. *In* Psychiatric Presentatins of Medical Illness: Somatopsychic Disorders. Edited by R.C. Hall. New York, Spectrum Publications, Inc., 1980.

40. Engel, G.L., and Romano, J.: Delirium, a syndrome of cerebral insufficiency. J. Chronic Dis *9*:260–277, 1959.

41. Varsamis, J.: Clinical management of delirium. *In* Psychiatric Clinics of North America. Symposium on Brain Disorders: Clinical Diagnosis and Management. Vol. 1. No. 1. Philadelphia, W. B. Saunders, 1978.

42. N.I.A. Task Force: Senility reconsidered: treatment possibilities for mental impairment in the elderly. JAMA *244*:259–263, 1980.

43. Hall, R.C.W., et al.: Physical illness manifesting as psychiatric disease. Arch Gen Psychiatry *2*:989–995, 1980.

44. Reifler, B.V., Larson, E., and Hanley, R.: Coexistence of cognitive impairment and depression in geriatric outpatients. Am J Psychiatry *139*:623–626, 1982.

45. Adams, R.D., and Victor, M.: Delirium and other acute confusional states. *In*: Harrison's Principles of Internal Medicine. 10th Ed. Edited by R.G. Petersdorf, et al. New York, McGraw-Hill, 1983.

46. Benson, F.: Positron emission tomography. Alzheimer's disease and related disorders. Mini White House Conference on Aging, January 15–16, Washington, D.C., U.S. Government Printing Office, 1981.

47. Blessed, G., Tomlinson, B.E., and Roth, M.: The association between quantitative measures of dementia and a senile change in the cerebral grey matter of elderly subjects. Br J Psychiatry *114*:797–811, 1968.

48. Schneck, M.K., Reisberg, R., and Ferris, S.H.: An overview of current concepts of Alzheimer's disease. Am J Psychiatry *139*:165–173, 1982.

49. Coyle, J.T., Price, D.L., and DeLong, M.R.: Alzheimer's disease: A disorder of cortical cholinergic innervation. Science *219*:1184–1190, 1983.

50. McGeer, P.L., et al.: Aging, Alzheimer disease and the cholinergic system of the basal forebrain. Neurology *34*:741–745, 1984.

51. Blass, J.P., and Weksler, M.C.: Toward an effective treatment of Alzheimer's disease. Ann Intern Med *98*:251–253, 1983.

52. Bondareff, W., Mountjoy, C.Q., and Roth, M.: Selective loss of neurons of origin of adrenergic projection to cerebral cortex (nucleus locus coeruleus) in senile dementia. Lancet *1*:783–784, 1981.

53. Rossor, M.N., et al.: Neuropeptides and neurotransmitters in cerebral cortex in Alzheimer disease. *In* Alzheimer's Disease: A Report of Progress in Research—Aging. Vol. 19, Edited by S. Corkin, et al. New York, Raven Press, 1982.

54. Katzman, R.: Delirium and dementia. *In* Merritt's Textbook of Neurology. 7th Ed. Edited by L.R. Rowland. Philadelphia, Lea & Febiger, 1984.

55. Jelliner, K.: Neuropathological aspects of dementia resulting from abnormal blood and cerebrospinal fluid dynamics. Acta Neurol Belg *76*:83–102, 1976.

55a. Wells, C.E.: Dementia. 2nd Ed. New York, Raven Press, 1977.

56. Katzman, R., and Terry, R.D.: The Neurology of Aging. Philadelphia, F.A. Davis, 1983.

57. Hachinski, V.C., et al.: Cerebral blood flow in dementia. Arch Neurol *32*:632–637, 1975.

58. Wells, C.E.: Pseudodementia. Am J Psychiatry *136*:895–900, 1979.

59. Folstein, M.F., Folstein, S.E., and McHugh, P.R.: ''Mini-Mental State'': A practical method for grading the cognitive state of patients for the clinician. J Psychiatr Res *12*:189–198, 1975.

60. Rudorfer, M.V., and Clayton, P.J.: Pseudodementia: use of the DST in diagnosis and treatment monitoring. Psychosomatics *23*:429–431, 1982.

61. McAllister, T.W., Ferrell, R.B., Price, T.R.P., and Neville, M.B.: The dexamethasone suppression test in two patients with

severe depressive pseudo-dementia. Am J Psychiatry *139*:479–481, 1982.

62. Alexopoulos, G.S., et al.: Dexamethasone suppression test. Limitations for use in geriatric psychiatric disorders. *In* Clinical and Psychopharmacological Studies in Psychiatric Disorders. Edited by G.D. Burrows and T.R. Norman. London, John Libbey, 1985.

63. Wolff, H.G., and Curran, D.: Nature of delirium and allied states. Arch Neurol Psychiatry *35*:1175–1215, 1935.

64. Posner, J.B.: Central causes of delirium, stupor, and coma. *In* Cecil Textbook of Medicine. 16th Ed. Edited by J.B. Wyngaarden and L.H. Smith, Philadelphia, W.B. Saunders, 1982.

65. American Psychiatric Association: Diagnostic and Statistical Manual of Psychiatric Disorders. 2nd Ed. (DSM II). Washington, D.C. 1968.

66. American Psychiatric Association: Diagnostic and Statistical Manual of Psychiatric Disorders. 3rd Ed. (DSM III) Washington, D.C., American Psychiatric Association, 1980.

67. Lipowski, Z.J.: Delirium: Acute Brain Failure in Man. Springfield, Ill., Charles C Thomas, 1980.

68. Engel, G.L., and Romano, J.: Delirium, a syndrome of cerebral insufficiency. J Chronic Dis *9*:260–277, 1959.

69. Moruzzi, G., and Magoun, H.W.: Brain stem reticular formation and activation of the EEG. Electroencephalog Clin Neurophysiol *1*:455–473, 1949.

70. Romano, L., and Engel, G.L.: Delirium: I. Electroencephalographic data. Arch Neurol Psychiatry *51*:356–377, 1944.

71. Victor, M., Adams, R.D., and Collins, G.H.: The Wernicke-Korsakoff Syndrome. Philadelphia, F.A. Davis, 1971.

72. Dreyfus, P.M.: Vitamin deficiencies. *In* Neurochemistry and Clinical Neurology. Edited by L. Battistin, G. Hashim, and A. Lujtha. New York, Alan R. Liss, 1980.

73. Dreyfus, P.M.: Nutritional disorders at the nervous system. *In* Cecil Textbook of Medicine. 16th Ed. Edited by J.B. Wyngaarden and L.H. Smith. Philadelphia, W.B. Saunders, 1982.

74. Dreyfus, P.M., and Geel, S.E.: Vitamin and nutritional deficiencies. *In* Basic Neurochemistry. 3rd Ed. Edited by R.W. Albers, G.J. Siegel, R. Katzman, and B.W. Agranoff. Boston, Little and Brown, 1982.

74a.Leonhard, R.: The Classification of Endogenous Psychosis. 5th Ed. New York, Irvington, 1979.

74b.Feighner, J.P., et al.: Diagnostic criteria for use in psychiatric research. Arch Gen Psychiatry *26*:57–63, 1972.

74c.Winokur, G., Behar, D., Vanvalkenburg, C., and Lowry, M.: Is a familial definition of depression both feasible and valid? J N Ment Dis *166*:764–768, 1978.

74d.McHugh, P.R., and Slavney, P.: The Perspectives of Psychiatry. Baltimore, Johns Hopkins University Press, 1984.

74e.Kraepelin, E.: Manic Depressive Insanity and Paranoia. Edinburgh, E & S Livingstone Publishers, 1921, pp. 61–74.

74f.Krouthammer, C., and Klerman, G.: Secondary mania. Arch Gen Psychiatry *35*:1333–1339, 1978.

74g.Marks, I., Lader, M.: Anxiety states (anxiety neurosis): A review. J Nerv Ment Dis *156*:3–18, 1973.

74h.Granville Grossman, K.L., and Turner, P.: The effect of propranolol on anxiety. Lancet *1*:788–790, 1966.

74i.Charney, D.S., Henninger, G.R., and Jatlow, P.I.: Increased anxiogenic effects of caffeine in panic disorder. Arch Gen Psychiatry *42*:233–243, 1985.

75. Myers, J.K., et al.: Six-month prevalence of psychiatric disordered in three communities. Arch Gen Psychiatry *41*:958–967, 1984.

76. Robins, L.N., et al.: Lifetime prevalence of specific psychiatric disorders in three sites. Arch Gen Psychiatry *41*:949–958, 1984.

77. Fifth Special Report to the U.S. Congress on Alcohol and Health from the Secretary of Health and Human Services, publication (ADM), Department of Health and Human Services, 1984, pp 84–1291.

78. Zucker, R., and Harford, T.: Natural survey of the demography of adolescent drinking practices. J Stud Alcohol *44*(6):974–985, 1983.

79. Substance Use Among New York State Public and Private School Students in Grades 7 Through 12, 1983. New York State Division of Substance Abuse Services, Sept. 1984.

80. Gold, M.S.: 800—Cocaine. New York, Bantam Books, 1984.

81. Gold, M.S., and Estroff, T.W.: The polysubstance abusing patient. *In* Handbook of Psychiatric Diagnostic Procedures. Edited by R.C.W. Hall. Spectrum Publications, Inc., 1984.

82. Niven, R.G.: Alcoholism—A problem in perspective. JAMA *252*:1912–1914, 1984.

83. DSM III: Diagnostic and statistical manual of mental disorders. Ed. 3. Washington, D.C., American Psychiatric Association, 1980.

84. Jaffe, J.H.: Opioid dependence. *In* Comprehensive Textbook of Psychiatry. 4th Ed. Edited by H.I. Kaplan and B.J. Sadock. Baltimore, Williams & Wilkins, 1984, pp 987–1003.

85. Goodwin, W.D.: Alcoholism and genetics. Arch Gen Psychiatry *42*:171–174, 1985.

86. Kaij, L.: Studies on the etiology and sequels of abuse of alcohol. Lund. Sweden, University of Lund, 1980.

87. Hrubec, Z., and Omenn, G.S.: Evidence of genetic predisposition to alcoholic cirrhosis and psychosis: Twin concordances for alcoholism and its biological end points by zygosity among male veterans. Alcoholism: Clin Exp Res *5*:207–215, 1981.

88. Frances, R.J., Timm, S., and Bucky, S.: Studies of familial and nonfamilial alcoholism: 1 demographic. Arch Gen Psychiatry *37*:564–566, 1980.

89. Frances, R.J., Bucky, S., and Alexopoulos, G.S.: Outcome study of familial and nonfamilial alcoholism. Am J Psychiatry *141*:11, November, 1984.

90. Korsten, M.A., and Lieber, C.S.: Hepatic and gastrointestinal complications of alcoholism. *In* The Diagnosis and Treatment of Alcoholism. Edited by J.H. Mendelson and N.K. Mello. New York, McGraw-Hill, 1979.

91. Blass, J.P., and Gibson, G.E.: Genetic factors in Wernicke-Korsakoff syndrome: Alcoholism *3*:126–134, 1979.

92. Fultz, R.L., et al. (eds.) GC/MS Assays for abused drugs in body fluid. Research Monograph Series No. 32. Rockville, Md., National Institute on Drug Abuse, 1980.

93. Gold, M.S., Pottash, A.L.C., and Extein, I.: The psychiatric laboratory. *In* Clinical Psychopharmacology. Edited by J.G. Bernstein. John Wright PSG Inc., 1984, pp 29–58.

94. Trill, E., Dristenson, H., and Fex, G.: Alcohol related problems in middle aged men with elevated serum gamma glutamyltransferase: A prevention medical investigation. J Stud Alcohol *45*(4):302–309, 1984.

95. Goodwin, D.W.: Alcoholism and Alcholic Psychoses. *In* Comprehensive Textbook of Psychiatry. 4th ed. Edited by H.I. Kaplan and B.J. Sadock. Baltimore, Williams & Wilkins, 1984. pp 1016–1025.

96. Isbell H., et al.: An experimental study of the etiology of ''rum fits'' and delirium tremens. Q J Study Alcohol *16*:1–13, 1955.

97. Thompson, W.L., Johnson, A.D., and Maddrey, W.: Diazepam and paraldehyde for treatment of severe delirium tremens: A controlled trial. Ann Intern Med *82*:176–180, 1975.

98. Minkoff, K.: II. A map of chronic mental patients. *In* The Chronic Mental Patient. Edited by J. Talbott. Washington, D.C., American Psychiatric Association, 1978, pp 11–37.

99. McCord, W., McCord, J., and Gudeman, J.: Origin of Alcohol. Stanford, California, Stanford University Press, 1960.

100. Vaillant, G.E.: The course of alcoholism and lessons for treatment. *In* Psychiatry Update *3*:311–319. Edited by L. Grinspoon. American Psychiatric Association Press, Washington, D.C., 1984.

101. Pettinati, H.N., Sugarman, A., and Maurer, M.S.: 4 Year MMPI changes in abstinent and drinking alcoholics. Alcoholism: Clin Exp Res *6*:487–494, 1982.

102. Schuckit, M.A.: Alcoholism and other psychiatric disorders. Hosp Community Psychiatry *34*:1022–1026.

103. Winokur, G.A., et al.: The division of depressive illness into depression spectrum disease and pure depressive illness. Int Pharmacopsychiatry *9*:5–13, 1974.

104. Wender, P.H., Reimherr, F.D., and Wood, D.R.: Attention deficit disorder (minimal brain dysfunction) in adults: A repli-

cation study of diagnosis in drug treatment. Arch Gen Psychiatry 38:449–456, 1981.

105. Tarter, R.E.: Psychosocial history in minimal brain dysfunction in differential drinking patterns of male alcoholics. J Clin Psychol 38:867–873, 1982.

106. Hindman, M., and Widem, P.: The multidisabled: emerging responses. Alcohol Health and Research Word 5(2):10, Winter 1980/81.

107. Kinsey, A.C., Pomeroy, W.B., and Martin, C.E.: Sexual Behavior in the Human Male. Philadelphia, W.B. Saunders, 1984.

108. Masters, W.H., and Johnson, V.E.: Human Sexual Inadequacy. London, Churchill, 1970.

109. Tuttle, W.P.: How good are activity recommendations given to cardiac patients? Am J Cardiol 15:99, 1964.

110. Reference deleted

111. Kenyon, F.E.: Studies in female homosexuality. IV Social and psychiatric aspects; V Sexual development, attitudes and experience. Psychiatry 114:1337–1350, 1968.

112. Kallman, F.J.: Comparative twin study of the genetic aspects of male homosexuality. J Nerv Ment Dis 115:283–98, 1952.

113. Bancroft, J.H.J.: Homosexuality in the male. Psychiatry, Special Publication, No. 9, 1975.

114. Bieber, I.: Homosexuality: A Psychoanalytic Study of Male Homosexuals. New York, Basic Books, 1962.

115. Young, W., Goy, R., and Phoenix, C.: Hormones and sexual behavior. Science 143:212–18, 1964.

116. Ehrhardt, A.A., Epstein, R., and Money, J.: Fetal androgens and female gender identity in the early treated androgenital syndrome. Johns Hopkins Med J 122:160–67, 1968.

GENERAL REFERENCES

MOVEMENT DISORDERS

Dyskinetic Movements

Baker, A.B., and Baker, L.H. (eds.): Clinical Neurology. Maryland, Harper & Row, 1978.

Baldessarini, R.J., et al.: Tardive Dyskinesia: Report of the American Psychiatric Association Task Force on Late Neurological Effects of Antipsychotic Drugs. Washington, D.C., American Psychiatric Association, 1980.

Baldessarini, R.J., et al.: The American Psychiatric Association Task Force: Late Neurological Effects of Antipsychotic Drugs. Am J Psychiatry 137:1163–1172, 1980.

Benson, D.F., and Blumer, D.: Psychiatric Aspects of Neurologic Disease. New York, Grune and Stratton, 1975.

Bliss, J., Cohen, D.J., and Freedman, D.X.: Sensory experiences of Gilles de la Tourette Syndrome. Arch Gen Psychiatry 37:1343–1347, 1980.

Brunn, R.D., et al.: A follow-up of 78 patients with Gilles de la Tourette's Syndrome. Am J Psychiatry 133:944–947, 1976.

Donaldson, I.M., and Cunningham, J.: Persisting neurologic sequelae of lithium carbonate therapy. Arch Neurol 40:747–751, 1983.

Fahn, S.: The clinical spectrum of motor tics. In Gilles de la Tourette Syndrome. Edited by A.J. Friedhoff and T.N. Chase. New York, Raven Press, 1982.

Gardos, G., Cole, J.O., and Tarsy, D.: Withdrawal syndromes associated with antipsychotic drugs. Am J Psychiatry 135:1321–1324, 1978.

Granacher, R.P., Jr.: Differential diagnosis of tardive dyskinesia: an overview. Am J Psychiatry 138:1288–1297, 1981.

Jankovic, J. (ed.): Neurologic Clinics—Symposium on Movement Disorders. Philadelphia, W.B. Saunders, 1984.

Jefferson, J.W., and Greist, J.H.: Primer of Lithium Therapy. Baltimore, Williams and Wilkins, 1977.

Jeste, D.V., et al.: Tardive dyskinesia—reversible and persistent. Arch Gen Psychiatry 36:585–590, 1979.

Jeste, D.V., and Wyatt, R.J. (eds): Neuropsychiatric Movement Disorders. Washington, D.C., American Psychiatric Press, 1984.

Kane, J.M., and Smith, J.M.: Tardive dyskinesia: prevalence and risk factors, 1959 to 1979. Arch Gen Psychiatry 39:473–481, 1982.

Kidd, K.K., Prusoff, B.A., and Cohen, D.J.: Familial pattern of Gilles de la Tourette Syndrome. Arch Gen Psychiatry 37:1336–1339, 1980.

Lidsky, T.I., Weinhold, P.M., and Levine, F.M.: Implications of basal ganglionic dysfunction for schizophrenia. Biol Psychiatry 14:3–12, 1979.

Lieberman, J.A., Kane, J.M., and Reife, R.: Neuromuscular effects of monoamine oxidase inhibitors. J. Clin Psychopharmacol 5:221–228, 1985.

Lippmann, S., Moskovitz, R., and O'Tuama, L.: Tricyclic-induced myoclonus. Am J Psychiatry 134:90–91, 1977.

Mukherjee, S., et al.: Tardive dyskinesia in psychiatric outpatients. Arch Gen Psychiatry 39:466–469, 1982.

Osifu, N.G.: Drug-related transient dyskinesias. Clin Pharmacol Ther 25:767–771, 1979.

Owens, D.G.C., Johnstone, E.C., and Frith, C.D.: Spontaneous involuntary disorders of movement: their prevalence, severity, and distribution in chronic schizophrenics with and without treatment with neuroleptics. Arch Gen Psychiatry 39:452–461, 1982.

Reisberg, B., and Gershon, S.: Side effects associated with lithium therapy. Arch Gen Psychiatry 36:879–887, 1979.

Todd, R., Lippmann, S., Manshadi, M., and Chang, A.: Recognition and treatment of rabbit syndrome, an uncommon complication of neuroleptic therapies. Am J Psychiatry 140:1519–1520, 1983.

Van Uitert, R.L., and Russakoff, L.M.: Hyperthyroid chorea mimicking psychiatric disease. Am J Psychiatry 136:1208–1210, 1979.

Wasserman, S., and Yahr, M.D.: Choreic movements induced by the use of methadone. Arch Neurol 37:727–728, 1980.

Tremors

Baker, A.B., and Baker, L.H. (eds.): Clinical Neurology. Maryland, Harper & Row, 1978.

Benson, D.F., and Blumer, D.: Psychiatric Aspects of Neurologic Disease. New York, Grune and Stratton, 1975.

Donaldson, I.M., and Cunningham, J.: Persisting neurologic sequelae of lithium carbonate therapy. Arch Neurol 40:747–751, 1983.

Fahn, S.: Differential diagnosis of tremors. In Medical Clinics of North America. Vol. 56. Edited by M.D. Yahr. Philadelphia, W.B. Saunders, 1972.

Granacher, R.P. Jr.: Differential diagnosis of tardive dyskinesia: an overview. Am J Psychiatry 138:1288–1297, 1981.

Jankovic, J. (ed.): Neurologic Clinics—Symposium on Movement Disorders. Philadelphia, W.B. Saunders, 1984.

Jefferson, J.W., and Greist, J.H.: Primer of Lithium Therapy. Baltimore, Williams and Wilkins, 1977.

Jeste, D.V., and Wyatt, R.J. (eds.): Neuropsychiatric Movement Disorders. Washington, D.C., American Psychiatric Press, 1984.

Reisberg, B., and Gershon, S.: Side effects associated with lithium therapy. Arch Gen Psychiatry 36:879–887, 1979.

Dystonia

Baker, A.B., and Baker, L.H. (eds.): Clinical Neurology. Maryland, Harper & Row, 1978.

Benson, D.F., and Blumer, D.: Psychiatric Aspects of Neurologic Disease. New York, Grune and Stratton, 1975.

Cavanaugh, J.J., and Finlayson, R.E.: Rhabdomyolysis due to acute dystonic reaction to antipsychotic drugs. J Clin Psychiatry 45:356–357, 1984.

Eldridge, R., and Fahn, S. (eds.): Advances in Neurology-Dystonia. New York, Raven Press, 1976.

Fahn, S., et al.: Hysterical dystonia, a rare disorder: report of five documented cases. Neurology 33(Suppl 2):161, 1983.

Granacher, R.P. Jr.: Differential diagnosis of tardive dyskinesia: an overview. Am J Psychiatry 138:1288–1297, 1981.

Jankovic, J. (ed.): Neurologic Clinics—Symposium on Movement Disorders. Philadelphia, W.B. Saunders, 1984.

Jankovic, J., and Ford, J.: Blepharospasm and orofacial-cervical dystonia: Clinical and pharmacological findings in 100 patients. Ann Neurol 13:402–411, 1983.

Schaaf, M., and Payne, C.A.: Dystonic reactions to prochlorperazine in hypoparathyroidism. N Engl J Med 275:991–995, 1966.

Neuroleptic Malignant Syndrome

Baker, A.B., and Baker, L.H. (eds.): Clinical Neurology. Maryland, Harper & Row, 1978.

Burke, R.E., et al.: Neuroleptic malignant syndrome caused by dopamine-depleting drugs in a patient with Huntington disease. Neurology 31:1022–1026, 1981.

Caroff, S.N.: The neuroleptic malignant syndrome. J Clin Psychiatry 41:79–83, 1980.

Caroff, S., Rosenberg, H., and Gerber, J.C.: Neuroleptic malignant syndrome and malignant hyperthermia. Lancet 1:244, 1983.

Delay, J., and Deniker, P.: Drug-induced extrapyramidal syndromes. In Handbook of Clinical Neurology: Diseases of the Basal Ganglia. Edited by P.J. Vinken and G.W. Bruyn. New York, Elsevier North Holland, 1968.

Eiser, A.R., Neff, M.S., and Slifkin, R.F.: Acute myoglobinuric renal failure—a consequence of the neuroleptic malignant syndrome. Arch Intern Med 142:601–603, 1982.

Fricchione, G.L., Cassem, N.H., Hooberman, D., and Hobson, D.: Intravenous lorazepam in neuroleptic-induced catatonia. J Clin Psychopharmacol 3:338–342, 1983.

Gelenberg, A.J., and Mandel, M.R.: Catatonic reactions to high-potency neuroleptic drugs. Arch Gen Psychiatry 34:947–950, 1977.

Granato, J.E., et al.: Neuroleptic malignant syndrome: successful treatment with dantrolene and bromocriptine. Ann Neurol 14:89–90, 1983.

Henderson, V.W., and Wooten, G.F.: Neuroleptic malignant syndrome: a pathogenetic role for dopamine receptor blockade? Neurology 31:132–137, 1981.

Itoh, H., et al.: Malignant neuroleptic syndrome—its present status in Japan and clinical problems. Folia Psychiatr Neurol Jpn 31:565–576, 1977.

Jessee, S.S., and Anderson, G.F.: ECT in the neuroleptic malignant syndrome: case report. J Clin Psychiatry 44:186–188, 1983.

Levenson, J.L.: Neuroleptic malignant syndrome. Am J Psychiatry 142:1137–1145, 1985.

Lew, T., and Tollefson, G.: Chlorpromazine-induced neuroleptic malignant syndrome and its response to diazepam. Biol Psychiatry 18:1441–1446, 1983.

Mann, S.C., and Boger, W.P.: Psychotropic drugs, summer heat and humidity, and hyperpyrexia: a danger restated. Am J Psychiatry 135:1097–1100, 1978.

May, D.C., et al.: Neuroleptic malignant syndrome: response to dantrolene sodium. Ann Intern Med 98:183–184, 1983.

McCarron, M.M., Boettger, M.L., and Peck, J.J.: A case of neuroleptic malignant syndrome successfully treated with amantadine. J Clin Psychiatry 43:381–382, 1982.

Meltzer, H.Y., Mrozak, S., and Boyer, M.: Effect of intramuscular injections on serum creatine phosphokinase activity. Am J Med Sci 259:42–48, 1970.

Morris, H.H., McCormick, W.F., and Reinarz, J.A.: Neuroleptic malignant syndrome. Arch Neurol 37:462–463, 1980.

Mueller, P.S., Vester, J.W., and Fermaglich, J.: Neuroleptic malignant syndrome—successful treatment with bromocriptine. JAMA 249:386–388, 1983.

Sechi, G., Tanda, F., and Mutani, R.: Fatal hyperpyrexia after withdrawal of Levodopa. Neurology 34:249–251, 1984.

Smego, R.A., and Durack, D.T.: The neuroleptic malignant syndrome. Arch Intern Med 142:1183–1185, 1982.

Tollefson, G.: A case of neuroleptic malignant syndrome: in vitro muscle comparison with malignant hyperthermia. J Clin Psychopharmacol 2:266–270, 1982.

Tollefson, G.D., and Garvey, M.J.: The neuroleptic syndrome and central dopamine metabolites. J Clin Psychopharmacol 4:150–153, 1984.

Toru, M., Matsuda, O., Makiguchi, K., and Sugano, K.: Neuroleptic malignant syndrome-like state following a withdrawal of antiparkinsonian drugs. J Nerv Ment Dis 169:324–327, 1981.

Weinberg, S., and Twersky, R.S.: Neuroleptic malignant syndrome. Anesth Analg 62:848–850, 1983.

Zubenko, G., and Pope, H.G., Jr.: Management of a case of neuroleptic malignant syndrome with bromocriptine. Am J Psychiatry 140:1619–1620, 1983.

EATING DISORDERS

Bruch, H.: Anorexia nervosa: therapy and theory. Am J Psychiatry 139:12, 1982.

Darby, P.L. Garfinkel, P.E., Garner, D.M., and Coscina, D.V.: Anorexia Nervosa: Recent Developments in Research. New York, Allan R. Liss, 1983.

Garner, D.M., and Garfinkel, P.E.: Body image in anorexia nervosa: measurement, theory and clinical implications. Int J Psychiatry Med 11:251, 1981.

Halmi, K.A.: Anorexia nervosa. In Clinical and Psychopharmacology. Edited by D.G. Grahame-Smith, H. Hippius, G. Winokur. Amsterdam, Excerpta Medica, 1982, p. 313.

Halmi, K.A.: The state of research in anorexia nervosa and bulimia. Psychiatr Dev 1:247, 1983.

Halmi, K.A., and Falk, J.R.: Common physiological changes in anorexia nervosa. Int J Eating Disorders 1:16, 1981.

Hsu, L.K., Crisp, A.H., and Harding, B.: Outcome of anorexia nervosa. Lancet 1:61, 1979.

Morgan, H.G., and Russell, G.F.M.: Value of family background and clinical features as predictors of long-term outcome in anorexia nervosa: Four year follow-up study of 41 patients. Psychol Med 5:355, 1975.

CHAPTER 17

SLEEP PROBLEMS

Charles P. Pollak, M.D.

Knowledge and interest in sleep disorders has been growing rapidly in the U.S. Currently, 42 sleep disorders centers have been certified by the Association of Sleep Disorders Centers. The development of the field has been stimulated by increasing awareness of previously unknown pathologic events that are limited to or occur predominately during sleep. Detection of these events requires the specialized sleep laboratories of sleep disorders centers, and the concentration of sleep disorders cases in sleep disorders centers, as well as the long-term follow-up of patients, has facilitated the training of a cadre of clinical polysomnographers with special expertise in sleep disorders who are now active in many medical centers.

Diagnostic Evaluation

The evaluation of a sleep disorders patient requires a complete history of the present illness, background data on the patient and family, and physical and laboratory examinations. There are also a few special procedures; a history should also be taken from the bed-partner or another family member whenever possible to determine the presence of significant behaviors such as stop-breathing episodes that may otherwise be missed. Occasionally, it may be useful for the patient to be observed during sleep by a family member; this observation may include a tape recording of breath sounds. Graphical sleep logs often contribute essential information, providing the physician with an overview of the sleep-wake pattern for ten or more days. (Sleep log forms are available from Metrodesign Associates, 81 S. Main St., Homer, N.Y. 13077.)

Polysomnography (PSG) is a generic term that refers to performing sleep recordings in a specially equipped laboratory. Many channels of physiologic data are recorded onto moving paper using a polygraph machine. The data obtained always includes the electroencephalogram (EEG, 1 or 2 channels), electro-oculogram (EOG, horizontal and sometimes vertical eye movements), and chin electromyogram (surface EMG, from mentalis muscle) to identify wakefulness and the stages of sleep. Most clinical recordings are performed for one or two nights. Recording daytime naps is useful when narcolepsy is suspected. Night-time recordings should also include the electrocardiogram (ECG lead II or equivalent), one or more measurements of breathing, and body movements, including movements of the legs. When sleep apnea is suspected, the measurements of breathing should include airflow measurements (using nasal and oral thermistors or thermocouples), assessment of respiratory effort (using chest and abdominal movement detectors) and respiratory gases (determining oxygen saturation by ear oximeter and establishing end-tidal carbon dioxide).

The patient's behavior during the night may be observed and recorded with video equipment sensitive to infrared illumination.[2]

Depending on the sleep disorder, specialized evaluations are often useful from such fields as psychiatry, neurology, clinical psychology, pulmonology, otolaryngology, and cardiology.

The integration and clinical interpretation of the broad physiologic profile requires the experience and training of a clinical polysomnographer.

The physician may encounter three broad categories of symptoms: difficulty initiating or maintaining sleep (insomnia), excessive daytime sleepiness (hypersomnia), and various experiences or events inappropriate to the sleeping state. Identifying the complaint at the start is important, because the chief complaint and its duration can indicate a narrow set of diagnostic possibilities to which further diagnostic steps can then be limited.

Complaints of insomnia, for example, can usually be classified as difficulty initiating sleep, difficulty maintaining sleep, and combinations thereof. A patient usually infers and complains of poor-quality sleep based on the way he feels on awakening or in the daytime. In such cases, the physician will do better to record the daytime symptoms themselves as the complaint, since daytime symptoms of fatigue, tiredness, and the like may be related to medical and psychiatric disorders not associated with sleep disturbance. Similarly, complaints of dependence of hypnotic drugs should be recorded as such, rather than as insomnia, since drug-dependent persons may actually sleep well but expereince sleep disturbance as a symptom of drug withdrawal whenever an attempt is made to reduce or eliminate the hypnotic.

Excessive daytime sleepiness (EDS) may be a problem in its own right, or it may be a symptom of underlying disease. EDS is nearly always present when an individual is driving, and many persons with narcolepsy and sleep apnea have had close calls or accidents. In comparison with other medical symptoms, EDS is unusually disabling because it affects thinking and performance all day long, in ways that masquerade as normal variations of alertness. The medical significance of EDS has therefore only recently begun to be appreciated.

Both sleeplessness and sleepiness may require symptomatic relief either temporarily (such as in a patient with sleep apnea awaiting surgical treatment) or permanently (in a patient with narcolepsy); initial emphasis, however, should be on uncovering the mechanism by which the symptom arises and, if possible, the symptom's cause. Knowledge of pathogeneses of disorders is available to varying degrees.

INSOMNIA

ACUTE DIFFICULTY INITIATING SLEEP

Difficulty falling asleep may be experienced at bedtime and after awakening during the sleep period. We refer in this section to difficulty sleeping at bedtime. The patient should be asked whether the problem is acute, intermittent or chronic. It may be considered acute if it has been present for 1 month or less.

Difficulty initiating sleep presumably involves the activation of brain stem arousal mechanisms; the hypnotic drugs used to treat these patients probably work through their sedative-tranquilizing effects. (If prescribed, such agents should not be administered for more than 1 to 2 months before the patient is re-evaluated.)

Intermittent sleep onset difficulty is usually related to a significant recent or anticipated life event, such as an unexpected death or an imminent wedding. Difficulty initiating sleep under such circumstances is probably universal. Indeed, its universality suggests that situational insomnia should be considered a normal psychophysiologic reaction instead of a disorder.

Acute insomnia also is usually easily related to a life event or situation. To decide whether medical management is appropriate, a more difficult judgment must be made: Is the insomnia an appropriate response, given the type and severity of the life event? Severe sleep reactions require that additional diagnostic possibilities be considered. These include the effects of drugs (caffeine, amphetamines, cocaine), drug withdrawal (sedative hypnotics, tranquilizers, propranolol), acute psychosis, mania, and phase shift of the sleep-wake cycle caused by travel across time zones or a new work schedule.

Diagnosis is made mainly by the patient's history. The patient's other physicians should be consulted to identify recent changes in health or in medical treatment.

RECURRENT DIFFICULTY INITIATING SLEEP

Intermittent sleep onset difficulty should suggest sleep schedule disturbance, hypnotic drug dependency, an affective disorder, and bouts of the restless legs syndrome (RLS).

Sleep logs kept by the patient at home may show a sleep schedule disturbance. Difficulty falling asleep is likely to occur when the patient retires earlier than the time for which his biologic rhythm of sleep and wakefulness is set. Retiring early is a feature of eastward travel, of certain work-shift rotations, and of anticipating the need to get up at an unusually early hour. (Changes in the sleep schedule can cause a disruption of sleep because of the inability of the biologic clock to respond fully to the imposed shift of schedules in the way a wristwatch can be instantly reset.)

Dependence on sedative hypnotic drugs is associated with withdrawal insomnia. Hence, dependent patients who periodically reduce or omit doses of such drugs may experience recurrent sleep onset difficulty. A sleep log can be helpful in making this diagnosis.

More commonly, sleep onset difficulties are not related to external events in any obvious way; rather, physiologic or psychologic endogenous factors predominate.

RLS is a chronic disorder of older adults that causes an agonizing, creeping feeling in the legs and an irresistible urge to move them. These feelings can make falling asleep impossible.[3] Because moving the legs can relieve the feeling, the patient usually gets out of bed to walk, pace, or jump on his legs. After several minutes, the restlessness subsides and the patient returns to bed. As he becomes physically quiet, however, the restlessness may return, and sleep onset may be delayed for hours. Fortunately, the symptoms often remit spontaneously for weeks, months, or years.

RLS is usually associated with periodic movements in sleep (PMS). These are highly periodic movements of one or both feet or violent withdrawals of the legs. The movements occur intermittently throughout sleep.[4] They may cause brief arousals or disturb the sleep of a bed-partner. They are easily detected during PSG by surface EMG electrodes placed over the anterior tibial muscles. Such a recording should be included in every PSG evaluation.

In selected cases of recurrent difficulty initiating sleep, PSG for two consecutive nights may be useful. Sleep is usually more disturbed on the first night of recording, the "first night effect"—itself an example of situational insomnia. In some cases the effect is exaggerated, a useful sign of sensitivity to novel situations. Such patients also report recurrent difficulty sleeping when away from home. The possibility of generalized anxiety disorder, or even panic disorder, should then be considered.

CHRONIC DIFFICULTY INITIATING SLEEP

The complaint of long-standing, nightly difficulty initiating sleep without difficulty maintaining sleep is unusual. Identifying this complaint is important, because it is the hallmark of the delayed sleep phase syndrome (DSPS), a chronobiologic (biologic rhythm) disorder that can be treated without the use of hypnotic drugs.[5]

An unusual work schedule and RLS should first be ruled out. The complaint should then be confirmed by the use of sleep logs, which show that the hour of retiring is quite late—2 A.M. or later. Attempts to retire earlier are associated with difficulty falling asleep, sometimes for several hours. This characteristic distinguishes the patient with DSPS from the phase-shifted normal sleeper (someone working a late shift, for example) who has reset the biologic clock to a late hour but has the capacity to reset it to an earlier hour. There may be a history of difficulty falling asleep even when early sleep hours have been harshly enforced, such as by Army basic training or certain boarding schools. Hypnotic drugs are likewise of little use in helping the patient sleep. The difficulty falling asleep may be wrongly attributed to the DSPS patient's tendency to ruminate while trying to fall asleep, which disappears when the syndrome has been successfully treated by nonpsychiatric means. Once sleep has been initiated, it is relatively solid; there is little or no difficulty maintaining sleep. Because of the late onset of sleep, there is great difficulty getting up in the morning; some patients have resorted to three or more alarm clocks and being splashed with cold water.

Similar but milder difficulties may be present in normal ''night people'' or ''night owls.'' In children, avoiding school may be a factor or complication. DSPS appears to be more common in young people, though it may persist to the middle years of life or later.

DSPS can be treated by a progressive delay of the phase of sleep (chronotherapy) until the desired phase is reached. (The capacity for delay but not advance of the sleep phase is what best distinguishes those with DSPS from those who are physiologically normal but have become adapted to a delayed schedule of sleep.)

CHRONIC DIFFICULTY MAINTAINING SLEEP

This is a somewhat unusual symptom category because most patients with sleep maintenance difficulty also develop difficulty falling asleep as the maintenance difficulty becomes chronic. A sleep log should be used to confirm the complaint; the patient awakens repeatedly but has little difficulty returning to sleep or falling asleep at bedtime. The cause is probably the inappropriate activation of phasic (short-term) arousal mechanisms.

Sleep apnea, which may interrupt sleep, may be predominantly obstructive or nonobstructive. In both forms, apnea or hypopnea events during sleep are ter-

minated by brief, partial arousals. In severe cases, hundreds of such arousals occur in a single night, yet few or none are recalled in the morning. Indeed, daytime sleepiness and not insomnia is usually the dominant symptom, but some patients do experience interruptions of sleep sufficiently intense or prolonged to complain of insomnia. The arousals may be associated with frightening sensations of choking or inability to breathe.

Narcolepsy is characteristically associated with nocturnal arousals. The arousals are brief and are usually less distressing than other symptoms of the disorder. PSG shows that PMS may also be associated with brief arousals.

Short arousals or microarousals are common in elderly patients. Some microarousals are related to sleep apnea or PMS. It is possible that such small events act as a nidus for more severe sleep disturbances when predisposing conditions such as pain, drug toxicity, or schedule disturbance develop.

Sleep logs and PSG are usually helpful in making a diagnosis. Indeed, sleep apnea and PMS-related microarousals require PSG for detection, and the diagnosis of narcolepsy also requires specialized laboratory testing. The laboratory evaluation of sleep apnea and narcolepsy will be described later.

CHRONIC DIFFICULTY INITIATING AND MAINTAINING SLEEP

This category includes those patients who complain of an inability to return to sleep after waking, waking too early, or poor quality of sleep. Most chronic insomniacs also have difficulty falling asleep at bedtime. This category of sleep difficulty produces striking sleep logs: bedtimes and morning arousal times are erratic; sleep latencies (delay from lights out to sleep onset) vary from minutes to many hours; awakenings occur at irregular intervals and for varying durations. Hypnotic drugs or alcohol are used at irregular times and amounts. Not surprisingly, the type and intensity of daytime symptoms also varies widely.[6] The irregularity of sleep and waking is itself a major source of distress; the insomniac never knows when sleep will develop.

The disorder usually involves the interaction of several factors; some are causative (depressive illness), whereas others are permissive (excessive time in bed) or reinforcing (drug toxicity/withdrawal, emotional reactions to sleeplessness). The complex of factors is referred to in the diagnostic system of the Association of Sleep Disorders Centers as psychophysiologic insomnia.[7] It is a common class of insomnia in large case-series of sleep disorders centers.[8]

The physician's challenge is to peel away each of

the factors until there is clinical resolution. A final assessment of the contribution of each factor to the pathogenesis is therefore best made *after* the completion of treatment.

Diagnostic considerations should begin with major depression, since it requires prompt psychiatric treatment. Insomnia is a common and distressing clinical feature of major depression. The sleep disturbances associated with depression include impaired sleep maintenance (early morning awakening), decreased stage 4 sleep, and shortened REM sleep latency (time from sleep onset to first REM sleep episode). The constellation of sleep abnormalities is fairly specific for depressive illness.[9] Insomnia is always distressing, but in the depressed patient lying awake with ruminations in the middle of the night it can be agonizing. Bipolar (manic-depressive) illness may also be associated with severe alterations of sleep amount and timing that are likely to be caused by abnormalities of the circadian timing system.[10]

Chronic anxiety can be associated with chronic or recurrent mixed insomnia. In our experience, the insomnia is milder than that associated with major depression and responds to tranquilizer therapy. PSG evaluation may be worthwhile to demonstrate the limited degree of sleep disturbance to the patient, but even mild sleep disturbances may be bothersome to obsessive personalities.

Hypnotics themselves may be a factor in the maintenance of insomnia. With chronic use, pharmacologic tolerance and psychologic dependence develop. Efforts to reduce dosage (by the patient or physician) may lead to temporary sleeplessness as a withdrawal effect; such rebound insomnia can occur on the same night a short-acting hypnotic is used. Long-acting hypnotics, on the other hand, may impair daytime alertness and judgment, especially in elderly patients.[11]

Most patients with chronic sleep onset and maintenance difficulties have irregular and inappropriate sleeping patterns. The irregularity of sleep is itself a major cause of distress: the patient never knows whether the night will be a "good one" or not and may grow anxious as bedtime approaches. Such anticipatory anxiety can, in turn, augment the sleeping difficulty. As another effect of unpredictable sleep, the patient may vary the hours of sleep in accordance with momentary expectations. It is likely that schedule irregularity also contributes to irregularity of sleep, especially if an excessive period of time is spent in bed trying to sleep. It is usually beneficial to impose a regular sleep schedule, with the time in bed limited to a maximum of 7 hours.

The aging process affects sleep in several ways: the number of arousals increases, sleep efficiency (sleep time as a percentage of time available for sleep) falls, total sleep time decreases, and the sleep stage organization and composition change.[12] The frequency of arousal-related physiologic events during sleep increases with age.[13] As a result of these factors, sleep is more "fragile" in elderly patients, and complaints of difficulty maintaining sleep and of awakening too early tend to predominate over difficulty falling asleep at the start of the sleep period.[14,15] Not surprisingly, sleep disorders centers report more objective PSG abnormalities in older patients, including RLS, periodic movements in sleep, and sleep-induced respiratory disorders.[16,17]

Aging may also reduce the capacity to maintain daytime wakefulness, perhaps because of the fragmentation of night-time sleep, or perhaps because of alterations in the central nervous control of the sleep-wake rhythm.[18,19]

Treatment of insomnia with hypnotic drugs is difficult in elderly patients. Elderly persons may not metabolize hypnotics rapidly enough to prevent excessive sedation, daytime hangover and day-to-day drug accumulation. They are likely to be using other drugs that may interact with hypnotics, and they may have medical illnesses that are partially responsible for the insomnia. It is therefore especially important to accurately diagnose the cause of sleep complaints in elderly patients before considering treatment.

Workup of patients at all ages should include a complete medical history, communication with other treating physicians and a review of records, a complete physical examination and laboratory screening profile, assessment by a psychiatrist or clinical psychologist, sleep logs (before and during treatment), frequent follow-up visits, and sometimes PSG. PSG is essential in patients age 60 and over. To re-emphasize, the usual sequence "first diagnosis, then treatment" is less effective than a continuous interaction of treatment measures (one at a time), followed by reassessment, then a new treatment. Most severe insomnias respond to basic measures, combined with an explanation of the causes of the problem and a therapeutic alliance with the patient that is based upon willingness to engage in trial and error.

EXCESSIVE DAYTIME SLEEPINESS (EDS)

EDS may or may not be pathologic, depending on its chronicity and its cause. Here we shall discuss chronic EDS, of the type associated with narcolepsy and severe sleep apnea. Recent or intermittent bouts of sleepiness are usually related to disruption of the sleep schedule in which the patient has been deprived of sleep or sleep has shifted to a new time of day.

When the patient uses terms such as "tiredness" and "fatigue" and episodes of daytime sleep are not part of the symptom picture, dysphoria of emotional origin, such as depression, and malaise of systemic medical origin should be considered.

EDS is chronic when it has been present for at least part of each day for a month or longer. It may be mild or severe enough to result in unwanted episodes of daytime sleep. EDS is most prominent during sedentary or tedious activities, including driving an automobile. It can be disabling because it affects virtually all activities, except possibly strenuous physical activity. The psychosocial effects of narcolepsy, for example, pervade all areas of life and exceed the disabling effects of epilepsy, probably because of persistent symptoms between episodes of sleep.[20]

EDS can be objectified with the multiple sleep latency test (MSLT). The MSLT is performed in a sleep laboratory, with small variations in the procedure at different laboratories. The patient should keep a sleep log for a week or more before the MSLT, and an all-night PSG should be performed to ascertain that the usual sleep pattern has been followed in the days before the test. Electrodes for sleep recording are applied around 9 A.M. At precisely 10 A.M., the patient is asked to lie down and go to sleep. The delay to sleep onset (sleep latency) is measured. After 20 minutes, the patient is gotten out of bed, even if no sleep occurred. No sleep is allowed until the next nap opportunity, at noon, and so on at 2 P.M. and 4 P.M. In pathologic EDS, the sleep latency for the five naps averages 5 minutes or less.

The causes of EDS include sleep deprivation, sleep-wake cycle disruption, and impairment of the arousal mechanisms. Most cases are caused by sleep apnea or narcolepsy.

SLEEP APNEA

Sleep apnea is a laboratory finding associated with several syndromes. A diminution (hypopnea) or cessation (apnea) of respiratory airflow occurs during sleep, resulting from reduced central nervous respiratory drive associated with a varying degree of upper airway obstruction. The obstruction is at the level of the oropharynx and can be seen with a fiberoptic endoscope.[21] In a PSG, the presence of obstruction is indicated by the simultaneous presence of respiratory thoracoabdominal respiratory movements when air-

flow, measured by nasal and oral thermistors or thermocouples, is diminished or absent. When obstruction is absent, the apnea is referred to as central or nonobstructive. When evidence of obstruction develops during the event, the apnea is termed mixed. When respiratory efforts are present throughout the apnea, they are termed obstructive. In most patients, and especially those with numerous apneas, more than one apnea type can be found. In severe cases, mixed apneas are usually the most frequent type of event.

Each hypopnea or apnea is terminated by a brief, partial arousal, accompanied by loud snoring, caused by a sudden inrush of air past a pharynx that is just reopening. The arousals, which interrupt the development of deep slow-wave sleep, are therefore as numerous as the respiratory events and may occur hundreds of times a night. EDS, which is a late symptom in the evolution of hypersomnia–sleep apnea syndrome, probably results from the frequent interruption and diminishment of nocturnal sleep.[22] Altered brain stem neurotransmitter metabolism caused by respiratory gas abnormalities may also be a contributing factor. Daytime carbon dioxide retention is *not* a necessary factor but may be present in those rare patients with primary alveolar hypoventilation syndrome. EDS should not be attributed to sleep apnea unless abundant apneas can be demonstrated polygraphically, because apneas with marked oxygen desaturation can be recorded in asymptomatic men.[23] Women are much less likely to show apneas during sleep. A single all-night recording is usually enough to establish the number and type of apneas.

Apneas of every type may be associated with oxygen desaturation, carbon dioxide retention, and transient bradycardia. Clinically significant sleep apnea in the adult is much more common in men. It usually develops in the sixth decade in men with long-standing snoring. In addition to age, obesity, nasopharyngeal obstruction, and use of respiratory depressants such as alcohol, major analgesics, and anesthetics increase the tendency to obstructive apnea during sleep.

SLEEP APNEA IN CHILDREN

Children may develop a syndrome of obstructive sleep apnea associated with EDS, polycythemia, and right-sided heart disease similar to that of adults. The usual cause is enlarged tonsils and adenoids; their role in the disorder can be demonstrated in the clinic by the temporary relief afforded by a nasopharyngeal tube.[24] Only some children with enlarged tonsils and adenoids develop sleep apnea, suggesting that individual structural airway or respiratory control factors contribute. The EDS may cause a mental retardation-like dullness, as well as retardation of growth and development.

Sudden infant death syndrome (SIDS) is characterized by unexpected death during sleep. Sleep apnea is one presumed mechanism and has been found in near-miss SIDS infants as well as in the siblings of SIDS infants. Recently, near-miss SIDS infants were found to later develop adenoidectomy-responsive obstructive sleep apnea, and the siblings of SIDS infants show respiratory control abnormality (periodic breathing to hypoxic stimulus).[25,26]

NARCOLEPSY

Narcolepsy is a chronic neurologic disorder with two major symptoms, EDS and cataplexy. The EDS of narcolepsy has not been shown to differ from that of sleep apnea. Although it can be severe, the EDS of narcolepsy does not occur in "attacks," that is, suddenly and without warning, except in those patients who are not aware of, or deny, a medical explanation and strenuously avoid napping. Narcolepsy appears during the teens or twenties but may begin as late as the forties. Once established, it persists for life.

The pathogenesis of EDS in narcolepsy is not yet understood. It is probably not a simple increase in the need for sleep or a decrease in some waking process, since nocturnal sleep is interrupted by awakenings that balance the interruptions of daytime wakefulness by napping. Thus, the entire sleep-wake cycle is disrupted.

Cataplexy is the sudden loss of muscle strength, tone, and reflexes in response to an emotion. Episodes are usually brief (a few seconds). The severity of cataplexy differs considerably from patient to patient. Mild episodes may consist of nothing more than a feeling of "rubbery legs" or of an inner feeling of being "drained." Observation may show slurring of speech, tremor of the jaw, or sinking on the legs. In a severe episode, the patient may fall to the floor almost completely paralyzed (except for eye movements and respirations), but not unconscious. The precipitating emotions are usually those of laughter and anger. Cataplexy is the pathognomonic feature of narcolepsy, but the episodes may be so mild and infrequent that they are not noticed.

The cause of cataplexy is thought to be the displacement of muscle atonia associated with normal REM sleep. Other symptoms of narcolepsy may also be REM components in an abnormal setting of wakefulness. These include sleep paralysis (also REM muscle atonia) and hypnagogic hallucinations (REM dreams).

Sleep paralysis is the brief inability to move upon awakening from sleep. Presumably, it signifies the carrying over of REM sleep atonia into wakefulness. Hypnagogic hallucinations are usually visual hallucinations experienced as one is falling asleep or, less often, waking up. Both symptoms may be related to an abnormal tendency of the narcoleptic patient to move back and forth directly between wakefulness and REM sleep. In these patients, sleep is characteristically initiated with an episode of REM sleep (sleep-onset REM period).

OTHER CAUSES OF EDS

Chronic EDS is occasionally found in those with busy schedules who allot too little time for sleep. Such patients are usually men in their prime years who at first may deny that they do not get enough sleep at night. A sleep log kept for a few weeks may show that the average subjective nightly sleep time is well under 7 hours. Sleep times may also be irregular. Increasing the sleep time and making it more regular may be highly effective, but the response can require several weeks to be detectable and 1 month or more to reach its maximum.

Drowsiness is a side effect of many drugs, but we have seen few cases of unexplained, chronic EDS that could be attributed to drug use alone. Exceptions are chronic use of hypnotics with long half-lives, such as flurazepam, and long-acting barbiturates used for seizure control. Special factors such as renal and hepatic disease and aging that may increase the elimination half-life of drugs should also be considered.

A tendency to sleep excessively may be associated with certain affective disorders. Patients with bipolar illness sleep excessively during the depressed phase, and hypersomnia is one of several predictors of the eventual development of mania in young depressive patients.[27] Recently, there has been described a group of bipolar patients with milder depressions associated with excessive sleeping, overeating, and carbohydrate craving that occur annually at the same time each year (seasonal affective disorder).[28] It is important to recognize this possibility, since nonpharmacologic treatment with bright light may be effective.

Diseases that are *not* likely to cause chronic EDS are brain tumors, hypoglycemia, and hypothyroidism.

DIAGNOSIS OF EDS

Workup of the patient with chronic EDS should begin with a precise description of the complaint: Has there been a daily tendency to fall asleep in inappropriate situations? If chronic EDS is described, the three most helpful clinical features for diagnosis are the sex of the patient and whether the patient snores or has cataplexy. A convincing description of cataplexy is practically tantamount to a diagnosis of narcolepsy. Since the disorder is lifelong, and because rare instances of malingering to obtain analeptic drugs have occurred, it is advisable to perform an MSLT in every case. The test is confirmatory if it shows a short mean sleep latency (less than 5 minutes) and 2 or more sleep-onset REM periods. In women, no further workup is necessary unless many symptoms of sleep apnea are present. In men, sleep apnea should be considered to be present in every case of chronic EDS, even if cataplexy is present, until being ruled out by all-night PSG. Narcolepsy may coexist with hypersomnia–sleep apnea syndrome, and many persons with narcolepsy have laboratory evidence, but not symptoms, of sleep apnea. In men with cataplexy, therefore, the most efficient evaluation consists of an all-night PSG followed by a MSLT the next day.

INAPPROPRIATE NIGHT-TIME EXPERIENCES

SNORING

Though mention of snoring formerly called up humorous associations, it has recently come to be recognized as a symptom with potential significance for health. It is caused by partial obstruction of oropharyngeal structures (palate, uvula, faucial pillars, tongue, and posterolateral pharyngeal walls), usually while sleeping in the supine position. Two forms of snoring may be distinguished. In the common variety, the characteristic motor-boat sound is not loud and is maximal in the supine position and minimal in the prone position. The sounds occur regularly with every breath, though periods of snoring may accompany position changes throughout the night. In snoring associated with obstructive sleep apnea, the sounds are loud enough to be heard from another room, and they occur in a periodic pattern: groups of several loud snores alternate with intervals of silence (apnea) that last 20 to 40 seconds. This form of snoring occurs in any position, though it also may be most prominent in the supine position.

The major significance of snoring is its association with sleep apnea. Nearly all patients with clinical apnea associated with periodic snoring have a long history of regular snoring. Clinicians have long used

Müller's maneuver (inspiratory effort against an airway occlusion) to reproduce in the examining room the pharyngeal closure associated with obstructive apneas during sleep. Recently, such closure has also been demonstrated at higher closing pressures in nonapneic snorers.[29] Thus, snoring is a physiological antecedent, as well as an earlier stage in the development of obstructive sleep apnea.[30]

All forms of snoring may be bothersome to a bed-partner, but marital strife usually has additional origins and does not justify surgical intervention.

NOCTURNAL CHOKING, GASPING, AND DYSPNEA

Unlike snoring, nocturnal choking, gasping, and dyspnea are usually complaints of the sleeper, not of the bed-partner. The sensation of choking may be extremely frightening, as the patient may sense he is about to die. When such events occur repeatedly, they may cause apprehension about going to sleep. One such patient insisted that his family remain awake and on guard all night.

Diagnostic possibilities include sleep apnea, paroxysmal nocturnal dyspnea caused by congestive heart failure, asthma, gastroesophageal reflux, and sleep terrors. Patients with obstructive sleep apnea may experience a sensation of choking in the back of the throat if they awaken during an obstructive episode. Rare patients describe inability to take a breath or expel a breath as they awaken from sleep. As with sensations of choking, the sensation usually disappears soon after full arousal. PSG should be carried out to rule out major sleep apnea. A PSG that contains a subjective event will of course be more valuable than one that does not, and the number of recordings should be planned with the frequency of subjective events in mind.

Unlike sleep apnea, congestive heart failure is usually associated with daytime symptoms such as dyspnea on physical exertion. Dyspnea of cardiac origin persists for at least several minutes—longer than the brief episodes associated with sleep apnea. The presence of heart failure should not rule out consideration of sleep apnea, because sleep apnea may contribute to heart failure. Furthermore, orthopnea of cardiac origin may be mimicked by position-dependent upper airway obstruction during sleep.

Gastroesophageal reflux of gastric contents may be associated with disturbed sleep, substernal discomfort, and difficulty breathing. It can be demonstrated in the sleep laboratory by monitoring episodic decreases of esophageal pH during sleep.[31]

Nocturnal asthma has been studied in adults and

children. It is occasionally responsible for dramatic respiratory emergencies during the night. Milder episodes disturb sleep but are not linked to a particular sleep stage.[32,33]

NIGHTMARES AND SLEEP TERRORS

Nightmares are dysphoric experiences associated with sleep. Many unrelated phenomena are involved. The bed-partners of patients with sleep apnea or narcolepsy often infer, from the patients' gesticulations and vocalizations during sleep, that they must be having nightmares. No dream may be reported by such patients when they awaken moments later. When frequent in older teenagers and adults, nightmares may be signs of major psychopathology, including schizophrenia, borderline personality, and schizotypal personality.[34] They are characteristic of post-traumatic stress disorder.[35] Nightmares may be associated with intensification of REM sleep, as occurs in states of alcohol or drug withdrawal, and are thought to represent disturbed dreams associated with REM sleep in most cases.[36]

Nightmares in children may actually be sleep terrors—sudden, intense episodes of behavioral and autonomic discharge occurring as the child emerges from deep non-REM sleep (sleep stage 4) early in the night. Cases cluster in certain families, along with related non-REM events such as nocturnal enuresis and somnambulism (sleep walking).[37] Although the child may refer vaguely to "monsters," the imagery and storyline of REM sleep–related nightmares is usually absent.

The intensity of sleep terrors is frightening to parents, who may require reassurance that the events are benign and, because the child is amnesic for the event, should have no lasting effect. In the rare child with known or suspected seizures, consideration should be given to nocturnal seizures as the cause of the sleep terrors.[38]

Sleep terrors can be diagnosed with confidence in the sleep laboratory. Two consecutive all-night recordings should be scheduled, since sleep terrors may be suppressed the first night in the laboratory, even in a child with nightly episodes. (It will probably be unproductive to study a child with fewer than 3 or 4 episodes a week.)

The child should be prepared by a prior visit to the laboratory. It is our practice to begin with a brief evaluation by a physician to determine the suitability of PSG. At the end of the visit, the child is taken to the laboratory and introduced to the technologist who will be present during the recording. The recording should include an augmented EEG montage for detection of seizure activity, standard EOG and EMG leads, ECG

respiratory monitoring, and video monitoring. The split screen technique should be employed if possible: a videotape recording is made of the child's behavior simultaneous with EEG activity. This technique is ideal for documenting and analyzing any significant events during sleep. The participation of a neurologist/electroencephalographer is useful.

The classic sleep terror consists of sitting up with a look of abject terror, calling out, tachypnea, and tachycardia. The episode typically arises suddenly out of stage 4 sleep, which is replaced by movement artifact. There should be no epileptiform EEG activity or slowing of the EEG after the event. Smaller episodes may be found, in which the polygraphic recording of stage 4 sleep is suddenly interrupted by movement artifact, but there is little behavioral manifestation.

SLEEP WALKING

Sleep walking, or somnambulism, represents the liberation of motor activity during sleep. During childhood, it is associated with incomplete arousal from non-REM sleep and may be a disorder of the arousal process.[39] Somnambulism in children may be heredofamilial, similar to nocturnal enuresis and sleep terrors. It is usually a transient problem, starting before age 10 and ending by age 15.[40] The prevalence is highest at 11 to 12 years.[41] Older teens and adults started walking at a later age and have more psychopathology. Episodes may not be related to deep non-REM sleep. The episodes in such patients may be intense: the patient often seems to be attempting to escape from some poorly described threat. There may be screaming and violent attacks against bedroom objects or, rarely, people. Nocturnal seizures are contrasted by more stereotyped, repetitive, and purposeless movements, and there is nearly always a history of daytime seizures (see section on nocturnal seizures, below).

For diagnostic certainty, PSG can be performed using sleep polygraphy and behavioral video monitoring.

NOCTURNAL ENURESIS

Nocturnal enuresis is micturition during sleep in a child 3 years or older who has achieved waking bladder control. Many of the comments made in reference to sleep terrors and sleep walking apply also to nocturnal enuresis. Nocturnal enuresis is a transient abnormality of childhood associated with non-REM sleep that may be heredofamilial in origin. It predominates in boys. A common misconception is that the voiding represents an overflow in a child that has had too much fluid to drink at bedtime. Voiding is caused by active detrusor contraction that develops inappropriately during the sleeping state.[42] Reduction of fluids at bedtime only causes the amount voided to be smaller.

Persistent nocturnal enuresis unresponsive to bladder training should prompt diagnostic consideration of urogenital malformations, sleep apnea, and nocturnal seizures. Sleep apnea is usually associated with snoring or other respiratory signs or symptoms during sleep. Seizures are usually not limited to sleep, but occur also during wakefulness.

REPETITIVE MOVEMENTS IN SLEEP

Body rocking, head rolling, and head banging (jactatio capitis nocturna) are common in early childhood. The normal child may engage in these stereotyped movements during the day, while going to sleep, or during sleep. Head banging is more common in boys.[43] Prolonged bouts of forceful movements after the age of 4 are more likely to be associated with autism, mental retardation, or emotional difficulties.

NOCTURNAL SEIZURES

Sleep potentiates seizures and is used for this purpose in diagnostic EEG laboratories. Slow-wave sleep is the most potent in this regard. It is not surprising, therefore, that many epileptics have a disproportionate number of seizures during sleep.[44] It is uncommon, however, for seizures to occur exclusively during sleep.[45] Nocturnal seizures may cause sleep-related events that usually have a nonepileptiform origin, such as enuresis and sleep terrors, as mentioned earlier. It is also worth mentioning that disturbance of the sleep-wake pattern is a common cause of break-through seizures and status epilepticus in epileptic patients.[46,47] The diagnosis of nocturnal seizures can be established by simultaneously recording epileptiform EEG activity and behavioral seizures, using the split screen video technique during a night's sleep.

NOCTURNAL HEADACHES

Patients with migraines commonly report the presence of a headache on awakening in the morning. Episodic cluster headache may be precipitated by nocturnal oxygen desaturation caused by sleep apnea, especially during REM sleep.[48] Milder headaches on awakening in the morning may be associated with obstructive sleep apnea, possibly because of carbon dioxide accumulation during sleep in some patients.

Several types of vascular nocturnal headache may be associated with REM sleep, including episodic cluster headache, chronic paroxysmal hemicrania, and, probably, common and classic migraine.[49]

NOCTURNAL CARDIAC ARRHYTHMIAS

Sleep apnea is commonly associated with slowing of the heart rate during the apneic phase, followed by mild tachycardia as arousal and resumption of breathing occurs. The resulting repetitive pattern of brady-tachycardia may be detected by overnight Holter ECG monitoring in such patients. When seen, this pattern should prompt an evaluation of symptoms (Is the patient sleepy? Does he snore loudly?), and a PSG evaluation that includes respiratory and oxygen saturation monitoring should be ordered.

In addition to brady-tachycardia, sleep apnea may be associated with unsustained ventricular tachycardia, sinus arrest lasting $2\frac{1}{2}$ to 13 seconds, and second-degree atrioventricular conduction block.[49]

Obstructive sleep apnea with oxygen desaturation may be common in men with coronary artery disease.[50] The clinical implications remain to be assessed. Arrhythmias also commonly occur during sleep in patients with chronic obstructive pulmonary disease, perhaps related to oxygen desaturation.[52] Asystole during REM sleep has been reported in apparently healthy young adults. It may be associated with syncope while the patient is ambulatory at night.[53]

IMPAIRED NOCTURNAL PENILE TUMESCENCE (NPT)

This sleep laboratory finding is widely used to help distinguish psychogenic from organogenic impotence.

REM sleep is accompanied by full, sustained erections in normal males. This nocturnal penile tumescence (NPT) may be detected throughout the life span, from infancy to old age.[54] It is part of the physiology of REM sleep and is not necessarily associated with erotic dreams. The nonpsychological nature of NPT is the basis for assuming that impaired NPT implies defective neurovascular mechanisms of erection, and thus that the origin of impotence is at least partially organic. This fact has indeed been demonstrated for diabetes,[55] but there is also evidence of impaired NPT in psychogenic forms of impotence.[56,57]

The evaluation of NPT should include both measurements of penile circumference changes during sleep (done with mercury strain gauges) and direct observation of at least one erection that is maximal, or close to maximal, for that individual. Observation is important because a wide range of circumference changes may be associated with tumescence that is adequate for intromission.

NPT findings should be interpreted only after adequate medical, neurologic, and urologic evaluation.[58]

REFERENCES

1. Guilleminault, C. (ed.): Sleeping and Waking Disorders: Indications and Techniques. Menlo Park, Addison-Wesley Publishing Co., 1982.

2. McGregor, P.A., Weitzman, E.D., and Pollak, C.P.: Polysomnographic recording techniques used for the diagnosis of sleep disorders in a Sleep Disorders Center. Am J EEG Technol 18:107–132, 1978.

3. Ekbom, R.A.: Restless legs syndrome. Neurology 10:868–873, 1960.

4. Coleman, R., Pollak, C., and Weitzman, E.: Periodic movements in sleep (nocturnal myoclonus): a case series analysis. Ann Neurol 8:416–421, 1979.

5. Weitzman, E.D., et al.: Delayed sleep phase syndrome. A chronobiological disorder with sleep-onset insomnia. Arch Gen Psychiatry 38:737–746, 1981.

6. Dement, W., Seidel, W., and Carskadon, M.: Issues in the diagnosis and treatment of insomnia. Psychopharmacology (Suppl) 1:11–43, 1984.

7. Association of Sleep Disorders Centers. Diagnostic Classification of Sleep and Arousal Disorders. 1st Ed. Prepared by the Sleep Disorders Classification Committee, H.P. Roffwarg, Chairman, Sleep 2:1–137, 1979.

8. Zorick, F., Kribbs, N., Roehrs, T., and Roth, T.: Polysomnographic and MMPI characteristics of patients with insomnia. Psychopharmacology (Suppl) 1:2–10, 1984.

9. Gillin, J.C., et al.: Successful separation of depressed, normal and insomniac subjects by sleep EEG data. Arch Gen Psychiatry 36:85, 1979.

10. Wehr, T.A., Gillin, J.C., and Goodwin, F.K.: Sleep and circadian rhythms in depression. In New Perspectives in Sleep Research. Edited by M. Chase. New York, Spectrum Publications, 1983.

11. Institute of Medicine. Report of a study: sleeping pills, insomnia, and medical practice. Washington, D.C., National Academy of Sciences, 1979.

12. Miles, L.E., and Dement, W.C.: Sleep and aging. Sleep 3:119–220, 1980.

13. Ancoli-Israel, S., Kripke, D.F., and Mason, W.J.: Obstructive sleep apnea in a senior population. Sleep Research 13:130, 1984.

14. Kales, A., et al.: Biopsychobehavioral correlates of insomnia, III: Polygraphic findings of sleep difficulty and their relationship to psychopathology. Int J Neurosci 23:43–55, 1984.

15. Roehrs, T., Lineback, W., Zorick, F., and Roth, T.: Relationship of psychopathology to insomnia in the elderly. J Am Geriatr Soc 30:312–315, 1982.

16. Roehrs, T., et al.: Age-related sleep-wake disorders at a sleep disorder center. J Am Geriatr Soc 31:364–370, 1983.

17. Coleman, R.M., et al.: Sleep-wake disorders in the elderly: polysomnographic analysis. J Am Geriatr Soc 29:289–296, 1981.

18. Carskadon, M.A., Brown, E.D., and Dement, W.C.: Sleep fragmentation in the elderly: relationship to daytime sleep tendency. Neurobiol Aging 3:321–327, 1982.

19. Weitzman, E.D.: Sleep and aging. In Neurology of Aging. Edited by R. Katzman and R.D. Terry. Philadelphia, F.A. Davis, 1982, pp 167–188.

20. Broughton, R.J., Guberman, A., and Roberts, J.: Comparison of the psychosocial effects of epilepsy and narcolepsy/cataplexy: a controlled study. Epilepsia 25:423–433, 1984.

21. Weitzman, E.D., et al.: The hypersomnia-sleep apnea syndrome: site and mechanism of upper airway obstruction. In Sleep Apnea Syndrome. Edited by C. Guilleminault. New York, Alan R. Liss, Inc., 1978, pp. 235–246.

22. Stepanski, E., et al.: Sleep fragmentation and daytime sleepiness. Sleep 7:18–26, 1984.

23. Block, A.J., Boysen, P.G., Wynne, J.W., and Hunt, L.A.: Sleep apnea, hypopnea and oxygen desaturation in normal subjects. A strong male predominance. N Engl J Med 300:513–517, 1979.

24. Kravath, R.E., Pollak, C.P., and Borowiecki, B.: Hypoventilation during sleep in children who have lymphoid airway obstruction treated by nasopharyngeal tube and T and A. Pediatrics 59:865–871, 1977.

25. Guilleminault, C., et al.: Five cases of near-miss sudden infant death syndrome and development of obstructive sleep apnea syndrome. Pediatrics 73:71–78, 1984.

26. Brady, J.P., and McCann, E.M.: Control of ventilation in subsequent siblings of victims of sudden infant death syndrome. J Pediatr 106:212–217, 1985.

27. Akiskal, H.S., et al.: Bipolar outcome in the course of depressive illness. Phenomenologic, familial, and pharmacologic predictors. J Affective Disord 5:115–128, 1983.

28. Rosenthal, N.E., et al.: Seasonal affective disorder. A description of the syndrome and preliminary findings with light therapy. Arch Gen Psychiatry 41:72–80, 1984.

29. Issa, F.G., and Sullivan, C.E.: Upper airway closing pressures in snorers. J Appl Physiol 57:528–535, 1984.

30. Lugaresi, E., et al.: Staging of heavy snorers' disease. A proposal. Bull Eur Physiopathol Respir 19:590–595, 1983.

31. Orr, W.C., Robinson, M.G., and Johnson, L.F.: Acid clearing during sleep in patients with esophagitis and controls. Gastroenterology 76:1213, 1979.

32. Kales, A., et al: Sleep studies in asthmatic adults: Relationships of attacks to sleep stage and time of night. J Allerg 41:164–173, 1968.

33. Kales, A., Kales, J.D., and Sly, R.M.: Sleep patterns of asthmatic children: All-night electroencephalographic studies. J Allerg 46:300–308, 1970.

34. Hartmann, E., et al.: A preliminary study of the personality of the nightmare sufferer: relationship to schizophrenia and creativity? Am J Psychiatry 138:794–797, 1981.

35. Terr, L.C.: Chowchilla revisited: the effects of psychic trauma four years after a school-bus kidnapping. Am J Psychiatry 140:1543–1550, 1983.

36. Fisher, C.J., Byrne, J., Edwards, T., and Kahn, E.: A psychophysiological study of nightmares. J Am Psychoanal Assoc 18:747–782, 1970.

37. Kales, A., et al.: Hereditary factors in sleepwalking and night terrors. Br J Psychiatry 137:111–118, 1980.

38. Montplaisir, J., et al.: Sleep and temporal lobe epilepsy: a case study with depth electrodes. Neurology 31:1352–1356, 1981.

39. Broughton, R.: Sleep disorders: Disorders of arousal? Science 159:1070–1078, 1968.

40. Kales, A., et al.: Somnambulism. Clinical characteristics and personality patterns. Arch Gen Psychiatry 37:1406–1410, 1980.

41. Klackenberg, G.: Somnambulism in childhood—prevalence, course and behavioral correlations. A prospective longitudinal study (6–16 years). Acta Paediatr Scand 71:495–499, 1982.

42. Gastaut, H., and Broughton, R.: A clinical and polygraphic study of episodic phenomena during sleep. Recent Adv Biol Psychiatry 7:197–221, 1964.

43. Sallustro, F., and Atwell, C.W.: Body rocking, head banging, and head rolling in normal children. J Pediatr 93:704–708, 1978.

44. Janz, D.: The grand mal epilepsies and the sleeping-waking cycle. Epilepsia 3:69–109, 1962.

45. Gibberd, F.B., and Bateson, M.C.: Sleep epilepsy: its pattern and prognosis. Br Med J 2:403–405, 1974.

46. Pratt, K.L., Mattson, R.H., Weikers, N.J., and Williams, R.: EEG activation of epileptics following sleep deprivation: A prospective analysis of 114 cases. Electroencephalogr Clin Neurophysiol 24:11–15, 1968.

47. Janz, D.: Conditions and causes of status epilepticus. Epilepsia 2:170–177, 1960.

48. Kudrow, L., McGinty, D.J., Phillips, E.R., and Stevenson, M.: Sleep apnea in cluster headache. Cephalalgia 4:33–38, 1984.

49. Dexter, J.D., and Weitzman, E.D.: The relationship of nocturnal headaches stage patterns. Neurology 20:513–518, 1970.

50. Guilleminault, C., Connolly, S.J., and Winkle, R.A.: Cardiac arrhythmia and conduction disturbances during sleep in 400 patients with sleep apnea syndrome. Am J Cardiol 52:490–494, 1983.

51. DeOlazabal, J.R., Miller, M.J., Cook, W.R., and Mithoefer, J.C.: Disordered breathing and hypoxia during sleep in coronary artery disease. Chest 82:548–552, 1982.

52. Flick, M.R., and Block, A.J.: Nocturnal vs diurnal cardiac arrhythmias in patients with chronic obstructive pulmonary disease. Chest 75:8–11, 1979.

53. Guilleminault, C., Pool, P., Motta, J., and Gillis, A.M.: Sinus arrest during REM sleep in young adults. N Engl J Med 311:1006–1010, 1984.

54. Karacan, I., Williams, R.L., Thornby, J.I., and Salis, P.J.: Sleep-related penile tumescence as a function of age. Am J Psychiatry 132:932–937, 1975.

55. Karacan, I., et al.: Nocturnal penile tumescence and diagnosis in diabetic impotence. Am J Psychiatry 135:191–197, 1978.

56. Fisher, C., et al.: Evaluation of nocturnal penile tumescence in the differential diagnosis of sexual impotence. A quantitative study. Arch Gen Psychiatry 36:431–437, 1979.

57. Roose, S.P., Glassman, A.H., Walsh, B.T., and Cullen, K.: Reversible loss of nocturnal penile tumescence during depression: a preliminary report. Neuropsychobiology 8:284–288, 1982.

58. Wasserman, M., Pollak, C.P., Spielman, A.J., and Weitzman, E.D.: The differential diagnosis of impotence: measurement of nocturnal penile tumescence. JAMA 243:2038–2042, 1980.

CHAPTER 18

DERMATOLOGIC PROBLEMS

Marie-Louise Johnson, M.D., Ph.D.

GENERAL PROBLEMS

When the skin is the source of the patient's complaint, most changes are visibly presented to the examiner; the physician and patient concurrently observe the problem. Pruritus and pain are the exceptions. These are subjective, and patients' thresholds vary; however, the presence and intensity of pruritus and pain can often be verified and add important information to the data base.

PRURITUS

Definition and Pathophysiologic Considerations

Pruritus is a cutaneous irritability that provokes scratching. A variety of stimuli, physical and chemical, can trigger mediators that act on a complex network of nerve endings thought to be the cutaneous receptor organ and localized at the dermo-epidermal junction in the superficially situated papillary dermis just tenths of a millimeter from the external environment. These receptors for itching are probably the same elements that perceive superficial cutaneous pain. There is an absence of itch, for example, in those individuals with congenital absence of cutaneous pain sensation.

Itch, however, cannot be said to be weak pain. Both itch and pain have a range of intensity, and are perceived as qualitatively different. Heating the skin to 41°C will block itch but augment pain. An eroded cutaneous segment of epidermis and papillary dermis will hurt, but it cannot itch. Histamine injected intracutaneously will produce not pain but itch, then a wheal, with both responses blocked by antihistamines. Endopeptidases such as in the spicules of cowage, the "itch powder" plant of Jamaica, will produce pruritus, as will other endopeptidases. Such well-localized, physiologically induced itch is thought to be conducted by the myelinated, rapidly conducting A fibers; poorly localized chronic itch is carried by unmyelinated, slowly conducting C fibers.

Lowered Itch Threshold. In what may be considered a hyperexcitable state, the most innocuous stimulus to the skin, whether chemical or physical, can provoke intense pruritus, a phenomenon attributed to malfunction of the superficial receptor system because of partial damage. Such a hyperexcitable state may be due to a disease process as in the eczematous change of atopic dermatitis, the cellular infiltrates of malignancy, or the deposited bile salts of obstructive biliary disease. It may be quite localized and the result of the topical application of a toxin, as from hairy spicules in "caterpillar dermatitis," or from its injection, as from the proboscis of the mosquito. By recognizing that minimal stimuli can trigger pruritus in such hyperexcited states, efforts to protect the skin will promote comfort and in some instances hasten resolution.

Recognizing other factors important in the lowering of the itch threshold will help in the assessment of the symptom and in broadly guiding therapy. Pruritus, whatever the cause, is more severe at night. Whether the distractions of the waking hours or the higher steroid levels of the diurnal variation serves to lessen daytime pruritus is not known. Raising the skin temperature, as with bedclothes or with exercise or high ambient temperature, aggravates itching. Vasodilatation, whether spontaneous or pharmacologically induced, suffuses and warms the skin with a similar consequence. Poorly hydrated, scaling, dry skin not only increases existing pruritus but can be the cause of pruritus de novo in elderly individuals or even in the young during winter.

Pyschic stress will also have its effect. Few dermatologic disorders are caused by the psyche, but most can be triggered or worsened by emotional stress. If from the first the psyche is suggested as having a role in the pruritus, all other causes must be evaluated and the significance of the psychic stress determined by exclusion.

Last, there are those who have inherited a lowered itch threshold, atopic individuals with the itch that when rubbed becomes rash. If such individuals have had infantile eczema and been recognized lifelong as atopic, they present no diagnostic problem. But the atopic diathesis is often subtle. The cause of itch in such patients will escape the examiner if there is no history elicited of previous rash, especially in flexural areas, or of respiratory allergies, asthma, or urticaria, and, if not in the patient, a history of such atopic manifestations in parents or siblings. Atopic individuals may have localized pruritus, typically of the hands or feet, but it can be generalized. Depending on the duration and intensity of the itch-scratch cycle, the skin may be excoriated, thickened, and hyperpigmented. The atopic diathesis presents a characteristic canvas upon which other pathologic change will be sketched; atopy should be recognized for the contribution it makes to the hyperexcitable state and the lowered threshold for pruritus of all other causes.

Normal Itch Threshold. Given normal skin and the average resistance to pruritus, the factors that produce itching are numerous, and wide ranging, from infestations to infiltrations.

Infestations. Infestations classically produce itch.

Scabies is the most intensely pruritic infection, with a notable night-time worsening and a suggestive anatomic distribution to finger web, wrists (flexor aspect), elbows (extensor surface), the anterior axillary folds, and around the areolae, umbilicus, and genitals, especially the penis. In unclean patients, tracks are found easily and the diagnosis proved by recovering the barely visible mite (Sarcoptes scabei var. hominis) from the blind end of the tunnel. In well-scrubbed patients, tracks may not be apparent and the mite difficult to find. Here the intensity of pruritus, indicated by scratching even during the distraction of the examination, along with the anatomic locations will be suggestive, and a 12-hour application of 1% lindane or 10% crotonotoluide with consequent relief of symptoms will prove diagnostic. Pruritus may smolder at a much diminished intensity for a week or so after treatment because of the persistence of mite products in the skin, but the immediate post-treatment relief, the contrast of pre- and post-treatment pruritus, is an affirmative test. A repeat application should be made in 7 days to ensure riddance of larvae that may have hatched from less vulnerable eggs.

With other infestations, the organism is easier to find if the search is directed correctly. Head lice (Pediculus humanus var. capitis) are easy to see because of their size but are short lived and hence scarce. They leave their characteristic nits tenaciously fastened to the hair. Difficult to pull free, the nits will not be confused with seborrheic scale. Pubic lice (Phthirius pubis), much more sluggish, will be found half buried in the hair follicle, mouth parts attached, in place for days. Most often found in the pubic area, crab lice can also involve the eyelashes, and infestations have been confused with pruritic blepharitis. The body louse (Pediculus humanus var. corporis) is harder to find unless the clothing seams are searched. Erythematous papules, excoriations, and ulcerations, especially in debilitated or downtrodden individuals, should lead to an inspection of garment seams.

Other erythematous pruritic papules occurring in a row, especially when each has a puncta, should raise the suspicion of arthropod bites. In the home, bed bugs (Cimex lectularius) living in crevices and moldings of heated buildings emerge to feed at night in the dark. In an infested room, a lighted lamp is protective. Spiders are not deterred by light and are common in old buildings and basements; unnoticed at the time of an asymptomatic bite, spider bites can have impressive sequelae with itch, burn, and, from some species, necrosis. As with all infestations, the exposure history and the cutaneous response will narrow the diagnostic possibilities.

Metabolic Causes. Metabolic causes of itching may be more subtle. Migratory pruritus with or without urticaria can be found in hyperthyroidism, but in fewer than 10% of cases. If the itch occurs in skin that is moist, pink, and fine, in a person with soft, thin, friable hair, the diagnosis is quite likely and easily confirmed by tests of thyroid function. Reduced thyroid function may also be associated with itching, but here the skin is thickened, yellow, coarse, and dry, with dryness contributing to the pruritus. It is the associated signs and symptoms, the hoarseness of the voice, the slowness of mentation and movement, that will point to hypothyroidism as a cause of the pruritus.

Because diabetes can be associated with itching, a glucose tolerance test should be done in patients with pruritus of obscure origin. Often the lower extremities and the anogenital area are involved, but the problem can be generalized. The predisposition to infection and the poor healing with injury may be associated with a hyperexcitable state and lowered itch threshold.

With renal failure pruritus occurs in as many as one third of patients; though it can be severe and intractable, it is a late finding, a challenge to therapy but not to diagnosis. The cause for the pruritus is unknown, although it is suggested that some dialyzable, high calcium, high phosphorus product accumulates in extracellular fluid and deposits calcium salts in the skin. While relief in such patients has been reported with subtotal parathyroidectomy, which reduces the hypercalcemia, an elevated serum calcium in the presence of normal renal function is not known to produce pruritus.

In obstructive biliary disease, the evidence for bile acids as the cause of itching is better established, although the mechanism remains unclear. The bile acid levels of the skin rather than serum levels correlate with the intensity of the pruritus. Specific effective treatment with cholestyramine, an anion exchange resin that binds bile salts, is directed at lowering the concentration of the bile salts in serum and skin.

Neoplastic Disorders. Neoplastic disorders can be associated with itching. Complaints of provoking pruritus with a warm bath or shower are not unusual for any pruritic problem, but classically bring to mind polycythemia vera, in which 20 to 50% of patients have severe itching or burning for 15 to 30 minutes after the exposure. It is the intensity and duration of the pruritus of polycythemia vera that sets it apart. It is sometimes lessened by lowering the hematocrit.

In the lymphoproliferative diseases pruritus is a significant symptom. Circumscribed or generalized, intermittent or continuous, mild or intense, it may precede the definitive clinical diagnosis by months, even years. Although it may remit sometimes with chemotherapy directed at the underlying malignancy, the pruritus may be unresponsive to all therapy and be so devastating as to provoke suicide. Generalized pruritus occurs in one quarter of the patients with Hodgkin's disease and is a common presenting complaint of patients with the T-cell lymphoma of mycosis fungoides or with leukemia or multiple myeloma. It rarely heralds other malignancies.

Allergens. Allergens are among the less threatening causes of pruritus but are quite debilitating if the offending agent is not identified. Medications are important contributors, especially when associated with eruption, but subclinical drug allergies occur; for example, opiates and amphetamines can produce pruritus without rash. A careful history should identify the allergen. Illicit drugs and marijuana must not be overlooked. Other ingestants are difficult to discriminate. List-keeping at times of exacerbation and label reading as well as elimination diets can be helpful.

Contact allergens, airborne or otherwise, such as cactus spicules and bird mites, can cause intense pruritus and must be suspected if they are to be identified. Rodents and birds that have nested in air conditioners in winter can be an easily overlooked source of airborne mites. So, too, are dried flowers and ferns or grain fed to animals.

Stasis dermatitis is a separate problem in which venous incompetence and edema are early signs along with pruritus. Hemosiderin is deposited in the skin, and an area of cyanotic erythema develops, occasionally with ulceration and more extensive pruritus and rash. Managing the early pruritus and venous incompetence would contain the entire problem.

Environmental Factors. Environmental factors are also to be considered. Blocking of the sweating mechanism, whether the result of high ambient humidity or adherent scale, causes trapped sweat to break into the skin. If the break is at the level of the superficial capillaries and nerves, redness and pruritus, or miliaria rubra, will be the result. Reducing the sweat flow with cooling and freeing the blocked sweat with keratolytics will ease the pruritus. Similarly, patients with atopic dermatitis sweat poorly, and lubricating their dry skin further blocks the sweating mechanism, aggravating the pruritus that is part of the disease.

Irritants in the environment, notably fiberglass insulation, with its myriad of fine glass spicules that traumatize the skin, can cause intense itching, as can caustic agents that dry and irritate. The mechanism is largely primary irritation with injury, triggering the mediators that work on the complex network of nerve endings.

Other Causes. There are, however, other disorders in which pruritus is a major symptom but the mechanism is unclear. An example is pregnancy. If the ges-

tation is not yet recognized, the itching could be a challenge. Most cases of pruritus in pregnancy are associated with variously classified rash, but in some 17% of pregnancies pruritus occurs alone. If intense generalized pruritus occurs, it tends to be late in the pregnancy.

Specific dermatologic conditions such as dermatitis herpetiformis, atopic dermatitis, and bullous pemphigoid can present with pruritus without rash. Only by suspecting the underlying diagnosis and waiting for confirmatory signs can the diagnosis be made; grouped vesicles over extensor aspects of the extremities or buttocks suggest dermatitis herpetiformis; flexural accentuation or appropriate history occurs in the atopic individual; and tense pruritic bullae or urticarial plaques indicate bullous pemphigoid.

Differential Diagnosis and Diagnostic Evaluation
(Table 18–1)

A cardinal rule in the examination of any patient is a complete assessment of the entire integument, scalp to toe. Only when this examination has been done can specific complaints and observations be interpreted.

The most common cause of itching is dry or xerotic skin. Whatever the reason for dryness, whether aging with its reduction in sebaceous gland activity or the warm, moistureless air of winter households, lubrication should relieve the symptom. If it does not or the skin was well lubricated at examination, then the search is on.

A localized pruritic area may be the continuation of the itch-scratch cycle initiated by a subclinical contact dermatitis or arthropod reaction. It may be the effect of irritation, allergy or psychic stress on such hyperexcitable sites as the eyelids or anogenital region. The differential is broad but the prognosis is good, for few life threatening problems present as localized pruritus. It is when the problem is generalized that concern is greater and intensity must be assessed. If the patient is scratching during the examination and there are extensive excoriations of the skin, the pruritus is severe; scabies or lymphoma must be considered. Immune-suppressed patients infested with scabies may not itch, while other patients with malignancy may itch, but not intensely. This limited differential is for intense pruritus.

Moderate or minimal generalized pruritus has a more extensive differential. The skin may be excoriated and, depending on the duration of the problem, may be thickened or lichenified. The clinician must always search for primary lesions. If none is found, providing symptomatic relief with lubrication, oral antihistamines, and a mentholated lotion should be attempted, with re-examination for primary lesions in 1 week. Senile xerosis and winter itch, even mild sub-

Table 18–1. Differential Diagnosis of Pruritus

Cutaneous Signs	Clinical Presentation	Tests
Extreme itch		
Scabies	Night-time worsening; anatomic distribution: finger webs, wrists (flexor aspect), elbows (exterior), anterior axillary folds, areolae, umbilicus, genitals	Identification of the mite, prompt response to lindane
	Tracks and mites in unscrubbed patients (less evident in fastidious patients)	
Lymphoma	Intensity (scratching during exam, excoriations) circumscribed or generalized; intermittent or continuous; may precede definitive diagnosis by months or years	Histology—blood smear
Hodgkin's disease		Bone marrow aspiration
Leukemia,		
Mycosis fungoides		
Multiple myeloma		
Moderate itch		
Generalized		
Metabolic diseases		
Hyperthyroidism	Moist, pink, fine skin; soft, thin, friable hair	Serologic tests of thyroid function
Hypothyroidism	Yellow, thick, coarse, dry skin; thinned eyebrows, hoarse voice	Serologic tests of thyroid function
Diabetes	Pruritus can be generalized or circumscribed (see below)	Abnormal glucose tolerance test
Renal failure	Occurs in one third of patients with diagnosed renal failure; can be severe and intractable	Elevated BUN
Obstructive biliary disease	Jaundice	Elevated serum bilirubin
Allergens	History of medications (including over-the-counter and illegal drugs); food diary, exposure history	Positive patch and scratch tests to specific allergens suggestive
Irritants	Exposure history	None
Pregnancy	17% of all pregnancies have itch without rash	Confirmation of pregnancy
Neoplastic change		
Polycythemia vera	Severe itching and burning 15 to 30 minutes after exposure to bath or shower	Elevated hematocrit
Localized		
Infestations		
Head lice	Nits, arthropods in scalp hair	Identifying arthropod
Crab lice	Pubic area, eyelashes	Identifying arthropod
Body lice	Erythematous papules, ulcerations, excoriations especially in "downtrodden" individuals	Identifying arthropod (check clothing seams)
Arthropod bites	Erythematous papules with puncta, exposure history	
Metabolic diseases		
Diabetes	Especially in lower extremities, anogenital area	Abnormal glucose tolerance test
Allergens	Erythema and vesicles	Positive patch test
Dermatologic conditions		
Dermatitis herpetiformis	Excoriated papules or grouped vesicles over extensor aspects of extremities or buttocks	Histology
Atopic dermatitis	Flexural accentuation	None
Bullous pemphigoid	Pruritic bullae or urticarial plaques	Histology—skin biopsy, tissue immunofluorescence
Mild itch		
Senile xerosis, winter itch	Dry skin, eczema craquelé	Response to lubrication

clinical contact dermatitis that has been continued through an itch-scratch cycle, will respond. If pruritus continues, the cause may be malignancy, a metabolic disorder, an allergy, or one of an array of idiopathic problems, including psychic stress. The continuing assessment requires a good review of systems; a complete blood count (white blood count and differential with sedimentation rate), along with a fasting blood sugar, tests of hepatic, renal, and thyroid function, and a routine urinalysis. Any suggested organ dysfunction gleaned from the history or physical examination must be pursued.

PAIN

Definition, Pathophysiologic Considerations, and Differential Diagnosis (Table 18–2)

Pain is a sensitivity of the skin that may be spontaneous or provoked by contact; it may be minimal or debilitating, interfering with sleep and all normal activity. Both pain and itch, as discussed above, are presumed to be gathered by the same cutaneous receptors and transmitted to the central nervous system by both myelinated A and unmyelinated B fibers.

Painful skin without exogenous trauma such as a

Table 18–2. Differential Diagnosis of Pain

Clinical Presentation	Dermatologic Condition	Tests
Intense pain—sudden onset, dermatome distribution; subsequent appearance of erythema and vesicles	Herpes zoster	Tzanck smear for multinucleated giant cells
Burning pain, usually involving extremities; history of incomplete nerve tract injury; skin may be warm, pink, and dry or cool and moist; no viral vesicles	Causalgia	None
Burning pain and vasodilatation; paroxysmal, no history of nerve damage	Erythromelalgia	None
	Primary: healthy individual	None
	Secondary: association with occlusive vascular disease, polycythemia vera, thrombocytopenia, gout	
Burning and erythema overlying an engorged, nodular, thickened vessel	Giant cell arteritis	Vessel biopsy
Burning pain and paresthesias of hands and feet, associated with keratotic blue-black vascular papules	Fabry's disease (angiokeratoma corporis diffusum)	Identification of the specific glycolipid in tissues secondary to galactosidase A deficiency

blow or burn is uncommon. When it occurs it is localized. The sudden onset of pain in dermatome distribution is considered herpes zoster until proved otherwise. The subsequent appearance of erythema and vesicles with a positive Tzanck smear will confirm the diagnosis. Herpes zoster infections may leave the skin normal or scarred with severe pain and sensitivity that may last several years. If the scar is not apparent and the history of active zoster vague, the symptom may be difficult to diagnose.

Burning pain, usually involving an extremity, and beginning after incomplete nerve tract injury, whether trauma or surgery, is known as causalgia. The involved skin may be warm, pink, and dry, or cool and moist from sweat, depending upon the hyperactivity or paralysis of the anatomic structures under autonomic control. There are no viral vesicles. There may be associated trophic changes of the epidermis and nails, and occasionally decalcification of underlying bone.

Causalgia must be distinguished from the vasodilatation and burning pain of erythromelalgia; the latter is paroxysmal and there is no history of antecedent damage to nerves. Primary erythromelalgia occurs in normal, otherwise healthy individuals; the secondary form is found in association with occlusive vascular disease, polycythemia vera, thrombocytopenia, or gout. Erythema and burning of the skin overlying an engorged, nodular or thickened vessel with diminished pulsations suggests arteritis and is most commonly diagnosed clinically when the temporal artery is involved.

In Fabry's disease (angiokeratoma corporis diffusum), burning pain and paresthesias of the hands and feet may be the presenting complaint before the appearance of the characteristic keratotic blue-black vascular papules. The pain may be brought on by environmental temperature extremes as well as by fever

and exertion. Usually the pain has a remittent pattern, but in some patients it may persist as a nagging discomfort. This sex-linked disorder of glycolipid storage is less severe in heterozygous females, who may have milder symptoms and it may go unrecognized unless the symptoms are interpreted in the light of the angiokeratomas or the associated vascular, ocular, neurologic, or renal changes that may result from storage of glycolipids in these various organs.

TEXTURE CHANGE (Table 18–3)

Scaling. A complaint of scaling, visibly sloughing keratin, which may or may not be associated with erythema, should be considered first for its extent. A localized patch of scale may result from mild, drying irritants such as caustic cleansing agents or from allergic sensitivity. A careful history and skin testing will help to differentiate the cause. The patch may be infectious, as from superficial fungi, evoking no erythematous response. A KOH (potassium hydroxide) test will show hyphae and distinguish such scale from that of a herald patch of pityriasis rosea, or from the classic round scaling hypopigmented patches on an adolescent arm or thorax that were once thought to be fungal but are now known to be a manifestation of a mild eczematous process, pityriasis alba. Without significance other than cosmetic, these lesions fade with time, responding poorly to any specific therapy.

Generalized scaling may be merely xerosis, skin dried by repeated cleansing without lubrication, further aggravated by high ambient temperature and low humidity as well as by the depleted moisture retention and lowered sebaceous gland activity of aging. Because of pruritus the skin may become excoriated and damaged, but even without itching, dry skin cracks,

Table 18–3. Differential Diagnosis of Cutaneous Texture Change

Cutaneous Signs	Dermatologic Condition	Supportive Observations	Tests
Localized scale			
Circumscribed, evenly distributed	Reaction to irritant	Patterned distribution	History
	Allergic sensitivity	Patterned distribution	Patch test
With active border, clearing center	Fungal infection	Anatomic distribution, e.g., body folds	KOH test, fungus culture
Herald patch—medallion lesions, Christmas tree configuration	Pityriasis rosea	Patient less than 40 years of age	None
Round, scaling, hypopigmented patches	Pitryriasis alba	Patient less than 10 years of age	None
Generalized scale			
Dry, excoriated, cracked	Xerosis	Occurring in elderly patients, in winter	None
Polyhedral, tenacious—involves face, scalp, sparing of flexural creases, hyperkeratotic palms, family history of dry skin, association with atopic diathesis and seasonal variation (improvement in summer, worsening in winter)	Ichthyosis vulgaris	Existing from childhood—autosomal dominant	Histology—absent granular layer
Severe, large, dark, tenacious scales; distribution: extensor and flexor surfaces of limbs; palms and soles normal; associated corneal opacities	X-linked ichthyosis	Present from birth or infancy	Histology—hyperkeratosis with granular layer
Erythematous, fissured skin, verrucous about joints; hair plastered down with scale, ectropion	Lamellar ichthyosis	Collodion-like membrane at birth; condition present from birth	Histology supportive, not diagnostic
Blisters, keratotic and verrucous skin, recurring bullae; normal hair and mucous membranes	Epidermolytic hyperkeratosis	Collodion-like membrane at birth; condition present from birth	Histology—large keratohyaline granules; vacuolated cells
Localized thickening			
Accentuation of skin markings in a plaque without distinct borders; distribution: common on legs and shoulders	Lichen simplex chronicus	Area easily reached by dominant hand	Histology—protective, curative effect of occlusive dressing
Nodular plaque: pink, tan, or brown; distribution: lower legs, especially pretibial aspect	Localized myxedema or amyloid	History of thyroid treatment, chronic illness	Histology—special stain for mucin or amyloid
Sudden onset of marked nonpitting induration of the skin; distribution: usually upper back and shoulders	Scleredema	Associated with mature-onset diabetes in obese patients	Biopsy supportive
Generalized thickening			
Skin thickened and dry with accentuated markings and hyperpigmentation	Atopic diathesis	History of atopy	None
Skin cold, dry, hyperkeratotic, ivory yellow	Hypothyroidism	Missing lateral third of eyebrows, alopecia	Tests of thyroid function
Skin puffy, pale, yellow, waxy	Myxedema	Tongue, lips thickened	Tests of thyroid function; histology—accumulated mucopolysaccharide
Nodular, associated with hyperpigmented macules	Neurofibromatosis of von Recklinghausen	Café au lait spots (more than 6), axillary freckles	Histology
Localized atrophy			
Thinning, wrinkling patches	Cicatrix	History of injury	Histology
Circumscribed, sclerotic plaque with ivory centers and lilac periphery, may be few or many	Morphea	None	Histology—biopsy
Atrophic lesions associated with telangiectasia and follicular plugging; carpet-tack scale	Lupus erythematosus	Increased SED rate, low WBC, occasionally positive ANA titer	Histology—biopsy
Ivory-white atrophic plaques in anogenital area; occasional hyperkeratinization, inflammation, and lichenification; may undergo malignant change	Lichen sclerosus et atrophicus	None	Histology—biopsy
Generalized atrophy			
Hidebound skin; may begin with rapid extension over the trunk and extremities or with acral sclerosis; tight skin, pinched facies, tapered, taut fingers with flexion contractures and ulcerations; cutaneous calcifications	Scleroderma	Raynaud's phenomenon, hyper-, hypo-, and depigmentation	Histology—biopsy

the normal cutaneous barrier is breached, and fissures admit bacteria. All older people are at risk, especially older diabetic patients. Lubricating the skin and using keratolytics to remove scale, if needed, is good preventive medicine.

If the generalized scale is polyhedral and tenacious, unresponsive to simple measures, the problem must be differentiated as congenital or acquired. If present from birth or early childhood the problem is one of the inherited disorders of keratinization, of which ichthyosis vulgaris is the most common. There is often a family history of dry skin, with great variation in the intensity of expression. The face and scalp are commonly involved, while the flexural surfaces, especially at the creases, may appear normal; the palms are hyperkeratotic and may have exaggerated skin markings. There is a frequent association with the atopic diathesis manifested as the respiratory component of hay fever or asthma, but also in its cutaneous expressions of frank eczema and urticaria. There is, as with all the ichthyoses, seasonal improvement in summer and worsening in winter.

The less common X-linked ichthyosis is more severe, with large, dark, tenacious scales covering the extensor and, somewhat less intensely, the flexor surfaces of the limbs; the palms and soles are normal. Associated corneal opacities are seen in affected males and, less often, in the female carrier. These opacities help in the differential diagnosis and detection of carriers; fortunately they do not limit vision.

Lamellar ichthyosis involves the entire cutaneous surface form birth, when there is usually a collodion-like membrane encasement. The skin throughout life is erythematous and fissured, somewhat verrucous about the joints. Hair is present, but plastered down in scale; there is a pathognomonic ectropion. Bacterial infection is a common problem in these patients, and interference with normal sweating makes them prone to hyperpyrexia.

Babies with epidermolytic hyperkeratosis may also be born with a collodion-like membrane and in addition have blisters. The skin becomes keratotic and verrucous, a change that may be generalized or limited, with bullae recurring periodically into adulthood. The hair and mucous membranes are normal.

The congenital ichthyoses other than ichthyosis vulgaris will be readily recognized as congenital problems and will not present the challenge of acquired ichthyosis. If the ichthyotic change is truly new and acquired there may be an underlying systemic problem, including malignancy, considered below.

Thickening. The most common localized form of thickening is the accentuation of skin markings in a plaque without distinct borders, lichen simplex chron-

icus. It may occur anywhere, the legs and shoulders being common areas. Frequent rubbing plays a significant causative role. Occluding the area will permit the skin to return to normal. If the plaque is more nodular, perhaps pink, tan, or brown, and the lower legs are involved, especially the pretibial aspect, localized myxedema or amyloid must be considered. A biopsy will distinguish between the two and will distinguish both from lichen simplex chronicus.

Scleredema is characterized by the appearance of marked, nonpitting induration of the skin, usually the upper back and shoulders. The skin has a woody, waxy appearance with no sharp demarcation from normal. If the problem is of long duration and associated with obesity, mature-onset diabetes should be suspected.

Generalized thickening of the skin is seen with generalized rubbing as found in the atopic diathesis. The skin is thickened and dry, with accentuation of skin markings and perhaps hyperpigmentation. There will be a history of atopy. By contrast, the patient with myxedema has skin that is pale, yellow, and waxy, a subtle change without history of rash. Histologic study will distinguish the two; appropriate tests of thyroid function will confirm the diagnosis of hypothyroidism.

Thickened skin that is nodular, especially if associated with hyperpigmented macules, is neurofibromatosis of von Recklinghausen. Although it should not be difficult to diagnose in its full clinical expression, in the younger patient or in the forme fruste of the disease there may be some uncertainty about the cutaneous or subcutaneous nodules. The pigmented lesions described under pigment aberrations below will confirm the clinical impression.

Atrophy. Thinned skin is atrophic. The change may be limited to the epidermis, leaving a transparent casing that may or may not retain skin markings, or the loss may be in the dermis, leaving normal skin color and markings over a depressed area. Localized atrophy that involves both epidermis and dermis may be the common post-traumatic scar, a cicatrix, or may be morphea, a circumscribed sclerotic plaque with an ivory center and lilac periphery. The lesions of morphea, usually few in number, may be several, or may even be quite numerous. When they occur in a linear fashion they may involve the extremities or the face as the coup de sabre lesion, which may rarely be associated with hemiatrophy of the face, a distressing, deforming loss of subcutaneous tissue, muscle, even bone.

The localized atrophy of lupus erythematosus may also be disfiguring. Found in long-standing lesions, it is associated with telangiectasia and follicular plugging. Such localized lesions are rarely supported by serologic evidence of lupus erythematosus or collagen disease; histologic examination is the best confirmatory test.

Other white atrophic plaques of note, while not common, may be seen in the genital area, where they may be symptomatic with tingling and tightness and on occasion undergo malignant change to squamous cell carcinoma. Identified as lichen sclerosus et atrophicus, it is characterized by white ivory plaques, sometimes with hyperkeratinization, and, in the anogenital area, often by inflammation and lichenification. Leukoplakia is a fairly common complication.

Generalized atrophic hidebound skin is seen in scleroderma. In its full expression it is easily recognized. While scleroderma may begin with rapid extension over the trunk and extremities, or, more insidiously and more commonly, with acral sclerosis and Raynaud's phenomenon, both forms may be severe and associated with visceral involvement. In the CRST syndrome variant of scleroderma, the triad of pulmonary hypertension, Raynaud's phenomenon, and telangiectasia is associated with the cutaneous changes of scleroderma: tight, thinned skin, pinched facies, and tapered, taut fingers with flexion contractures and ulcerations. Subsequently there will be evidence of cutaneous calcifications and pigmentary changes, diffuse hyperpigmentation, localized hyper- and hypopigmentation, and areas of perifollicular pigmentaiton appearing in patches devoid of pigment.

PIGMENTATION

Skin color is derived from four biochromes: two of the epidermis, brown melanin and the yellow carotenoids; and two of the dermis, red oxyhemoglobin and blue-red reduced hemoglobin. These biochromes beneath an epidermis that varies in the thickness of its protective keratin from lips to soles will, in association with underlying vessels, color the skin. Spasm or suffusion of the dermal vessels will cause blanch, blush, or the tricolor change of Raynaud's phenomenon, showing clearly that physiologic mechanisms effect color change.

So, too, will pigments have their effect, those exogenously derived, such as B-carotene from plants, or those endogenously produced, such as bilirubin or the carotenoids. Metals such as silver, bismuth, and mercury can be deposited in the skin to give a blue-gray hue to the integument. A similar blue-gray discoloration of the pinna, occasionally more extensive, is seen in ochronosis or alkaptonuria. In this inborn error of homogentisic acid metabolism, deposits of polymers of homogentisic acid in the tissues are manifest as pigment changes in the ears and are readily identified in the black urine of such patients. Parenteral gold

therapy is rarely, but strikingly, associated with hyperpigmentation about the eyes and on areas exposed to the sun.

All these pigment changes must be recognized for what they connote—a current underlying obstructive problem causing an elevated serum bilirubin; an ongoing metabolic problem such as diabetes, hypothyroidism, or unrecognized pernicious anemia in which there may be carotenemia; and a previous but permanent "tatoo" from medicinally prescribed metals such as silver, bismuth, and gold that are now deposited in the tissues.

The most significant contributor to skin color, however, is melanin through the epidermal melanin unit that controls melanin synthesis. The melanosome, a cellular organelle produced within the melanocyte, contains the melanin formed after the tyrosine-tyrosinase reaction. Transferred to keratinocytes, which in turn transport them to the skin surface, melanosomes profoundly affect human skin color through their number, size, type, and distribution.

Melanocytes vary in concentration over the body, with the skin of the head and forearm having double the number of the rest of the skin, except the scrotum and foreskin. There is no difference in distribution or total numbers among races. There are, however, morphologic differences and varying concentrations of melanosomes in the several stages of melanosome development (I through IV) in the perikarya of the melanocytes and its dendrites, and there are also changes both before and after ultraviolet light exposure.

How is pigment in the given patient to be assessed? The signal of underlying disease need not be of recent appearance. A life-long marker, ignored because of familiarity, may be exactly the sign that gives significance to a symptom.

Pigment aberrations as related to systemic disease are considered in detail below, leaving the present section to provide an overview for identifying and charting observed color change. The extent of change and its duration are to be considered first. Focal change may be present from birth, as in a giant hairy nevus or nevus flammeus; it may be acquired, as some dysplastic nevi are, genetically determined but appearing later in life. Focal color may be environmentally produced, as with a tatoo, whether by design or accident. Generalized pigment change may come from without or within. The skin color observed will be the sum of the individual's own melanin density and the exogenous and endogenous factors that will modify its hue.

If there has been change in color and the color is brown or black, melanin formation has contributed, probably through melanocyte-stimulating hormone (MSH) or ACTH, perhaps through deposits of hemosiderin, as in hemochromatosis, and rarely by homogentisic acid. If the color is red there may be vascular change with persistent suffusion, as in carcinoid, but the clinician must consider the effect of dyes in medications such as clofazimine used in the treatment of leprosy. Sunburn erythema, even with exquisite photosensitivity, should be recognized from its distribution as light-induced, and the redness as reflecting burn. If the skin is yellow, bilirubin is the most common cause and the sclerae are yellow. Endogenous carotenoids, elevated in 10% of patients with diabetes mellitus and in hypothyroidism, will give a yellow color, as will exogenous β-carotenes and quinacrine; the sclerae are normal in color. If the color is gray or blue, silver, bismuth, or mercury or perhaps hemosiderin, as in hemochromatosis, may have been deposited in the skin.

RASH (Table 18–4)

To this point the descriptive data of the skin have been limited to texture and color. Rash, which constitutes the bulk of dermatologic tomes, should not prove a stumbling block to diagnosis. The distribution of the problem is apparent on examination of the entire skin, and a pattern may be evident. If it is dermatomal, the diagnosis may be herpes zoster, nevus, or vitiligo. A clothing pattern should bring a contact dermatitis to mind, for example, a rash where the shirt was or, conversely, a rash where the shirt was not, in which the clothing was protective and spared the skin as from an airborne contactant. There may be an anatomic pattern of involvement, such as the seborrheic areas, the scalp, chest, genitalia, and umbilicus. The problem may be generalized or may have special characteristics. It may be violaceous, as seen in the collagen diseases; purpuric, as seen in leukocytoclastic vasculitis or in the blood dyscrasias; or hemorrhagic from minimal trauma, as seen in senile purpura or amyloidosis.

If the lesions are macular, that is, if they cannot be distinguished by the finger with eyes closed, the problem may be infectious, as in viral infections, or drug induced. The viral exanthems may be accompanied by clinically helpful manifestations, such as Koplik's spots (measles) and occipital lymphadenopathy rubella).

If the lesions are papular and there are systemic symptoms, an infectious cause is more likely, although papular drug rashes may have associated fever and systemic manifestations. The exanthems may also be pustular, vesicular, or petechial. Identifying the primary lesion may help (Table 8–5), but serologic screening may provide the only definitive answer. Petechial lesions may be seen in subacute bacterial endocarditis as well as typhoid fever, the rickettsial diseases, and thrombocytopenia. Bacterial infections, such as those caused by the gonococcus, may present a characteristic tender hemorrhagic papule surmounted by a small pustule that may go undetected or be mistaken for a puncta. Associated fever, chills, and arthralgias with periarticular tenderness or evidence of frank tenosynovitis suggest gonococcemia.

Urticarial eruptions are probably a greater challenge. In an infectious process or drug allergy, the history and the laboratory examinations may help. Drugs can be discontinued; viral infections will subside. Quite often such is not the case with hives. Apart from medications and foods, the allergens of the environment capable of inducing an urticarial response are too numerous to list. Faced with the patient with urticaria but reassured by examination that there is no respiratory distress or by history that there is no likelihood of hereditary or acquired angioedema, the physician should make every effort to suppress the urticarial response while attempting to establish the cause.

All oral and inhaled medications are suspect, even those used for many years; formulations and preservatives can change. A careful history should be taken of the circumstances of the outbreak, foods eaten, places attended, and activities undertaken in the preceding 12 hours. Vitamins, suppositories, and douches are commonly ignored as potential allergens; so, too, are aerosols, hair sprays, and perfumes.

Among medications, penicillin is the most likely to produce an urticarial eruption; among foods, shellfish, chocolate, strawberries, tomatoes, and nuts are most likely.

Vesicular eruptions may be infectious, such as from the viruses of herpes simplex or herpes zoster varicella; proof is afforded by a Tzanck smear, in which multinucleated giant cells will confirm that the vesicle is viral in origin. When the patient has erythema and intense pruritus the problem is probably contact dermatitis. If a plant is the allergen, as in poison ivy dermatitis, the oleoresin will have brushed the skin and the vesicles and erythema will occur in linear streaks. Atopic dermatitis in the small child may be vesicular and weeping, but the eczematous process in the adult is more apt to be a nummular eczema (grouped vesicles, in coin shaped patches of wide distribution) or dermatitis herpetiformis, in which the vesicles are characteristically distributed over extensor surfaces, the buttocks, and shoulders may be so minute as to be missed. Pruritus is marked. The association of dermatitis herpetiformis with gluten enteropathy makes it of particular interest.

Table 18—4.   Differential Diagnosis of Rash

Cutaneous Signs	Dermatologic Condition	Tests
Distribution		
Dermatome	Herpes zoster	Tzanck smear
	Nevus	Histology—melanocytes
	Vitiligo	Histology—absence of melanocytes (may be present in new lesion, but then disappear)
Clothing pattern	Contact dermatitis	Patch test
Anatomic pattern	Seborrheic dermatitis	None
Texture		
Macular lesions	Viral rash	Antibody titers
	Drug rash	History and challenge
Papular lesions	Viral rash	Antibody titers
	Drug rash	History and challenge
	Bacterial infection	Culture
	Exanthems	Viral antibody studies
	Infections	Culture
Pustular lesions		
Around hair follicles on face, or over buttocks, back	Pustular acne	None—culture sterile for pathogens Histology if in doubt
On hands or feet	Pustular bacterid or pustular psoriasis	Histology—sterile pustules
Generalized, confluent "lakes of pus"	Von Zumbusch psoriasis	Histology
	Tinea pedis	KOH/culture
Vesicular rash	Exanthems	Viral antibody studies
Infectious	Herpes simplex, herpes zoster	Tzanck smear
With erythema, pruritus	Contact dermatitis	Patch test
With erythema in linear streaks	Rhus dermatitis (plant)	History, distribution (patch test not needed)
With weeping, in child	Atopic dermatitis	None
With eczematous process, adult	Nummular eczema	Histology
Grouped vesicles, wide distribution		
Grouped vesicles, often symmetrical, over extensor surface, buttocks, and shoulders, with pruritus	Dermatitis herpetiformis	Histology
Petechial rash	Exanthems	Serologic tests
	Subacute bacterial endocarditis	Blood cultures
	Typhoid, rickettsial diseases	Serologic studies
	Thrombocytopenia	Depressed platelets
Urticarial rash	Allergic to medications, ingestants, environment	History, challenge, patch tests, scratch tests
Bullous rash		
Blisters localized or widespread with erythema	Infectious: staphylococcus, streptococcus, bullous impetigo	Culture
Blistering on normal base	Pemphigus, pemphigoid	Histology—biopsy and immunofluorescence
Plaques and papulosquamous eruptions		
With silvery scale and multiple lesions	Psoriasis	Histology
	Generalized neurodermatitis	Histology
	Photodermatitis	Histology—distribution
With collarette of fine scale and skin-line orientation of medallion-shaped lesions	Pitryiasis rosea	None
With a paucity of scale	Tinea, lichen planus, Bowen's disease	Histology, KOH/culture

Table 18–5. Cutaneous Lesions in Certain Viral and Rickettsial Infections

Macules/Papules	Vesicles/Pustules	Petechiae
Rubella	Varicella	ECHO 9 virus
Rubeola	Generalized zoster	Coxsackie A5, A9 virus
ECHO 9, 16 virus	Herpes simplex	Infectious mononucleosis
Coxsackie A5, A9, A16, B5 virus	Coxsackie A and B virus	Rubella
Reovirus	Reovirus 2	
Arbovirus	ECHO 4 virus	
Hepatitis	Orf	
Infectious mononucleosis	Mycoplasma pneumoniae	
Rickettsiae	Rickettsial pox	

Bullae, if not friction or arthropod induced, leave a differential between infection with staphylococcus or streptococcus, that is, a bullous impetigo or the blistering diseases such as pemphigus and pemphigoid. These will not be diagnosed unless considered, and must be sorted out by biopsy and immunofluorescence.

Pustular lesions, if they occur around hair follicles on the face or over the buttocks, are apt to be infectious. The exception is pustular acne, in which the pustules may contain some organisms but are not primarily an infectious problem. Sterile pustules are more of a challenge. On the hands or feet they may represent a pustular bacterid or pustular psoriasis. They may be generalized and confluent in lakes of pus in the Von Zumbusch form of psoriasis, a potentially fatal disease. Occasionally tinea pedis can present as a pustule, but KOH preparations corroborate the clinical impression of fungous infection.

Plaques on the skin and papulosquamous eruptions are generally considered to represent psoriasis by the layman and often by the nondermatologist physician. Psoriasis is probably the correct diagnosis, in cases with silvery scale and multiple lesions, but generalized neurodermatitis or photodermatitis must be considered. In pityriasis rosea with characteristic but less impressive papulosquamous lesions, the collarette of fine scale and skin line orientation of medallion shaped erythematous plaques would suggest the correct diagnosis. When papulosquamous lesions are few, tinea, lichen planus, and Bowen's disease, which is squamous cell carcinoma in situ, must be considered but are apt to be misdiagnosed. The importance of scrapings for fungus and biopsies for diagnostic confirmation cannot be underestimated.

HAIR ABNORMALITIES

Hair loss and hair in excess can both be devastating problems. Male-pattern alopecia is the most common problem of loss. Even in women diffuse hair loss with crown thinning can be seen after the climacteric or earlier, probably related to hormonal levels and genetic predisposition.

Less common but of considerable concern is the impressive hair fall of telogen effluvium. Stressful situations, physical or psychic, can cause actively growing hair to assume suddenly a resting phase. Some 2 to 3 months after the insult, the hair bulb begins to grow actively, producing new hair and dislodging the old. This process is normal for some 10 to 20% of hairs at any given time but is a stunning surprise when the hair fall exceeds 50 or 60%. Root bulb examination will show the characteristic ball of the club hair in resting phase, and the patient can be reassured that hair is growing and will become evident within 6 weeks.

Hair loss that is circumscribed, alopecia areata, is of greater concern. In those past puberty, some 80% will recover from the initial episode, but in any patient with extensive loss, the prognosis is more guarded. About 20% of all patients with alopecia areata have a family history of the disease.

Excessive hair growth may be genetically determined or may come from the friction of rubbing. It has been associated with such drugs as phenytoin and with dermatomyositis and multiple sclerosis. In women, excessive growth of terminal hairs has been associated with elevated levels of androstenedione. The sudden appearance of lanugo hair, initially over the face and ultimately generalized, is associated with underlying malignant disease.

NAIL ABNORMALITIES

Nail inspection should include the paronychial tissue. Any inflammatory change, infectious or eczematous, will have its effect on the nail matrix and cause dystrophy to some degree. The nail itself should then be examined for lifting, loosening, surface contour change, as with pitting or pterygium, pigmentation, and changes in the vascular bed. Comparisons should be made between toe and finger nails and among all nails.

Common nail dystrophies include linear leukonychia, the white spots that result from abnormal keratinization, and Beau's lines, horizontal grooves in the nail plate which are associated with systemic stress that decreases the size of the nail matrix with consequent thinning. Longitudinal striations become more apparent in the nails of the older patient, as does thickening, a general hypertrophy from trauma common to toe nails.

Of the infectious processes, those caused by fungi and yeasts are fairly common, occurring as a primary event and opportunistically in damaged nails. Individuals with persistent and extensive glabrous skin involvement with a Trichophyton or Epidermophyton species may over years develop nail involvement; initially a foot problem, this process may infect the hands and finger nails if the fungus burden is excessive or if there are predisposing factors such as trauma or immersion. Yeast infections other than in body folds classically involve the hands, producing web maceration and paronychial infection with erythema, tenderness, and often a yeasty odor. Dishwashers and janitors are at occupational risk.

Nails also share in the systemic disease process and can provide corroborative evidence for diagnosis. Pitting of the nails is common in psoriasis but is also seen in lichen planus and alopecia areata. The appearance of an ''oil droplet'' lesion under the nail is pathognomonic for psoriasis, and winged lifting and central dipping of the nail is common. Thickening and friability may be seen in psoriasis and fungous infection; opportunistic fungi can also infect psoriatic nails. Paronychial involvement if present will not help in the diagnosis, since psoriatic fingers may be erythematous and edematous. If, however, the paronychia and glabrous skin appear normal and there has been no antifungal therapy, psoriasis is more likely. Onycholysis without cutaneous disease may indicate hyperthyroidism.

Pterygia are destructive of nails; they are seen in lichen planus and may support a diagnosis of tuberous sclerosis.

Color changes in the nail may be caused by external factors, but the keratin of the hands need not share in the stain if the cause was a nail lacquer or if the time interval permitted the glabrous skin to clear. Among endogenous causes are the metabolic disorders such as the white nail of hypoalbuminemia, the yellow nail of lymphedema, and the half-and-half nails of renal and liver disease, in which the proximal portion of the nail is white and the distal aspect a normal pink color. Blue lunulae are seen in patients with hepatolenticular degeneration and with argyria.

Of all pigment changes, the brown longitudinal streak is of greatest concern. Commonly found in the nails of hyperpigmented individuals, its sudden appearance in a light-complexioned individual means a melanocytic nevus with risk of melanoma. A biopsy should be done.

MOUTH, LIPS, AND TONGUE ABNORMALITIES (Table 18–6)

The mouth and the entire gastrointestinal tract share in responses to systemic change. Through the endoscope, the lesions of leukocytoclastic vasculitis can be seen in the gastric mucosa, but even without intubation, inspection of the mouth may reveal much about nutrition, medications taken, and infectious, neoplastic, or pigmentary problems. It may provide corroborative evidence for the systemic diseases that have characteristic lesions of the oral mucosa.

The lips share in the perioral cutaneous changes of contact dermatitis manifested by scaling with or without erythema, and sometimes with edema and vesiculation (Table 18–7). They are exposed to the sun and may show the acute change of burn and blister, even to the flaring of a herpes simplex infection, but more commonly they show the blanched and white atrophic change of chronic actinic damage. Found more on the lower lip, which is less shielded from the sun, local areas of induration and ulceration are a sign of premalignant if not frank malignant change; only a biopsy will determine the extent of change. In lichen planus, white lacy infiltrates involve the lips, but the suggestion of lilac color and the presence of classic lesions in the mouth or elsewhere will help differentiate the problem from actinic cheilitis.

The lips will show vascular changes and transmit the blue color of reduced blood oxygenation whether caused by congenital heart disease or the normal physiologic shunt of the blue-lipped, shivering child in cold lake water. A blue-black macule or papule of the lips that is compressible is a phlebectasia, a dilated vein of nothing but cosmetic significance.

Lips may also show pigment change. The freckle-like macules of Peutz-Jeghers syndrome may extend into the mouth and are important for their association with gastrointestinal polyposis. These pigmentary changes will occur around the mouth and over the dorsa of the fingers, where freckles are uncommon except in the red-headed freckler. Unlike true freckles, which show a distal diminution in concentration, the pigmented macules of Peutz-Jeghers syndrome are more numerous and intense distally; acral involvement may be the only involvement of the digits.

Within the mouth, pigment can be a striking and significant observation. Varying widely with racial dif-

Table 18–6. Differential Diagnosis of Conditions of the Mouth

Cutaneous Sign	Dermatologic Association	Tests
Pigment change		
Gray—brown/black, blue, black	Ingestion of heavy metals: lead, bismuth, silver, mercury	Histology—special stain
Yellow	Antimalarials	
Yellow	Dietary carotene	Serum level elevated
Yellow, hair lightened	Phenothiazines, cholestatic jaundice	Serum bilirubin elevated
	Metabolic problems	
Yellow	Elevation of serum bilirubin	Serum levels elevated
Slate-gray/brown	Elevation of serum iron	Serum levels elevated
Brown-black (melanin)	Addison's disease	Serum cortisol
	Melanocytic nevi (oral melanoma)	Biopsy
Yellow-brown to black, with thickening of filiform papillae of tongue	Lingua nigra (black hairy tongue)	Biopsy
Inflammation and ulceration		
White curd exudate on erythematous base	Candidiasis—especially in frail adult, premature neonate, diabetic, pregnant, or immunosuppressed patient	Smear and stain
Edematous, erythematous denuded mucosa; vesicles coalesced into yellowish plaques with erosion	Herpes simplex	Tzanck smear and culture, serologic tests
	Erythema multiforme	None
	Behçet's syndrome	None
Ulcerations	Aphthae (canker sores)	None
	Trauma	Histology, inspection
	Syphilis	Serologic test
	Histoplasmosis	Skin test and culture
	Lesions secondary to blood dyscrasias, agranulocytosis or leukemia, diabetes, methotrexate therapy, uremia	Blood and bone marrow studies; history—test of renal impairment
	Pemphigus	Histology—immunofluorescence
Circumscribed lesions		
White lacy change involving buccal mucosa, lips, tongue	Lichen planus	Histology—biopsy
Silvery white, scarred, with erythema and erosion	Lupus erythematosus	Histology, ANA
Leathery plaque on mandibular gingiva and alveolar mucosa, mandibular sulcus, buccal mucosa	Leukoplakia	Histology
Serpiginous patches of atrophic erythematous mucosa surrounded by margin of hypertrophy and whitish keratin ridge	Geographic tongue	Histology, documented migration
Yellow waxy nodules, purpuric macules and papules on large tongue	Amyloid	Histology—special stains
Vascular lesions		
Pinpoint to 3 mm, becoming spidery with age	Hereditary hemangiomas	Histology
Larger lesions, flat, without spidery legs	Angiokeratomas of Fabry's disease, mat telangiectasia of scleroderma	Histology
Soft, bumpy, rubbery neuromas of lips, tongue, buccal mucosa	Congenital neuromas; associated with pheochromocytoma and medullary adenocarcinoma of the thyroid, marfanoid habitus	Histology
Translucent or pink cyst on mucosal surface of lower lip	Mucocele	Histology
Pink, friable, easily eroded	Pyogenic granulomata	Histology
Malignancies		
Erythematous plaques	Erythroplasia of Queyrat	Histology
Indurated ulcerations	Squamous cell carcinoma	Histology

Table 18–7. Differential Diagnosis of Lesions of the Lips

Cutaneous Signs	Dermatologic Condition or Diagnosis	Tests
Scaling, erythema, edema, vesiculation	Contact dermatitis	Patch tests, occlusive protection
Vesicles, blisters	Herpes simplex	Tzanck smear for multinucleated giant cells
	Erythema multiforme	Biopsy
	Pemphigus, benign mucous membrane pemphigoid	Biopsy, H & E, histologic and serologic immunofluorescence
Blanching, atrophy	Actinic damage, previous injury	Biopsy
Local areas of induration and ulceration (usually lower lip)	Premalignant or malignant change	Biopsy
Lacy white infiltration	Lichen planus	Biopsy
Pigmented macules	Peutz-Jeghers syndrome	None
Blue-black papule	Venous phlebectasia	Diascopy

ferences, the routine inspection of the mouth of every patient will give the examiner some feeling for the range of normal. Abnormal pigment may come from the tatoo of an amalgam filling or, as in the skin, from the systemic ingestion of heavy metals, antimalarials, phenothiazines, and dietary carotenes. Lead and other heavy metals from industrial exposure are frequently deposited at the gingival margin, perhaps fostered by low-grade inflammatory change when oral hygiene is poor. Bismuth and mercury tend to be more diffusely deposited, as is silver, giving a dusky, almost cyanotic look in argyria. Medicinal painting, as with silver nitrate (Argyrol), can cause a circumscribed stain, as may nicotine from smoking, while the exogenous stains of chewed tobacco and betel nuts are usually more extensive. Metabolic problems that lead to an elevation of serum bilirubin or iron may color the oral mucous membrane.

Melanin, the most significant contributor to skin color, can serve, by pigment increase in the oral mucosa, as a signal of melanocyte stimulation. As such it may be a sensitive and early indicator of Addison's disease but is not pathognomonic. The melanin pigment is commonly found on the buccal mucosa and tongue but may appear anywhere within the mouth and may be related to trauma, as at the interdental line. It will then occur in streaks or blotches and should be distinguished from a melanocytic nevus. While uncommon, nevi of the oral mucosa do occur, most often in the palatal and maxillary mucosae, the sites of predilection for 80% of orai melanoma. Any melanocytic lesion of the mouth suspected of being a nevus should be assessed histopathologically.

If pigment that is yellow-brown to jet black is seen with thickness of the filiform papillae of the tongue, the diagnosis is lingua nigra or black hairy tongue—asymptomatic unless the papillae are so long that they cause gagging. The cause is uncertain and is variously attributed to oxidizing agents, oral antibiotics, and excessive smoking.

If the mouth is inflamed and sore, the problem may be of recent onset, chronic, or recurrent. The most common diagnosis suspected but often incorrectly made is candidiasis. Since Candida albicans is a normal inhabitant of the mouth, its presence on smear and culture from the oral lesion is not surprising, but there must be a fit between the clinical and mycologic findings. The white curd exudate must occur on an erythematous base, indicating active yeast infection, and the patient must be vulnerable to such infection. The premature neonate, the frail adult debilitated from senility or malignancy or an individual who is diabetic, pregnant, or immunosuppressed are all predisposed to oral candidiasis. If the patient has none of these disorders and the problem is stubborn it may be a herald of AIDS.

The initial exposure to herpes simplex may produce in the mouth the sudden onset of an edematous, erythematous denuded mucosa on which vesicles have coalesced into yellowish plaques with erosion. There may be systemic symptoms including fever, and lymphadenopathy, but no history of fever blisters. Usually a disease of childhood or young adults, such erosive stomatitis must be distinguished from erythema multiforme and Behçet's syndrome. Viral cultures help to distinguish among the diagnoses, but erythema multiforme can be a reaction to herpes simplex infection. Characteristic target lesions elsewhere on the skin, with or without erosions of the vaginal mucosa, suggest erythema multiforme. Both Behçet's syndrome and erythema multiforme may include eye involvement.

The more common oral lesions of Behçet's syndrome are the superficial grayish erosions suggestive of aphthous stomatitis, or canker sores. Aphthae, which can be more extensive and necrotic tend to be recurrent, familial, and stress related.

In assessing oral ulcerations, especially those in patients without systemic manifestations, the differential diagnosis must include trauma and uncommon infection. Dentures, broken teeth, and dental procedures, hot foods or those with sharp bones, and chemicals such as aspirin can cause injury. Infectious agents can also produce erosions, for example, the chancre of syphilis, or the lingual ulcer of histoplasmosis. History, inspection, and appropriate dark-field examination or culture will help to select among the causes and distinguish such ulcerations from those secondary to blood dyscrasias, such as agranulocytosis or leukemia, the metabolic problems of diabetes or uremia, or chemotherapeutic agents such as methotrexate. Pemphigus may also cause oral erosions, sometimes antedating associated cutaneous lesions for as long as 2 years. The diagnosis must first be suspected to be identified histopathologically and by immunofluorescence.

Of the infiltrative or nodular circumscribed lesions of the mouth, the change may be in the mucosa or the vascular or glandular bed beneath. The white lacy change of lichen planus, which involves the buccal mucosa as well as the lips and often the tongue, must be distinguished from the lesion of lupus erythematosus, which is characteristically more silvery white and scarred, sometimes with erythema and erosion. Both must be distinguished from the circumscribed leathery plaque of leukoplakia, occurring often on the mandibular gingiva and alveolar mucosa, in the mandibular sulcus, or on the buccal mucosa. Although most oral leukoplakia is said to remain benign, some do develop into invasive carcinoma and biopsy must be performed on all, innocent as they may appear.

By contrast, geographic tongue is usually of considerable concern to the examiner with its serpiginous patches of atrophic erythematous mucosa surrounded by a margin of hypertrophy and whitish keratin ridge. The atrophy represents loss of filiform papillae and tends to migrate, as documented by biopsy from an area of change that subsequently appears as normal tongue. Asymptomatic and of unknown cause, variously attributed to vitamin deficiency and emotional stress, it is important to be recognized for what it is, and to be distinguished from leukoplakia and lichen planus.

Lesions of substance and surface change may be infiltrative around the blood vessels and in the connective tissue, as in amyloid. The infiltrated tongue of primary amyloidosis may become enormously large. Yellow waxy nodules may be noted and there may be a hemorrhagic component, so that purpuric macules and papules are scattered among the nodules of amyloid. A biopsy with special stains for amyloid will confirm the diagnosis.

Vascular lesions of the mouth include the hemangiomas of hereditary familial telangiectasia that involve skin and mucous membranes as well as the gastrointestinal and genitourinary tract. From pinpoint to 3 mm in size, they may with age become spidery. Unexplained hemorrhage in a patient with such lesions suggests hemangioma as the source of the bleeding. Such hemangiomas must be distinguished from the angiokeratomas of Fabry's disease which are 0.1- to 3-mm purple-red macules or papules, and from the mat telangiectasia of scleroderma, which are larger, flat, and without spidery legs.

Firm excrescences of the hard palate or inner aspect of the mandible are developmental abnormalities, bony exostoses that are of no concern. If the overlying mucosa is taut it may be easily traumatized. By contrast, mucosal neuromas of the lips, tongue, and buccal mucosa are softer and of rubbery consistency. Present from childhood and recognized as an inherited albeit rare problem, their association with the Marfan diathesis, pheochromocytoma, and medullary carcinoma of the thyroid should not be overlooked. A more common tumefaction of the mouth is the mucocele, a retention cyst of the mucous glands found anywhere, but commonly on the mucosal surface of the lower lip; they are translucent or pink, asymptomatic, and may occasionally be confused with pyogenic granuloma, a pink, friable, and easily eroded lesion. Common to the buccal mucosa, pyogenic granulomas are a benign neoplastic response to injury.

Lesions of grave concern in the mouth are the erythematous plaques and any indurated ulceration. The brightly erythematous, raised surface of erythroplasia of Queyrat is an intraepithelial squamous cell carcinoma that must be proved by biopsy and treated as a true malignancy. Any indurated lesion that is ulcerated is squamous cell carcinoma until proven otherwise, for such lesions account for 95% of all malignant tumors of the mouth. Compared to malignancy of the skin, squamous cell carcinoma of the oral cavity is a grave disease with significant mortality. Constant assessment of the mouth with biopsy of suspicious lesions is good preventive medicine.

INDICATIONS OF SYSTEMIC DISEASE

ACANTHOSIS NIGRICANS

Skin that is velvety, spongy, and creased with a black-brown color in the axillae, groin, or nuchal folds is unmistakably acanthosis nigricans. Tending to be bilateral and symmetrical, it can involve any body fold or may be generalized. Although cosmetically disturbing, acanthosis nigricans is neither symptomatic nor malignant. The focus is on its implications. In the prepubescent child the finding is rarely of significance, but in the postpubescent individual, while it may merely be associated with obesity or be a manifestation of an inherited cutaneous disorder, it may be a sign of endocrinopathy or malignancy. The cutaneous sign is a clue and does not reflect by extent or intensity the benignity or seriousness of the associated disease.

When present from birth, the cutaneous changes of acanthosis nigricans are considered a nevoid genodermatosis that may spread or intensify at puberty, after which it may persist or regress. Transmitted in an irregular dominant way, it is never associated with malignancy. Similarly, when seen as part of a syndrome such as congenital lipodystrophy, a recessively inherited disorder, the dermatologic manifestation is present at birth or from childhood and malignancy is not a concern.

Nor is malignancy a concern when the cutaneous change occurs in dark-complexioned, obese individuals in whom it is aggravated by excessive sweat and friction in the body folds; this finding, unassociated with malignancy, is sometimes called pseudoacanthosis nigricans. Such a ''benign'' manifestation may follow the ingestion of corticosteroids, diethylstilbestrol, or nicotinic acid. The appearance and disappearance of acanthosis nigricans has been correlated with the use of oral contraceptives and has been reported to remit in the insulin-resistant diabetic patient as glucose intolerance lessens. The appearance of the cutaneous sign in an adult is nonetheless of concern, of gravest concern for malignancy, which is considered below, but important also for adrenal insufficiency, Cushing's syndrome, acromegaly, Stein-Leventhal syndrome, and various pituitary and hypothalamic tumors.

ICHTHYOSIS

Skin that is rough and dry with scale in angular sheets that tend to turn up at the edge suggests ''fish skin.'' The scale may be fine and adherent with follicles plugged with keratin or may be large, loose, and polyhedral. There is no erythema and the palms and soles may or may not be thickened.

When present from birth or childhood, the problem is undoubtedly an inherited disorder of retained keratin that may be of lifelong morbidity to the individual but not important as an indicator of systemic disease. Even when associated with metabolic disorders, such as Ref-

sum's disease, in which there is an inability to break down phytanic acid with consequent tissue accumulation and polyneuritides, the problem and its ichthyotic change present early in life. It is the ichthyosis of recent onset that should alert the physician to underlying systemic change. Because decreased humidity and lubrication, as well as the drying effects of aging skin, may make pre-existing ichthyotic changes more apparent under certain conditions, the onset of dry scaling skin must be assessed to ascertain if it is truly new.

Underlying malignancy, considered below, can certainly provoke the sudden appearance of ichthyosiform changes in the skin, but patients with hypothyroidism may have such changes along with carotenemia and alopecia; in individuals with pre-existing ichthyosis and hypothyroidism the ichthyotic skin problems tend to worsen. Diets deficient in essential fatty acids, such as those that might be used in hyperalimentation, can evoke ichthyotic change within a week's time; these changes reverse when the essential fatty acids are restored. Such ichthyosiform scaling has also been associated with the administration of nicotinic acid, triparanol, and butyrophenones, all chemicals that inhibit normal lipid synthesis.

Marked scaling of the skin, including the trunk and lower extremities, has been observed in sarcoid. It can occur in leprosy, especially lepromatous leprosy, a challenging underlying problem often overlooked in the differential diagnosis in the Western world.

ERYTHRODERMA

Ichthyosiform Erythroderma

When dryness and scaling of the skin are associated with erythema and the appearance is explosive, malignancy is the first consideration, as elaborated below. Certain antecedent dermatologic conditions, however, notably psoriasis but even lichen planus, may, with physical insult or psychic stress, extend to exfoliation; the history of plaque lesion and distribution in addition to the stigmata of scalp and nail involvement or buccal mucosal involvement in the case of lichen planus should help in identifying the cause of the generalized dermatitis.

A diffuse eruption with scale, occasionally denuded or pustular, frequently tender, should raise the possibility of necrolytic migratory erythema and pancreatic glucagonoma. Fatigue, weight loss, and the recent onset of diabetes would be additional supportive data. Determination of an elevated serum glucagon level would confirm the diagnosis.

Exfoliative Erythroderma

When the scale is not like "fish skin" but fine, and a generalized erythema is the major finding, we are presented with an exfoliative erythroderma, a smoldering continuing reaction to a drug or contactant, perhaps a manifestation of atopy or seborrheic dermatitis that has progressed to a generalized reaction. Underlying systemic disease, apart from malignancy, is not likely. Many allergens, however, are overlooked, such as those bound to vitamins or other over-the-counter oral medications, or those absorbed from suppositories, vaginal lubrications and douches, spermicidal jellies, and intrauterine devices, to cite a few examples.

The exfoliative erythroderma nonetheless may have been induced by an untoward reaction to sunlight, and the whole array of photosensitivity reactions and what they portend must be considered. In such instances the patient should have a history of an increased reaction to ultraviolet light and an initial rash in sun-exposed areas with sparing of the eyelids and submental area.

PHOTOSENSITIVITY

Light as a precipitating or aggravating factor in the course of an eruption may or may not be obvious to a patient. Diffuse erythema, as in a sunburn, is readily suspected as being light-related. However, discrete erythematous patches with or without scar, hives, and vesicles without erythema may not be suspected as light-related. The description, duration, and circumstances of a rash are important to elicit as is the distribution. Light-sensitive eruptions arise where the light strikes more intensely: the forehead, nose, eartips, the back of as well as the "V" of the neck, and the dorsal aspect of the hands and feet. By contrast, the submental area is spared, as are the eyelids and the webs of the fingers.

The normal reaction to ultraviolet light will vary with the intensity of the radiation and the protective melanin of the exposed skin, ranging from an imperceptible change to severe burn and blister formation with progressive cumulative damage that includes malignancy. Such photosensitivity is not our concern here; neither will we consider the exaggerated response to sunlight that characterizes those with defects in DNA repair and replication, or the polymorphous photodermatitis, that exquisite sensitivity to sunlight that is manifested by an eruption of papules and vesicles in spring sunlight but that diminishes somewhat by summer through acquired tolerance. In all these photosensitivities, genetic predisposition is an important documented dimension with specific defects identified, except in the case of the polymorphous light eruption.

Table 18–8.   Classification of Porphyrias

Tissue Origin	Type
Erythropoietic	Erythropoietic porphyria
	Erythropoietic protoporphyria
	Erythropoietic coproporphyria
Hepatic	Acute intermittent porphyria
	Variegate porphyria
	Hereditary coproporphyria
	Porphyria cutanea tarda

(From Harber, Leonard C., and Bickers, David R.: Photosensitivity Diseases: Principles of Diagnosis and Treatment. Philadelphia, W.B. Saunders, 1981, p. 198, with permission.)

Such responses to sunlight are important to be recognized for what they are and sorted out from those photosensitivities derived from an underlying acquired problem that makes the individual more light sensitive. While some of these may have a genetic predisposition, they become manifest only under specific circumstances or with challenge.

Metabolites

PORPHYRINS

When intermediates of porphyrin metabolism accumulate excessively in the skin resulting from abnormalities of heme synthesis, light reacts with the porphyrins to produce both acute and chronic cutaneous change. Porphyrins absorb light at the 400 nm range to become photoactivated and biologically reactive, capable of damaging if not destroying living cells. Excitation of porphyrins in the presence of oxygen has been shown to induce the formation of lipid peroxidase and hydrogen peroxide, both destructive to cell membranes. Hence the membrane is especially vulnerable, but also vulnerable are the intracellular organelles, the cholesterol and fatty acids, and even the amino acids.

The porphyrias have been differentiated by the pattern of porphyrin or porphyrin precursor in the tissues, urine, or feces. Several have distinctive cutaneous manifestations permitting a diagnosis on clinical observation alone. The table adapted by Harber and Bickers lists the various porphyrias (Table 18–8). The eythropoietic types, erythropoietic porphyria (EP) and erythropoietic protoporphyria (EPP), have classic cutaneous signs and are recognized from infancy or early childhood. In EP, vesicles, bullae, and erosions in association with hypertrichosis and hypermelanosis lead to scarring with mutilating deformities of the ears, nose, and hands. These cutaneous changes occur in association with pink teeth and pink urine. In EPP the photosensitivity is less severe, but from childhood there is an erythematous, edematous response to sun, occasionally purpura, with the development of waxy scars on the nose and hands with thickening of sun-exposed skin. Stinging and burning of the skin during light exposure is a disturbing symptom and a frequent complaint.

For present purposes it is porphyria cutanea tarda (PCT) that deserves the greater focus. Skin fragility with bullae or erosions appearing on the dorsa of the hands, and possibly the forehead or scalp of the older balding patient, might be missed as a manifestation of porphyria. Even the dark urine may go unnoticed. Hypertrichosis of the face, typically in a periorbital distribution with mottled diffuse hyperpigmentation, can be an associated finding and may be the presenting complaint, especially in women. The average patient is in the third or fourth decade, rarely younger. Urinary uroporphyrins and coproporphyrins are excreted and an orange-red fluorescence can be detected by simple Wood's light examination of the acidified urine. A negative urine fluorescence does not rule out the diagnosis and a qualitative test of stool porphyrins should be done. About two thirds of the patients have increased total body iron stores, elevating the serum iron and hepatocellular iron; about one quarter have diabetes or a diabetic glucose tolerance curve.

Precipitating factors in PCT include alcohol, estrogens, hexachlorobenzene, and chlorinated phenols. Ethanol induces amino levulinic acid (ALA) synthetase, which is important in the biosynthetic pathway of heme but whose role in inducing PCT in susceptible individuals is not known, nor is it understood why estrogens taken by women as contraceptives or as hormonal supplements or by men with prostatic cancer as adjunctive therapy are associated with an increased incidence of PCT. Perhaps the most tantalizing data come from the "epidemic" of PCT-like signs and symptoms that occurred in southeast Turkey after the ingestion of wheat treated with the fungicide hexachlorobenzene. Those affected were mostly children of diverse ethnic groups, showing a porphyrin excretion pattern similar to that produced by ethanol or estrogens. All of these precipitating factors as well as iron could cause an increase in hepatic porphyrinogenesis, but the clinical expression of PCT probably depends on factors both genetic and environmental. PCT should be held distinct from acute intermittent porphyria (AIP), which is characterized by acute abdominal pain and neurologic symptoms and is frequently familial but lacking in photosensitivity or cutaneous signs. Those individuals with features of both AIP and PCT have been classified as having mixed or variegate porphyria. A final sorting among the porphyrias must await the identification of specific genetic defects.

DISORDERED TRYPTOPHAN METABOLISM

Pellagra occurs when the diet is deficient in niacin, as in alcoholics or in populations with maize as their major nutritional source. Its cutaneous manifestation presents as an erythematous, vesicular dermatitis in light-exposed areas, progressing to intense hyperpigmentation and desquamation, a leathery appearance with powdery scale. The eruption is precipitated by sun exposure. While the role of niacin deficiency is unclear, a similar light-induced change has been noted in patients on antituberculosis therapy with isoniazide, presumably because it interferes with niacin by competitive inhibition.

In Hartnup disease, a rare inherited amino aciduria with mental retardation, there is a transport defect of tryptophan with failure of absorption from the gastrointestinal tract and renal tubule. Because tryptophan is metabolized through kinurenines to niacin, the diminished tryptophan results in depleted niacin, and photosensitivity with pellagrous skin changes develops. Similarly, utilizing available tryptophan for the excessive production of serotonin, as occurs in the carcinoid syndrome with metastases, permits a consequent interference with niacin formation, a plausible explanation for the photosensitivity and pellagrous skin changes reported in some patients with carcinoid.

Exogenous Agents

If the light sensitivity is neither genetically determined nor related to recognized metabolites and is not due to one of the collagen diseases for which there are appropriate and helpful tests, the identification of the causal agent becomes a greater challenge. The chemicals in our environment, those we ingest and those that we (often unwittingly) apply topically, are legion, many capable of evoking reactions when the exposure is associated with ultraviolet light.

Phototoxic reactions occur without a recognized immune mechanism and are a dose-related response common to a large number of people on first exposure. Antimicrobial therapy, as with sulfonamides or demeclocycline; colorings in medications or fruits, as with acridine; psychotherapeutic drugs such as phenothiazines; the sulfonylurea hypoglycemic agents; the thiazide diuretics; the antifungal agent griseofulvin—all these may, on the patient's exposure to light, induce a photosensitivity that is characterized by burning, prompt erythema with edema reaching a maximum intensity in 24 hours, followed by desquamation and hyperpigmentation. Fortunately, the sensitivity does not persist.

Photoallergic reactions depend on a demonstrable immune mechanism. Occurring in a small number of those exposed, the dose-response relationship is not as apparent, and imperceptible quantities of allergen or light may be sufficient to evoke the response. Occasionally prompt and urticarial, the reaction can appear after 24 hours or more, is often persistent, and may show cross-photosensitivity. The photoreactions to the topical application of sulfonamides, to the halogenated salicylanilides, and to chlorpromazine are among the few examples of true photoallergy.

When plant contact and light exposure combine to cause a rash, the term phytophotodermatitis is used. The plant substance involved is probably one or more of the naturally occurring psoralen compounds, the furocoumarins, found in the plant kingdom and used in photochemotherapy. The response is a phototoxic reaction with the psoralen absorbed into the skin, activated by long-wave ultraviolet light, producing erythema even to bulla formation and subsequent hyperpigmentation. Vegetable harvesters and cannery workers exposed to crushed plants are at risk of phytophotodermatitis from parsley, celery, fennel, dill, parsnips, and carrots; bartenders are at risk from Persian limes.

In the search for the cause of a photodermatitis, the diagnosis must first be suspected. The patient is the best resource and guide. A detailed assessment of the work place, of leisure activities, and of causal ingestants and occasional medicaments must be made to elicit all possible exposure to chemicals, plants, and the array of sources of ultraviolet light, including welding arcs and fluorescent bulbs. All oral medications must be reviewed, with suppositories not overlooked; all topical applications must be listed, including soaps, cosmetics, and sunscreens. By alerting the patient and involving the family in the search for an offending substance the chance of identification is greater, because the focused concern of the family may reveal an unsuspected agent or even a family tendency toward photosensitivity.

Photoaggravated Conditions

SYSTEMIC LUPUS ERYTHEMATOSUS (SLE)

If the eruption is merely an exaggerated sunburn or hives in response to sun exposure but is associated with symptoms of fatigue, an underlying collagen disease should be sought. Perhaps the most significant, if not the most symptomatic, of adult-onset photosensitivities, lupus erythematosus, can be provoked and exacerbated by ultraviolet light with an action spectrum in the 300-nm range (UVB). In fact, about one third of patients with systemic lupus erythematosus will have some photosensitivity. Abundant laboratory testing of blood and tissue is available to assess the clinical impression of SLE. Although no one test is

specific, high antinuclear antibody (ANA) titers with a peripheral pattern of staining, especially in patients with active skin lesions, are significant. If there are no antinuclear antibodies, anti-Ro cytoplasmic antibody may support the diagnosis. Direct immunofluorescent studies of cutaneous tissue obtained from lesional or nonlesional skin can be quite helpful. A band of fluorescent skin at the dermo-epidermal junction or basement membrane is a positive test and reflects deposits of IgG or IgM antibody.

SUNLIGHT

The role of sunlight in dermatomyositis and scleroderma has not been established. Although dermatomyositis has a classic heliotrope rash about the eyes and elsewhere, and in some patients the dermatitis does seem to be activated by sunlight, the provocation is not as obvious or consistent as in SLE. The hyperpigmentation of scleroderma may be intensified by ultraviolet light exposure.

With a concern for photosensitivity as an indicator of systemic disease, herpes simplex, common and commonly recognized as provoked by sunlight, would not seem to have a place. However, with underlying atopic dermatitis, lymphoma, or immunosuppression and with a response to sunlight that is erythematous but intensely vesicular, the possibility of viral origin may be overlooked. A positive Tzanck smear would establish the vesicle as viral.

There are in addition several miscellaneous dermatologic conditions such as Darier-White's disease (keratosis follicularis) and Hailey-Hailey disease (benign familial pemphigus) that are very much aggravated by sunlight, although heat with sweating and maceration may also have its effects. The first manifestation of Darier-White's disease, for example, may appear after sun exposure; if the differential diagnosis does not include the evoking of an underlying cutaneous disease, the search for other causes would be endless. In this instance the eruption is not a diffuse erythema or a vesicular to bullous contact dermatitis, but greasy keratotic papules in a sun-exposed distribution.

PIGMENTARY ABERRATIONS

Many pigmentary signs are subtle and lost in the wide range of normal variability. Even when sought as a clue, a specific pigment change may appear so innocuous that the clinician is reluctant to gather it into the data base. The rule should be to study the skin always, in every ill person and in every healthy person examined, checking, questioning, comparing, testing, and taking a skin biopsy whenever in doubt.

Table 18–9. Differential Diagnosis of Pigmentary Aberrations

Cutaneous Signs	Dermatologic Associations	Supportive Observations	Tests
Hypopigmentation			
Generalized			
Pigment diminished or lacking	Albinism	Nystagamus, photophobia	Positive dopa reaction
Pigmentary dilution of skin, hair, eyes	Phenylketonuria	Mental retardation without treatment	Ferric chloride test of urine, blood—hyper-phenylalaninemia
Pigmentary fading—white spots	Vitiligo	Normal eye color, poliosis	Histology-biopsy; melanocytes absent from long-standing lesions
	Leukoderma	History of chemical/toxic exposure	None
Skin normal in texture, lacks pigment	Hansen's disease	Lesional hypoesthesia, palpable ulnar, posterior-auricular, and peroneal nerves	Histology—biopsy
Circumscribed			
White forelock, amelanotic areas, hyperpigmented macules	Partial albinism	From birth, no extension	Positive dopa reaction (negative in white macules)
Unilateral macules, circular or rectangular on trunk or lower abdomen	Nevus depigmentosus	Dermatomal distribution	Positive dopa reaction (positive—less reactive)
"Ash leaf" or polygonal hypomelanosis	Tuberous sclerosis	Seizures, subungual fibromas, shagreen patch	Examination under Wood's light
Poorly circumscribed hypomelanosis	Sarcoidosis	Granulomatous lesions	Positive dopa reaction
Depigmented macules—legs, neck, face, arms, abdomen, over bony prominences, with or without hyperpigmentation	Pinta	History of antecedent copper-red, then slate-blue lesions	Treponemes in early lesions
Amelanotic areas	Chemical depigmentation	Acquired; history of exposure	Biopsy
Depigmented or hypopigmented atrophic areas with halo	Yaws	Children	Treponeme
Depigmented pretibial skin	Onchocerciasis	Leopard appearance	Biopsy—filaria
Depigmented areas following inflammation			
With atrophy and telangiectasia	Lupus erythematosus	Photosensitivity, serologic abnormalities	Serologic tests, histology
With woody induration	Scleroderma	Raynaud's phenomenon, hypercalcinosis	Histology
With fine scale and indistinct border, especially on face and upper arms of pubertal children and adolescents	Pityriasis alba	Family history of atopy	Negative KOH
Hypo- and hyperpigmentation, round macular and raised pink to tan scaling lesions	Tinea versicolor	Rarely, endocrine dysfunction	Negative KOH, Wood's light examination
Large hypopigmented areas	Resolved psoriasis	Nail stigmata, scalp scaling	Wood's light examination (verifies hypo-, not depigmentation)
Hyperpigmentation			
Generalized			
Brown/black	Addison's disease, pituitary or other brain tumors		Tests of adrenal and pituitary function, CT scan
Bronze, slate-gray, or brown/black	Hemochromatosis	Cirrhosis, diabetes	Histology—test for liver function, glucose tolerance
Gray/black	Whipple's intestinal lipodystrophy	Spared mucous membranes	
Yellow	Primary biliary cirrhosis		Elevated billirubin
Yellow	Vitamin B_{12} or folate deficiency	Hypersegmented PMNs	Carotenemia
Yellow/red	Drug therapy		History, recurrence with challenge

Table 18—9. Continued

Cutaneous Signs	Dermatologic Associations	Supportive Observations	Tests
Circumscribed			
Congenital blue spots			
In sacral area, indistinct margins	Mongolian spots		Histology
About eye, surrounding skin	Nevus of Ota (1st and 2nd branches trigeminal nerves)	None	Histology
	Nevus of Ito—posterior supra- clavicular and lateral tra- cheal cutaneous nerves		
Acquired blue spots	Melanoma, vascular lesion, dermal nevus	None	Histology—biopsy
Acquired tan or brown, black, red, white, blue spots	Melanoma	Family history supportive	Dermal melanocytes, biopsy
Acquired tan, brown, black spots	Ephelides (ephelides of the axillary vault—neurofibromatosis)		
Café au lait spots (more than 6)	Von Recklinghausen's disease (neurofibromatosis)		Histology of nodule
Greasy tan to brown/black macular lesions	Seborrheic keratoses	Family history	Biopsy
Pigment in whorls	Incontinentia pigmenti	Blisters at birth	

Pigment problems will be considered below as they present clinically, whether circumscribed or diffuse, whether deficient, overproduced, or a combination of both, whether congenital or acquired.

When pigment is deficient, a Wood's light examination will establish whether any pigment persists: is the skin completely without pigment (amelanotic) or just lighter in color (hypomelanotic)? Is it uniform in its pigment loss? Has the deficiency been present from birth, or could it have gone unnoticed? Has the skin lost pigment or become depigmented? Is there a family history?

Similar questions can be asked about hyperpigmented skin, such as whether it is circumscribed or diffuse, variegated or evenly pigmented, congenital or acquired. It is on these clinical observations that distinctions and identifications will be made, and underlying systemic disease considered (Table 18—9).

Hypopigmentation

GENERALIZED

Albinism. When pigment is diminished or lacking entirely in a generalized distribution from birth, the differential is among the various types of albinism, a hypomelanosis or amelanosis limited to eyes and skin or to the eyes alone. There are six types of oculocutaneous albinism, classified by tyrosinase activity and extent of the melanin deficiency in skin and eyes, related to melanogenetic pathways and the relative concentration of melanosome stages in the hair bulb. Although most albinos have diminished visual acuity, so severe as to qualify as legal blindness, underlying

disease is not a problem except in the Chédiak-Higashi syndrome, a rare form of oculocutaneous albinism in which there is an increased susceptibility to infection and in some cases the development of a lymphoreticular-like malignancy. These patients present to the physician in childhood with recurrent staphylococcal and streptococcal infections. The skin color is light cream to slate gray; the hair is light blond to brunette. Consanguinity is a factor in almost half the reported cases.

A generalized pigmentary dilution of skin, hair, and eyes is also part of phenylketonuria, an autosomal recessive disorder of phenylalanine metabolism with a block in the conversion of phenylalanine to tyrosine. The pigmentary defect may be absence or decrease of tyrosine or tyrosinase or an inhibition of the tyrosine to melanin pathway by phenylalanine. Infants screened at birth can be preserved from severe mental retardation by restricting dietary phenylalanine, the only therapy. Untreated patients have multiple neurologic abnormalities; both treated and untreated patients have structural abnormalities such as kyphosis and spina bifida and may have the cutaneous changes of acrocyanosis and scleroderma. They have a shortened life expectancy.

While the patient with phenylketonuria and mental retardation will probably have been diagnosed in childhood, the metabolic cause of the retardation and its associated pathologic changes may be forgotten after years of institutional confinement. With the current release from institutional living of a number of retarded adults, blond, blue-eyed retarded individuals coming under the care of a physician should be suspected of having phenylketonuria and checked for multiple abnormalities, both neurologic and cardiac.

Vitiligo. When pigment is lacking in a generalized fashion but has been observed to fade either universally or by the appearance of ever-increasing numbers of "white spots," the diagnosis is probably vitiligo. Leukoderma secondary to chemical or toxic destruction of the melanocytes might be considered but would involve some history of exposure. Hansen's disease with depigmentation would be distinguished by lesional hypoesthesia as well as other findings such as palpable ulnar, great auricular, and common peroneal nerves.

Vitiligo occurs in 1% of the population and is often familial, with onset at any age from birth to the eighties but a peak appearance between the first and fourth decades. In half the patients it is noted before age 20. It may be localized or generalized, even limited to mucous membranes; it may be segmentally distributed or scattered, with a tendency to occur at body orifices. Scalp hair may become depigmented with or without a loss of pigment in the underlying scalp. In the extremely light complexioned individual its presence may go unnoticed.

The course of vitiligo is unpredictable. In established lesions, melanocytes disappear; in newer lesions, repigmentation may occur spontaneously but not to a cosmetically satisfactory extent. When there is repigmentation it occurs as interrupted macules around hair follicles where melanocytes are still nested in the hair bulb.

In general, the patient with vitiligo can be reassured about health and longevity. One third will have prematurely gray hair; ocular pigmentation is usually normal, but iris and retinal pigmentary abnormalities occur more frequently than in the normal population. Thyroid dysfunction, hyperthyroidism, toxic goiter, and thyroiditis are more frequently found in patients with vitiligo, but myxedema and thyroid carcinoma are not.

Pernicious anemia occurs more often in patients with vitiligo. In one study it was concluded that it was found 30 times more frequently in such patients compared to the general population. In those with pernicious anemia, vitiligo is variously reported as occurring in 2 to 11%.

Diabetes mellitus is also found more commonly; both the juvenile and late-onset types are reported in 1 to 7% of patients with vitiligo; of all individuals with diabetes, about 5% have vitiligo. In patients with Addison's disease, vitiligo occurs in 2%, and I have personally cared for a patient with vitiligo, hyperthyroidism, Addison's disease, and circulating antibodies for parietal cells. At least 26 cases of multiglandular disease are reported associated with vitiligo. Alopecia areata and associated adrenal, thyroid, parietal cell, and smooth muscle antibodies are variously observed in as many as 16% of patients with vitiligo.

CIRCUMSCRIBED

Congenital. In partial albinism, the circumscribed absence of pigment, even one small macule, if new, may represent the onset of vitiligo, but there are other considerations. The first question is whether the observed white spot is new or was present from birth. Piebaldism, or partial albinism, is characterized by a white forelock and amelanotic areas, some with hyperpigmented macules. As an autosomal dominant condition, it occurs in less than 1 in 20,000 births. Except for occasional deafness or heterochromia irides, there are no associated defects.

Other circumscribed areas of congenital amelanotic skin include nevus depigmentosus. Usually unilateral, the circular or rectangular macules present on the trunk or lower abdomen of generally healthy individuals, although there have been reports of seizure disorders and mental retardation.

Nevus depigmentosus is to be distinguished from the "ash leaf" or polygonal hypomelanosis that occurs, if not at birth, then soon after. It is the hallmark of tuberous sclerosis, a neurocutaneous syndrome that affects the skin and central nervous system, the eyes, and, less commonly, the heart, lungs, kidneys, and bones. Every newborn at risk and every newborn with seizures should be examined under Wood's light for the hypomelanotic lesions. Their presence in an infant with seizures is considered pathognomonic of the diagnosis of tuberous sclerosis. Recognizing such lesions in the asymptomatic or undiagnosed adult is of value in genetic counseling.

Acquired. Although suggested in the differential diagnosis of vitiligo, which may begin as circumscribed hypomelanotic areas and is acquired, similar amelanotic lesions may result from chemical depigmentation. Phenol derivatives and sulfhydryl compounds are common causes, as are antioxidants such as the monobenzylether of hydroquinone. Tannery workers and those in rubber manufacturing are at risk. Localization of the leukoderma and history of exposure will make the diagnosis.

Many cutaneous conditions characterized by inflammation leave hypopigmented and totally depigmented areas. Patients with lupus erythematosus, for example, can be impressively depigmented, initially with atrophy and telangiectasia, and may have an inactive residuum of lightened or white skin, usually with some continuing evidence of atrophy. In scleroderma, as well, there may be areas of depigmentation, but if it is associated with extensive hyper- and hypopigmentation as well as woody induration, the diagnosis is evident. In these collagen diseases the underlying disorder will be recognized; the pigment aberration will not be the presenting complaint.

Not so with pityriasis alba, a common hypomelanotic problem with a fine scale and indistinct border that occurs on the face and upper arms of pubertal children and adolescents. It is of cosmetic concern with no associated underlying disease, but it may be a manifestation of the atopic diathesis. The eczematous changes of atopic dermatitis can result in areas of hypopigmentation, probably as a postinflammatory change thought to be vasoconstrictive, enhanced by the shielding effect of scale and edematous epidermis against ultraviolet light.

Such minimal circumscribed hypopigmentation must be distinguished from tinea versicolor, characterized by hyper- and hypopigmentation. The round, scaling lesions, macular to minimally raised and pink to tan, caused by the superficial fungus Pityrosporon orbiculare (Malassezia furfur) interfere with tyrosinase activity, hence the hypopigmentation. The accumulated scale accounts for the hyperpigmented areas, and the combination of hyper- and hypopigmented areas with mild erythema accounts for the name T. versicolor. The problem is common and of no systemic consequence; it has been seen to appear and disappear without topical therapy but related to systemic corticosteroids given for other reasons. If the Pityrosporon infection is active, the organism can be identified by its morphological appearance on the KOH preparation and may even fluoresce a brick-red color under Wood's light examination. If only residual hypopigmentation can be seen, the diagnosis should be suspected from the configuration and distribution (thorax, upper arms, possibly neck), although resolved guttate psoriasis or parapsoriasis are in the differential diagnosis. Psoriasis vulgaris would leave larger hypopigmented areas. All hypopigmented areas will repigment if the skin remains free of the papulosquamous problem or infection and if vitiligo is not an accompanying diagnosis.

In other areas of the world the differential diagnosis of hypomelanotic macules extends to pinta, yaws, endemic syphilis, and kala-azar. Leprosy, which will not be diagnosed unless considered, would leave hypopigmented macules that are usually less distinct and are hypoesthetic.

Hyperpigmentation

GENERALIZED

Generalized racial color differences are expressed by genotypic variations that have their effect on the fine structure of the melanocyte. At birth the epidermal-melanin unit is set; the pigmentation of the individual may darken somewhat through infancy and with ultraviolet light exposure, but basically it will remain until aging lightens the skin with the disappearance of melanocytes, or unless modified by endogenous or exogenous forces.

The factors from within with most dramatic impact on pigment are the pituitary hormones, alpha- and beta-MSH, and ACTH, which can produce hyperpigmentation through darkening mechanisms that are not well understood in man. In Addison's disease, decreased cortisol levels result in increased production of MSH and ACTH with consequent hyperpigmentation. Pituitary tumors and other tumors producing polypeptides of analogous structure cause hyperpigmentation that is indistinguishable from Addison's disease, including brown or blue-black macules of the gingiva and buccal mucosa. There may also be linear nail hyperpigmentation.

Diffuse hyperpigmentation is seen in hemochromatosis, associated with deposits of melanin and hemosiderin in the skin. The color may be bronze, slate-gray, or brown-black and can appear before the cirrhosis or diabetes. In Whipple's intestinal lipodystrophy and in primary biliary cirrhosis, diffuse hyperpigmentation may be noted. It has also been reported with vitamin B_{12} and folate deficiency.

Exogenous agents in the form of drug therapy, such as busulfan, 5-fluorouracil, and cyclophosphamide, can cause diffuse hyperpigmentation. It can also be seen as a postinflammatory phenomenon in those who have had an exfoliative erythroderma or a chronic pruritic dermatitis, as in the atopic diathesis.

The deepening of skin pigment without obvious cause warrants a close assessment of the adrenal-pituitary axis and the brain itself, because there have been reports of mottled hyperpigmentation associated with brain tumors other than those arising in the pituitary.

CIRCUMSCRIBED

Circumscribed hyperpigmentation is more of a spectrum of pigment presentation and hence is a greater challenge diagnostically. Many lesions of focalized hypermelanosis, such as a residuum of a thermal burn, need merely to be identified, for they neither herald nor reflect underlying disease.

Blue spots, indicative of the depth of melanin in the skin, the so-called Mongolian spots, are seen more in oriental and black individuals but also in caucasians. Comprised of dermal melanocytes, they are usually found in the sacral area but can occur anywhere, appearing at birth or shortly thereafter. They are of no concern. An acquired blue spot, however, though perhaps a vascular lesion or a benign dermal nevus, should undergo biopsy to rule out melanoma.

Other circumscribed pigmented lesions such as ephelides or seborrheic keratoses are usually of no significance. Ephelides are a common response to ultraviolet light of certain light-complexioned individuals. Ephelides associated with exquisite sun sensitivity may be an indicator of xeroderma pigmentosum and defective excision repair of induced pyrimidine dimers of DNA or, in one subset, defective S-phase DNA synthesis. Patients are at risk for neurologic abnormalities as well as cutaneous malignancies induced by the effects of ultraviolet light on DNA repair. Ephelides of the axilla, especially in the vault, where they could not be provoked by sunlight, are a sign of neurofibromatosis, as reliable a sign as the more obvious café au lait spot. These larger, evenly pigmented but irregularly shaped macules are a diagnostic clue, and six or more indicate the diagnosis of von Recklinghausen's disease, even in the absence of neurofibromas. Seborrheic keratoses, the greasy, tan to brown, "tacked on" or macular benign lesions of the skin, mostly a cosmetic nuisance and occasionally pruritic, may, when they appear in an eruptive fashion over a period of several months, be associated with visceral malignancy, (Leser-Trélat sign) (see Table 18–12).

Pigment in whorls suggests incontinentia pigmenti, which affects mostly females and is inherited. An inflammatory vesicobullous phase present at birth and perhaps persisting for months is followed by a verrucous change and by pigmentation, which may fade completely by age twenty or may persist as faint brown to slate-gray configurations. The disorder, of unknown cause, is associated with an array of abnormalities, of which ocular and neurologic disorders are the most common; mental retardation occurs in 10% or more. The whorled hallmark on the skin is a signal to search for underlying associated disease, and to proceed with genetic counseling.

INDICATIONS OF MALIGNANCY

The epidermis can undergo malignant change with cells that metastasize and kill, as in squamous cell carcinoma; it can also support malignant growth, as it supports the T cell in the lymphoma of mycosis fungoides, or supports metastatic cells from visceral organs; most importantly, it can respond to the visceral presence of tumor with cutaneous signs that are a challenge to explain.

CUTANEOUS MALIGNANCY

Plaques or nodules of the skin that enlarge rapidly, especially if they ulcerate, should be suspected as being malignant and should undergo biopsy. The anatomic location ought not influence the decision. While basal cell and squamous cell carcinoma occur classically on light-exposed and damaged skin, they may occur anywhere. The nodular exophytic basal cell that is a pearly translucent papule or has a rolled pearly border, often with fine telangiectatic vessels, is easy to see and identify; the depressed, atrophic, waxy, morphea-type basal cell is less easily detected and hence often unrecognized for the malignancy that it is.

Any of these lesions appearing on young, unblemished skin, which does occur though rarely, would be easily spotted as new and abnormal. But skin cancers are more common in the older population, in whom the background epidermis is often atrophic, telangiectatic, mottled with fading pigment, and sprinkled with the benign barnacles of aging: seborrheic keratoses, intradermal nevi, senile lentigines, cherry hemangiomas, and an assortment of acrochordon or skin tags, a perfect camouflage for the malignant lesions.

Skin inspection must be thorough and the hand lens is indispensable in assessing the surface and quality of the many lesions of elderly skin. Red scaling patches are often overlooked as tumor and are most frequently labeled psoriasis. An intraductal adenocarcinoma of the breast or Paget's disease may present as a marginated scaling lesion about the nipple or areola and go unappreciated for the breast malignancy it is. Superficial spreading basal cells and squamous cell carcinoma in situ will also present as asymptomatic erythematous patches. Differentiated by histologic recognition of the malignant cell, the contained squamous cell carcinoma of Bowen's disease may be an indicator of underlying visceral malignancy, especially if it occurs on protected skin.

But what of changes in younger, actinically damaged skin? Apart from patients with tyrosinase deficiency (albinism) or defects in DNA repair (xeroderma pigmentosum), the skin of the light-complexioned, blue-eyed freckler is most at risk. Telangiectasia, ephelides, and erythematous blotches, some with scale, indicate prior actinic exposure and resulting damage. In those who have had acne, therapeutic x-ray may have compounded the damage. All patients with evidence of significant acne by scar or with continuing activity should be queried about x-ray therapy, not only for its implications for cutaneous malignancy, but also for neoplasm of the thyroid. The risk of malignant change obtains for all skin that has undergone radiation therapy for any reason.

Basal cell carcinomas can erode and kill by extension and invasion; they can also metastasize. More common than squamous cell carcinoma, they occur in a younger age group and may be multiple. A patient with one type of carcinoma is at greater risk of developing another. In the diagnosis of a basal cell carcinoma, trichoepithelioma should be considered; this is a fairly common benign epidermal nevoid tumor. If the basal cell tumor is pigmented, a melanoma should be considered. The histology will distinguish among these several lesions.

Squamous cell carcinoma occurring in the older age group, often arising in association with actinic keratoses, is ill-defined and may be multicentric in origin and invasiveness. When arising on protected skin it may be a signal of visceral malignancy, especially of the bronchus or of the urinary tract if there is a history of arsenic ingestion such as from tonics or Fowler's solution. The nodular ulcerative variety of squamous cell carcinoma arising de novo on normal-appearing skin is rapidly invasive and frequently metastatic. It must be distinguished from a keratoacanthoma, a rather common cutaneous neoplasm that is variably aggressive but disappears spontaneously. The diagnosis on clinical and histopathologic grounds can be difficult; when it is, the therapy should be a complete and wide excision.

Plaques, with or without ulceration, often with the configuration of a large fixed urticarial lesion and a history of a psoriasiform pruritic dermatitis, suggest mycosis fungoides, a T-cell lymphoma. Rarely is a tumefaction alone the presenting complaint. Biopsies from plaques or tumors will confirm the diagnosis.

Nodules with and occasionally without pigment may be nodular melanoma. Representing a small fraction of all melanoma, they underscore the need for identifying common skin lesions in order to suspect and perform a biopsy on those that are unusual. Seborrheic keratoses and intradermal and compound nevi should be recognized for what they are and distinguished from the macular or barely palpable melanocytic nevus. Any congenital or acquired melanocytic nevus that has undergone change in that it appears to have smudging of pigment or variegated color with depigmented areas, or seems to have provoked an erythematous response or tingling sensation is to be suspected of having undergone malignant change.

In neurofibromatosis of von Recklinghausen, the skin nodules may cover the entire integument, but the sudden enlarging of any one tumor should be considered malignant degeneration until proven otherwise. Such malignant change occurs in 2 to 5% of those with neurofibromatosis, and the tumors become neurofibrosarcomas. In the central neural system such patients may have astrocytomas, glioblastomas, or meningiomas.

Firm to hard nodules in the skin, if fixed, may represent a direct lymphatic extension of malignant cells, as from lung or bone. The primary tumor can be assumed to be of considerable size. By contrast, a freely movable nodule, in the skin or just beneath it, may be the first indication of underlying malignancy. Of all patients with metastatic disease, some 3 to 5% have metastases to the skin. Breast malignancy is most common and may present as the impressive inflammatory breast plate of cutaneous metastases. Tumors of the stomach, lung, uterus, and kidney may also metastasize to the skin, as may, less often, those arising in the colon, prostate, ovary, or testicle. If the tumors metastasize to the abdominal wall, the more common primary sites are the lung, stomach, and kidney in men, and the ovary in women; metastasis to the scalp is from the lung, kidney, or breast; metastasis to the thorax is from the lung or breast; metastasis to the face is from the oropharynx; and metastasis to the extremities, melanoma.

Pink to purple papules of the skin progressing to nodules that ulcerate suggest a myelomonocytic leukemia. An ulcerated cutaneous infiltrate with a greenish discoloration is most likely the chloroma of acute granulocytic leukemia. Deeper nodules, dermal or subcutaneous, may be cellular aggregates of histiocytic lymphoma. Biopsy will identify these cutaneous extensions and metastases as malignant even though the primary site may not at first be evident. Livid or dusky blebs exuding fluid with chemistries characteristic of lymph are lymphangiosarcoma. Usually representing a second primary malignancy, lymphangiosarcoma develops in a chronically edematous extremity such as an edematous arm, the sequela of a radical mastectomy.

CUTANEOUS MANIFESTATIONS ASSOCIATED WITH MALIGNANCY

Of great interest and greater challenge is the array of cutaneous signs and symptoms that are not the malignancy itself but are associated with it. For some signs the association is clear, as is the cause, such as in the darkening associated with the circulating MSH and ACTH-like polypeptides of oat cell carcinoma of the lung. For others the association is not clear, as in the dermatomyositis that presents even before a breast carcinoma can be detected. Concurrent start, parallel course, and a uniformity in the type of associated neoplasm give credence to the association. The skin may

Table 18–10. Cutaneous Indicators of Malignancy According to Lesion—Frequent Association

Cutaneous Lesion or Change	Sign, Syndrome, or Disease
Discrete lesions	
Adenomas: multiple sebaceous adenomas of trunk	Torre's syndrome
Angiomas	von Hippel-Lindau disease
Cysts: epidermal inclusion cysts and sebaceous cysts on scalp and face (trunk)	Gardner's syndrome
Macules, papules, nodules:	
Multiple reddish brown or yellow macules, papules, or nodules	Urticaria pigmentosa
Macules urticate	
Warty papules and nodules on central face; oral mucosa, hands, and dorsal forearms	Cowden's disease
Neuromas: multiple neuromas of lips, eyelids, nares, and anterior two thirds of tongue (pink nodules)	Multiple endocrine neoplasia type III
Seborrheic keratoses: sudden development of a large number of seborrheic keratoses	Leser-Trélat sign
Hair	
Hypertrichosis: long, fine, silky hair on face and other sites normally clinically hairless (does not involve palms and soles)	Acquired hypertrichosis lanuginosa
Poliosis	Ataxia-telangiectasia
Pigment change	
Hyperpigmentation	
Heavily pigmented macules or erythroderma	Urticaria pigmentosa
Hyperpigmentation (gray-black) on legs, forearms, trunk, with hyperkeratosis; or yellow-brown pigmentation on forehead, back, wrists, thighs	Carcinoid
Hyperpigmentation of perineum, buttocks, groin, lower abdomen, lower extremities	Necrolytic migratory erythema
Confluent hyperpigmented, hyperkeratotic verrucosities in body folds, especially axillae, nipples, and umbilicus	Acanthosis nigricans
Purpura: purpura on skin and mucous membranes	Wiskott-Aldrich syndrome
Telangiectasia	
Telangiectasia on bulbar conjunctiva, ears, eyelids, cheeks, limbs	Ataxia-telangiectasia
Telangiectasias on face and upper trunk	Carcinoid
Rash	
Erythema	
Heliotrope erythema on eyelids, upper cheeks, forehead, temples, scalp	Dermatomyositis
Irregular wavy bands with peculiar gyrate or serpiginous outline, with marginal desquamation on trunk, neck, and extremities	Erythema gyratum repens
Texture change	
Acrosclerosis: acrosclerosis with or without osteolysis and papular skin lesions	Vinyl chloride disease
Calcification: cutaneous calcification	Dermatomyositis
Dermatitis	
Generalized symmetrical dermatitis, initially eczematous, over perineum, buttocks, and extremities	Necrolytic migratory erythema
Erythematous areas with central blister formation progressing to central crusting and healing, followed by hyperpigmentation (see above)	
Eczema: eczematous lesions on scalp, face, flexures, and buttocks	Wiskott-Aldrich syndrome
Edema: edema of hands and arms	Dermatomyositis
Keratoderma: diffuse keratoderma of palms and soles	Acanthosis nigricans
Plaques	
Erythematous to gray-white plaque that may be scaly, crusted, ulcerated, or papillary on vulva or perianal area	Extramammary Paget's disease
Scaly bluish red plaques over knuckles	Dermatomyositis
Sebaceous activity: increased sebaceous activity on face and scalp	Acquired pachydermoperiostosis
Thickening: skin of forehead and scalp thickened and thrown into folds; skin of hands and feet thickened	Acquired pachydermoperiostosis

have shared with the viscera in a carcinogenic exposure, as with arsenic, or in an inherited predisposition, as in the Peutz-Jeghers-Touraine syndrome; it may be a change associated with a metabolic product of the malignancy, as in amyloid with multiple myeloma or in necrolytic migratory erythema with a functioning glucagonoma of the pancreas. Many times the association is impressive but the reason obscure, as in acquired pachydermoperiostosis, a rare dermatosis that may be associated with underlying bronchogenic carcinoma. Whatever the cause of the cutaneous marker, the early detection of an otherwise unsuspected ma-

Table 18–11. Cutaneous Indicators of Malignancy According to Lesion—Occasional Association

Cutaneous Lesion or Change	Sign, Syndrome, or Disease
Discrete lesions	
Basal cell carcinoma: multiple basal cell carcinomas	Nevoid basal cell carcinoma syndrome
Bullae	
Bullae, erosions, and leukoplakia of mucous membranes; palms and soles form bullae with trauma	Dyskeratosis congenita
Bullae, bleeding, and crusting provoked by sunlight	Bloom's syndrome
Cysts: epidermoid cysts	Nevoid basal cell carcinoma syndrome
Macules	
Axillary freckles	Neurofibromatosis (von Recklinghausen's disease)
White macular areas	
Brown-black, discrete macular lesion 2 to 5 mm	Peutz-Jeghers-Touraine syndrome
Nevi	
Sebaceous nevus—circumscribed, slightly raised, hairless plaques of orange-yellow that become verrucous and nodular in puberty	Congenital nevi
Bathing trunk nevus or other congenital pigmented nevus—dark brown, irregular, raised surface with small mamillary projections (may have hair, well-defined margins)	
Nevus verrucosus and nevus unius lateris—skin-colored or yellow-brown with rough, warty surface, more often on limbs and trunk	
Nodules	
Multiple tumors that may be small to large and soft to firm; most numerous on trunk and limbs	Neurofibromatosis (von Recklinghausen's disease)
Tender subcutaneous erythematous nodules, on lower legs and thighs (occasionally)	Nodular liquefying panniculitis
Successive crops of tender, linear, and oval nodules affecting large and small vessels throughout the body	Thrombophlebitis migrans
Nodules in auditory meatus and body flexures	Systemic amyloidosis (secondary)
Papules	
Small pink papule slowly enlarges to form a ring, as the central area flattens and fades; may attain diameter of 6 to 8 cm; appears on buttocks, thighs, upper arms	Erythema annulare centrifugum
Small, glistening papules on eyelids, central area of face, lips, and tongue	Systemic amyloidosis (secondary)
Small, firm, pink, moderately pruritic papules or nodules on dorsa of hands, forearms, scalp, face, ears, trunk, and mucosa of lip; fluctuates in severity	Reticulohistiocytoma
Adenoma sebaceum—firm, discrete, yellow or telangiectatic papules 1 to 10 mm; extend from nasolabial fold, occasionally in the ear; periungual fibroma and smooth, firm, flesh-colored excrescences emerging from nail beds (5 to 10 mm)	Tuberous sclerosis
Ulcers: leg ulcers	Werner's syndrome
Hair	
Alopecia	Acquired ichthyosis
Early balding	Werner's syndrome
Hirsutism	Cushing's syndrome
Hypopigmentation	
Lightened color	Chédiak-Higashi syndrome
Poliosis	Tuberous sclerosis, Werner's syndrome
Nails	
Dystrophic nails, suppurative paronychia	Dyskeratosis congenita
Periungual fibroma and firm, flesh-colored excresences emerging from nail beds (5 to 10 mm)	Tuberous sclerosis
Pigment change	
Ash-leaf spot	Tuberous sclerosis
Café au lait spots	Neurofibromatosis (von Recklinghausen's disease)
Hyperpigmentation	
Discrete mucocutaneous pigmentation, including lips, face, buccal mucosa, hands	Peutz-Jeghers-Touraine syndrome

Table 18–11. Continued

Cutaneous Lesion or Change	Sign, Syndrome, or Disease
Fine reticulate gray-brown pigment on neck and thighs and involving greater trunk with telangiectasias; face is red and atrophic with irregular macular pigmentation	Dyskeratosis congenita
Hypopigmentation: lightened color of skin and hair	Chédiak-Higashi syndrome
Pruritus: small, firm, pink, moderately pruritic papules (see above)	Reticulohistiocytoma
Rash	
Erythema	
Generalized erythematous skin with scaling	Erythroderma exfoliativum
Erythema of the face most pronounced in butterfly area—may involve margins of eyelids, forehead, and ears	Bloom's syndrome
Texture change	
Atrophy	
Red, atrophic face	Dyskeratosis congenita
Atrophic shiny skin on hands and feet	
Striae	Cushing's syndrome
Keratosis	
Hyperkeratotic palms and soles	Acquired ichthyosis
Late-onset keratosis palmaris et plantaris; diffuse palmar and plantar hyperkeratosis with hyperhidrosis	Tylosis
Pitting: "pits" of palms and soles	Nevoid basal cell carcinoma syndrome
Plaques	
Well-demarcated, slightly raised plaque that is erythematous and indurated; may have fine scale (face, neck, head)	Alopecia mucinosa
Shagreen patch—irregular, soft, elevated plaque in lumbosacral area	Tuberous sclerosis
Leonine facies due to plaques	Systemic amyloidosis (secondary)
Thickening	
Elephantiasis neuromatosa—wrinkled and pendulous skin with overgrowth of subcutaneous tissue along nerve trunk with diffuse neurofibromatosis (rare)	Neurofibromatosis (von Recklinghausen's disease)
Scleroderma-like changes	Werner's syndrome
Xerosis	
Generalized dry, cracking skin, usually starts at legs	Acquired ichthyosis
Hypohidrotic palms and soles	Dyskeratosis congenita

Table 18–12. Cutaneous Indicators of Malignancy According to Malignancy—Frequent Association

Lesion, Syndrome, or Disease	Malignancy
Acanthosis nigricans	Adenocarcinoma of stomach, pancreas, colon, lung, breast, uterus, ovary, rectum, cystic and hepatic ducts
Acquired hypertrichosis lanuginosa	Bronchus, gallbladder, rectum, bladder
Acquired pachydermoperiostosis	Bronchus, stomach, esophagus, thymus, mesothelioma
Ataxia-telangiectasia (inherited disorder; autosomal recessive)	Reticulum cell sarcoma, lymphosarcoma, Hodgkin's disease, gastric
Carcinoid	Metastatic carcinoids
Cowden's disease (inherited disorder; dominant inheritance)	Breast, thyroid, female reproductive
Dermatomyositis (40 years or older)	Breast, lung, gastrointestinal tract, genitourinary system, lymphoma
Erythema gyratum repens	Breast, lung, tongue
Extramammary Paget's disease	Rectum, cutaneous, adnexal tumors
Gardner's syndrome (inherited disorder; dominant inheritance)	Colon
Leser-Trélat sign	Carcinoma of stomach
Multiple endocrine neoplasia type III (inherited disorder; dominant inheritance)	Thyroid, pheochromocytoma
Necrolytic migratory erythema	Glucagonoma
Torre's syndrome	Gastrointestinal
Urticaria pigmentosa	Mast cell leukemia, systemic mastocytosis
Vinyl chloride disease	Angiosarcoma
von Hippel-Lindau disease	Hypernephroma, pheochromocytoma
Wiskott-Aldrich syndrome (inherited disorder; sex-linked recessive)	Reticuloendothelial

Table 18–13.   Cutaneous Indicators of Malignancy According to Malignancy—Occasional Association

Lesion, Syndrome, or Disease	Malignancy
Alopecia mucinosa	Mycosis fungoides, lymphomas
Acquired ichthyosis	Hodgkin's disease
Bloom's syndrome (inherited disorder; autosomal recessive)	Leukemia
Chédiak-Higashi syndrome (inherited disorder; autosomal recessive)	Lymphoma
Congenital nevi	Melanoma; basal cell epithelioma, squamous cell carcinoma
Cushing's syndrome	Oat cell of lung, pituitary, hypothalamus, adrenal
Dyskeratosis congenita (inherited disorder; sex-linked recessive)	Carcinoma develops in area of leukoplakia (squamous cell)
Erythema annulare centrifugum	Variable; skin lesions reported to disappear with excision of malignancy and to reappear with recurrence or metastases
Erythroderma exfoliativum	Lymphoma, lung, rectum, leukemia
Neurofibromatosis (von Recklinghausen's disease) (inherited disorder; dominant inheritance)	Sarcomas, pheochromocytomas, astrocytomas, gliomas
Nevoid basal cell carcinoma syndrome (inherited disorder; dominant inheritance)	Medulloblastoma, fibrosarcoma of jaw
Nodular liquefying panniculitis (with pancreatitis)	Pancreatic carcinoma
Peutz-Jeghers-Touraine syndrome (inherited disorder; dominant inheritance)	Malignancy proximal to ligament of Treitz
Reticulohistiocytoma	Sarcoma, gastric, colon, lung
Systemic amyloidosis (secondary)	Multiple myeloma
Thrombophlebitis migrans	Lung, pancreas, breast, colon, stomach
Tuberous sclerosis (inherited disorder; dominant inheritance)	Brain, rhabdomyoma
Tylosis (inherited disorder; dominant inheritance)	Esophageal
Werner's syndrome (inheritied disorder; autosomal recessive)	Sarcoma; meningioma

lignancy reinforces the value of such signs. I have grouped them according to frequent or only occasional association with the dermatologic lesion as guide to those varied diagnoses that may be associated with a specific malignancy (Tables 18–10, 18–11, 18–12, and 18–13). Several have been reviewed above for recognition and for association with nonmalignant disease; of these, some, such as acanthosis nigricans and dermatomyositis, need further consideration under malignancy.

The two symptoms of pruritus and pain are not tabulated because their special focus as an indicator of underlying malignant change is so limited. Intense pruritus is a signal of significance only for lymphoma, Hodgkin's disease, leukemia, and occasionally multiple myeloma. Initially pruritus may be localized with burning sensations, then generalized and unremitting. The skin will be damaged by scratching but there will be no primary lesions. With the leukemias and T-cell lymphoma, cutaneous infiltration and erythema may change the cutaneous response into an exfoliative erythroderma. Mild pruritus may also be a prodromal symptom for the lymphoma/leukemia group and for visceral malignancies of the gastrointestinal tract, lung, ovaries, and prostate, but the many causes of mild itching lessen its value as an indicator of malignant change.

Cutaneous pain is important only as it relates to herpes zoster. Extensive or disseminated varicella infection is a feared painful and not uncommonly lethal complication of widespread malignancy and immu-

nosuppression. As a signal of unsuspected malignancy it probably has no role, but even limited herpes zoster, especially if the patient is older or debilitated, warrants a thorough system review and routine laboratory studies. Cutaneous burning pain often precedes the viral vesicles and, whether or not in a dermatome, should serve as a warning of the presence of possible infection and as a reason to withhold chemotherapy until the infection is resolved.

The ichthyosiform changes of the skin associated with malignancy are acquired and are occasionally associated with erythroderma; they will be recognized as of late onset and distinct from the congenital inherited ichthyoses. Of the various reported cases associated with malignancy, a high percentage had Hodgkin's disease, but other lymphomas have been seen, as well as metastatic disease from breast and lung. In most cases the sign is not a herald, although in one instance it is said to have preceded the disease by 7 years.

The acanthosis nigricans that appears with malignancy may precede the clinical recognition of the malignant change in 20% of cases, be concurrent in 60%, and follow it in 20%. The cutaneous sign has been observed to disappear after therapy for the malignancy, only to reappear with reactivation of the tumor. The gastrointestinal tract is the most common site of malignant change, with two thirds of tumors occurring in the stomach; less often the malignancy may be in the ovaries, prostate, breast, or lung. Rarely, acanthosis nigricans is associated with lymphoma. The tumors are usually aggressive and rapidly fatal.

Pachydermoperiostosis and erythema gyratum repens are rare, dramatic changes of the skin associated with thickening and underlying malignancy. Pachydermoperiostosis, characterized by heavy folded skin, enlarged extremities, and clubbed fingers with thickened palms, may be familial and as such is of great cosmetic concern, but has no medical implications. When acquired, however, pachydermoperiostosis may be associated with bronchogenic carcinoma, usually in men over 40 years of age. Acral changes may precede the recognition of the cancer, but the hypertrophic osteoarthropathy and striking facial changes usually appear when the malignancy is advanced. Erythema gyratum repens presents as thickened erythematous serpiginous bands resembling burled wood, extending over trunk and extremities. It is associated with adenocarcinoma of the breast and lung, and with malignancies of the oral pharynx.

A far more subtle sign is the initial presentation of dermatomyositis. Whereas weakness may be an early complaint, some 25% of patients first have cutaneous changes that may go unnoticed. The erythema of the scalp and eyelids may be confused with seborrheic dermatitis, but the blue-red heliotrope color and the paucity of scale are not characteristic of seborrheic dermatitis. Later, the extension of blotchy, blue-red erythema of the forehead and malar eminences, with or without periorbital edema, and the blue-red plaques of Gottron over the dorsa of the fingers at the interphalangeal joints will reinforce the clinical impression. The association of dermatomyositis with malignancy is accepted but its frequency is variously reported, depending on criteria for the dermatologic diagnosis and the intensity of tumor search. The correlation is best for the older age group, with the gastrointestinal tract as the predominant site of malignant change, especially colon and stomach. The cutaneous change and muscle weakness may disappear with the successful treatment of tumor, only to reappear with tumor recurrence. All adults with dermatomyositis require close scrutiny for indications of underlying tumor, and in those over 40 years the search should be aggressive.

Superficial thrombophlebitis, especially if migratory on the trunk or extremities, should raise the question of malignancy, especially of the pancreas. Deeper veins may also be involved, with multiple embolic phenomena. Thrombophlebitis may be a sign of malignancy of any of the viscera and has been observed in lymphomas and Hodgkin's disease.

Peculiar to the glucagonoma of the pancreas is an erythematous, scaling, erosive dermatitis of the intertriginous areas and flexural aspect of the extremities, often tender, and sometimes associated with stomatitis. Diagnostically it can be confused with pustular psoriasis of the von Zumbusch type and the oral lesions can be confused with candidiasis. This necrolytic migratory erythema is associated with elevated levels of circulating glucagon. It is surmised that glucagon and related gastrointestinal polypeptides similar to glucagon are the cause of the cutaneous change, but other metabolic abnormalities resulting from malabsorption and zinc deficiency may be at fault. So debilitating is the disease that characteristic skin lesions both clinically and histopathologically, even in the presence of normal serum glucagon levels, warrant an aggressive search for tumor, even to laparotomy.

Tables 18–10, 18–11, 18–12, and 18–13 review the array of dermatological lesions, the syndromes and signs they represent, and the malignancies with which they may be associated, some often, others less so. The spectrum should underscore the importance of scrutinizing and sampling the skin, the one organ system so readily available for inspection and biopsy as it shares in the effects of genetic, environmental, metabolic, and malignant aberrations that involve the body as a whole.

GENERAL REFERENCES

Braverman, I.M.: Skin Signs of Systemic Disease. 2nd Ed. Philadelphia, W.B. Saunders, 1981.
Fitzpatrick, T.B., et al. (eds.): Dermatology in General Medicine. 3rd Ed. New York, McGraw-Hill Book Company, 1987.
Harber, L.C., and Bickers, D.R.: Photosensitivity Diseases, Principles of Diagnosis and Treatment. Philadelphia, W.B. Saunders, 1981.
Johnson, M.L.: Skin diseases: cutaneous manifestations of internal malignancy. In Cecil Textbook of Medicine. Edited by J.B. Wyngaarden and L.H. Smith. Philadelphia, W.B. Saunders, 1982.
Johnson, M.L., and Roberts, J.: Skin conditions and related need for medical care among persons 1–74 years, United States 1971–1974. Vital and Health Statistics Series 11, No 212, 1979.
Moschella, S.L., Pillsbury, D.M., and Hurley, H.J., Jr.: Dermatology. Philadelphia, W.B. Saunders, 1975.
Rook, A., Wilkinson, D.S., and Ebling, F.G.: Textbook of Dermatology. 3rd Ed. Oxford, Blackwell Scientific Publications, 1979.

CHAPTER 19

NUTRITIONAL PROBLEMS

Harvey L. Katzeff, M.D.

WEIGHT LOSS

DEFINITION

Abnormal weight loss is loss of 10% or more of body weight within 6 months or a weight/height index less than 80% of standard.

PATHOPHYSIOLOGIC CONSIDERATIONS

Weight loss can pertain to loss of water, fat, or lean body tissue. In the initial phase of any hypocaloric diet, extracellular volume is lost as water in conjunction with a sodium diuresis. In addition, the utilization of liver and muscle stores of glycogen (100 g) as a calorie source releases 1 kg of intracellular water, which is also excreted. During the initial adaptation to undernutrition, the body uses both fat and protein stores as calories. If there are no added stresses to the body and protein intake is adequate (0.8 g of protein/day per kg body weight), protein stores can be maintained after 4 to 6 weeks of moderate undernutrition.[1] During chronic undernutrition, secretion of hormones such as triiodothyronine (T_3), cortisol, and norepinephrine and epinephrine decreases.[2] This decrease in hormonal secretion leads to a fall in protein catabolism and promotes maintenance of lean body tissues. Marasmus refers to chronic underfeeding with maintenance of adequate proteins stores for liver protein synthesis and cell-mediated immunity.

Weight loss in an individual who also has an acute or chronic illness may lead to more severe and dangerous consequences of malnutrition. During an acute stress, there is an increase in the secretion of cortisol and catecholamines and inhibition of insulin secretion.[3] The increased secretion of these hormones promotes protein catabolism, and the weight loss in these individuals includes a severe loss of nitrogen. This state, protein-calorie malnutrition, denotes a failure of the liver to maintain protein synthesis. Decreases in serum albumin and other liver-synthesized proteins and suppressed cell-mediated immunity produce significant increases in medical and surgical morbidity.[4]

Loss of weight may also occur because of malabsorption of food intake. Loss of appropriate pancreatic or intestinal enzymes, damage to the absorptive surface of the small intestine, infection, abnormal intestinal motility, or rapid transit time of food in the gut all may impair calorie absorption.

Alterations in energy expenditure may produce weight loss and utilization of both fat and protein as calories. This situation frequently occurs in thyrotoxicosis and pheochromocytoma. Other disturbances in metabolism may produce a selective loss of muscle and other protein stores. These include hypercortisolism, glucagonomas, and some types of neoplastic diseases.

DIFFERENTIAL DIAGNOSIS AND DIAGNOSTIC EVALUATION

A complete history and physical examination should readily identify a chronic or acute malnourished state. Studies have shown that the nutritional assessments of patients by clinicians performing only history and physical examinations were similar to the nutritional assessments of patients performed by clinicians also using laboratory tests.[5] Table 19–1 indicates the more frequently used laboratory tests. The serum albumin and transferrin levels in blood are indicators of liver synthetic ability, although both false positive and false negative tests may occur because of other disease states. The blood lymphocyte count and delayed skin hypersensitivity tests are additional indicators of protein-calorie malnutrition but are also abnormal during cancer chemotherapy. Mean arm circumference, urinary creatinine excretion, and blood urea nitrogen levels indicate protein intake and muscle stores of protein. These tests are helpful in determining the severity of the malnourished state but cannot determine the cause of malnutrition.

Table 19–2 divides sources of weight loss into three main categories—decreased calorie intake, malabsorption, and hypermetabolic states.

The patient history is of utmost importance in determining which of the causes of weight loss to investigate. Inadequate caloric intake causes weight loss in the majority of patients. Anorexia, nausea and vomiting, and other GI complaints invariably lead to decreased food intake. These symptoms, although referable to the GI tract, may have other causes such as chronic renal insufficiency or hypercalcemia.

Malabsorption that produces weight loss is often associated with steatorrhea; patients with such problems soon learn to avoid fatty foods, however, and may not have diarrhea on presentation to the physician. Malabsorption of certain carbohydrates may produce a severe osmotic diarrhea, as will an injury to the intestinal lining. If surgery has been performed on the GI tract, bacterial overgrowth or decreased absorptive surfaces may produce malabsorption.

Hypermetabolic states frequently can be diagnosed on physical examination. The classic symptoms of thy-

Table 19—1. Laboratory Tests of Nutritional Assessment

Test	Function of Test	Disease State
Serum albumin	Measures visceral protein stores	Low in liver disease, nephrotic syndrome, protein-losing enteropathy
Serum transferrin	Measures visceral protein stores	Transfusions raise levels; low in liver disease
Serum lymphocyte count	Measures immune response	Chemotherapy, primary lymphomas
Delayed hypersensitivity	Measures T-cell function	Chemotherapy, primary lymphomas
Skinfold thickness	Measures fat stores	
Mean arm muscle circumference	Measures somatic protein stores	
Urinary creatinine excretion	Measures muscle protein stores	
Serum urea nitrogen	Measures level of protein intake	Low in liver disease

Table 19—2. Differential Diagnosis of Weight Loss

Decreased Calorie Intake	Malabsorption	Hypermetabolic
Chronic illness	Small intestine injury	Hyperthyroidism
Chronic fevers and infection	Pancreatic insufficiency	Endogenous
Chronic obstructive pulmonary disease	Diabetes mellitus	Exogenous
Congestive heart failure	Short-bowel syndrome	Drug-induced
Chronic liver disease	Radiation enteritis	Theophylline
Chronic renal insufficiency	Bacterial overgrowth	Amphetamines
Inflammatory bowel disease	Alcoholism	Pheochromocytoma
Connective tissue disorders		Malignancy
Neoplastic diseases		Ectopic hormone section
Localised		Maladaptation to starvation
Metastatic		
Gastrointestinal disease		
Hypogeusesthesia, glossitis, depapillation		
Esophageal motility disorders		
Delayed gastric emptying		
Dumping syndromes		
Chronic diarrheal syndromes		
Drugs		
Narcotics		
Antineoplastic agents		
Theophylline derivatives		
Antibiotics		
Vitamin deficiencies		
Thiamin		
Riboflavin		
Folate and vitamin B_{12}		
Zinc		
Endrocrinopathies		
Hypercalcemia		
Hypothyroidism		
Panhypopituitarism		
Adrenal insufficiency		
Neurologic illness		
Dementia		
Cerebral infarctions		
Parkinson's disease		
Aging		
Psychiatric illness		
Anorexia nervosa		
Depression		
Psychotic thought disorders		
Poverty		

rotoxicosis are easy to diagnose, although apathetic hyperthyroidism may be difficult to spot. Resting tachycardia may be the only somatic sign of which a patient may be aware.

Weight loss is frequently characterized by a deficiency of nutrients other than calories and protein. Table 19–3 lists some of the physical findings and abnormal laboratory tests observed for each of these nutritional deficiencies. These abnormalities are usually observed, not as classic single abnormalities, but as a polynutritional deficiency with numerous abnormalities.

WEIGHT GAIN

DEFINITION

Abnormal weight gain is an increase in weight greater than 5 kg in less than 6 months.

PATHOPHYSIOLOGIC CONSIDERATIONS

Weight gain can be produced by an increase in calorie intake, an increase in weight gain efficiency, or an increase in total body fluids. As with weight loss, the rate of weight gain and the composition of the tissue mass will be determined by the cause. The weight gained because of calorie ingestion in excess of caloric expenditure is mostly fat, along with some lean tissue mass. The proportion of fat to muscle that is added depends on several factors. The most important factor appears to be genetic; some individuals naturally gain more muscle mass than others during weight gain.[6] Athletes have known for years that overfeeding and exercise produces an increase in muscle mass with little or no increase in fat mass. Although many individuals increase their intake of protein to gain muscle mass, the protein requirements for gain of lean body tissue in healthy individuals is 1.5 g of protein per kg body weight. Exercise without an increase in calorie intake also decreases fat mass but may increase lean body tissue, with the net result being little change in total body weight.

Hormones also influence the composition of weight gain. Androgens stimulate muscle mass increase and are often used inappropiately by athletes to improve athletic performance. Estrogens stimulate adipose tissue deposition in certain regions of the body including breasts, hips, and thighs.

Other hormones such as cortisol, epinephrine, and glucagon are often increased during stress in protein-calorie malnourished patients. When these patients are overfed in order to replenish their bodies' protein and fat stores, the extra calories are frequently stored as fat. Preliminary studies indicate that refeeding protein-depleted patients may require higher protein intakes (2 to 4 g of protein per kg body weight) in addition to extra carbohydrate and lipid calories.[7]

Increased weight gain efficiency in certain individuals has been proposed as a defect that may predispose them toward obesity. The Neel hypothesis states that many human beings are alive today because their ancestors were more efficient in storing as fat the calories that were ingested.[8] These people were better able to survive the frequent famines that existed in agricultural societies. In modern industrial societies, where food is abundant and physical activity less, people can become obese as a maladaptation to their environment. Long-term overfeeding studies in humans suggest that lean and obese individuals have different abilities to gain excess weight.[6]

Hypothyroidism decreases resting energy expenditure and free water clearance by the kidney and will predispose individuals to both fat deposition and water retention. Hypercortisolism will stimulate fat deposition in adipocytes only in certain areas, producing the pathognomonic sign of truncal obesity with decreased or normal lean body tissue. Excess insulin concentration in blood, either endogenous or exogenous will increase triglyceride esterification and deposition and will increase protein synthesis. Insulin will also stimulate the appetite to prevent hypoglycemia.

An increase in both extra- and intracellular body fluids can produce a significant weight gain. Both decreased free water clearance by the kidney and hyperaldosteronism will produce excess fluid retention. Decreased oncotic pressure in blood secondary to hypoalbuminemia will cause a loss of fluid into the extravascular space and produce secondary aldosteronism. Lymphatic obstruction can often produce massive fluid retention because the lymphatic system returns almost 50% of the extracellular fluid to the blood.

DIFFERENTIAL DIAGNOSIS

The differential diagnosis is divided into changes in food intake, weight gain efficiency, and fluid retention (Table 19–4). The history and physical examination are important in sorting the possible causes of weight gain. The most common cause of weight gain is excessive food intake without any obvious cause, except possibly psychologic. Using medications such as corticosteroids or L-dopa that stimulate appetite and over-

Table 19–3. Clinical Features of Nutritional Deficiencies

Deficiency	Physical Findings	Laboratory Abnormalities
Protein	Edema Hair—sparse, depigmented Skin—dry, scaly Nail ridging Mouth—cheilosis Hepatomegaly	Decreased serum albumin Decreased total lymphocyte count Absent delayed hypersensitivity Normocytic, normochromic anemia Low total serum calcium
Calorie	Decreased subcutaneous fat stores Decreased muscle mass Nonedematous	Low serum triiodothyronine Low serum transferrin Low urinary creatinine/height ratio Hypothermia
Vitamin A	Hair—coarse, sparse Pruritus Follicular keratosis Conjunctival xerosis and keratomalacia Night blindness	Decreased retinol-binding protein levels in serum
Thiamin (B_1)	Peripheral neuropathy Myopathy Anorexia and constipation Congestive heart failure Myelopathy Subacute cerebellar degeneration Wernicke's encephalopathy	Decreased red blood cell transketolase activity
Riboflavin (B_2)	Angular stomatitis Glossitis and cheilosis Seborrheic dermatitis Corneal vascularization	Decreased erythrocyte glutathione reduc- tase activity
Niacin	Pigmentation, desquamation Cheilosis Glossitis Dementia Diarrhea Peripheral neuropathy Myelopathy	Normochromic, normocytic anemia Decreased serum tryptophan Nonspecific colitis
Pyridoxine (B_6)	Perioral cheilosis Weight loss, anorexia Depression Peripheral neuropathy	Sideroblastic anemia (pyridoxine-respon- sive)
Folate and B_{12}	Fatigue Macroglossia and glossitis Icterus and pallor Diarrhea (folate) Constipation (B_{12}) Peripheral neuropathy (B_{12}) Ataxia and dementia (B_{12})	Megaloblastic bone marrow Low serum B_{12} Low serum folate Increased serum LDH High serum iron, increased iron stores
Ascorbic acid (Vitamin C)	Scurvy Fatigue Skin and mucosal hemorrhages Sjögren's syndrome Poor wound healing	Subperiosteal hemorrhages
Vitamin D	Bone pain Kyphosis	Increased serum alkaline phosphatase Hypophosphatemia Low serum $1,25(OH)_2$-D_3 Low serum 25-OH-D_3 Decalcified bone Pseudofractures

Table 19–3.   Clinical Features of Nutritional Deficiencies (Continued)

Deficiency	Physical Findings	Laboratory Abnormalities
Vitamin E	Hemorrhages	Impaired red cell survival Creatinuria
Vitamin K	Hemorrhage	Increased prothrombin time
Calcium	Tetany Osteopenia Seizures	Hyperphosphatemia Increased serum PTH Prolonged QT interval (ECG)
Phosphorus	Muscle weakness Renal calculi	Osteomalacia Hemolytic anemia Hypercalciuria
Magnesium	Seizures Anorexia Nausea	Hypocalcemia Decreased serum PTH Hypokalemia
Iron	Weakness Fatigue Poor exercise tolerance	Decreased serum iron Normal or increased binding capacity
Serum total iron	Plummer-Vinson syndrome	Hypochromic, microcytic anemia Increased platelet counts
Iodine	Goiter	Hypothyroidism
Copper	Wilson's disease Neurologic disturbances Keyser-Fleischer rings Hepatic cirrhosis	Decreased ceruloplasmin levels Aminoaciduria Renal tubular acidosis
Zinc	Growth retardation Acrodermatitis enteropathica Hypogeusesthesia	Hypopituitarism Hypogonadism

using insulin in attempting to lower blood glucose levels in type II diabetes are common causes of iatrogenic weight gain. Many obese patients complain of increased weight gain efficiency ("low metabolism"), but studies indicate that only a small percentage (<5%) have diseases such as hypothyroidism or Cushing's disease that may promote obesity. An increase in weight of greater than 2 to 3 pounds per week suggests fluid retention, especially in patients with chronic diseases.

DIAGNOSTIC EVALUATION

The history and physical examination will be able to differentiate excessive fat deposition from excessive fluid retention. The rate of weight gain, medication usage, chronic illnesses, and family history are important pieces of information. Signs and symptoms of hypothyroidism that may be significant include oligomenorrhea, changes in hair and skin texture, a decrease in mental acuity, and delayed relaxation phase

Table 19–4.   Differential Diagnosis of Weight Gain

Increase in Calorie Intake	Increase in Weight Gain Efficiency	Increase in Fluid Retention

Increased hunger sensation
  Hypothalamic obesity
  Reaction to stress
  Hypoglycemia
    Increased endogenous insulin secretion
    Excessive exogenous insulin therapy
  Drugs
    L-dopa
  Phenothiazines
    Anabolic steroid usage
    Exogenous corticosteroid administration
  Hyperthyroidism
  Acromegaly
	Decreased energy expenditure
	  Hypothyroidism
	Decreased lean body tissue
	  Aging process
	  Cushing's disease
	  Refeeding after low-calorie
	    diet
	Insulin resistance, insulinoma, genetic predisposition
		Dependent edema
		  Congestive heart failure
		  Hyperaldosteronism
		  Obesity-associated
		  Oral contraceptive
		    agents
		Hypoalbuminemia
		  Nephrotic syndrome
		  Chronic liver disease
		  Protein-losing enteropathy
		  Lymphatic obstruction

of the deep tendon reflexes. Hypercortisolism is observed in conjunction with hypertension, impaired glucose tolerance, truncal obesity, and skin changes. One of the more difficult diagnostic challenges in medicine is insulinoma, the symptoms of which are insidious and may not produce classic hypoglycemic symptoms. The chief complaint may be hunger at night in association with weight gain and can be diagnosed only with appropriate laboratory testing.

The physical examination will provide information on the presence of dependent edema, congestive heart failure, or both. The distribution of fat, presence of a buffalo hump, and purple striae are important in the diagnosis of hypercortisolism. Delay relaxation of the deep tendon reflexes is classic for hypothyroidism. Lymphatic obstruction may be present when a single extremity is edematous or the entire lower body is markedly edematous in the absence of hypoalbuminemia.

Laboratory tests are required to determine the presence or absence of disorders such as hypothyroidism and hypercortisolism. Usually, obtaining a total T_4 level and TSH level in the blood will screen for hypothyroidism. The screening process for Cushing's disease is more complicated. Most commonly, suppression of the morning serum cortisol level after a 1-mg dexamethasone overnight suppression test indicates that Cushing's disease is not present. The diagnosis of insulinoma can be made only by providing that hypoglycemia is present with an inappropriate blood insulin concentration. This test most commonly requires a fast that may extend to 72 hours. About 90% of individuals with insulinomas will develop hypoglycemia within 24 hours, 95% by 48 hours, and 99% by the end of 72 hours and exercise.

When excessive fluid retention is the cause of the weight gain, a biochemical blood screen will often provide the answers to the cause. The presence of hypoalbuminemia is the first question to answer. Another possibility is the presence of proteinuria, which should be determined by a 24-hour urine collection.

NEUROLOGIC MANIFESTATIONS OF NUTRITIONAL DISORDERS

DEFINITION

Certain nutritional deficiencies such as of thiamin or B_{12} produce specific neurologic syndromes. Al-though specific deficiencies of one nutrient can occur, nutrient deficiences most frequently are multiple and occur in chronically malnourished individuals. Alcoholism is frequently the cause of the poor intake of nutrients, but syndromes such as Wernicke's disease may also occur in other settings of malnutrition.

PATHOPHYSIOLOGIC CONSIDERATIONS

Normal function of the nervous system requires a continuous supply of nutrients as metabolic fuels and adequate vitamin stores for proper metabolism. Deficiency of one or more nutrients or vitamins can produce diffuse abnormalities of neurologic function such as metabolic encephalopathy or specific deficits such as peripheral neuropathy. Cells of the central and peripheral nervous system are differentially sensitive to metabolic derangements or deficiencies. One example is thiamin deficiency, which affects only cells of the wall of the third ventricle and specific brain stem sites.[9]

Diffuse cerebral dysfunction, either encephalopathy or seizures, can be produced by either a deficiency or an excess of minerals or vitamins. Minerals such as calcium, magnesium, sodium, or heavy metals are usually concentrated within a narrow normal range; concentrations outside the normal range alter the cell membrane potential and may produce abnormal membrane conduction leading to diffuse dysfunction or seizures.

The central nervous system utilizes glucose as its main fuel source, requiring 100 to 120 g/day. Therefore, the cofactors used in metabolizing glucose such as thiamin, riboflavin, pyridoxine, and niacin are essential for normal brain cell function. Vitamin B_{12} deficiency also damages myelin and may produce a peripheral neuropathy and posterior spinal column degeneration. Central nervous system effects include thought disorders such as paranoid ideation.

DIFFERENTIAL DIAGNOSIS

Several nutritional causes of diffuse cerebral dysfunction produce encephalopathy or seizures (Table 19–5). These causes have been divided into chemical deficiency and chemical excess. As previously explained, normal ranges for cations such as sodium, calcium, or magnesium are usually narrow because they directly affect the membrane potential of the neurons. Cranial nerve abnormalities are usually confined to single nerves or nerve groups. Vitamin A deficiency is a well-known cause of night blindness, and acute thiamin deficiency (Wernicke's syndrome) produces abnormal function of the third, fourth, and sixth cranial nerves.

Since peripheral nerves also require glucose as their

Table 19–5.   Neurologic Manifestations of Nutritional Disorders

Encephalopathy and seizures	Cranial nerve abnormalities
Chemical deficiency states	Vitamin A deficiency
Vitamin B$_{12}$ deficiency	Lead intoxication
Vitamin E deficiency	Thiamin deficiency
Hypoglycemia	
Hypomagnesemia	Cerebellar disorders
Hypocalcemia	Thiamin deficiency
Niacin deficiency	Niacin deficiency
Pyridoxine deficiency in children	Pantothenic acid deficiency
Protein-calorie malnutrition	Chronic alcohol ingestion
Thiamin deficiency	
	Peripheral neuropathy
Chemical excess	Arsenic intoxication
Aluminum dementia	Thiamin deficiency
Chronic alcohol ingestion	Pantothenic acid deficiency
Vitamin A intoxication	Pyridoxine deficiency
Hypercalcemia	B$_{12}$ deficiency
Heavy metal poisoning	Niacin deficiency
Arsenic, lead, bismuth	
	Myopathy
Metabolic abnormalities	Hypokalemia
Hepatic encepalopathy	Alcohol ingestion
Metabolic alkalosis	Arsenic poisoning
Metabolic acidosis	

energy source, deficiency of B vitamins and the other cofactors of the Krebs cycle will produce neuropathy. In addition, heavy metals such as arsenic and mercury may produce damage to peripheral nerve tissue.

DIAGNOSTIC EVALUATION

Nutritional deficiencies usually produce abnormalities in both the central and peripheral nervous systems, a circumstance uncommon for other diseases. Thus, nutritional deficiencies should be considered when individuals present with polyneuropathy and central nervous system findings. In addition, subacute encephalopathies and optic nerve atrophy may also have nutritional deficiencies as the cause. In many cases, obvious malnutrition is associated with the other nutrient deficiencies, but alcoholism may obscure calorie deprivation. Thus, in individuals who otherwise appear well-nourished, alcohol use can precipitate a crisis such as nutritional amblyopia or Wernicke's encephalopathy.

DERMATOLOGIC SIGNS OF NUTRITIONAL DISORDERS

The skin has been called the window to the body, and many nutritional diseases are associated with skin abnormalities. Because the cells of the skin are replaced every 5 days, nutritional deficiencies are more apparent in this organ than others. The abnormalities produced in skin, as with other organs, may not be specific to deficiencies of a single nutrient. Protein deficiency alone produces many of the same skin and oral mucosa abnormalities as deficiency of the B vitamins (Table 19–6). The dietary history as well as the medical history is important in determining the cause of the abnormality. Skin biopsy may be helpful in the diagnosis, but frequently a good history and physical examination will lead to the diagnosis.

NUTRITIONAL ANEMIA

DEFINITION

Nutritional deficiencies of iron, vitamin B$_{12}$, and folate are frequent causes of anemias. It has been estimated that 95% of megaloblastic anemias are due to deficiencies of vitamin B$_{12}$, folate, or both, and that iron deficiency is the major source of microcytic anemias.[10]

PATHOPHYSIOLOGIC CONSIDERATIONS

A vitamin or mineral deficiency can be secondary to one of several factors; it can result from nutrient

Table 19–6. Dermatologic Signs of Nutritional Disorders

Abnormalities	Nutritional Deficiencies
Hair abnormalities	
Coarse and sparse	Protein-calorie malnutrition
	Vitamin A deficiency
Loss of color	Copper deficiency
Alopecia	Zinc deficiency
Kinky	Copper deficiency
Eyes	
Corneal neovascularization	Riboflavin deficiency
Oral cavity	
Cheilosis	Riboflavin deficiency
	Thiamin deficiency
	Iron deficiency
Angular stomatitis	Niacin deficiency
	Riboflavin deficiency
	Pyridoxine deficiency
	Iron deficiency
Gingivitis	Dilantin therapy
	Ascorbic acid deficiency
Glossitis	Riboflavin deficiency
	Iron deficiency
	Vitamin B_{12} or folate deficiency
	Pyridoxine deficiency
	Niacin deficiency
Papillary atrophy of the tongue	Vitamin B_{12} or folate deficiency
	Riboflavin deficiency
	Iron deficiency
Skin	
Abnormal pigmentation	Excess carotene ingestion
	Vitamin B_{12} deficiency
	Niacin deficiency
	Riboflavin deficiency
	Biotin deficiency
Dermatitis	Niacin deficiency
	Zinc deficiency
	Arsenic poisoning
	Biotin deficiency
Seborrhea	Pyridoxine deficiency
	Niacin deficiency
	Riboflavin deficiency
	Intertrigo
	Pyridoxine deficiency
Eczema	Zinc deficiency
Pruritus	Vitamin A deficiency
Petechiae-purpura	Ascorbic acid deficiency
	Vitamin K deficiency

Table 19–7. Differential Diagnosis of Nutritional Anemias

Anemia	Abnormality
Iron deficiency anemia	
Inadequate intake	Hypocaloric diet
	Food faddism
	Pica
	Alcoholism
Impaired absorption	Gastric achlorhydria
	Gastrectomy
	Rapid intestinal transit time
	Alkaline antacid ingestion
	Pica
Increased excretion	Pathologic bleeding increased menstrual blood loss, hematochezia, hematuria
	Proteinuria
	Hemoglobinuria
	Hemolysis secondary to artificial valve placement
Impaired utilization	Anemia of chronic disease, sideroblastic anemia
	Hereditary absence of transferrin
	Pulmonary hemosiderosis
	Paroxysmal nocturnal hemoglobinuria
Increased requirements	Pregnancy
	Lactation
B_{12} deficiency	
Inadequate intake	Alcoholism
	Poverty
	Total vegetarian diet
Impaired absorption	Impaired intrinsic factor activity
	Abnormal protein
	Atrophic gastritis
	Gastrectomy
	Small intestine
	Loss of ileal function
	Steatorrhea
	Inflammatory bowel disease
	Tropical and nontropical sprue
	Calcium chelating agents
	Blind loop syndrome
Increased excretion	Liver disease
Impaired utilization	Protein-calorie malnutrition
	Chronic illness
	Abnormal B_{12} binding protein
	Enzyme activity deficiency
Increased requirements	Hyperthyroidism
	Pregnancy
	Malignancy
Folate deficiency	
Inadequate intake	Poor diet
	Chronic alcoholism
Impaired absorption	Upper small-bowel disease
	Pancreatic insufficiency
	Foods
	Drugs
Impaired utilization	Folic acid antagonists
	Antibiotics
	Cancer chemotherapy
	B_{12} deficiency
	Alcohol
	Enzyme deficiency
Increased requirements	Pregnancy
	Lactation
	Malignancy
	Hyperthyroidism
Copper deficiency	Inadequate intake
	Protein-calorie malnutrition
	Increased excretion
	Nephrotic syndrome

deficiency caused by decreased intake, impaired absorption, or increased excretion; from impaired utilization; and from increased requirements. Abnormalities in uptake, utilization, or requirements have been reported for each of the three nutrients (Table 19–7). Diagnosing the cause of megaloblastic anemias is important because treatment with folate may improve the anemia of B_{12} deficiency but not overcome the neurologic deficits. It is equally important to diagnose the cause of iron deficiency because occult bleeding is a frequent and potentially serious cause of iron deficiency.

DIFFERENTIAL DIAGNOSIS AND DIAGNOSTIC EVALUATION

The large red cells of nutritional megaloblastic anemia are oval. Ovalocytes have to be differentiated from macrocytes of macrocytosis caused by hypothyroidism and liver disease and other anemias such as hemolytic anemia, sideroblastic anemia, or hypoplastic anemia. In addition, leukopenia with hypersegmented polymorphonuclear neutrophils (B_{12} only) and thrombocytopenia are also present. Intestinal megaloblastosis secondary to either B_{12} or folate deficiency can produce malabsorption of both B_{12} and folate and a low serum level of both. Only vitamin B_{12} deficiency produces methylmalonic aciduria.

To test for adequacy of B_{12} stores and the ability of the body to absorb B_{12}, administration of radiolabeled B_{12} with and without intrinsic factor should discriminate between the various abnormalities that may occur.

There are several causes of microcytic anemias, including iron deficiency, thalassemia, and the sideroblastic anemias. The serum iron and iron binding capacity of the serum in addition to the blood smear will frequently provide the correct diagnosis. Bone marrow aspiration with iron stains will tell whether iron is present and whether it is being utilized. More importantly, once the diagnosis of iron deficiency is established, the discovery of its cause is paramount. A diet history is useful in determining oral intake, and a history of prior gastric surgery may be important. What is most important is to determine whether there is pathologic bleeding and, if so, what is its source. Occult malignancies are just one cause of iron deficiency but should not be overlooked.

BONE PAIN

DEFINITION

Bone pain is almost always a sign of underlying disorder. It can be as minor as a bone bruise secondary to trauma or as serious as a pathologic fracture secondary to metastatic disease. Bone pain should be investigated until a reason for the pain is discovered. Bone pain is a frequent complaint in elderly individuals, and the causes are many but often treatable. Several important nutritional causes of bone pain can be diagnosed and will be discussed in this section.

PATHOPHYSIOLOGIC CONSIDERATIONS

Bone is composed of living cells and connective tissue organized in a matrix that is then calcified with calcium hydroxyapatite crystals. A defect in calcification is called osteomalacia in adults and rickets in children. Osteomalacia produces weak bones, bone pain, and gait disturbances. Normal mineralization of bone requires an adequate amount of both calcium and phosphate in the extracellular bone fluid, a positive or neutral calcium and phosphate balance, and a normal parathyroid hormone level in blood. Vitamin D is required for normal absorption of both calicum and phosphate from the gut and for maintaining a positive calcium balance. If any of these factors is not correct, osteomalacia may ensue. Primary vitamin D deficiency caused by lack of food intake or sunlight is rare in the U.S., but malabsorption, liver disease (for conversion of vitamin D_3 to 25-OH-D_3), or renal disease (for conversion of 25-OH-D_3 to 1,25 $(OH)_2$-D_3) may alter vitamin D metabolism.

A decrease in bone matrix with normal calcification is called osteoporosis. It is now recognized as a major source of morbidity in elderly patients.[11] Osteoporosis occurs when the rate of bone accretion is less than the rate of bone resorption. When osteoporosis is severe enough to be seen as decreased bone mass on x-ray, approximately 30 to 50% of the tissue has been resorbed. At least two possible defects can cause osteoporosis: a low rate of bone accretion and an acceleration of bone resorption. Both defects have been described in various forms of osteoporosis.

Decreased bone accretion appears to be the major defect in the most common form, senile or postmenopausal osteoporosis. Women are usually in a positive calcium balance and enlarge the bulk of their skeletons until the end of their fourth decade. Men, probably because of their anabolic hormones, have heavier skeletons and stay in a positive calcium balance until their later decades. After menopause, women tend to lose calcium unless their calcium intake is at least 1200 mg/day,[12] most likely because of estrogen deficiency and possibly an alteration of vitamin D metabolism. High-turnover osteoporosis has a variety of causes (Table 19–8).

DIFFERENTIAL DIAGNOSIS AND DIAGNOSTIC EVALUATION

When dealing with bone pain it is important to determine whether the disease process has affected just

Table 19–8. Differential Diagnosis of Bone Pain

Abnormality	Defect
Mineralization defect of bone	Osteomalacia
	Decreased vitamin D activity
	Inadequate intake
	Malabsorption
	Lack of sunlight
	Defect in 25-hydroxylation, chronic
	liver disease
	Impaired 1,25-hydroxylation
	Genetic—vitamin D–resistant rickets
	Chronic renal failure
	Tumors
	Hypercalcemia
	Hyperparathyroidism
	Primary
	Parathyroid adenoma
	Parathyroid hyperplasia
	Ectopic PTH secretion
	Ectopic non-PTH substances
	Immobilization
	Milk-alkali syndrome
	Vitamin D intoxication
Decreased bone mass	Decreased bone accretion
	Aging
	Estrogen deficiency in women
	Turner's syndrome
	Premature ovarian failure
	Bilateral oophorectomy
	Increased bone resorption
	Hyperthyroidism
	Glucocorticoids
	Immobilization
	Diabetes mellitus
	Vitamin C deficiency
	Increased dietary phosphate intake
	Chronic heparin therapy

one area or whether there is diffuse bone involvement. The performance of a complete history and physical examination is imperative because diseases of the GI tract, endocrine system, and hematopoietic system, renal disease, and steroid usage may provide important information as to the cause of the bone pain. A complete biochemical profile, CBC, Bence Jones protein check, serum parathyroid hormone level, and both 25-OH-D$_3$ and 1,25-OH-D$_3$ levels may be required to determine whether the problem is abnormal mineralization, decreased bone mass, or a combination of the two.

The x-ray findings of osteomalacia and osteoporosis are distinct, and if the disease process is advanced, the diagnosis of the two entities is not difficult. If osteomalacia is present, determining whether an abnormality of vitamin D intake, absorption, or conversion is warranted. Sometimes a renal phosphate leak may lead to hypophosphatemia and osteomalacia. Hypercalcemia may produce bone pain if hyperparathyroidism is the cause.

If x-rays and blood tests are not conclusive of the type of bone abnormality present, a tetracycline-labeled bone biopsy may be required. Tetracycline is incorporated into bone in a manner similar to calcium and is fluorescent under the appropriate light source. This test will determine whether there is abnormal mineralization or accelerated resorption in the bone.

NUTRITIONAL DISORDERS OF ELDERLY PATIENTS

The causes of many of the nutritional problems encountered by elderly individuals are socioeconomic (Table 19–9). The poverty level at which many elderly people live does not allow them to buy high-quality, protein rich foods. Difficulty in food shopping and preparing hot meals lead to the ingestion of simple

Table 19–9. Nutritional Disorders of Elderly Patients

Nutrient	Abnormality	Cause
Calories	Low intake	Poverty Dementia Inability to masticate Impaired taste
Protein	None	None
Carbohydrate	Impaired glucose tolerance	Increased insulin resistance
Fat	None	None
Calcium	Osteopenia	Decreased calcium intake
Iron	Iron deficiency	Decreased absorption secondary to atrophic gastritis
Folate	Folate deficiency	Decreased oral intake
Ascorbic acid	Ascorbic acid deficiency	Decreased oral intake

foods such as breads and cookies, which are low in protein.

In addition, health problems common in elderly people may prevent an adequate food intake. Loss of teeth and poorly fitting dentures deter individuals from eating solid foods. Short-term memory loss is frequent in dementia, and afflicted individuals may forget to eat and may not ingest adequate protein and calories. Arthritis may prevent a person from preparing and cooking properly, and medications can produce anorexia. Elderly men and especially women increase their risk of developing osteoporosis because many are lactose intolerant and will not drink milk or eat dairy products.

Evidence indicates that elderly individuals require fewer total calories to maintain their weight because there is a loss of lean tissue mass with age.[13] This loss occurs even in spite of continued physical activity. Protein utilization does not appear to change, however, and protein requirements are still proportional to body weight (0.8 to 1.0 g/kg). Calcium intake is frequently below what is recommended, especially for postmenopausal women (1200 mg/day), and supplements are often required. There does not appear to be increased requirements for any of the other vitamins or minerals in elderly individuals, and supplementation should be reserved for those individuals whose diets are deficient.

CANCER-RELATED EFFECTS ON NUTRITIONAL STATUS

The most common nutritional problem encountered in cancer patients is weight loss. Inadequate calorie and protein intake may be secondary to a variety of causes (Table 19–10). Anorexia is a common complaint of many cancer patients, and they often note that breakfast is the only meal that they can complete. Anorexia usually occurs in the setting of metastatic diseases, but primary tumors such as pancreatic carcinoma and hepatocellular carcinoma also can produce anorexia. Anorexia is also a frequent complication of both chemotherapy and radiation therapy. Chemotherapy can in addition produce xerostomia, nausea, and vomiting, which will reduce oral intake of food.

Cancer cells directly and indirectly promote protein catabolism.[14] Secretion of ectopic hormones and other factors may alter liver amino acid metabolism to allow the tumor to utilize preferentially the available amino acid pool for protein synthesis. Fat stores are also used, as both the tumor and host require calories for energy metabolism.

Mineral deficiencies are a common complication of chronic diarrhea or chemotherapy. Also, certain chemotherapeutic agents interfere with vitamin metabolism such as the activity of methotrexate on folate metabolism, and may produce vitamin deficiencies. All these problems can be corrected and are best prevented when nutritional support is provided early in the course of treatment.

DRUG-NUTRIENT INTERACTIONS

Medications have both direct and indirect effects on nutrient metabolism. They can interfere with absorption, inhibit normal nutrient activity, or increase the body's requirements for specific nutrients. These effects can be either the primary drug effect or a sec-

Table 19–10.   Cancer-Related Effects on Nutritional Status

Nutrient Deficiency	Cause

Calories	Cancerous cachexia—decreased intake of calories
	  Anorexia
	  Radiation effects
	    Decreased taste and xerostomia
	    Radiation enteritis
	  Chemotherapy
	  Chronic diarrhea
	    Zollinger-Ellison syndrome
	    Verner-Morrison syndrome (wDH$_A$ syndrome)
	  Hypercalcemia-induced anorexia
	  Short-bowel syndrome

Protein	Protein-calorie malnutrition of host as tumor preferentially utilizes amino acids Increased protein catabolism due to ectopic ACTH secretion or exogenous steroid therapy Increased protein losses—protein-losing enteropathies Decreased protein absorption—chronic steatorrhea
Fat	Increased lipolysis of adipose tissue stores
Folate	Folate deficiency caused by folic acid antagonists
B$_{12}$	Increased serum but not tissue levels in hematopoietic malignancies
B$_6$	Deficient in Hodgkin's disease
Potassium, magnesium, zinc	Deficiencies observed during chronic diarrhea
Malnutrition, most nutrient deficiencies	Primary tumors of the GI tract or pancreas caused by obstruction or malabsorption

Malnutrition	Surgical therapy of GI tumors
	  Dumping syndrome
	  Bacterial overgrowth in blind loop of bowel
	  Short-bowel syndrome

ondary, nonintended effect of drug therapy. Almost every drug has either primary or secondary effects on nutrient metabolism, and physicians should be aware of these potentially serious complications. A partial list of drug-nutrient interactions is shown in Table 19–11.

VITAMIN INTOXICATION

With the tremendous public interest in nutrition and many self-styled nutritionists claiming that nutritional therapy can prevent or cure diseases, vitamin intoxication has risen dramatically in the past decade. The recommended daily allowance (RDA) of vitamins and minerals is calculated to provide the daily requirements of vitamins and minerals for the adult population. It is usually greater than the minimum requirements but well within the safe range for all the nutrients. Problems occur when quantities greater than ten times the RDA are ingested. At this intake level, these vitamins

have pharmacologic actions that may be distinct from their normal metabolic actions.

Vitamin C at doses greater than 20 times the RDA has been given enormous publicity as a cure for both the common cold and for cancer. While the evidence for the curative effects of vitamin C has not held up to rigorous testing, side effects do occur. They are related to the fact that vitamin C is an acid excreted by the kidney. Oxalate stones and interference in the measurement of glucosuria have been reported (Table 19–12).

Fat-soluble vitamins may cause problems related to their long half-life in the body. Chronic administration of vitamin D may produce hypercalcemia after a period of months because of the build up of vitamin D stores in fat tissues. Similar problems may occur with excess vitamin A intake. An orange discoloration of the skin is produced over time by excessive ingestion of vitamin A, which is stored in body tissues.

It used to be thought that the water-soluble B vitamins were safe even at excessive doses because they could not be stored in excessive amounts, but new data indicates that this is not the case. Niacin intake, as

Table 19–11. Drug-Nutrient Interactions

Drug	Effect on Nutrient
Antacids	Aluminum salts inhibit phosphate absorption
	Calcium, iron, and thiamin may be malabsorbed
Antibiotics	
Neomycin	Precipitates bile acids
	Impairs fat-soluble vitamin absorption
Oxacillin	Causes fat and fat-soluble vitamin malabsorption
Isoniazid	Produces B_6 deficiency
Sulfonamides	Decreases gut bacterial folic acid and vitamin K production
Tetracyclines	Binds to calcium in gut, prevents absorption
Anticoagulants	
Coumarin	Causes vitamin K deficiency
Anticonvulsants	
Phenytoin	Increases folate requirements
	Increases hepatic elimination of vitamin D
Barbiturates	Increase folate requirements
Primidone	Increases vitamin C and K requirements because of acceleration of vitamin degradation
Antihypertensives	
Thiazides	Potassium, magnesium, zinc, vitamin C depletion
Hydralazine	Vitamin B_6 antagonist
Aspirin	Increases vitamin C excretion
Chemotherapeutic agents	
Actinomycin D	Impairs calcium absorption
Methotrexate	Folic acid antagonist
Glucocorticoids	Inhibit vitamin D utilization
	Cause hypokalemia
	Increase protein requirements
	Increase B_1 and B_{12} requirements
Hypolipemic agents	
Cholestyramine	Bile sequestration, may cause fat-soluble vitamin deficiency
Colestipol	
Niacin	In doses utilized, may cause liver dysfunction
Mithramycin	Produces hypocalcemia
Digitalis	Interferes with thiamin utilization
	Hypokalemia
Ethanol	Increases requirements for vitamin B_6, folate, magnesium, and zinc
	Associated with dietary thiamin deficiency
Mineral oil	May produce fat-soluble vitamin deficiency

Table 19–12. Signs and Symptoms of Excessive Vitamin Intake

Vitamin	Dose	Effect
Vitamin A	>10,000 U/day	Fatigue, malaise Dementia Anorexia, GI disturbances Hydrocephalus Liver failure
Riboflavin (B_2)		Interferes with methotrexate
Niacin	750 mg/day	Hepatitis, cholestatic jaundice Hyperuricemia and gout
	3 g/day	Cardiac arrhythmias
Pyridoxine (B_6)	2 g/day	Sensory neuropathy Interferes with l-dopa
Folic acid	5 to 15 mg/day	Interferes with anticonvulsant therapy May mask B_{12} deficiency
Vitamin C	1000 mg/day	Nausea, diarrhea Impairs vitamin A activity Oxalate renal stones False positive and false negative urinary glucose test Interferes with Warfarin therapy

Vitamin D	10,000 U/day	Hypercalcemia
		  Anorexia
		  Constipation
		  Renal stones
		  CNS dysfunction

Vitamin E	1200 U/day	Thrombophlebitis Pulmonary emboli Hypertension Gynecomastia Infertility GI disturbances Interference with vitamin K

little as 500 mg/day, can produce a peripheral neuropathy.[15] Obtaining the patient's trust and a good dietary history will frequently identify the problem.

REFERENCES

1. Owen, O.E., et al.: Liver and kidney metabolism during prolonged starvation. J Clin Invest 48:574, 1969.
2. Cahill, G.F., Jr.: Starvation in man. N Engl J Med 282:668, 1970.
3. Crim, M.C., and Munro, H.N.: Protein-energy malnutrition and endocrine function. In Endocrinology. Edited by L.J. DeGroot, et al.: New York, Grune and Stratton, 1979, pp 1987–2000.
4. Baker, J.P.,et al.: Nutritional assessment: a comparison of clinical judgement and objective measures. N Engl J Med 306:969, 1982.
5. Mullen, J.L., et al.: Reduction of operative morbidity and mortality by combined preoperative and postoperative nutritional support. Ann Surg 192:604, 1980.
6. Sims, E.A.H.: Experimental obesity, dietary-induced thermogenesis and their clinical implications in obesity. Clin Endocrinol Metab 5:377, 1976.
7. Long, C.L., et al.: Whole body protein synthesis and catabolism in septic man. Am J Clin Nutr 30:1340, 1977.
8. Neel, J.V.: Diabetes mellitus: a thrifty genotype rendered detrimental by "progress." Am J Hum Genet 14:353, 1962.
9. Sturman, J.A., and Rivlin, R.S.: Pathogenesis of brain dysfunction in deficiency of thiamine, riboflavin, pantothenic acid, or vitamin B_6 p425. In Biology of Brain Dysfunction. Edited by G.E. Gaul. New York, Plenum Press, 1975.
10. Wintrobe, M.M., et al.: Clinical Hematology. 7th Ed. Philadelphia, Lea & Febiger, 1974.
11. Heany, R.P., et al.: Calcium nutrition and bone health in the elderly. Am J Clin Nutr 36:986, 1982.
12. Osteoporosis. National Institues of Health Consensus Development Conference Statement 5:3, 1984. Washington, D.C., NIH.
13. Tzankoff, S. and Norris, H.: Effect of muscle mass decrease on age-related BMR changes. J Appl Physiol 43:1001, 1977.
14. Lundholm, K., et al.: Skeletal muscle metabolism in patients with malignant tumour. Eur J Cancer 12:465, 1976.
15. Schaumberg, A., et al.: Sensory neuropathy from pyridoxine abuse. N Engl J Med 309:445, 1983.

CHAPTER 20

OPHTHALMOLOGIC PROBLEMS

Murk-Hein Heinemann, M.D. and D. Jackson Coleman, M.D.

Ophthalmologic problems usually manifest themselves within a narrow range of signs and symptoms, but the implications of these findings to the physician are broad. Commonly, pain, visual disturbances, and external abnormalities such as redness, either singly or in combination, alert the patient that something is wrong. The physician must assess these clinical findings not only in terms of what the specific ocular problem is and whether the problem requires referral to an ophthalmic specialist, but also in terms of the patient's general medical condition. For example, an intraocular hemorrhage may result from a solely ocular problem such as vitreous detachment or may be due to a systemic disorder such as diabetes mellitus.

The diagnosis may be problematic for two reasons; first, because the number of presenting signs and symptoms is so small, the differential diagnosis of ocular problems is complex; second, because the eye is small and anatomically complex, physical examination often becomes frustrating for the general physician if he lacks access to the sophisticated diagnostic instruments available to the ophthalmologist. Careful evaluation of clinical history, measurement of the visual acuity, and examination with a hand light and ophthalmoscope, however, can provide a great deal of useful information about specific ocular disorders as well as ocular complications of systemic disease.

The most important part of the ocular physical examination, whether the physician is evaluating the patient within the context of a generalized medical problem such as diabetes or for a specific ocular problem such as injury, is the measurement of visual acuity. By convention, visual acuity is designated by two numbers, the first (numerator) representing the distance between the patient and the test image, usually 20 feet or 6 meters, and the second (denominator) representing the distance at which the test image subtends an angle of arc of 5 minutes. The Snellen letter "E" is constructed in such a way that each part of the letter subtends 1 minute of arc. Because visual acuity testing depends on many factors that may affect the final result, such as the patient's intelligence and motivation and the environment in which the test is performed, the physician who is not working in a controlled environment with standardized equipment is at a disadvantage. Awareness of the variables that can affect visual acuity testing is therefore of great importance. Many patients, because of age, mental status, or education, are not able to read; in these cases, test objects such as the "illiterate E" should be used.

If the vision is profoundly reduced, the patient may have only light perception (with or without projection), hand motion, or finger counting vision. Many patients may have reduced vision because of amblyopia or "lazy eye," the result of strabismus or refractive error. When the patient to be tested is confined to bed it may be possible to test acuity only of near vision. In this situation, presbyopia must be taken into account. A 50-year-old patient may have 20/20 vision at a distance but have reduced near vision because he is not wearing a reading spectacle that corrects for the decreased accommodative ability associated with age.

When testing visual acuity it is important to establish whether the patient has a refractive error. Whenever possible, visual acuity testing should be done with the patient wearing his glasses, although refractive error may change, as in diabetes mellitus of recent onset or high-dose corticosteroid therapy. Refractive error can easily be neutralized by having the patient look through a small pinhole device. If the patient's vision improves, a refractive error is present. Vision may also be reduced when opacities of the ocular media such as cataract or vitreous hemorrhage are present. A pinhole and a +2.50 diopter lens that will compensate for presbyopia are useful instruments for visual acuity testing, especially when testing must be done at the bedside.

Once the assessment of visual acuity has been made, the visual field of each eye should be evaluated by means of confrontation with a test object. When abnormalities of the optic nerve are suspected, using a red object as the test object may uncover a more subtle field defect that may be present. In addition, a red object can be used to evaluate the patient's ability to sense color. Asymmetry in the patient's ability to see a red object (color desaturation or dyschromatopsia) suggests disorder of the optic nerve or macula.

The next step in the examination of the eyes is to systematically examine the external ocular structures, eye movements, and pupillary reflexes. Once the symmetry of the lids and orbits has been established, ruling out problems such as exophthalmos and ptosis, the physician should perform a careful examination of the eyelids and adnexal structures. When a foreign body is suspected it is important to evert the upper and lower lids to expose the tarsal conjunctiva. Examination of the extraocular movements can uncover problems with isolated extraocular muscles and abnormalities of voluntary and involuntary conjugate movements (pursuit and saccade) and vestibulo-ocular reflexes.

Although the anterior segment of the eye is best examined with a slit lamp, much information can be obtained by inspection using a hand light and small magnifying lens such as a convex (high plus) lens of a direct ophthalmoscope. The pattern of conjunctival and episcleral injection, the clarity and condition of the cornea, the depth and condition of the anterior chamber, the size, shape and reactivity of the pupil, and the clarity of the lens and ocular media can all be assessed with these simple instruments.

Examination of the vitreous and retina is then performed with the direct ophthalmoscope. The color, contour, and symmetry of the optic nerves should be noted. The condition of the retinal arterioles and venules as well as the presence of vascular abnormalities such as hemorrhages, cotton-wool spots, and exudates can be evaluated. The physician can examine the macula by having the patient fixate on the light source of the ophthalmoscope.

LOSS OF VISION

Loss of visual acuity, whether occurring abruptly or over a long period of time, is indicative of ocular or neurologic disease or dysfunction. Evaluation of loss of vision must include a careful history. Questions should be asked regarding whether the visual loss was sudden or slowly progressive, or accompanied by other symptoms such as headache or diplopia. The physician should determine if there are underlying medical problems such as diabetes mellitus or hypertension, if the visual loss is permanent or intermittent or if there is a family history of ocular disease such as glaucoma, age-related macular degeneration, or cataract.

SUDDEN LOSS OF VISION

Definition

Sudden loss of vision is visual loss occurring over a period of seconds or minutes. It is an ophthalmic emergency that must be evaluated and treated within minutes of onset. Critical to the evaluation of sudden visual loss is the patient history. Acute, profound vision loss is usually caused by arteriolar occlusive disease of the retinal circulation. Intermittent sudden visual loss, amaurosis fugax, may be due to cerebrovascular insufficiency, migraine, hyperviscosity states, systemic vasculitis, retinal venous occlusions, neurologic problems, and ocular toxicity.

Pathophysiologic Considerations (Table 20-1)

Sudden monocular visual loss, whether transient or permanent, is often caused by impairment of the ocular circulation. Conditions that disrupt the intraretinal or optic nerve circulation can profoundly and often irreversibly destroy vision. Often such visual loss is a manifestation of a systemic disease process such as

Table 20-1. Causes of Sudden Visual Loss

Retinal artery embolism
  Carotid atheroma
  Platelet thrombi
  Cholesterol

Vasculitis
  Giant cell arteritis
  Periarteritis nodosa
  Takayasu's disease

Ischemia
  Ischemic optic neuropathy
  Ophthalmic migraine
  Hypotension

Retinal venous occlusive disease
  Central retinal vein occlusion
  Branch retinal vein occlusion

Retinal hemorrhage
  Diabetes mellitus
  Thrombocytopenia

Vitreous hemorrhage
  Vitreous separation with avulsion of retinal vessel
  Diabetes mellitus
  Sickle-cell disease
  Anemias

Optic neuropathy
  Demyelinating diseases
  Ischemia
  Vasculitis

embolization of the intraretinal circulation from cardiac or vascular plaques. The retina and the optic nerve are particularly sensitive to any disruption of their normal blood flow. The inner retinal layers are vascularized primarily by the central retinal artery and its branch arterioles, while the outer layers, including the photoreceptors, depend on the choroidal circulation. The optic nerve receives its blood supply from branches of the central retinal artery and from the pial plexus and distally is also vascularized by the ciliary circulation. Intermittent visual loss may be caused by transient vasoconstriction, as in the case of ophthalmic migraine; cerebrovascular insufficiency, as in the case of occlusive carotid artery disease or mitral valve prolapse; disorders of the blood, such as anemia and sickle-cell disease; and, finally, by generalized hyper- or hypotension. Impairment of optic nerve function as seen with multiple sclerosis and other demyelinating processes may also cause transient, and often profound, monocular visual loss.

Differential Diagnosis

Profound sudden visual loss must be considered as resulting from occlusion of the central retinal artery until proven otherwise. Occlusion of the central retinal artery may be caused by emboli or may be the result of a vasculitis, as seen in giant cell arteritis (temporal arteritis). In these cases, visual acuity may be reduced to mere light perception or worse. All or part of the visual field may be involved. If the visual loss is less sudden and the visual loss less pronounced, venous occlusive disease should be considered. In older patients, hypertension and atherosclerosis are prominent contributors to the development of retinal venous occlusions, whereas in younger people primary inflammation of the venules may be a precipitating cause.

Damage to the optic nerve, whether on an ischemic or inflammatory basis, can cause acute visual loss. Ischemic optic neuropathy is a common complication of atherosclerosis, diabetes mellitus, and giant cell arteritis. Demyelinating diseases can on rare occasions be complicated by sudden and profound vision loss.

A large or total retinal detachment can cause acute loss of vision and should be suspected in patients with high myopia or history of antecedent ocular trauma.

A vitreous hemorrhage complicating underlying diabetic or sickle cell retinopathy or caused by a vitreous detachment with avulsion of a retinal vessel may be another cause of visual loss. Less commonly, transient vasoconstriction caused by ophthalmic migraine (with or without accompanying cephalalgia) can cause sudden visual loss that only rarely is permanent.

Diagnostic Evaluation

Sudden loss of vision is an ophthalmic emergency. If the visual loss occurs over a matter of seconds and the visual loss is profound, i.e., entails loss of light perception, ischemia of the retina or optic nerve should be suspected. Once the visual acuity has been evaluated, confrontation visual fields should be performed on each eye. Examination of the pupils will often reveal anisocoria and afferent pupillary defects complicating retinal artery occlusions and optic neuropathies. Occlusion of the central retinal artery causes generalized edema of the nerve fiber layer. The characteristic cherry-red spot that can be seen with the ophthalmoscope is caused by the lack of edematous nerve fibers in the area immediately overlying the macula. Often, optic nerve swelling and narrowing of the retinal arterioles can also be discerned.

Arterial emboli of the retinal circulation are characteristic. Cholesterol emboli are often mobile and appear yellowish and highly refractile. Calcium fragments are usually off-white, whereas platelet thrombi may be virtually transparent or dull white.

Ischemic damage to the optic nerve may be more difficult to appreciate ophthalmoscopically, but often swelling or hyperemia of the disk can be demonstrated. Atrophic changes of the optic nerve head such as pallor or optic atrophy manifest themselves much later.

Cloudy media may suggest a vitreous hemorrhage.

Retinal detachments, when large and bullous, are easy to identify but may be obscured by overlying vitreous hemorrhage.

Treatment of arteriolar occlusions is effective when instituted before development of irremediable ischemia of the retina. Retinal damage from ischemia develops as early as 9 minutes following onset, but therapeutic intervention within up to 45 minutes may salvage some vision. The immediate goals of treatment are to reduce intraocular pressure in order to enhance arteriolar perfusion and to dislodge the embolus distally in the retinal circulation. If a central retinal artery occlusion is suspected and immediate referral to an ophthalmologist is not possible, the patient should be treated with ocular massage (to reduce intraocular pressure) and inhalation therapy with 5% carbon dioxide (to promote vasodilatation). When giant cell arteritis is suspected, a systemic workup including sedimentation rate is mandatory. The prompt administration of high-dose corticosteroids, while rarely restoring lost vision, may preserve what vision remains and protect the other eye.

Examination of the retina may also reveal the presence of retinal hemorrhage and edema characteristic of venous occlusions. While a central retinal vein occlusion with massive retinal hemorrhage and edema causes severe visual loss, branch vein occlusions with far more subtle findings can also cause severe visual impairment if the macula is involved.

RAPIDLY PROGRESSIVE LOSS OF VISION

Definition

Rapidly progressive loss of vision is visual loss occurring over a period of hours or days. Many of the entities discussed as causes of sudden visual loss may also cause less abrupt changes in vision if the ischemic or inflammatory processes in question are incomplete or more slowly progressive.

Pathophysiologic Considerations and Differential Diagnosis (Table 20–2)

Whereas sudden visual loss is usually caused by conditions that disrupt circulation to the retina or optic nerve, a variety of ocular disorders can cause less abrupt loss of vision. Infection and edema of the cornea may severely compromise vision. The cornea is normally maintained in a state of relative dehydration, which ensures clarity of vision, and any condition that compromises the integrity of the corneal epithelium or endothelium may cause corneal clouding. Such corneal decompensation is often seen following anterior segment trauma or surgery. Corneal infections and ulcers caused by bacterial, fungal, or viral organisms may

Table 20–2. Causes of Rapidly Progressive Loss of Visual Acuity

Corneal diseases
    Corneal infection or ulceration
    Corneal edema

Anterior chamber diseases
    Acute angle closure glaucoma
    Anterior uveitis

Vitreous disorders
    Hemorrhage
    Posterior uveitis

Retinal diseases
    Retinal detachment
    Macular hemorrhage and neovascularization
    Posterior uveitis and retinochoroiditis

Optic nerve diseases
    Ischemia
    Inflammation
    Toxicity
    Severe papilledema

damage the corneal epithelium and stroma. Some diseases such as herpetic keratitis and herpes zoster ophthalmicus are accompanied by uveitis, which can compromise the corneal endothelium as well. Corneal edema may also be caused by acute angle closure glaucoma, which will be discussed separately.

Severe uveitis may cause deposition of precipitates on the corneal endothelium and lens but may also involve the posterior structures of the eye. Posterior uveitis caused by Toxoplasma gondii or sarcoidosis, for example, may cloud the vitreous and damage the retina and choroid, a process that can severely affect vision.

Retinal detachment may cause sudden visual loss but more commonly progresses more slowly. Critical not only to management but also to prognosis is involvement of the macula in the detachment. Macular detachment causes severe loss of vision and compromises functional visual recovery even after successful surgery for retinal detachment.

Disruption of normal macular function is a common complication of age-related macular degeneration and retinal vascular diseases such as diabetes mellitus. In some patients with macular degeneration, subretinal neovascularization may cause rapidly progressive visual loss. Prompt recognition of this condition may make treatment with photocoagulation feasible in selected cases. Diabetic patients with long-standing disease may suffer rapidly progressive visual loss from hemorrhage, tractional detachment of the macula, or severe macular edema.

Inflammation, toxicity, and ischemia of the optic nerve may also cause rapidly progressive visual loss, as discussed above.

SLOWLY PROGRESSIVE LOSS OF VISION

Definition

Slowly progressive loss of vision may be defined as visual loss occurring over a period of months or years.

Pathophysiologic Considerations and Differential Diagnosis (Table 20–3)

Slowly progressive degeneration or disease of any part of the eye may cause slowly progressive loss of vision. Among adults, cataract, age-related macular degeneration, chronic open angle glaucoma, and complications of diabetes mellitus are frequent causes of reduced visual acuity. These important conditions will be discussed separately.

Opacifications of the cornea occur as the result of a number of hereditary dystrophies. More commonly, chronic epithelial changes occurring as a result of dry eye (Sjögren's syndrome) can gradually reduce vision.

Although age-related macular degeneration and diabetes mellitus cause the majority of slowly progressive visual loss of retinal origin, hereditary and acquired tapetoretinal degenerations may also cause visual loss. Retinitis pigmentosa and many other rare retinal and choroidal hereditary degenerations may cause gradual visual loss. More commonly, normal retinal function is adversely affected by a variety of drugs such as chloroquine and phenothiazines.

Abnormalities of the optic nerve, especially optic nerve compression, are an important cause for slowly progressive visual loss. The presence of functional pupillary abnormalities, changes in the visual field, and pallor or atrophy of the optic disk all suggest optic nerve compression when occurring over a prolonged period of time.

Table 20–3. Causes of Slowly Progressive Loss of Vision

Corneal diseases
    Hereditary corneal dystrophies
    Keratitis sicca

Chronic open angle glaucoma

Cataract

Retinal diseases
    Age-related macular degeneration
    Diabetic retinopathy
    Toxic retinopathies
    Hereditary tapetoretinal degenerations

RED EYE

DEFINITION

Red eye is a common ocular sign. It may be an isolated finding or may be accompanied by pain, discharge, and loss of visual acuity. Red eye is caused by hyperemia of the external ocular structures, specifically the conjunctiva, episclera, and sclera, or by subconjunctival hemorrhage.

PATHOPHYSIOLOGIC CONSIDERATIONS

Red eye is an extremely common manifestation of eye disease. In the majority of cases, mild allergies, nonspecific inflammation, and conjunctival infection are the underlying causes. For this reason it is easy for the physician to overlook more serious problems. Depending on the underlying cause, different patterns of conjunctival and episcleral vascular injection can be seen. If only the branches of the anterior ciliary circulation are involved, ciliary or limbal flush occurs. In this situation, redness is confined to the limbal area, that is, the area where the cornea meets the sclera. Such ciliary injection is usually accompanied by varying degrees of ocular pain, visual disturbances, and photophobia and is usually a sign of extraocular inflammation (episcleritis or scleritis), intraocular inflammation (uveitis), or corneal disease. Red eye caused by diffuse hyperemia of the more superficial conjunctival vessels is usually a manifestation of conjunctival inflammation or infection, i.e., conjunctivitis. Although the conjunctiva may be quite inflamed, other ocular structures are usually not involved and visual acuity remains normal. It should be remembered, however, that viral and bacterial infections of the conjunctivae may progress to involve the cornea as well, in which case the visual acuity may be adversely affected.

Differential Diagnosis (Table 20–4)

Subconjunctival hemorrhages appear as localized or diffuse, intensely red areas, vascular detail often being obscured. They usually occur unilaterally and spontaneously, often after coughing or vomiting. Hemorrhages may also complicate thrombocytopenia or anticoagulant therapy. Patients with hypertension often have recurrent hemorrhages. Some types of bacterial and viral conjunctivitis may have associated subconjunctival hemorrhages.

Conjunctivitis can be caused by a wide variety of bacteria. In these cases the conjunctival injection is often accompanied by mucopurulent discharge. Common gram-positive organisms are species of staphylococcus and pneumococcus, whereas hemophilus species are the most common gram-negative bacteria. Diphtheroids and streptococcus species may cause pseudomembranous conjunctivitis. Gonococcal conjunctivitis is characterized by the production of copious amounts of greenish discharge and severe periocular swelling. Because of the risk of corneal involvement in these cases, prompt diagnosis and treatment is essential.

Nonbacterial conjunctivitis can be caused by infection of the conjunctivae by viruses, fungi, parasites, and rickettsial and chlamydial organisms. Epidemic keratoconjunctivitis (EKC) is a highly contagious form of conjunctivitis caused by adenovirus species. Another common form of nonbacterial conjunctivitis is inclusion conjunctivitis, so-called swimmers' eye, caused by chlamydial infection. Another chlamydial infection of great importance is trachoma, which initially presents as a follicular conjunctivitis and, if left untreated, can cause severe, irremediable ocular damage.

The herpes simplex virus (HSV) can infect the eye and deserves special mention. Initially presenting as a painful, red-eye herpetic keratoconjunctivitis, HSV can cause severe corneal scarring. Inappropriate treatment of this disorder with topical corticosteroid preparations or a delay in instituting topical antiviral therapy can have disastrous results. Hence, topical corticosteroids should never be used in the treatment of red eye if the diagnosis is uncertain. Topical application of fluorescein to the cornea may reveal the typical dendritic ulcer. Decreased corneal sensitivity, photophobia, and severe pain characterize ocular HSV infection.

External ocular infections frequently complicate contact lens wear. Patients should always be asked if they use contact lenses. Amoebic keratoconjunctivitis is now recognized as a frequent complication of extended wearing of contact lenses.

Iritis or inflammation of the iris and anterior uveal tract is another cause of red eye. In the majority of cases there is no identifiable cause, and making the diagnosis may be extremely difficult without the aid of a slit lamp. In severe cases the pupil may be irregular and sluggishly reactive, and an inflammatory reaction in the anterior chamber may be noted. Iritis may complicate infections such as herpes zoster ophthalmicus, syphilis, and tuberculosis. Sarcoidosis and rheumatic disorders such as ankylosing spondylitis are sometimes complicated by iritis.

Table 20–4. Common Signs and Symptoms Associated with Red Eye

Condition	Pattern of Injection	Visual Acuity	Pain	Pupils	Discharge
Conjunctivitis	Superficial	Intact	Mild	Unaffected	Often purulent
Uveitis	Limbal and episcleral vessels	Reduced	Photophobia	Often poorly reactive	Tearing
Acute glaucoma	Limbal and episcleral vessels	Reduced	Severe	Fixed	Tearing
Subconjunctival hemorrhage	Diffuse redness	Intact	None	Unaffected	None

Episcleritis, or inflammation of the superficial scleral coat of the eye, may cause redness and localized tenderness but usually does not affect visual acuity. Episcleritis is usually a localized phenomenon, but many collagen vascular diseases such as rheumatoid arthritis, systemic lupus erythematosus, periarteritis nodosa, and inflammatory bowel disease may have episcleritis as an associated sign. Most cases of episcleritis are self-limited and responsive to topical corticosteroid therapy. Deeper inflammation of the sclera, scleritis, may complicate collagen diseases or may be associated with exogenous or endogenous infections. Scleritis may cause severe pain and can be sight-threatening if significant scleral thinning results.

EXOPHTHALMOS

DEFINITION

Exophthalmos refers to abnormal protuberance of one or both eyes. The term proptosis is sometimes used when the problem is unilateral. Exophthalmos is a common manifestation of orbital disease that may be due to an inflammatory process, mass lesion, or vascular abnormality. Although many types of instruments (exophthalmometers) are available to measure anterior displacement of the eye relative to the orbital rim, a simple method to detect exophthalmos is to view the eyes over the patient's brow from above and behind. An exophthalmometer should be used to quantify the degree of exophthalmos present, especially when comparative measurements will be taken.

PATHOPHYSIOLOGIC CONSIDERATIONS

Once the degree of exophthalmos has been determined, associated signs and symptoms should be noted. Of particular importance are visual acuity, extraocular movements, bruits, pulsations, and the degree of retropulsion. Visual acuity can be affected for several reasons. Pressure on or damage to the optic nerve by tumor or an inflammatory process can cause decreased vision as well as such other signs of optic nerve dysfunction as afferent pupillary defects and visual field defects. A mass behind the eye exerting pressure anteriorly can induce a significant amount of farsightedness, which may manifest itself as increasing difficulty with reading if the axial length of the eye is shortened sufficiently. Striations of the posterior pole, choroidal folds, can sometimes be seen with the ophthalmoscope in these situations.

Because the volume of the orbit is small and finite (roughly 25 to 30 cc), mass lesions and orbital inflammations can mechanically restrict the movement of the eye, as in the case of myositis seen in Graves' disease. Extraocular muscles can also be affected if the oculomotor, trochlear, or abducent nerves are damaged. Disease or injury to the orbital apex or superior orbital fissure may involve the trigeminal nerve as well, and hence corneal sensitivity should be tested. Abnormalities of venous drainage of the orbit such as carotid-cavernous sinus fistula can cause severe orbital congestion, engorgement of superficial vessels, and orbital bruits.

DIFFERENTIAL DIAGNOSIS

In adults the most common cause of unilateral and bilateral exophthalmos is thyroid disease. The infiltrative ophthalmopathy may be the only manifestation of Graves' disease but more commonly is associated with hyperthyroidism and thyroid gland hyperplasia. Up to 20% of patients may be euthyroid (ophthalmic Graves' disease). Edema and cellular infiltration by lymphocytes and other white blood cells can cause enlargement of the extraocular muscles, especially the inferior rectus muscle. In addition to exophthalmos, other im-

Table 20—5. Ophthalmic Signs and Symptoms in Graves' Disease (Werner Classification, 1969)

Class	
0	No signs or symptoms
1	Only signs, no symptoms (i.e., conjunctival redness or lid edema, retraction, or lag)
2	Soft tissue involvement with signs and symptoms
3	Proptosis
4	Extraocular muscle involvement
5	Corneal exposure changes
6	Optic nerve dysfunction (compression)

portant clinical features of ocular involvement in Graves' disease include lid retraction (which may simulate exophthalmos), lid lag, periorbital edema, and epibulbar injection. Severe orbital involvement can cause compression of the optic nerve, which can cause reduced vision and even blindness (Table 20–5).

Among adults a wide variety of tumors and inflammations as well as orbital trauma can cause exophthalmos (Table 20–6). In addition, thyroid disease and acute and chronic inflammations of the orbit are common causes of exophthalmos. Important among these is idiopathic orbital pseudotumor, a chronic nongranulomatous inflammation with highly variable histologic characteristics sometimes associated with abnormalities of immunoglobulins. This benign condition may present clinically like a neoplasm but can usually be managed by corticosteroid therapy.

Orbital cellulitis caused by bacterial infection is a common complication of trauma or of adjacent infection of the eyelids or ethmoid simuses. An especially virulent and dangerous acute suppurative cellulitis is that caused by phycomycosis (mucormycosis) in diabetic patients. Chronic granulomatous inflammations caused by tuberculosis, aspergillosis, and sarcoidosis may also be encountered.

A wide variety of neoplastic disorders can cause exophthalmos. Important among these are hemangioma, benign and malignant lymphoid tumors such as lymphoma and benign lymphoid hyperplasia, meningioma, and dermoid. Tumors of the lacrimal gland may also cause exophthalmos. Secondary tumors of the orbit may be metastatic or, more commonly, may be direct extensions of malignancies from the eye (melanoma), brain (meningioma), eyelids (basal cell car-

Table 20—6. Common Causes of Orbital Disease in Adults

Thyroid disease
Orbital cellulitis
Trauma
Inflammatory pseudotumor
Benign and malignant lymphoid tumors
Hemangioma
Secondary orbital tumors
Metastatic tumors

cinoma, squamous cell carcinoma), or sinuses (carcinoma). In adult males, prostate and lung cancer metastasize to the orbit, while among females, breast cancer is a more common source of orbital metastasis.

DIAGNOSTIC EVALUATION

Radiographic and ultrasonographic imaging techniques are of particular value in evaluating orbital disorders. Plain-film x-rays, when obtained in specific projections such as Caldwell's, Waters', base, optic nerve, and lateral views, can offer specific information regarding certain anatomic sites within the orbit, such as the superior orbital rim, the orbital floor, and the optic foramen. For evaluation of orbital soft tissue as well as bone imaging, techniques such as the CT scan, ultrasonography, and MRI, especially when used in conjunction, are extremely valuable in evaluating a broad range of orbital diseases and injuries.

GLAUCOMA

ACUTE ANGLE CLOSURE GLAUCOMA

Definition (Table 20–7)

Acute angle closure glaucoma is an uncommon form of glaucoma in which the intraocular pressure is rapidly elevated by obstruction of the normal outflow channels in the anterior chamber angle by the iris root.

Pathophysiologic Considerations

Aqueous humor is produced by the ciliary epithelium covering the ciliary body. The aqueous then courses through the pupil to be drained through the

Table 20—7. Classification of Glaucoma

Primary
  Open angle
    Ocular hypertension (elevated IOP without optic nerve or visual field changes)
    Open angle glaucoma
    Low-tension glaucoma (normal IOP with optic nerve and visual field changes)
  Angle closure

Secondary
  Trauma
  Inflammation
  Steroid therapy
  Postsurgical

trabecular meshwork, which is positioned just anterior to the iris root. In patients with narrow anterior chamber angles the iris root can be displaced anteriorly, blocking access to the trabecular meshwork and causing elevation of the intraocular pressure. In most cases the disease is caused by an inherited defect of the normal anatomic configuration of the anterior chamber angle. Attacks of angle closure glaucoma may be precipitated by dilation of the pupils. Patients who have narrow anterior chamber angles or who are highly hyperopic should have their pupils dilated only under supervision of an ophthalmologist.

Differential Diagnosis

Typically, angle closure glaucoma presents with severe pain and redness of the eye, often accompanied by nausea and reduced vision. The cornea eventually becomes hazy because of edema and the pupil may become immobile. Unlike other causes of red eye, acute glaucoma is accompanied by reduced vision, no significant discharge, a hard and tender eyeball, and a cloudy cornea.

Diagnostic Evaluation

Markedly increased intraocular pressure is the hallmark of angle closure glaucoma. Typically the intraocular pressure may be in excess of 50 mm Hg (normal range is 10 to 20 mm Hg). Intraocular pressure may be measured with a Schiotz tonometer. Other features of angle closure glaucoma include corneal clouding, shallowing of the anterior chamber, and immobility of the pupil.

OPEN ANGLE GLAUCOMA

Definition

Glaucoma may be defined as a chronic elevation of the intraocular pressure that results in damage to the optic nerve and retinal nerve fiber layer. Damage to the optic nerve may result in changes to the central and peripheral visual fields and may cause visual loss and eventual blindness if left untreated.

Pathophysiologic Considerations

Open angle glaucoma is caused by reduced outflow of aqueous humor. In contrast to angle closure glaucoma, the anterior chamber in open angle glaucoma is of normal depth and the anterior chamber angle is open. It is believed that reduction of outflow facility is caused by defects within the trabecular meshwork and drainage pathway.

Chronic elevation of intraocular pressure causes characteristic degeneration of the optic nerve (disk cupping). In most cases the onset and progression of the disease is insidious until large changes in the visual field become noticeable to the patient. Large fluctuations of intraocular pressure may, in some cases, cause headache and visual disturbances such as halos around bright lights. Open angle glaucoma is more common in patients with a positive family history, in patients over the age of 40, and among blacks.

Diagnostic Evaluation

Because of its insidious nature, open angle glaucoma is a serious public health hazard. The prevalence of the disease may be as high as 2% of the population over age 40. Intraocular pressures should be taken during any ophthalmic evaluation, and patients over the age of 40 should have their pressure measured yearly. As glaucoma frequently occurs at an earlier age in blacks, these patients should be encouraged to have the intraocular pressure checked routinely when in their thirties.

Not all patients with elevated intraocular pressure have glaucoma, and normal intraocular pressure does not guarantee that glaucoma cannot develop. The diagnosis of glaucoma is usually made on the basis of many pressure measurements, to account for diurnal variation of intraocular pressure, changes in the contour of the optic nerve head (disk cupping), and changes in the visual field as measured by perimetry.

CATARACT

DEFINITION

Cataract may be defined as an opacity of the lens. Most cataracts result in only partial opacification of the lens, usually involving the nucleus, cortex, or posterior subcapsular region singly or in combination. A total opacification of the lens is termed a mature cataract. Immature cataracts, when they reduce vision significantly, are removed routinely.

PATHOPHYSIOLOGIC CONSIDERATIONS
(Table 20–8)

Progressive changes within the lens contribute to the development of senile cataract. As it ages, the human lens gradually becomes more rigid, increases in size, and gradually accumulates pigment, a process called nuclear sclerosis. Such changes in the nucleus

Table 20—8. Classification of Cataract

Senile
Congenital
Developmental
Traumatic
Toxic
    Corticosteroids
    Electromagnetic radiation
Metabolic
    Diabetes
    Hypocalcemia
    Galactosemia
Secondary
    Glaucoma
    Uveitis
    Retinal detachment
    Ocular neoplasm

of the lens are a common cause of reduced vision in older patients. Cataracts may also develop in the cortical region of the lens and apear as wedge shaped opacities.

Cataracts can develop as complications of a variety of diseases, traumas, and toxic agents. Metabolic disorders such as diabetes mellitus, galactosemia, and hypocalcemia are often complicated by cataracts. Regional sensitivity of the lens to toxic agents is demonstrated by the typical posterior subcapsular cataracts that develop after prolonged corticosteroid use or as a complication of radiation therapy. Trauma to the eye may cause cataract, especially if the integrity of the lens capsule is compromised. Cataracts may also be complications of long-standing retinal detachment, uveitis, or intraocular neoplasm.

DIAGNOSTIC EVALUATION

Opacities of the lens can often be detected with the ophthalmoscope, but evaluation of the lens is best achieved with a slit lamp biomicroscope. Although a cataract may cause visual loss, other factors such as age-related macular degeneration may also contribute to the patient's visual difficulty.

AGE-RELATED MACULAR DEGENERATION

DEFINITION

Age-related macular degeneration (ARMD) is a progressive degenerative condition of the macula and un-

derlying retinal pigment epithelium that can result in loss of central visual acuity. In the U.S., ARMD is the most common cause of legal blindness in the over-65 age group.

PATHOPHYSIOLOGIC CONSIDERATIONS

Macular degeneration may be caused by progressive atrophy of the retina and underlying choriocapillaris or by degeneration of the pigment epithelium and associated membrane that can lead to the formation of subretinal fibrovascular membranes, profoundly affecting central vision. Most of the profound central visual loss in patients with ARMD is caused by these membranes and the hemorrhages that accompany them. In some cases subretinal membrane formation and neovascularization can be controlled with laser treatment. No treatment is available for the atrophic form of ARMD.

DIFFERENTIAL DIAGNOSIS

Macular function can be adversely affected by a variety of diseases. Because of the extreme functional importance of the macula, even a minute abnormality can have a profound effect on the central visual acuity.

Cystoid macular edema (CME) is caused by accumulation of fluid in the macula as a result of abnormal vascular permeability. This abnormal permeability may occur as a complication of intraocular surgery, especially cataract surgery. CME also can complicate retinal vascular disorders such as diabetes mellitus, venous occlusions, and severe hypertension.

Macular hemorrhage is a common complication of ARMD but is also seen in a variety of vascular and hematologic disorders. Even small hemorrhages can cause profound visual loss if they involve the fovea centralis.

The macula may also be damaged by infections such as toxoplasmosis and histoplasmosis, both of which commonly involve the posterior pole of the eye. Chronic posterior uveitis may be complicated by macular dysfunction.

DIAGNOSTIC EVALUATION

Macular function can be assessed in a number of ways, including measurement of visual acuity, evaluation of the central visual field, and color vision testing. Patients with macular disease frequently complain of distorted central acuity, metamorphopsia, or central scotoma. The detection of entoptic phenomena and two-point discrimination may also be useful in evaluating macular function.

The macular microcirculation is best evaluated using fluorescein angiography of the fundus. The presence of macular edema and neovascular membranes (which may be amenable to treatment) can be detected using this technique.

SWOLLEN OPTIC NERVE HEAD

DEFINITION

Swelling of the optic nerve head is an important clinical sign that may be seen in a wide variety of ocular, neurologic, and systemic conditions. Swelling may be caused by anatomic variations, ischemia, inflammation, infiltration, or intracranial pressure changes.

PATHOPHYSIOLOGIC CONSIDERATIONS AND DIFFERENTIAL DIAGNOSIS (Table 20–9)

Disk swelling that is caused by elevations of the intracranial pressure is known as papilledema. Both obstruction of normal axoplasmic flow and stagnation of normal venous return have been implicated as possible causes of papilledema.

The optic nerve may become swollen as a result of inflammation or ischemia. Localized inflammation of the optic nerve head may be caused by demyelinating disease or posterior uveitis or may be idiopathic. Visual acuity is usually affected. In older patients or those with vascular disease such as diabetes or hypertension, ischemia or infarction of the optic nerve head may cause swelling.

The optic nerve may be the site of leukemic, lymphomatous, or metastatic infiltrates. Orbital tumors such as optic nerve glioma or nerve sheath meningioma may cause disk swelling.

DIAGNOSTIC EVALUATION

Papilledema is usually characterized by bilateral, although often asymmetrical, optic disk swelling. Visual acuity is normal and the visual fields full, although enlargement of the blind spots may be present. In contrast, most ischemic, inflammatory, infiltrative, and toxic causes of optic disk swelling cause visual loss with associated visual field defects and signs of optic nerve dysfunction such as afferent pupillary defects.

In addition to measurement of visual acuity and visual fields, evidence for additional neurologic dysfunction should be sought, specifically external ophthalmoplegia and pupillary abnormalities. If an orbital or infiltrative process is suspected, orbital ultrasonography, CT scan, and MRI may be useful.

DIABETIC RETINOPATHY

DEFINITION

Diabetic retinopathy is the most common cause of retinal vascular disease, and its prevalence is a function of the duration of illness. In the U.S., diabetic eye complications are the most common cause of legal blindness in patients under the age of 65. By convention, diabetic retinopathy is classified as being either background or proliferative, depending on the degree and nature of the retinal vascular changes.

PATHOPHYSIOLOGIC CONSIDERATIONS

The earliest manifestations of diabetic retinopathy are venous dilation and the appearance of small microaneurysms. These findings are often accompanied by small intraretinal hemorrhages and hard exudates. As the damage to the retinal capillaries progresses, further leakage and exudation can be appreciated. Eventually, areas of capillary closure and nonperfusion develop, leading to retinal ischemia. It is important to recognize this ischemic, preproliferative phase because it sets the stage for neovascularization, which preceded fibrovascular proliferation and vitreous hemorrhage. Signs of ischemia include venous beading, soft exudates, which are microinfarctions of the nerve fiber layer, and intraretinal microvascular abnormalities.

The proliferation of new blood vessels at the optic disk and elsewhere in the retina is an ominous development. The neovascular vessels leak and are prone to cause hemorrhages that, depending on their extent, can dramatically reduce vision. The associated fibrovascular proliferation that accompanies neovascularization and hemorrhage can cause destructive tractional retinal detachments.

Severe visual loss can also occur in patients without significant proliferative retinopathy if they develop macular edema. Macular edema and exudative maculopathy is a common complication of background retinopathy in patients with type II diabetes mellitus.

Table 20–9. Causes of Optic Disk Swelling

Developmental and congenital
  Farsightedness (hyperopia)
  Hyaline bodies of nerve head
  Myelinated nerve fibers

Elevated intracranial pressure
  Intracranial neoplasm
  Cerebral hemorrhage
  Encephalitis/meningitis
  Pseudotumor cerebri
  Trauma

Optic nerve disease
  Inflammatory
    Optic neuritis
    Retinochoroiditis
  Neoplasia
    Primary
      Glioma
      Hemangioma
    Metastatic/infiltrative
  Vascular
    Ischemic optic neuropathy
    Retinal vein occlusion
    Giant cell arteritis

Intraocular disease
  Uveitis
  Low intraocular pressure (post-traumatic/postsurgical)

Orbital disease
  Neoplasm
  Thyroid eye disease
  Inflammation
    Orbital pseudotumor
    Orbital cellulitis

Systemic disease
  Diabetes
  Hypertension
  Blood dyscrasias
  Collagen diseases
  Toxic
    Corticosteroids
    Carbon monoxide
    Lead
    Methanol

DIAGNOSTIC EVALUATION

Because of the progressive nature of diabetic retinopathy, patients should be followed closely. The development of macular edema and diabetic retinopathy are dependent on the duration of the diabetes in both adult-onset and juvenile-onset disease. For this reason, the longer the patients have the disease, the more carefully they should be followed. With few exceptions, proliferative retinopathy is uncommon within the first 10 years in juvenile-onset disease and 8 years in adult-onset patients.

Timely panretinal photocoagulation, which destroys the ischemic retinal foci, has been shown to be an effective treatment of proliferative diabetic retinopa-thy. The presence of disk neovascularization or of hemorrhage with neovascularization elsewhere in the retina is a prominent risk factor. Prompt referral to a retinal specialist of patients with preproliferative or proliferative diabetic retinopathy is recommended.

ANISOCORIA

DEFINITION

Anisocoria is an asymmetry in the size of the pupils and is often an important sign of pupillary and neurologic dysfunction. Up to 20% of the normal population may have some degree of anisocoria.

PATHOPHYSIOLOGIC CONSIDERATIONS

Pathologic anisocoria may be caused by unilateral miosis, mydriasis, or pupillary immobility. Miosis may be caused by the topical application of parasympathomimetic agents such as pilocarpine, a drug often used in the treatment of glaucoma. Disruption of the sympathetic nervous system is an important cause of miosis. Miosis accompanied by ptosis, enophthalmos, and anhidrosis, known as Horner's syndrome, may be congenital or acquired. In the congenital form, heterochromia is often an associated finding. Acquired Horner's syndrome may be caused by lesions to the pre- and postganglionic fibers of the sympathetic tracts.

Unilateral mydriasis may be caused by the intentional or inadvertent use of topical parasympatholytic agents such as atropine, or by the use of sympathomimetic drugs such as phenylephrine or cocaine. Damage to the oculomotor nerve (CNIII) as the result of elevated intracranial pressure is an important cause of anisocoria, which often precedes more generalized external ophthalmoplegia. A fixed and dilated pupil is sometimes encountered in diabetic patients and in those with optic neuropathy.

Another important cause of a unilaterally fixed and dilated pupil is the tonic pupil, which when accompanied by diminished patellar reflexes is known as Adie's syndrome. This condition, thought to be due to dysfunction of the ciliary ganglion, is most commonly seen in young adult women. Although the pupil reacts poorly to light, some accommodative response is usually present. Pharmacologic tests can facilitate diagnosis.

DIAGNOSTIC EVALUATION

If the anisocoria is greater in low light than in bright light, unilateral miosis is present. The diagnosis of Horner's syndrome can usually be made on the basis of associated signs such as ptosis, enophthalmos, and anhidrosis. If the diagnosis remains in doubt, topical application of 4% cocaine solution will cause dilation of a normal pupil but will fail to dilate a pupil with a lesion to the sympathetic tract. In order to distinguish between a pre- and postganglionic lesion, a 1% solution of hydroxyamphetamine is applied (at least 12 hours after the use of topical cocaine). Hydroxyamphetamine does not directly affect the adrenergic receptors, and the pupil will dilate only when the postganglionic fibers are intact. A common cause of central Horner's syndrome is intrathoracic tumor.

If the anisocoria is more pronounced in bright light, the differential diagnosis includes paralytic mydriasis, tonic pupil, or internal ophthalmoplegia. The tonic pupil will constrict, albeit slowly, during accommodation and will usually manifest marked hypersensitivity to parasympathomimetic agents such as ⅛% pilocarpine. Light-near dissociation, which is a feature of the dilated tonic pupil, is also a feature of the miotic Argyll Robertson pupil. In these cases, the light reflex is diminished while the accommodative reflex remains intact. Although light-near dissociation with a miotic pupil is the hallmark of syphilis, a wide variety of neurologic conditions such as multiple sclerosis can cause it.

GENERAL REFERENCES

LOSS OF VISION

Liversedge, C.A., and Smith, V.H.: Neuromedical and ophthalmic aspects of central retinal artery occlusion. Trans Ophthalmol Soc UK 82:571, 1982.

Henkind, P., and Gold, D.H.: Ocular manifestations of rheumatologic disorders. Rheumatology 4:13, 1973.

Mancall, I.T.: Occlusion of the central retinal vein. Arch Ophthalmol 46:675, 1951.

RED EYE

Havener, W.H.: Synopsis of Ophthalmology. St. Louis, C.V. Mosby, 1979, pp 358–384.

Thygeson, P., and Kimura, S.J.: The cytology of external ocular disease. Am J Ophthalmol 39:137, 1955.

Patterson, A., and Jones, B.R.: Management of ocular herpes. Trans Ophthalmol Soc UK 87:59, 1967.

Oh, J.O. (ed.): Herpes virus infections. Surv Ophthalmol 21:81, 1976.

EXOPHTHALMOS

Grove, A.S.: Evaluation of exophthalmos. N Engl J Med 292:1005, 1975.

Henderson, J.W., and Farrow, G.M.: Summary of 465 consecutive orbital tumors. In Orbital Tumors. Edited by J.W. Henderson. Philadelphia, W.B. Saunders, 1973.

Werner, S.C.: Orbital changes in Graves's disease. In Clinical Ophthalmology. Vol. 2. Edited by T.D. Duane. Philadelphia, Harper and Row, 1983.

ACUTE ANGLE CLOSURE GLAUCOMA

Duane, T.D. (ed.): Clinical Ophthalmology. Vol. 3. Hagerstown, MD, Harper and Row, 1981, chapter 52, pp 1–45.

Kirsch, R.E., and Anderson, D.R.: Clinical recognition of glaucoma cupping. Am J Ophthalmol 75:442, 1973.

Kolker, A.E., and Hetherington, J.J. (eds.): Becker-Shaffer's Diagnosis and Therapy of the Glaucomas. 4th ed. St. Louis, C.V. Mosby, 1976.

Simmons, R.J., and Dallow, R.L.: Primary angle closure glaucoma. In Clinical Ophthalmology. Vol. 3. Edited by T.D. Duane. Hagerstown, Md., Harper & Row, 1986, pp 1–31.

OPEN ANGLE GLAUCOMA

Moses, R.A.: Intraocular pressure. In Adler's Pathology of the Eye. 6th Ed. Edited by R.A. Moses. St. Louis, C.V. Mosby, 1975, p. 179.

Schwartz, B.: Primary open angle glaucoma. In Clinical Ophthalmology. Vol. 3. Edited by T.D. Duane. Hagerstown, Md., Harper & Row, 1986.

CATARACT

Jaffe, N.S.: Cataract Surgery and its Complications. 4th edition. St. Louis, C.V. Mosby, 1984.

Kinoshita, J.H., Kador, P., and Catiles, M.: Aldose reductase in diabetic cataracts. JAMA 246:257, 1981.

AGE-RELATED MACULAR DEGENERATION

Maumenee, A.E., and Emory, J.M.: An anatomic classification of diseases of the macula. Am J Ophthalmol 74:594, 1972.

Gass, J.D.M.: Drusen and disciform macular detachment. Arch Ophthalmol 90:206, 1973.

SWOLLEN OPTIC NERVE HEAD

Hedges, T.R.: Papilledema: Its recognition and relation to intracranial disease. Surv Ophthalmol 19:201, 1975.

Henkind, P., Charles, N., and Pearson, J.: Histopathology of ischemic neuropathy. Am J Ophthalmol 69:78, 1970.

DIABETIC RETINOPATHY

Davis, M.D., et al.: Natural evolution. In Current Diagnosis and Management of Chorioretinal Diseases. Edited by F.A. L'Esperance. St. Louis, C.V. Mosby, 1977, p. 192.

The Diabetic Retinopathy Study Research Group: Photocoagulation treatment of proliferative retinopathy: Clinical application of DRS findings. Ophthalmology 88:583–600, 1981.

L'Esperance, F.A., and James, W.A., Jr.: Diabetic Retinopathy: Clinical Evaluation and Management. St. Louis, C.V. Mosby, 1981.

ANISOCORIA

Thompson, H.S., and Pihey, S.F.J.: Unequal pupils. A flow chart for sorting out the anisocorias. Surv Ophthalmol 21:45–48, 1976.

CHAPTER 21

EAR, NOSE, THROAT, AND NECK PROBLEMS

Robert W. Selfe, Jr., M.D.

Disease of the head and neck lends itself to clinical diagnosis by the internist because most of the sources of disorder are accessible to physical examination. Only the paranasal sinuses, inner ear, esophagus, and soft tissues of the neck cannot be directly evaluated by a physical examination. Expertise in physical examination of the head and neck varies among physicians and among specialists. No distinction will be made in this discussion regarding who should perform various aspects of the physical examination of the head and neck or when special referral should be considered.

EARACHE (OTALGIA)

DEFINITION

Earache is defined as pain that a patient describes as being in or around the ear.

PATHOPHYSIOLOGIC CONSIDERATIONS AND DIFFERENTIAL DIAGNOSIS

The three general sources of otalgia are the external ear, the middle ear, and referred pain. The fact that many cranial nerves contribute to the sensory supply of the middle and external ear and that several muscle groups are attached to the temporal bone make referred pain a difficult diagnostic challenge.

A number of disease processes produce earache. Table 21–1 shows the most common causes of earache according to the site of the disorder.

DIAGNOSTIC EVALUATION

The patient history should be very specific; the patient should be asked to carefully describe the location and character of the pain.

In the physical examination, the physician should be aware that rarely does a patient have otalgia from an external ear source when the external ear is normal on physical examination; that rarely does pain from the middle ear source occur in the setting of a normal eardrum; and that investigation of referred pain requires an extensive and complete head and neck examination.

Inspection and manipulation of the external ear (auricle and external ear canal) will reveal evidence of nearly all external ear sources of otalgia. Inspection of the eardrum including evaluation of the position and

Table 21–1. Causes of Earache

External ear
  Otitis externa
  Trauma, foreign body
  Impacted cerumen
  Dermatologic conditions of external ear canal
  Herpes zoster oticus
Middle ear
  Acute otitis media
  Serous otitis media
  Barotitis media
  Eustachian tube dysfunction
  Chronic otitis media with or without cholesteatoma
  Middle ear tumor, glomus, etc.
Referred pain (Rule of T's)
  Tongue
  Teeth
  Temporomandibular joint
  Tonsil
  Tumor
    Oral cavity
    Pharynx
    Neck
  Thyroid
  Throat

mobility of the eardrum will reveal nearly all sources of middle ear otalgia. Investigation of a source of referred pain requires visualization of the mucosal surfaces of the oral cavity, pharynx, and larynx and vigorous palpation of the neck and oral cavity with special attention to the muscles of the temporomandibular joint and the stylohyoid complex. No specific laboratory studies will help explain otalgia not diagnosed on a physical exam. These cases will be considered for referral to a specialist (otorhinolaryngologist and/or neurologist).

DISCHARGE (OTORRHEA)

DEFINITION

Otorrhea is defined as any discharge from the external auditory meatus.

PATHOPHYSIOLOGIC CONSIDERATIONS AND DIFFERENTIAL DIAGNOSIS

Discharge from the external auditory meatus may consist of cerumen, blood, pus, or cerebrospinal fluid (CSF). The presence of any of these fluids may be indicative of a pathologic state (Table 21–2).

Table 21–2. Causes of Otorrhea

Cerumen
  Abnormal in volume or consistency
Blood
  Trauma to external canal skin
  Trauma to temporal bone and middle ear
  Trauma to tympanic membrane
  Tumor of external canal or middle ear
Pus
  Otitis externa
  Otitis media with perforation of tympanic membrane
  Mastoiditis with perforation of tympanic membrane
CSF
  Perforation of tympanic membrane and violation of
    the temporal bone and meninges secondary to
    trauma, cholesteatoma, or tumor

Table 21–3. Causes of Hearing Loss

External ear
  Cerumen
  Infection
  Foreign body
  Tumor
Middle ear
  Acute otitis media
  Chronic otitis media with or without cholesteatoma
  Serous otitis media, adhesive otitis media, eustachian tube dys-
    function
  Barotitis media
  Otosclerosis
  Congenital deformity of middle ear
  Trauma to eardrum or middle ear
  Tumor of middle ear
Inner ear
  Congenital
  Traumatic
    Temporal bone fracture
  Infection
    Mumps, measles, lues, etc.
  Degeneration
    Presbycuses
  Miscellaneous
    Meniere's disease
    Noise trauma
    Ototoxic trauma

DIAGNOSTIC EVALUATION

Inspection of the external ear canal and tympanic membrane will suggest most causes of otorrhea. It is very unusual to have middle ear disease and external ear disease at the same time. An intact tympanic membrane indicates that the discharge originated in the external canal and is secondary to a dermatologic condition of the external canal (such as otitis externa and eczematoid otitis externa); if the eardrum is not intact and has a tear or perforation, the discharge is most likely from the middle ear or mastoid system and usually represents either infection or tumor of the middle ear or mastoid. Clear watery discharge in the presence of a perforation of an eardrum should be investigated for the presence of CSF.

HEARING LOSS

DEFINITION

Hearing loss is defined as a change in the perception of sounds as determined by the patient.

PATHOPHYSIOLOGIC CONSIDERATIONS AND DIFFERENTIAL DIAGNOSIS

Hearing loss may be caused by a block in the transmission of sound to the tympanic membrane, a dysfunction of the transmission of sound by the middle ear system, or damage to the inner ear (cochlear hair cells or cochlear nerve).

Table 21–3 shows various causes of hearing loss on the basis of different pathophysiologic processes and the site of involvement.

DIAGNOSTIC EVALUATION

The patient history should include efforts to determine whether the loss is acute, chronic and stable, chronic and progressive, or fluctuating. The history should include any symptoms associated with hearing loss, such as tinnitus and vertigo.

The physical examination should be directed toward identifying external or middle ear sources of the symptom and evaluating the symmetry, nature (conductive versus sensorineural), and range of the loss (primary high frequency, primary low frequency, all frequencies). Physical examination of the external ear and the eardrum will reveal most of the causes of conductive hearing loss; otosclerosis and middle ear deformities may not be identified on physical exam. The inner ear can be examined only by laboratory investigations (such as audiogram and x-ray). In general, a bilateral symmetrical loss of hearing is less serious, less treatable, and less urgent than an asymmetrical loss, which may be treatable and may imply a serious pathologic disorder.

Aside from inspection of the external ear and eardrum, the best way to evaluate hearing in a clinical examination is with tuning forks that range from a frequency of 512 to 4098 Hz. With some practice in using Weber's test, the Rinne test, and the Schwabach test, the clinician can develop reasonable expertise in evaluating hearing. This kind of clinical evaluation will give significantly more information than the watch-tick or whisper tests, which are frequently misleading.

The initial physical examination either will reveal a treatable disease in the external or middle ear that should be treated prior to further investigation, or will suggest that physical structures are normal and will indicate further investigation of the hearing, involving a complete audiologic evaluation. Basic audiologic evaluation is designed to measure accurately the degree of hearing loss and the frequencies of loss. Basic audiology will also separate conductive hearing loss from sensorineural hearing loss and suggest whether the sensorineural hearing loss is cochlear or retrocochlear. The configuration of the loss may also suggest the cause.

Further investigation of hearing loss beyond basic audiology is usually reserved for cases that may represent serious or treatable disease. Further investigation may include brain stem–evoked audiometry, electronystagmography, and radiologic study of the temporal bone and cerebellar-pontine angle.

DIZZINESS

DEFINITION

Dizziness is not a clearly defined symptom; in general it refers to a patient's perceived abnormal relationship to his environment. Dizziness can be separated into three types of sensations—light-headedness, imbalance, and vertigo. Vertigo is defined as a patient's abnormal orientation to the environment, usually associated with a sensation of motion. (See Chapter 15.)

Table 21–4. Causes of Dizziness/Vertigo

Labyrinthitis
Vestibular neuronitis (epidemic labyrinthitis, infectious labyrinthitis)
Serous labyrinthitis
Circumscribed labyrinthitis
Purulent labyrinthitis
Meniere's disease
Trauma to inner ear
Round window rupture or fistula
Miscellaneous

PATHOPHYSIOLOGIC CONSIDERATIONS AND DIFFERENTIAL DIAGNOSIS (Table 21–4)

The labyrinthine portion of each inner ear responds to a change in physical position, primarily to a change in linear or rotational acceleration or deceleration. The two sides give equal and opposite responses to these position changes, and each side generates a constant "tonal discharge" when there is no position change. An imbalance between the two sides produces an abnormal sensation of position change (vertigo). The patient will usually describe a sensation of motion at rest (unbalanced "tonal" discharge) and an exaggerated sensation of motion, described as a spinning sensation, with position change. If loss of function of the labyrinth is symmetrical, the patient will describe a vague sense of inadequate information about the body position in relationship to the environment (imbalance).

DIAGNOSTIC EVALUATION

A meticulous patient history and description of the symptom is extremely important in the clinical investigation of a patient complaining of dizziness. The physician should request that the patient describe the symptom repeatedly to try to define the symptom. Classifying the patient's symptom as light-headedness, imbalance, or vertigo may be revealing; vertigo is frequently secondary to otologic disease, imbalance is sometimes secondary to otologic disease, and light-headedness is rarely secondary to otologic disease. The history should also determine any associated symptoms (e.g., otologic symptoms).

The clinical examination should include evaluation of the external and middle ear, although this investigation frequently proves normal. An abnormal external or middle ear may or may not be related to the patient's complaint of dizziness. The physical examination should include evaluation of the cochlear aspect of the inner ear (tuning fork test) and evaluation of indirect evidence of labyrinthine dysfunction (the presence or absence of nystagmus, with or without position change). All cranial nerves should be examined and cerebellar function should be evaluated. Associated ear symptoms or abnormal physical findings in the external or middle ear should lead to further otoneurologic evaluation. Lack of physical abnormality in the setting of a description of vertigo with or without nystagmus should lead to further otoneurologic investigation. Additional otologic investigation should include complete audiology, electronystagmography, and, possibly, radiologic studies and neurologic consultation.

TINNITUS

DEFINITION

Tinnitus is a sound perceived by the patient.

PATHOPHYSIOLOGIC CONSIDERATIONS AND DIFFERENTIAL DIAGNOSIS

Tinnitus is occasionally caused by abnormalities in the external or middle ear or is secondary to irritation of the external or middle ear. Tinnitus in most cases is secondary to damage to the hair cells of the cochlear nerve or the eighth cranial nerve.

All of the diseases listed under the differential diagnoses of ear pain, hearing loss, and dizziness can also be causes of tinnitus.

DIAGNOSTIC EVALUATION

Investigation of tinnitus will usually require a complete physical examination of the external ear and middle ear and audiologic studies. The primary purpose for investigating tinnitus is to rule out serious or treatable diseases. Tinnitus can rarely be treated unless it is secondary to ototoxic drug use or irritation to the middle or external ear. Almost all cases are secondary to damage to the hair cells in the cochlear nerve or to filaments of the eighth cranial nerve.

SORE THROAT

DEFINITION

Sore throat is a sensation of pain or discomfort located in the pharynx, frequently exaggerated by the act of swallowing.

PATHOPHYSIOLOGIC CONSIDERATIONS AND DIFFERENTIAL DIAGNOSIS (Table 21–5)

The pain is almost always secondary to some alteration of the mucosa (inflammation, irritation, ulceration, metabolic change, tumor, etc.). Occasionally the mucosa is normal and the pain is secondary to a neu-

Table 21–5. Causes of Sore Throat

Inflammation
  Pharyngitis
    Bacterial or viral
    Ulcerative (herpes angina)
    Fungal (thrush)
    Mononucleosis
  Tonsillitis
  Epiglottitis
  Abscess
    Peritonsillar
    Retropharyngeal
    Parapharyngeal
Irritation
  Smoking
  Inhaled irritants
  Mouth breathing
  Hiatal hernia reflex
  Abnormal drainage
    Dental
    Sinus infection
Neurologic
  Glossopharyngeal neuralgia
Tumor
  Benign or malignant tumor of oral cavity or pharynx
Miscellaneous
  Eagles syndrome
  Foreign body
  Stylohyoid syndrome

ralgia (glossopharyngeal neuralgia) or a musculoskeletal neuralgia (Eagles syndrome).

DIAGNOSTIC EVALUATION

Most acute inflammatory sources of sore throat can be determined by routine history and physical examination of the pharynx. It is helpful to have the patient point out the location of the pain; some sore throats are revealed to be neck pain. Throat culture, CBC, and heterophil testing may be helpful in determining therapy for pharyngitis.

Sore throats that are not secondary to acute or chronic pharyngitis require a more detailed history (including the location, type, and other characteristics of the pain) and a complete inspection of the entire oral cavity, nasopharynx, oropharynx, hypopharynx, and neck. This inspection may require endoscopy. X-rays are usually not helpful unless they are used to confirm a suspected diagnosis (such as elongated styloid process). Those patients not diagnosed should undergo repeated head and neck examinations if not responsive to management of symptoms.

DYSPHAGIA

DEFINITION

Dysphagia is a perceived or observed difficulty swallowing. (See Chapter 12.)

PATHOPHYSIOLOGIC CONSIDERATIONS AND DIFFERENTIAL DIAGNOSIS (Table 21–6)

The symptom may originate anywhere from the oral cavity to the stomach. The cause of the symptom is secondary to neuromuscular or intraluminal mechanical obstruction or is caused by extraluminal distortion of the upper digestive tract.

DIAGNOSTIC EVALUATION

The history and physical examination should include inspection of the hypopharynx and cranial nerves. If the diagnosis is not suggested by the history and physical examination, the physician should obtain an esophagogram. The radiologist should be advised that the study is being performed for a complaint of dysphagia and should pay special attention to the pharynx, cervical esophagus, and gastroesophageal junction. The choice of cinefluoroscopy or rapid sequence films can then be determined by the radiologist. Endoscopy with or without biopsy and manometric studies should follow the esophagogram, as indicated.

Table 21–6.   Causes of Dysphagia

Neuromuscular
  Cranial nerve palsies, brain stem dysfunction
  Achalasia
    Cricopharyngeal achalasia (with or without Zenker's diverticulum)
    Gastroesophageal
  Miscellaneous
    Muscular abnormalities
    Collagen vascular disease
    Scleroderma
Mechanical
  Intraluminal
  Tumor of oral cavity, pharynx, or esophagus
  Hypertrophy of Waldeyer's ring (tonsils and adenoids)
    Foreign body
    Congenital webs
    Traumatic stenosis
  Extraluminal
    Mediastinal mass, abnormal vasculature
    Parapharyngeal mass or abscess

HOARSENESS

DEFINITION

Hoarseness is an alteration in the voice as perceived by the patient.

PATHOPHYSIOLOGIC CONSIDERATIONS AND DIFFERENTIAL DIAGNOSIS (Table 21–7)

Hoarseness is caused by some change in the vocal cord mass (diffuse swelling or an isolated abnormality) or by a change in the neuromuscular function (palsy, cricoarytenoid dysfunction, pure muscular dysfunction).

DIAGNOSTIC EVALUATION

Hoarseness of more than 1 or 2 weeks' duration should be investigated by inspection of the vocal cords. Indirect, fiberoptic, or rigid direct laryngoscopy will be required, as indicated by the individual case. Further investigation will be directed by the findings on laryngoscopic examination.

Table 21–7.   Causes of Hoarseness

Altered vocal cord mass
  Diffuse
    Laryngitis
    Mixed edema, amyloidosis
  Isolated
    Polyps (nodules)
    Granuloma, fibroma
    Contact ulcer
    Tumor (benign of malignant)
Altered neuromuscular function
  Vocal cord palsy (recurrent and/or superior laryngeal nerve)
  Cricoarytenoid dysfunction
  Rheumatoid involvement
  Traumatic
  Traumatic laryngeal stenosis
  Myasthenia
    Specific (myasthenia gravis)
    Nonspecific secondary to general muscle weakness
  Atrophy

EPISTAXIS

DEFINITION

Epistaxis is a pure bloody discharge from the nasal cavity.

Table 21–8. Causes of Epistaxis

"Pure epistaxis" (bleeding from an isolated, exposed blood
  vessel with no associated illness as a contributing factor)
Clotting (bleeding disorder)
Trauma
Foreign body
Tumor

PATHOPHYSIOLOGIC CONSIDERATIONS AND DIFFERENTIAL DIAGNOSIS

The source of bleeding is usually an isolated, exposed, and ulcerated vessel or a mucosal abnormality (such as tumor or mucosal inflammation in association with a clotting abnormality) (Table 21–8).

DIAGNOSTIC EVALUATION

Of nosebleeds, 90% are pure epistaxis, and 90% of pure epistaxis nosebleeds are anterior nosebleeds. Pure epistaxis can almost always be diagnosed by inspection of the nasal cavity (in 80 to 90% of cases the bleeding site is the anterior nasal septum). Those cases not identified as pure epistaxis or diagnosed by initial inspection of the nasal cavity and nasopharynx (foreign body, tumor of nasal cavity, tumor of nasopharynx) will require a hematologic evaluation or radiologic evaluation (sinus x-rays, angiogram, CT scan).

NASAL OBSTRUCTION

DEFINITION

The patient describes obstruction of airflow through the nose.

PATHOPHYSIOLOGIC CONSIDERATIONS AND DIFFERENTIAL DIAGNOSIS (Table 21–9)

Obstruction to nasal airflow can be caused by abnormal anatomy (deviated nasal septum, choanal atresia, nasal fracture), mucosal edema (rhinitis), or abnormal mass (polyp, tumor, foreign body).

DIAGNOSTIC EVALUATION

Complete inspection of the nasal cavity will identify or exclude most causes of nasal obstruction except for chronic nonspecific rhinitis. Specific diagnosis of chronic nonspecific rhinitis can be very frustrating; the

Table 21–9. Causes of Nasal Obstruction

Abnormal anatomy
  Deviated nasal septum
  Nasal fracture
  Choanal stenosis—atresia
  Anterior valve dysfunction (usually traumatic or postsurgical)
Mucosal edema
  Rhinitis
    Infectious
    Allergic
    Vasomotor
  Mucosal disease—granulomatous (Wegener's granulomatosis, lethal midline granuloma)
  Mucosal—turbinate hypertrophy
Abnormal mass
  Polyps
  Foreign body
  Adenoid hypertrophy
  Tumor (benign or malignant)

investigation may include sinus x-rays, allergy evaluation, and mucosal biopsy.

NASAL DISCHARGE (RHINORRHEA)

DEFINITION

Rhinorrhea is defined as an abnormal discharge from the nasal cavity.

PATHOPHYSIOLOGIC CONSIDERATIONS AND DIFFERENTIAL DIAGNOSIS (Table 21–10)

Rhinorrhea can result from excessive production or diminished drainage of normal secretions. Watery rhinorrhea can represent a CSF fistula. Purulent rhinorrhea can result from an inflammation of the nasal cavity or sinuses. Bloody rhinorrhea (blood-tinged mucoid discharge) can be secondary to any of the causes of rhinorrhea but is more likely to represent a significant pathologic process.

DIAGNOSTIC EVALUATION

History and physical examination of the nasal cavity and nasopharynx will reveal the cause of 50 to 75% of cases of rhinorrhea. Those cases not diagnosed by the initial patient history and physical examination may require extensive investigation including analysis of

Table 21–10. Causes of Rhinorrhea

Clear mucoid
  Obstructive drainage
    Choanal atresia
    Tumor of nasal cavity, nasopharynx
    Decreased mucociliary flow (cystic fibrosis, sicca syndrome)
  Excess secretion
    Viral rhinitis
    Allergic rhinitis
    Vasomotor rhinitis
    Nonspecific rhinitis
Purulent
  Viral rhinitis
  Bacterial rhinitis, sinusitis
  Chronic rhinitis, granulomatous disease
  Foreign body
Watery
  CSF fistula
Bloody
  Tumor
    Nasal cavity
    Sinus
    Nasopharynx
  Chronic granulomatous disease of mucosa (lethal midline granuloma, Wegener's granulomatosis)

Table 21–11. Causes of Facial Pain

Sinus disease
  Acute
  Chronic
Dental disease
Headache
  Muscular
  Vascular (migraine, cluster)
Neuralgia
  Trigeminal
  Glossopharyngeal
  Tympanic
  Sphenopalatine
  Vidian
  Postherpetic
  Geniculate

the abnormal discharge (culture, chemical, microscopic), sinus x-rays, allergy evaluation, and mucosal biopsy. Of cases, 10 to 25% may not result in a specific diagnosis; symptoms should be treated and the entire investigation repeated, as indicated.

FACIAL PAIN

DEFINITION

Facial pain is pain perceived by the patient in the region of the face.

PATHOPHYSIOLOGIC CONSIDERATIONS AND DIFFERENTIAL DIAGNOSIS

Most all facial pain is mediated by the cranial nerves and is caused by an abnormality of the mucosa, muscle, vessels, or skeletal structure supplied by these nerves (Table 21–11).

DIAGNOSTIC EVALUATION

Facial pain associated with acute sinusitis can usually be suspected by the patient history (history of boring aching pain localized at a specific sinus, rarely symmetrical, associated with nasal symptoms, worse during daytime hours) and confirmed by examination (inflamed nasal mucosa, purulent discharge from meatus of involved sinus, and tenderness of involved sinus). Facial pain associated with chronic sinus disease, if isolated to a single sinus, can usually be diagnosed by patient history and physical examination. Facial pain associated with chronic pansinusitis may be more ill-defined, less localized, and more symmetrical and may have diffuse nonspecific intranasal mucosal abnormalities. Meticulous evaluation of the middle meatus may suggest sinus disease. Sinus x-rays are required in these cases. CT scan may be helpful in cases with subtle physical findings and nonspecific plain x-ray findings. Facial pain associated with a normal intranasal exam and normal sinus x-ray is very rarely related to nasal or sinus disease. If sinus disease is unlikely, facial pain should be evaluated from a neurologic or dental perspective.

NECK MASS

DEFINITION

There is no good definition of an abnormal neck mass because a neck mass is abnormal only as it relates to the experience of the examiner. Some neck masses defined as abnormal by the patient are normal anatomy to the examining physician. In general, a mass that is 2 cm in size and does not represent a variation of normal anatomy requires diagnostic evaluation.

Table 21–12. Causes of Neck Mass

Congenital
  Cyst
    Thyroglossal duct cyst
    Branchial cleft cyst
    Dermoid cyst
  Vascular
    Hemangioma
    Lymphangioma
Infectious
  Cervical adenitis (acute or chronic)
  Neck abscess
  Sialadenitis (parotid, submaxillary)
  Thyroiditis
Tumor
  Benign
    Thyroid
    Parotid
    Submaxillary
    Mesenchymal
      Chordoma
      Neurogenic
      Muscular
      Lipoma
      Paraganglioma
  Malignant
    Primary
      Thyroid
      Parotid
      Submaxillary gland
      Mesenchymal
      Lymphoma
    Secondary
      Metastasis to cervical nodes from head
        and neck primary or from other pri-
        mary tumors

PATHOPHYSIOLOGIC CONSIDERATIONS AND DIFFERENTIAL DIAGNOSIS (Table 21–12)

A mass can be the result of a congenital anomaly (cyst, vascular anomaly), an infection involving a glandular or lymphatic structure in the neck, or a tumor involving a glandular, lymphatic, or soft-tissue structure of the neck.

DIAGNOSTIC EVALUATION

A neck mass should be characterized according to its location, consistency, symptoms, and history. The mass should be localized to a geographic position in the neck (e.g., anterior versus lateral neck; anterior, deep, or posterior to sternocleidomastoid muscle; above or below hyoid) and localized as it relates to other palpable structures in the neck (adherent to or adjacent to a glandular structure). Its consistency should be defined as cystic, soft, hard, mobile, immobile, or multinodular. Symptoms that may be di-

rectly related to the mass include pain, tenderness, or dysfunction of associated structures (cranial nerve palsy, limited mobility of local structures); associated symptoms are primarily those symptoms related to the mouth, pharynx, larynx, nose, or ears. The history should include the duration of the mass and any change or fluctuation over time.

After adequate preliminary evaluation and classification of the mass is completed, some presumptive diagnoses can be considered. In cases in which adenopathy is a part of the presumptive diagnosis, the next step should be complete visualization of the mucosal surface of the upper aerodigestive tract for possible primary infectious or primary tumor sources of secondary disease in the neck. This visualization may require endoscopy and may include random biopsies. In cases in which adenopathy is not a part of the differential diagnosis, a complete visualization of the upper aerodigestive tract may still be indicated to search for possible occult abnormalities of the neck mass. Those cases with a strong presumptive diagnosis of conditions related to glandular or mesenchymal structures in the neck will require further radiologic studies (thyroid scan, sonogram, CT scan, angiogram, MRI) as indicated.

All cases that are not adequately explained by the investigations above require histologic diagnosis. Fine-needle aspiration cytology is a useful step and when diagnostic tissue is obtained has a 90% accuracy rate. Fine-needle aspiration can be helpful in planning therapy but is required if radical therapy is planned. Histologic confirmation should be considered if conservative management is planned (followed with repeated examination and thyroid suppression therapy).

GENERAL REFERENCES

Ballenger, J.J.: Diseases of the Nose, Throat, Ear, Head and Neck. 13th Ed. Philadelphia, Lea & Febiger, 1985.
Batsakis, J.G.: Tumors of the Head and Neck. 2nd Ed. Baltimore, Williams & Wilkins Co., 1979.
DeWeese, D.D., and Saunders, W.H.: Textbook of Otolaryngology. 6th Ed. St. Louis, The C.V. Mosby Co., 1982.
Goodhill, V.: Ear-Diseases, Deafness and Dizziness. Hagerstown, Harper & Row, 1979.
Hughes, G.B.: Textbook of Clinical Otology. New York, Thieme-Stratton, 1985.
Lee, K.J.: Differential Diagnosis—Otolaryngology. New York, Arco Publishing Co., 1978.
Paparella, M.M., and Shumrick, D.A.: Otolaryngology. 2nd Ed. Vols. 1, 2, 3. Philadelphia, W.B. Saunders Co, 1980.
Wood, R.P., and Northern, J.L.: Manual of Otolaryngology. Baltimore, Williams & Wilkins, 1979.

CHAPTER 22

MISCELLANEOUS PROBLEMS

A.H. Samiy, M.D.

TONGUE MANIFESTATIONS OF SYSTEMIC DISEASE

DEFINITION

Many systemic diseases are associated with changes in the tongue. *Glossitis* is an inflammation of the tongue often associated with redness and smoothness caused by atrophy and edema of the papillae. *Glossodynia* refers to a painful tongue. *Glosspyrosis* is a painful burning of the tongue. *Macroglossia* refers to an enlargement of the tongue.

Patients often examine their own tongues at the slightest suggestion of illness and expect that the physician will examine the oral cavity when they are ill. This expectation is not inappropriate, for the tongue often serves as an indicator of disease, though it is seldom diagnostic of a specific disease. The most effective detection of systemic disorders by examination of the tongue can be achieved only when the clinician is thoroughly familiar with the normal variations and local diseases of the tongue.

PATHOPHYSIOLOGIC CONSIDERATIONS

Patients sometimes become concerned when they first notice one or two of the large circumvallate papillae on the dorsum of the tongue. Eight to twelve of these papillae are arranged in an inverted "V" fashion, forming the posterior boundary of the dorsum of the tongue. Atrophic changes do not occur in these papillae.[1]

Mushroom shaped fungiform papillae are found on the entire tongue surface but at greater density near the tip and lateral surfaces. These papillae are involved in atrophic and inflammatory changes in a variety of systemic conditions. Filiform or hairlike papillae are the most numerous and are uniformly distributed. The high metabolic activity and growth or turnover rates of fungiform and fusiform papillae make these papillae an early indicator of problems impairing this continuous rapid repair. When we remember that this rapid turnover is true of the entire gastrointestinal tract mucosa, it becomes clear why the tongue is referred to as the window of the digestive system and the mirror of the stomach.[2] The constant hydration of the GI tract and the oral mucosa, combined with the rapid rate of cell removal, ensures that the tongue will be a more rapid and sensitive reflector of disorder than the drier, more slowly replaced cells such as those of the skin.

Table 22–1. Causes of Macroglossia

Symmetrical generalized enlargement
  Pituitary tumors (acromegaly)
  Hypothyroidism
  Amyloidosis
  Lead poisoning
  Glycogen storage disease
  Down's syndrome
  Food allergies
  Serum sickness
  Vitamin B_{12} deficiency

Asymmetrical localized enlargement
  Neurofibromatosis
  Hemangiomas
  Hematomas
  Lymphangiomas
  Malignancies

DIFFERENTIAL DIAGNOSIS AND DIAGNOSTIC EVALUATION

Adequate examination of the tongue can be accomplished quickly but must include assessment of the tongue's size, shape, color, and muscular tone, the condition of the papillae, and the presence of any lesions. Many physicians omit the simple process of slipping on a glove and palpating the tongue and oral structures, but this procedure is mandatory in the patient who smokes. Palpation can detect unsuspected lesions and offers considerably more information about the nature of a lesion being evaluated. Patients are often startled when the examiner palpates their tongue and mouth tissues, a procedure that affords an additional opportunity to emphasize the risks of smoking.

Macroglossia. Symmetrical enlargement of the tongue is seen in a number of systemic diseases (Table 22–1).[3-6] Pituitary tumors, which secrete excessive growth hormone, result in an active overgrowth of the soft tissues, and patients soon present with the familiar features of acromegaly. The pressure of this enlargement combined with the overgrowth of cartilage and bony structures results in prognathism, malocclusion, and widely spaced teeth that tilt outward. A simple glucose suppression of the serum growth hormone makes an excellent screening test for this metabolic disturbance.

Hypothyroidism of a degree severe enough to produce cretinism or adult myxedema results in macroglossia from extensive interstitial or extravascular edema fluid. Thyroid function tests will quickly confirm the diagnosis. Speech impediment can be quite severe from the combined problems of tongue enlargement, poor tongue muscle function, and vocal cord involvement with similar changes.

Amyloidosis (primary), which is a systemic disease of uncertain cause and is often associated with chronic inflammatory diseases, may cause significant macro-glossia from amyloid accumulation in the tongue tissue. Biopsy of the tongue or gingiva frequently helps confirm the disease.[3]

Lead poisoning (plumbism) from chronic exposure to lead can result in lingual enlargement, and actual collections of lead sulfide are found in the oral tissues.[3] Another disorder, glycogen storage disease (von Gierke's disease), is a severe metabolic disturbance resulting from a deficiency of hepatic glucose-6-phosphatase. The subsequent deposition of glycogen in body cells enlarges the cells of many tissues, including the tongue, to such an extent that the organ itself is enlarged. Hypoglycemia is a serious associated consequence. Another disorder associated with an enlarged tongue, Down's syndrome, is usually recognized in infancy. Some genetic mosaic patterns, however, are unrecognized until well into adulthood.

Food allergies and other antigens can produce dramatic life threatening swelling of oral cavity tissues, manifesting in a symptom complex called angioneurotic edema. Serum sickness, which again relates to an antigen-antibody reaction, also enlarges the tongue with edema fluid. Vitamin B_{12} deficiency, which is seen mostly in older adults, can produce an edematous, erythematous enlarged tongue. Vitamin B_{12} deficiency in the geriatric population is much more frequent than once suspected—perhaps as much as 10%. Enlarged tongues often have serrated or notched edges from pressure on the teeth, though this finding may be seen in tongues of normal size, especially if the teeth are widely spaced.

Asymmetrical enlargement is more suggestive of local oral disorder, although some growths can reflect systemic or multisystem disease such as neurofibromatosis. Lymphangiomas and hemangiomas, as well as local and metastatic malignancies, must be included in the differential diagnosis.

Surface Problems. Hairy tongue, a condition in which the tongue is covered with coarse papillae that look like hairs, is an impressive finding for patient and physician alike. It results from hyperkeratoses and elongation of the filiform papillae. Color varies from gray to brown to black. A history of recent antibiotic therapy is frequently elicited, but the condition does occur spontaneously and is most commonly seen in young males. Antibiotics may change the oral flora and result in overgrowth of pigment-producing bacteria and fungi. Heavy smokers and patients who have undergone head and neck irradiation are more apt to develop a hairy tongue. The oral dryness associated with radiation suggests that changes in the composition and volume of saliva contribute to the disorder. Good oral hygiene, including brushing the surface of the

tongue with a soft toothbrush, corrects the problem, which is also associated with hyperplasia and lack of normal desquamation.

Scrotal or fissured tongue is diagnosed when there are numerous furrows on the dorsum of the tongue. The cause is not known and no treatment is required.

Glossitis. Geographic tongue, or benign migratory glossitis, consists of irregularly shaped, fairly sharply demarcated patches of the tongue. Desquamation of the filiform papillae has occurred and the central portion of the lesion is inflamed and smooth, while the periphery is lined by a thin white or cream-colored band. These patches migrate for weeks or months, even disappearing and reappearing. No treatment is needed; geographic tongue is not associated with any other health problems, though it may occasionally be mildly symptomatic.

Allergic Glossitis. Many different drugs can produce glossitis of the tongue along with other systemic signs of allergy. Two common drugs are penicillin and phenolphthalein.

Glossitis Venemata. This is a contact allergy produced most commonly by such substances as dentifrices, candy, cough drops, and mouthwashes.

Nutritional Glossitis. Malnutrition of a generalized nature produces glossitis, though the glossitis may be related to specific deficiencies associated with the poor nutrition.

Riboflavin (vitamin B_2) deficiency often causes the tip of the tongue to look smooth and, when advanced, makes the tongue magenta. Cheilosis occurs with riboflavin deficiency, as well.

Folic acid deficiency has many similarities to pernicious anemia, described in detail below.

Nicotinic acid (niacin) deficiency often results in a burning sensation with desquamation and soreness of the tongue. Chronic niacin deficiency results in pellagra with other skin symptoms, dementia, and diarrhea.

Kwashiorkor is associated with glossitis and generalized edema. Glossitis is seen quite early in the severely protein-deficient, malnourished patient.

Pernicious anemia (vitamin B_{12} deficiency) results frequently in glossitis of the tongue and is probably the most important of all manifestations of the disease. The tongue becomes beefy red and smooth, and it is almost always sore and painful. The telltale macrocytic anemia and achlorhydria assist in diagnosis. Plummer-Vinson syndrome often presents with severe glossitis and is associated with chronic iron deficiency and esophageal webbing.

Fatty acids including linoleic acid, which the body is unable to synthesize, are essential in the diet as precursors of the prostaglandins. In patients deficient in fatty acids, the oral mucosa and tongue can suffer from the same findings described in the skin; these include increased capillary fragility and cell permeability. The tongue presents with glossitis, while the skin becomes thick and dry and scaly.

Glossodynia and Glossopyrosis. A painful or burning tongue is a common symptom in both local and systemic disease. The same diseases producing these symptoms produce glossitis; the overlap may approach 100% as glossitis increases in severity (Table 22–2). Glossodynia and sometimes glossopyrosis are seen not uncommonly in elderly patients. It is difficult to determine which nutritional and physiologic changes contribute the most to these disorders. Estrogen deficiency may contribute to this diffuse erythema and shininess of the entire oral mucosa, just as it does to atrophy of the vaginal mucosa.[6]

Ulcerations. Any of the atrophic or denuding conditions may increase the risk of infection. Ulceration is the most common expression of systemic disease in the oral cavity. Most infections of the tongue result in ulcerations, though certainly not all ulcerations represent infections. Nevertheless, the presence of actual ulcerations should immediately raise questions about a number of serious underlying diseases, while steering the physician away from many others (Table 22–2).[3–6]

Many of the sexually contracted diseases may present with or are associated with lesions on the tongue. Syphilis may cause painful lesions in the mouth in all three of its stages. The chancre is characteristic of primary syphilis and develops at the site of initial infection. It is often a crateriform lesion and may have a clean, shiny center or may be covered with an exudate when in the mouth. It is surrounded by induration, and regional nodes are often enlarged. History of exposure is critical and certainly the most cost-effective diagnostic approach. Dark-field microscopy is difficult to perform, and serology may be negative very early in the disease. Even more complicating, the primary lesion can heal in 2 to 3 weeks, leading both the clinician and the patient into a false sense of security.

Secondary oral syphilis lesions are painful, serpiginous, superficial ulcerations and can be associated

Table 22–2. Signs and Symptoms Associated with Diseases of the Tongue

Condition	Glossitis	Glossodynia and Glossopyrosis	Ulceration
General			
Alcohol	+	+	−
Atrophied mucosa with estrogen deficiency	+	+	−
Dermatomyositis	−	+	−
Drug allergies	+	+	−
Geographic tongue	+	+ −	−
Highly seasoned food	−	+	−
Hot food	+	+	−
Mercury and gold	+	+	−
Scrotal tongue	−	−	−
Smoking	+ −	+ −	+ −
Stevens-Johnson syndrome	+	+	+
Xerostomia	+	+	−
Nutrition			
Folic acid deficiency	+	+	−
Iron deficiency	+	+	−
Kwashiorkor syndrome	+	+	−
Malnutrition, general	+	+	−
Nicotinic acid deficiency	+	+	−
Pernicious anemia	+	+	−
Pregnancy	+	+ −	−
Pyridoxine deficiency (vitamin B$_6$)	+	+	−
Riboflavin deficiency	+	+ −	−
Sprue	+	+	−
Infection			
Fungus, especially Monilia	+	+	+
Gonorrhea	−	+	+
Herpes viruses	−	+	+
Scarlet fever (strawberry tongue)	−	+	−
Syphilis	+	+	+

with a papular rash, fever, and lymphadenopathy. The tertiary lesion is a gumma, which later appears in the tongue as an area of necrosis. During its earlier formation, it is easily confused with a tumor.

The syphilitic tongue is characterized by deep longitudinal furrows that become sore and irritated from trapped food particles. Incidence of cancer of the tongue is increased in these patients.

Gonococcal infections and the more frequent viral lesions of herpes also affect the tongue. The oral cavity harbors many other neisserial microorganisms that are indistinguishable from N. gonorrhea on smear.

Tuberculous ulcers present most frequently with pain or dysfunction at the involved site, though some patients report that the initial lesion is painless.[4] These lesions frequently have sparse organisms, and smearing the lesions for acid-fast bacilli does not satisfactorily rule out the disease.

The oral cavity is highly susceptible to infections and ulcerations with both agranulocytosis and acute leukemia. The toxicity of systemic cancer chemotherapy frequently is first visualized here, again because of the high metabolic rate and rapid cell turnover.

DISORDERS OF TASTE

DEFINITION

Disorders of taste may have several different forms and intensities. Ageusia (absence of taste), hypogeusia (decreased perception of taste), cacogeusia (foul or perverted taste), and dysgeusia (distorted perception of taste) are the most commonly encountered disturbances of taste.

PATHOPHYSIOLOGIC CONSIDERATIONS

Taste is the interpretation of orally ingested materials as determined by taste buds on the tongue, palate, and throat. Salivary proteins such as the zinc-containing gustin determine the capacity to discriminate ingested materials. The interpretation of taste is based on combinations of the four basic taste sensations—sweet, sour, bitter, and salty. Taste discrimination is rarely effective in the presence of impaired smell.

Various pharmacologic and toxicologic agents, disease states, and nutritional disorders alter taste buds and the interpretation of ingested material. Any abnormality that interferes with the direct contact of the

Table 22–3.   Differential Diagnosis of Hypogeusia and Aegusia

Endocrine disorders
  Cushing's syndrome
  Hypothyroidism
  Diabetes mellitus
  Gonadal dysgenesis
  Pseudohypoparathyroidism
  Dysautonomia
Systemic disorders
  Renal failure
  Cirrhosis of the liver
  Hepatitis
  Sjögren's syndrome
Local disorders
  Neoplasia of the mouth
  Laryngectomy
  Radiation therapy
  Glossitis
  Thermal burn
Neurologic disorders
  Ear trauma
  Surgery of the head
  Familial dysautonomia
  Parkinson's disease
  Multiple sclerosis
  Head trauma
  Nerve injury
    Lingual nerve
    Chorda tympani
    Glossopharyngeal nerve
  Bell's palsy
Toxicologic agents
  Pyrethrins
  Carbon monoxide
  Cocaine
  Gasoline
  Penicillamine
  DMSO (dimethylsulfoxide)
  Spironolactone
Nutritional disorders
  Niacin deficiency
  Copper deficiency
  Nickel deficiency
  Zinc deficiency
Psychiatric disorders
  Hysteria

Adapted from Goldfrank, L., et al. (eds.): Goldfrank's Toxicologic Emergencies. 3rd Ed. Norwalk, Ct., Appleton-Century-Crofts, 1986, p. 522.

substance to be tasted at the level of the gustatory cells of the tongue, the facial (VII) nerve (the anterior two thirds of the tongue), or the glossopharyngeal (IX) nerve (the posterior third of the tongue) will dramatically affect taste.

DIFFERENTIAL DIAGNOSIS

The differential diagnosis of various forms of taste disorders are shown in Tables 22–3, 22–4, and 22–5.

Table 22–4. Differential Diagnosis of Cacogeusia

Gastrointestinal diseases
    Inflammatory and neoplastic diseases
        Esophagus
        Stomach
Pulmonary diseases
    Lung abscess
    Bronchiectasis
Systemic diseases
    Sarcoidosis
Local disorders
    Gingival disease
    Dental disease
    Lingual disease

Adapted from Goldfrank, L., et al. (eds.): Goldfrank's Toxicologic Emergencies. 3rd Ed. Norwalk, Ct., Appleton-Century-Crofts, 1986, p. 522.

Table 22–3 shows the various causes of hypogeusia and ageusia. A number of local disorders involving the tongue and mouth such as neoplasia, glossitis, and thermal or radiation burn may result in a diminution of taste. Several systemic diseases, notably chronic renal failure, cirrhosis of the liver, and Sjögren's syndrome, may be associated with altered perception of taste. A number of endocrine disorders, including Cushing's syndrome, hypothyroidism, diabetes mellitus, and three rare congenital diseases, gonadal dysgenesis, pseudohypoparathyroidism, and dysautonomia, should be considered in the differential diagnosis. Neurologic disorders such as Parkinson's disease, multiple sclerosis, or trauma or surgery of the lingual nerve, chorda tympani, or glossopharyngeal nerves may be associated with a reduced perception of taste.

Foul or perverted taste may be seen with local disorders of the mouth, particularly of the tongue, gingiva, and teeth (Table 22–4). Chronic pulmonary infections such as lung abscess and bronchiectasis and neoplastic and inflammatory diseases of the upper gastrointestinal tract may produce perception of foul taste. Metallic taste is a common symptom in cacogeusia, often associated with exposure to toxins (Table 22–5).

Table 22–5. Agents Causing Metallic Taste

Acetaldehyde
Arsenicals
Cadmium
Copper
Mercury
Iron
Iodine
Lead
Disulfiram

Adapted from Goldfrank, L., et al. (eds.): Goldfrank's Toxicologic Emergencies. 3rd Ed. Norwalk, Ct., Appleton-Century-Crofts, 1986, p. 522.

Table 22–6. Differential Diagnosis of Dysgeusia

Hereditary
    Capacity to distinguish phenylthiourea
CNS disorders
    Uncinate lesions
    Horner's paratrigeminal syndrome
Drugs/toxins/foods
    Griseofulvin
    Captopril
    DMSO (dimethylsulfoxide)
    Nicotine
    Artichokes
    Quinine
Pregnancy
Glossitis
Miscellaneous
    Dengue fever
    Hypozincemia

Adapted from Goldfrank, L., et al. (eds.): Goldfrank's Toxicologic Emergencies. 3rd Ed. Norwalk, Ct., Appleton-Century-Crofts, 1986, p. 522.

The differential diagnosis of dysgeusia includes the hereditary capacity to taste phenylthiourea, local diseases of the tongue, zinc deficiency, exposures to toxins and drugs, and CNS disease (Table 22–6). Dysgeusia may also be seen during pregnancy.

DIAGNOSTIC EVALUATION

A complete history and careful examination of patients with the symptom of disturbed taste is essential in the diagnostic evaluation. In all forms of disordered taste, a careful history of drug intake and exposure to chemicals or toxins should be elicited. In patients with symptoms of cacogeusia a careful history with regard to disulfiram use or ethanol abuse is important. Exposure to arsenicals, cadmium, copper, mercury, iron, iodine, and lead should be considered. Because nutritional deficiencies may produce symptoms of disturbed taste, a dietary and nutritional history must be obtained.

Although there are few helpful specific findings on physical examination, a complete physical examination with careful evaluation of the head and neck, particularly of the mouth, is essential, particularly in detecting diseases of gingiva, teeth, tongue, and oropharynx. Careful neurologic examination must include evaluation of cranial nerves and evidence of recent trauma or surgery of the head.

Very few specific laboratory tests or other diagnostic procedures are available in the differentiation of various causes of taste disorder. If endocrine disorders such as Cushing's disease and hypothyroidism are under consideration, however, appropriate diagnostic studies should be carried out. Taste stimulation tests with sodium chloride, dilute hydrochloric acid, sucrose, and urea may define specific taste symptoms.

DISORDERS OF SMELL

DEFINITION

Alteration in perception of smell is not an uncommon clinical problem. Patients may present with a variety of symptoms, including hyposmia (decreased perception of smell), anosmia (loss of smell), dysosmia (distorted perception of smell), cacosmia (sensation of foul smell), and parosmia (sensation of smell without stimulus).

PATHOPHYSIOLOGIC CONSIDERATIONS

Olfactory receptor sites receive messages from various odor particles that stimulate the olfactory mucosal receptor cells. The olfactory mucosae have a more diverse sensory capacity than the tongue, allowing for the discrimination of numerous odors, which are the stimuli leading to the perception of smell. The most sensitive olfactory epithelium lies at the roof of the nasal cavity. These nerve endings (rods) with synapses generate impulses to nerve fibers that perforate the cribriform plate of the ethmoid bone leading to the olfactory bulb. Any interruption of this pathway leads to a pathologic state. It is important to remember that the olfactory capability is symmetrically distributed and that unilateral disease of the receptive pathways or nasopharynx will not usually be noted by the patient.

The causes of all the disorders of smell are quite similar. Various pharmacologic and toxicologic agents, disease states, and nutritional disorders may lead to decreased, absent, or distorted perceptions of smell.

DIFFERENTIAL DIAGNOSIS

The differential diagnosis of various causes of disorders of smell is extensive. A number of entities including systemic diseases or local disorders involving the nasopharynx, nutritional deficiencies, and exposure to toxic agents may be involved in decrease or loss of smell (Table 22–7). Local reactions resulting in impaired perception include allergic rhinitis, nasal polyposis, sinusitis, upper respiratory tract infections, and asthma. In addition, infections such as viral hep-

Table 22–7. Differential Diagnosis of Hyposmia and Anosmia

Chronic diseases
  Cirrhosis of the liver
  Renal failure
Endocrine diseases
  Cushing's syndrome
  Diabetes mellitus
  Gonadal dysgenesis (Turner's syndrome)
  Hypogonadotropic hypogonadism (Kallmann's syndrome)
  Hypothyroidism
  Primary amenorrhea
  Pseudohypoparathyroidism
Hereditary
  Capacity to distinguish hydrocyanic acid
  Cystic fibrosis
Infection
  Viral hepatitis
  Influenza
  Leprosy
Local disorders
  Allergic rhinitis
  Nasal polyposis
  Sinusitis
  Bronchial asthma
  Adenoid hypertrophy
  Inflammatory—upper respiratory infections
  Laryngectomy
  Sarcoidosis (local manifestation of systemic disease)
  Sjögren's syndrome (local manifestation of systemic disease)
Neurologic disorders
  Head trauma
  Multiple sclerosis
  Parkinson's disease
  Frontal lobe tumors
Nutritional deficiencies
  Vitamin B_{12}
  Zinc
Toxicologic
  Cadmium
  Hydrogen sulfide

Adapted from Goldfrank, L., et al. (eds.): Goldfrank's Toxicologic Emergencies. 3rd Ed. Norwalk, Ct., Appleton-Century-Crofts, 1986, p. 614.

atitis and influenza may lead to a diminished perception of smell. Neurologic disorders such as head trauma, multiple sclerosis, Parkinson's disease, and frontal lobe tumors may be associated with diminished smell. Nutritional disorders such as vitamin B_{12} and zinc deficiency may also lead to diminished smell. Chronic diseases such as renal failure and cirrhosis of the liver may be associated with decreased perception of smell. Cushing's syndrome, hypothyroidism, diabetes mellitus, and other endocrine disorders also occur with hyposmia and anosmia. Toxicologic agents such as cadmium or hydrogen sulfide poisoning may lead to diminished perception of smell. Certain rare individuals lack the hereditary capacity to smell particular toxins such as hydrocyanic acid.

Table 22–8.   Differential Diagnosis of Dysosmia, Cacosmia, and Parosmia

Drugs and toxins
  Amebicides/antihelmintics
    Metronidazole
  Anesthetics, local
  Antiepileptic
    Phenytoin
    Carbamazepine
  Antihistamines
  Antihypertensives
    Captopril
    Diazoxide
  Antimicrobials
  Anti-inflammatory/antirheumatics
    Allopurinol
    Colchicine
    Gold
    D-penicillamine
    Phenylbutazone
  Antithyroid agents
    Methimazole
    Methylthiouracil
    Propylthiouracil
  Dental
    Toothpastes
  DMSO (dimethylsulfoxide)
  Diuretics
    Ethacrynic acid
  Insecticides
  Levodopa
  Lithium
  Nicotine
  Opioids
  Sympathomimetics
  Vitamin D
Endocrine diseases
  Addison's disease
Neurologic diseases
  Temporal lobe epilepsy

Adapted from Goldfrank, L., et al. (eds.): Goldfrank's Toxicologic Emergencies. 3rd Ed. Norwalk, Ct., Appleton-Century-Crofts, 1986, p. 614.

Table 22–8 shows the differential diagnosis of distorted perception of smell. Toxicologic agents are the most common causes of distorted perception of smell. In addition, a broad range of pharmacologic agents such as antimicrobial agents, antithyroid drugs, dimethylsulfoxide (DMSO), diuretics, L-dopa, lithium, nicotine, opioids, sympathomimetic agents, vitamin D, and toothpaste may be associated with disturbances of smell. Occasionally, temporal lobe epilepsy and, rarely, Addison's disease may manifest with altered perception of smell.

DIAGNOSTIC EVALUATION

A careful history and complete physical examination are essential in the diagnosis of patients presenting with abnormal perception of smell. In taking the history, the physician should make a special effort to obtain information about medications and exposure to toxins. In the physical examination, the physician should pay particular attention to evaluation of the nasopharynx and oropharynx. A careful search for the physical findings associated with endocrinopathies such as Cushing's syndrome, hypothyroidism, and diabetes mellitus is essential. Patients should also have a thorough neurologic examination.

There are no specific laboratory studies to help in determining the causes of smell disturbances. However, appropriate laboratory tests for detection of various systemic diseases and endocrine disorders should be performed. Neurologic evaluation may require additional studies such as electroencephalogram for temporal lobe epilepsy.

The most reliable method to evaluate the functioning of the olfactory receptor sites is specific odor identification tests. Aromatic volatile substances that are known to the patients can be used to test functional capacity. Pungent or noxious odors such as ammonia should not be used because their use tests not the olfactory nerve but the trigeminal nerve.

ODOR

Odor is an important clinical sign that has been used since ancient times in the diagnosis of various diseases. Most clinicians are aware of more familiar odors, such as acetone with ketoacidosis, fish or musty odor with hepatic failure, and putrid odor with anaerobic infection. Table 22–9 shows an extensive list of odors that are encountered in a number of diseases or with exposure to toxic agents or drugs.

CLINICAL SIGNS OF POISONING

(Table 22–10)

TOXICOLOGIC SYNDROMES

(Table 22–11)

Table 22—9. Diagnostic Odors

Odor	Toxin, Drug, or Disease Process
Acetone (sweet, like Russet apples)	Lacquer, ethanol, isopropyl alcohol, chloroform; ketoacidosis
Acrid (pear-like)	Paraldehyde, chloral hydrate
Alcohols (fruit-like)	Ethanol, isopropyl alcohol
Ammoniacal	Uremia
Bitter almonds	Cyanide (in choke-cherry, apricot pits)
Carrots	Cicutoxin
Coal gas (stove gas)	Carbon monoxide (odorless but associated with coal gas)
Disinfectants	Phenol, creosote
Eggs (rotten)	Hydrogen sulfide, mercaptans, disulfiram (Antabuse)
Feculent	Intestinal obstruction, esophageal diverticulum
Fish or raw liver (musty)	Hepatic failure, zinc phosphide, hypermethioninemia, trimethyl-aminuria
Fruit-like	Amyl nitrite, ethanol, isopropyl alcohol
Garlic	Phosphorus, tellurium, arsenic (breath and perspiration), parathion, malathion, selenium, dimethylsulfoxide (DMSO), thallium
Halitosis	Acute illness, poor oral hygiene
Mothballs	Camphor-containing products
Peanuts	RH-787 (Vacor)
Pepper-like	O-chlorobenzylidene malonic dinitrile
Pungent aromatic	Ethchlorvynol (Placidyl)
Putrid	Anaerobic infections
Rope (burned)	Marijuana
Shoe polish	Nitrobenzene
Sweating feet	Isovaleric acid acidemia
Tobacco (stale)	Nicotine
Violets	Urinary turpentine
Wintergreen	Methyl salicylate

Adapted from Goldfrank, L., et al. (eds.): Goldfrank's Toxicologic Emergencies. 3rd Ed. Norwalk, Ct., Appleton-Century-Crofts, 1986, pp. 60–63.

Table 22–10. Clinical Signs of Poisoning

Sign or Symptom	Drugs or Toxins
Abdominal colic	Arsenic, caffeine, botanical irritant toxins, lead, mushrooms, thallium, colchicine, food poisoning, organophosphates, drug withdrawal, laxatives
Ataxia	Hypoglycemia, carbon monoxide, phenytoin, benzodiazepines, ethanol, lithium
Bradycardia	Digitalis, ethyl gasoline, mushrooms, sedative hypnotics, opioids, organophosphates, clonidine, beta blockers, calcium channel blockers, quinidine
Bradypnea/hypoventilation	Anesthetics, carbon monoxide, cyanide, ethanol, opioids, sedative hypnotics
Bullae/vesicles	Carbon monoxide, sedative hypnotics (ethychlorvynol, barbiturates)
Conjunctivitis	Marijuana
Constipation	Lead, opioids, thallium (severe)
Diaphoresis	Amphetamines, ASA, barbiturates, LSD, mushrooms, organophosphates, snake bites, hypoglycemia, cocaine
Diarrhea	Organophosphates, opioid withdrawal, arsenic, iron, boric acid (blue-green), lithium, botanical irritant toxins
Dry mouth	Amphetamines, anticholinergics, opioids, thallium
Gum discoloration	Lead, mercury, bismuth, arsenic
Hallucinations	Ethanol intoxication/withdrawal, LSD, mescaline, amphetamines, cocaine, phencyclidine
Hypertension	Amphetamines, lead, nicotine, sympathomimetic agents, tricyclic antidepressants, thyroid supplements, phencyclidine
Hyperthermia	Amphetamines, anticholinergics, ASA, cocaine, ethanol, LSD, PCP, thyroid supplements, dinitrophenol
Hypotension	Antihypertensive agents, nitrites, nitrates, opioids, phenothiazines, sedative hypnotics, beta blockers, calcium channel blockers
Hypothermia	Carbon monoxide, ethanol, opioids, sedative hypnotics, phenothiazines, hypoglycemia, H_2S, HCN, clonidine, butyrophenones
Lacrimation	Organophosphates, opioid withdrawal, noxious gases
Metabolic acidosis (anion gap)	ASA, methanol, uremia, diabetes, paraldehyde, phenformin, lactic acidosis, isoniazid, iron, ethanol, ethylene glycol, toluene
Miosis	Opioids, organophosphates, phenothiazines, pilocarpine
Mydriasis	Atropine, LSD, amphetamines, drug withdrawal, cocaine, botulism, anticholinergic agents, glutethimide, meperidine, dextromethorphan
Needle marks	Opioids, PCP, phencyclidine, amphetamines, cocaine
Nystagmus	Alcohol, ASA, barbiturates, carbon dioxide, phenytoin, quinine, phencyclidine, cocaine, ethchlorvynol, glutethimide

Table 22–10. *Continued*

Sign or Symptom	Drugs or Toxins
Odor	
Ammoniacal	Uremia
Garlic	Arsenic, phosphorus, thallium, parathion, malathion, selenium, DMSO
Carrots	Cicutoxin
Bitter almonds	Cyanides (silver polish)
Acetone	Isopropyl alcohol, methanol, ASA, chloroform, ketoacidosis
Pungent aromatic	Ethchlorvynol
Disinfectants	Phenol, creosote
Violets	Turpentine
Shoe polish	Nitrobenzene
Coal gas	Carbon monoxide
Mothballs	Camphor
Wintergreen	Methyl salicylates
Peanuts	Vacor
Pear-like	Chloral hydrate, paraldehyde
Eggs (rotten)	Hydrogen sulfide, mercaptans, disulfiram
Fish or raw liver (musty)	Hepatic failure, zinc phosphide
Fruit-like	Amyl nitrite, ethanol, isopropyl alcohol
Pepper-like	O-chlorobenzylidene malonic dinitrile
Purpura	ASA, snake and spider bites, warfarin
Radiopaque ingestions	Chloral hydrate, heavy metals (As, Pb, Fe), iodides, CCl_4, psychotropics (phenothiazines, tricyclic antidepressants), enteric-coated medication (salicylates) (chewable or liquid iron preparations are not radiopaque)
Red skin	Boric acid, carbon monoxide, cyanide, anticholinergic agents (atropine, scopolamine)
Salivation	Mercury, mushrooms, strychnine, organophosphates, arsenic, physostigmine (anticholinesterases)
Tachycardia	Alcohols, arsenic, nicotine, atropine, ASA, amphetamines, caffeine, cocaine, thyroid supplements, anticholinergic agents
Tachypnea/hyperventilation	Ethanol, methanol, ethylene glycol, amphetamines, ASA, carbon monoxide, camphor, CNS stimulants, cocaine, hydrocarbons
Tinnitus	ASA, furosemide, heavy metals, kanamycin, quinine, streptomycin
Tremor	Thyroid medication, cocaine, sympathomimetic agents, carbon monoxide, parathion, phenothiazines, mercury, ethanol, lithium, arsenic
Vision disturbance	Botulism, parathion, methanol, digitalis, vitamin A, quinidine

Modified after unpublished works of Arena, J., Becker, C., Done, A., and Rumack, B. Adapted from Goldfrank, L., et al. (eds.): Goldfrank's Toxicologic Emergencies. 3rd Ed. Norwalk, Ct., Appleton-Century-Crofts, 1986, pp. 60–63.

Table 22–11. Toxicologic Syndromes

Drug or Toxin	Signs and Symptoms
Amphetamines	Track marks; toxic psychosis; hyperthermia; dilated pupils (reactive); heatstroke, flushing, diaphoresis; increased blood pressure; active bowel sounds
Antifreeze (ethlyene glycol)	Metabolic acidosis; renal failure; hypocalcemia; calcium oxalate crystals in urine
Arsenic	Garlicky breath; profuse diarrhea; polyneuropathy; abnormal kidney, ureter, and bladder; vomiting, abdominal pain; arrhythmias, cutaneous abnormalities
Barbiturates	Bullae; slightly constricted pupils; coma, hyporeflexia; hypothermia; disconjugate eye movement; respiratory depression
Boric acid	Lobster-red skin; severe acidosis; coma; blue-green diarrhea; convulsions
Botulism	Epidemic; vertigo; ptosis; muscle weakness; sore throat; dilated pupils; ophthalmoplegia; dysphagia
Brominism	Acne; dementia/psychosis; hyperchloremia; cation gap
Carbon monoxide	Epidemic (family illness); charcoal burning, coma seizures; coal gas odor; headache, nausea, vomiting; bullae
Cocaine	Perforated nasal septum; psychosis; skin tracks; dilated pupils (reactive); hyperthermia, diaphoresis, seizures, agitation, tremor
Cyanide	Bitter almond odor; coma; convulsions; abnormal ECG
Digitalis	Visual disturbances; abnormal ECG; delirium; nausea
Disulfiram	Flushing; circulatory collapse; pulsating headache
Ethchlorvynol	Hypotension; bradycardia; pungent aromatic odor; pink or green gastric aspirate
Fluoride	Roach powder; decreased potassium, magnesium; tetany (hypocalcemia)
Heroin	Track marks; coma; miosis; hypotension; bradycardia
Hydrocarbons	Pulmonary edema; tinnitus; ventricular fibrillation; lipoid pneumonia; convulsions
Iron	Pregnant mother; diarrhea; hematemesis; abdominal pain; abnormal ECG; coma; radiopaque material; metabolic acidosis
Isopropyl alcohol	Gastritis; coma; acetonemia, ketonuria; normoglycemia
Lead	Severe abdominal pain; milky vomiting; hypertension; convulsions; peripheral neuropathy
Lithium	Confusion, seizures; weakness, tremor, ataxia, diarrhea; renal abnormalities, diabetes; QT prolongation, arrhythmias, leukocytosis
Mercury	Stomatitis; colitis; ataxia; gingivitis; nephrotic syndrome
Methadone	Miosis; bradycardia; transient response to naloxone; coma; hypoventilation; hypotension
Methaqualone	Increased reflexes; coma; hypotension, bradycardia; tonic-clonic spasms
Methyl alcohol	Alcoholic patient; decreased vision; hyperventilation; metabolic acidosis
Organophosphates	Miotic pupils; cramps; salivation; urination; fasciculations; sialorrhea; bronchorrhea; lacrimation; defecation; garlic odor
Paraquat	Pseudodiphtheria; oropharynx burning; vomiting; acute renal failure; headache; diarrhea, pleural effusion
Phencyclidine (PCP)	Muscle twitching; prolonged psychosis, agitation, miosis, bidirectional nystagmus; track marks; tachycardia; hypertension
Phenothiazines	Postural hypotension; miosis; abnormal abdominal x-ray (radiopaque substance); hypothermia; tremor; increased QT interval
Salicylates	Hyperventilation; fever, diaphoresis, tinnitus; vomiting, agitation; bleeding
Strychnine	Stiff neck; status epilepticus; signs of intravenous drug use
Thallium	Alopecia; personality change; peripheral neuropathy; retrobulbar neuritis
Tricyclic antidepressants	Vasodilation; ileus; response to physostigmine, lilliputian hallucinations; dilated pupils (unreactive); supraventricular arrhythmia; convulsions, agitation; dry mucosa, axilla

Modified after the works of Arena, J., Becker, C., Done, A., and Rumack, B. Adapted from Goldfrank, L., et al. (eds.): Goldfrank's Toxicologic Emergencies. 3rd Ed. Norwalk, Ct., Appleton-Century-Crofts, 1986, pp. 60–63.

REFERENCES

1. Keyes, K.S.: Diseases of the tongue. *In* Burket's Oral Medicine: Diagnosis and Treatment. Edited by M. Greenberg. Philadelphia, J.B. Lippincott, 1984.
2. Zehm, S.: Inflammation of the oral cavity. *In* Otolaryngology. Edited by G.M. English. Philadelphia, Harper & Row, 1984.
3. Gardner, A.F.: Alterations in the tongue accompanying systemic diseases. *In* Pathology of Oral Manifestations of Systemic Diseases. Edited by A.F. Gardner. New York, Hafner Publishing Co., 1972.
4. McNulty, J.S.: Granulomatous and venereal diseases of the oral cavity. *In* Otolaryngology. Edited by G.M. English. Philadelphia, Harper & Row, 1984.
5. Ferguson, C.F.: Pharyngeal manifestations of systemic disease. *In* Pediatric Otolaryngology. Vol. II. Edited by C.F. Ferguson and E.L. Kendig. Philadelphia, W.B. Saunders, 1972.
6. Lyons, D.C.: Oral and Facial Signs and Symptoms of Systemic Diseases. Springfield, Charles C Thomas, Publisher, 1968.

GENERAL REFERENCES

Schiffman, S.S.: Taste and smell in disease. N Engl J Med *308*:1275–1279, 1337–1343, 1983.
Thawley, S.E.: Disorders of taste and smell. South Med J *71*:267–270, 1978.

APPENDIX

```
┌─────────────────────────────────────┐
│                                      │
│        REFERENCE VALUES FOR          │
│     COMMON LABORATORY TESTS          │
│                                      │
└─────────────────────────────────────┘
```

The following tables list the reference ranges for laboratory tests in common use. Unless otherwise specified, the tables indicate the central 95% confidence limits for a healthy mixed adult population in the fasting state. There is considerable variation among clinical laboratories in the choice of methods, instruments and reagents, and reference ranges vary accordingly. This variation is especially true for enzyme assays and immunologic tests. Consequently, test results provided by an individual laboratory may not be comparable to the reference ranges listed here. Usu-

ally, a patient's test results should be evaluated only by comparing them with the normal ranges provided by the laboratory that performed the test. Other problems in the interpretation of laboratory test results are discussed in Chapter 7.

The International System of Units (SI) has been gaining increasing recognition, particularly in Europe, and the World Health Organization has recommended general use of this system by the medical community. In the U.S., acceptance of the SI system in clinical medicine has been delayed by a lack of agreement on the use of certain units, particularly those requiring the abandonment of familiar units for denoting amount of substance (mole) and enzyme activity (katal). The following tables reflect the general recommendations of the American National Metric Council.[1,11]

Abbreviations: B = whole blood; Erc = erythrocyte; P = plasma; S = serum; vP = venous plasma.

Table 1. Serum, Plasma, or Blood Values

Test	Reference Range	
	Conventional	SI Units
Acetone (qualitative) [B,S]	Negative	Negative
Acid phosphatase, prostatic Men [S]	<0.9 U/L	<0.9 U/L
Acid phosphatase, total [S]	0–5.4 U.L	0–90 nkat/L
Alanine aminotransferase (SGPT, ALT) [S]	0–45 U/L	0–0.75 μkat/L
Albumin [S]	3.3–5.2 g/dl	33–52 g/L
Alkaline phosphatase [S]	30–115 U/L	0.5–1.92 μkat/L
Alpha-1-antitrypsin [S]	200–400 mg/dl	2–4 g/L
Alpha-fetoprotein [S]	<5.0 ng/ml	<5 μg/L
Aluminum [S]	3–10 μg/L	111–370 nmol/L
Amino acids [P]		
Alanine	209–659 μmol/L	209–659 μmol/L
Arginine	21–137 μmol/L	21–137 μmol/L
Aspartic acid	0–24 μmol/L	0–24 μmol/L
Citrulline	0–55 μmol/L	0–55 μmol/L
Cystine	48–141 μmol/L	48–141 μmol/L
Glutamic acid	14–192 μmol/L	14–192 μmol/L
Glutamine + asparagine	413–690 μmol/L	413–690 μmol/L
Glycine	120–553 μmol/L	120–553 μmol/L
Histidine	31–106 μmol/L	31–106 μmol/L
Isoleucine	35–97 μmol/L	35–97 μmol/L
Leucine	71–175 μmol/L	71–175 μmol/L
Lysine	82–236 μmol/L	82–236 μmol/L
Methionine	6–39 μmol/L	6–39 μmol/L
Ornithine	29–125 μmol/L	29–125 μmol/L
Phenylalanine	37–115 μmol/L	37–115 μmol/L
Serine	67–193 μmol/L	67–193 μmol/L
Taurine	27–168 μmol/L	27–168 μmol/L
Threonine	79–246 μmol/L	79–246 μmol/L
Tryptophan	0–73 μmol/L	0–73 μmol/L
Tyrosine	21–87 μmol/L	21–87 μmol/L
Valine	116–315 μmol/L	116–315 μmol/L
Ammonia [vP]		
Men	18–54 μmol/L	18–54 μmol/L
Women	12–50 μmol/L	12–50 μmol/L
Amylase [S]	20–100 U/L	0.33–1.67 μkat/L
Arsenic (as As) [B]	0.2–6.2 μg/dl	0.03–0.83 μmol/L
Aspartate aminotransferase (SGOT, AST) [S]	10–50 U/L	0.16–0.83 μkat/L

Table 1. Continued

Test	Reference Range	
	Conventional	*SI Units*
Bicarbonate [B,P,S]	24–32 mEq/L	24–32 mmol/L
Bilirubin [S]		
Total	0.1–1.2 mg/dl	2–21 µmol/L
Direct	0–0.3 mg/dl	0–5 µmol/L
Indirect	0.1–0.9 mg/dl	2–15 µmol/L
C1 esterase inhibitor [S]	Present	Present
Calcium [S]		
Total	8.5–10.5 mg/dl	2.12–2.52 mmol/L
Ionized	2.3–2.8 mEq/L	1.15–1.42 mmol/L
Carcinoembryonic antigen [P]	<5 ng/ml	<5 µg/L
Carotenes [S]	40–200 µg/dl	0.75–3.7 µmol/L
Ceruloplasmin [S]	24–48 mg/dl	240–480 mg/L
Chloride [S]	96–106 mEq/L	96–106 mmol/L
Cholesterol [S]		
Total (low risk)	140–240 mg/dl	3.6–6.2 mmol/L
HLD fraction		
Men	30–70 mg/dl	0.8–1.8 mmol/L
Women	30–85 mg/dl	0.8–2.2 mmol/L
Citrate [S]	1.7–3.0 mg/dl	88–156 µmol/L
Complement [S]		
Total	22–40 CH$_{50}$ U/ml	22–40 CH$_{50}$ kU/L
C3	83–177 mg/dl	0.83–1.77 g/L
C4	15–45 mg/dl	0.15–0.45 g/L
Copper [S]		
Men	70–140 µg/dl	11–22 µmol/L
Women	85–155 µg/dl	13–24 µmol/L
Creatine phosphokinase (CK) [S]		
Total		
Men	0–123 U/L	0–2.05 µkat/L
Women	6–61 U/L	0.10–1.02 µkat/L
CK-MB fraction	<16 U/L	<0.27 µkat/L
	<3% of total	<.03
Creatinine [S]	0.6–1.4 mg/dl	53–124 µmol/L
Creatinine clearance [S,U]	70–140 ml/min	1.17–2.33 mL/s
Cryoglobulin [S]	<0.12 mg/ml	<0.12 g/L
Cyanide [B]	<0.1 mg/L	<3.84 µmol/L
Erythropoietin [S]	4–26 mU/ml	4–26 U/L
Ferritin [S]	10–275 ng/ml	10–275 µg/L
Fluoride [S]	0.01–0.10 mg/L	0.5–5.3 µmol/L
Folate [S]	2–20 ng/ml	4.5–45 nmol/L
Galactose screen [P]	Negative	Negative
Gamma-glutamyl transpeptide (GGT) [S]	5–50 U/L	0.08–0.83 µkat/L
Gastrin [S]	<200 pg/ml	<200 ng/L
Glucose [S]	70–110 mg/dl	3.9–6.1 mmol/L
Haptoglobin [S]	25–200 mg/dl	0.25–2.00 g/L
Histamine [B]	3–9 µg/dl	30–90 µg/L
Immunoglobulins [S]		
IgA	50–390 mg/dl	0.5–3.9 g/L
IgE	10–42 U/ml	25–100 µg/L
IgG	630–1600 mg/dl	6.3–16 g/L
IgM	50–340 mg/dl	0.5–3.4 g/L
IgD	0.5–3.0 mg/dl	5–30 mg/L
Insulin [S]	5–25 µU/ml	36–179 pmol/L
Iron [S]		
Total	50–150 µg/dl	9–27 µmol/L
Binding capacity	235–450 µg/dl	42–81 µmol/L
Saturation	15–55%	0.15–0.55

Table 1.   Serum, Plasma, or Blood Values (Continued)

Test	Reference Range	
	Conventional	SI Units
Lactate (as lactic acid) [B]	5–20 mg/dl	0.56–2.2 mmol/L
Lactate dehydrogenase [S]		
Total	60–210 U/l	1.00–3.50 μkat/L
Isoenzymes		
Fraction 1	17–27%	0.17–0.27
Fraction 2	28–38%	0.28–0.38
Fraction 3	19–27%	0.19–0.27
Fraction 4	5–16%	0.05–0.16
Fraction 5	5–16%	0.05–0.16
Lead [B]	<50 μg/dl	<2.4 μmol/L
Leucine aminopeptidase [S]	15–33 U/L	0.25–0.55 μkat/L
Lipase [S]	23–208 U/L	0.38–3.47 μkat/L
Lysozyme [S]	5–15 μg/ml	5–15 mg/L
Magnesium [S]	1.6–2.7 mg/dl	0.66–1.1 mmol/L
Mercury [B]	<1.0 μg/dl	<50 nmol/L
5′-Nucleotidase [S]	1–11 U/L	0.02–0.18 μkat/L
Osmolality [S]	275–295 mOsm/kg	275–295 mmol/kg
Phosphate, inorganic (as phosphorus) [S]	2.5–4.5 mg/dl	0.80–1.45 mmol/L
Potassium [S]	3.5–5.0 mEq/L	3.5–5.0 mmol/L
Protein [S]		
Total	6–8.5 g/dl	60–85 g/L
Albumin	3.0–5.0 g/dl	30–50 g/L
Globulin	2.1–3.3 g/dl	21–33 g/L
Protein electrophoresis [S]		
Albumin	47–71%	0.47–0.71
Alpha-1-globulin	2.7–5.8%	0.027–0.058
Alpha-2-globulin	5.1–12%	0.051–0.12
Beta-globulin	4.5–15.7%	0.045–0.157
Gamma-globulin	11.3–24%	0.113–0.24
Pyruvate (as pyruvic acid) [B]	0.3–0.9 mg/dl	34–102 μmol/L
Sodium [S]	135–145 mEq/L	135–145 mmol/L
Transferrin [S]	215–400 mg/dl	2.15–4.0 g/L
Triglycerides [S]	10–160 mg/dl	0.11–1.83 mmol/L
Urate (as uric acid) [S]	2.2–7.7 mg/dl	130–460 μmol/L
Urea nitrogen [S]	10–24 mg/dl	3.6–8.6 mmol/L
Vitamins		
Vitamin A (retinol) [S]	30–95 μg/dl	1.0–3.3 μmol/L
Vitamin B_1 (thiamin hydrochloride) [B]	1.6–4.0 μg/dl	47.4–118 nmol/L
Vitamin B_6 (pyridoxal phosphate) [P]	3.6–18 ng/ml	22–108 nmol/L
Vitamin B_{12} (cyanocobalamin) [S]	160–950 pg/ml	118–700 pmol/L
Vitamin C (ascorbic acid) [S]	0.2–2.0 mg/dl	11–110 μmol/L
Vitamin D, 25-OH [S]	10–80 ng/ml	25–200 nmol/L
Vitamin D, 1,25-OH_2 [S]	20–76 pg/ml	48–182 pmol/L
Vitamin E [S]	0.5–1.0 mg/dl	12–23 μmol/L
Zinc [S]	50–150 μg/dl	7.6–23 μmol/L

Table 2.   Hematologic Values

Test	Reference Range Conventional	SI Units
Acid hemolysis test [B]	Negative	Negative
Coagulation factor activity [P]		
Factor II	60–150%	0.60–1.50
Factor V	50–150%	0.50–1.50
Factor VII	50–150%	0.50–1.50
Factor VIII	50–150%	0.50–1.50
Factor VIII–related antigen	40–230%	0.4–2.3
Factor VIII multimers	Normal	Normal
Factor IX	60–150%	0.60–1.50
Factor X	50–150%	0.50–1.50
Factor XI	50–150%	0.50–1.50
Factor XII	50–150%	0.50–1.50
Factor XIII	Stable clot	
Factor inhibitors	Negative	Negative
Ristocetin cofactor (von Willebrand factor)	50–160%	0.50–1.60
Coagulation screening tests		
Bleeding time (template)	2.5–9.5 min	2.5–9.5 min
Euglobulin lysis time [P]	>2 h	>2 h
Fibrin degradation products [S]	<10 µg/ml	<10 mg/L
Fibrin D-dimers [P]	<0.5 µg/ml	<0.5 mg/L
Fibrinogen [P]	170–440 mg/dl	1.7–4.4 g/L
Partial thromboplastin time, activated (PTT) [P]	24–35 s	24–35 s
Plasminogen [P]		
Immunoreactive	7.6–17.8 mg/dl	
Activity	73–122%	0.73–1.22
Prothrombin time (PT) [P]	10–12 s	10–12 s
Reptilase time [P]	13–20 s	13–20 s
Russell's viper venom time [P]	24–37 s	24–37 s
Thrombin time [P]	24–35 s	24–35 s
"Complete blood count"		
Erythrocyte (RBC) count [B]		
Men	$4.4–5.8 \times 10^6/\mu l$	$4.4–5.8 \times 10^{12}/L$
Women	$3.9–5.5 \times 10^6/\mu l$	$3.9–5.5 \times 10^{12}/L$
Hematocrit (Packed cell volume, Hct, PCV) [B]		
Men	40–51%	0.40–0.51
Women	35–47%	0.35–0.47
Hemoglobin (Hb) [B]		
Men	13.5–17.3 g/dl	135–173 g/L
Women	11.6–15.8 g/dl	116–158 g/L
Leukocyte (WBC) count [B]	$3.9–11.7 \times 10^6/dl$	$3.9–11.7 \times 10^{12}/L$
Mean cell hemoglobin (MCH) [Erc]	26–34 pg	26–34 pg
Mean cell hemoglobin concentration (MCHC) [Erc]	31.5–36 g/dl	315–360 g/L
Mean cell volume (MCV) [Erc]	80–100 fl	80–100 fl
Erythrocyte enzymes [Erc]		
Adenosine deaminase	0.6–1.7 U/g Hb	0.6–1.7 U/g Hb
Adenylate kinase	199–317 U/g Hb	199–317 U/g Hb
Aldolase	1.5–4.9 U/g Hb	1.5–4.9 U/g Hb
Diphosphoglyceromutase	3.5–6.1 U/g Hb	3.5–6.1 U/g Hb
Enolase	3.7–7.1 U/g Hb	3.7–7.1 U/g Hb
Glucose-6-phosphate dehydrogenase	5.1–11.5 U/g Hb	5.1–11.5 U/g Hb
Glucosephosphate isomerase	39–83 U/g Hb	39–83 U/g Hb
Glutathione peroxidase	21–40 U/g Hb	21–40 U/g Hb
Glutathione reductase	5.0–9.4 U/g Hb	5.0–9.4 U/g Hb
Glyceraldehyde phosphate dehydrogenase	142–310 U/g Hb	142–310 U/g Hb
Hexokinase	1.0–2.5 U/g Hb	1.0–2.5 U/g Hb
Monophosphoglyceromutase	26–49 U/g Hb	26–49 U/g Hb

Table 2. Hematologic Values (Continued)

Test	Reference Range	
	Conventional	SI Units
Phosphofructokinase	6.3–15.7 U/g Hb	6.3–15.7 U/g Hb
Phosphoglucomutase	4.3–6.7 U/g Hb	4.3–6.7 U/g Hb
6-Phosphogluconic dehydrogenase	7.2–10.3 U/g Hb	7.2–10.3 U/g Hb
Phosphoglycerate kinase	248–392 U/g Hb	248–392 U/g Hb
Pyrimidine-5'-nucleotidase	102–175 mU/g Hb	102–175 mU/g Hb
Pyruvate kinase	11–19 U/g Hb	11–19 U/g Hb
Triose phosphate isomerase	1.3–2.9 kU/g Hb	1.3–2.9 kU/g Hb
Erythrocyte sedimentation rate (Westergren) [B]	0–15 mm/h	0–15 mm/h
Folate [Erc]	>200 ng/ml	>450 nmol/L
Free erythrocyte porphyrin [B]	<40 μg/dl	<400 μg/L
Glycerol lysis time (GLT$_{50}$) [B]		
Immediate	26–73 s	26–73 s
After incubation	17–36 s	17–36 s
Hemoglobin components [B]		
Carboxyhemoglobin		
Nonsmokers	<2%	<0.02
Smokers	<10%	<0.10
Glycosylated hemoglobin		
(Hemoglobin A$_{1c}$)	3.4–6.1%	0.034–0.061
Hemoglobin electrophoresis (qualitative)	Hb A	Hb A
Hemoglobin A$_2$	<3.5%	<0.035
Hemoglobin F	<1.0%	<0.01
Methemoglobin	<3.0%	<0.03
Sickle preparation	Negative	Negative
Leukocyte alkaline phosphatase (LAP) [B]	20–100 score	20–100 score
Leukocyte differential count [B]		
Relative values		
Neutrophils	42–78%	0.42–0.78
Bands	0–5%	0–0.05
Lymphocytes	16–51%	0.16–0.51
Monocytes	0–10%	0–0.10
Eosinophils	0–6%	0–0.06
Basophils	0–2%	0–0.02
Absolute values		
Neutrophils	$1.8–8.4 \times 10^3/\mu l$	$1.8–8.4 \times 10^9/L$
Lymphocytes	$1.1–4.6 \times 10^3/\mu l$	$1.1–4.6 \times 10^9/L$
Monocytes	$0–1.0 \times 10^3/\mu l$	$0–1.0 \times 10^9/L$
Eosinophils	$0–0.6 \times 10^3/\mu l$	$0–0.6 \times 10^9/L$
Basophils	$0–0.6 \times 10^3/\mu l$	$0–0.2 \times 10^9/L$
Lymphocytes, T [B]		
T-helper/suppressor ratio	1.1–2.8	1.1–2.8
T-helper cells	30–49%	0.30–0.49
T-suppressor cells	14–37%	0.14–0.37
Osmotic fragility [B]		
Immediate		
10% lysis	0.44–0.55% NaCl	4.4–5.5 g/L NaCl
50% lysis	0.40–0.50% NaCl	4.0–5.0 g/L NaCl
90% lysis	0.36–0.48% NaCl	3.6–4.8 g/L NaCl
After incubation		
10% lysis	0.54–0.66% NaCl	5.4–6.6 g/L NaCl
50% lysis	0.47–0.58% NaCl	4.7–5.8 g/L NaCl
90% lysis	0.37–0.54% NaCl	3.7–5.4 g/L NaCl
Paroxysmal nocturnal hemoglobinuria (PNH)		
screening test [S]	Negative	Negative
Platelet count [B]	$180–400 \times 10^3/\mu l$	$180–400 \times 10^9/L$
Protoporphyrin [Erc]	<50 μg/dl	<0.90 μmol/L
Reticulocyte count [B]		
Relative	0.5–2.0%	0.005–0.02
Absolute	$25–100 \times 10^3/\mu l$	$25–100 \times 10^9/L$

Table 3. Urine Values

Test	Reference Range	
	Conventional	*SI Units*
Amino acids		
Alanine	60–800 µmol/d	60–800 µmol/d
Cystine	20–130 µmol/d	20–130 µmol/d
Glutamic acid	55–270 µmol/d	55–270 µmol/d
Glutamine + asparagine	410–1560 µmol/d	410–1560 µmol/d
Glycine	160–4200 µmol/d	160–4200 µmol/d
Histidine	130–2100 µmol/d	130–2100 µmol/d
Isoleucine	18–210 µmol/d	18–210 µmol/d
Leucine	21–200 µmol/d	21–200 µmol/d
Lysine	48–640 µmol/d	48–640 µmol/d
Methionine	20–95 µmol/d	20–95 µmol/d
Phenylalanine	24–190 µmol/d	24–190 µmol/d
Serine	160–700 µmol/d	160–700 µmol/d
Taurine	63–2300 µmol/d	63–2300 µmol/d
Threonine	85–440 µmol/d	85–440 µmol/d
Tyrosine	40–270 µmol/d	40–270 µmol/d
Valine	14–51 µmol/d	14–51 µmol/d
Amylase	<14 U/h	<14 U/h
	<500 U/L	<500 U/L
Arsenic	<100 µg/L	<1.3 µmol/L
Arylsulfatase A	<0.3 U/L	<0.3 U/L
Calcium	100–300 mg/d	2.5–7.5 mmol/d
Chloride	110–250 mEq/L*	110–250 mmol/L*
Citrate	140–940 mg/d	0.73–4.89 mmol/d
Copper	0–50 µg/d	0–0.8 µmol/d
Creatinine	0.9–1.9 g/d	8.0–16.8 mmol/d
Delta aminolevulinic acid	1.0–7.0 mg/d	8–53 µmol/d
Fluoride	<1.0 mg/L	<53 µmol/L
Glucose	66–165 mg/d	0.37–0.92 mmol/d
Hemosiderin	Negative	Negative
Homovanillic acid	<15 mg/d	<82 µmol/d
5-Hydroxyindoleacetic acid (5-HIAA)		
Qualitative	Negative	Negative
Quantitative	2–8 mg/d	10.5–42 µmol/d
Iron	<300 µg/d	<5.4 µmol/d
Lead	<80 µg/L	<0.4 µmol/L
Magnesium	15–300 mg/d	0.6–12 mmol/d
Melanin (qualitative)	Negative	Negative
Mercury	<20 µg/L	<0.1 µmol/L
Metanephrines		
Metanephrine	45–285 µg/d	0.23–1.45 µmol/d
	35–235 µg/g creatinine	20–135 µmol/mol creatinine
Normetanephrine	110–470 µg/d	0.6–2.6 µmol/d
	105–335 µg/g creatinine	65–207 µmol/mol creatinine
Nitrogen	4.7–19 g/d	0.34–1.4 mol/d
Osmolality	50–1200 mOsm/kg	50–1200 mmol/L
Oxalate	<41 mg/d	<0.46 mmol/d
Phosphorus	0.4–1.3 g/d*	13–42 mmol/d*
Porphobilinogen (qualitative)	Negative	Negative
Porphyrins		
Coproporphyrins	28–132 µg/d	43–202 nmol/d
Uroporphyrins	0–30 µg/d	0–36 nmol/d
Potassium	40–65 mEq/d*	40–65 mmol/d*
Protein	<150 mg/d	<150 mg/d

Table 3.   Urine Values (Continued)

Test	Reference Range	
	Conventional	SI Units
Routine urinalysis		
Bilirubin	Negative	Negative
Color	Light yellow to amber	Light yellow to amber
Glucose	Negative	Negative
Ketones	Negative	Negative
Leukocyte esterase	Negative	Negative
Microscopic examination		
Erythrocytes	0/high power field	0/high power field
Leukocytes	0–2/high power field	0–2/high power field
Casts	0/low power field	0/low power field
Nitrites	Negative	Negative
Occult blood	Negative	Negative
pH	4.5–8.0	4.5–8.0
Protein—qualitative	Negative	Negative
Specific gravity	1.002–1.030	1.002–1.030
Sodium	130–200 mEq/d*	130–200 mmol/d*
Urea nitrogen	10–20 g/d	167–333 mmol/d
Uric acid	250–750 mg/d	1.5–4.5 mmol/d
Urine concentration test	1.025–1.030 specific gravity	1.025–1.030 specific gravity
Urine dilution test	1.001–1.003 specific gravity	1.001–1.003 specific gravity
Urobilinogen	<1:32 dilution	<1:32 dilution
Vanillylmandelic acid (VMA)	0.1–8 μg/mg creatinine	0.06–4.6 μmol/mol creatinine
Zinc	0.15–1.3 mg/d	2.3–20 μmol/d

*Output varies with diet

Table 4.   Cerebrospinal Fluid Values

Test	Reference Range	
	Conventional	SI Units
Albumin	7.5–39 mg/dl	75–390 mg/L
Cell count	0–5 lymphocytes/μl	0–5 × 10⁶ lymphocytes/L
Glucose	40–75 mg/dl	2.2–4.2 mmol/L
	>55% of serum level	>0.55 serum level
Glutamine	8–16 mg/dl	0.55–1.1 mmol/L
IgG	≤5.1 mg/dl	≤51 mg/L
IgG Index	0.23–0.64	0.23–0.64
Lactate (as lactic acid)	10–25 mg/dl	1.1–2.8 mmol/L
Protein, total	15–45 mg/dl	150–450 mg/L

APPENDIX 853

Table 5. Endocrine Values

Test	Reference Range	
	Conventional	SI Units
Adrenocorticotropic hormone (ACTH) [P]		
0800 h	25–100 pg/ml	5–22 pmol/L
1600 h	<50 pg/ml	<11 pmol/L
Aldosterone [U] (on sodium intake 100 mmol/d)	4–20 µg/d	11–55 nmol/d
Androstenedione [S]	50–410 ng/dl	1.7–14.3 nmol/L
Catecholamines		
Plasma		
Total	140–730 pg/ml	0.8–4.3 nmol/L
Epinephrine	<60 pg/ml	<0.33 nmol/L
Norepinephrine	120–680 pg/ml	0.7–4.0 nmol/L
Urine		
Total	0–115 µg/d	0–670 nmol/d
Epinephrine	0–20 µg/d	0–110 nmol/d
Norepinephrine	0–95 µg/d	0–560 nmol/d
Cortisol [P]	5–23 µg/dl (A.M.)	138–630 nmol/L
Basal	3–13 µg/dl (P.M.)	83–360 nmol/L
Post-ACTH	≥2-fold increase	≥2-fold increase
Dehydroepiandrosterone (DHEA), total [S]		
Men	1.7–4.2 ng/ml	6–15 nmol/L
Women		
Nonpregnant	2.0–5.2 ng/ml	7–18 nmol/L
Pregnant	0.5–12.5 ng/ml	2–43 nmol/L
Dehydroepiandrosterone sulfate [S]		
Men	2.0–3.3 µg/ml	5.2–8.7 µmol/L
Women		
Premenopausal	0.8–3.4 µg/ml	2.1–8.8 µmol/L
Postmenopausal	0.1–0.6 µg/ml	0.3–1.6 µmol/L
Term pregnancy	0.2–1.2 µg/ml	0.6–3.0 µmol/L
11-Deoxycortisol (Compound S) [S]		
Basal	<0.5 µg/dl	<15 nmol/L
Postmetyrapone	>8 µg/dl	>230 nmol/L
Estrogens [S]		
Estradiol		
Men	12–40 pg/ml	40–150 pmol/L
Women		
Prepubertal	<10 pg/ml	<0.04 nmol/L
Early follicular phase	10–90 pg/ml	0.04–0.33 nmol/L
Late follicular phase	100–400 pg/ml	0.37–1.47 nmol/L
Luteal phase	50–150 pg/ml	0.18–0.55 nmol/L
Postmenopausal	<30 pg/ml	<0.11 nmol/L
Estrone	40–100 pg/ml	0.15–0.37 nmol/L
Follicle stimulating hormone (FSH) [S]		
Men	2–17 mU/ml	2–17 U/L
Women	4–20 mU/ml	4–20 U/L
Growth hormone (HGH) [S]	0–8 ng/ml	0–8 µg/L
17-Hydroxycorticosteroids (Porter-Silber) [U]		
Men	3–15 mg/d	8.3–41 µmol/d
Women	2–12 mg/d	5.5–33 µmol/d

Table 5.   Endocrine Values (Continued)

Test	Reference Range	
	Conventional	SI Units
17-Hydroxyprogesterone [S]		
Men	0.2–1.8 ng/ml	0.6–5.5 nmol/L
Women		
Follicular phase	0.2–0.8 ng/ml	0.6–2.4 nmol/L
Luteal phase	0.8–3.0 ng/ml	2.4–9.1 nmol/L
Postmenopausal	0.04–0.5 ng/ml	0.1–1.5 nmol/L
Insulin [S]	5–25 μU/ml	36–179 pmol/L
17-Ketosteroids [U]		
Men	8–24 mg/d	28–83 μmol/d
Women	5–15 mg/d	17–52 μmol/d
Long-acting thyroid stimulator (LATS) [S]	Nondetectable	Nondetectable
Luteinizing hormone (LH) [S]		
Men	4–18 mU/ml	4–18 U/L
Women	5–25 mU/ml	5–25 U/L
Pregnanediol [U]		
Men	0.6–1.5 mg/d	1.9–4.7 μmol/d
Women		
Follicular phase	0.5–1.5 mg/d	1.6–4.7 μmol/d
Luteal phase	2.0–7.0 mg/d	6.2–22 μmol/d
Postmenopausal	0.2–1.0 mg/d	0.6–3.1 μmol/d
Pregnanetriol [U]	<2.0 mg/d	<5.9 μmol/d
Progesterone [S]		
Men	0.1–0.3 ng/ml	0.3–1.0 nmol/L
Women		
Follicular phase	0.3–0.8 ng/ml	1.0–2.5 nmol/L
Luteal phase	4–20 ng/ml	13–64 nmol/L
Postmenopausal	0.03–0.3 ng/ml	0.1–1.0 nmol/L
Prolactin [S]		
Men	0–15 ng/ml	0–15 μg/L
Women	0–20 ng/ml	0–20 μg/L
Renin [P]		
Sodium intake 100 mmol/d		
Recumbent position	0–2.1 ng/ml/h	0–0.58 ng/(L·s)
Upright position	0.9–4.5 ng/ml/h	0.25–1.25 ng/(L·s)
Sodium intake <10 mmol/d		
Recumbent position	1.5–5.4 ng/ml/h	0.42–1.50 ng/(L·s)
Upright position	1.8–10.2 ng/ml/h	0.50–2.83 ng/(L·s)
Testosterone [S]		
Men	300–1000 ng/dl	10–35 nmol/L
Women	20–80 ng/dl	0.7–2.8 nmol/L
Thyroid stimulating hormone (TSH) [S]	0.8–5.0 μU/ml	0.8–5.0 mU/L
Thyroxine [S]		
Free (FT_4)	0.6–1.8 ng/dl	8–23 pmol/L
Total (T_4)	5–12 μg/dl	64–154 nmol/L
Triiodothyronine (T_3), total [S]	80–170 ng/dl	1.2–2.6 nmol/L

Table 6. Therapeutic and Toxic Values

| Test | Reference Range | |
	Therapeutic	Toxic
Acetaminophen [P]	5–21 mg/L	>300 mg/L 4 hours after ingestion >50 mg/L 12 hours after ingestion
Amikacin [S]		
Peak	20–30 mg/L	>30 mg/L
Trough		>8 mg/L
Amiodarone (and metabolite N-des- methylamiodarone) [S]	1.0–2.5 mg/L	
Amitriptyline (and metabolite nor- triptyline) [S]	120–250 µg/L	>500 µg/L
Barbiturates [B]		
Amobarbital	3–12 mg/L	>12 mg/L
Butabarbital	2–14 mg/L	>30 mg/L
Butalbital	1–5 mg/L	>7 mg/L
Pentabarbital	1–5 mg/L	>5 mg/L
Phenobarbital	15–40 mg/L	>40 mg/L
Secobarbital	1–5 mg/L	>40 mg/L
Thiopental	7–130 mg/L	
Carbamazepine [S]	4–8 mg/ml	
Chloramphenicol [S]	10–20 mg/L	
Cimetidine [S]	0.5–2.5 mg/L	
Clonazepam [S]	10–80 µg/L	
Cyclosporine A [S]	50–400 µg/L	
Desipramine [P]	50–300 µg/L	>500 µg/L
Diazepam [P]	0.5–2.0 mg/L	>3.0 mg/L
Digitoxin [P]	10–30 µg/L	15–50 µg/L
Digoxin [P]	0.5–1.5 µg/L	>2.0 µg/L
Disopyramide [P]	2.0–5.0 mg/L	
Doxepin [P]	100–300 µg/L	>500 µg/L
Ethanol [P]		
Legal intoxication		>100 mg/dl
Coma		>500 mg/dl
Ethosuximide [P]	40–100 mg/L	
Gentamicin [S]		
Peak	5–8 mg/L	>10 mg/L
Trough		>2 mg/L
Gold [S]	38–500 µg/dL	>500 µg/dl
Lidocaine [P]	1.5–5.0 mg/L	
Lithium [S]	0.5–1.5 mmol/L	>2 mmol/L
Methanol [P]		>100 mg/L
Nortriptyline [P]	50–140 µg/L	>300 µg/L
Phenytoin [P]	10–20 mg/L	>20 mg/L
Procainamide [P]	4–8 mg/L	>16 mg/L
Quinidine [P]	1–4 mg/L	
Salicylate [S]	15–30 mg/dl	>30 mg/dl
Theophylline [P]	10–20 mg/L	>30 mg/L
Tobramycin [S]		
Peak	4–8 mg/L	>10 mg/L
Trough	<2 mg/L	>2 mg/L
Tocainide [S]	4–10 mg/dl	
Valproic acid [P]	50–100 mg/L	>100 mg/L
Vancomycin [S]		
Peak	15–35 mg/L	
Trough	<10 mg/L	

NORMAL HEMODYNAMIC VALUES

Table 7

Pressures	
Chamber	Pressures (mm Hg)
Right atrium (mean)	≤6
Right ventricle	15–30/≤6
Pulmonary artery	15–30/4–12
Mean pulmonary artery	10–20
Mean pulmonary arterial wedge	4–12
Left atrium (mean)	≤12
Left ventricle	100–140/≤12
Aorta	100–140/60–80

Volumes	
Left ventricle	
End diastole	70–100 ml/M^2
End systole	25–35 ml/M^2
Ejection fraction	55–80%
Cardiac index	2.8–4.2 L/M^2/min
A-V$_{02}$ difference	≤5.0 vol %

Blood Oxygen Values		
Chamber	O$_2$ Content (vol %)	O$_2$ Saturation (%)
Superior vena cava	14.0 ± 1	70 ± 5
Inferior vena cava	16.0 ± 1	80 ± 5
Right atrium (mean)	15.0 ± 1	75 ± 5
Right ventricle (mean)	15.2 ± 1	75 ± 5
Pulmonary artery	15.2 ± 1	75 ± 5
Systemic artery	18.9 to 19.3	94 to 96
Arteriovenous difference	3 to 5	

Normal Values for Echocardiographic Measurements*		
M-Mode Echocardiography		
	Range (cm)	Mean (cm)
Right ventricular dimension (flat)	0.7–2.3	1.5
Right ventricular dimension (left lateral)	0.9–2.6	1.7
Left ventricular dimension (flat)	3.7–5.6	4.7
Left ventricular dimension (left lateral)	3.5–5.7	4.7
Posterior left ventricular wall thickness	0.6–1.1	0.9
Intraventricular wall thickness	0.6–1.1	0.1
Left atrial dimension	1.9–4.0	2.9
Aortic root dimension	2.0–3.7	2.7

Two-Dimensional Echocardiography	
	Range
Left ventricular diameter-diastole	3.6–5.2 cm
Left ventricular diameter-systole	2.3–3.9 cm
Left atrial diameter	2.1–3.7 cm
Left ventricular volume-diastole	95.5 ± 19.4 ml/M^2
Left ventricular volume-systole	38.6 ± 9.5 ml/M^2
Left ventricular ejection fraction	60%

*From Feigenbaum, H.: Echocardiography. 4th Ed. Philadelphia, Lea & Febiger, 1986, p. 621.

```
┌─────────────────────────────────────┐
│                                     │
│      PULMONARY FUNCTION TEST        │
│             VALUES                  │
│                                     │
└─────────────────────────────────────┘
```

Table 8

Normal Values for a 45-year-old man
Height 69"—Weight 160 lbs

First sec vc (Fev$_1$) (L)	3.97
Vital capacity (vc) (L)	4.9
Fev$_1$/vc %	81.0
Peak exp fl rte (L/sec)	9.08
Flow-50% vc (L/sec)	5.53
Flow-25% vc (L/sec)	2.59
Peak insp fl rate (L/sec)	
Max br cap—calc (L/min)	159

Lung Volumes (Plethysmography)

Tot lung cap (L)	6.63
Residual vol (L)	2.05
RV/TLC	0.31
Func res cap (L)	3.76
Airway resist (cm H$_2$O/L/sec)	(NL = 0.8–2.4)
Sp cond airway (L/sec/cm H$_2$O/L)	(NL >.12)

Normal Values for a 45-year-old woman
Height 65"—Weight 160 lbs

First sec vc (Fev$_1$)(L)	2.92
Vital capacity (vc) (L)	3.54
Fev$_1$/vc %	82.0
Peak exp fl rate (L/sec)	6.24
Flow-50% vc (L/sec)	4.13
Flow-25% vc (L/sec)	2.18
Peak insp fl rte (L/sec)	
Max br cap—calc (L/min)	117

Lung Volumes (Plethysmography)

Tot lung cap (L)	5.19
Residual vol (L)	1.79
RV/TLC	0.34
Func res cap (L)	2.91
Airway resist (cm H$_2$O/L/sec)	(NL = 0.8–2.4)
Sp cond airway (L/sec/cm H$_2$O/L)	(NL >.12)

REFERENCE LABORATORY VALUES FOR IMPORTANT NUTRIENTS

Table 9

Nutrient	Test	Normal Values
Albumin	Serum	3.5–5.0 g/dl
Vitamin A	Serum	20–80 µg/dl
Thiamin (B_1)	Plasma	10–64 ng/dl
Riboflavin (B_2)	Red cell ketolase activity	0.9–1.3 activity units
Pyridoxine (B_6)	Plasma (as phosphate)	3.0–18.0 mg/ml
Vitamin (B_{12})	Serum	200–900 pg/ml
Folate	Serum	4.0–20.0 ng/ml
	Red cell	140–700 ng/ml
Ascorbic acid (Vitamin C)	Serum	0.2–2.0 mg/dl
Vitamin D		
25-OH	Serum	10–55 ng/ml
1,25-OH_2	Serum	20–76 pg/ml
Vitamin E	Serum	5–20 µg/ml
Copper	Serum	70–155 µg/dl
	Urine	20–65 µg/24 h
Iodine	Serum—inorganic	0.5–1.0 µg/dl

REFERENCES

1. Beeler, M.F.: SI units and the AJCP. Am J Clin Pathol 87:140, 1987.
2. Beutler, E.: Red Cell Metabolism. A Manual of Biochemical Methods. 3rd Ed. Orlando, Grune & Stratton, Inc., 1984.
3. Clinical Laboratories Manual, San Francisco General Hospital Medical Center, San Francisco, 1986.
4. Clinical Laboratories Manual, University of California Hospitals and Clinics, San Francisco, 1986.
5. Gottfried, E.L., and Nigro, F.A.: SMAC panel and blood count reference values based on executive health survey. Clin Chem 28:1556, 1982.
6. Gottfried E.L. (ed): Laboratory Reference Values. New York, Hospital-Cornell Medical Center Lab Report 6:3, 1980.
7. Lippert H., and Lehmann, H.P.: SI Units in Medicine. Baltimore, Urban & Schwarzenberg, 1978.
8. Powsner, E.R., et al.: Committee report: Quantities and units: SI. National Committee for Clinical Laboratory Standards 3:97, 1983.
9. Scully, R.E., McNeely, B.U., and Mark, E.J. (eds.): Case records of the Massachusetts General Hospital. Normal reference laboratory values. N Engl J Med 314:39, 1986.
10. Tietz, N.W. (ed): Clinical Guide to Laboratory Tests. Philadelphia, W.B. Saunders Co., 1983.
11. Young, D.S.: Implementation of SI units for clinical laboratory data. Ann Intern Med 106:114, 1987.

INDEX

Page numbers followed by "f" indicate figures; numbers followed by "t" indicate tables.

INDEX

Cancer *(Continued)*
  skin signs associated with, 128t, 129, 784-789
    basis for association, 784-785, 788
    discrete lesions, 785t, 786t
    frequent associations, 785t, 787t
    hair, 785t, 786t
    occasional associations, 786-787t, 788t
    in pancreatic glucagonoma, 789
  testicular failure in, 499
  thrombophlebitis as sign, 789
  tumor lysis syndrome, 122-123
  weight loss in, 127, 802, 803t
Candidiasis
  in diabetes, 160
  disseminated, 160
  esophagitis, odynophagia in, 538
  IgE elevation in, 74
  mucocutaneous, 78
  oral cavity, 772t, 773
Capgras' syndrome, 701
Capillary microscopy, in scleroderma, 589t
Capsulitis, adhesive, 634
Captopril test, 259
Caput medusa, 561
Carbon monoxide poisoning, 842t
  inadequate tissue oxygenation in, 189
Carcinoid syndrome, 124, 442-444
  cardiomyopathy in, 239
  clinical presentation, 443
  diagnostic evaluation, 444
  differential diagnosis, 443-444
  flushing in, 646
  pathophysiology, 442
  physical findings, 647
Carcinoid tumors
  carcinoid syndrome due to, 442-444
  hormone production by, 124, 442
Cardiac arrest, 248-250
Cardiac catheterization
  in constrictive pericarditis, 243
  in ischemic heart disease, 231
  in pulmonary hypertension, 248
Cardiac output
  decreased, fatigue related to, 187-189, 187t
  increased demand causing fatigue, 189
Cardiac tamponade. *See also* Pericardial effusion
  in cancer, 120
  cardiogenic shock after myocardial infarction distinguished from, 246
  pathophysiology, 241
  physical findings, 241
Cardiogenic shock, 245-246
Cardiomegaly, 225-227
Cardiomyopathy
  classification, 237, 237t
  constrictive pericarditis distinguished from, 243
  dilated, 237-238
  drugs causing, 239
  hypertrophic, 238-239
    chest pain in, 192
    differential diagnosis, 238-239
    echocardiography in, 238
    pathophysiology, 238
  ischemic, 237-238
  after myocarditis, 237
  obstructive versus nonobstructive, 238
  pathophysiology, 237-238
  restrictive, 239
  sudden death in, 249
  toxins causing, 239

ventricular tachycardia in, 223
Cardiovascular disorders, 186-250. *See also* Heart; Vascular disorders
  in anorexia nervosa, 726
  arterial pulse abnormalities in, 203-205
  bruits in, 214-215
  cardinal manifestations, 186t
  chest pain in, 190-195
  cyanosis in, 207-208
  extracardiac sounds in, 216-217
  fatigue in, 186-190, 187t
  normal hemodynamic values, 856t
  swelling in, 200-201, 200t
  syncope, 197-198, 197t
  weakness in, 646
Carey-Coombs murmur, 212
Carotenemia, 767
Carotid artery disease
  aneurysm, 356
  bruit, 214
  diagnostic evaluation, 683
  transient ischemic attacks, 681-683
Carotid sinus hypersensitivity, 679
Carpal tunnel syndrome, 633-634
  clinical features, 610t
  definition, 633
  diagnostic evaluation, 633-634
  pathophysiology, 633
Cartilage
  degeneration, 574t
  joint pain due to disorders, 605-607
  polychondritis, 598
Cataplexy, in narcolepsy, 753
Cataract, 815-816
  classification, 816t
  definition, 815
  diagnostic evaluation, 816
  pathophysiology, 815-816
Catatonia, malignant neuroleptic syndrome in, 718
Catecholamines
  normal laboratory values, 853t
  pheochromocytoma secreting, 262, 476
    plasma levels, 479, 480t
    platelet levels, 482
    urinary levels, 479, 480t
  synthesis and degradation, 481f
Catheters, sepsis associated with, 152, 153t
Cats, infections related to, 136t
Cauda equina syndrome, 664
Causalgia, 661, 764
Cellulitis, orbital, 396, 397, 814
Central nervous system
  altered mental change. *See* Consciousness, altered
  in cancer, 118-119
    diagnostic evaluation, 119
    differential diagnosis, 118-119
    pathophysiology, 118
  diabetes insipidus due to disorders, 309
  hypercalcemia effect on, 408-409
  in hypernatremia, 307
  hypertensive encephalopathy, 255
  in hyponatremia, 304
  in porphyrias, 440t
  in precocious puberty, 522, 522t, 523
  and sudden cardiac arrest, 249-250
  syncope disorders, 197t, 199
  in vomiting, 546, 546t
Central venous pressure, ascites related to, 565, 565t
Cephalosporins

allergy, 46-47
  cross-reactivity with penicillin, 46-47
Cerebellar disease
  gait in, 672
  subacute degeneration in cancer, 119t
  tremor in, 691, 716
Cerebral arteriography
  in comatose patient, 670
  in transient ischemic attack, 683
Cerebral blood volume, headache due to increase, 659
Cerebral edema, management, 668-669
Cerebral hemorrhage, in cancer, 118
Cerebral infarction
  in cancer, 118
  in rheumatic disease, 620t
  thalamic and parietal syndromes after, 662
Cerebral ischemia, conditions associated with, 682t
Cerebrospinal fluid (CSF)
  in AIDS, 164
  in amnestic syndrome, 711
  electrophoretic analysis, 25
  low pressure causing headache, 660
  normal laboratory values, 852t
  protein determination, 23-24
  in rhinitis, 63
Cerebrovascular disease. *See also* Cerebral infarction
  dementia in, 704
  sexual dysfunction in, 740
  vertigo in, 666
Cervical root pain syndromes, 663
  carpal tunnel syndrome, 633
  in shoulder pain, 635
Cervix
  infertility disorders, 512
  mucus, and fertility, 512, 514-515
CH50, 84
Chagas' disease, 237
Challenge test, in hypersensitivity pneumonitis, 68
Chediak-Higashi leukocyte anomaly, 92
Chediak-Higashi syndrome, 82
  oculocutaneous albinism in, 780
Cheilosis, 799t
Chemotaxis
  complement role in, 84
  deficiency, 81-82, 82t
Chemotherapy
  CNS effects, 118-119
  nutritional disorders due to, 802, 804t
  pulmonary toxicity, 126, 127t
Chest. *See also* Lung
  breathing pattern abnormalities, 171
  examination, 10-11
  mediastinal mass, 181-183
Chest pain, 190-195
  angina pectoris, 190-191. *See also* Angina pectoris
    pathophysiology, 191-192
  aortic, 192-193
  cardiac causes, 190-192
  classification, 190t
  diagnostic evaluation, 541
  differential diagnosis, 7, 192-195
  differentiating gastrointestinal from cardiac origin, 541
  in dysphagia, 537
  esophageal, 194-195, 538, 541
  etiology, 171, 172t
  in gastrointestinal disease, 194-195

laboratory tests in, 457t, 459t, 464-467
metapyrone test in, 459t, 466-467
obesity distinguished from, 256
obesity in, 437-438, 463
osteoporosis in, 445
pathophysiology, 462-463
psychiatric disorders in, 463
radiography in, 464-465, 467
skin in, 463
C wave, 206, 207
Cyanide poisoning, 842t
Cyanosis, 174-175
in cardiovascular disorders, 175, 207-208
central, 207-208
definition, 207
differential, 208
in Eisenmenger complex, 234
in lung disease, 175
pathophysiology, 174, 207-208
peripheral, 207
physical examination in, 174-175
in Raynaud's phenomenon, 207
right-to-left shunt causing, 233-234
Cyclothymic disorder, 724
Cyproheptadine suppression test, 261
Cystic fibrosis, rhinitis with, 63
Cystinuria, 295-296
calculi in, 298
Cystitis, 272
Cysts, kidney, 294
Cytosine arabinoside, lung toxicity, 127t

Darier's sign, 58, 443
Darier-White's disease, 778
Data base, 3-5. See also Clinical data base
Data processing, in diagnosis, 5-6
Decerebrate rigidity, 668, 669
Decorticate responses, 669
Deformities, joint, 628-629
Dehydration
in alcoholism, 736
with hyponatremia, 305, 305f, 306
Dehydroepiandrosterone, factors determining, 494t, 495
Deja vu, 699
Delirium, 706-709
in alcohol withdrawal, 735-736, 735t
amnestic syndrome distinguished from, 711
brain pathology in, 708
clinical features, 706-707
definition, 667, 706
delusions in, 701
dementia distinguished from, 703
diagnostic evaluation, 708-709
etiology, 708t
laboratory tests in, 709
movement disorder in, 707
pathophysiology, 707-708
in sedative withdrawal, 736, 736t
supratentorial mass causing, 709
Delirium tremens, 735-736, 735t
hallucinations in, 700, 701
Delta-aminolevulinic acid. See delta-Aminolevulinic acid
Delusions, 701-702
in alcoholism, 702
in amphetamine psychosis, 701-702
classification, 701, 701t
definition, 701
with depression, 719
differential diagnosis, 701-702

grandiose, 722
with hallucinations, 719
in organic brain syndrome, 701
paranoid, 701-702
pathophysiology, 701
in schizophrenia, 701
Dementia, 683-684, 703-706
Alzheimer's disease causing, 683-684, 704
amnestic syndrome distinguished from, 711
benign forgetfulness distinguished from, 705-706
in cancer, 119t
in cerebrovascular disease, 704
clinical presentation, 703-704
definition, 683, 703
delirium distinguished from, 703
delusions in, 701
in depression, 705, 706
diagnostic evaluation, 684, 705-706
during dialysis, 684
differential diagnosis, 684, 704-705, 704t
drugs causing, 705
and gait disorder, 705
Huntington's chorea causing, 705
mental retardation distinguished from, 703
metabolic causes, 705
multi-infarct, 684, 705
normal pressure hydrocephalus causing, 705
pathophysiology, 683-684, 704
pseudodementia of depression distinguished from, 684
psychiatric disorders causing, 705
Dengue, rash in, 138t
Deoxycorticosterone test, 260
11-Deoxycortisol, in congenital adrenal hyperplasia, 494t, 495
Depersonalization, 697-698
Depersonalization disorder, 698
Depression, 718-722
brain pathology in, 721-722
classification, 719-720, 719t
clinical features, 719
Cushing's syndrome distinguished from, 464
definition, 718-719
dementia in, 705, 706
determination of need for hospitalization, 721
diagnostic criteria, 719, 719t
differential diagnosis, 721-722, 721t
distinguishing psychiatric etiology from medical illness, 696
drugs causing, 721
endocrine disorders causing, 720-721
endogenous, 719-720
hereditary basis, 721
insomnia in, 751
neurotransmitters role in, 720
in nutritional disorders, 721
pathophysiology, 720-721
primary versus secondary, 720
pseudodementia distinguished from true dementia, 684
psychotic, 719, 720
unipolar versus bipolar, 720, 723
Derealization, 697-698
definition, 698
differential diagnosis, 698
with illusion, 699
pathophysiology, 698
Dermatitis. See Atopic dermatitis; Contact dermatitis
Dermatographism, 58

Dermatomes, 662
Dermatomyositis
in cancer, 119t, 128t, 789
clinical features, 574t, 596
diagnostic tests in, 589-590t
eye involvement, 622t
laboratory tests in, 592t
pattern of organ involvement in, 575
sunlight influence on, 778
Devices, bacteremia associated with, 152, 153t
Dexamethasone suppression test
in Cushing's syndrome, 458t, 464, 466, 467
in dementia, 706
false-positive results, 466
high-dose, 466
in hyperandrogenicity, 494t, 496
low-dose, 466
overnight, 466
Diabetes insipidus. See also Antidiuretic hormone
ACTH deficiency masking, 338
central, 308-309, 309t
clinical presentation, 310
diagnostic evaluation, 310-314, 311f
differential diagnosis, 312-314
distinguishing central from nephrogenic, 307, 308f, 310-313, 311f
etiology, 309t
hypernatremia in, 307
nephrogenic, 309, 309t
osmolality determination in, 310
plasma ADH in, 312
polyuria due to, 308, 309t
primary, 308
trauma causing, 308-309
water deprivation test in, 310-312
Diabetes mellitus, 416-424. See also Hyperglycemia
in aldosteronism, 471
arteriosclerosis in, 417
arthropathy in, 603
ataxia in, 672
bladder dysfunction in, 418-419
candidiasis in, 160
in children, 422
classification, 416-417
complications, 417-420
definition, 416
diagnostic studies in, 420-422
fasting glucose in, 420-421
foot in, 419
gastrointestinal tract in, 418
glucose tolerance test in, 421
in hemochromatosis, 423
hyperkalemia in, 317-318
hyperosmolar, nonketotic coma in, 420
diagnosis, 423
hypoglycemia in, 423
immunodeficiency in, 160
impotence in, 419, 504
infections in, 157, 419
insulin-dependent, 416
clinical features, 417
pathogenesis, 416
physical examination, 417
ketoacidosis, 419-420
diagnosis, 422-423
kidney in, 293-294, 418
lactic acidosis in, 423
lipoatrophic, 424
metabolic complications, 419-420
diagnosis, 422-423

definition, 536, 826
diagnostic evaluation, 536-537, 826
differential diagnosis, 826t
etiology, 536t
odynophagia with, 537
pathophysiology, 536, 536t, 826
Dyspnea, 169-171, 195-196
with cough, fever and malaise, 66-68
definition, 169, 195
differential diagnosis, 195-196
etiology, 169-170, 170t
in heart disease, 195-196
history-taking on, 170
myocardial ischemia causing, 190
pathophysiology, 169-170, 195
physical examination in, 170-171
pleural effusion distinguished from
    pulmonary embolism in, 125
in sleep, 754-755
with wheezing, 63-66. See also Asthma
Dysprosody, 687
Dystonia, 691, 716-717
classification, 716
clinical presentation, 716
definition, 716
differential diagnosis, 716-717
drugs causing, 716
hereditary, 717
hysteria distinguished from, 717
oromandibular, 716
tardive, 716-717

Eagles syndrome, 825
Ear
abnormalities related to disorders, 9-10
discharge from, 822-823, 823t
hearing loss, 823-824, 823t
pain, 822, 822t
referred pain to, 822t
tinnitus, 825
vertigo, 824, 824t
Earache, 822, 822t
Eating disorders, 726-729
anorexia nervosa, 726-727
bulimia, 727-729
sudden death in, 728
Eaton-Lambert syndrome, 119, 119t, 689
Ebstein's anomaly, opening snap in, 216
Echocardiography
applications, 15
in cardiac tamponade, 120
in fever of unknown origin, 146
in hypertrophic cardiomyopathy, 238
for left ventricular function, 230
in mitral valve prolapse, 236
normal measurements, 856t
in pericardial effusion, 241
in pulmonary hypertension, 247
Eclampsia, 297
pulmonary edema in, 245
Ecthyma gangrenosum, 158, 160
Edema, 199-201
in allergic disorders, 201
in congestive heart failure, 200
definition, 199
in extremities, 12
of feet and ankles, 200-201
in heart failure, 244
hormonal imbalances causing, 201
with hyponatremia, 305, 305f
in kidney disease, 200

in liver disease, 200
in lymphatic disorders, 201
in nephrotic syndrome, 271
pathophysiology, 199-201
in pregnancy, 200-201
weight gain due to, 794, 797
Ehlers-Danlos syndrome, 604
Eisenmenger complex, 234
Ejaculation
disorders, 504
physiology, 503
premature, 504, 740
retarded, 740
retrograde, 504
Elation, 722-724
Elderly
benign forgetfulness distinguished from
    dementia in, 705-706
gait disturbances in, 671-672
hypertension in, 263
insomnia in, 751
macular degeneration in, 816-817
myxedema coma in, 375
nocturnal arousal in, 750
nutritional disorders in, 801-802, 802t
osteoporosis in, 800
perceptual disorders in, 703
pruritus in, 70
skin cancer in, 783-784
sleep disorders in, 751
substance abuse in, 738-739
Electrocardiogram (ECG)
aberrancy, 223
ambulatory monitoring in ischemic heart
    disease, 191, 230-231
in coronary artery disease, 191
exercise testing with, 229
in hyperkalemia, 318
in hypokalemia, 315
in hypothermia, 651
in ischemic heart disease, 228-231
in mitral valve prolapse, 236
in myocardial infarction, 192
in pancreatitis, 195
in pericarditis, 228
in rheumatic disease, 576t
Electrodiagnostic testing, in carpal tunnel
    syndrome, 633
Electroencephalogram (EEG)
in comatose patient, 671
in delirium, 709
in eating disorders, 728
night recording in sleep disorders, 748
in perceptual disturbances, 702-703
in seizures, 681
Electrolytes. See Fluid and electrolytes; and
    under each electrolyte
Electromyogram (EMG)
in dermatomyositis and polymyositis, 590t
in diabetes mellitus, 419
Electronystagmography, in vertigo, 666
Elephantiasis, 201
Elliptocytes, 90
Emergency care
history-taking in, 3-4
laboratory tests, 35-36
of unconscious patient, 668-669
Emphysema, mediastinal, extracardiac sounds
    in, 216-217
Empty sella syndrome, 353-354
ENA, antibodies against, 580t

Encephalopathy. See also Consciousness,
    altered
delirium, 706-709
EEG in, 671
hepatic, 567
hypertensive, 255
metabolic, 667
    diagnosis, 668
nutritional deficiency causing, 797, 798t
Wernicke's, 705
Endocarditis
fever of unknown origin due to, 142
history-taking in, 142
laboratory tests in, 593t
nonbacterial thrombotic, in cancer, 120
Endocrine disorders
in anorexia nervosa, 726
in cancer, 121-125
constipation in, 554t
in depression, 720-721
impotence due to, 503t, 504
multiple neoplasia syndromes in cancer,
    122, 124
normal laboratory values, 853-854t
osteoporosis in, 445t
smell abnormalities in, 837t
swelling in, 201
taste abnormalities in, 835t
Endometriosis, infertility related to, 512
Endomyocardial fibrosis, 239
Endoscopy. See also Esophagoscopy
in dyspepsia, 545-546
in dysphagia, 537
Enterovirus infections, rash in, 140t
Enthesopathy, 573t
Enuresis, 755-756
Enzymes
in anorexia nervosa, 726
in dermatomyositis and polymyositis, 589t
in red blood cells, 849-850t
serum normal values, 846-848t
Eosinophil(s)
in anaphylaxis, 40
in asthma, 65-66
in pleural fluid, 181
Eosinophil chemotactic factor, 94
Eosinophilia, 70-73, 94-95, 94t
in allergic disorders, 70, 71, 94t
with angioedema, 73
definition, 70, 94
diagnostic evaluation, 71, 94-95
differential diagnosis, 71-73, 72t, 94t
in fever of unknown origin, 146, 147t
in gastrointestinal disease, 72, 72t
hypereosinophilic syndrome, 71-72
IgE elevation with, 70, 70t
in immunodeficiency, 72, 72t
in infections, 137, 141t
in leukemia, 71
nonallergic rhinitis with, 62
in parasite infections, 94t
pathophysiology, 70-71, 94
pulmonary infiltrates with, 71
radiotherapy causing, 73
in rheumatic disease, 582
Eosinophilic chemotactic factor of anaphylaxis,
    40
Eosinophilic granuloma, 71
Eosinophilic granulomatous vasculitis, 596
Ephelides, 783
Epidermolytic hyperkeratosis, 765t, 766
Epilepsy, 679-681. See also Seizures

Epinephrine
  plasma levels in pheochromocytoma, 479,
    480t
  provocative test in carcinoid syndrome, 444
Episcleritis, 59, 813
Epistaxis, 10, 826-827, 827t
  in hypertension, 257
Equilibrium, physiology, 665
Equinus, 628
Eructation, 547-548
Erythema gyratum, in cancer, 789
Erythema multiforme, 55-56
  conditions associated with, 617t
  rash in, 139t
Erythema nodosum, 597-598
  systemic diseases associated with, 598,
    598t, 617t
Erythrocyte sedimentation rate (ESR)
  in back pain, 637, 637t
  in fever of unknown origin, 146, 147t
  in hospital-acquired fever, 151-152
  in infections, 139, 141t
  in rheumatic disease, 580, 584t, 585t,
    592-593t
Erythrocytosis, 97-98
  diagnostic evaluation, 97-98
  differential diagnosis, 98f
  pathophysiology, 97, 97f
Erythroderma, 775-776
  exfoliative, 776
  ichthyosiform, 775
Erythromelalgia, 764
Erythroplasia of Queyrat, 774
Erythropoietin, increased production, 97f
Esophagitis
  Candida, odynophagia in, 538
  chest pain in, 194-195
  odynophagia in, 537-538
  reflux, 538-541
    diagnostic evaluation, 539-541, 540f
    esophageal pH in, 539
    esophagoscopy in, 540
    pathophysiology, 538-539, 539t
Esophagoscopy
  in dysphagia, 537
  in esophagitis, 538, 540
Esophagus
  bleeding from, 556t
  chest pain disorders, 541
  dysphagia, 536-537
  manometric studies
    in dysphagia, 537
    in heartburn, 540-541
    in rheumatic disease, 587t
    in scleroderma, 589t
  varices causing gastrointestinal bleeding,
    556
Estradiol, in hypogonadism, 487t, 501t
Estrogen
  gynecomastia related to, 506, 507
  normal laboratory values, 853t
  progesterone test with, 487t
  and weight gain, 794
Ethchlorvynol intoxication, 842t
Euphoria, 722-724
Ewart's sign, 241
Examination. See Physical examination
Exercise
  anaphylaxis related to, 55
  claudication after, 201-202
  growth hormone stimulation test after, 340t
  urticaria in, 58

Exercise tests
  accuracy, 229
  contraindications, 229
  interpretation, 15
  in ischemic heart disease, 229
Exfoliative dermatitis, in cancer, 128t
Exophthalmos, 395-398, 813-814
  definition, 813
  diagnostic evaluation, 398, 814
  differential diagnosis, 397-398, 813-814
  etiology, 396t
  in Graves' disease, 395
  neoplasms causing, 396, 396t, 814
  pathophysiology, 395-396, 813
  pseudoexophthalmos distinguished from,
    398
  unilateral, 397
  vascular shunts causing, 396
Extracardiac sounds, 216-217, 216t
Extremities
  claudication, 201-202
  dorsal root pain disorders, 663
  examination, 12
  pain syndrome, 661
  Raynaud's phenomenon, 202-203
Eye, 808-819
  in albinism, 780
  anisocoria, 818-819
  cataract, 815-816
  in comatose patient, 669-670
  corneal deposits, 10
  in diabetes mellitus, 417-418, 817-818
  difficulty in diagnosing disorders, 808
  exophthalmos, 395-398, 813-814
  in fever of unknown origin, 145t
  fourth cranial nerve disorder, 677
  glaucoma, 814-815
  in Graves' disease, 376, 377, 396-397, 813-
    814, 814t
  in hypertension, 257
  macular degeneration, 816-817
  optic nerve disorders, 673-675
  optic nerve head swelling, 817, 818t
  physical examination, 10, 808
    with ophthalmoscope, 808-809
    visual acuity, 808
    visual fields, 808
  red, 812-813, 813t
    definition, 812
    differential diagnosis, 812-813, 813t
    in glaucoma, 815
    pathophysiology, 812
  refractive error, 808
  in rheumatic disease, 617t, 622t, 612-613,
    622t
  in sella enlargement, 357-358
  in Sjogren's syndrome, 632
  subconjunctival hemorrhage, 812
  third cranial nerve disorders, 675-677
  in thyrotoxicosis, 396
  visual loss, 809-811
Eye movements, in comatose patient, 670

Fabry's disease
  angiokeratoma of, 774
  burning pain in, 764
Face
  pain, 658-661, 828, 828t. See also
    Headache
  weakness, 677-678
Facial nerve, 677-678

Bell's palsy, 678
Failure to thrive, 347, 350
Fainting, 199, 678-679. See also Syncope
Faintness, weakness distinguished from, 645
Fallopian tube, patency determination in
    infertility, 513t, 515
False negative result, 24-25
False positive result, 24-25
  number of tests increasing likelihood, 29
Familial Mediterranean fever, laboratory tests
    in, 593t
Family history, 8
Fanconi's syndrome, 296
  phosphaturia in, 449
  proximal renal tubular acidosis in, 275
Farmer's lung, 66
Fasting
  glucose metabolism in, 424-425
    in diabetes, 420-421
  hypoglycemia in, 425-426
    diagnosis, 427, 428f, 429
Fat. See also Lipid disorders
  fecal levels in malabsorption, 550
Fatigue, 186-190, 640-645
  alcohol causing, 641, 645
  algorithm for diagnostic approach, 642-644f
  definition, 186, 640
  diagnostic evaluation, 641-645
  differential diagnosis, 640-641
  diseases associated with, 641t
  drugs causing, 641t
  etiology, 186-187, 187t
  in fever of unknown origin, 143, 144t
  pathophysiology, 640
    in cardiovascular disease, 187-190, 187t
  psychologic disorder causing, 643, 645
  sleepiness distinguished from, 752
  weakness distinguished from, 645
Fatty acid deficiency
  ichthyosis associated with, 775
  tongue changes in, 833-834
Fear, anxiety distinguished from, 724
Feces
  in abdominal pain, 543
  characteristics in diarrhea, 553
  leukocytes in, 552-553
    with rectal bleeding, 558
  normal sodium loss in, 302
  normal water loss in, 302
  occult blood in, 559
  potassium in, 314
  quantitative fat measurement, 550
Felty's syndrome, 630
Femoral artery, bruit, 214-215
Fertility, physiologic requirements, 510. See
    also Infertility
Fever. See also Infections
  with abdominal pain, 542-543
  as adaptive defense mechanism, 133
  camel-back, 132, 134t
  in cancer, 126-127
  diagnostic approach to, 132-166
  double quotidian, 132, 134t
  drug, 150, 153-154, 154t
  hectic, septic, 132, 134t
  hospital-acquired, 148-155
    diagnostic evaluation, 150-155
    differential diagnosis, 149-150, 149t
    history-taking in, 150
    laboratory tests in, 151-152
    pathophysiology, 149
    physical findings in, 150-151

differential diagnosis, 699-701
drugs causing, 700-701
gustatory, 700, 700t
nonpathologic, 699-700
olfactory, 673, 700, 700y
organic, 699
pathophysiology, 699
in poisoning, 840t
sleep related to, 699
tactile, 700, 700t
visual, 700, 700t
Hallucinogens, 700-701
intoxication, 734, 734t
Haloperidol. *See* Neuroleptics
Halothane, jaundice due to, 563
Hamman's sign, 194, 214t, 216-217
Hansen's disease, hypopigmentation in, 781
Hartnup disease, 295-296
photosensitivity in, 777
Hashimoto's thyroiditis. *See* Thyroiditis,
    Hashimoto's
Headache, 658-660
in brain tumor, 659
cluster, 658-659
definition, 658
diagnostic evaluation, 660
differential diagnosis, 658t
distinguishing tension from migraine type,
    659
extracranial sources, 658-659
in fever of unknown origin, 143, 144t
in hypertension, 257
with increased cerebral blood volume, 659
increased intracranial pressure causing, 659
intracranial sources, 658, 659-660
low CSF pressure causing, 660
after lumbar puncture, 660
in meningitis, 659
migraine, 658
muscle contraction type, 659
nocturnal, 756
pathophysiology, 658
in temporal arteritis, 659-660
tension, 659
Head and neck, 822-829
examination, 10
Head banging, 756
Head injury, diabetes insipidus after, 308-309
Health care costs, 20, 21f
Hearing loss, 823-824, 823t
diagnostic evaluation, 823-824
pathophysiology, 823
Heart, 186-250. *See also* Cardiovascular
    disorders
arrest, 248-250
arrhythmias, 218-223. *See also* Arrhythmias
auscultation, 11
automaticity in, 218
in cancer, 119-121
in carcinoid syndrome, 443
chest pain of, 190-192
congenital disease
    in adult, 231-234
    classification, 231-232, 231t
    diagnostic approach to, 231-232
    fatigue in, 188
    inadequate tissue oxygenation in, 189-190
in diabetes mellitus, 417
enlargement, 225-227
    chest x-ray in, 226-227
    definition, 225
    differential diagnosis, 226, 226t

physical examination, 225-226
fatigue related to, 187-190, 187t
myocarditis and cardiomyopathy, 236-239.
    See also Cardiomyopathy
normal hemodynamic values, 856t
palpitations, 196-197
physical examination, 11, 225-226
point of maximal impulse, 225-226
radionuclide imaging, 16
in rheumatic disease, 618t
tamponade. *See* Cardiac tamponade
in thyrotoxicosis, 377
tumor
    fatigue in, 188
    filling sound in, 217
valvular disease, fatigue in, 188
Heart block, 223-225
AV node block, 224-225
complete, 224-225
congenital, 234
fatigue in, 189
pathophysiology, 224-225
sinoatrial, 224
syncope in, 198
Heartburn, 538-541. *See also* Esophagitis,
    reflux
algorithm for diagnostic approach, 540f
definition, 538
diagnostic evaluation, 539-541, 540f
pathophysiology, 538-539, 539t
Heart failure, 243-245
acute, 244-245, 244t
asthma distinguished from, 66
chronic, 244t, 245
classification, 244, 244t
congestive, 243-244
definition, 243-244
hypokinetic pulse in, 205
internal jugular vein examination in, 206
pathophysiology, 244-245
sleep apnea causing, 754
swelling in, 200
wheezing in, 174
Heart murmurs, 210-214
Austin Flint, 212
cardiopulmonary, 213
classification, 210t
continuous, 212-213
definition, 210
diastolic, 210t, 211-212
ejection, 210-211, 210t
eponymic, 213-214, 214t
holosystolic, 211
in pregnancy, 213
regurgitant, 211-212
rumbles, 212
systolic, 210-211, 210t
to-and-fro, 213
venous hum distinguished from, 212
whoop or honk, 211
Heart sounds, 208-209
clicks and snaps, 215-216, 215t
extracardiac, 216-217
filling sounds, 217-218
gallop, 217-218
of gastrointestinal origin, 217
pathophysiologic considerations, 209
in right bundle branch block, 209
second
    physiologic splitting, 209
    reverse splitting, 209

splitting, click distinguished from, 215-
    216
splitting, 209
Heart surgery
constrictive pericarditis after, 242
pericardial effusion after, 240
Heat
disorders, 652-654
regulation, 651-652
urticaria due to, 58
Heatstroke, 652
neuroleptic malignant syndrome
    distinguished from, 718
Heberden's nodes, 574t, 627
Heerfordt's syndrome, 157
Helminth infections, eosinophilia in, 71, 72t
Hemangioma
in oral cavity, 772t, 774
of synovium, 607
Hemarthroses, 625t
Hematemesis. *See also* Gastrointestinal
    bleeding
definition, 555
diagnostic approach, 557, 557f
hemoptysis distinguished from, 175-176
pathophysiology, 555
Hematochezia. *See also* Gastrointestinal
    bleeding
definition, 555
diagnostic evaluation, 557-559, 558f
pathophysiology, 555
Hematologic disorders, 90-117
anemia, 98-104
in anorexia nervosa, 726
blood smear abnormalities, 90-92
coagulation, 110-112
diagnostic approach, 90
eosinophilia in, 71-72, 72t
erythrocytosis, 97-98
leukocyte disorders, 92-97
lymphocytosis in, 96t
monocytosis in, 97t
myelodysplastic syndromes, 112-113
myeloproliferative disorders, 113-115. *See
    also* Leukemia
neutrophilia, 92-93, 92t
normal laboratory values, 849-850t
platelets, 104-110
pruritus in, 69t, 70
in rheumatic disease, 576t, 580-582, 584t,
    618t
Hematuria, 268-269
in Alport's syndrome, 295
classification by etiology, 268, 268t
definition, 268
diagnostic studies in, 269
history-taking in, 268-269
in IgA nephropathy, 286-287
microscopic, 139, 142t
pathophysiology, 268
and rheumatic disease, 620t
Heme, production from porphyrins, 438-439,
    439f
Hemianopsia, homonymous, 674
Hemiballismus, 691
Hemiparesis, gait in, 671
Hemiplegia, 688
Hemoccult test, 559
Hemochromatosis
arthropathy in, 601-602
diabetes mellitus in, 423
diagnosis, 602

distinguishing psychologic from organic cause, 506
endocrine disorders causing, 503t, 504
etiology, 503t
history-taking in, 504
laboratory tests in, 505
nocturnal penile tumescence in, 756-757
pathophysiology, 502-504
physical examination in, 504-505
psychologic disorder causing, 504
Incontinentia pigmenti, 780t, 783
Infant, hypercalcemia in, 408
Infections. *See also* Fever
  adrenal insufficiency due to, 454
  in AIDS, 163-164, 164t
  anergy in, 81t
  animals related to, 133, 136t
  arthritis associated with, 574t, 599-601. *See also* Arthritis, septic
  depression in, 721
  in diabetes mellitus, 419
  diagnostic evaluation in febrile patient, 132-142
  eosinophilia in, 71, 72t, 137, 141t
  erythema nodosum associated with, 598t
  erythrocyte sedimentation rate in, 139, 141t
  fever of unknown origin, 142-148
  foreign travel related to, 133, 135t
  history-taking in, 133
  hospital-acquired, 148-155
    definition, 148-149
    diagnostic evaluation, 150-155
    differential diagnosis, 149-150, 149t
    history-taking in, 150
    laboratory tests in, 151-152
    pathophysiology, 149
    physical findings in, 150-151
    radiography in, 152-153
  IgE elevation in, 74, 74t
  in immunocompromised host, 155-166
    differential diagnosis, 156-159
    meningitis, 157, 157t
    pathophysiology, 155-156, 156t
  in immunodeficiency disorders, 76t
  jaundice related to, 563
  in joints, 574t, 599-601
  laboratory tests in, 135, 137, 139, 141-142t
  in leukemia
    acute lymphatic, 162, 162t
    acute myelogenous, 161-162, 161t
    chronic lymphatic, 162-163, 163t
  leukocyte count in, 137, 141t
  in leukopenia, 93t, 157-159
  liver function tests in, 139, 142t
  lymphadenopathy in, 133, 135, 137t
  lymphocytosis in, 96t
  myocarditis, 236-237, 236t
  neck mass in, 829t
  nosocomial, 148-155. *See also under* hospital-acquired *above*
  pericarditis due to, 242, 242t
  physical examination in, 133, 135
  skin lesions in, 135, 138-140t
  splenomegaly in, 110t, 135, 137t, 569t
  syndrome approach to, 133
  tongue changes in, 834t
  urinalysis in, 139, 142t
  urticaria in, 57
Infertility, 510-516
  definition, 510
  diagnostic evaluation, 512-516
  etiology, 511t

female, 511-512
  algorithm for diagnostic approach, 515-516, 518f
  cervical factors, 512
  documenting ovulatory function in, 514
  history-taking in, 512
  inadequate luteal phase causing, 511-512
  ovulatory disorders causing, 511-512
  pelvic inflammatory disease causing, 512
  postcoital test, 513t, 514-515
  tube patency determination, 513t, 515
  uterine factors, 512
male, 510-511
  algorithm for diagnostic approach, 515, 516f, 517f
  in cryptorchidism, 510-511
  history-taking in, 512
  in Klinefelter's syndrome, 510
  mumps causing, 511
  in myotonia dystrophica, 511
  in Reifenstein's syndrome, 510
  semen analysis in, 512, 513t, 514
  sexual dysfunction causing, 511
  varicocele causing, 510
  pathophysiology, 510-512
Inflammation
  in musculoskeletal disorders, 575, 578-579t. *See also* Arthritis
  noninflammatory joint disorder distinguished from, 576t
Inflammatory bowel disease
  arthropathy
    diagnostic tests in, 588t, 592t
    spine and peripheral joint involvement, 621t
  diagnostic evaluation, 544
Inhibin, 499, 499f
Insect sting, 52-53, 52f
  management approaches, 53t
Insomnia, 749-751
  anxiety causing, 751
  classification, 748
  depression causing, 751
  diagnostic approach, 750-751
  drug-induced, 749, 751
  in elderly, 751
  initiating and maintaining sleep, 750-751
    acute difficulty, 749
    chronic difficulty, 749-750
    recurrent difficulty, 749
  life events related to, 749
  restless legs syndrome causing, 749
  treatment, 751
  withdrawal, 749
Inspection, 9-11
Insulin
  allergy, 48-49, 48t
  C peptide level, 429
  in glucose homeostasis, 424-425
  hypoglycemia due to, 426
    in ACTH evaluation, 341t
    in growth hormone test, 340t
  provocative stimulation tests, 429
  serum levels in fasting hypoglycemia, 427, 429
  surreptitious administration, 426, 429
Insulin-dependent diabetes mellitus, 416. *See also* Diabetes mellitus
Insulin-like activity, nonsuppressible, 125
Insulinoma
  diagnosis, 429
  hypoglycemia in, 124, 425-426

obesity in, 438
  weight gain in, 797
Insulin suppression test, 429
Insulin tolerance test
  in adrenal insufficiency, 459t, 460
  in Cushing's syndrome, 459t
Intellectual function, 683-688. *See also* Cognitive disorders
Intervertebral disc. *See* Disc disease
Interviewing. *See* History-taking
Intestinal obstruction. *See* Gastrointestinal tract, obstruction
Intracranial pressure, increased
  headache due to, 659
  management, 668-669
  papilledema in, 674
Intraocular pressure, in glaucoma, 815
Intravenous therapy, sepsis associated with, 152, 153t
Iodine
  deficiency
    clinical features, 796t
    goiter due to, 384
    hypothyroidism due to, 369
  hyperthyroidism due to, 376, 383
  hypothyroidism due to suppressive effect, 369
  plasma determination in thyrotoxicosis, 382
  radioactive
    hypothyroidism after therapeutic use, 369
    scanning, in thyroid solitary nodule, 391
    uptake, in thyrotoxicosis, 382
Iodocholesterol adrenal scanning, 261
Iritis, 812
Iron
  deficiency, 799t
    anemia, 98t, 800
    clinical features, 796t
    diagnostic features, 99-100, 99t
    in elderly, 802t
    importance of determining cause, 800
    sequential diagnostic workup, 33-34
    thalassemia trait distinguished from, 33
  intoxication, 842t
Irritable bowel syndrome
  bloating in, 548
  constipation in, 555
  diagnostic evaluation, 544
  diarrhea in, 553
Ischemia, abdominal pain of, 542
Ischemic heart disease, 227-231. *See also* Coronary artery disease
  clinical presentation, 228
  definition, 227
  echocardiography in, 230
  electrocardiogram in, 228-229
  exercise testing in, 229
  Holter monitoring in, 230-231
  pathophysiology, 227
  physical findings, 228
  point of maximal impulse in, 225
  radiography in, 229-231
  radionuclide imaging in, 230
  risk factors for, 228
Isopropyl alcohol intoxication, 842t
Itching, 760-763. *See also* Pruritus

Jaccoud's syndrome, 628
Jakob-Creutzfeldt disease
  dementia in, 705
  dyskinetic movements in, 714